CLINICAL, INTERVENTIONAL, *and* INVESTIGATIONAL THROMBOCARDIOLOGY

Fundamental and Clinical Cardiology

Editor-in-Chief
Samuel Z. Goldhaber, M.D.
Harvard Medical School
and Brigham and Women's Hospital
Boston, Massachusetts

CLINICAL, INTERVENTIONAL, and INVESTIGATIONAL THROMBOCARDIOLOGY

Edited by

RICHARD C. BECKER
Duke University Medical Center, Durham, North Carolina, U.S.A.

ROBERT A. HARRINGTON
Duke University Medical Center, Durham, North Carolina, U.S.A.

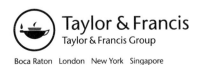

Taylor & Francis
Taylor & Francis Group

Boca Raton   London   New York   Singapore

Published in 2005 by
Taylor & Francis Group
6000 Broken Sound Parkway NW, Suite 300
Boca Raton, FL 33487-2742

International Standard Book Number-10: 0-8247-5419-0 (Hardcover)
International Standard Book Number-13: 978-0-8247-5419-8 (Hardcover)

Library of Congress Cataloging-in-Publication Data

Catalog record is available from the Library of Congress

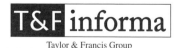

Taylor & Francis Group
is the Academic Division of T&F Informa plc.

**Visit the Taylor & Francis Web site at
http://www.taylorandfrancis.com**

Series Introduction

Marcel Dekker, Inc., has focused on the development of various series of beautifully produced books in different branches of medicine. These series have facilitated the integration of rapidly advancing information for both the clinical specialist and the researcher.

My goal as editor-in-chief of the Fundamental and Clinical Cardiology Series is to assemble the talents of world-renowned authorities to discuss virtually every area of cardiovascular medicine. In the current monograph, has / have edited a much-needed and timely book. Future contributions to this series will include books on molecular biology, interventional cardiology, and clinical management of such problems as coronary artery disease and ventricular arrhythmias.

Samuel Z. Goldhaber

*Dedicated to our families and
to our colleagues at
Duke University Medical Center,
the Duke Clinical Research Institute,
and throughout the world.*

Foreword

The last 50 years have witnessed remarkable growth in our understanding of the underlying pathophysiology of cardiovascular disease. Furthermore, the ability of physicians to diagnose and treat patients with cardiovascular disorders has expanded in step with the enlarging knowledge concerning the causes of heart and vascular disease. Effective therapy for patients with these disorders depends on the clinician's ability to formulate an accurate diagnosis. It is equally important for the clinician to understand the pathological processes that produce the specific condition that has been diagnosed. Once both of these factors have been clearly formulated in the mind of the physician, an effective therapeutic strategy can be selected. Recently, basic and clinical investigation has helped to define the role played by abnormalities of thrombosis in the etiology of a variety of cardiovascular diseases. What has become increasingly clear from this research is that abnormalities in the clotting system often play critically important roles in the development of cardiovascular illness. Since many of these research developments are new and are often published in non-cardiovascular journals, the task undertaken by Drs. Becker and Harrington is particularly important, to produce a text for cardiologists that would elucidate the connection between disorders of clotting and cardiovascular disease. The result of their collaborative effort has been an outstanding collection of contributions from the leading authorities in this new field of thrombocardiology.

The initial chapters of this book clarify the basic, underlying scientific principles of this new interdisciplinary field. Next, a number of areas of clinical pharmacology, applicable to thrombocardiology, are reviewed. Finally, various aspects of the clinical presentation of various cardiovascular diseases, their diagnosis, therapy, as well as the most recent relevant clinical research findings are discussed in light of the new knowledge brought to bear by this new field. Drs. Becker and Harrington are to be congratulated for this monumental new work: in scope, originality, and insight, no other cardiology text currently available is comparable. I look forward to seeing the new discipline of thrombocardiology grow and prosper, and I anticipate that this textbook will become a classic in the cardiology literature.

Joseph S. Alpert, M.D.
Robert S. and Irene P. Flinn Professor of Medicine
Head, Department of Medicine
University of Arizona Health Science Center
Tucson, Arizona, U.S.A.

Preface

The active translation of scientific knowledge to safe, effective, widely available and implementable patient care represents a bidirectional, coordinated effort among clinicians, scientists, clinician-scientists, industry, governmental and private-sector funding agencies and deliverers at multiple levels of healthcare. In essence, the foundation for developing new treatments and management strategies is a hybrid of recognized needs, discovery, and modalities of application to individuals most likely to derive benefit. This requires awareness, diversity, communication, and an environment that nurtures a meaningful interaction between those skilled at the bench, clinicians with a gift at the bedside, and a messenger or master facilitator (translational scientist) who understands both disciplines in the context of a larger universe. Applied inquiry is an overriding and sustaining theme for success.

The Practice of Clinical, Interventional, and Investigational Thrombocardiology links fundamental concepts, patient care and applied research, creating a mosaic of related fields into a working paradigm for discovery, innovation and practical solutions. Having experienced several decades of medial specialization and subspecialization, driven by a rapidly expanding knowledge base at the cellular and molecular levels, we believe that the time has come to center our attention on a multidisciplinary approach to both cardiovascular disease prevention and its treatment. This philosophy, beyond offering a unified approach to healthcare delivery, can be applied seamlessly to broader constructs for education, professional training and investigating common illnesses and, through collaborative networks, rare disorders by providing an integrated and dynamic platform that stresses biology, physiology, pharmacology, genomics, proteomics, entrepreneurship and evidence obtained through validated scientific methods.

The basis of collaboration and for establishing a trusting relationship both within the academic community and between its scholarly representatives and the lay public is integrity. The ethical obligation (or "universal good" at which actions and choices are to be aimed) surrounding scientific research underlies an indelible cornerstone to human conduct that was summarized eloquently over 2,000 years ago by Aristotle during lectures to his students at the Lyceum in Athens:

> *A man must believe in basic truths more than the conclusion. Moreover, if a man sets out to acquire the scientific knowledge that comes through demonstration, he must have a better knowledge of the basic truths and a firmer conviction of them than the connection that is being demonstrated. For indeed the conviction of pure science and the virtue of those dedicated to it must forever be unshakable.*

It is our sincerest hope that we have succeeded, with the unconditional support and unfettered patience of our section editors and contributing authors, to illustrate in a succinct and practical manner the logical progression of ideas and distinguishing sequence of events which underlie a system of science created on affirmative syllogisms and an ethos committed thus – "Bench to Bedside to Bench . . ."

Richard C. Becker, M.D.
Robert A. Harrington, M.D.
Durham, North Carolina
2005

Contents

Contributors

Mary Amato
Massachusetts College of Pharmacy and Health Sciences, Boston, Massachusetts, U.S.A.

Elliott M. Antman
Brigham & Women's Hospital, Boston, Massachusetts, U.S.A.

Dale Ashby
New York University School of Medicine and the Cardiovascular Research Foundation, New York, New York, U.S.A.

Eve Aymong
New York University School of Medicine and the Cardiovascular Research Foundation, New York, New York, U.S.A.

Jorge M. Balaguer
University of Massachusetts Medical School, Worcester, Massachusetts, U.S.A.

Richard C. Becker
Duke Clinical Research Institute, Durham, North Carolina, U.S.A.

Christoph Bode
University Hospital, Freiburg, Germany

Edwin Bovill
University of Vermont, Burlington, Vermont, U.S.A.

William Brennan, Jr.
Massachusetts College of Pharmacy and Health Sciences, Boston, Massachusetts; Hartford Hospital, Hartford, Connecticut; University of Connecticut School of Pharmacy, Storrs, Connecticut, U.S.A.

Michael F. Caron
Hartford Hospital, Hartford, Connecticut; University of Connecticut School of Pharmacy, Storrs, Connecticut, U.S.A.

John Carr
Boston University School of Medicine, Boston, Massachusetts, U.S.A.

Youssef G. Chami
Harper University Hospital, Wayne State University, Detroit, Michigan, U.S.A.

James H. Chesebro
Mayo Clinic, Jacksonville, Florida, U.S.A.

Mauricio G. Cohen
The University of North Carolina at Chapel Hill, Chapel Hill, North Carolina, U.S.A.

Michael D. Cooper
Mayo Clinic, Jacksonville, Florida, U.S.A.

George Danges
New York University School of Medicine and the Cardiovascular Research Foundation, New York, New York, U.S.A.

Paul Dobesh
St. Louis College of Pharmacy, St. Louis; and St. Luke's Hospital, Chesterfield, Missouri, U.S.A.

Alisha Dunn
Massachusetts College of Pharmacy and Health Sciences, Boston, Massachusetts; Hartford Hospital, Hartford, Connecticut; University of Connecticut School of Pharmacy, Storrs, Connecticut, U.S.A.

Paul Edwards
Harper University Hospital, Wayne State University, Detroit, Michigan, U.S.A.

Michael E. Farkouh
New York University School of Medicine and the Cardiovascular Research Foundation, New York, New York, U.S.A.

James J. Ferguson
Texas Heart Institute at St. Luke's Episcopal Hospital, Baylor College of Medicine, The University of Texas Health Science Center at Houston, Houston, Texas, U.S.A.

Marcus Flather
The Royal Brompton Hospital, London, England

James B. Froehlich
University of Massachusetts Medical School, Worchester, Massachusetts, U.S.A.

Noyan Gokce
Boston University School of Medicine, Boston, Massachusetts, U.S.A.

Christopher B. Granger
Duke Clinical Research Institute, Durham, North Carolina, U.S.A.

Kamal Gupta
St. Luke's Episcopal Hospital, Texas Heart Institute, Baylor College of Medicine, The University of Texas Health Science Center at Houston, Houston, Texas, U.S.A.

Christoph Hehrlein
University Hospital, Freiburg, Germany

Robert C. Hendel
Rush-Presbyterian–St. Luke's Medical Center, Chicago, Illinois, U.S.A.

Ik-Kyung Jang
Massachusetts General Hospital, Harvard Medical School, Boston, Massachusetts, U.S.A.

James S. Kalus
Hartford Hospital, Hartford, Connecticut; University of Connecticut School of Pharmacy, Storrs, Connecticut, U.S.A.

Sekar Kathiresan
Massachusetts General Hospital, Harvard Medical School, Boston, Massachusetts, U.S.A.

Robert V. Kelly
The University of North Carolina at Chapel Hill, Chapel Hill, North Carolina, U.S.A.

Dean J. Kereiakes
The Lindner Center Research & Education and The Ohio Heart Health Center, Cincinnati, Ohio, U.S.A.

Todd C. Kerwin
Rush-Presbyterian–St. Luke's Medical Center, Chicago, Illinois, U.S.A.

Scott Kinlay
Cardiovascular Division, Brigham Women's Hospital, Boston, Massachusetts, U.S.A.

David M. Larson
Ridgeview Medical Center, Waconia, Minnesota; and Minneapolis Heart Institute Foundation, Minneapolis, Minnesota, U.S.A.

Joseph Loscalzo
Boston University School of Medicine, Boston, Massachusetts, U.S.A.

Briain D. MacNeill
Massachusetts General Hospital, Harvard Medical School, Boston, Massachusetts, U.S.A.

Kenneth G. Mann
University of Vermont, Burlington, Vermont, U.S.A.

Wojciech Mazur
The Lindner Center Research & Education and The Ohio Heart Health Center, Cincinnati, Ohio, U.S.A.

Brian McBride
Hartford Hospital, Hartford, Connecticut; University of Connecticut School of Pharmacy, Storrs, Connecticut, U.S.A.

Clive A. Meanwell
The Medicines Company, Parsippany, New Jersey, U.S.A.

Roxana Mehran
New York University School of Medicine and the Cardiovascular Research Foundation, New York, New York, U.S.A.

David J. Moliterno
Division of Cardiovascular Medicine, Gill Heart Institute, University of Kentucky, Lexington, Kentucky, U.S.A.

David A. Morrow
Brigham & Women's Hospital, Boston, Massachusetts, U.S.A.

Karen Moulton
Vascular Biology, Children's Hospital; Cardiovascular Division, Brigham Women's Hospital, Boston, Massachusetts, U.S.A.

Debabrata Mukherjee
Division of Cardiovascular Medicine, Gill Heart Institute, University of Kentucky, Lexington, Kentucky, U.S.A.

Craig R. Narins
University of Rochester School of Medicine and Dentistry, Rochester, New York, U.S.A.

E. Magnus Ohman
The University of North Carolina at Chapel Hill, Chapel Hill, North Carolina, U.S.A.

Abdallah G. Rebeiz
Duke Clinical Research Institute, Durham, North Carolina, U.S.A.

Thomas L. Rihn
University Pharmacotherapy Associates, LLC, and Duquesne University School of Pharmacy, Pittsburgh, Pennsylvania, U.S.A.

Michael J. Rohrer
University of Massachusetts Medical School, Worcester, Massachusetts, U.S.A.

Frederick L. Ruberg
Boston University School of Medicine, Boston, Massachusetts, U.S.A.

Aaron Satran
Rush-Presbyterian–St. Luke's Medical Center, Chicago, Illinois, U.S.A.

Maarten L. Simoons
University Hospital Rotterdam, Rotterdam, The Netherlands

Sarah Spinler
Cost-Effective Drug Selection: Injectable Anticoagulants

Gordon J. Vanscoy
University Pharmacotherapy Associates, LLC, Pittsburg Veterans Affairs Health System, and university of Pittsburgh School of Pharmacy, Pittsburgh, Pennsylvania, U.S.A.

C. Michael White
Hartford Hospital, Hartford, Connecticut; University of Connecticut School of Pharmacy, Storrs, Connecticut, U.S.A.

Harvey D. White
Green Lane Hospital, Auckland, New Zealand

J. Michael Wilson
St. Luke's Episcopal Hospital, Texas Heart Institute, Baylor College of Medicine, The University of Texas Health Science Center at Houston, Houston, Texas, U.S.A.

Cheuk-Kit Wong
Green Lane Hospital, Auckland, New Zealand

Philip Wong
Massachusetts General Hospital, Harvard Medical School, Boston, Massachusetts, U.S.A.

Joanna J. Wykrzykowska
Massachusetts General Hospital, Harvard Medical School, Boston, Massachusetts, U.S.A.

John J. Young
The Lindner Center Research & Education and The Ohio Heart Health Center, Cincinnati, Ohio, U.S.A.

Kathleen Brummel Ziedins
University of Vermont, Burlington, Vermont, U.S.A.

I. SCIENTIFIC PRINCIPLES

1-1

Coagulation Factors and Fibrinolysis

Kathleen Brummel Ziedins, Kenneth G. Mann, and Edwin Bovill
University of Vermont, Burlington, Vermont, U.S.A.

I. INTRODUCTION

Blood has intrigued people since ancient times when the transformation of fluid blood to a gel-like mass as it escaped the body was a source of recurrent speculation (1). The earliest reference to bleeding disorders dates back to the fifth-century A.D. Babylonian Talmud, which cautioned that if two male children had died of bleeding after circumcision, the third must not be circumcised (2). The realization that clots stem blood loss did not occur until the beginning of the eighteenth century (1,3) Prior to this some observers hypothesized that blood clotted because it cooled upon exposure to air or that it dried as it left the body (4). It was not until the nineteenth century that the existence of thrombin, the key enzyme in coagulation, was recognized (1).

Paul Morawitz in 1905 proposed the classic theory of coagulation (5). He established that in the presence of calcium and thromboplastin, prothrombin was converted to thrombin, which in turn converted fibrinogen to the fibrin clot. These clotting factors were then assigned Roman numerals: factor I (fibrinogen), factor II (prothrombin), factor III (thromboplastin factor), and factor IV (calcium) (6). As more coagulation factors were introduced, they were assigned consecutive Roman numerals. Due to the potential complexity of the system, the activated forms have been distinguished by a lowercase "a" after their Roman numeral designation. Therefore, the activated form of factor V became known as factor Va.

Today we base our descriptions of the sequences of events leading to fibrin clot formation upon concepts introduced by Davie and Ratnoff in 1964 (7,8). They conceived of blood coagulation as a cascade or waterfall in which a set of sequential, multistep reactions share a similar mechanism in which an inactive zymogen precursor protein is converted to an active enzyme in a chain of reactions that results in thrombin generation. Generation of the active enzyme requires an enzyme-cofactor complex, a surface, and divalent calcium ions (Ca^{2+}). While most facets of these initial descriptions are still valid today, the emerging concept of coagulation and fibrinolysis centers on a complex network of highly interwoven concurrent processes that occur to maintain hemostasis (Fig. 1). Procoagulant and fibrinolytic events occur simultaneously, with many positive and negative feedback loops to regulate the processes. The procoagulant cascade, as observed in the routine screening tests (prothrombin time and activated partial thromboplastin time), includes two arms, the intrinsic (contact) pathway and the extrinsic (tissue factor) pathway, with each of the sources of initiation leading to thrombin generation.

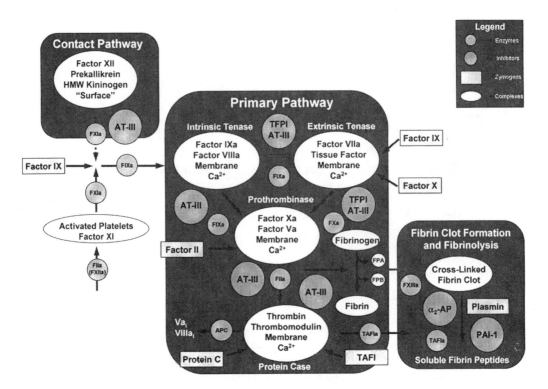

Figure 1   Overview of hemostasis. (a) There are two pathways to initiate coagulation: the contact, intrinsic pathway (shown on the left) and the primary extrinsic pathway (shown on the right). These multicomponent processes are illustrated as either enzymes, inhibitors, zymogens, or complexes. The contact pathway has no known bleeding etiology associated with it, thus this path is considered accessory to hemostasis. Upon injury to the vessel wall, tissue factor, the cofactor for the extrinsic tenase complex, is exposed to circulating factor VIIa (FVIIa) and forms the vitamin K–dependent complex the extrinsic tenase. Factor IX and factor X are converted to their serine proteases factor IXa (FIXa) and factor Xa (FXa), which then form the intirinsic tenase and the prothrombinase complexes, respectively. The combined actions of the intrinsic and extrinsic tenase and the prothrombinase complexes lead to an explosive burst of the enzyme thrombin (FIIa). In addition to its multiple procoagulant roles, thrombin also acts in an anticoagulant capacity when combined with the cofactor thrombomodulin in the protein Case complex. The product of the protein Case reaction, activated protein C (APC), inactivates the cofactors factors Va (FVa$_i$) and VIIIa (FVIIIa$_i$). The cleaved species, FVa$_i$ and FVIIIa$_i$, no longer support the respective procoagulant activities of the prothrombinase and intrinsic tenase complexes. Once thrombin is generated through procoagulant mechanisms, thrombin cleaves fibrinogen, releasing fibrinopeptide A and B (FPA and FPB) and activates factor XIII (FXIIIa) to form a cross-linked fibrin clot. Thrombin-thrombomodulin also activates thrombin-activatable fibrinolysis inhibitor, which slows down fibrin degradation by plasmin. The procoagulant response is downregulated by the stoichiometric inhibitors tissue factor pathway inhibitor (TFPI) and antithrombin III (AT-III). TFPI serves to attenuate the activity of the extrinsic tenase trigger of coagulation. AT-III directly inhibits FIIa, FIXa, and FXa. The accessory pathway provides an alternate route for the generation of FIXa. Thrombin has also been shown to activate factor XI. The fibrin clot is eventually degraded by plasmin, yielding soluble fibrin peptides.

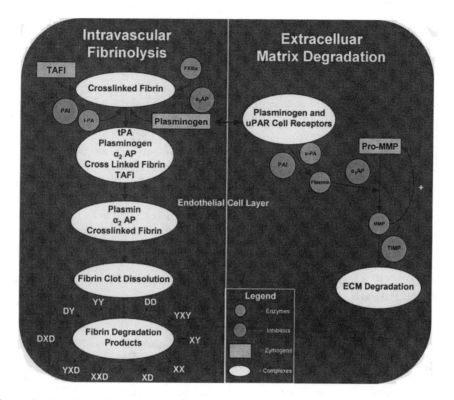

Figure 1 Overview of hemostasis *(Continued)*. (b) Schematic of the dynamic interaction between the proteins and inhibitors of intravascular fibrinolysis and extracellular matrix degradation. Cross-linked fibrin formation (Fig. 1a) is integrated with fibrin clot dissolution and degradation of its products. Two fibrinolysis pathways are shown; an intravascular and an extracellular matrix, separated by an endothelial cell layer. The enzymes, inhibitors, zymogens, and complexes are illustrated in a simplified form to show this multicomponent process. The key proteins of the fibrinolytic system (left panel) are plasminogen, the plasminogen activator tissue-type plasminogen activator (t-PA), plasminogen activator inhibitor (PAI), α_2-antiplasmin (α_2-AP), and thrombin-activatable fibrinolysis inhibitor (TAFI), and the transglutaminase activated factor XIII (FXIIIa). t-PA and plasminogen both bind to the fibrin surface, cross-linked by FXIIIa, where t-PA is an effective catalyst of plasminogen activation to plasmin. Initially, plasmin proteolysis of fibrin generates new, higher-affinity binding sites for plasminogen, setting up an amplifying loop of plasminogen activation. Formation of activated TAFIa results in removal plasmin-generated COOH-terminal lysine residues, thus suppressing the rate of fibrin lysis. Opposing these events are antifibrinolytic mechanisms. Soluble and cross-linked α_2-AP complexes with plasmin, rendering it inactive. PAI rapidly reacts with t-PA, reducing the concentration of the plasminogen activator. Fibrin degradation occurs by cleavage at the D-E-D domains of fibrin polymers by plasmin to yield a variety of polymers as illustrated (for a definition of the fibrin fragments formed, see Fig. 3). Plasminogen can cross the endothelial cell layer and become converted to plasmin by the urokinase-type plasminogen activator (u-PA) (right panel). Plasmin can convert latent matrix metalloproteinases (Pro-MMP) to its active form (MMP). MMPs themselves can act in a positive feedback mechanism to convert pro-MMP to more MMP and ultimately degrading the extracellular matrix. Plasmin-mediated effects are inhibited by PAI and α_2-AP, whereas MMP-mediated effects are inhibited by tissue inhibitors (TIMP)

This chapter will review basic hemostatic and fibrinolytic mechanisms as a foundation for a description of recent insights into the pathophysiology of hemostasis and thrombosis. These new insights have arisen from the deployment of novel experimental model systems that are bridging the gap between relatively crude clinical testing modalities such as the prothrombin time and the activated partial thromboplastin time, and the elegant enzymological assessment of isolated hemostatic proteins in purified systems. These new models range from systems assessing real time clot formation in vivo to computer simulations that incorporate the enzymological characteristics of the multitude of complex steps in hemostasis in silico. Following a description of experiments focused on the mechanisms of normal hemostasis; results of experiments from the application of these model systems in clinical settings ranging from hemophilia to differential effects of platelet inhibition on platelet glycoprotein IIIa PL^{A1}/PL^{A2} variants will be discussed. Following an overview of its molecular components, the hemostatic system will be described below as comprised of four phases: initiation, propagation, termination, and elimination.

II. INTRINSIC AND EXTRINSIC PATHWAYS TO THROMBIN GENERATION

Discoveries that have extended our inventory of blood coagulation proteins and the concepts of connectivity and control of hemostatic mechanisms were made possible by the ease of attaining and studying blood and from the fact that mothers almost always note with alarm when their child is bleeding excessively. Many hemorrhagic diseases were identified through clinical observations, including hemophilia A (factor VIII deficiency) (9,10), hemophilia B or Christmas disease (factor IX deficiency) (11,12), hemophilia C (factor XI deficiency), parahemophilia or proaccelerin deficiency (factor V deficiency), Stuart factor disease (factor X deficiency), and serum prothrombin conversion accelerator deficiency (factor VII deficiency). These plasma protein deficiencies represent defects in both the extrinsic tissue factor pathway and the intrinsic pathway. However, no bleeding is associated with deficiencies of factor XII, prekallikrein, and high molecular weight kininogen in the contact pathway. Therefore, these factors cannot be the primary route for the generation of factor IXa that is part of the intrinsic factor X–activating complex following the perforation of a blood vessel. The identification of the contact factors as components of the intrinsic pathway was due to the artifactual activation of these factors by the negatively charged borosilicates in the glass tubes used by early hemostasis investigators.

The primary physiological route for the generation of thrombin is through the tissue factor pathway. Vitamin K–dependent proteins play a central role in both the generation and the inhibition of thrombin generation. The vitamin K–dependent protein family includes the zymogen procoagulant factors VII, IX, X, and prothrombin and the anticoagulants protein C, protein S, and protein Z. They are part of a family of serine proteases (except for protein S and protein Z) related to the trypsin and chymotrypsin superfamily. Vitamin K is essential to the biosynthesis of these clotting factors by participating in the cyclic oxidation and reduction of the enzyme that converts 9 to 13-amino-terminal glutamic acid residues to gamma-carboxyglutamic acid residues (Gla). This posttranslational modification to form Gla residues adds a net negative charge to the molecules that enables the vitamin K–dependent proteins to interact with Ca^{2+} and a membrane surface. Preventing the formation of Gla residues by coumarin derivatives, which are chemically similar in structure to vitamin K, is the basis for anticoagulant therapy. The resultant Gla-deficient, vitamin K–dependent proteins cannot bind Ca^{2+} normally and thus do not function in the surface-dependent reactions of hemostasis. This is also the basis for the antico-agulant activity of sodium citrate, a calcium chelator, in the common blue-top vacuum tube used for clinical laboratory testing of clotting activity.

The activated forms of these vitamin K–dependent proteins/zymogens are the serine protease enzyme components of the macromolecular complexes of vitamin K–dependent proteins and their cofactors. These complexes are commonly referred to by their substrate, thus factor X is activated to factor Xa by the "tenase" complex comprised of factor VIIIa and factor IXa. Three procoagulant complexes are formed on the nega-tively charged membrane surfaces of cells such as endothelial cells, monocytes, and platelets: the extrinsic tenase (factor VIIa–tissue factor), the intrinsic tenase (factor IXa–factor VIIIa), and the prothrombinase (factor Xa–factor Va) complex. One anticoag-ulant complex is formed: the protein Case (thrombin–thrombomodulin) (Fig. 1a). When the enzyme is associated with its respective cofactor on an appropriate membrane surface with Ca^{2+}, the specific reactions occur at an enhanced rate 10^5- to 10^6-fold greater than the enzyme–substrate combination alone. One way to visualize the importance of the assembly of these macromolecular complexes in the formation of the hemostatic plug is to note that it takes a healthy person about 2 minutes for his or her blood to clot, whereas without the cofactor and membrane present it would take the enzyme alone approxi-mately 1.9 years to form a blood clot.

III. INITIATION

Initiation of the tissue factor pathway occurs when circulating factor VIIa comes in con-tact with its integral membrane cofactor, tissue factor, on a membrane surface to form the extrinsic tenase complex. This complex is referred to as extrinsic because it contains tissue factor, a protein not normally present in an active form in the circulation. Controversy does exist over the source and presentation of active tissue factor and whether functional tissue factor circulates in blood (13–16). The factor VIIa that is pre-sent circulating in the plasma (0.1 nM) does not possess the appropriate catalytic machinery to display the serine protease–active site unless it is bound to its cofactor, tissue factor (17,18). The mechanism of the initial activation of the factor VII zymogen is unclear. The single-chain zymogen factor VII can be converted to its two-chain serine protease form by a single cleavage at Arg^{152}-Ile^{153}, yielding the same molecular weight product of 50,000 Da (Table 1). This cleavage can be catalyzed by several proteases, including thrombin (19), factor IXa (20), factor Xa (19), autoactivation by factor VIIa (18), factor XIIa (21), and factor VII–activating protease (22). The function of the extrinsic tenase complex is to activate a fraction of the circulating zymogens, factors IX and X, to their serine protease forms (23–26) in order to, in essence, "prime the pump." Factor X (Mr = 59,000) is the more efficient substrate, requiring a single cleavage at Arg^{194}-Ile^{195} to form the 46,500 Da serine protease factor Xa. The factor IX zymogen (Mr = 55,000) is competitive with factor X and requires a two-step process with sequen-tial cleavages at Arg^{145}–Ala^{146} (factor IXα) and Arg^{180}-Val^{181} (factor IXαβ or factor IXa), releasing a 35-residue activation peptide (27,28) for full biological activity. Both of these cleavages are catalyzed by factor VIIa–tissue factor (24,29) or factor XIa (30,31). Factor IX has also been shown in vitro to be cleaved by factor Xa at Arg^{145} on phospholipid membrane surfaces (32), producing the inactive precursor factor IXα and increasing the overall rate of factor IXa production by tissue factor–factor VIIa. Both cleavage sites in factor IX, Arg^{145} and Arg^{180}, have been identified as single-point muta-tions in hemophilia B (33).

Table 1 Procoagulant, Anticoagulant, and Fibrinolytic Proteins, Inhibitors, and Receptors

Protein	Mr (kDa)	Plasma concentration (nmol/L)	(µg/mL)	Plasma $t_{1/2}$ (days)	Clinical manifestation[a] H	T	Functional classification
Procoagulant proteins and receptors							
Factor XII	80	500	40	2–3	–		Protease zymogen
HMW Kininogen	120	670	80		–		Cofactor
LMW Kininogen	66	1300	90				Cofactor
Prekallikrein	85/88	486	42				Protease zymogen
Factor XI	160	30	4.8	2.5–3.3	+/–		Protease zymogen
Tissue Factor	44			N/A			Cell-associated cofactor
Factor VII	50	10	0.5	0.25	+	+/–	VKD protease zymogen
Factor X	59	170	10	1.5	+		VKD protease zymogen
Factor IX	55	90	5	1	+		VKD protease zymogen
Factor V	330	20	6.6	0.5	+	+	Soluble procofactor
Factor VIII	285	0.7	0.2	0.3–0.5	+	–	Soluble procofactor
WF	255	Varies	10		+		Platelet adhesion carrier for FVIII (monomer)
Factor II	72	1400	100	2.5	+	–	VKD protease zymogen
Thrombin	37						VKD serine protease
Fibrinogen	340	7400	2500	3–5	+	+/–	Structural protein cell Adhesion
Factor XIII	320	94	30	9–10	+	+/–	Transglutaminase zymogen

Anticoagulant proteins, inhibitors, and receptors

Protein C	62	65	4	0.33		+	Proteinase zymogen
Protein S	69	300	20	1.75		+	Inhibitor/cofactor
Protein Z	62	47	2.9	2.5	+/−		Cofactor
Thrombomodulin	100	N/A	N/A	N/A			Cofactor/modulator
Tissue Factor Pathway Inhibitor	40	1–4	0.1	6.4×10^{-4}–1.4×10^{-3}			Proteinase inhibitor
Antithrombin-III	58	3400	140	2.5–3	+		Proteinase inhibitor
Heparin Cofactor II	66	500–1400	33–90	2.5		+/−	Proteinase inhibitor

Fibrinolytic proteins, inhibitors, and receptors

Plasminogen	88	2000	200	2.2			Proteinase zymogen
t-PA	70	0.07	0.005	0.00167			Proteinase zymogen
μ-PA	54	0.04	0.002	0.00347			Proteinase zymogen
TAFI	58	75	4.5	0.00694		+	Carboxypeptidase
PAI-1	52	0.2	0.01	<0.00694			Proteinase inhibitor
PAI-2	47/60	<0.070	<0.005	—			Proteinase inhibitor
α2-Antiplasmin	70	500	70	2.6	+		Proteinase inhibitor
μPAR	55						Cell membrane receptor

VKD: vitamin K–dependent proteins;
[a]Clinical phenotype; the expression of either hemorrhagic or thrombotic phenotype in deficient individuals.
H, Hemorrhagic disease/hemophilia; T, thrombotic disease/thrombophilia: +, presence of phenotype; −, absence of phenotype; ±, some individuals present with the phenotype and others do not.

IV. PROPAGATION

Once generated, the limited amounts of factor Xa produced (~10 pM) (34) by the extrinsic tenase bind to available membrane sites and convert picomolar amounts of prothrombin to thrombin (35–37). Although this process is inefficient, it is essential to the acceleration of coagulation by activating membrane surfaces on cells such as platelets and activating the procofactors factor VIII (38) and factor V (39), allowing the initial formation of the intrinsic tenase (factor IXa–factor VIIIa) and prothrombinase (factor Xa–factor Va) complexes (Fig. 1a). Once the intrinsic tenase complex is formed, it activates the majority of factor Xa (32,40) by being kinetically more efficient (50-fold) than the extrinsic tenase complex (tissue factor–factor VIIa). The serine protease factor Xa then combines with its cofactor factor Va on a membrane surface to form the prothrombinase complex, which catalyzes the conversion of prothrombin to thrombin, the key enzyme in coagulation. Prothrombinase is 300,000-fold more active than the enzyme factor Xa alone in activating thrombin.

V. TERMINATION

All the proteins and complexes are under tight regulation at each stage to ensure an appropriate hemostatic response. Termination of the response depends on two complementary inhibitory anticoagulant processes to eliminate the procoagulant activity: one stoichiometric (antithrombin III and tissue factor pathway inhibitor, TFPI) and the other the dynamic inactivation of the procoagulant cofactors factor Va and factor VIIIa by activated protein C (APC). Antithrombin III and tissue factor pathway inhibitor largely regulate the ultimate amount of thrombin produced.

Antithrombin III is a member of the serpin proteinase inhibitory family and is present in plasma at a concentration (3.4 µM) higher than any of the potential target coagulation enzymes generated by the tissue factor pathway. Despite its name, antithrombin III has a broad spectrum of inhibitory activity, primarily inhibiting thrombin, factor Xa, factor IXa, factor VIIa–tissue factor, factor XIa, and factor XIIa (41–43). The general mechanism of inhibition is the formation of a tight, equimolar (1:1) complex with its serine protease target. Antithrombin III also displays antiproliferative and anti-inflammatory properties that primarily derive from its ability to inhibit thrombin. Deficiency of antithrombin III is associated with thromboembolic disease (44–47).

TFPI (Table 1) circulates in plasma at a low concentration of 0.1 µg/mL (~2.4 nM) and is the principal stoichiometric inhibitor of the extrinsic pathway (factor VIIa–tissue factor) of coagulation. It is also releasable from the vasculature by the action of heparin (48). The TFPI mechanism allows the factor VIIa–tissue factor complex to initiate factor Xa formation but then suppresses high levels of factor Xa product formation by this complex. TFPI is the principal regulator of the initial thrombin generated during the initiation phase (34). The mechanism involves a rapid interaction between TFPI and the factor Xa active site, followed by localization of the complex to the membrane surface. Once surface bound, the factor Xa–TFPI complex rapidly inactivates tissue factor–factor VIIa to form a stable quaternary complex (49–51). The interaction of TFPI with the factor Xa product complex is of critical importance in downregulating the activity of the extrinsic tenase, the factor VIIa–tissue factor procoagulant trigger (52–55). The end result of these stoichiometric mechanisms is to shut down the extrinsic pathway procoagulant initiator. The cooperation of the inhibitors antithrombin III and TFPI provides an activation threshold for the initiation phase of blood coagulation.

Similar cooperative inhibition is seen with the dynamic activated protein C (APC) system. The activity of this anticoagulant pathway is directly dependent on the level of thrombin production. The vitamin K–dependent protein C–activating complex, or protein Case, is a membrane-dependent complex formed between thrombin and its cofactor, the constituitive endothelial cell membrane protein thrombomodulin (Fig. 1a). Protein C is cleaved by thrombin at the Arg[169]-Lys[170] bond, releasing an 11,000 Da activation peptide and forming APC (Mr = 51,000) (56,57). APC inactivates the cofactor for the prothrombinase complex, factor Va, via a sequential series of proteolytic cleavages, inhibiting the generation of thrombin. APC also cleaves and inactivates the cofactor for the intrinsic tenase complex, factor VIIIa, although the spontaneous dissociation and consequent inactivation of factor VIIIa are likely the physiological regulator of factor Xa generation. The inactivation of the cofactors eliminates the procogulant complexes and attenuates thrombin production. The rates of APC inactivation of factors Va and VIIIa are enhanced by protein S. APC also has a profibinolytic effect due to a carboxypeptidase B–like enzyme known as thrombin activatable fibrinolysis inhibitor (TAFI). TAFI is activated by protein Case (thrombin–thrombomodulin) and acts to prolong clot lysis (58,59). APC cleavage of factor Va inhibits thrombin generation, reducing thrombin–thrombomodulin–mediated TAFI activation (60).

VI. ELIMINATION/FIBRINOLYSIS

The pathological thrombus restricting blood flow is structurally composed of aggregated platelets and crosslinked fibrin. The steps in thrombin generation of a crosslinked fibrin clot are shown diagrammatically in Figure 2 and fully described in Sec. IX. Other plasma proteins and blood cells are also trapped within the clot. Clot formation is integrated with clot dissolution by plasmin to maintain hemostatic balance. The traditional view of the plasminogen system centered on its role in the dissolution of fibrin. It has become clear that the plasminogen system has, in fact, two roles: (a) tissue-type plasminogen activator (t-PA) generates plasmin at the fibrin surface and governs fibrin homeostasis, and (6) urokinase-type plasminogen activator (u-PA) binds to a cellular u-PA receptor (u-PAR) and generates pericellular plasmin, which plays an important role in tissue remodeling and cellular migration. The latter function is, to a great extent, mediated by plasmin activation of matrix metalloproteinases (MMP), which degrade extracellular matrix (ECM). t-PA and u-PA are secreted by vascular endothelial cells and regulated by cellular cytokines and components produced during the clotting cascade, including thrombin.

In the absence of fibrin, t-PA is a poor enzyme. However, both t-PA and plasminogen bind to the fibrin surface, with a resulting 100-fold enhancement in plasminogen activation. Thus, t-PA activation of fibrinolysis is primarily initiated by and localized to fibrin. Plasmin digests fibrin in a pattern that produces a collection of degradation products, including a fragment X, fragment Y, and the core fragment D and fragment E (Fig. 1b).

The first step in degrading fibrin is the removal of the α chains, thus exposing the coils. As these coils are cleaved, different sized fragments are released (61). Fibrinogen is represented as a trinodular structure (D-E-D domains), with each E domain and D domain separated by a coiled domain. Upon formation of fibrin, the crosslinks occur between alternating molecules of fibrin at the D domain (D=D). Plasmin degrades fibrin releasing various sized fragments, of which the smallest is the D=D or D-dimer (Mr = 180,000). The largest of these fragments is the XXD, where X=D-E-D, with a mass of 595,000 Da (62,63). Figure 3 presents a diagrammatic representation of products of fibrinolysis. D-dimer has been identified in the blood of patients with various thrombotic or thrombolytic disorders.

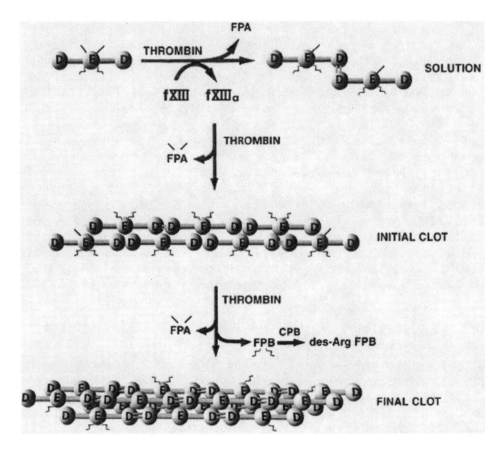

Figure 2 Schematic representation of whole blood fibrin formation. Thrombin at the beginning of clot formation simultaneously acts upon fibrinogen (D-E-D) and factor XIII (fXIII). A portion (~40%) of fibrinopeptide A (FPA) is released from fibrinogen, and an initial clot is formed from the complementary overlap of the exposed sites between the E and D domains of adjacent molecules. Activated factor XIII (fXIIIa) simultaneously cross-links adjacent D domains (D=D). Thus, the initial soluble fibrin clot is composed of fibrinogen, fibrin and γ-γ dimers with fibrinopeptide B (FPB) still attached. The initial clot is continuously acted upon by thrombin, releasing the remaining FPA and some of the FPB to yield a final clot with the majority of FPB still attached. The released FPB is selectively acted upon by a carboxypeptidase B–like enzyme (CPB) cleaving the carboxyl terminal arginine to produce des-Arg FPB. The significance of this cleavage is still unclear. (From Ref. 86.)

Fibrinolysis is regulated primarily by PAI-1, PAI-2, α_2-antiplasmin, and TAFI. The plasminogen activator inhibitors and α_2-antiplasmin are members of the Serpin family of serine protease inhibitors. The antagonism between PAI-1 and the plasminogen activators, two-chain u-PA (K_{assoc} 1.6×10^8 $M^{-1}s^{-1}$) and two-chain t-PA (K_{assoc} 3.7×10^8 $m^{-1}s^{-1}$) provides for a threshold response of the fibrinolytic process in much the same way as the procoagulant/anticoagulant balance provides an activation threshold for the clotting process (64). α_2-Antiplasmin is the primary inhibitor of plasmin. Plasmin, when bound through its lysine-binding sites to fibrin, reacts more slowly with α_2-antiplasmin than when free in solution because α_2-antiplasmin interacts with plasma plasmin by binding to the lysine-binding sites. In contrast, α_2-antiplasmin, bound covalently by factor XIIIa to the Aα chain of fibrin, blocks plasmin binding and appears to decrease plasminogen activation.

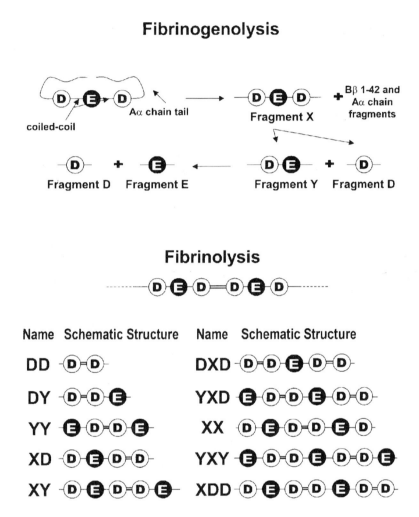

Figure 3 Fibrinogenolysis and fibrinolysis. Fibrinogen is represented as a trinodular structure (D-E-D domains). Each E-domain and D-domain is separated by a coiled-coil domain. The Aα chain tail is shown as a line. Plasmin digests fibrinogen, yielding various fragments, the largest of which is fragment X. Fragment X contains the two D-domains, the E-domain, and the α-helical coiled-coils but lacks the C-termini of the Aα chains and the peptide Bβ chains. Fragment Y consists of the central E-domain connected by the coiled-coil to one of the terminal D-domains. Fragment Y can be further degraded by cleavage of the coiled-coil domain to release a second D-domain and fragment E. The domain composition of the monomer units of degraded fibrin are indicated by the circles containing a "D" or an "E." Intermolecular cross-links between the γ chains are shown as thicker lines connecting the D regions. The structures of the various sized fragments of cross-linked fibrin monomers resulting from plasmin proteolysis of fibrin are presented. The process of fibrinolysis is shown in Figure 1b.

TAFI is a natural inhibitor of fibrinolysis and exists in plasma as a zymogen with a Mr of 58,000 and a plasma concentration of 75 nM (58,59). TAFI is thought to circulate in blood in complex with plasminogen. Activation of TAFI requires the cleavage of the zymogen at Arg[92] yielding a carboxypeptidase B–like enzyme of 35,000 Da. The primary physiological activator of TAFI is thrombin–thrombomodulin (65,66). TAFIa catalyzes the removal of basic amino acids (i.e., lysines and arginines) from the carboxy termini of polypeptides, specifically of fibrin. As carboxy-terminal lysine residues are being exposed in fibrin through the initial degradation by plasmin, TAFIa removes these residues. The fibrin fragments formed constituted a positive feedback loop for plasminogen activation by t-PA. Removing these residues downregulated the number of plasminogen-binding sites and the overall rate of plasmin generation and clot lysis. Thus, TAFIa functions as an antifibrinolytic factor by suppressing the positive feedback pathway of fibrinolysis.

The elimination phase begins the process of tissue repair by dissolving the fibrin-platelet clot generated in the earlier phases of hemostasis. The damaged vascular tissue requires plasmin not only to clear the fibrin clot but also to initiate removal of damaged tissue to allow for cell migration into the injured area (67,68). Plasmin activates a variety of matrix metalloproteinases that degrade subendothelial matrix components and extricate the damaged tissue (68,69). These processes mark the beginnings of the final stages of the hemostatic response, repair and regeneration.

The importance of the tight regulation of these processes is perhaps best illustrated by malfunctions of the hemostatic response. An inappropriate response can lead to one of two opposing, but equally undesirable outcomes. Failure to form a sufficient hemostatic plug to arrest blood flow subsequent to vascular injury can result in pathological hemorrhage. Excessive clot formation or failure to efficiently lyse a clot may result in thrombosis with consequent vascular obstruction. Under normal circumstances, the vascular endothelium together with the aforementioned positive and negative feedback loops within the procoagulant pathways prevent these negative outcomes by actively controlling the coagulation process until a triggering stimulus of sufficient magnitude threatens vascular integrity. Initiation of the procoagulant response also initiates the fibrinolytic response, as described above, simultaneously with repair and regeneration processes. The thromboresistant properties of the vascular endothelium (not covered by this chapter) include t-PA and u-PA release, thrombin–thrombomodulin activation of protein C, the heparin sulfate glycocalyx, prostacyclin release, and nitric oxide generation. In contrast, perturbation of endothelial cells by various agents including thrombin, endotoxin, interferon gamma (IFN-γ), hypoxia, and assorted cytokines can induce a range of procoagulant responses. These procoagulant responses include tissue factor expression, von Willebrand factor release/surface expression, specific surface binding of procoagulant enzymes, platelet-activating factor expression, and PAI-1 release. The role of the endothelium in hemostasis and thrombosis has been reviewed by Hajjar (70).

VII. MODELS OF THROMBIN GENERATION

The focal point of hemostasis is the generation of thrombin. The dynamics of thrombin generation and the significance of this process in defining hemorrhagic and thrombotic phenotypes has been explored in our laboratory through various techniques, including in vitro assays (71–73), para vivo assays (36,74), in vivo assays (75,76), and computational models (34,77).

To understand the process of following thrombin generation utilizing different techniques, a brief description of several of these methods is shown below. Each of the model systems used has specific benefits and limitations. All of the model systems display thrombin generation after tissue factor initiation of the hemostatic reaction with a similar profile (34,37,74,75,78).

1. The first model is an in vitro model (synthetic plasma), which attempts to mimic coagulation utilizing a mixture of all the procoagulant vitamin K–dependent proteins and their cofactors and the stoichiometric inhibitors and is termed a synthetic plasma model. The reaction takes place at 37°C and contains the procoagulants factors VII/VIIa, IX, X, V, VIII, and prothrombin, the anticoagulants antithrombin III and TFPI, and a membrane source of either natural (i.e., platelets) or synthetic membranes (i.e., phosphatidyl choline/phosphatidyl serine) (35,37,78–84). The reaction is started by the addition of relipidated tissue factor.

2. The primary tissue factor pathway of coagulation is visualized without the interference of the contact pathway by performing para vivo studies in which the contact pathway is suppressed by the use of corn trypsin inhibitor (CTI). Whole blood is obtained by phlebotomy and maintained in CTI at 37°C and induced to clot by the addition of a fixed amount of membrane relipidated tissue factor (36,74,85–91). Since this is whole blood, the vascular component is absent.

3. The most biologically relevant model is an in vivo bleeding time model (Simplate) of the hemostatic system, in which whole blood exuding from a microvascular wound is sequentially sampled for relevant product formation (75,76,92,93). The vascular component is present, and an injury induced by the device is the source of tissue factor initiation in the circulation.

4. Finally, computer simulations of the coagulation system based on the ensemble of published and estimated rate constants, mechanisms, and concentrations of the procoagulants factors VII/VIIa, IX, X, V, VIII, and prothrombin and the anticoagulants antithrombin III and TFPI were developed to rapidly determine the fate of the protein products (34,77,94,95). Computer simulations using Speed Rx software is the least expensive, most rapid, and most convenient method of analysis. Because it is a numerical model (in silico model), it can provide insight into the regulation of reaction mechanisms occurring at concentrations of intermediates and products that may not be measured by current technology (i.e., $<10^{-19}$ M).

Different techniques being used by others to explore mechanisms of hemostatic competence are the thrombogram or endogenous thrombin potential (measures thrombin generation from recalcified citrated plasma initiated with tissue factor) (73), the thromboelastogram (measures fibrin clot formation and fibrinolysis) (96), and the activated clotting time (measures clotting in a tissue factor based model) (97).

The intricate blood coagulation mechanisms that govern thrombin generation can be categorized into four distinct phases for analysis: initiation of coagulation, clot formation, propagation of thrombin formation, and termination of the procoagulant response. These phases are analyzed in the next sections utilizing the models described above.

VIII. INITIATION OF COAGULATION

The hemostatic system is relatively quiescent if vascular damage is not present; however, if vascular injury does occur, a measured response is triggered with platelet and fibrin deposition proportionate to the degree of damage. Platelets play a major role in the blood coagulation response. Activated platelets provide the membrane surfaces upon which coagulation enzyme complexes can be anchored, assembled, and expressed. The activated platelet membrane therefore adds both an initiating and a limiting component to the extent of a coagulation reaction. More vascular damage produces more anchored activated platelets, and more activated membrane allows the assembly of more coagulation enzymes, which ultimately results in increased fibrin formation.

When the vascular system is perturbed, the initial stages of the hemostatic response are triggered. The principal player is the extrinsic tenase complex, which is composed of a cell membrane, tissue factor exposed by vascular damage or cytokine stimulation, and plasma factor VIIa. This complex activates low levels of the zymogens factor X and factor IX to their respective enzymes factor Xa (~10 pM) and factor IXa (~1 pM). Once generated, the limited amounts of factor Xa produced bind to available membrane sites and convert picomolar amounts of prothrombin to thrombin (35–37). This time period in which factor Xa directly generates picomolar amounts of thrombin is referred to as the initiation phase of blood coagulation. During the initiation phase, circulating blood cells and procoagulant proteins are activated, the procoagulant elements necessary for the full procoagulant response are generated, and a preliminary fibrin network is formed.

In an analysis of a whole blood para vivo model of coagulation, an initial time course of thrombin generation (based on thrombin–antithrombin III complex formation) and of the protein products of its catalytic activities illustrates that most procoagulant responses to thrombin occur during the initiation phase before fibrin clot formation (74) (Fig. 4). The small amount of thrombin that is generated during this phase (~10–25 nM) is able to activate platelets (500 ± 0.2 pM), factor XIII (800 ± 0.3 pM), factor V (800 ± 0.3 pM), and factor VIII and release fibrinopeptide A (1.3 ± 0.4 nM) and fibrinopeptide B (1.7 ± 0.5 nM) from fibrinogen to form fibrin. Less than 0.2% of the final thrombin produced is required to achieve the activation of its primary substrates in blood. Many of these products are required to provide the catalysts that generate the bulk of thrombin (~95%) during the propagation phase of the reaction (74,98).

IX. CLOT FORMATION

Fibrinogen is the plasma precursor of fibrin. Fibrinogen is composed of six polypeptide chains [two Aα (Mr = 66,500), two Bβ (Mr = 52,000), and two γ chains (Mr = 46,500)] that form two symmetrical half-molecules (three chains each) with the amino termini crosslinked to each other. Fibrinogen circulates in plasma at a concentration of 7 μM and a Mr of 340,000 (Table 1). The outside two domains of fibrinogen are comprised of the Bβ and γ chains and designated domain D. The central domain that contains the amino termini of all the chains is designated domain E (Fig. 2). From x-ray crystallographic data, one molecule of fibrinogen has a trinodular structure aligned as D-E-D domains.

The description of fibrinogen activation and fibrin assembly has been based on studies using citrated plasmas or purified proteins. The three main players in fibrinogen-to-fibrin conversion are the enzyme thrombin, the substrate fibrinogen, and the crosslinking tranglutaminase factor XIII. The kinetics of fibrinogen cleavage by thrombin results in the hydrolysis of Arg-Gly bonds removing small, polar amino-terminal pieces (fibrinopeptides, FP) from the α and β chains (99,100). Cleavage by thrombin at the Arg[16]-Gly[17] bond of the Aα chain releases FPA and forms fibrin I. The release of two FPA peptides exposes a site in the E domain that has a complementary overlap with a site in the D domain to form overlapping fibrils. Subsequent cleavage of the Arg[14]-Gly[15] bond by

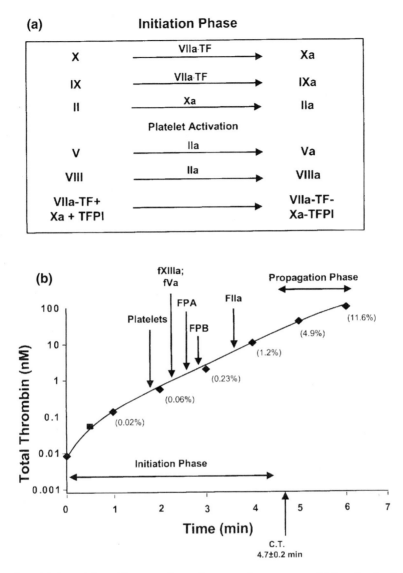

Figure 4 Initiation of thrombin generation and procoagulant response. (a) Low levels of thrombin are required to initiate clot formation (initiation phase) and trigger the coagulation cascade response (propagation phase). The enzymes, cofactors, and inhibitors act together to generate a hemostatic response that can be divided into an initiation phase and propagation/termination phase. During the initiation phase, factors X and IX are converted to their respective serine proteases, factor Xa and factor IXa; low levels of thrombin are subsequently generated by factor Xa. This thrombin can then activate platelets and procofactors factors V and VIII, which stimulate further thrombin generation during the propagation phase. Thrombin generation is attenuated by shutting down the initiation phase via stoichiometric inhibitor of the extrinsic Xase complex, tissue factor pathway inhibitor (TFPI). (b) Time course of early thrombin-antithrombin III (total thrombin) complex formation from whole blood coagulation of 35 individuals is presented: y axis, total thrombin concentrations are shown on a log scale. Arrows indicate the time and total thrombin concentration at which each of the indicated events [osteonectin (OSN) release, a marker of platelet activation, factor XIII activation (fXIIIa), fibrinopeptide A (FPA) release, fibrinopeptide B (FPB) release, and prothrombin activation] has entered a phase of rapid activation. The percentage of total thrombin present at the point of activation is shown in parentheses. Beginning of the propagation phase coincides with the clot time (CT). (From Ref. 75.)

thrombin releases FPB to form fibrin II, presumably increasing lateral aggregation of the protofibrils. This is thought to be a requirement for the transglutaminase factor XIII to begin crosslinking adjacent chains (101). Only the Aα chain and the γ chain [which has donor (Gln[398]) and acceptor (Lys[406]) sites] participate in crosslinking of adjacent glutamyl and lysyl residues by factor XIIIa (102). No residues in the Bβ chain participate in crosslink formation. The process of fibrin formation and polymerization is demonstrated in Figure 2.

To understand the in vivo process of fibrin formation, a para vivo model with nonanticoagulated blood has recently been used (86). Differences in the pattern of fibrin formation based on fibrinopeptide release were detected when compared to previous models (103–106). In this experimental model, cleavage of FPA and subsequent clot formation occur just before the propagation phase of thrombin generation. At the point of visual clot formation, virtually all fibrinogen (and some product already crosslinked) disappears from the fluid phase of the reaction. Thus, the clot appears to be a mixture composed of fibrin I (incomplete cleavage of fibrinogen) and fibrinogen (Fig. 2). The insoluble material present in the fibrin clot is virtually all crosslinked by factor XIIIa, whose activation is nearly simultaneous with FPA removal. Therefore, the transglutaminse factor XIIIa is available to crosslink the γ chains of the initial fibrinogen/fibrin I clot. In purified systems, it has been observed that FPB removal precedes the crosslinking reaction. However, in whole blood the B peptide antigen epitope is found associated with the β chain after clot formation has occurred. FPB release proceeds at a slower rate than FPA release, occurs after γ-γ dimer formation, and only reaches approximately 38% of its theoretical maximum value.

In a whole blood para vivo study, the concentrations of thrombin required for initial fibrin formation were calculated to be 0.8 ± 0.3 nM for factor XIII activation, 1.3 ± 0.4nM for FPA release, and 1.7 ± 0.5 nM for FPB release (74). These processes all occur during the initiation phase of thrombin generation, prior to a visual clot time. By visual clot time, 50% of FPA has already been released and ~50% of factor XIII has been activated, suggestive of soluble fibrinogen/fibrin products. FPB release occurs later, with only ~15% released prior to visual clot time. At visual clot time approximately 10–25 nM thrombin is present compared to the ultimate total of 851 ± 53 nM at the end of the propagation phase. It thus appears that there is ongoing fibrin formation within the preliminarily crosslinked fibrin/fibrinogen clot following visible clot formation and factor XIII–mediated cross linkage.

Fibrin clot–based assays are commonly utilized in the clinical diagnosis of bleeding disorders. Two in vitro plasma tests, prothrombin time and activated partial thromboplastin time, segregate the coagulation process into tissue factor–initiated or surface contact factor processes, respectively. The activated partial thromboplastin time initiates coagulation by the introduction of a negatively charged foreign surface such as diatomaceous earth and measures only the biological constituents intrinsic to plasma. This assay is sensitive to isolated or combined deficiencies of factor XII, high molecular weight kininogen, prekallikrein, factor XI, factor VIII, factor IX, factor X, factor V, prothrombin, and fibrinogen. The prothrombin time assay, based on initiating coagulation via an extrinsic tissue factor source (thromboplastin), is sensitive to isolated or combined deficiencies of factor VII, factor X, factor V, prothrombin, and fibrinogen. Although these in vitro clotting assays help us establish a basis for hemostasis, it is not always mirrored by human pathology associated with bleeding or thrombosis. For example, when individuals with hemophilia A (factor VIII deficiency) are studied in a para vivo whole blood model, their clot times, although slightly prolonged, are not significantly different from those of healthy individuals (Fig. 5). The major difference is in the total amount and rate of thrombin generation

Propagation / Termination Phase

(a)

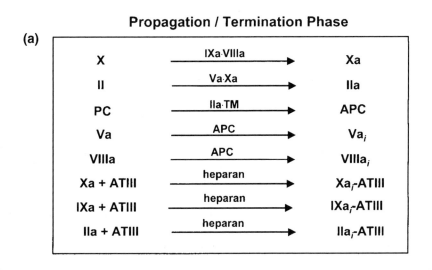

(b)

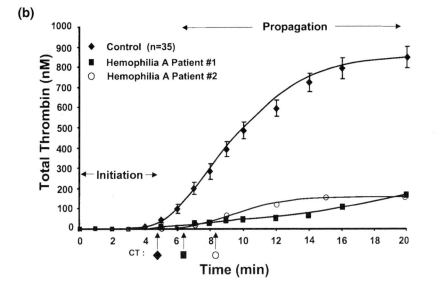

Figure 5 Propagation and termination of thrombin generation. (a) During the propagation phase the majority of thrombin is generated from activation of factor X by factor IXa–factor VIIIa (intrinsic tenase complex) and subsequent formation of the prothrombinase complex (factor Va–factor Xa). Thrombin that is formed then downregulates itself by binding to thrombomodulin (TM) and activating protein C (APC), which inactivates cofactors for the intrinsic tenase (factor IXa) and prothrombinase complex (factor Va). The stoichiometric inhibitor antithrombin III (AT III) inhibits the serine proteases factor Xa, factor IXa, and factor IIa (thrombin). Heparins and heparin sulfates potentiate these reactions and are used in treatment of thrombosis. (b) A time course of thrombin–antithrombin III formation during whole blood coagulation initiated with 5 pM tissue factor (74). Data represent means ± SEM for 35 individuals; thrombin-antithrombin levels reach maximum levels of 900 nM ($\blacklozenge$). Clot time (CT) is shown below, with the symbols for each curve. Thrombin generation is divided into two phases: an initiation phase and propagation phase. When two hemophilia A patients were studied ($\blacksquare$, $\bigcirc$), clot time is delayed and propagation phase of thrombin generation is not present (85, 90). By not having factor VIIIa present, the intrinsic tenase complex is unable to generate the additional factor Xa required for the burst or propagation phase of thrombin generation.

during the propagation phase. This difference would not be recognized with the use of a whole blood clot-based assay, since the endpoint is the clot and the propagation phase does not begin until after clot formation.

X. PROPAGATION OF THROMBIN FORMATION

Assembly of the multicomponent procoagulant complexes on the membrane surface triggers the propagation of the coagulation response that we observed to occur after clot formation. The net result of the activities of the intrinsic and extrinsic tenase complexes is to generate greater amounts of factor Xa for the formation of the prothrombinase complex. The prothrombinase complex (factor Xa–factor Va–membrane Ca^{2+}) converts prothrombin to thrombin in an explosive manner. This rapid burst of thrombin is required to sustain the procoagulant response by participating in multiple processes, including activating platelets, factors V, VIII, VII and XI, cleaving fibrinogen to form fibrin, and activating factor XIII and TAFI. Therefore, the propagation phase generates explosive thrombin, builds a stable crosslinked fibrin-platelet clot, and stems blood loss.

Important to the formation of the prothrombinase complex is the generation of factor Xa. Factor Xa is a unique regulatory enzyme in that it is formed through both the intrinsic tenase and the extrinsic tenase complexes. Under normal conditions, factor Xa is the rate-limiting component of the prothrombinase complex. The other components of the complex, platelets (membrane surface–binding sites) and the cofactor (factor Va), are activated rapidly to produce a surplus that is ready for action. The coagulation mechanism can become sensitive to factor V or platelets when confronted with congenital deficiencies, thrombocytopenia, platelet pathology, or pharmacological interventions[107].

After the initial factor Xa generated via the factor VIIa–tissue factor complex during the initiation phase is downregulated by TFPI, additional factor Xa is generated by the intrinsic tenase complex (factor IXa–factor VIIIa–membrane Ca^{2+}). The relative factor Xa generation by these complexes is illustrated in a computational model shown in Figure 6. Initially, the concentration of the factor VIIa–tissue factor complex is higher than the concentration of the factor VIIIa–factor IXa complex, which requires activation and assembly. As time progresses, the contribution of the intrinsic tenase complex exceeds the extrinsic tenase complex in generating factor Xa. The intrinsic tenase complex is kinetically more efficient and activates factor X at a 50- to 100- fold higher rate than the extrinsic tenase complex (32,40,108). The intrinsic pathway burst of factor Xa generation overcomes the levels of factor Xa inhibitors such as TFPI and achieves maximal prothrombinase activity and propagation of the procoagulant response. The bulk of thrombin (~95%) is formed during the propagation phase, after fibrin clot formation as seen in the para vivo model shown in Figure 5. Without the intrinsic tenase complex being formed, as occurs in situations like hemophilia A or B, factor Xa is not generated in levels sufficient to produce the propagation phase of thrombin generation (Fig. 5) (74,85,90).

XI. TERMINATION

Termination of the thrombin-generating reaction is essential to eliminate the procoagulant response and clot formation. Thrombin inhibition is the ultimate result of complex formation with the stoichiometric inhibitors antithrombin III and TFPI. A computational (in

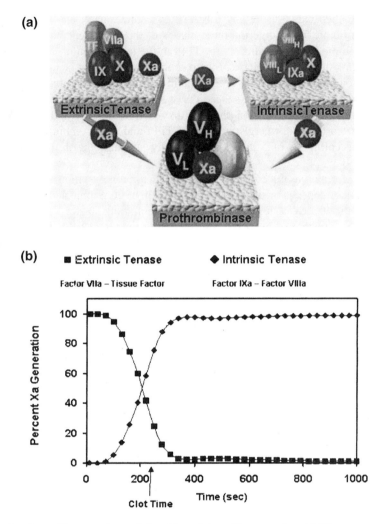

Figure 6 Factor Xa generation and the effect of thrombin generation. (a) Three procoagulant complexes are illustrated: extrinsic tenase, intrinsic tenase, and the prothrombinase. Each membrane complex consists of a vitamin K–dependent serine protease [factor VIIa (FVIIa), factor IX/IXa (FIX/FIXa) or prothrombin/thrombin (II/IIa)] and a soluble or cell surface–associated cofactor [factor VIIIa (heavy and light chain VIII_H and VIII_L) and factor Va (heavy and light chain V_H and V_L) and tissue factor (TF)]. Each serine protease is shown in association with the appropriate cofactor protein and zymogen substrate(s) on the membrane surface. The membrane serves as a scaffold for the coagulation reactants, enhancing the reaction rates by 10^5–10^6-fold. When vascular damage or inflammatory cytokine activation occurs, TF becomes exposed to flowing blood and FVIIa. The formed extrinsic tenase complex activates the circulating serine protease zymogens FIX and FX. FIXa becomes the serine protease for the intrinsic tenase complex with its cofactor FVIIIa, and activates FX to its active serine protease FXa. FXa formed from either the extrinsic tenase or intrinsic tenase activates II to IIa on the prothrombinase complex. (Courtesy Vermont Business Graphics.). (b) Computer simulation of the time course of factor Xa generation upon activation of the factor VIIa–tissue factor pathway. Factor Xa concentrations are expressed as % of maximum for the extrinsic Xase (■, tissue factor – factor VIIa) (100% ≅ 10 pM) and % of maximum for the intrinsic Xase (◆, factor IXa – factor VIIIa) (100% ≅ 1 nM). The factor Xa that is initially produced is via the extrinsic tenase complex. After clot time the majority of factor Xa generated is via the intrinsic Xase. The clot time represents the time point in the computer simulation where calculated thrombin levels are comparable to thrombin levels (~10 nM) measured in clotting whole blood. (From Ref. 34.)

silico model) in silico model using physiological concentrations of antithrombin III and TFPI as seen in Figure 7 illustrate the three phases of thrombin generation. Utilizing in vitro and in silico models, the main role for TFPI in the termination of thrombin generation is in inhibiting the initiation phase of the reaction, thus delaying factor Xa generation (34,109). The stoichiometric inhibitor antithrombin III is a general serpin inhibitor that in an in silico model produces the bell-shaped curve seen in Figure 7. The major effect of antithrombin III is on the propagation phase of the reaction. In silico and in vitro experiments demonstrated that the synergistic effect of TFPI and antithrombin III between the tissue factor concentrations of 5 and 1 pM virtually attenuate the thrombin formation response (34,109).

The initial formation of a clot in a low tissue factor concentration model similar to most in vivo settings depends on the generation of 10–30 nM thrombin and is easily downregulated by TFPI, whereas at high tissue factor concentrations, factor VIIa–tissue factor generate factor Xa rapidly and mask the contribution of the factor VIIIa–factor IXa complex in clot endpoint assays. This is the case for the prothrombin time in which the initiator, thromboplastin (tissue factor and phospholipid), is chosen to produce a clot time of 11–15 seconds. This corresponds to a tissue factor concentration of >20 nM. In our whole blood studies, a concentration of 5 pM tissue factor is used, which produces a clot time of approximately 5 minutes. Therefore, in situations like hemophilia A, the prothrombin time does not reflect a change in clot time in this well-established hemorrhagic disease because

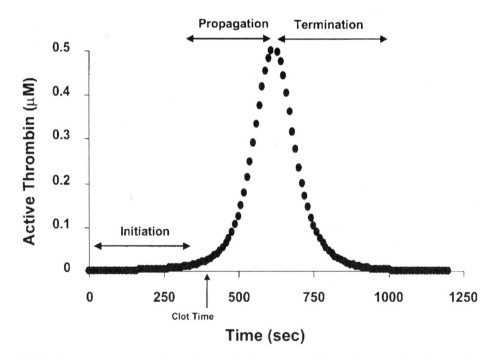

Figure 7 Computer simulation of the termination phase of thrombin generation. An in silico model illustrating the termination phase of thrombin generation shown as active thrombin versus time. The mean physiological concentrations of the procoagulants, factors VII/VIIa, II, IX, X, V, VIII, and the anticoagulants antithrombin III and tissue factor pathway inhibitor. Coagulation is initiated with a stimulus of 5 pM tissue factor. Clot time is seen at the onset of the propagation phase.

of the overwhelming impact of the large concentrations of thromboplastin used in the assay. An in vivo analogue of this phenomenon is the success of large doses of recombinant factor VIIa in the treatment of hemophiliacs with inhibitors. Thus, the major defect in the hemophilias occurs after clot time during the propagation phase of thrombin generation, which is dramatically decreased (Fig. 5).

XII. PHENOTYPIC PROFILES OF THE INITIATION, CLOT FORMATION, AND PROPAGATION PHASES

Although the initiation and propagation phases of thrombin generation were separated for discussion, they are intricately intertwined and essential to the hemostatic response. Fibrin clot formation occurs at the juncture of the initiation and propagation phases of the reaction. Most of our past knowledge about hemorrhagic syndromes has been confined to the associations of bleeding pathology with thrombin formation during the initiation phase and clot formation because of the nature of clinical screening assays (e.g., PT, PTT). Utilizing the synthetic plasma or para vivo model, we have determined what kind of effect certain proteins, congenital deficiencies, or therapeutic regimens have on either the initiation or the propagation phase (Table 2). The anticoagulant antithrombin III has a major influence on the propagation phase, directly inhibiting thrombin and other serine proteases (34,109), whereas the anticoagulant TFPI has a major effect on the initiation phase of the reaction, downregulating the initial generation of factor Xa from the extrinsic tenase (factor VIIa–tissue factor) complex (34,109). Protein C and thrombomodulin influence the propagation phase (80).

Table 2 Major Effects on Thrombin Generation Phases

Agent	Initiation	Propagation	Ref.
Par vivo / synthetic plasma assays			
Antithrombin III	No effect	Effect	34,109
TFPI	Effect	No effect	34,109
PC/TM	No effect	Effect	80
TRAP	No effect	No effect	107
PGE$_1$	Effect	Effect	107
IIb-IIIa antagonists	No effect	Effect	107
Aspirin	No effect	No effect	107
Warfarin	Effect	Effect	117
Hemophilia A (FVIII)	No effect	Effect	85,90,91
Hemophilia B (FIX)	No effect	Effect	90,91
Hemophilia C (FXI)	Effect[a]	Effect[a]	81,85
Parahemophilia (FV)	Effect	Effect	
Factor VII (−)	Effect	Effect	131
In vivo simplate assay			
Aspirin	Effect	Effect	75
Simastatin	Effect	Effect	92
PL^{A2} vs. PL^{A1}	Effect	Effect	76
PL^{A1} + aspirin	Effect	Effect	76
PL^{A2} + aspirin	No effect	No effect	76

[a] Seen only at low tissue factor concentrations.
F: factor.

Platelet activation is not ordinarily the rate-limiting step in the tissue factor pathway to thrombin generation (87). Thus, as anticipated, when platelets are preactivated with the thrombin receptor activation peptide (TRAP) in a para vivo model, there is no effect on thrombin generation during the initiation or the propagation phase (107). These results reinforce the conclusion that in the tissue factor–initiated reaction in normal blood, platelet and factor V activation are not the limiting factors of the tissue factor–induced thrombin generation during the initiation phase (36,37). Rather, factor Xa appears to be the limiting component of the thrombin-generating prothrombinase complex (37). In contrast to TRAP, PGE_1, a natural prostanoid that inhibits intracellular release of stored Ca^{2+} and platelet activation by the upregulation of adenylate cyclase to form cAMP (110), has strong effects on both phases (107). These para vivo results suggest that PGE_1 suppresses the formation of platelet membrane sites, which are required for complex assembly, making thrombin generation during the initiation and propagation phases platelet dependent. These results with PGE_1 are similar to para vivo studies with whole blood from thrombocytopenic patients with platelet counts less than 11,000/mL (87). Analogs of PGE_1 have been shown to be useful in controlling pulmonary hypertension (111).

Integrelin or abciximab inhibitors of the glycoprotein IIbIIIa complex on the platelet surface are designed to block the interactions between fibrinogen and platelets, thus suppressing the formation of platelet aggregates (112). In para vivo studies with these antibodies, the major effect is seen as a suppressed propagation phase of thrombin generation (107). This inhibition of thrombin generation during the propagation phase by the platelet antagonists probably accounts for the antithrombotic effect of these agents.

Aspirin has proven effective in secondary prevention of coronary artery disease (CAD). Its efficacy has been ascribed to its antiplatelet action through inhibiting thromboxane A_2 (TxA_2)–mediated platelet aggregation (113). Experiments with aspirin have no effect in whole blood para vivo experiments on either the initiation or propagation phases of thrombin generation (107). This suggests that aspirin's therapeutic effect does not arise primarily from direct modulation of platelet procoagulant function in the tissue factor pathway to thrombin generation. Second, thrombin, a potent platelet agonist, may override the weak inhibitory effects of aspirin via the TxA_2 pathway. Conversely, in the in vivo bleeding time model examining the effect of aspirin using the Simplate bleeding time method, a suppressant effect is seen on both the initiation and propagation phases (75). These results suggest that aspirin has an effect at the vascular/platelet interface.

Coumadin (warfarin) is used to treat/prevent venous thromboembolism, systemic thromboembolic disorders, and arterial thrombosis and is the most frequently prescribed oral anticoagulant in the United States (114,115). Coumadin has a reasonably predictable onset and duration of action along with excellent bioavailability. Coagulation inhibition via warfarin therapy can be affected by many variables that differ among individuals taking similar doses, including liver function in the synthesis of the clotting factors, enhancement/suppression of anticoagulant effects from interactions with other medications, and dietary intake/absorption of vitamin K (116). Monitoring warfarin therapy by prothrombin times (PTs) standardized by the international normalized ratio (INR) is the presently accepted monitoring tool. When stably anticoagulated individuals are studied over time on coumadin therapy in a para vivo model, the initiation and propagation phases of thrombin generation are extremely variable, with an increase in the initiation phase and a decreased propagation phase seen (117). The extent of these alterations is not predicted by the INR, which is monitored by the clot endpoint PT assay, pointing to the need for monitoring tools that better reflect the physiology of clot formation.

When individuals with hemophilia A (factor VIII) or hemophilia B (factor IX) are studied in both the synthetic plasma and para vivo models, the major influence is on the propagation phase of thrombin generation (85,90,91). It is during this phase that 95% of thrombin is generated after fibrin clot formation (74). When hemophilia C (factor XI deficiency) is studied in either a para vivo model with natural hemophilia C blood (85) or a synthetic plasma model (81), the significance of factor XI deficiency is only prominent at the lowest tissue factor concentrations. At moderate concentrations of tissue factor (5–10 pM) congenital factor XI deficiency has little or no effect on thrombin generation (85). When the tissue factor concentration is changed to 1–2 pM, the initiation phase is extended, the clot time increased, and the propagation phase decreased. This variability is possibly a reflection of the dimension of the tissue factor stimulus associated with the vascular lesion. Parahemophilia (factor V deficiency) and factor VII deficiency have a major influence on both phases, and in some instances no thrombin is generated during a 20-minute time period. Interestingly, factor V–deficient mice die in utero, but individuals with less than 1% factor V are living (118–120).

Pharmacological interventions and genetic influence on thrombin generation during the initation and propagation phases were tested using the in vivo bleeding time blood model (Table 2). Statins like 3-hydroxy-3-methylglutaryl coenzyme A (HMG-CoA) reductase inhibitors (e.g., Simvastatin) have been shown to be effective in the prevention of CAD by reducing cholesterol levels (121,122), stabilizing atherosclerotic plaques, improving endothelial function, and enhancing fibrinolysis and antithrombotic actions (123,124). Individuals on Simvastatin were tested with the in vivo bleeding time model before and after treatment (92). Results showed a decreased activation of prothrombin during both phases that was independent of the lipid-lowering effect. This effect on blood coagulation may be due to suppressed isoprenoid production, which are substrates for posttranslational modification of numerous intracellular proteins, leading to decreased expression of tissue factor in the endothelium and/or subendothelium (125).

In vivo bleeding time blood studies have been conducted on individuals with the glycoprotein PL^{A1}, PL^{A2} platelet receptor polymorphism before and after low-dose aspirin ingestion (76) (Table 2). Glycoprotein IIb-IIIa molecules play an important role in platelet aggregation and adhesion and determining efficient thrombus formation (126). A common glycoprotein IIbIIIa polymorphism is characterized by a thymidine-to-cytosine transition at nucleotide 1565, which results in Leu33-to-Pro substitution, defining the Pl^{A1} and Pl^{A2} alleles, respectively (127). The Pl^{A2} allele is present in 20–30% of the European population (128) and is associated with a 2.8-fold increase in the risk of the first myocardial infarction. Sudden cardiac death was reported to occur more frequently in the Pl^{A2} carriers (129). Experiments with the in vivo bleeding time blood model demonstrated that the presence of the Pl^{A2} allele is associated with enhanced thrombin formation during both phases and that the Pl^{A2} carriers exhibited impaired anticoagulant action of aspirin (76). This study provides evidence that in the Pl^{A2} carriers compared to the Pl^{A1A1} homozygotes, thrombin is generated more rapidly at sites of microvascular injury and that this difference between genotypes becomes more pronounced by aspirin. Therefore, individuals possessing the Pl^{A2} polymorphism may have life-long procoagulant effects as well as muted antithrombotic effects of aspirin. These experiments demonstrate that for the evaluation of hemorrhagic risk or antithrombotic effect, both the initiation and propagation phases of thrombin generation as well as genotype are important for diagnosis and treatment. As a consequence, a clot endpoint–based assay is unable to display both these parameters.

Interestingly, the G20210A prothrombin polymorphism has been associated with both an increased risk for venous thrombosis and higher prothrombin levels (130). In

(a)   **(b)**

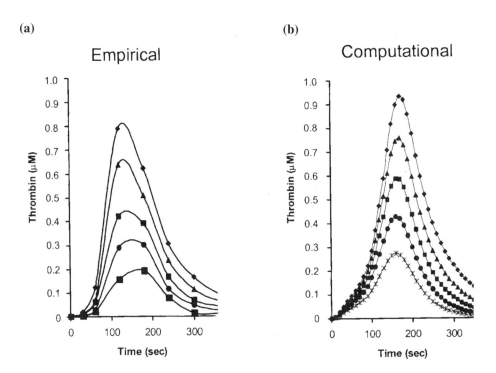

Figure 8 Empirical and computational simulation of thrombin generation. The extent of thrombin generation for reaction mixtures containing various levels of prothrombin ranging from 50% (stars) to 150% (filled diamonds). (a) An empirical or in vitro synthetic plasma system is illustrated with varying prothrombin concentration from 50 to 150%. (b) A numerical simulation of thrombin generation corresponding to the same conditions as the empirical system is seen. (From Ref. 34.)

in vitro studies, altering the plasma prothrombin concentration within the range of 50–150% (Fig. 8a) is enough to change the propagation phase of thrombin generation (83). When the concentration is over 100% the propagation phase increases, and when the concentration is below 100% the propagation phase decreases. A numerical simulation of these prothrombin concentrations has the same result (Fig. 8b) (34). The only other protein that has a great effect on the propagation phase when the concentration is varied between 50 and 150% is antithrombin III (83). Most of the other proteins do not have an individual effect, but when combined effects are considered, they can have a significant influence. Interestingly, what is considered a normal or healthy coagulation protein level extends over a range of 50 – 150% of the mean plasma value. In complex diseases, like CAD, our accepted notion of "normal" appears to need serious reassessment.

XIII. CONCLUSION

Recent advances in the dynamic assessment of the clot formation process, from initiation to termination, have shed new light on such conditions as the hemophilias, thrombophilias, and anticoagulant therapy. All of these conditions have in common the fact that the affected patient's hemostatic system is deviated markedly from normal. In contrast, an important insight to be gained from these dynamic new analytical tools is the wide variation in "normal" hemostasis, which has been essentially invisible to our routine screening tools and factor assays. We have shown major differences, for example, in the propagation phase of thrombus formation, with variation of hemostatic factors like prothrombin and antithrombin III within the normal range. The vast majority of patients who suffer from venous or arterial thrombosis have hemostatic systems that fall within the normal range, and yet thrombosis is the major cause of death in western countries. These normal variations can be initially assessed by in silico computer simulations based on theoretical constructs or clinical data sets and then tested in a range of para vivo to in vivo systems. A test or tests that would predict the propensity for thrombosis in these normal populations has been for some time the Holy Grail of hemostasis testing. The dynamic testing modalities reviewed in this chapter, and tests like them, appear to have the potential to fill this important clinical need.

REFERENCES

1. Ratnoff OD. The evolution of knowledge about hemostasis. In: Ratnoff OD, Forbes CD, eds. Disorders of Hemostasis. Philadelphia: W.B. Saunders Company; 1996:1–22.
2. Brinkhous KM. A short history of hemophilia, with some comments on the word "hemophilia." In: Brinkhous KM, Hemker HC, eds. Handbook of Hemophilia. New York: Elsevier Publishing Company; 1975.
3. Owen CA. Older concepts of blood coagulation. In: Nichols WL, Bowie EJ, eds. A History of Blood Coagulation. Rochester, MN: Mayo Foundation for Medical Education and Research; 2001:7–16.
4. Nichols WL, Bowie EJ, eds. A History of Blood Coagulation. Rochester, MN: Mayo Foundation for Medical Education and Research; 2001.
5. Morawitz P. Die Chemie der Blutgerrinnung. Ergebn Physiol. 1905; 4:307.
6. Wright IS. The nomenclature of blood clotting factor. Thromb Diath Haemost. 962; 7:381–388.
7. MacFarlane RG. An enzyme cascade in the blood clotting mechanism and its function as a biochemical amplifier. Nature. 1964; 202:498–499.
8. Davie EW, Ratnoff OD. Waterfall sequence for intrinsic blood clotting. Science. 1964; 145:1310–1312.
9. Patek AJ, Taylor F. Hemophillia II: some properties of a substance obtained from normal plasma effective in accelerating the clotting of hemophilic blood. J Clin Invest. 1937; 113–124.
10. Brinkhous KM. Clotting defect in hemophilia: deficiency in a plasma factor required for platelet utilization. Proc Soc Exp Bio Med. 1947; 66:117–120.
11. Schulman II. Hemorrhagic disease in an infant due to deficiency of a previously undescribed clotting factor. Blood. 1952; 7:794–807.
12. Biggs R, Douglas AS, MacFarlane RG. Christmas disease: a condition previously mistaken for hemophilia. Br Med J. 1952; 2:1384.
13. Giesen PL, Rauch U, Bohrmann B, et al. Blood-borne tissue factor: another view of thrombosis. Proc Natl Acad Sci USA. 1999; 96:2311–2315.
14. Osterud B. The role of platelets in decrypting monocyte tissue factor. Semin Hematol. 2001; 38:2–5.
15. Zillmann A, Luther T, Muller I, et al. Platelet-associated tissue factor contributes to the collagen-triggered activation of blood coagulation. Biochem Biophys Res Commun. 2001; 281:603–609.
16. Bogdanov VY, Balasubramanian V, Hathcock J, Vele O, Lieb M, Nemerson Y. Alternatively spliced human tissue factor: a circulating, soluble, thrombogenic protein. Nat Med. 2003; 9:458–462.

17. Neuenschwander PF, Fiore MM, Morrissey JH. Factor VII autoactivation proceeds via interaction of distinct protease- cofactor and zymogen-cofactor complexes. Implications of a two-dimensional enzyme kinetic mechanism. J Biol Chem. 1993; 268:21489–21492.

18. Lawson JH, Krishnaswamy S, Butenas S, Mann KG. Extrinsic pathway proteolytic activity. Methods Enzymol. 1993; 222:177–195.

19. Radcliffe R, Nemerson Y. Activation and control of factor VII by activated factor X and thrombin. Isolation and characterization of a single chain form of factor VII. J Biol Chem. 1975; 250:388–395.

20. Seligsohn U, Osterud B, Brown SF, Griffin JH, Rapaport SI. Activation of human factor VII in plasma and in purified systems: roles of activated factor IX, kallikrein, and activated factor XII. J Clin Invest. 1979; 64:1056–1065.

21. Kisiel W, Fujikawa K, Davie EW. Activation of bovine factor VII (proconvertin) by factor XIIa (activated Hageman factor). Biochemistry. 1977; 16:4189–4194.

22. Romisch J, Feussner A, Vermohlen S, Stohr HA. A protease isolated from human plasma activating factor VII independent of tissue factor. Blood Coagul Fibrinolysis. 1999; 10:471–479.

23. Krishnaswamy S, Field KA, Edgington TS, Morrissey JH, Mann KG. Role of the membrane surface in the activation of human coagulation factor X. J Biol Chem. 1992; 267:26110–26120.

24. Osterud B, Rapaport SI. Activation of factor IX by the reaction product of tissue factor and factor VII: additional pathway for initiating blood coagulation. Proc Natl Acad Sci USA. 1977; 74:5260–5264.

25. Jesty J, Silverberg SA. Kinetics of the tissue factor-dependent activation of coagulation factors IX and X in a bovine plasma system. J Biol Chem. 1979; 254:12337–12345.

26. Morrison SA, Jesty J. Tissue factor-dependent activation of tritium labeled factor IX and factor X in human plasma. Blood. 1984; 63:1338–1347.

27. Braunstein KM, Noyes CM, Griffith MJ, Lundblad RL, Roberts HR. Characterization of the defect in activation of factor IX Chapel Hill by human factor XIa. J Clin Invest. 1981; 68:1420–1426.

28. Griffith MJ, Breitkreutz L, Trapp H, et al. Characterization of the clotting activities of structurally different forms of activated factor IX. Enzymatic properties of normal human factor IXa alpha, factor IXa beta, and activated factor IX Chapel Hill. J Clin Invest. 1985; 75:4–10.

29. Jackson CM, Nemerson Y. Blood coagulation. Annu Rev Biochem. 1980; 49:765–811.

30. Baglia FA, Sinha D, Walsh PN. Functional domains in the heavy-chain region of factor XI: a high molecular weight kininogen-binding site and a substrate-binding site for factor IX. Blood. 1989; 74:244–251.

31. Kurachi K, Fujikawa K, Schmer G, Davie EW. Inhibition of bovine factor IXa and factor Xabeta by antithrombin III. Biochemistry. 1976; 15:373–377.

32. Lawson JH, Mann KG. Cooperative activation of human factor IX by the human extrinsic pathway of blood coagulation. J Biol Chem. 1991; 266:11317–11327.

33. Giannelli F, Green PM, High KA, et al. Haemophilia B: database of point mutations and short additions and deletions—fourth edition, 1993. Nucleic Acids Res. 1993; 21:3075–3087.

34. Hockin MF, Jones KC, Everse SJ, Mann KG. A model for the stoichiometric regulation of blood coagulation. J Biol Chem. 2002; 277:18322–18333.

35. Lawson JH, Kalafatis M, Stram S, Mann KG. A model for the tissue factor pathway to thrombin. I. An empirical study. J Biol Chem. 1994; 269:23357–23366.

36. Rand MD, Lock JB, van't Veer C, Gaffney DP, Mann KG. Blood clotting in minimally altered whole blood. Blood. 1996; 88:3432–3445.

37. Butenas S, van ', V, Mann KG. Evaluation of the initiation phase of blood coagulation using ultrasensitive assays for serine proteases. J Biol Chem. 1997; 272:21527–21533.

38. Neuenschwander PF, Morrissey JH. Deletion of the membrane anchoring region of tissue factor abolishes autoactivation of factor VII but not cofactor function. Analysis of a mutant with a selective deficiency in activity. J Biol Chem. 1992; 267:14477–14482.

39. Monkovic DD, Tracy PB. Activation of human factor V by factor Xa and thrombin. Biochemistry. 1990; 29:1118–1128.

40. Ahmad SS, Rawala-Sheikh R, Walsh PN. Components and assembly of the factor X activating complex. Semin Thromb Hemost. 1992; 18:311–323.

41. Olson ST, Bjork I, Shore JD. Kinetic characterization of heparin catalyzed and uncatalyzed inhibition of blood coagulation proteinases by antithrombin. Methods Enzymol. 1993; 222:525–559.

42. Olson ST, Shore JD. Demonstration of a two-step reaction mechanism for inhibition of alpha-thrombin by antithrombin III and identification of the step affected by heparin. J Biol Chem. 1982; 257:14891–14895.

43. Casu B, Oreste P, Torri G, et al. The structure of heparin oligosaccharide fragments with high anti-(factor Xa) activity containing the minimal antithrombin III-binding sequence. Chemical and 13C nuclear magnetic-resonance studies. Biochem J. 1981; 197:599–609.

44. Harper PL, Luddington RJ, Daly M, et al. The incidence of dysfunctional antithrombin variants: four cases in 210 patients with thromboembolic disease. Br J Haematol. 1991; 77:360–364.

45. Thaler E, Lechner K. Antithrombin III deficiency and thromboembolism. Clin Haematol. 1981; 10:369–390.

46. Demers C, Ginsberg JS, Hirsh J, Henderson P, Blajchman MA. Thrombosis in antithrombin-III-deficient persons. Report of a large kindred and literature review. Ann Intern Med. 1992; 116:754–761.

47. Hathaway WE. Clinical aspects of antithrombin III deficiency. Semin Hematol. 1991; 28:19–23.

48. Novotny WF, Brown SG, Miletich JP, Rader DJ, Broze GJ, Jr. Plasma antigen levels of the lipoprotein-associated coagulation inhibitor in patient samples. Blood. 1991; 78:387–393.

49. Huang ZF, Wun TC, Broze GJ, Jr. Kinetics of factor Xa inhibition by tissue factor pathway inhibitor. J Biol Chem. 1993; 268:26950–26955.

50. Hamamoto T, Yamamoto M, Nordfang O, Petersen JG, Foster DC, Kisiel W. Inhibitory properties of full-length and truncated recombinant tissue factor pathway inhibitor (TFPI). Evidence that the third Kunitz-type domain of TFPI is not essential for the inhibition of factor VIIa-tissue factor complexes on cell surfaces. J Biol Chem. 1993; 268:8704–8710.

51. Wesselschmidt RL, Girard TJ, Likert KM. Tissue factor pathway inhibitor: the carboxyterminus is required for optimal inhibition of factor Xa. Blood. 1992; 779:2004–2010.

52. Rapaport SI. The extrinsic pathway inhibitor: a regulator of tissue factor-dependent blood coagulation. Thromb Haemost. 1991; 66:6–15.

53. Broze GJ, Jr., Warren LA, Novotny WF, Higuchi DA, Girard JJ, Miletich JP. The lipoprotein-associated coagulation inhibitor that inhibits the factor VII-tissue factor complex also inhibits factor Xa: insight into its possible mechanism of action. Blood. 1988; 71:335–343.

54. Sandset PM, Sirnes PA, Abildgaard U. Factor VII and extrinsic pathway inhibitor in acute coronary disease. Br J Haematol. 1989; 72:391–396.

55. Sandset PM, Warn-Cramer BJ, Rao LV, Maki SL, Rapaport SI. Depletion of extrinsic pathway inhibitor (EPI) sensitizes rabbits to disseminated intravascular coagulation induced with tissue factor: evidence supporting a physiologic role for EPI as a natural anticoagulant. Proc Natl Acad Sci USA. 1991; 88:708–712.

56. Kisiel W. Human plasma protein C: isolation, characterization, and mechanism of activation by alpha-thrombin. J Clin Invest. 1979; 64:761–769.

57. Kisiel W, Canfield WM. Snake venom proteases that activate blood coagulation factor V. Methods Enzymol. 1981; 80:275–285.

58. Nesheim M. Fibrinolysis and the plasma carboxypeptidase. Curr Opin Hematol. 1998; 5:309–313.

59. Bajzar L. Thrombin activatable fibrinolysis inhibitor and an antifibrinolytic pathway. Arterioscler Thromb Vasc Biol. 2000; 20:2511–2518.

60. Bajzar L, Nesheim ME, Tracy PB. The profibrinolytic effect of activated protein C in clots formed from plasma is TAFI-dependent. Blood. 1996; 88:2093–2100.

61. Gaffney PJ, Brasher M. Subunit structure of the plasmin-induced degradation products of crosslinked fibrin. Biochim Biophys Acta. 1973; 295:308–313.

62. Hudry-Clergeon G, Patural L, Suscillon M. Identification d'un complexe (D-D)E dans les produits de degradation de la fibrine bovine stabilisee par lè factor XIII. Pathol Biol. 1974; 22 (suppl.):47–52.

63. Gaffney PJ, Lane DA, Kakkar VV, Brasher M. Characterisation of a soluble D dimer-E complex in crosslinked fibrin digests. Thromb Res. 1975; 7:89–99.64. Loskutoff DJ, Sawdey M, Mimuro J. Type 1 plasminogen activator inhibitor. In: Coller B, ed. Progress in Hemostasis and Thrombosis. Philadelphia: W.B. Saunders; 1988:87–115.

65. Cote HC, Bajzar L, Stevens WK, et al. Functional characterization of recombinant human meizothrombin and Meizothrombin(desF1). Thrombomodulin-dependent activation of protein C and thrombin activatable fibrinolysis inhibitor (TAFI), platelet aggregation, antithrombin-III inhibition.

66. Bajzar L, Morser J, Nesheim M. TAFI, or plasma procarboxypeptidase B, couples the coagulation and fibrinolytic cascades through the thrombin thrombomodulin complex. J Biol Chem. 1996; 271:16603–16608.

67. Collen D. Ham-Wasserman lecture: role of the plasminogen system in fibrin- homeostasis and tissue remodeling. Hematology (Am Soc Hematol Educ Program). 2001; 1–9.

68. Ellis V, Pyke C, Eriksen J, Solberg H, Dano K. The urokinase receptor: involvement in cell surface proteolysis and cancer invasion. Ann NY Acad Sci. 1992; 667:13–31.

69. Lijnen HR. Plasmin and matrix metalloproteinases in vascular remodeling. Thromb Haemost. 2001; 86:324–333.

70. Hajjar KA. The endothelium in thrombosis and hemorrhage. In: Loscalzo J, Schafer AI, eds. Thrombosis and Hemorrhage. Philadelphia: Lippincott Williams & Wilkins; 2003.

71. Quick AJ. The prothrombin time in haemophilia and in obstructive jaudice. J Biol Chem. 1935; 109:73–74.

72. Al Dieri R, Peyvandi F, Santagostino E, et al. The thrombogram in rare inherited coagulation disorders: its relation to clinical bleeding. Thromb Haemost. 2002; 88:576–582.

73. Hemker HC, Beguin S. Phenotyping the clotting system. Thromb Haemost. 2000; 84:747–751.

74. Brummel KE, Paradis SG, Butenas S, Mann KG. Thrombin functions during tissue factor-induced blood coagulation. Blood. 2002; 100:148–152.

75. Undas A, Brummel K, Musial J, Mann KG, Szczeklik A. Blood coagulation at the site of microvascular injury: effects of low-dose aspirin. Blood. 2001; 98:2423–2431.

76. Undas A, Brummel K, Musial J, Mann KG, Szczeklik A. Pl(A2) polymorphism of beta(3) integrins is associated with enhanced thrombin generation and impaired antithrombotic action of aspirin at the site of microvascular injury. Circulation. 2001; 104:2666–2672.

77. Jones KC, Mann KG. A model for the tissue factor pathway to thrombin. II. A mathematical simulation [published erratum appears in J Biol Chem 1995 Apr 14; 270(15):9026]. J Biol Chem. 1994; 269:23367–23373.

78. van't Veer C, Kalafatis M, Bertina RM, Simioni P, Mann KG. Increased tissue factor-initiated prothrombin activation as a result of the Arg506 → Gln mutation in factor VLEIDEN. J Biol Chem. 1997; 272:20721–20729.

79. van't Veer C, Mann KG. Regulation of tissue factor initiated thrombin generation by the stoichiometric inhibitors tissue factor pathway inhibitor, antithrombin- III, and heparin cofactor-II. J Biol Chem. 1997; 272:4367–4377.

80. van't Veer C, Golden NJ, Kalafatis M, Mann KG. Inhibitory mechanism of the protein C pathway on tissue factor-induced thrombin generation. Synergistic effect in combination with tissue factor pathway inhibitor. J Biol Chem. 1997; 272:7983–7994.

81. van't Veer C, Golden NJ, Kalafatis M, Simioni P, Bertina RM, Mann KG. An in vitro analysis of the combination of hemophilia A and factor V(LEIDEN). Blood. 1997; 90:3067–3072.

82. van't Veer C, Butenas S, Golden NJ, Mann KG. Regulation of prothrombinase activity by protein S. Thromb Haemost. 1999; 82:80–87.

83. Butenas S, Mann KG. "Normal" thrombin generation. Blood. 1999; 94:2169–2178.

84. van't Veer C, Golden NJ, Mann KG. Inhibition of thrombin generation by the zymogen factor VII: implications for the treatment of hemophilia A by factor VIIa. Blood. 2000; 95:1330–1335.

85. Cawthern KM, van't Veer C, Lock JB, DiLorenzo ME, Branda RF, Mann KG. Blood coagulation in hemophilia A and hemophilia C. Blood. 1998; 91:4581–4592.

86. Brummel KE, Butenas S, Mann KG. An integrated study of fibrinogen during blood coagulation. J Biol Chem. 1999; 274:22862–22870.

87. Butenas S, Branda RF, van't Veer C, Cawthern KM, Mann KG. Platelets and phospholipids in tissue factor-initiated thrombin generation. Thromb Haemost. 2001; 86:660–667.

88. Holmes MB, Schneider DJ, Hayes MG, Sobel BE, Mann KG. A novel, bedside, tissue factor-dependent clotting assay permitting improved assessment of combination antithrombotic and antiplatelet therapy. Circulation. 2000.

89. Butenas S, Cawthern KM, van't Veer C, DiLorenzo ME, Lock JB, Mann KG. Antiplatelet agents in tissue factor-induced blood coagulation. Blood. 2001; in press.

90. Butenas S, Brummel KE, Branda RF, Paradis SG, Mann KG. Mechanism of factor VIIa-dependent coagulation in hemophilia blood. Blood. 2002; 99:923–930.

91. Butenas S, Brummel KE, Paradis SG, Mann KG. Influence of factor VIIa and phospholipids on coagulation in "acquired" hemophilia. Arterioscler Ther 2003.

92. Undas A, Brummel KE, Musial J, Mann KG, Szegedi G. Simvastatin depresses blood clotting by inhibiting activation of prothrombin, factor V, factor XIII and by enhancing factor Va inactivation. Circulation. 2001; 103:2248–2253.

93. Undas A, Brummel KE, Musial J, Mann KG, Szczeklik A. Aspirin alters the cardioprotective effects of the Factor XIII Val34Leu polymorphism. Circulation. 2003; 107: 17–20.

94. Adams TE, Everse SJ, Mann KG. Predicting the pharmacology of thrombin inhibitors. J Thromb Haemost. 2003; in press.

95. Mann KG. How much factor V is enough? [comment]. Thromb Haemost. 2000; 83:3–4.

96. Hartert HS. The phsical and biological constants of thrombelastography. Biorheology. 1962; 1:31–39.

97. Holmes MB, Schneider DJ, Hayes MG, Sobel BE, Mann KG. Novel, bedside, tissue factor-dependent clotting assay permits improved assessment of combination antithrombotic and antiplatelet therapy. Circulation. 2000; 102:2051–2057.

98. Mann KG, Butenas S, Brummel KE. The dynamics of thrombin formation. Arterioscler Thromb Vasc Biol. 2003; in press.

99. Bailey K, Bettelheim FR, Lorand L, Middlebrook WR. Action of thrombin in the clotting of fibrinogen. Nature. 1951; 167:233–234.

100. Blomback B. Studies on the action of thrombotic enzymes on bovine fibrinogen as measured by N-terminal analysis. Arkiv Kemi. 2003; 12:321.

101. Lorand L, Chenoweth D, Domanik RA. Chain pairs in the crosslinking of fibrin. Biochem Biophys Res Commun. 1969; 37:219–224.

102. Jenkins GR, Seiffert D, Parmer RJ, Miles LA. Regulation of plasminogen gene expression by interleukin-6. Blood. 1997; 89:2394–2403.

103. Mosesson MW. The roles of fibrinogen and fibrin in hemostasis and thrombosis. Semin Hematol. 1992; 29:177–188.

104. Shafer JA. CRC Critical Reviews. Clin Lab Sci. 1988; 26:1–4.

105. Blomback B. Fibrinogen and fibrin—proteins with complex roles in hemostasis and thrombosis. Thromb Res. 1996; 83:1–75.

106. Ng AS, Lewis SD, Shafer JA. Quantifying thrombin-catalyzed release of fibrinopeptides from fibrinogen using high-performance liquid chromatography. Methods Enzymol. 1993; 222:341–358.

107. Butenas S, Cawthern KM, van't Veer C, DiLorenzo ME, Lock JB, Mann KG. Antiplatelet agents in tissue factor-induced blood coagulation. Blood. 2001; 97:2314–2322.

108. Mann KG, Krishnaswamy S, Lawson JH. Surface-dependent hemostasis. Semin Hematol. 1992; 29:213–226.

109. van't Veer C, Mann KG. Regulation of tissue factor initiated thrombin generation by the stoichiometric inhibitors tissue factor pathway inhibitor, antithrombin- III, and heparin cofactor-II. J Biol Chem. 1997; 272:4367–4377.

110. Schroit AJ, Zwaal RF. Transbilayer movement of phospholipids in red cell and platelet membranes. Biochim Biophys Acta. 1991; 1071:313–329.

111. Okano Y, Yoshioka T, Shimouchi A, Satoh T, Kunieda T. Orally active prostacyclin analogue in primary pulmonary hypertension. Lancet. 1997; 349:1365.

112. Coller BS, Peerschke EI, Scudder LE, Sullivan CA. A murine monoclonal antibody that completely blocks the binding of fibrinogen to platelets produces a thrombasthenic-like state in normal platelets and binds to glycoproteins IIb and/or IIIa. J Clin Invest. 1983; 72:325–338.

113. Patrono C. Aspirin as an antiplatelet drug. N Engl J Med. 1994; 330:1287–1294.

114. Breckenridge A. Oral anticoagulant drugs: pharmacokinetic aspects. Semin Hematol. 1978; 15:19–26.

115. O'Reilly RA. Vitamin K and the oral anticoagulant drugs. Annu Rev Med. 1976; 27:245–261.

116. Cosgriff SW. The effectiveness of an oral vitamin K in controlling excessive hypothrombinemia during anticoagulant therapy. Ann Intern Med. 1956; 45:14–22.

117. Brummel KE, Paradis SG, Branda RF, Mann KG. Oral anticoagulation thresholds. Circulation. 2001; 104:2311–2317.

118. Cui J, O'Shea KS, Purkayastha A, Saunders TL, Ginsburg D. Fatal haemorrhage and incomplete block to embryogenesis in mice lacking coagulation factor V. Nature. 1996; 384:66–68.

119. Mann KG, Kalafatis M. Factor V: a combination of Dr Jekyll and Mr Hyde. Blood. 2003; 101:20–30.

120. Girolami A, Simioni P, Scarano L, Girolami B, Marchiori A. Hemorrhagic and thrombotic disorders due to factor V deficiencies and abnormalities: an updated classification. Blood Rev. 1998; 12:45–51.

121. LaRosa JC, He J, Vupputuri S. Effect of statins on risk of coronary disease: a meta-analysis of randomized controlled trials. JAMA. 1999; 282:2340–2346.

122. Maron DJ, Fazio S, Linton MF. Current perspectives on statins. Circulation. 2000; 101:207–213.

123. Blumenthal RS. Statins: effective antiatherosclerotic therapy. Am Heart J. 2000; 139:577–583.

124. Rosenson RS, Tangney CC. Antiatherothrombotic properties of statins: implications for cardiovascular event reduction. JAMA. 1998; 279:1643–1650.

125. Colli S, Eligini S, Lalli M, Camera M, Paoletti R, Tremoli E. Vastatins inhibit tissue factor in cultured human macrophages. A novel mechanism of protection against atherothrombosis.

126. Calvete JJ. Clues for understanding the structure and function of a prototypic human integrin: the platelet glycoprotein IIb/IIIa complex. Thromb Haemost. 1994; 72:1–15.

127. Newman PJ, Derbes RS, Aster RH. The human platelet alloantigens, Pl^{A1} and Pl^{A2}, are associated with a leucine33/proline33 amino acid polymorphism in membrane glycoprotein IIIa, and are distinguishable by DNA typing. J Clin Invest. 1989; 83:1778–1781.

128. Sperr WR, Huber K, Roden M, et al. Inherited platelet glycoprotein polymorphisms and a risk for coronary heart disease in young central Europeans. Thromb Res. 1998; 90:117–123.

129. Mikkelsson J, Perola M, Laippala P, Penttila A, Karhunen PJ. Glycoprotein IIIa Pl(A1/A2) polymorphism and sudden cardiac death. J Am Coll Cardiol. 2000; 36:1317–1323.

130. Poort SR, Rosendaal FR, Reitsma PH, Bertina RM. A common genetic variation in the 3'-untranslated region of the prothrombin gene is associated with elevated plasma prothrombin levels and an increase in venous thrombosis. Blood. 1996; 88:3698–3703.

131. Brummel-Zedins K, Rivard GE, Pouliat RL, Bateras S, Grssel M, Parhami-Serem B, Mann KG, Factor VIIIa replacement therapy in factor VII deficiency. J Thrombo Haemost 2004; 21:1735–1744.

2-1

Vascular Thromboresistance and the Genetics of Thrombotic Risk

Frederick L. Ruberg and Joseph Loscalzo
Boston University School of Medicine, Boston, Massachusetts, U.S.A.

I. INTRODUCTION

Thrombosis is best defined as pathological hemostasis. Classically, the etiology of thrombosis was first elucidated by Virchow in 1856 as dependent upon the presence of either blood stasis, endothelial injury, and/or hypercoagulability. While stasis and injury are self-explanatory, hypercoagulability is a vague term that refers to a congenital or acquired pathological state favoring thrombus formation. The regulation of coagulation is a carefully orchestrated balance between pro- and antithrombotic factors derived from the vascular endothelium and circulating blood. Thrombosis results when a shift in that hemostatic equilibrium occurs that favors coagulation, and a "hypercoagulable state" refers to this bias on a continual basis. Interestingly, the initiating mechanisms that elicit thromboses in the venous and arterial system appear to be different. Venous thrombosis is principally predicated upon blood stasis and is influenced by the presence of a hypercoagulable state. Clinically, venous thromboses are manifest as lower extremity deep venous thrombosis (DVT) and pulmonary embolism (PE) or in situ thromboses of the hepatic, renal, mesenteric, pulmonary, or cerebral venous systems. Conversely, arterial thromboses most commonly occur in the setting of endothelial injury resulting from a preexisting atherosclerotic lesion. Arterial thrombotic events are also influenced by the presence of a hypercoagulable state; however, there appears an intriguing segregation among the hypercoagulable factors that favor arterial and venous thrombosis. The clinical manifestations of atherothrombosis include peripheral vascular disease (infrainguinal, aortic/mesenteric, subclavian, or carotid systems), cerebrovascular disease, and coronary artery disease.

As introduced previously, the hypercoagulable state is a poorly defined clinical entity that encompasses inherited and acquired alterations in the balance of hemostasis that favors thrombosis. Acquired conditions that favor the development of thrombosis include pregnancy and estrogen replacement, malignancy, cigarette smoking, and the development of anti-phospholipid antibodies. Inherited abnormalities that favor thrombosis may result from single nucleotide polymorphisms (SNPs) or insertion/deletion mutations in key regulators of platelet function, factors in the coagulation/fibrinolytic cascade, and endothelium-derived proteins. The phenotypic results of these mutations are myriad, including both alterations in expression levels and loss or gain of function. In this review we will examine the genetic aspects of hypercoagulability through a systematic examination of each relevant defined mutation that promotes arterial and venous thrombosis and its resultant phenotypic and clinical implications.

II. MECHANISMS OF HEMOSTASIS

Hemostasis involves a carefully balanced interplay among factors that favor and oppose the autoregulated cessation of blood flow, including platelet function, the coagulation cascade, the regulation of the propagating thrombus, and ultimately fibrinolysis. Thrombosis occurs when this equilibrium is shifted toward coagulation. A brief review of the relevant factors is, therefore, appropriate.

Hemostasis following vascular injury is predicated first (primary hemostasis) upon platelet adhesion to the site of injury, followed by platelet activation and aggregation. This process is integral to atherothrombosis as endothelial injury results from the development and destabilization of the atherosclerotic plaque. Now understood as a chronic inflammatory process, atherosclerosis is defined by the infiltration of inflammatory cells, including T-cell lymphocytes and macrophages, and cholesteryl ester into the subendothelium of the arterial wall. The luminal surface of the developing atherosclerotic plaque consists of a fibrous cap of collagen, matrix proteins, and fibroblasts superimposed upon a lipid core. Rupture of this fibrous cap and exposure of the thrombogenic plaque core to circulating blood is the pathophysiological process understood as plaque destabilization. The molecular cues that prompt destabilization are now being identified and likely involve expression of matrix metalloproteinases and signaling events between macrophages and T-cell lymphocytes in part via the CD40-CD40 ligand system (1–3).

Erosion of the cap of the atherosclerotic plaque exposes a subendothelial matrix that is intensely thrombogenic owing to the high levels of expression of both tissue factor (TF) and von Willebrand factor (vWF) by the cells surrounding the lipid core. Platelets adhere to the disrupted plaque via a bridging complex of glycoproteins (GP) including GPIbα, GPIbβ, GPIX, and GPV (expressed on platelet surface in 2:2:2:1 stoichiometry), and the vessel wall–expressed vWF. (4) This Ib-IX-V-vWF complex firmly adheres the platelet to the site of injury and resists disruption of the platelet lawn by shear stress. Binding of vWF occurs via the GPIbα component, an important molecule that also contains a binding site for thrombin and is linked to the platelet cytoskeleton via its cytoplasmic domain. Platelets are then activated by vWF binding and thrombin, as well as by thromboxane A_2 (TxA_2), adenosine 5′-diphosphate (ADP), and serotonin (5). Platelet activation then promotes a calcium-dependent conformational change in the platelet GP IIb/IIIa, exposing a binding site for fibrinogen, thereby resulting in platelet aggregation. GPIIb/IIIa is a heterodimeric integrin composed of two subunits, α_{IIb} and β_3. Activation by one of the aforementioned agonists results in modifications to the cytoplasmic domain of GPIIb/IIIa, prompting a conformational change in the extracellular domain that exposes and Arg-Gly-Asp (RGD)–binding site with a high affinity for fibrinogen (5). Two important endothelium-derived substances serve to inhibit platelet activation. Endothelium-derived nitric oxide (NO•), synthesized by the conversion of L-arginine to L-citrulline by the endothelial isoform of the enzyme nitric oxide synthase (eNOS), inhibits platelet activation, as well as adhesion and aggregation, by increasing platelet cyclic guanosine-monophosphate (cGMP) and by inhibiting phophoinositol-3-kinase (PI-3 kinase) (6,7). Platelet activation and aggregation (but not adhesion) are also inhibited by prostacyclin (PGI_2), an eicosanoid produced from the metabolism of arachidonic acid by the enzyme prostacyclin synthase. PGI_2 inhibits platelet activation by increasing platelet cyclic adenosine-monophosphate (cAMP) (8). Additionally, endothelial cells express ecto-ADPase (CD39), an enzyme that impairs ADP-dependent platelet activation by metabolizing ADP derived from activated platelets to 5′-AMP (9).

Concurrent with platelet adhesion and activation, the coagulation cascade (secondary hemostasis) is also initiated by the exposure of circulating blood to the subendothelial matrix and specifically to TF. TF is a membrane-bound glycoprotein expressed by endothelial cells and macrophages under conditions of vessel injury. In atherothrombosis, TF is inappropriately expressed and, hence, thrombosis in inappropriately initiated (10). TF activates circulating clotting factor VII, which in turn activates factor IX. Factor IXa then activates factor X on a phospholipid surface, with factor VIIIa as an accelerating cofactor. Factor Xa then cleaves prothrombin (factor II) to thrombin (factor IIa), a process accelerated by factor Va. Factor V is converted to its active form through the action of thrombin itself. Thrombin also cleaves the Aα and Bβ chains of fibrinogen to form soluble fibrin monomer. As previously mentioned, thrombin further serves to activate platelets and endothelial cells. Fibrin then polymerizes in end-to-end and staggered side-to-side noncovalent associations, resulting in the formation of an insoluble fibrin thrombus. Covalent cross linking of fibrin occurs under the control of factor XIIIa, a process that is slow kinetically and serves to stabilize the nascent thrombus over time. Activated platelets bound to fibrin via GPIIb/IIIa as well as other clotting factors and fibrinolytic factors are incorporated into the developing thrombus (11).

Thrombus propagation is controlled concurrent with its formation by a number of circulating and endothelium-derived substances. Circulating tissue factor pathway inhibitor (TFPI) binds and inactivates the complex of TF, factor VIIa, and factor Xa. Circulating anti-thrombin III (ATIII), a serine protease inhibitor, binds and inactivates factors IXa, Xa, and IIa. Endothelium-derived NO• inhibits endothelial and macrophage TF expression, as well as platelet activation. Heparan sulfate is a proteoglycan expressed on the EC surface that accelerates the inhibitory activity of ATIII approximately 2000-fold. Thrombomodulin, a membrane-bound glycoprotein expressed on the EC surface, binds thrombin and circulating factors C and S, resulting in the generation of activated protein C (APC). APC then binds and proteolytically cleaves factors V and VIII, thereby slowing thrombus formation.

Clot dissolution also proceeds concurrent with thrombus formation. The fibrinolytic enzyme plasmin is produced by the proteolytic cleavage of plasminogen by tissue-type plasminogen activator (t-PA) or urokinase-type plasminogen activator (u-PA). Plasminogen activators act upon both circulating and clot-bound plasminogen and are themselves recruited into the developing thrombus, an important point in the regulation of fibrinolysis, as in so doing the developing thrombus facilitates its own dissolution. Fibrin crosslinking, however, obscures binding sites for t-PA/u-PA and protects the thrombus from lytic degradation. Endothelium-derived plasminogen activator inhibitors (PAI-1 and PAI-2) bind and inhibit t-PA/u-PA and thereby regulate the fibrinolytic process. Fibrinolysis is also regulated by thrombin-activable fibrinolysis inhibitor (TAFI), a circulating glycoprotein also known as procarboxypeptidase U or plasma procarboxypeptidase B, which is activated by the thrombin-thrombomodulin complex. TAFI cleaves the carboxyterminal lysine from fibrin, thereby interfering with plasminogen binding and slowing fibrinolysis (12). Finally, circulating α_2-antiplasmin binds and inhibits plasmin (11).

III. OVERVIEW OF GENETIC DETERMINANTS OF THROMBOSIS

The inheritance of a particular genotype does not necessarily correspond to or predict the development of a thrombotic phenotype, despite retrospective analysis predicting an association. Clearly, interactions with other genes and environmental factors ultimately promote thrombosis however, the presence of some of these genetic risk factors may be seen as predisposing one to the development of a venous or atherothrombotic event. Interestingly, the majority of the genetic risk factors discussed below have been associated with either venous or arterial thrombosis, but rarely both. While one can understand why, for example, a platelet glycoprotein mutation may predispose one to athero- but not venous thrombosis, as platelets are clearly integral to the former but probably not the latter, precisely why a mutation in a clotting factor (such as the factor V Leiden mutation) would be strongly associated with venous but weakly associated with arterial thrombosis remains less clear. This difference may reflect the divergent pathobiological processes that participate in thrombosis within these two vascular systems.

IV. COAGULATION PROTEINS

A. Protein C, Protein S, and Antithrombin III

Inherited deficiencies in protein C, protein S, and antithrombin III have long been associated with venous thrombosis but are not felt to be associated with atherothrombotic disease (13). They are included here for completeness.

B. Factor V

Clotting factor V is a 300 kDa glycoprotein synthesized by the liver that participates in the coagulation cascade by accelerating the conversion of prothombin to thrombin. In 1994, a single nucleotide polymorphism (G → A) was first reported in the factor V gene at position 1691 (14). This G1691A mutation results in the substitution of a glutamine for an arginine at position 506 of the factor V protein. First associated with venous thrombosis in the Leiden Thrombophilia Study, the mutation became known as factor V Leiden (15). Factor V Leiden is thought to promote thrombosis by conferring resistance to APC. APC regulates thrombus propagation by inhibition of the clot-accelerating activity of factor V. Similar to wild-type factor V, factor V Leiden is activated normally by thrombin, but resists inactivation by APC and, thus, promotes thrombosis. Interestingly, factor V itself is also an anticoagulant, as it participates in factor VIIIa degradation through a complex with protein S and APC. To accomplish this end, factor V must be cleaved at position 506. Factor V Leiden resists cleavage at 506, and, hence, its participation as an anticoagulant is diminished. Precisely which mechanism predominates in vivo remains unclear. APC resistance also has been observed in the absence of the factor V Leiden mutation and has been linked to a restriction enzyme-defined haplotype of factor V termed HR2 (4).

Factor V Leiden is a common polymorphism occurring with a prevalence of 5% in the white population (interestingly nearly absent in the African American population), suggesting a genetic founder effect occurring approximately 20,000–30,000 years ago. Its association with venous thromboembolic (VTE) disease (deep venous thrombosis and pulmonary embolism) has now been demonstrated in numerous large case-control retrospective trials ,including the aforementioned Leiden Thrombophilia Study and in the nonpopulation-based prospective U.S. Physicians Health Study (16). In the latter the estimated relative risk for VTE was 2.7 for heterozygotes carrying the factor V Leiden mutation . It remains controversial whether factor V Leiden itself increases the risk of recurrent venous thrombosis [although studies exploring co-inheritance of factor V

Leiden and other mutations suggests an increased risk (17)] or whether individuals with the mutation who have not had a thrombotic event are definitely at increased risk (18,19). One recently published, population-based prospective trial (the Longitudinal Investigation of Thromboembolism Etiology, or LITE) demonstrated an increased odds ratio of 3.7 for the development of VTE in carriers of factor V Leiden vs. noncarriers, as well as an association of factor V Leiden with recurrent VTE events (20). Homozygosity for the HR2 haplotype in the absence of factor V Leiden was also associated with a five-fold increased risk of VTE in this study. Factor V Leiden has also been associated with the development of cerebral venous thrombosis (21). Conversely, only a weak association has been demonstrated between factor V Leiden and cerebral atherothrombosis (stroke) (22). The Study of Myocardial Infarction Leiden (SMILE), a retrospective case-control trial of patients with MI, demonstrated a small increased risk of factor V Leiden for MI (23), while other trials, including the U.S. Physicians Health Study, have failed to detect an association between factor V Leiden and MI or stroke (16). The association between factor V Leiden and MI appears to be strengthened by interaction with other mutations or environmental factors such as smoking (23). Recent trials have bolstered this negative result, failing to detect an association between factor V Leiden and sudden cardiac death (24). Thus, while factor V Leiden is an important and rather common risk factor for venous thrombosis, its association with atherothrombotic disease is, at best, weak. This finding reflects the complexity of the thrombotic process and speaks to the importance of other factors in the determination of atherothrombotic as compared to venous thrombotic events.

C. Prothrombin

In the latter half of the 1990s, following identification of factor V Leiden, a second important thrombophilic mutation was identified in the 3' untranslated region of the gene coding for prothrombin, a 72 kDa zymogen that is the direct precursor to thrombin (25). This polymorphism, occurring at position 20210 (G → A), does not alter the pro-thombin gene product per se, but is associated with increased expression levels of the protein. Initial small studies estimated that the increased risk for venous thrombosis among carriers of the A allele was 2.7- to 3.8-fold higher than among noncarriers (25). This thrombophilic predisposition, with a prevalence of 2% in the white population, was confirmed in the larger Leiden Thrombophilia Study, estimating a 2.8-fold increased risk for carriers of the A allele. The precise mechanism by which the G20210A mutation increases prothrombin levels remains unclear; however, one potential mechanism involves an increased efficiency of polyadenylation of mRNA transcripts (4). This polymorphism, like factor V Leiden, has also been associated with an increased risk of cerebral venous thrombosis (26). In a conflicting study, the prospective U.S. Physicians Health Study identified only a nonsignificant, weak association between G20210A and VTE (relative risk of 1.7), despite a high population prevalence of 3.9% of the A allele (27). The association between G20210A and recurrent VTE remains unclear; however, retrospective studies have suggested that co-inheritance of G20210A and factor V Leiden does connote an increased risk of recurrent VTE (17). In a comparison of the two mutations, it appears that factor V Leiden connotes a greater risk of VTE than prothrombin G20210A. As with factor V Leiden, the association between G20120A and atherothrombotic events remains less well defined. The SMILE study did demonstrate a small but significant increased risk of MI for carriers of the G20210A mutation, an effect enhanced by environmental factors including smoking

(23); however, this result was again not reproduced by the U.S. Physicians Health Study (27). It appears, therefore, that the G20210A mutation is not strongly linked to the development of atherothrombotic events.

D. Factor XIII

Factor XIII is a 320 kDa protransglutaminase composed of a tetrameric structure of 2A and 2B subunits that accelerates the formation of fibrin crosslinks, which stabilize the developing thrombus and provide protection from both shear-stress and fibrinolysis. Factor XIII, following cleavage and activation by thrombin, facilitates covalent interactions between glutamyl and lysyl residues in the γ chain of fibrin. Deficiency in factor XIII results in a bleeding diathesis (4). Within the gene for the 75 kDa A subunit, at least 20 mutations have been identified relating to factor XIII deficiency that result in absence of the A subunit. In addition, four SNPs have also been identified, the most extensively studied of which results in a leucine-for-valine substitution at position 34 of the A subunit (Val34Leu). This substitution is only three amino acid residues away from the thrombin cleavage activation site at position Arg37-Gly38. Interestingly, the Leu34 allele has been associated with a protective effect against thrombosis in small retrospective trials (although the benefit seems to depend on homozygosity) (28). One potential mechanism for this finding involves enhanced activation of factor XIII by thrombin and more efficient crosslinking of fibrin (29). The significance of the role of factor XIII Val34Leu in the general population in relation to thrombosis, as well as its interaction with thrombophilic mutations, is the subject of ongoing investigation.

The association of factor XIII and atherothrombosis has also been evaluated in a limited fashion, with the Leu34 allele less commonly associated with a history of MI in retrospective trials (24). The large, population-based, prospective Atherosclerosis Risk in Communities (ARIC) trial, however, failed to demonstrate an association between Val34Leu genotype and atherothrombotic disease (30).

E. Thrombomodulin

Thrombomodulin, a 100 kDa EC surface protein that binds thrombin and proteins C and S to liberate APC, has been shown to contain two polymorphisms: one at position 445, resulting in an alanine-to-valine substitution, and another at position 25, resulting in an alanine-to-threonine substitution. While not affecting protein expression levels, both have been weakly associated with MI in limited trials (31). Data from the ARIC trial reflect that thrombomodulin levels are inversely proportional to the development of coronary artery disease, suggesting that measurement of this protein may be a useful tool in the prediction of CAD (32). Further study of polymorphisms that may affect thrombomodulin expression level is, therefore, appropriate.

F. APC Receptor

Recently, the receptor for activated protein C (APC), a 43-kDa endothelial cell surface protein, has been shown to harbor a 23 bp insertion polymorphism in exon 3 of the molecule, resulting in truncation of the translated gene. Early evidence suggests an association between this genotype and venous thrombosis, while its role in the generation of atherothrombosis remains unknown (33).

G. Factor VIII

Elevated levels of factor VIII (an acceleration cofactor for factor X formation) have also been identified with VTE (34). Although the genetics of this process have yet to be elucidated, known polymorphisms in the factor VIII or vWF genes do not seem to affect the risk for thrombosis (35).

H. Fibrinogen

Fibrinogen is a 340 kDa glycoprotein that consists of three nonidentical peptide subunits connected by disulfide linkages. The genes coding for the three subunits reside on choromosome 4, and each has promotor regions containing TATA or CAAT boxes and response elements that confer tissue-specific and factor-enhanced expression, including upregulation of transcription in the presence of interlukin-6 (IL-6) and hepatic nuclear factor-1 (HNF-1) (4). These response elements are felt to mediate the acute-phase upregulation of fibrinogen in the setting of inflammation, a finding of particular importance as increased levels of fibrinogen have been linked to atherothrombosis. This association between elevated levels of fibrinogen and MI/stroke has been noted in numerous, large, retrospective clinical trials (36,37). Interestingly, elevated fibrinogen has also been associated with cigarette smoking, perhaps through this same pro-inflammatory mechanism, a finding that almost certainly contributes to the prothrombotic effects of smoking (38,39). While the determination of fibrinogen expression level is likely heritable and influenced by environmental factors, a number of polymorphisms have been identified in each of the subunit genes, the most interesting of which is a G → A SNP at position 455 in the 5′ promoter region of the β subunit. Also known by its restriction enzyme site (*Hae*III), this polymorphism is in close proximity to the response elements to IL-6 and HNF-1. Extensively studied, the –455A genotype has been consistently associated in retrospective trials with elevated fibrinogen levels; however, a direct association between –455A and atherothrombosis remains less clear (40). In the Etude Cas-Temoins sur l'Infarctus du Myocarde (ECTIM), a retrospective trial of patients with MI, 10 polymorphisms of the β gene were identified and found to occur in linkage disequlibrium; however, multivariate analysis suggested that the G455A polymorphism was independently associated with fibrinogen levels, although this result was noted only in smokers (41). This finding was supported by the European Atherosclerosis Research Study (EARS) (42). Analysis of data from the REGRESS trial, an angiographic trial of pravastatin, demonstrated an association between the –455A genotype and fibrinogen level and suggested an association with progression of angiographically documented CAD (43). Conversely, the large population-based Copenhagen City Heart Trial determined that while the –455A mutation was associated with elevated fibrinogen levels, it was not a predictor of the development of ischemic heart disease (44). In addition, a recently published meta-analysis suggested that the –455A genotype connoted a decreased risk of MI (45). Thus, while the –455A polymorphism is associated with elevated fibrinogen levels, it is not clearly associated with the development of the disease phenotype.

Another β gene polymorphism detected by the *Bcl*I restriction enzyme in the 3' region of the gene has been studied and, while not associated with fibrinogen level, has been associated with MI in a reanalysis of the GISSI-2 study (46). Finally, a polymorphism in the α chain (Thr312Ala) was evaluated in the ECTIM study and found not to be associated with disease (41).

I. Factor VII

Factor VII is a 48 kDa vitamin K–dependent zymogen that is synthesized by the liver in its inactive form and subsequently activated by exposure to TF and factor Xa. Initial evidence linking elevated factor VII levels and atherothrombosis was obtained in the prospective Northwick Park Heart Study (36), but, two subsequent trials, the Prospective Cardiovascular Munster (PROCAM) trial (47) and the Edinburgh Artery Study (48), failed to detect a significant association. Nevertheless, five polymorphisms have been identified that are generally associated with variations in expression of factor VII (4). The most important of these is a SNP in exon 8 that results in glutamine-for-arginine substitution at position 353 of the factor VII protein. The Gln353 allele has been associated with 20% lower levels of factor VII (49). The conclusions of subsequent studies evaluating the association of Arg353 with atherothrombosis have been inconsistent. In the ECTIM study, Arg353 was associated with elevated factor VII levels, but there was no difference in allele frequency between cases (subjects with MI) and controls (50). This result was supported by two smaller case-control trials. Conversely, the Dutch SMILE trial identified the previously observed association between factor VII level and MI, but found that the Arg353 allele was associated with a reduced, rather than increased, risk for MI (51). Alternatively, an analysis drawn from the GISSI-2 population identified an increased risk of MI with the Arg353 allele (52). These disparate conclusions may result from differences in subject selection and the prevalence of other, as yet unidentified, disease modifying genes or haplotypes. Suffice it to say factor VII, like fibrinogen, has been linked to atherothrombosis, but the currently identified polymorphisms, while themselves linked to factor expression level, have not been definitively shown to correlate with disease.

V. FIBRINOLYTIC PROTEINS

A. Plasminogen Activator Inhibtor-1

Fibrinolysis of the established thrombus occurs through the action of plasmin, an enzyme formed from the cleavage of plasminogen by t-PA. t-PA is principally inhibited by the endothelium-derived PAI-1, a 50 kDa member of the serine protein inhibitor (SERPIN) family. PAI-1 expression is induced by a diverse number of substances, including thrombin; inflammatory mediators such as TNF-α; growth factors such as IGF-1 and TGF-β; lipids such as lipoprotein(a) and fatty acids; insulin; angiotensin II; and endotoxin. PAI-1 has a 30-minute half-life, but is stabilized through vitronectin binding (53). The central role of the fibrinolytic system in the development of atherothrombosis was suggested by the observation that low plasma fibrinolytic activity was associated with the development of MI and sudden cardiac death (54,55). Indeed, retrospective trials have demonstrated elevated circulating PAI-1 levels in patients with MI, recurrent MI, and, particularly, in patients with MI before the age of 40 years (56,57). In addition, PAI-1 has been demonstrated by histochemical staining in *postmortem* studies of atherosclerotic plaques, particularly in diabetic patients (58). An interesting association between elevated PAI-1 levels and type II diabetes mellitus has been identified, particularly in subjects with the metabolic syndrome (typified by dyslipidemia, hypertension, diabetes, and central obesity) (59). This observation may, in part, be the result of the hyperinsulinemic state of type II diabetes, as the Framingham Offspring Study demonstrated an association between PAI-1 and insulin levels (60,61). Alternatively, lipids may interact directly with the transcriptional regulation of the PAI-1 gene itself (53).

The PAI-1 gene contains a common polymorphism within its promoter region of a 4 guanine bp insert (4G) or a 5 guanine bp insert (5G) that lies 675 bp upstream from the site of transcriptional initiation. The 4G/4G genotype is associated with approximately 25% higher levels of PAI-1 expression as compared to the 4G/5G or 5G/5G genotypes, perhaps because the 4G allele binds an enhancer factor, whereas the 5G allele binds both enhancer and suppressor factors (62). Hypertriglyceridemia is also associated with higher PAI-1 levels in persons with the 4G/4G genotype, a finding possibly related to a potential triglyceride response element adjacent to the insertion site (63).

In addition to its association with higher PAI-1 expression levels, the 4G genotype has also been directly linked to atherothrombotic disease. In a number of small retrospective trials of patients with known MI, the 4G allele was disproportionately represented — a finding supported in additional trials of patients with angiographically demonstrated coronary disease (64–66). A larger, retrospective trial of healthy subjects also detected an association between the 4G allele and MI, with an estimated odds ratio of 1.6 (67); however, larger trials, such as the ECTIM (68), SMILE (69), and the U.S. Physicians Health Study (70), among others, have failed to detect an association between the 4G allele and MI (71). A recently published meta-analysis demonstrated a positive but weak association between PAI-1 genotype and MI (72). While it is intriguing to implicate the 4G genotype with enhanced PAI-1 expression, particularly in diabetics with elevated trigylcerides, the evidence from clinical trials in sum suggests only a weak association with atherothrombotic events.

B. t-PA

Tissue plasminogen activator is a 70 kDa proteinase expressed by endothelial cells that converts plasminogen to the active fibrinolytic enzyme, plasmin. Elevated levels of t-PA have been associated with an increased risk of MI (perhaps counterintuitively) in large prospective and retrospective trials (73,74) This finding may be a reflection of the chronic inflammatory process of atherosclerosis or simply a marker of increased fibrinolytic activity, a finding linked to atherothrombosis by the aforementioned Northwick Park Heart Study. More recently, the plasma ratio of t-PA to PAI-1 (t-PA:PAI-1) has been suggested as an indicator of a prothrombotic state and linked to atherothrombotic events (75,76). While a polymorphism at position 7351 (T → C) has been identified and associated with increased t-PA expression level and first MI (77), further study is necessary to clarify the role of this mutation in atherothrombotic disease.

VI. PLATELET GLYCOPROTEIN POLYMORPHISMS

Mutations in platelet proteins have thus far been associated primarily with atherothrombosis, an observation likely owing to the requisite role the platelet plays in the initiation of atherothrombotic events. To date, correlations between platelet glycoprotein mutations and venous thrombosis have not been definitively demonstrated.

A. GPIb

Platelet GPIb is a heterodimeric protein that consists of a 140 kDa α subunit and a 25 kDa β subunit joined by a disulfide linkage. These proteins are noncovalently associated with two other platelet surface glycoproteins, GPV and GPIX, and together form a linkage complex for vWF that mediates platelet binding to the subendothelial matrix.

Two polymorphisms in GPIbα that affect protein structure and one that affects expression have attracted attention. First, a SNP at position 434 (C → T) resulting in a threonine-to-methionine substitution at position 145 (the Ko polymorphism) has been suggested to associate with coronary artery disease but has not been substantiated to do so (78). Second, a variable number of tandem repeats insert (VNTR) of 39 bp coding for a 13-amino-acid insert into the glycosylated region of the molecule has been identified. The insert can be present in one to four copies (termed A, B, C, or D), thus elongating the subunit and facilitating interactions with the subendothelium. The data linking this mutation to atherothrombosis are conflicting, as one small retrospective study demonstrated an association between coronary and cerebrovascular disease (OR of 2.8) for the C/B genotype, while another trial did not (79). Finally, a SNP (T → C) at position −5 from the ATG start codon (Kozak sequence) may increase surface expression of GPIbα, an observation attributed to increased translational efficiency of mRNA transcripts (80). The data thus far gathered are conflicting. One large case-control trial of 1000 patients with known CAD demonstrated an association between the C allele and unstable angina was well as adverse events following PTCA (81). The Kozak polymorphism has also been associated with the development of ischemic stroke (82); however, a larger trial of patients undergoing PTCA demonstrated no association between the C allele and ischemic events (83).

B. GPIIb/IIIa

Platelet glycoprotein IIb/IIIa is a 240 kDa member of the integrin family of adhesion molecules composed of two subunits, α_{IIb} and β_3. Many polymorphisms have been identified in the genes encoding the two subunits, 18 of which are thought to be involved in the pathogenesis of Glanzmann thrombasthenia (4); however, within the gene for the β_3 subunit, a SNP at position 1565 (T → C) resulting in a proline-to-leucine substitution at position 33 has been identified (84). The wild type (Leu33 or PLA1) is found in approximately 85% of the white population, and the mutant form (Pro33 or PLA2) is present in the remaining 15%. In 1996, the first association between PLA2 and MI was identified in a retrospective study of patients admitted to a coronary care unit. PLA2 was overrepresented in patients with MI, suggesting a 2.8-fold increased risk of coronary artery disease for carriers of this genotype (85). Furthermore, when subjects under the age of 60 were analyzed, an OR of 6.2 was determined. This finding of an association between the PLA2 genotype and MI in young men has been supported by additional trials (86). PLA2 was also associated with the development of sudden cardiac death in the Helsinki Sudden Death Study, with an OR of 2.5 for patients below the age of 50 years (87). Interestingly, histopathologic evidence from this trial suggested increased frequencies of plaque fissure and complex atherosclerotic lesions among carriers of PLA2, and increased association of PLA2 with fatal coronary thrombosis (88). PLA2 has also been associated with an increased risk of in-stent thrombosis and peri-procedural death following stenting (89). Mechanistically, it has been hypothesized that the PLA2 mutation may alter the outside-in signaling function of GPIIb/IIIa (90), and may affect platelet-fibrinogen interactions (91). In contrast to these positive associations between PLA2 and atherothrombosis, large clinical trials failed to show any association between PLA2 and MI, stroke, or venous thrombosis (92). Furthermore, a recently published meta-analysis reached the same conclusions (93). Studies of platelets in PLA2 homozygotes have failed to show any difference in function when compared to PLA1 controls, particularly in ADP sensitivity, fibrinogen or vitronectin binding, aggregation, or thrombus formation (94). Finally, another trial of patients undergoing coronary angiography demonstrated only a weak association between PLA2 and the severity of coronary disease or subsequent MI (95).

C. GPIa

The GPI receptor is a heterodimeric platelet glycoprotein that functions as a ligand for collagen and is expressed at relatively low densities on the platelet surface; up to a 10-fold variation in collagen affinity has been noted among different individuals, which suggests variation in receptor expression levels (78). Theoretically, increased receptor density might facilitate increased platelet binding to subendothelial collagen in the ruptured plaque. Two SNPs (C807T and G873A) that do not result in amino acid substitutions as well as a third that does (lysine for glutamic acid) have been identified with equivocal associations to myocardial infarction and stroke (96–98). The association between receptor density and genotype has not been definitively demonstrated.

A polymorphism in platelet glycoprotein VI, a surface molecule that contributes to platelet-collagen interaction similar to GPIa, that results in a serine substitution for proline (T13254C) has been associated with an increased risk of MI, particularly in women and non-smokers. The functional significance of this mutation has yet to be definitively evaluated (99).

VII. ENZYME/RECEPTOR POLYMORPHISMS

A. Methytetrahydrofolate Reductase and Homocysteine

Methytetrahydrofolate reductase (MTHFR) is a key enzyme in the remethylation pathway that clears homocysteine (HCY) from the circulation. HCY, a sulfhydryl amino acid formed during the metabolism of methionine, has been associated with an increased risk of both arterial as well as venous thrombosis, although the risk for atherothrombosis appears greater. HCY is metabolized, in part, by methionine synthase, an enzyme that utilizes the cofactors vitamin B_{12} and N^5-methyl-tetrahydrofolate. MTHFR is required for the regeneration of the latter co-factor. The mechanism by which HCY promotes thrombosis most likely involves the potentiation of oxidant stress and the development of increased levels of reactive oxygen species (ROS). HCY is auto-oxidized in the plasma, leading to increased concentrations of ROS such as superoxide ($\bullet O_2$-) and hydrogen peroxide (H_2O_2). HCY also downregulates expression of the important cellular antioxidant enzyme, glutathione peroxidase-1. Oxidant stress results in endothelial cell activation and injury, as well as smooth muscle proliferation (7,100).

A SNP at position 667 (C → T) of the MTHFR gene, resulting in a alanine-to-valine substitution, has been identified and associated with decreased steady-state levels of the molecule owing to increased thermolability (101). This relatively common allele results in elevated HCY levels, the degree of which seems to be inversely proportional to folate intake (102). While some studies have suggested a link between C667T and venous thrombosis (particularly in homozygotes), the results have not been broadly verified (103,104). Similarly, the evidence linking C677T to atherothrombotic disease has also been equivocal. A small, retrospective Israeli trial of 169 patients with angiographically documented CAD or MI who were evaluated for C667T genotype demonstrated that homozygosity for the TT genotype was associated with premature (<45 years of age) CAD (105). Conversely, a similarly sized U.S. trial of patients with angiographically defined CAD failed to demonstrate a significant association between atherothrombotic disease and genotype (106), while genotype and HCY levels were associated—a finding

Table 1 Summary of Polymorphisms Relevant to Atherothrombotic Disease

Gene and polymorphism	Phenotype	Association with atherothrombosis
Clotting factors		
Factor V		
G1691A (Arg506Gln, Leiden)	APC resistance	Weak itself, but may connote increased risk with other factors
HR2 halplotype	APC resistance	Strong independent predictor of VTE
Prothrombin		
G20210A	Altered expression	Weak to absent itself, but may connote increased risk with other factors; moderate independent predictor of VTE
Factor XII		
Val34Leu	Altered activation	34Leu allele may be protective against MI
Thrombomodulin		
Ala25Thr	Unclear	25Thr may be weakly associated with MI
APC receptor		
23-bp insertion	Truncated gene product	May be associated with VTE; relation to atherothrombosis unclear
Fibrinogen β chain		
G455A (*HaeIII*)	Altered expression	Both associated with elevated fibrinogen levels but inconsistent association with atherohrombosis
BclI	Altered expression	
Factor VII		
Arg353Gln	Altered expression	353Gln associated with lower levels of factor VII but inconsistent association with atherothrombosis
Thrombolytic factors		
PAI–1		
-675 4G/5G	Altered expression	4G allele associated with elevated PAI-1 levels (particularly in diabetics), but inconsistent association with atherothrombosis
t-PA		
T7351C	Altered expression	Preliminary data suggest association with increased t-PA levels and first MI

Platelet glycoproteins		
GP Ib		
C434T (Met145Thr)	Altered expression	Potentially associated with increased risk of MI and increased post-PCI complications but inconsistent results
VNTR (39 bp inertion)		
T-5C (Kozak)		
GP IIb/IIIa		
Leu34Pro or PL^{A2}	Altered function	Potentially associated with increased risk of MI, increased sudden death, but inconsistent results
GP Ia		
C807T and G873A	Unclear	Equivocal association with MI
GP VI		
T13254C	Unclear	Few data, suggestion of increased association with MI
Enzyme/receptor system		
MTHFR		
C667T	Altered half-life	Conflicting results, while associated with elevated homocysteine levels, likely not strongly associated with disease
GPx-3		
A-943C, T-928C		
A-862T, T-569C, T-519C, A-303T, T-65C	Unclear	Associated with premature stroke, unclear association with MI
eNOS		
G894T (Gln298Asp)	Altered function	Associated with MI and coronary spasm as well as altered endothelial function
T-786C, A-922G, T-1468A	Altered expression	
ACE		
287 bp insertion-deletion	Unclear	Conflicting results, itself likely a weak predictor of MI but may connote increased risk in conjunction with other mutations
Angiotensin		
T235	Unclear	Unclear, perhaps associated independently with MI
AII receptor		
A1166C	Unclear	Conflicting results, may connote increased risk if inherited with ACE D mutation

similar to the conclusions of the U.S. Physicians Health Study (107) and the REGRESS trial (108). The association between C667T and stroke are similarly equivocal, with some trials suggesting that homozygosity for the T allele is a risk factor for juvenile stroke (<45 years) and others not (109). In summary, while elevated HCY levels seem clearly associated with atherothrombosis and venous thrombosis, the presence of C667T, while associated with elevated plasma HCY levels, is not clearly associated with the development of disease.

B. Glutathione Peroxidases

Endothelial cell oxidant stress is a fundamental mechanism underlying the process of atherothrombosis. Reactive oxygen species such as superoxide ($\bullet O_2^-$) and hydrogen peroxide (H_2O_2), produced in the setting of hypertension, diabetes mellitus, and cigarette smoking, result in the oxidative inactivation of critical cellular enzymes and proteins. ROS also reduce the supply of bioavailable nitric oxide (NO$\bullet$) through oxidation of NO$\bullet$ to peroxynitrite (ONOO-), itself a potent oxidant. ROS are countered by cellular antioxidants, the most important of which is glutathione (7). Glutathione peroxidases (GPx) reduce hydrogen peroxide and lipid peroxides to water and lipid alcohols, respectively, and in so doing oxidize glutathione (GSH) to glutathione disulfide (GSSG). In this way, GPx play a critical role in the maintenance of the oxido-reductive balance of the cell. Hyperhomocysteinemia decreases GPx-1, the most prevalent isoform of the enzyme, a deficiency of which is associated with endothelial dysfunction (110,111). A deficiency of GPx-3, the plasma isoform, has been associated with premature stroke, a finding attributable to decreased platelet responsiveness to NO$\bullet$ (112). Within GPx-3, seven linked promoter polymorphisms (A-943C, T-928C, A-862T, T-569C, T-519C, A-303T, and T-65C) have been identified and associated with premature stroke (7). Importantly, these polymorphisms define a NaPb-type that reduces promoter activity. To date, no assessment of GPx polymorphisms and coronary atherothrombosis has been made. Further studies examining co-inheritance of GPx polymorphisms and the MTHFR C677T mutation seem appropriate.

C. Nitric Oxide Synthase

Nitric oxide insufficiency, manifest as decreased bioavailable NO$\bullet$, results from both oxidative inactivation of NO$\bullet$ by ROS and decreased NO$\bullet$ production. Vascular NO$\bullet$ is generated by the oxidative conversion of L-arginine to L-citrulline by the endothelial isoform of nitric oxide synthase (eNOS). Recently, attention has turned to polymorphisms within the eNOS gene that might affect expression level and thus, NO$\bullet$ production and might be associated with atherothrombotic disease. Three linked polymorphisms within the 5'-flanking region of eNOS (T-786C, A-922G, and T-1468A) have been defined and associated with coronary artery spasm and MI (113,114). The T786C polymorphism was associated with a 50% reduction in eNOS promotor activity. In addition, a SNP within the coding region of eNOS (G $\rightarrow$ T at position 894 resulting in aspartate for glutamine at residue 298) has also been identified and linked to atherothrombotic disease (115). Homozygosity for the 298Asp allele, as studied in the Cambridge Heart AntiOxidant Studies (CHAOS and CHAOS II) of patients with angiographically defined CAD or recent MI, was associated with a fourfold increased risk of CAD and a twofold increased risk of MI (116). This mutation has also been associated with carotid atherosclerosis (117).

Studies of endothelial function as detected by flow mediated brachial artery dilatation suggest a deleterious effect of 298Asp in patients who smoke (118). Further study of this potentially important mutation is warranted.

D. ACE D

The renin-angiotensin-aldosterone axis is one of the principal homeostatic mechanisms that maintain blood pressure. Angiotensin II (AII) a potent vasoconstrictor and regulator of vascular smooth muscle migration, is formed following cleavage of angiotensin I by angiotensin-converting enzyme (ACE). AII has also been recently shown to affect the endothelial cell oxido-reductive state directly by modulation of ROS-producing enzymes, such as NAD(P)H oxidase (119). ACE also degrades bradykinin, a mediator whose effects counter those of AII in that it promotes vasodilation and inhibits smooth muscle proliferation partly through the generation of endothelial NO. Inhibitors of ACE and AII are potent antihypertensives and have been shown to have beneficial effects when applied in a wide range of disease processes, including left ventricular dysfunction, coronary artery disease, and diabetic nephropathy. Owing to its central role in cardiovascular disease, as well as the utility of inhibitors of this system in preventing disease progression, the genes for ACE and AII have been examined for mutations that might be associated with atherothrombotic disease progression. In the early 1990s, attention turned to a 287 bp insertion/deletion polymorphism within exon 16 of the ACE gene, termed ACE I (insertion) and ACE D (deletion), resulting in three genotypes II, DD, or ID (120). The genotypic frequency in the general population is approximately 20% for II, 50% for ID, and 30% for DD (121). The ACE D allele has been associated with increased ACE activity and, thus, has been investigated for its association with atherothrombosis (122). Initial studies linked the ACE D mutation with an increased risk of both CAD and MI, especially in subjects with "low-risk" characteristics (nonsmoker, nondiabetic, etc.) (123). Further support for ACE D and CAD for "lower-risk" patients was obtained in a 2200-patient retrospective trial that demonstrated an association between the D allele and CAD only in patients younger than 62 years (121). Additional data have identified ACE D as a significant risk factor for CAD and MI in women (124), for recurrent events following MI (125), and have suggested that co-inheritance of ACE D with PLA2 increases atherothrombotic risk (126). Conversely, the prospective U.S. Physicians Health study failed to detect an association between ACE genotype and CAD or MI (127). A meta-analysis of 18 published trials supports a weak association between inheritance of the ACE D genotype and MI (128). In summary, the association between ACE D and atherothrombotic disease appears inconsistent, as multiple trials have yielded divergent conclusions, perhaps owing to differences in subject selection or sample size.

A mutation within the gene coding for a receptor for AII (the angiotensin II subtype I receptor, or AT1R) has been identified at position 1166 (A → C), and while initial evidence linked this mutation to CAD and MI, especially if co-inherited with ACE D, subsequent trials have yielded negative results (129). Finally, evaluation of a SNP within the angiotensinogen gene (T235) has suggested an independent association with CAD (130). Given the disparate results of numerous studies of genes within the angiotensin-angiotensin receptor system, one must conclude that an association between genotype and disease has not been definitely shown and, if it does exist, is most likely weak.

VIII. CONCLUSION

The elucidation of a strong genetic predisposition that favors the development of atherothrombotic disease remains an unrealized goal of cardiovascular medicine. Genetic epidemiology, particular in light of the completion of the human genome project, holds considerable promise as efforts to define the numerous heritable risk factors that contribute to a family history of atherothrombotic disease are now yielding results. The polymorphisms detailed above have been evaluated and correlated, to varying degrees, with the development of atherothrombosis. Two common observations seem to emerge from these single candidate gene studies. First, while a particular factor may be associated with disease (for example, an elevated fibrinogen level), and while a mutation may be associated changes in the level of activity, the mutation itself need not necessarily correlate with disease. This finding underscores the inherent complexity of polygenic and environmental contributions that ultimately result in a particular disease phenotype. Second, while a genotype may connote risk for venous thrombosis, it is not necessarily associated with atherothrombosis — a finding likely related to the different pathophysiological processes that bring about thrombosis within the two domains of the vasculature. As with defined polymorphisms associated with venous thrombosis, each identified polymorphism that is correlated with atherothrombosis contributes to our understanding of the hypercoagulable state and may ultimately merit consideration in disease screening, secondary prevention, or treatment selection.

ACKNOWLEDGMENT

Supported in part by NIH Grants HI55993, HL58976, and HL61975.

REFERENCES

1. Libby P, Ridker PM, Maseri A. Inflammation and atherosclerosis. Circulation 2002; 105:1135–1143.
2. Peng DQ, Zhao SP, Li YF, Li J, Zhou HN. Elevated soluble CD40 ligand is related to the endothelial adhesion molecules in patients with acute coronary syndrome. Clin Chim Acta 2002; 319:19–26.
3. Henn V, Slupsky JR, Grafe M, et al. CD40 ligand on activated platelets triggers an inflammatory reaction of endothelial cells. Nature 1998; 391:591–594.
4. Lane DA, Grant PJ. Role of hemostatic gene polymorphisms in venous and arterial thrombotic disease. Blood 2000; 95:1517–1532.
5. Kroll MK, Sullivan R. Mechanisms of Platelet Activation. In: Loscalzo J, and Schafer A, eds. Thrombosis and Hemorrhage Second Ed. Philadelphia, PA: Williams and Wilkins, 1998:261–291.
6. Pigazzi A, Heydrick S, Folli F, Benoit S, Michelson A, Loscalzo J. Nitric oxide inhibits thrombin receptor-activating peptide-induced phosphoinositide 3–kinase activity in human platelets. J Biol Chem 1999; 274:14368–14375.
7. Loscalzo J. Nitric oxide insufficiency, platelet activation, and arterial thrombosis. Circ Res 2001; 88:756–762.
8. Loscalzo J. Endothelial injury, vasoconstriction, and its prevention. Tex Heart Inst J 1995; 22:180–184.
9. Gayle RB, 3rd, Maliszewski CR, Gimpel SD, et al. Inhibition of platelet function by recombinant soluble ecto-ADPase/CD39. J Clin Invest 1998; 101:1851–1859.

10. Wilcox JN, Smith KM, Schwartz SM, Gordon D. Localization of tissue factor in the normal vessel wall and in the atherosclerotic plaque. Proc Natl Acad Sci USA 1989; 86:2839–2843.

11. Rosenberg RD, Aird WC. Vascular-bed-specific hemostasis and hypercoagulable states. N Engl J Med 1999; 340:1555–1564.

12. Bajzar L, Manuel R, Nesheim ME. Purification and characterization of TAFI, a thrombin-activable fibrinolysis inhibitor. J Biol Chem 1995; 270:14477–14484.

13. Folsom AR, Aleksic N, Wang L, Cushman M, Wu KK, White RH. Protein C, antithrombin, and venous thromboembolism incidence: a prospective population-based study. Arterioler Thromb Vasc Biol 2002; 22:1018–1022.

14. Bertina RM, Koeleman BP, Koster T, et al. Mutation in blood coagulation factor V associated with resistance to activated protein C. Nature 1994; 369:64–67.

15. Koster T, Rosendaal FR, de Ronde H, Briet E, Vandenbroucke JP, Bertina RM. Venous thrombosis due to poor anticoagulant response to activated protein C: Leiden Thrombophilia Study. Lancet 1993; 342:1503–1506.

16. Ridker PM, Hennekens CH, Lindpaintner K, Stampfer MJ, Eisenberg PR, Miletich JP. Mutation in the gene coding for coagulation factor V and the risk of myocardial infarction, stroke, and venous thrombosis in apparently healthy men. N Engl J Med 1995; 332:912–917.

17. De Stefano V, Martinelli I, Mannucci PM, et al. The risk of recurrent deep venous thrombosis among heterozygous carriers of both factor V Leiden and the G20210A prothrombin mutation. N Engl J Med 1999; 341:801–806.

18. Ridker PM, Miletich JP, Stampfer MJ, Goldhaber SZ, Lindpaintner K, Hennekens CH. Factor V Leiden and risks of recurrent idiopathic venous thromboembolism. Circulation 1995; 92:2800–2802.

19. Simioni P, Prandoni P, Lensing AW, et al. The risk of recurrent venous thromboembolism in patients with an Arg506–>Gln mutation in the gene for factor V (factor V Leiden). N Engl J Med 1997; 336:399–403.

20. Folsom AR, Cushman M, Tsai MY, et al. A prospective study of venous thromboembolism in relation to factor V Leiden and related factors. Blood 2002; 99:2720–2725.

21. Brey RL, Coull BM. Cerebral venous thrombosis: role of activated protein C resistance and factor V gene mutation. Stroke 1996; 27:1719–1720.

22. Longstreth WT, Jr, Rosendaal FR, Siscovick DS, et al. Risk of stroke in young women and two prothrombotic mutations: factor V Leiden and prothrombin gene variant (G20210A). Stroke 1998; 29:577–580.

23. Doggen CJ, Cats VM, Bertina RM, Rosendaal FR. Interaction of coagulation defects and cardiovascular risk factors: increased risk of myocardial infarction associated with factor V Leiden or prothrombin 20210A. Circulation 1998; 97:1037–1041.

24. Reiner AP, Rosendaal FR, Reitsma PH, et al. Factor V Leiden, prothrombin G20210A, and risk of sudden coronary death in apparently healthy persons. Am J Cardiol 2002; 90:66–68.

25. Poort SR, Rosendaal FR, Reitsma PH, Bertina RM. A common genetic variation in the 3'-untranslated region of the prothrombin gene is associated with elevated plasma prothrombin levels and an increase in venous thrombosis. Blood 1996; 88:3698–3703.

26. Reuner KH, Ruf A, Grau A, et al. Prothrombin gene G20210–>a transition is a risk factor for cerebral venous thrombosis. Stroke 1998; 29:1765–1769.

27. Ridker PM, Hennekens CH, Miletich JP. G20210A mutation in prothrombin gene and risk of myocardial infarction, stroke, and venous thrombosis in a large cohort of US Men. Circulation 1999; 99:999–1004.

28. Catto AJ, Kohler HP, Coore J, Mansfield MW, Stickland MH, Grant PJ. Association of a common polymorphism In the factor XIII gene with venous thrombosis. Blood 1999; 93:906–908.

29. Trumbo TA, Maurer MC. Examining thrombin hydrolysis of the factor XIII activation peptide segment leads to a proposal for explaining the cardioprotective effects observed with the factor XIII V34L mutation. J. Biol. Chem. 2000; 275:20627–20631.

30. Aleksic N, Ahn C, Wang Y-W, et al. Factor XIIIA Val34Leu polymorphism does not predict risk of coronary heart disease: the Atherosclerosis Risk in Communities (ARIC) Study. Arterioscler Thromb Vasc Biol 2002; 22:348–352.

31. Doggen CJ, Kunz G, Rosendaal FR, et al. A mutation in the thrombomodulin gene, 127G to A coding for Ala25Thr, and the risk of myocardial infarction in men. Thromb Haemost 1998; 80:743–748.

32. Salomaa V, Matei C, Aleksic N, et al. Soluble thrombomodulin as a predictor of incident coronary heart disease and symptomless carotid artery atherosclerosis in the Atherosclerosis Risk in Communities (ARIC) Study: a case-cohort study. Lancet 1999; 353:1729–1734.

33. Van de Water NS, French JK, McDowell J, Browett PJ. The endothelial protein C receptor (EPCR) 23bp insert in patients with myocardial infarction. Thromb Haemost 2001; 85:749–751.

34. Koster T, Blann AD, Briet E, Vandenbroucke JP, Rosendaal FR. Role of clotting factor VIII in effect of von Willebrand factor on occurrence of deep-vein thrombosis. Lancet 1995; 345:152–155.

35. Kamphuisen PW, Eikenboom JC, Rosendaal FR, et al. High factor VIII antigen levels increase the risk of venous thrombosis but are not associated with polymorphisms in the von Willebrand factor and factor VIII gene. Br J Haematol 2001; 115:156–158.

36. Meade TW, Mellows S, Brozovic M, et al. Haemostatic function and ischaemic heart disease: principal results of the Northwick Park Heart Study. Lancet 1986; 2:533–537.

37. Wilhelmsen L, Svardsudd K, Korsan-Bengtsen K, Larsson B, Welin L, Tibblin G. Fibrinogen as a risk factor for stroke and myocardial infarction. N Engl J Med 1984; 311:501–505.

38. Folsom AR. Hemostatic risk factors for atherothrombotic disease: an epidemiologic view. Thromb Haemost 2001; 86:366–373.

39. Tuut M, Hense HW. Smoking, other risk factors and fibrinogen levels. Evidence of effect modification. Ann Epidemiol 2001; 11:232–238.

40. Humphries SE, Cook M, Dubowitz M, Stirling Y, Meade TW. Role of genetic variation at the fibrinogen locus in determination of plasma fibrinogen concentrations. Lancet 1987; 1:1452–1455.

41. Behague I, Poirier O, Nicaud V, et al. ß Fibrinogen gene polymorphisms are associated with plasma fibrinogen and coronary artery disease in patients with myocardial infarction: the ECTIM study. Circulation 1996; 93:440–449.

42. Humphries SE, Ye S, Talmud P, Bara L, Wilhelmsen L, Tiret L. European Atherosclerosis Research Study: genotype at the fibrinogen locus (G-455–A ß-Gene) is associated with differences in plasma fibrinogen levels in young men and women from different regions in europe: evidence for gender-genotype-environment interaction. Arterioscler Thromb Vasc Biol 1995; 15:96–104.

43. de Maat MP, Kastelein JJ, Jukema JW, et al. -455G/A polymorphism of the ß-fibrinogen gene is associated with the progression of coronary atherosclerosis in symptomatic men: proposed role for an acute-phase reaction pattern of fibrinogen. Arterioscler Thromb Vasc Biol 1998; 18:265–271.

44. Tybjarg-Hansen A, Agerholm-Larsen B, Humphries SE, Abildgaard S, Schnohr P, Nordestgaard BG. A common mutation (G-455 → A) in the beta-fibrinogen promoter is an independent predictor of plasma fibrinogen, but not of ischemic heart disease. A study of 9,127 individuals based on The Copenhagen City Heart Study. J Clin Invest 1997; 99:3034–3039.

45. Boekholdt SM, Bijsterveld NR, Moons AH, Levi M, Buller HR, Peters RJ. Genetic variation in coagulation and fibrinolytic proteins and their relation with acute myocardial infarction: a systematic review. Circulation 2001; 104:3063–3068.

46. Zito F, Di Castelnuovo A, Amore C, D'Orazio A, Donati MB, Iacoviello L. Bcl I polymorphism in the fibrinogen ß-chain gene is associated with the risk of familial myocardial infarction by increasing plasma fibrinogen levels: a case-control study in a sample of GISSI-2 patients Arterioscler Thromb Vasc Biol 1997; 17:3489–3494.

47. Junker R, Heinrich J, Schulte H, van de Loo J, Assmann G. Coagulation factor VII and the risk of coronary heart disease in healthy men Arterioscler Thromb Vasc Biol 1997; 17:1539–1544.

48. Smith FB, Lee AJ, Fowkes FG, Price JF, Rumley A, Lowe GD. Hemostatic factors as predictors of ischemic heart disease and stroke in the Edinburgh Artery Study. 1997; 17:3321–3325.

49. Lane A, Cruickshank JK, Mitchell J, Henderson A, Humphries S, Green F. Genetic and environmental determinants of factor VII coagulant activity in ethnic groups at differing risk of coronary heart disease. Atherosclerosis 1992; 94:43–50.

50. Lane A, Green F, Scarabin PY, et al. Factor VII Arg/Gln353 polymorphism determines factor VII coagulant activity in patients with myocardial infarction (MI) and control subjects in Belfast and in France but is not a strong indicator of MI risk in the ECTIM study. Atherosclerosis 1996; 119:119–127.

51. Doggen CJ, Manger Cats V, Bertina RM, Reitsma PH, Vandenbroucke JP, Rosendaal FR. A genetic propensity to high factor VII is not associated with the risk of myocardial infarction in men. Thromb Haemost 1998; 80:281–285.

52. Iacoviello L, Di Castelnuovo A, de Knijff P, et al. Polymorphisms in the coagulation factor vii gene and the risk of myocardial infarction. N Engl J Med 1998; 338:79–85.

53. Kohler HP, Grant PJ. Plasminogen-activator inhibitor type 1 and coronary artery disease. N Engl J Med 2000; 342:1792–1801.

54. Juhan-Vague I, Pyke SDM, Alessi MC, Jespersen J, Haverkate F, Thompson SG. Fibrinolytic factors and the risk of myocardial infarction or sudden death in patients with angina pectoris. Circulation 1996; 94:2057–2063.

55. MacCallum PK, Cooper JA, Howarth DJ, Meade TW, Miller GJ. Sex differences in the determinants of fibrinolytic activity. Thromb Haemost 1998; 79:587–590.

56. Hamsten A, de Faire U, Walldius G, et al. Plasminogen activator inhibitor in plasma: risk factor for recurrent myocardial infarction. Lancet 1987; 2:3–9.

57. Hamsten A, Wiman B, de Faire U, Blomback M. Increased plasma levels of a rapid inhibitor of tissue plasminogen activator in young survivors of myocardial infarction. N Engl J Med 1985; 313:1557–1563.

58. Sobel BE, Woodcock-Mitchell J, Schneider DJ, Holt RE, Marutsuka K, Gold H. Increased plasminogen activator inhibitor type 1 in coronary artery atherectomy specimens from type 2 diabetic compared with nondiabetic patients: a potential factor predisposing to thrombosis and its persistence. Circulation 1998; 97:2213–2221.

59. Juhan-Vague I, Roul C, Alessi MC, Ardissone JP, Heim M, Vague P. Increased plasminogen activator inhibitor activity in non insulin dependent diabetic patients—relationship with plasma insulin. Thromb Haemost 1989; 61:370–373.

60. Meigs JB, Mittleman MA, Nathan DM, et al. Hyperinsulinemia, hyperglycemia, and impaired hemostasis: the Framingham Offspring Study. JAMA 2000; 283:221–228.

61. Bastard JP, Pieroni L, Hainque B. Relationship between plasma plasminogen activator inhibitor 1 and insulin resistance. Diabetes Metab Res Rev 2000; 16:192–201.

62. Dawson SJ, Wiman B, Hamsten A, Green F, Humphries S, Henney AM. The two allele sequences of a common polymorphism in the promoter of the plasminogen activator inhibitor-1 (PAI-1) gene respond differently to interleukin-1 in HepG2 cells. J Biol Chem 1993; 268:10739–10745.

63. Eriksson P, Nilsson L, Karpe F, Hamsten A. Very-low-density lipoprotein response element in the promoter region of the human plasminogen activator inhibitor-1 gene implicated in the impaired fibrinolysis of hypertriglyceridemia. Arterioscler Thromb Vasc Biol 1998; 18:20–26.

64. Dawson S, Hamsten A, Wiman B, Henney A, Humphries S. Genetic variation at the plasminogen activator inhibitor-1 locus is associated with altered levels of plasma plasminogen activator inhibitor-1 activity. Arterioscler Thromb 1991; 11:183–190.

65. Mansfield MW, Stickland MH, Grant PJ. Plasminogen activator inhibitor-1 (PAI-1) promoter polymorphism and coronary artery disease in non-insulin-dependent diabetes. Thromb Haemost 1995; 74:1032–1034.

66. Ossei-Gerning N, Mansfield MW, Stickland MH, Wilson IJ, Grant PJ. Plasminogen activator inhibitor-1 promoter 4G/5G genotype and plasma levels in relation to a history of myocardial infarction in patients characterized by coronary angiography. Arterioscler Thromb Vasc Biol 1997; 17:33–37.

67. Margaglione M, Cappucci G, Colaizzo D, et al. The PAI-1 gene locus 4G/5G polymorphism is associated with a family history of coronary artery disease. Arterioscler Thromb Vasc Biol 1998; 18:152–156.

68. Ye S, Green FR, Scarabin PY, et al. The 4G/5G genetic polymorphism in the promoter of the plasminogen activator inhibitor-1 (PAI-1) gene is associated with differences in plasma PAI-1 activity but not with risk of myocardial infarction in the ECTIM study. Etude CasTemoins de I'nfarctus du Mycocarde. Thromb Haemost 1995; 74:837–841.

69. Doggen CJ, Bertina RM, Cats VM, Reitsma PH, Rosendaal FR. The 4G/5G polymorphism in the plasminogen activator inhibitor-1 gene is not associated with myocardial infarction. Thromb Haemost 1999; 82:115–120.

70. Ridker PM, Hennekens CH, Lindpaintner K, Stampfer MJ, Miletich JP. Arterial and venous thrombosis is not associated with the 4G/5G polymorphism in the promoter of the plasminogen activator inhibitor gene in a large cohort of US men. Circulation 1997; 95:59–62.

71. Anderson JL, Muhlestein JB, Habashi J, et al. Lack of association of a common polymorphism of the plasminogen activator inhibitor-1 gene with coronary artery disease and myocardial infarction. J Am Coll Cardiol 1999; 34:1778–1783.

72. Iacoviello L, Burzotta F, Di Castelnuovo A, Zito F, Marchioli R, Donati MB. The 4G/5G polymorphism of PAI-1 promoter gene and the risk of myocardial infarction: a meta-analysis. Thromb Haemost 1998; 80:1029–1030.

73. Thompson SG, Kienast J, Pyke SD, Haverkate F, van de Loo JC, The European Concerted Action on Thrombosis and Disabilities Angina Pectoris Study Group. Hemostatic factors and the risk of myocardial infarction or sudden death in patients with angina pectoris. N Engl J Med 1995; 332:635–641.

74. Wiman B, Andersson T, Hallqvist J, Reuterwall C, Ahlbom A, deFaire U. Plasma levels of tissue plasminogen activator/plasminogen activator inhibitor-1 complex and von Willebrand factor are significant risk markers for recurrent myocardial infarction in the Stockholm Heart Epidemiology Program (SHEEP) study. Arterioscler Thromb Vasc Biol 2000; 20:2019–2023.

75. Vaughan DE, Rouleau J-L, Ridker PM, Arnold JM, Menapace FJ, Pfeffer MA. Effects of ramipril on plasma fibrinolytic balance in patients with acute anterior myocardial infarction. Circulation 1997; 96:442–447.

76. Barua RS, Ambrose JA, Saha DC, Eales-Reynolds L-J. Smoking is associated with altered endothelial-derived fibrinolytic and antithrombotic factors: an in vitro demonstration. Circulation 2002; 106:905–908.

77. Ladenvall P, Johansson L, Jansson JH, et al. Tissue-type plasminogen activator—7,351C/T enhancer polymorphism is associated with a first myocardial infarction. Thromb Haemost 2002; 87:105–109.

78. Kandzari DE, Goldschmidt-Clermont. Platelet polymorphisms and ischemic heart disease: moving beyond traditional risk factors. J Am Coll Cardiol 2001; 38:1028–1032.

79. Gonzalez-Conejero R, Lozano ML, Rivera J, et al. Polymorphisms of platelet membrane glycoprotein ibalpha associated with arterial thrombotic disease. Blood 1998; 92:2771–2776.

80. Afshar-Kharghan V, Li CQ, Khoshnevis-Asl M, Lopez JA. Kozak sequence polymorphism of the glycoprotein (GP) Ibralpha gene is a major determinant of the plasma membrane levels of the platelet GP Ib-IX-V complex. Blood 1999; 94:186–191.

81. Meisel C, Afshar-Kharghan V, Cascorbi I, et al. Role of Kozak sequence polymorphism of platelet glycoprotein Ib alpha as a risk factor for coronary artery disease and catheter interventions. J Am Coll Cardiol 2001; 38:1023–1027.

82. Baker RI, Eikelboom J, Lofthouse E, et al. Platelet glycoprotein Ibalpha Kozak polymorphism is associated with an increased risk of ischemic stroke. Blood 2001; 98:36–40.

83. Santoso S, Zimmermann P, Sachs UJ, Gardemann A. The impact of the Kozak sequence polymorphism of the glycoprotein Ib alpha gene on the risk and extent of coronary heart disease. Thromb Haemost 2002; 87:345–346.

84. Newman PJ, Derbes RS, Aster RH. The human platelet alloantigens, PlA1 and PlA2, are associated with a leucine33/proline33 amino acid polymorphism in membrane glycoprotein IIIa, and are distinguishable by DNA typing. J Clin Invest 1989; 83:1778–1781.

85. Weiss EJ, Bray PF, Tayback M, et al. A polymorphism of a platelet glycoprotein receptor as an inherited risk factor for coronary thrombosis. N Engl J Med 1996; 334:1090–1094.

86. Carter AM, Ossei-Gerning N, Wilson IJ, Grant PJ. Association of the platelet PlA polymorphism of glycoprotein IIb/IIIa and the fibrinogen Bß 448 polymorphism with myocardial infarction and extent of coronary artery disease. Circulation 1997; 96:1424–1431.

87. Mikkelsson J, Perola M, Laippala P, Penttila A, Karhunen P. Glycoprotein IIIa PlA1/A2 polymorphism and sudden cardiac death. J Am Coll Cardiol 2000; 36:1317–1323.

88. Mikkelsson J, Perola M, Laippala P, et al. Glycoprotein IIIa PlA polymorphism associates with progression of coronary artery disease and with myocardial infarction in an autopsy series of middle-aged men who died suddenly. Arterioscler Thromb Vasc Biol 1999; 19:2573–2578.

89. Kastrati A, Koch W, Gawaz M, et al. PlA polymorphism of glycoprotein IIIa and risk of adverse events after coronary stent placement. J Am Coll Cardiol 2000; 36:84–89.

90. Vijayan KV, Goldschmidt-Clermont PJ, Roos C, Bray PF. The Pl(A2) polymorphism of integrin beta(3) enhances outside-in signaling and adhesive functions. J Clin Invest 2000; 105:793–802.

91. Feng D, Lindpaintner K, Larson MG, et al. Platelet glycoprotein IIIa PlA polymorphism, fibrinogen, and platelet aggregability: The Framingham Heart Study. Circulation 2001; 104:140–144.

92. Ridker PM, Hennekens CH, Schmitz C, Stampfer MJ, Lindpaintner RU. PIA1/A2 polymorphism of platelet glycoprotein IIIa and risks of myocardial infarction, stroke, and venous thrombosis. Lancet 1997; 349:385–388.

93. Zhu MM, Weedon J, Clark LT. Meta-analysis of the association of platelet glycoprotein IIIa PlA1/A2 polymorphism with myocardial infarction. Am J Cardiol 2000; 86:1000–1005.

94. Bennett JS, Catella-Lawson F, Rut AR, et al. Effect of the Pl(A2) alloantigen on the function of beta(3)–integrins in platelets. Blood 2001; 97:3093–3099.

95. Anderson JL, King GJ, Bair TL, et al. Associations between a polymorphism in the gene encoding glycoprotein IIIa and myocardial infarction or coronary artery disease. J Am Coll Cardiol 1999; 33:727–733.

96. Santoso S, Kunicki TJ, Kroll H, Haberbosch W, Gardemann A. Association of the platelet glycoprotein Ia C807T gene polymorphism with nonfatal myocardial infarction in younger patients. Blood 1999; 93:2449–2453.

97. Benze G, Heinrich J, Schulte H, et al. Association of the GPIa C807T and GPIIIa PlA1/A2 polymorphisms with premature myocardial infarction in men. Eur Heart J 2002; 23:325–330.

98. Kroll H, Gardemann A, Fechter A, Haberbosch W, Santoso S. The impact of the glycoprotein Ia collagen receptor subunit A1648G gene polymorphism on coronary artery disease and acute myocardial infarction. Thromb Haemost 2000; 83:392–396.

99. Croft SA, Samani NJ, Teare MD, et al. Novel platelet membrane glycoprotein VI dimorphism is a risk factor for myocardial infarction. Circulation 2001; 104:1459–1463.

100. Welch GN, Loscalzo J. Homocysteine and atherothrombosis. N Engl J Med 1998; 338:1042–1050.

101. Kang SS, Passen EL, Ruggie N, Wong PW, Sora H. Thermolabile defect of methylenetetrahydrofolate reductase in coronary artery disease. Circulation 1993; 88:1463–1469.

102. Christensen B, Frosst P, Lussier-Cacan S, et al. Correlation of a common mutation in the methylenetetrahydrofolate reductase gene with plasma homocysteine in patients with premature coronary artery disease. Arterioscler Thromb Vasc Biol 1997; 17:569–573.

103. Salomon O, Rosenberg N, Zivelin A, et al. Methionine synthase A2756G and methylenetetrahydrofolate reductase A1298C polymorphisms are not risk factors for idiopathic venous thromboembolism. Hematol J 2001; 2:38–41.

104. Fujimura H, Kawasaki T, Sakata T, et al. Common C677T polymorphism in the methylenete-trahydrofolate reductase gene increases the risk for deep vein thrombosis in patients with pre-disposition of thrombophilia. Thromb Res 2000; 98:1–8.

105. Mager A, Lalezari S, Shohat T, et al. Methylenetetrahydrofolate reductase genotypes and early-onset coronary artery disease. Circulation 1999; 100:2406–2410.

106. Anderson JL, King GJ, Thomson MJ, et al. A mutation in the methylenetetrahydrofolate reductase gene is not associated with increased risk for coronary artery disease or myocardial infarction. J Am Coll 1997; 30:1206–1211.

107. Ma J, Stampfer MJ, Hennekens CH, et al. Methylenetetrahydrofolate reductase polymor-phism, plasma folate, homocysteine, and risk of myocardial infarction in US physicians. Circulation 1996; 94:2410–2416.

108. Kluijtmans LA, Kastelein JJ, Lindemans J, et al. Thermolabile methylenetetrahydrofolate reductase in coronary artery disease. Circulation 1997; 96:2573–2577.

109. Madonna P, de Stefano V, Coppola A, et al. Hyperhomocysteinemia and other inherited pro-thrombotic conditions in young adults with a history of ischemic stroke. Stroke 2002; 33:51–56.

110. Weiss N, Zhang Y-Y, Heydrick S, Bierl C, Loscalzo J. Overexpression of cellular glutathione peroxidase rescues homocyst(e)ine-induced endothelial dysfunction. Proc Nat'l Acad Sci (USA) 2001; 98:12503–12508.

111. Weiss N, Heydrick S, Zhang Y-Y, Bierl C, Cap A, Loscalzo J. Cellular redox state and endothelial dysfunction in mildly hyperhomocysteinemic cystathionine {beta}-synthase-defi-cient mice. Arterioscler Thromb Vasc Biol 2002; 22:34–41.

112. Kenet G, Freedman J, Shenkman B, et al. Plasma glutathione peroxidase deficiency and platelet insensitivity to nitric oxide in children with familial stroke. Arterioscler Thromb Vasc Biol 1999; 19:2017–2023.

113. Nakayama M, Yasue H, Yoshimura M, et al. T-786–>C Mutation in the 5'-flanking region of the endothelial nitric oxide synthase gene is associated with coronary spasm. Circulation 1999; 99:2864–2870.

114. Nakayama M, Yasue H, Yoshimura M, et al. T-786–>C mutation in the 5'-flanking region of the endothelial nitric oxide synthase gene is associated with myocardial infarction, especially without coronary organic stenosis. Am J Cardiol 2000; 86:628–634.

115. Colombo MG, Andreassi MG, Paradossi U, et al. Evidence for association of a common variant of the endothelial nitric oxide synthase gene (Glu298—>Asp polymorphism) to the presence, extent, and severity of coronary artery disease. Heart 2002; 87:525–528.

116. Hingorani AD, Liang CF, Fatibene J, et al. A common variant of the endothelial nitric oxide synthase (Glu298 → Asp) is a major risk factor for coronary artery disease in the UK. Circulation 1999; 100:1515–1520.

117. Lembo G, De Luca N, Battagli C, et al. A common variant of endothelial nitric oxide syn-thase (Glu298Asp) is an independent risk factor for carotid atherosclerosis. Stroke 2001; 32:735–740.

118. Leeson CP, Hingorani AD, Mullen MJ, et al. Glu298Asp endothelial nitric oxide synthase gene polymorphism interacts with environmental and dietary factors to influence endothelial function. Circ Res 2002; 90:1153–1158.

119. Mollnau H, Wendt M, Szocs K, et al. Effects of angiotensin II infusion on the expression and function of NAD(P)H oxidase and components of nitric oxide/cGMP signaling. Circ Res 2002; 90:E58–65.

120. Rigat B, Hubert C, Alhenc-Gelas F, Cambien F, Corvol P, Soubrier F. An insertion/deletion polymorphism in the angiotensin I-converting enzyme gene accounting for half the variance of serum enzyme levels. J Clin Invest 1990; 86:1343–1346.

121. Gardemann A, Fink M, Stricker J, et al. ACE I/D gene polymorphism: presence of the ACE D allele increases the risk of coronary artery disease in younger individuals. Atherosclerosis 1998; 139:153–159.

122. Cambien F, Poirier O, Lecerf L, et al. Deletion polymorphism in the gene for angiotensin-con-verting enzyme is a potent risk factor for myocardial infarction. Nature 1992; 359:641–644.

123. Gardemann A, Weiss T, Schwartz O, et al. Gene polymorphism but not catalytic activity of angiotensin I–converting enzyme is associated with coronary artery disease and myocardial infarction in low-risk patients. Circulation 1995; 92:2796–2799.
124. Schuster H, Wienker TF, Stremmler U, Noll B, Steinmetz A, Luft FC. An angiotensin-converting enzyme gene variant is associated with acute myocardial infarction in women but not in men. Am J Cardiol 1995; 76:601–603.
125. Yoshida M, Iwai N, Ohmichi N, Izumi M, Nakamura Y, Kinoshita M. D allele of the angiotensin-converting enzyme gene is a risk factor for secondary cardiac events after myocardial infarction. Int J Cardiol 1999; 70:119–125.
126. Bray PF, Cannon CP, Goldschmidt-Clermont P, et al. The platelet PlA2 and angiotensin-converting enzyme (ACE) D allele polymorphisms and the risk of recurrent events after acute myocardial infarction. Am J Cardiol 2001; 88:347–352.
127. Lindpaintner K, Pfeffer MA, Kreutz R, et al. a prospective evaluation of an angiotensin-converting-enzyme gene polymorphism and the risk of ischemic heart disease. N Engl J Med 1995; 332:706–712.
128. Samani NJ, Thompson JR, O'Toole L, Channer K, Woods KL. A meta analysis of the association of the deletion allele of the angiotensin converting enzyme gene with myocardial infarction. Circulation 1996; 94:708–712.
129. Steeds RP, Wardle A, Smith PD, Martin D, Channer KS, Samani NJ. Analysis of the postulated interaction between the angiotensin II sub-type 1 receptor gene A1166C polymorphism and the insertion/deletion polymorphism of the angiotensin converting enzyme gene on risk of myocardial infarction. Atherosclerosis 2001; 154:123–128.
130. Katsuya T, Koike G, Yee TW, et al. Association of angiotensinogen gene T235 variant with increased risk of coronary heart disease. Lancet 1995; 345:1600–1603.

2-2

Vascular Biology and Pathobiology in Acute Coronary Syndromes

Noyan Gokce, John Carr, and Joseph Loscalzo
Boston University School of Medicine, Boston, Massachusetts, U.S.A.

The vascular system serves as more than a simple passive conduit for blood flow. Rather, cellular elements in the vessel wall actively participate in the homeostatic functions of the vasculature that maintain vascular integrity and sustain normal circulation. The vascular endothelium, in particular, plays a critical role in the regulation of vessel physiology through elaboration of antiatherogenic paracrine factors that maintain vascular tone, inhibit platelet activation and inflammatory cell adhesion, promote fibrinolysis, and modulate vascular cell proliferation. Under pathological conditions, phenotypic changes occur in endothelial cells that impair normal homeostasis and promote a vasospastic, prothrombotic, and proinflammatory milieu, thus supporting atherothrombogenesis and clinical cardiovascular events (1). In this chapter we will briefly summarize normal homeostatic functions of blood vessels. We will then discuss the role of vascular dysfunction in mechanisms of atherogenesis and acute coronary syndromes and consider therapeutic implications.

I. NORMAL VASCULAR PHYSIOLOGY

A. Anatomy

Muscular arteries are comprised of three layers termed the intima, media, and adventitia. The intima consists of a single monolayer of endothelial cells resting on a basement membrane in direct contact with circulating blood that serves as a mechanical barrier and modulates vascular function. The intima represents the initial site of atheroma development (2). Separated by an internal elastic lamina, the media is comprised predominantly of smooth muscle cells embedded in extracellular matrix that regulate vascular tone in response to endothelium-derived and humoral stimuli. In addition to responding to vasoactive signals, smooth muscle cells have the potential to proliferate and synthesize growth factors and cytokines that modulate extracellular matrix composition and vascular growth relevant to atherosclerosis. The adventitia represents the outermost layer of the vessel wall harboring nutrient vessels (vasa vasorum), nerves, fibroblasts, and dense collagenous and fibroelastic tissue.

B. Endothelial Control of Vascular Tone, Thrombosis, and Inflammation

A critical function of vascular cells involves regulation of blood flow and vascular tone. Endothelial cells modulate vasomotor function through local release of endothelium-derived dilator and constrictor substances that exert a dynamic influence on vascular tone (3). Endothelial production of nitric oxide (NO), in particular, plays a critical role in the regulation of arterial relaxation in humans. Nitric oxide is synthesized in endothelial cells from the conversion of L-arginine to L-citrulline through the tightly regulated activity of endothelial nitric oxide synthase (eNOS). Agonists for endothelium-derived nitric oxide (EDNO) release include acetylcholine, catecholamines, substance P, and platelet-derived factors, such as serotonin and adenosine 5'-diphosphate, that act through specific receptors on endothelial cells (4,5). Shear stress on the endothelial surface from increased blood flow also serves as an important stimulus for NO production (6). Nitric oxide maintains basal vascular tone and relaxes vascular smooth muscle, promoting vasodilation through soluble guanylyl cyclase activation and consequent increases in intracellular cyclic 3'5'-guanosine monophosphate (cGMP) concentration (7,8). In addition to its vasodilator properties, NO evokes antiatherogenic actions through inhibition of platelet activation, leukocyte adhesion, and vascular smooth muscle migration and proliferation. EDNO synthesis or bioactivity is impaired in patients with cardiac risk factors and atherosclerosis (9). The endothelium may compensate for loss of EDNO action by increasing production of other dilator substances involved in regulation of vascular tone, including bradykinin, prostacyclin, carbon monoxide, and endothelium-derived hyperpolarizing factor (10). Conversely, endothelial cells may also synthesize and release vasoconstrictor substances including angiotensin II (AT II), endothelin (11), prostaglandin H_2, and endothelium-derived constricting factor(s) that antagonize EDNO action (12). In pathological conditions, augmented production of these mediators produces a dynamic imbalance that favors vasospasm, luminal narrowing, and reduced blood flow and tissue ischemia.

Vascular cells also play a critical role in the regulation of fibrinolysis and thrombosis. The endothelium serves as a mechanical barrier to circulating platelets and procoagulant factors that are activated following exposure to subendothelial matrix components, such as tissue factor (TF), collagen, and von Willebrand factor (vWF), leading to platelet deposition and thrombosis (13). In addition to its barrier function, the normal endothelium actively releases factors that prevent platelet adhesion and aggregation including EDNO, prostacyclin (PGI_2), and ectoADPase/CD39 (14). Endothelial cells also express antithrombotic factors, including thrombomodulin, heparan and dermatan sulfates, and tissue factor pathway inhibitor (TFPI), and release fibrinolytic agents, such as tissue-type plasminogen activator (t-PA), that limit thrombosis and favor fibrinolysis (15). Activated or dysfunctional endothelial cells may, however, also produce procoagulant and antifibrinolytic factors, such as TF and plasminogen activator inhibitor-1 (PAI-1), respectively, that are upregulated in atherosclerosis and disease states such as hypertension, diabetes mellitus, and hypercholesterolemia (16,17). The local vascular balance of TFPI/TF and t-PA/PAI–1 has the potential to determine the propensity for intravascular thrombosis in response to vascular injury and the ensuing extent of luminal occlusion and tissue infarction.

The inflammatory response is strongly implicated in the pathogenesis of atherosclerosis and plaque rupture (18,19). Monocyte adhesion to the vascular wall represents the earliest lesion in atherosclerosis. Normally, intact endothelium serves as a barrier to subendothelial leukocyte entry and limits monocyte-endothelial interactions through EDNO release. As will be discussed, in response to cytokines and other pathogenic stimuli, endothelial cell expression of surface integrins and adhesion molecules, such as intracellular adhesion molecule-1 (ICAM-1) and vascular cell adhesion molecule-1 (VCAM-1), facilitates proinflammatory processes.

II. VASCULAR DYSFUNCTION AND ATHEROTHROMBOSIS

A. Endothelial Dysfunction and Altered Vasomotion

Endothelial dysfunction defines a pathophysiological state in which normal regulation of vascular homeostasis is deficient. In the presence of cardiovascular risk factors such as diabetes mellitus, hypercholesterolemia, and hypertension, endothelial cells adopt a maladaptive phenotype that contributes to not only the initial stages of the atherogenic process, but also to the subsequent clinical activity of more advanced lesions. One of the key features of impaired vascular function under pathological conditions is impairment in endothelium-derived NO bioactivity (9). This functional abnormality is present in the earliest stages of atherosclerosis long before occlusive plaques develop and is evident in peripheral arteries of children with risk factors as early as the teenage years (20). In patients with atherosclerosis, intracoronary infusion of acetylcholine, which serves as an endothelium-dependent stimulus for NO release, evokes blunted dilator responses or overt "paradoxical" vasoconstriction owing to ineffective EDNO action (5). The dilator response to exogenous nitroglycerin, which reflects non–endothelium-dependent vascular smooth muscle relaxation, is generally preserved, at least in early phases of atherosclerosis, providing evidence for a functional abnormality specific to the endothelium. Paradoxical responses are elicited in overtly atherosclerotic, as well as mildly diseased vessels, whereas vasodilation is observed in normal arteries, providing evidence for impaired EDNO action early in the atherosclerotic process. Vasodilator responses to other stimuli, such as serotonin and shear stress, are also reduced in diseased vessels.

There is growing mechanistic evidence that loss of EDNO action represents a unifying pathophysiological abnormality shared by several cardiac risk factors that contributes to the atherosclerotic process itself. Inhibition of NO synthesis promotes endothelial monocyte adhesion (21) and worsens atherosclerotic lesions in cholesterol-fed rabbits (22). Endothelium-dependent vasodilation is lost in patients with hypercholesterolemia (9) and improves with lipid-lowering therapy (23). In patients with diabetes mellitus, EDNO-dependent coronary and peripheral vascular responses are impaired early in atherosclerosis (24,25) and correlate with severity of diabetes and glycemic control. Acute hyperglycemia impairs vasomotion possibly through additional upregulation of vasoconstrictor prostanoids (26). Insulin stimulates EDNO release, and its deficiency or resistance has the potential to blunt NO bioaction (27). Vasomotor abnormalities in diabetes also extend to blunted vascular smooth muscle cell response to NO.

Similarly, patients with hypertension also exhibit reduced agonist-mediated vascular reactivity in the forearm and coronary circulations (28–30). N-Monomethyl-L-arginine (L-NMMA) blunts resting flow less in hypertensives, suggesting additional impairment in basal EDNO action (31). Normotensive offspring of hypertensive patients have reduced vascular responses to acetylcholine, providing evidence for a mechanistic defect in NO activity in certain forms of hypertension (32). Impaired NO release and increased endothelin and AT II activity may enhance vasoconstriction. Cigarette smoking also causes a dose-related and reversible alteration in vasomotor function that is similarly observed with passive secondary exposure (33,34). Basal and stimulated NO production is blunted in association with cigarette use, possibly related to reduced NO bioavailability. Abnormalities in the NO pathway are also operative in the vascular diathesis of more recently recognized risk factors such as hyperhomocysteinemia (35). Impaired EDNO-dependent dilation is characteristic of individuals with elevated homocysteine levels and improves with interventions, such as folate, that reduce plasma homocysteine (36).

Derangements in EDNO action and vasomotor dysfunction, linked to the pathophysiology of a number of cardiovascular risk factors, likely play a mechanistic role in clinical manifestations of coronary disease. Impaired vasomotor reserve in patients with fixed anatomical stenoses may result in reduced blood flow or provoke vasospasm leading to tissue ischemia and angina. Studies in patients with stable angina provide evidence that this mechanism is operative in activities of daily living. For example, individuals with coronary artery disease (CAD) exhibit paradoxical coronary vasoconstriction when subjected to commonly encountered stimuli, such as exercise, exposure to cold, and mental stress (37). Such abnormal vascular responses have the potential to provoke clinical symptoms in patient with otherwise non–flow-limiting stenoses (38).

B.   Endothelial Dysfunction and Prothrombosis

Atheromatous plaque disruption and subsequent intraluminal thrombosis underlie the predominant mechanisms of acute coronary syndromes. Thrombogenesis requires complex interactions involving the vascular endothelium, platelets, and the coagulation cascade. Intimal injury and exposure of subendothelial matrix components to circulating blood triggers a series of events initiated by platelet adhesion and aggregation at the site of localized injury. Subsequent tissue factor-mediated activation of the coagulation cascade and rapid generation of fibrin intermeshed with aggregating platelets produce an occlusive thrombus. Dysfunctional endothelium may potentiate the extent of localized thrombosis through enhanced expression of prothrombotic factors including PAI-1, tissue factor, and factor V. Tissue factor, a transmembrane glycoprotein that binds factor VII, thereby promoting factor X activation and thrombin generation, in particular, plays a critical role in determining plaque thrombogenicity. Under normal conditions, endothelial cells express minimal TF, which is upregulated following endothelial activation in response cytokines and atherogenic stimuli (39). Tissue factor expression is increased in atheromatous plaques, and elevated plasma levels are observed in patients with acute coronary syndromes. EDNO reduces TF expression, and thus, impaired EDNO release has the potential to enhance prothrombosis (40). Tissue factor pathway inhibitor expressed by vascular endothelial cells, represents another major regulator of TF-mediated procoagulant activity. Overexpression of TFPI reduces thrombus formation following vascular injury, and impaired endogenous TFPI activity supports atherosclerosis and thrombogenesis (41). TFPI co-localizes with TF in atherosclerotic plaques, suggesting an important role for TFPI /TF balance in the regulation of procoagulant activity in the vascular wall (42,43).

Endogenous fibrinolytic properties of normal endothelium are also impaired in disease conditions through increased expression of PAI-1 and decreased bioavailability of endothelium-derived t-PA. Patients with hypercholesterolemia exhibit reduced fibrinolytic activity (44), and exposure of endothelial cells to cholesterol potentiates PAI-1 release (16). PAI-1 expression is increased in atherosclerotic lesions, and plasma concentrations are elevated in patients with acute myocardial infarction (45). Endothelial control of fibrinolysis is also disturbed in individuals with hypertension, possibly due to angiotensin II–mediated PAI-1 production (46). Hyperinsulinemia and glucose intolerance are also associated with increased PAI-1 activity (47). Cigarette smoking is linked to impaired substance P–induced t-PA release in vivo in humans (48) and concomitant downregulated TFPI production (49). Altogether, impaired endothelial regulation of fibrinolysis and reduced local t-PA/PAI-1 balance, common to several cardiovascular risk factors, are likely to play an important pathogenic role in mechanisms of atherothrombosis.

Abnormalities in vascular endothelial phenotype are also important in regulation of platelet function. Reduced endothelial NO and prostacyclin enhance platelet adhesion and activation. The importance of vascular NO in preventing atherothrombosis is supported by animal studies demonstrating that inhibition of NO synthase promotes intravascular platelet accumulation (50). In human coronary arteries, the platelet-inhibitory effect of nitric oxide is reduced in parallel with endothelium-dependent vasodilation, further providing evidence for a regulatory role of EDNO in platelet behavior (51). Endothelial dysfunction also facilitates platelet-endothelial interactions through upregulated expression of vWF and surface adhesion molecules, such as P-selectin, that mediate platelet adhesion at sites of vascular injury and atherosclerosis. A well-established association exists between elevated vWF and P-selectin levels in individuals with coronary artery disease, hypercholesterolemia, hypertension, and inflammatory vascular disease, supporting a pathophysiological role of endothelial dysfunction in mechanisms of dysregulated platelet function and prothrombosis (52–54).

C. Oxidative Stress and Vascular Dysfunction

A dominant mechanism of impaired EDNO action appears to relate to increased oxidative stress, defined as an imbalance between endogenous oxidants and antioxidants in favor of the former (55). Vascular cells generate reactive oxygen species, such as superoxide anion (O_2^-), hydroxyl radicals (OH·), and hydrogen peroxide (H_2O_2), that play an important role in the regulation of endothelial phenotype (56). An important mechanism of reduced vascular nitric oxide bioaction relates to its oxidative inactivation by superoxide or lipid peroxyl radicals and consequent elimination of its biological activity (57). Vascular production of superoxide is increased in atherosclerosis and in association with cardiovascular risk factors, such as hypercholesterolemia, diabetes mellitus, hypertension, and cigarette use (58,59). An important source of O_2^- appears to be the membrane-associated nicotinamide adenine dinucleotide (phosphate) [NADH/NAD(P)H] oxidase enzyme complex (60). The activity of NADH/NADPH oxidases in vascular endothelial and smooth muscle cells is driven by angiotensin II, thrombin, tumor necrosis factor-α (TNF-α), and platelet-derived growth factor (PDGF). Angiotensin II, in particular, serves as a potent stimulus for increased oxidase activity, which may represent a pathophysiological link between the renin-angiotensin system and cardiovascular disease.

There is growing evidence that oxidative stress contributes to other mechanisms of vascular dysfunction. Reactive oxygen species, particularly superoxide and hydrogen peroxide, participate in vascular cell signaling that modulate proatherogenic transduction pathways (61). For example, expression of proinflammatory cell-surface molecules by the transcriptional regulatory protein nuclear factor kappa B (NF-κB) is sensitive to intracellular redox status (62). NF-κB is also important in proliferative signals involved in vascular smooth muscle cell growth, vascular remodeling, and atherogenesis. Oxidant species also modulate intracellular kinase and caspase activities important for cell proliferation and apoptosis. Collectively, an imbalance of NO-mediated versus oxidant-mediated signals may define vascular cell phenotype and support atherothrombogenesis (Fig. 1). In support of these mechanisms, patients with clinical evidence of endothelial dysfunction and vascular oxidative stress experience a greater incidence of cardiovascular events (63).

Another important mechanism of oxidative stress relates to lipid peroxidation and proatherogenic modification of low-density lipoprotein (LDL) (64). Fatty streaks and diffuse intimal thickening characterize the earliest manifestation of atherosclerosis, repre-

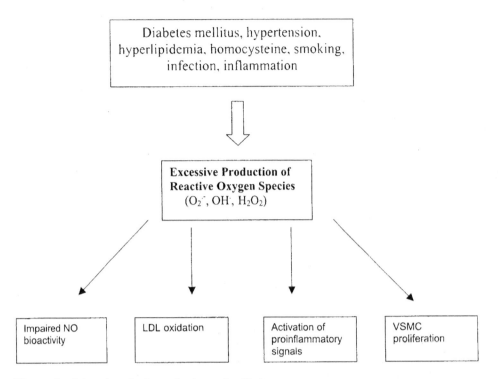

Figure 1   Atherothrombotic mechanisms of oxidative stress.

senting subendothelial accumulation of cholesterol-laden macrophages termed foam cells. Many lines of evidence suggest that circulating LDL cholesterol requires oxidative alteration in the vessel wall prior to its incorporation into, and accumulation within, foam cells. The "oxidative modification hypothesis of atherosclerosis" refers to the central role of oxidized LDL (ox-LDL) in the atherosclerotic process and provides the basis for a mechanistic link between hypercholesterolemia and vascular disease. Although mechanisms of LDL oxidation in vivo are incompletely understood, endothelial cells, vascular smooth muscle cells (VSMCs), and monocytes are collectively able to oxidize LDL (65). Local generation of peroxynitrite as a product of superoxide and NO metabolism also plays a role in lipid peroxidation, protein nitration, and oxidative modification of LDL. In addition to fueling lipid accumulation in foam cells within the atheroma, ox-LDL contributes to vascular dysfunction and plaque formation by other mechanisms. Oxidized LDL stimulates expression of monocyte chemotactic protein-1 (MCP-1) and ICAM-1, thereby facilitating monocyte recruitment and adhesion to the vessel wall (66). Further, ox-LDL inactivates nitric oxide (67), is directly cytotoxic to endothelial cells (68), stimulates smooth muscle cell proliferation, and upregulates TF and PAI-1 expression that have the potential to fuel atherothrombotic events (69,70).

D.   Vascular Dysfunction and Inflammation

There is considerable evidence to suggest that inflammation plays a causal role in atherosclerotic lesion development and, as will be discussed, subsequent activity of more advanced unstable lesions responsible for acute coronary syndromes (71). Infiltration of circulating monocytes into the vascular subendothelium represents a very early event in atherosclerosis. Normally, a quiescent endothelium limits vascular inflammation through downregulation of proinflammatory signals and release of paracrine factors such as nitric oxide (72,73). Increased endothelial expression of cell-surface ligands is critical to supporting vascular cell-leukocyte interactions (74). In the response-to-injury hypothesis of atherosclerosis, altered biochemical forces, atherogenic stimuli, or infection elicit phenotypic changes in endothelial cells that become "activated" and begin to express cell-surface ligands, such as VCAM-1, ICAM-1, and selectins, that support monocyte recruitment (75,76). Oxidized LDL and regulatory protein NF-kB are important in promoting proinflammatory signals. Adhesion molecule expression occurs in specific sites of the arterial tree, such as branch points and bifurcations, where laminar flow is impaired and alterations in shear stress downregulate NO activity (77).

Facilitated by monocyte chemotactic protein-1 and macrophage colony-stimulating factor, leukocytes that adhere to endothelium migrate into the vessel wall, localize subendothelially, and develop into lipid-rich foam cells. Foam cells produce a wealth of growth factors, cytokines, and mitogenic signals that, in turn, recruit VSMCs, further support endothelial dysfunction, and induce proliferative responses leading to lesion propagation and generation of more advanced fibrofatty plaques (18). Infiltration of T cells into vascular lesions similarly orchestrates release of proinflammatory cytokines that modulate atheroma development (78). In a slowly evolving process, lesions progress to mature plaques composed of a necrotic lipid core, VSMCs, and inflammatory elements covered by connective tissue and dysfunctional endothelial cells.

E. Role of Vascular Dysfunction in Acute Coronary Syndromes

Atherosclerotic lesions remain clinically silent for decades prior to precipitating acute coronary syndromes, such as myocardial infarction and unstable angina. It was previously largely believed that gradual growth of atherosclerotic plaques progressively encroach on the vascular lumen, producing arterial occlusion and coronary events. A shift in paradigm occurred following pathological studies, demonstrating that over 90% of acute infarcts result from an occlusive coronary thrombus overlying a small intimal tear or fissure on the surface of a previously nonobstructive atheromatous lesion (79,80). Critical information provided by these studies has consistently demonstrated that, in fact, atherosclerotic plaques typically grow by outward expansion in the vascular wall in a process termed remodeling (81). We now understand that acute plaque rupture or fissuring with subsequent subendothelial hemorrhage, platelet deposition, and intraluminal thrombosis rather than progressive atheroma growth represent the essential mechanisms of acute coronary events (82). Confirming this mechanism, angiographic studies demonstrated that two thirds of plaques responsible for acute coronary syndromes evolve from antecedent stenoses that were rarely flow limiting and only mild to moderately obstructive (83–85). Thus, most lesions at risk for future rupture are frequently missed by angiography, which only provides information about the vascular lumen rather than the pathogenic atherosclerotic process involving the vessel wall.

We now understand that the mere anatomical presence of an atherosclerosis lesion does not relate to its propensity for precipitating an acute myocardial infarction. Rather, physical disruption of a vulnerable plaque, and exposure of its highly thrombogenic lipid core and subendothelial matrix components with subsequent platelet deposition and activation of the coagulation cascade represent the mechanistic underpinnings of thrombotic vascular occlusion. Mechanisms of lesion activation remain incompletely understood, but transition of stable plaques to unstable vulnerable lesions prone to rupture most likely relate to a fundamental lapse in vascular homeostasis (Fig. 2). As a central regulator of vas-

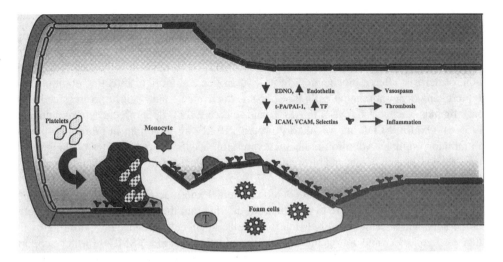

Figure 2   Mechanisms of vascular dysfunction and atherothrombosis.

cular biology and pathobiology, abnormalities in endothelial function and impaired endogenous antiatherogenic mechanisms likely play a significant role in these events (86).

Several features distinguish vulnerable plaques from those that are stable (Table 1). Vulnerable plaques have a large lipid core, thin fibrous cap, reduced mechanical strength, a paucity of VSMCs, and abundant inflammatory cells including lymphocytes and macrophages concentrated in shoulder regions at sites of typical lesion rupture (78,87,88). The inflammatory process plays a critical role in the dynamic remodeling and evolution of atheromatous lesions. T lymphocytes, in particular, orchestrate a series of proinflammatory signals that destabilize plaques. Among other actions, T cells release lymphokine gamma interferon (IFN-γ) which inhibits VSMC collagen synthesis and promotes release of proteolytic agents, including matrix metalloproteinases (MMPs) (89). Matrix metalloproteinases include a family of enzymes, such as collagenase, gelatinase, and stromelysin, that degrade collagen, glycosaminoglycans, and elastin, thereby reducing tensile strength of plaques and jeopardizing the integrity of the protective fibrous cap. Expression of matrix metalloproteinases is upregulated by ROS and inflammatory cytokines, including interleukin-1 (IL-1) and TNF-α (90).

Cytokine crosstalk within vascular cells further amplifies the immune response through upregulation of adhesion molecule expression and consequent monocyte recruitment and foam cell accumulation within plaques. Functional changes also occur in activated VSMCs that lose their contractile phenotype and contribute to the progression of plaque development through synthesis and release of degradative enzymes, growth factors, and cytokines. Endothelial cells and VSMCs undergo apoptosis in response to inflammatory mediators, further weakening plaques. The central role of inflammation in acute coronary syndromes is supported by human clinical studies linking elevated plasma levels of C-reactive protein (CRP), serum amyloid A protein, and interleukin-6 (IL-6) as biomarkers of inflammation to increased cardiovascular events (19,91,92). There is growing interest in the clinical utilization of CRP as a tool to identify individuals at increased risk for cardiovascular syndromes, given the limitations of conventional angiography for this purpose.

Oxidative stress may also play a role in plaque behavior (93). NADH/NAD(P)H oxidase activity and superoxide generation are increased in shoulder regions of atheromatous lesions (94) which relates to enhanced local AT II activity, as evidenced by increased

Table 1 Characteristics of Vulnerable Plaques

Morphological
  Large lipid core
  Thin fibrous cap
  Mechanical injury
    Erosion
    Ulceration
    Fissuring
  Increased inflammatory cells
  Reduced VSMC content
Inflammatory
  Increased immune response
    Macrophages/Foam cells
    T-lymphocytes
    Leukocytes
    B-lymphocytes
  Upregulated cytokine release
    IFN-γ
    IL-1
    TNF-α
    CD40 ligand
  Matrix metalloproteinase expression
    Collagenase
    Gelatinase
    Elastase
Thrombotic
  Reduced t-PA/PAI-1
  Impaired EDNO
  Tissue factor expression
  Increased platelet adhesion

expression of angiotensin converting enzyme in unstable atherosclerotic plaques. In this regard, AT II may be viewed as a potential proinflammatory mediator. Reactive oxygen species participate in collagen matrix metabolism through activation of matrix metalloproteinases. Oxidant-driven matrix metalloproteinase expression is increased in shoulder regions where their activity produces collagen degradation and increases the propensity for plaque rupture. Excessive production of oxygen-derived radicals further fuels LDL oxidation and lipid accumulation. Reactive oxygen species also modulate caspase activity, which plays a role in apoptotic signals leading to endothelial cell loss and plaque destabilization (95).

While plaque composition and inflammatory activity are important determinants of plaque behavior, other components of vascular dysfunction, such as dysregulation of vasomotor tone, are also important in the ultimate clinical expression of acute coronary syndromes. For example, impaired endothelial dilator function may increase the risk for plaque rupture through loss of flow-mediated dilation and increased coronary vasoconstriction in response to catecholamines, thereby augmenting mechanical shear stress at plaque sites (96,97). Following plaque rupture, activation of platelets and local generation of platelet-derived factors, such as serotonin and thrombin, may promote vasoconstriction as a result of ineffective counterregulatory EDNO release. Enhanced endothelial release of angiotensin, endothelin-1, and prostanoids may also fuel this process (98,99). Vasospasm superimposed on vascular thrombosis may impair arterial flow, jeopardize vascular patency, and aggravate ischemia. There is clinical evidence that this mechanism is operative in the human coronary circulation. The vasoconstrictor response to acetylcholine in the infarct-related coronary artery is significantly greater than in similarly stenosed uninvolved vessels (100). In patients with coronary syndromes sufficiently stabilized to undergo provocative studies, patients with unstable angina exhibit more severe coronary vasoconstriction during ergometric bicycle exercise and cold pressor testing as compared to subjects with stable angina (101).

Other aspects of vascular dysfunction may contribute to the clinical expression of acute coronary syndromes through dysregulation of the fibrinolytic and prothrombotic balance. Plaque composition is an important factor in the ensuing thrombotic response that closely relates to TF expression. Dysfunctional endothelial cells and monocytes augment TF expression in response to TNF-α and IL-1, and activated T-cell CD40 ligand also serves as a powerful stimulus for TF upregulation (102). Local release of cytokines also produce phenotypic alterations in endothelial cells that upregulate PAI-1, and reduce t-PA release, further supporting a prothrombotic state (103). Enhanced endothelial cell PAI-1 expression also relates to increased local AT II activity (104). Impaired EDNO and prostacyclin release enhances platelet-endothelial interactions (50,105). Evidence exists that plaque rupture or superficial erosion formation occurs not infrequently in asymptomatic individuals; the local, prevailing hemostatic and fibrinolytic balance may be a critical determinant of the fate of a medical event.

F. Vascular Dysfunction and Clinical Studies

Several recent outcome studies provide the strongest evidence for a pathophysiological link between vascular endothelial dysfunction and cardiovascular events. In a study of 157 patients with nonobstructive coronary artery disease by angiography, patients with impaired endothelium-dependent vasodilation of coronary resistance and conduit arteries were more likely to experience cardiovascular events over a 28-month follow-up period than were those without dysfunction (106). A similar study examined coronary vasomotor responses to acetylcholine, nitroglycerin, increased flow, and sympathetic activation by cold pressor testing in 147 patients undergoing cardiac catheterization (107). Over a median follow-up period of 7.7 years, patients with impaired vasomotor function were at higher risk for adverse events, including death, unstable angina, myocardial infarction, stroke, and revascularization. The predictive value of vascular dysfunction was independent of traditional risk factors and atherosclerotic lesion burden. Similarly, in a sizable study involving 308 patients with a 46-month follow-up period, ischemic events were more prevalent in patients with blunted coronary vascular responses, and endothelium-dependent vasodilation predicted events even in patients with angiographically normal coronary arteries (108). These studies of the coronary circulation provide important clinical evidence for a link between vascular dysfunction and acute cardiovascular syndromes.

Assessment of endothelial function in peripheral arteries also appears to provide prognostic information about cardiac risk. Hypertensive patients with blunted forearm microvascular responses are more likely to experience adverse outcomes than are those without abnormal microvessel responses (109). Similarly, coronary artery disease patients with reduced forearm vasodilator responses to intra-arterial acetylcholine developed more cardiovascular events over a 4.5-year follow-up period than did those without reduced responses (63). Impaired endothelial function independently predicts perioperative cardiac events in patients undergoing vascular surgery (110). Overall, these findings suggest that vascular dysfunction is central to the pathophysiology of integrated atherothrombotic events, and assessment of endothelial function may serve as a barometer of vascular health and a determinant of cardiovascular risk.

III. THERAPEUTIC IMPLICATIONS

Based upon our current understanding of the vascular pathobiology of atherothrombosis and the central role of endothelial dysfunction in this process, therapeutic modulation of vascular endothelial function represents an attractive goal. A consistent body of evidence from large clinical trials demonstrates that treatment with hydroxymethylglutaryl coenzyme A reductase inhibitors, or statins, reduce cardiovascular events in a broad spectrum of individuals (111–113). Despite dramatic reductions in lipids and clinical events with statin treatment, minimal changes occur in the angiographic appearance of coronary lesions over time (98). These findings suggest that qualitative modification of plaques or improved vascular function may represent operative mechanisms for the observed clinical benefit of this class of drugs. Indeed, clinical studies of statin therapy demonstrate that EDNO action improves in vessels of hypercholesterolemic patients within days of treatment, and this effect is sustained with more prolonged therapy (114,115). There is evidence that statin therapy also improves other aspects of vascular dysfunction owing to their "pleiotropic" actions in the vascular wall (116). For example, statins have direct antioxidant properties and may reduce LDL oxidation. Lipid-lowering therapy reduces adhesion molecule expression, monocyte chemotaxis and matrix metalloproteinase synthesis, and upregulation of NF-kB, proinflammatory cytokines, and CRP (117,118). With regard to antithrombotic actions, statins increase t-PA production, lower PAI-1 production, and inhibit TF expression. Overall, improvement in vasodilator, antithrombotic, and anti-inflammatory functions of the vascular endothelium likely plays a role in plaque stabilization and the beneficial effects of statins.

Numerous clinical studies demonstrate that angiotensin, converting enzyme (ACE) inhibitor therapy also offers similar beneficial effects on vascular function and improves cardiovascular outcomes (119). In the TREND study, 6-month treatment with ramipril improved coronary vasomotion in patients with CAD, and similar salutary effects of ACE inhibitors noted on EDNO action were evident in other disease states such as diabetes mellitus and hypertension (120). Downregulation of AT II has the potential to alter vascular tone favorably through reduced vasoconstriction and endothelin expression. Increased bradykinin bioavailability may also play a role in enhanced EDNO action with ACE inhibition therapy. The link between AT II and NAD(P)H oxidase activity suggests that ACE inhibitors may also act as antioxidants, in part by attenuating superoxide generation, thereby augmenting EDNO action. ACE inhibitor therapy may also limit peroxynitrite generation and lipid peroxidation, lower activation of redox-sensitive proinflammatory signals, and interrupt growth promoting and proatherogenic stimuli (121). With regard to antithrombotic actions, ACE inhibitors reduce PAI-1 activity and enhance bradykinin-mediated t-PA release. Many of these beneficial vascular effects also appear to extend to treatment with AT II receptor antagonists.

Other strategies aimed at endothelial "passivation" and improving vascular function have the potential to influence cardiovascular outcomes favorably. Interventions such as exercise, smoking cessation, and L-arginine and flavonoid supplementation have been shown to improve endothelial function. The apparent central role of oxidant stress in mechanisms of vascular dysfunction has generated considerable interest in antioxidant treatment. Antioxidant trials to date, predominantly with vitamin E, have been disappointing, in part attributed to limited in vivo activity of vitamin E against diverse ROS-mediated cellular processes (122,123). Studies investigating different antioxidant-treatment regimens are currently ongoing. Aspirin therapy may interrupt atherothrombogenic mechanisms through anti-inflammatory actions, and through its antiplatelet action aspirin may exert antioxidant effects by reducing the generation of platelet-derived ROS.

IV. CONCLUSION

The vascular endothelium plays a critical role in homeostatic mechanisms of vascular function. Loss of vasodilator, anti-inflammatory, and antithrombotic actions of the endothelium contributes to the pathophysiology of atherosclerosis and clinical cardiovascular syndromes. Identification and treatment of individuals with cardiac risk factors and impaired vascular function are likely to attenuate atherosclerosis progression and reduce the risk of adverse cardiovascular events.

REFERENCES

1. Gokce N, Keaney JFJ, Vita JA: Endotheliopathies: Clinical manifestations of endothelial dysfunction, in Loscalzo J, Shafer AI (eds): Thrombosis and Hemorrhage. Philadelphia: Williams and Wilkins, 1998, pp 901–924.
2. Ross R: The pathogenesis of atherosclerosis—an update. N Engl J Med 1986; 314:488–500.
3. Vane JR, Anggard EE, Botting RM: Regulatory functions of the vascular endothelium. N Engl J Med 1990; 323.27–36.
4. Golino P, Piscione F, Willerson JT, Capelli-Bigazzi M, Focaccio A, Villari B, Indolfi C, Russolillo E, Condorelli M, Chiarello M: Divergent effects of serotonin on coronary artery dimensions and blood flow in patients with coronary atherosclerosis and control patients. N Engl J Med 1991; 324:641–648.
5. Ludmer PL, Selwyn AP, Shook TL, Wayne RR, Mudge GH, Alexander RW, Ganz P: Paradoxical vasoconstriction induced by acetylcholine in atherosclerotic coronary arteries. N Engl J Med 1986; 315:1046–1051.
6. Cox DA, Vita JA, Treasure CB, Fish RD, Alexander RW, Ganz P, Selwyn AP: Atherosclerosis impairs flow-mediated dilation of coronary arteries in humans. Circulation 1989; 80:458–465
7. Moncada S, Higgs A: The L-arginine nitric oxide pathway. N Engl J Med 1993; 329:2002–2012.
8. Ignarro LJ: Endothelium-derived nitric oxide: actions and properties. FASEB 1989; 3:31–36.
9. Vita JA, Treasure CB, Nabel EG, McLenachan JM, Fish RD, Yeung AC, Vekshtein VI, Selwyn AP, Ganz P: Coronary vasomotor response to acetylcholine relates to risk factors for coronary artery disease. Circulation 1990; 81:491–497.
10. Cohen RA, Vanhoutte PM: Endothelium-dependent hyperpolarization: Beyond nitric oxide and cyclic GMP. Circulation 1995; 92:3337–3349.
11. Yanagisawa M, Kurihara H, Kimura S, Tomobe Y, Kobayashi M, Mitsui Y, Yazaki Y, Goto K, Masaki T: A novel potent vasoconstrictor peptide produced by vascular endothelial cells. Nature 1988; 332:411–415.
12. Luscher TF, Vanhoutte PM: Endothelium-dependent contractions to acetylcholine in the aorta of the spontaneously hypertensive rat. Hypertension 1986; 8:344–348.
13. Coller BS: Platelets and thrombolytic therapy. N Engl J Med 1990; 322:33–42.
14. Marcus AJ, Broekman MJ, Drosopoulos JHF, Islam KN , Islam N, Gayle RB, Maliszewski CR: Thromboregulation by endothelial cells. Significance for occlusive vascular diseases. Arterioscler Thromb Vasc Biol 2001; 21:178–182.
15. Hekman CM, Loskutoff DJ: Fibrinolytic pathways and the endothelium. Semin Thromb Hemost 1987; 13:514–527.
16. Stiko-Rahm A, Wiman B, Hamsten A, Nillson J: Secretion of plasminogen activator inhibitor-1 from cultured umbilical vein endothelial cells is induced by very low density lipoprotein. Arteriosclerosis 1990; 10:1067–1073.

17. Palermo A, Bertalero P, Pizza N, Amelotti R, Libretti A: Decreased fibrinolytic response to adrenergic stimulation in hypertensive patients. J Hypertens 1989; 7:S162–S163.

18. Ross R: Atherosclerosis—an inflammatory disease. N Engl J Med. 1999; 340:115–126.

19. Libby P, Ridker PM, Maseri A: Inflammation and atherosclerosis. Circulation 2002; 105:1135–1143.

20. Sorensen KE, Celermajer DS, Georgakopoulos D, Hatcher G, Betteridge DJ, Deanfield JE: Impairment of endothelium-dependent dilation is an early event in children with familial hypercholesterolemia and is related to the lipoprotein (a) level. J Clin Invest 1994; 93:50–55.

21. Tsao PS, McEvoy LM, Drexler H, Butcher EC, Cooke JP: Enhanced endothelial adhesiveness in hypercholesterolemia is attenuated by l-arginine. Circulation 1994; 89:2176–2182.

22. Cayatte AJ, Palacino JJ, Horten K, Cohen RA: Chronic inhibition of nitric oxide production accelerates neointima formation and impairs endothelial function in hypercholesterolemic rabbits. Arterioscler Thromb 1994; 14:753–759.

23. Dupuis J, Tardif JC, Cernacek P, Theroux P: Cholesterol reduction rapidly improves endothelial function after acute coronary syndromes : The RECIFE (Reduction of Cholesterol in Ischemia and Function of the Endothelium) Trial. Circulation 1999; 99:3227–3233.

24. Nitenberg A, Valersi P, Sachs R, Dali M, Aptecar E, Attali JR: Impairment of coronary vascular reserve in and ACH-induced coronary vasodilation in diabetic patients with angiographically normal coronary arteries and normal left ventricular systolic function. Diabetes 1993; 42:1017–1025.

25. Johnstone MT, Creager SJ, Scales KM, Cusco JA, Lee BK, Creager MA: Impaired endothelium-dependent vasodilation in patients with insulin-dependent diabetes mellitus. Circulation 1993; 88:2510–2516.

26. Williams SB, Goldfine AB, Timimi FK, Ting HH, Roddy MA, Simonson DC, Creager MA: Acute hyperglycemia attenuates endothelium-dependent vasodilation in humans in vivo. Circulation 1998; 97:1695–1701.

27. Scherrer U, Randin D, Vollenweider P, Vollenweider L, Nicod P: Nitric oxide release accounts for insulin's vascular effects in humans. J Clin Invest. 1994; 94(6):2511–2515.

28. Treasure CB, Klein JL, Vita JA, Manoukian SV, Renwick GH, Selwyn AP, Ganz P, Alexander RW: Hypertension and left ventricular hypertrophy are associated with impaired endothelium-mediated relaxation in human coronary resistance vessels. Circulation 1993; 87:86–93.

29. Panza JA, Quyyumi AA, Brush JE, Epstein SE: Abnormal endothelium-dependent vascular relaxation in patients with essential hypertension. N Engl J Med 1990; 323:22–27.

30. Gokce N, Holbrook M, Duffy SJ, Demissie S, Cupples Biegelsen E, Keaney JFJ, Loscalzo J, Vita JA: Effects of race and hypertension on flow-mediated and nitroglycerin-mediated dilation of the brachial artery. Hypertension 2001; 38:1349–1354.

31. Panza JA, Casino PR, Kilcoyne CM, Quyyumi AA: Role of endothelium-derived nitric oxide in the abnormal endothelium-dependent vascular relaxation of patients with essential hypertension. Circulation 1993; 87:1468–1474.

32. Taddei S, Virdis A, Mattei P, Chiadoni L, Sudano I, Salvetti A: Defective L-arginine-nitric oxide pathway in offspring of essential hypertensive patients. Circulation 1996; 94:1298–1303.

33. Kugiyama K, Yasue H, Ohgushi M, Motoyama T, Kawano H, Inobe Y, Hirashima O, Sugiyama S: Deficiency in nitric oxide bioactivity in epicardial coronary arteries of cigarette smokers. J Am Coll Cardiol 1996; 28:1161–1167.

34. Celermajer DS, Adams MR, Clarkson P, Robinson J, McCredie R, Donald A, Deanfield JE: Passive smoking and impaired endothelium-dependent arterial dilatation in healthy young adults. N Engl J Med 1996; 334:150–154.

35. Tawakol A, Omland T, Gerhard M, Wu JT, Creager MA: Hyperhomocyst(e)inemia is associated with impaired endothelium-dependent vasodilation in humans. Circulation 1997; 95:1119–1121.

36. Woo KS, Chook P, Lolin YI, Sanderson JE, Metreweli C, Celermajer DS: Folic acid improves arterial endothelial function in adults with hyperhomocystinemia. J Am Coll Cardiol 1999; 34:2002–2006.

37. Yeung AC, Vekshtein VI, Krantz DS, Vita JA, Ryan TJ, Jr., Ganz P, Selwyn AP: The effect of atherosclerosis on the vasomotor response of coronary arteries to mental stress. N Engl J Med. 1991; 325:1551–1556.

38. Egashira K, Inou T, Hirooka Y, Yamada A, Urabe Y, Takeshita A: Evidence of impaired endothelium-dependent coronary vasodilatation in patients with angina pectoris and normal coronary angiograms. N Engl J Med 1993; 328(23):1659–1664.

39. Semeraro N, Colucci M: Tissue factor in health and disease. Thromb Haemost 1997; 78:759–764.

40. Yang Y, Loscalzo J: Regulation of tissue factor expression in human microvascular endothelial cells by nitric oxide. Circulation 2000; 101:2144–2148.

41. Westrick RJ, Bodary PF, Xu Z, Shen Y-C, Broze GJ, Eitzman DT: Deficiency of tissue factor pathway inhibitor promotes atherosclerosis and thrombosis in mice. Circulation 2001; 103:3044–3046.

42. Kato H: Regulation of functions of vascular wall cells by tissue factor pathway inhibitor. Basic and clinical aspects. Aterioscler Thromb Vasc Biol 2002; 22:539–548.

43. Crawley J, Lupu F, Westmuckett AD, Severs NJ, Kakkar VV, Lupu C: Expression, localization, and activity of tissue factor pathway inhibitor in normal and atherosclerotic human vessels. Arterioscler Thromb Vasc Biol 2000; 20:1362–1373.

44. Andersen P, Arnesen J, Hjermann I: Hyperlipoproteinemia and reduced fibrinolytic activity in healthy coronary high-risk men. Acta Med Scand 1981; 209:199–202.

45. Hamsten A, Wiman B, de Faire U, Blomback M: Increased plasma levels of a rapid inhibitor of tissue plasminogen activator in young survivors of myocardial infarction. N Engl J Med 1985; 313:1557–1563.

46. Vaughan DE, Lazos SA, Tong K: Angiotensin II regulates the expression of plasminogen activator inhibitor-1 in cultured endothelial cells. A potential link between the renin-angiotensin system and thrombosis. J Clin Invest 1995; 95(3):995–1001.

47. Nordt TK, Sawa H, Fujii S, Sobel BE: Induction of plasminogen activator inhibitor type-1 (PAI-1) by proinsulin and insulin in vivo. Circulation 1995; 91:764–770.

48. Newby DE, Wright RA, Labinjoh C, Ludlam CA, Fox KA, Boon NA, Webb DJ: Endothelial dysfunction, impaired endogenous fibrinolysis, and cigarette smoking. A mechanism for arterial thrombosis and myocardial infarction. Circulation 1999; 99:1411–1415.

49. Barua RS, Ambrose JA, Saha DC, Eales-Reynolds L-J: Smoking is associated with altered endothelial-derived fibrinolytic and antithrombotic factors. An in vivo demonstration. Circulation 2002; 106:905–908.

50. Loscalzo J: Nitric oxide insufficiency, platelet activation, and arterial thrombosis. Circ Res 2001; 88:756–762.

51. Andrews NP, Husain M, Dakak N, Quyyumi AA: Platelet inhibitory effect of nitric oxide in the human coronary circulation: impact of endothelial dysfunction. J Am Coll Cardiol 2001; 37:510–516.

52. Lip GY, Blann A: von Willebrand factor: a marker of endothelial dysfunction in vascular disorders? Cardiovasc Res 1997; 34:255–265.

53. Barbaux S, Blankenberg S, Rupprecht HJ, Francomme C, Bickel C, Hafner G, Nicaud V, Meyer J, Cambien F, Tiret L, for the AtheroGene Group: association between P-selectin gene polymorphisms and soluble P-selectin levels and their relation to coronary artery disease. Arterioscler Thromb Vasc Biol 2001; 21:1668–1673.

54. Davi G, Romano M, Mezzetti A, Procopio A, Iacobelli S: Increased levels of soluble p-selectin in hypercholesterolemic patients. Circulation 1998; 97:953–957.

55. Oxidative stress and vascular disease. In: Keaney, J.F. Jr., editor. Dordrecht: Kluwer Academic Publishers, 2000.

56. Kojda G, Harrison DG: Interactions between NO and reactive oxygen species: pathophysiological importance in atherosclerosis, hypertension, diabetes, and heart failure. Cardiovasc Res 1999; 43:562–571.

57. Gryglewski RJ, Palmer RM, Moncada S: Superoxide anion is involved in the breakdown of endothelium-derived vascular relaxing factor. Nature 1986; 320:454–456.

58. Rajagopalan S, Kurz S, Munzel T, Tarpey M, Freeman BA, Griendling KK, Harrison DG: Angiotensin II-mediated hypertension in the rat increases vascular superoxide production via membrane NADH/NADPH oxidase activation. J Clin Invest 1996; 97:1916–1923.

59. Ohara Y, Peterson TE, Harrison DG: Hypercholesterolemia increases endothelial superoxide anion production. J Clin Invest 1993; 91:2546–2551.

60. Griendling KK, Sorescu D, Ushio-Fukai M: NADP(H) oxidase. Role in cardiovascular biology and disease. Circ Res 2000; 86:494–501.

61. Kunsch C, Medford RM: Oxidative stress as a regulator of gene expression in the vasculature. Circ Res 1999; 85:753–766.

62. Valen G, Yan Z, Hansson GK: Nuclear factor kappa-B and the heart. J Am Coll Cardiol 2001; 38:307–314.

63. Heitzer T, Schlinzig T, Krohn K, Meinertz T, Munzel T: Endothelial dysfunction, oxidative stress, and risk of cardiovascular events in patients with coronary artery disease. Circulation 2001; 104:2673–2678.

64. Witztum JL, Steinberg D: Role of oxidized low density lipoprotein in atherogenesis. J Clin Invest 1991; 88:1785–1792.

65. Steinberg D, Parthasarathy S, Carew TE, Khoo JC, Witztum JL: Beyond cholesterol. Modifications of low-density lipoprotein that increase its atherogenicity. N Engl J Med 1989; 320:915–924.

66. Navab M, Imes SS, Hama SY, Hough GP, Ross LA, Bork RW, Valente AJ, Berliner JA, Drinkwater DC, Laks H, Fogelman AM: Monocyte transmigration induced by modification of low density lipoprotein in cocultures of human aortic wall cells is due to induction of monocyte chemotactic protein 1 synthesis and is abolished by high density lipoprotein. J Clin Invest. 1991; 88:2039–2046.

67. Chin JH, Azhar S, Hoffman BB: Inactivation of endothelium-derived relaxing factor by oxidized lipoproteins. J Clin Invest 1992; 89:10–18.

68. Nègre-Salvayre A, Pieraggi MT, Mabile L, Salvayre R: Protective effect of 17–beta-estradiol against the cytotoxicity of minimally oxidized LDL to cultured bovine aortic endothelial cells. Atherosclerosis 1992; 99:207–217.

69. Berliner JA, Heinecke JW: The role of oxidized lipoproteins in atherogenesis. Free Radic Biol Med 1996; 20:707–727.

70. Penn MS, Chui M, Winokur AL, Bethea J, Hamilton TA, DiCorleto PE, Chisolm GM: Smooth muscle cell surface tissue factor pathway activation by oxidized low-density lipoprotein requires cellular lipid peroxidation. Blood 2000; 96:3056–3063.

71. Libby P: Current concepts of pathogenesis of acute coronary syndromes. Circulation 2001; 104:365–372.

72. Wang BY, Candipan RC, Arjomandi M, Hsiun PT, Tsao PS, Cooke JP: Arginine restores nitric oxide activity and inhibits monocyte accumulation after vascular injury in hypercholesterolemic rabbits. J Am Coll Cardiol 1996; 28:1573–1579.

73. Kubes P, Suzuki M, Granger DN: Nitric oxide: an endogenous modulator of leukocyte adhesion. Proc Natl Acad Sci U.S.A. 1991; 88:4651–4655.

74. Ikeda U, Takahashi M, Shimada K: Monocyte-endothelial cell interactions in atherogenesis and thrombosis. Clin Cardiol 1998; 21:11–14.

75. O'Brien KD, Allen MD, McDonald TO, Chait A, Harlan JM, Fishbein D, McCarty J, Ferguson M, Hudkins K, Benjamin CD, Ross R: Vascular cell adhesion molecule-1 is expressed in human coronary atherosclerotic plaques. Implications for the mode of progression of advanced coronary atherosclerosis. J Clin Invest 1993; 92:945–951.

76. Nelken NA, Coughlin SR, Gordon D, Wilcox JN: Monocyte chemoattractment protein-1 in human atheromatous plaques. J Clin Invest 1991; 88(4):1121–1127.

77. Tsao PS, Buitrago R, Chan JR, Cooke JP: Fluid flow inhibits endothelial adhesiveness: nitric oxide and transcriptional regulation of VCAM-1. Circulation 1996; 94:1682–1689.

78. Libby P: Molecular basis of the acute coronary syndromes. Circulation 1995; 91:2844–2850.

79. Shah PK, Forrester JS: Pathophysiology of acute coronary syndromes. Am J Cardiol 1991; 68:16C–23C.

80.   Mizuno K, Satomura K, Miyamoto A, Arakawa K, Shibuya T, Arai T, Kurita A, Nakamura H, Ambrose J: Angioscopic evaluation of coronary artery thrombi in acute coronary syndromes. N Engl J Med 1992; 326:287–291.

81.   Glagov S, Weisenberg E, Zarins CK, Stankunavicius R, Kolettis GJ: Compensatory enlargement of human atherosclerotic coronary arteries. N Engl J Med 1987; 316:1371–1375.

82.   Rentrop KP: Development and pathophysiological basis of thrombolytic therapy in acute myocardial infarction, part I, 1912–1977: the controversy over the pathogenic role of thrombus in acute myocardial infarction. J Intervent Cardiol 1998; 11:255–263.

83.   DeWood MA, Spores J, Notske R, Mouser LT, Burroughs R, Golden MS, Lang HT: Prevalence of total coronary occlusion during the early hours of transmural myocardial infarction. N Engl J Med. 1980; 303:897–902.

84.   Ambrose JA, Winters SL, Stern A, Eng A, Teichholz LE, Gorlin R, Fuster V: Angiographic morphology and the pathogenesis of unstable angina pectoris. J Am Coll Cardiol 1985; 5:609–616.

85.   Giroud D, Li JM, Urban P, Meier B, Rutishauser W: Relation of the site of acute myocardial infarction to the most severe coronary arterial stenosis at prior angiography. Am J Cardiol 1992; 69:729–732.

86.   Kinlay S, Ganz P: Relation between endothelial dysfunction and the acute coronary syndrome: implications for therapy. Am J Cardiol 2000; 86 (suppl):10J-14J.

87.   Lee RT, Libby P: The unstable atheroma. Arterioscler Thromb Vasc Biol 1997; 17:1859–1867.

88.   Falk E: Why do plaques rupture? Circulation 1992; 86(suppl III):III-30.

89.   Galis ZS, Sukhova GK, Lark MW, Libby P: Increased expression of matrix metalloproteinases and matrix degrading activity in vulnerable regions of human atherosclerotic plaques. J Clin Invest 1994; 94:2493–2503.

90.   Saren P, Welgus HG, Kovanen PT: TNF-alpha and IL-beta selectively induce expression of 92–kDa gelatinase by human macrophages. J Immunol 1996; 157:4159–4165.

91.   Ridker PM, Buring JE, Shih J, Matias M, Hennekens CH: Prospective study of C-reactive protein and the risk of future cardiovascular events among apparently healthy women. Circulation 1998; 98:731–733.

92.   Ridker PM, Rifai N, Pfeffer MA, Sacks FM, Moye LA: Inflammation, pravastatin, and the risk of coronary events after myocardial infarction in patients with average cholesterol levels. Circulation 1998; 98:839–844.

93.   Davies MJ: Reactive oxygen species, metalloproteinases, and plaque stability. Circulation 1998; 97:2382–2383.

94.   Sorescu D, Weiss D, Lassegue B, Clempus R, Szocs K, Sorescu G, Valppu L, Quinn M, Lambeth J, Vega J, Taylor W, Griendling KK: Superoxide production and expression of Nox family proteins in human atherosclerosis. Circulation 2002; 105:1429–1435.

95.   Irani K: Oxidant signaling in vascular cell growth, death, and survival. A review of the roles of reactive oxygen species in smooth muscle and endothelial cell mitogenic and apoptotic signaling. Circ Res 2000; 87:179–183.

96.   Vita JA, Treasure CB, Yeung AC, Vekshtein VI, Fantasia GM, Fish RD, Ganz P, Selwyn AP: Patients with evidence of coronary endothelial dysfunction as assessed by acetylcholine infusion demonstrate marked increase in sensitivity to constrictor effects of catecholamines. Circulation 1992; 85:1390–1397.

97.   Loree HM, Kamm RD, Stringfellow RG, Lee RT: Effects of fibrous cap thickness on peak circumferential stress in model atherosclerotic vessels. Circ Res 1992; 71:850–858.

98.   Levine GN, Keaney JFJ, Vita JA: Cholesterol reduction in cardiovascular disease: clinical benefits and possible mechanisms. N Engl J Med 1995; 332:512–521.

99.   Cardillo C, Kilcoyne CM, Cannon RO, III, Panza JA : Increased activity of endogenous endothelin in patients with hypercholesterolemia. J Am Coll Cardiol 2000; 36:1483–1488.

100. Okumura K, Yasue H, Matsuyama K, Ogawa H, Morikami Y, Obata K, Sakaino N: Effect of acetylcholine on the highly stenotic coronary artery: difference between the constrictor

response of the infarct-related coronary artery and that of the noninfarct-related artery. J Am Coll Cardiol 1992; 19:752–758.

101. Bogaty P, Hackett D, Davies G, Maseri A: Vasoreactivity of the culprit lesion in unstable angina. Circulation 1994; 90:5–11.

102. Libby P: Coronary artery injury and the biology of atherosclerosis: inflammation, thrombosis, and stabilization. Am J Cardiol 2000; 86 (suppl):3J-9J.

103. Hanss M, Collen D: Secretion of tissue-type plasminogen activator and plasminogen activator inhibitor by cultured human endothelial cells: modulation by thrombin, endotoxin, and histamine. J Lab Clin Med 1987; 109:97–104.

104. Vaughan DE, Lazos SC: Angiotensin II induces plasminogen activator inhibitor (PAI-1) in vitro. Circulation 1992; 86(suppl 1):I-557.

105. Radomski MW, Palmer RM, Moncada S: Endogenous nitric oxide inhibits human platelet adhesion to vascular endothelium. Lancet 1987; 2(8567):1057–1058.

106. Suwaidi JA, Hamasaki S, Higano ST, Nishimura RA, Holmes DR, Lerman A: Long-term follow-up of patients with mild coronary artery disease and endothelial dysfunction. Circulation 2000; 101:948–954.

107. Schachinger V, Britten MB, Zeiher AM: Prognostic impact of coronary vasodilator dysfunction on adverse long- term outcome of coronary heart disease. Circulation 2000; 101:1899–1906.

108. Halcox JPJ, Schenke W, Zalos G, Mincemoyer R, Prasad A, Waclawiw MA, Nour KRA, Quyyumi AA: Prognostic value of coronary vascular endothelial dysfunction. Circulation 2002; 106:653–658.

109. Perticone F, Ceravolo R, Pujia A, Ventura G, Iacopino S, Scozzafava A, Ferraro A, Chello M, Mastroroberto P, Verdecchia P, Schillaci G : Prognostic significance of endothelial dysfunction in hypertensive patients. Circulation 2001; 104:191–196.

110. Gokce N, Keaney JF Jr, Hunter LM, Watkins MT, Menzoian JO, Vita JA: Risk stratification for postoperative cardiovascular events via noninvasive assessment of endothelial function. A prospective study. Circulation 2002; 105:1567–1572.

111. Scandinavian Simvastatin Survival Study Group: Randomized trial of cholesterol lowering in 4444 patients with coronary heart disease: The Scandinavian Simvastatin Survival Study (4S). Lancet 1994; 344:1383–1389.

112. Sacks FM, Pfeffer MA, Moye LA, Rouleau JL, Rutherford JD, Cole TG, Brown L, Warnica JW, Arnold JMO, Wun CC, Davis BR, Braunwald EB: The effect of pravastatin on coronary events after myocardial infarction in patients with average cholesterol levels. N Engl J Med 1996; 335:1001–1009.

113. Heart Protection Study Collaborative Group: MRC/BHF Heart Protection Study of cholesterol lowering with simvastatin in 20,536 high-risk individuals: a randomised placebo-controlled trial. Lancet 2002; 360:7–22.

114. Tsunekawa T, Hayashi T, Kano H, Sumi D, Matsui-Hirai H, Thakur NK, Egashira K, Iguchi A: Cerivastatin, a Hydroxymethylglutaryl coenzyme A reductase inhibitor, improves endothelial function in elderly diabetic patients within 3 days. Circulation 2001; 104:376–379.

115. Treasure CB, Klein JL, Weintraub WS, Talley JD, Stillabower ME, Kosinski AS, Zhang J, Boccuzzi SJ, Cedarholm JC, Alexander RW: Beneficial effects of cholesterol-lowering therapy on the coronary endothelium in patients with coronary artery disease. N Engl J Med 1995; 332:481–487.

116. Laufs U, La Fata V, Plutzky J, Liao JK: Upregulation of endothelial nitric oxide synthase by HMG CoA reductase inhibitors. Circulation 1998; 97:1129–1135.

117. Takemoto M, Liao JK: Pleiotropic effects of 3–Hydroxy-3–methylglutaryl coenzyme A reductase inhibitors. Arterioscler Thromb Vasc Biol 2001; 21:1712–1719.

118. Ridker PM, Rifai N, Pfeffer MA, Sacks F, Braunwald E: Long-term effects of pravastatin on plasma concentration of C-reactive protein. Circulation 1999; 100:230–235.

119. Yusuf S, Sleight P, Pogue J, Bosch J, Davies R, Dagenais G: Effects of an angiotensin-converting-enzyme inhibitor, ramipril, on cardiovascular events in high-risk patients. The Heart

Outcomes Prevention Evaluation Study Investigators [see comments] [published erratum appears in N Engl J Med 2000 Mar 9; 342(10):748]. N Engl J Med. 2000; 342:145–153.

120. Mancini GB, Henry GC, Macaya C, O'Neill BJ, Pucillo AL, Carere RG, Wargovich TJ, Mudra H, Luscher TF, Klibaner MI, Haber HE, Uprichard AC, Pepine CJ, Pitt B: Angiotensin-converting enzyme inhibition with quinapril improves endothelial vasomotor dysfunction in patients with coronary artery disease. The TREND (Trial on Reversing ENdothelial Dysfunction) Study. Circulation 1996; 94:258–265.

121. Munzel T, Keaney JF Jr. Are ACE inhibitors a "magic bullet" against oxidative stress? Circulation 2001; 104:1571–1574.

122. Yusuf S, Dagenais G, Pogue J, Bosch J, Sleight P: Vitamin E supplementation and cardiovascular events in high-risk patients. The Heart Outcomes Prevention Evaluation Study Investigators. N Engl J Med 2000; 342:154–160.

123. Anonymous: Dietary supplementation with n-3 polyunsaturated fatty acids and vitamin E after myocardial infarction: results of the GISSI-Prevenzione trial. Gruppo Italiano per lo Studio della Sopravvivenza nell'Infarto Miocardico. Lancet 1999; 354:447–455.

3-1

Thrombogenic Aspects of Atherosclerosis

Michael D. Cooper and James H. Chesebro
Mayo Clinic Jacksonville, Jacksonville, Florida, U.S.A.

The understanding of the pathogenesis of unstable angina and acute myocardial infarction has advanced greatly over the past two decades. Because of these advances, many effective new treatment strategies have been developed. Despite these significant advances, ischemic heart disease remains the number one cause of mortality in the world (1). It is known that the vast majority of acute coronary syndromes are due to thrombosis developing on a culprit atherosclerotic plaque (2). These vulnerable lesions upon which thrombosis occurs have certain characteristics, including a large cholesterol-containing lipid core, a thin fibrous cap, and an increased number of lipid-filled macrophages (foam cells) (3). The mechanism from which coronary arterial thrombosis occurs takes on two main forms. The most common form is plaque disruption, accounting for approximately three quarters of cases (4). A tear in the cap exposes circulating blood to the highly thrombogenic lipid core, leading to thrombus formation on the plaque itself, then into the arterial lumen. The second mechanism responsible for coronary artery thrombosis is endothelial erosion, accounting for the remaining one quarter of thrombotic episodes. In this circumstance, denudation and erosion of the endothelium lead to thrombus formation on the plaque surface.

Many complex factors alter the thrombotic milieu, all of which can be divided into three major categories, first described by Virchow more than 100 years ago. These include vascular endothelial injury (arterial wall substrate), increased shear force that pushes platelets against the arterial wall (rheology), and hypercoagulability of blood (systemic factors). (Table 1). This chapter focuses on these factors and how they are affected by atherothrombotic risk factors such as cholesterol, diabetes, and smoking.

I. RHEOLOGY

The degree of platelet deposition is directly related to the velocity of arterial blood flow and inversely related to the third power of the luminal radius. This phenomenon has been demonstrated experimentally using the Badimon ex vivo perfusion chamber (5,6). Using this system, different substrates can be exposed to circulating blood at various shear rates. The thrombus burden and rate of thrombus development are also dependent on the depth of vessel-wall injury. When mild injury (above the internal elastic lamina) is simulated using deendothelialized aorta, blood flowing at low shear rates produces maximal platelet deposition in 5–10 minutes, resulting in only one or two layers of platelets. At high shear rates that mimic a stenosed coronary artery, higher platelet deposition occurs, again

Table 1 Risk Factors for Thrombosis

Rheology

High shear rates—stenotic coronary arteries, endothelial dysfunction, vasoconstriction
Oscillatory shear stress—bifurcation of arteries, plaque irregularities
Slow blood flow or stasis—intimal dissection, aneurysms

Arterial wall substrate

Atherosclerosis
Large lipid core and tissue factor content
Mural thrombus is highly thrombogenic
High concentration of macrophages

Systemic factors

Catecholamines (smoking, stress, pain, surgery, cocaine)
Lipids (high LDL, Lp(a), triglycerides, and low HDL)
Diabetes
Fibrinogen
Impaired fibrinolysis (increased PAI-1)
Tissue factor (present in mural thrombus within 5 min of formation)

Source: Adapted from Ref. 3.

peaking at 5–10 minutes, but then decreasing after longer exposure, suggesting a transient and labile thrombosis in this setting (6).

After deep arterial wall injury (below the internal elastic lamina), simulated with collagen type I fibers from pig tendon or arterial wall media from porcine aorta, platelet deposition is two orders of magnitude greater (>100×) than with mild injury, platelet thrombi remain adherent, and occlusion can occur in 10–20 minutes (7). If vascular injury is held constant, increasing stenosis increases platelet deposition. The area of greatest platelet deposition occurs at the apex, or the peak of the stenosis (8). Just distal to the apex is the recirculation zone, an area where blood decelerates after accelerating through the stenotic region. This segment of the coronary artery, with low shear rates, activates fibrin. While fibrin(ogen) deposition remains maximal at the apex, it is less dependent on high shear rates, thus significantly depositing in the recirculation zone (9). This difference between platelets and fibrinogen gives thrombus a platelet-rich head attached to the subendothelium or to smooth muscle cells in deeply injured artery, and a largely fibrin- and red cell–containing tail extending distally in the arterial lumen (10).

As platelet deposition is increased with increasing stenosis, thrombus formation alone stimulates further formation of thrombus via its rheological forces (and substrate and blood changes as outlined below). These rheological forces include both physical obstruction causing stenosis and vasoconstriction. Vasoconstriction, which may be due to thrombin generated within thrombus or on cell membranes, catecholamines, substances released from platelets (thromboxane A_2 or serotonin), or damaged artery (endothelin), also increases shear force and hence increases platelet deposition. Thrombolysis, whether pharmacological or endogenous, increases luminal diameter, improving rheology and decreasing platelet deposition.

II. ARTERIAL WALL SUBSTRATE

The arterial wall substrate is composed of the normal wall layers—the intima, tunica media, and adventitia—as well as the components of the atherosclerotic plaque. Atherosclerotic plaques are composed of two main components: a core of soft, lipid-rich, atheromatous material and an outer cap composed of collagen-rich tissue. Certain features of an atherosclerotic plaque make it vulnerable to rupture and subsequent thrombosis. These include a large atheromatous core, a thin fibrous cap, inflammation within the cap, and cap fatigue (4).

While most stable plaques are chiefly composed of hard fibrous tissue, ruptured plaques tend to have a more significant lipid core. When comparing plaque composition in disrupted coronary plaques to intact plaques, the lipid core occupied 32% and 5–12% of the plaques, respectively (11). The lipid core is rich in cholesterol and its esters and is usually soft, like gruel (12). This soft, deformable core is not capable of carrying circumferential stress, and the stress is therefore redistributed onto the fibrous cap (13). Because of this redistribution, fibrous cap thickness is another important factor for plaque stability. Caps that are thin and uneven are unable to carry stress and are more susceptible to rupture (14).

Inflammation within the cap causes further weakening and makes it more prone to rupture. This has been tested in vitro and in vivo, with in vitro studies demonstrating reduced tensile strength of aortic fibrous caps in regions with foam cell infiltration (15). In a study comparing coronary specimens from patients with unstable angina versus stable angina, macrophage content was significantly higher (16% vs. 5%) in the former than the latter (16). Macrophages weaken the cap by degrading extracellular matrix via phagocytosis and by secreting proteolytic enzymes, such as metalloproteinases. Metalloproteinases are capable of degrading all components of connective tissue matrix, including collagen (2). Cap fatigue is another factor that leads to plaque disruption. A repetitive, steady load or stress can lead to a weakened cap and eventually cause the cap to fracture. This can result from cyclic bending, flexion, stretching, and compression of the cap (4).

The relative thrombogenicity of the different arterial wall substrates has been studied using ex vivo and in vitro perfusion models. Of the three layers of the normal arterial wall, the adventitia, which normally contains tissue factor to initiate the coagulation cascade, is the most thrombogenic, followed by the tunica media, which does not normally contain tissue factor, and finally the intima (3). Deep arterial injury below the internal elastic lamina into the smooth muscle cells (containing prothrombin) of the media produces macroscopic (visible) mural thrombus. Endothelial denudation without stenosis produces only a single layer of platelets.

Of the atherosclerotic components, the lipid-rich core is the most thrombogenic, as the amount of thrombus formed can be up to six times greater than on foam cell-rich matrix or collagen-rich matrix (17). The thrombogenicity of each component may, in part, be related to its relative amount of tissue factor, a protein that initiates the coagulation cascade and thrombin generation. Tissue factor interacts with factor VII, which subsequently activates factor X, leading to conversion of prothrombin to thrombin. The highest content of tissue factor is found in the lipid-rich core, followed by adventitia, atherosclerotic tunica media, foam cell-rich matrix, collagen-rich matrix, and atherosclerotic intima (18). The high thrombogenic potential of the adventitia and arterial media may account for the greater proliferative response that occurs after deep (below the elastic lamina) arterial injury in comparison to superficial (subendothelial) injury as previously demonstrated in vivo in pigs (19). In addition, mural thrombus contains tissue factor within 5 minutes of formation and thus stimulates more thrombin generation (20).

III. SYSTEMIC FACTORS

There are several important systemic factors that can provide the proper milieu for thrombosis. These include increased amounts of circulating catecholamines, low-density lipoprotein (LDL) cholesterol, triglycerides, lipoprotein (a) [Lp(a)], homocysteine, fib-

Table 2 Major Contributions to Thrombosis from Coronary Risk Factors

	Rheology	Substrate	Blood
Dyslipidemia	Vasoconstriction due to endothelial dysfunction Cholesterol releases endothelin (vasoconstrictor)	Increased tissue factor Increased lipid core Apoptosis	LDL enhances thrombus growth LDL reduction reduces thrombus growth by 20%
Diabetes	Vasoconstriction due to endothelial dysfunction Greater plaque burden decreases intraluminal radius	Increased tissue factor Increased lipid core Apoptosis Glycosylated collagen	Greater degree of dyslipidemia Increased PAI-1 Increased F1.2 Increased FPA
Smoking	Vasoconstriction due to endothelial dysfunction Causes catecholamines release—further vasoconstriction	Increased tissue factor Increased macrophages Apoptosis	Increased catecholamines Shortens platelet survival

PAI-1, plasminogen activator inhibitor-1; F1.2, prothrombin fragment 1.2; FDA, fibrinopeptide A.

rinogen, and also the presence of smoking and diabetes (Table 2). Many of these risk factors for coronary artery disease and thrombosis are of particular clinical importance because they can be modified pharmacologically and by lifestyle changes.

A. Catecholamines

High levels of circulating catecholamines increase vasospasm (worsen rheology and shear force) and also potentiate platelet activation and thrombus growth. Using a porcine model, it has been demonstrated that an epinephrine surge, in the absence of local vasoconstriction, stimulates platelet interaction with a damaged arterial wall (21). Evidence exists that platelet activity is increased during stress and in smokers (22), a finding that may be related to the increased levels of catecholamines. Catecholamines may also be the cause of cocaine-induced thrombosis.

B. Lipids

The dyslipidemias have clearly been associated with the development of atherosclerosis, increased thrombotic events,and acute coronary syndromes. These include high levels of LDL cholesterol and Lp(a) or low levels of high-density lipoprotein (HDL) cholesterol. Lowering LDL cholesterol has been shown to reduce coronary events in both primary prevention (23) and secondary prevention trials (24,25). The mechanism for this reduction in cardiovascular events is multifactorial, involving rheology, substrate, and blood factors. Several trials involving patients treated with lipid-lowering therapy have demonstrated reduced coronary arterial disease progression as well as plaque regression (26,28). However, the degree of plaque regression demonstrated angiographically has been quite small. Despite this seemingly modest effect, lipid lowering has been shown to greatly reduce cardiovascular events, especially in patients with known coronary artery disease. This is likely due to changes in the arterial wall substrate of high-risk atheromatous lesions. Lipid lowering decreases the number of lipid-laden macrophages and decreases the size of the highly thrombogenic lipid core (29).

1. LDL Cholesterol

LDL cholesterol causes endothelial dysfunction and thus vasoconstriction. Lowering of LDL cholesterol with no change in rheology or substrate decreases arterial thrombus formation of flowing blood by 20% (30).

The thrombogenic lipid core of atherosclerotic plaques is predominantly composed of LDL cholesterol. After LDL cholesterol is oxidized by endothelial cells, it is responsible for recruitment of monocytes, which further oxidize LDL, then bind with it to create foam cells, or lipid-laden macrophages. These cells, discussed earlier, promote further endothelial injury and may lead to plaque disruption and thrombus formation (31). The size of the lipid core is an essential determinant of plaque stability. In a study from Davies et al. more than 90% of aortic plaques that underwent thrombosis had a lipid pool that occupied more than 40% of the plaque (32).

2. HDL Cholesterol

Clinically, increases in HDL cholesterol have been shown, like reduction in LDL, to significantly improve cardiovascular outcomes (33). The Helsinki Heart Study, in which patients received gemfibrozil for 5 years, showed a 34% reduction in cardiovascular endpoints with an increase in HDL cholesterol by an average of 10%. LDL cholesterol and triglycerides were decreased in this study by 10% and 35%, respectively. Other studies have shown that increasing HDL provides additional benefit to reduction in LDL alone (34). Increased HDL cholesterol likely reduces cardiac events because of its plaque-stabilizing effects. It inhibits LDL oxidation, removes LDL from the vessel wall and the foam cell, and promotes reverse cholesterol transport (35). This emphasizes the importance of raising HDL while lowering LDL cholesterol in the treatment of dyslipidemia, which has been well documented in the HATS study (36). In summation of studies, each decrease in LDL cholesterol by 1 mg% reduces cardiovascular risk by 1% per year. Each increase in HDL cholesterol by 1 mg% reduces cardiovascular events by 2–4% per year.

3. Lipoprotein (a)

Lipoprotein (a) is similar in structure to LDL cholesterol and is another important risk factor for ischemic heart disease and coronary thrombosis. Lp(a) is composed of two principal constituents, an apo B100 lipoprotein linked by a disulfide bridge to apoprotein (a) [apoc(a)] (37). The apo(a) portion of Lp(a) is structurally very similar (75–90% homology) to human plasminogen. Lp(a) has been shown to compete with plasminogen and t-PA for fibrin binding, thus reducing t-PA's catalytic ability that fibrin binding facilitates (38). This competitive inhibition of plasminogen appears to increase the risk of thrombotic events in patients, which is consistent with the opposing effects of thrombosis and lysis; blocking of one process enhances the other. Thus it is desirable to block thrombosis so as to enhance lysis of thrombus, which may occur by endogenous mechanisms.

C. Homocysteine

Plasma homocysteine has been linked to coronary thrombosis and has become another modifiable risk factor in patients with coronary artery disease. A recent angiographic study of patients presenting with acute coronary syndromes showed a significant positive correlation between plasma homocysteine levels and coronary thrombus burden (39). The mechanism behind this association is unclear, but several explanations have been proposed. Activation of coagulation occurs, as elevated levels of homocysteine are associated with elevated factor VIIa and thrombin generation (measured by F1.2) in patients presenting with acute coronary syndromes (40). Other possible mechanisms include vascular endothelial toxicity, increased von Willebrand factor, activation of factor V, and impaired endothelial-dependent vasodilation (41).

D. Smoking

Smoking is associated with an increased risk of myocardial infarction and sudden death (40) that has been linked with thrombosis (42). In a study of 113 men with coronary artery disease who died suddenly, men who died of acute thrombosis were more likely to be smokers (75%) compared with men who died of stable plaque (44%) (43). The increased risk of thrombosis in patients who smoke can be related to the three major influences on thrombosis. Enhanced catecholamine release increases vasoconstriction and thus shear force (rheology). In a study using an ex vivo perfusion chamber to compare platelet thrombus formation before and after smoking two cigarettes, platelet thrombus formation increased by 64% and plasma epinephrine increased more than twofold after smoking (42). Smoking increases tissue factor expression from atherosclerotic plaques in the arterial wall (44). Finally, the increased catecholamine release enhances platelet aggregation, shortens platelet survival, and thus increases the risk of thrombosis (22).

E. Diabetes

Cardiovascular death accounts for a disproportionately high percentage of total mortality in diabetic patients. The increased risk of myocardial infarction in diabetic patients is multifactorial, but thrombosis plays a key role. The presence of diabetes can alter all three major factors that influence thrombosis.

Rheology is affected because of greater plaque burden, which reduces luminal diameter. In addition, vasoconstriction occurs because endothelium-dependent relaxation, which normally occurs in response to hypoxia, is impaired in the setting of diabetes (45).

Arterial wall substrate is larger and exhibits greater thrombogenicity in diabetics. Diabetics have larger lipid cores in coronary plaques (46) and have a greater concentration of tissue factor in the lipid core (47). This correlates with the greater event rate and greater severity of cardiovascular events in diabetics. A likely mechanism is increased thrombin generation. Another factor appears to be glycosylated collagen, which is more thrombogenic than nonglycosylated collagen (3).

Finally, systemic factors play an important role in the increased thrombogenicity seen in diabetes. Increased levels of plasminogen activator inhibitor-1 (PAI-1) are present in states of hyperinsulinemia (48,49). Since PAI-1 is the principal inhibitor of tissue-type plasminogen activator, this may account for the finding that diabetics had lower reperfusion rates than nondiabetics in several thrombolytic trials (50,51). Platelet reactivity and aggregability and arterial thrombus formation of flowing blood are also increased in the presence of diabetes (52,53). This combination of local (rheology and substrate) and systemic factors acts to shift the balance of thrombosis and thrombolysis toward thrombosis in diabetic patients.

IV. THROMBIN

Thrombin, a procoagulant enzyme, plays a central role in thrombus formation, growth, maintenance, consolidation, and dissolution and continues to be produced in mural thrombus. Understanding this role is critical in understanding thrombogenesis (Fig. 1).

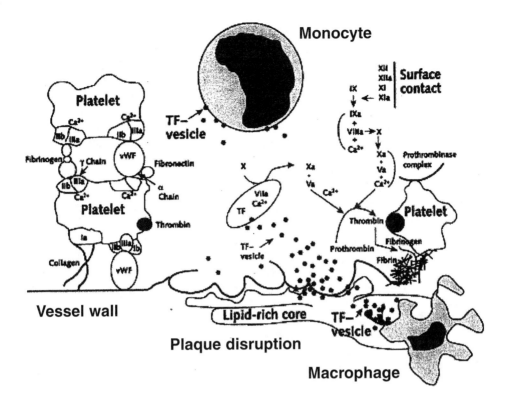

Figure 1 Biochemical interactions between platelets and vessel wall (left). Platelets bind to vessel wall via collagen and vonWillebrand factor, which leads to steric conformation changes and exposure of high-affinity binding site for fibrinogen (cross-bridging). Tissue factor release from macrophages and the lipid-rich core activates coagulation and leads to thrombin generation (right).Thrombin further activates platelets, activates factor V to Va, which generates more thrombin, converts fibrinogen to fibrin, and cross-links fibrin. (From Ref. 61).

Thrombin has various distinct functions, including increased platelet activation (even in minute amounts) and platelet thrombus formation, conversion of fibrinogen to fibrin, activation of factor V and factor VIII (which further induces thrombin generation), stabilization of the fibrin polymer, and binding to endothelial cell thrombomodulin (54). Thrombin generation is more extensive after deep arterial injury than it is after mild injury (55). This may be related to relative tissue factor concentrations of the different arterial wall layers. The central role of thrombin in thrombus formation has been demonstrated experimentally by the ability of hirudin, a direct, specific, and potent thrombin inhibitor, to completely block the formation of mural thrombus after deep arterial injury (56,57). After mural thrombus is formed it is highly thrombogenic, and it expresses large amounts of thrombin and factor Xa bound to fibrin. Thrombin is also necessary for the maintenance of platelet cohesion after thrombus is formed, and finally for consolidation of thrombus, by inducing cross-linking of fibrin via activation of factor XIII to XIIIa.

Thrombin generation can be measured using prothrombin fragment 1.2 (F1.2), a polypeptide released from prothrombin during conversion to thrombin, or fibrinopeptide A (FPA), a peptide cleaved from fibrinogen during conversion to fibrin (58). These coagulation proteins have been found to have an impact on prognosis in acute coronary syndromes, again indicating the central role of thrombin. In a cross-sectional study, FPA levels were five times higher in patients who died from sudden cardiac death than in those dying from other causes (59). In a prospective cohort study of patients with unstable angina, an abnormally elevated plasma fibrinopeptide A level, signifying activation of the hemostatic mechanism, was associated with an increased risk of further cardiac events (60). In another study of patients presenting with unstable angina and acute myocardial infarction, F1.2 and FPA levels were expectedly elevated on presentation. After 6 months, F1.2 levels had fallen significantly, whereas FPA levels remained elevated, suggesting a continued hypercoagulable state without persistent generation of thrombin (61). Those data provides further evidence for the central role that thrombin plays in thrombosis and acute coronary syndromes.

Figure 2 summarizes the actions of thrombin and how thrombin begets thrombin to perpetuate arterial thrombosis in the coagulation cascade, on the arterial wall, and via blood cells. Activator complexes of coagulation factors assemble on cell membranes and negatively charged phospholipids (e.g., on the lipid gruel of disrupted plaques and on apoptotic cells). In the prothrombinase complex this increases thrombin generation 278,000 times. The induction of tissue factor (TF) in the arterial wall and blood by thrombin plays a major role in thrombin generation, as do the coronary risk factors, which increase TF via LDL-C in macrophages and the lipid core, diabetes, which further increases TF in arterial plaques, and smoking, which induces TF in the arterial wall. Thrombin also stimulates neointimal proliferation in the arterial wall via induction of oncogenes and genes, mitogenic stimulation of smooth muscle cells, chemotaxis of monocytes, and platelet activation with release of growth factors [platelet-derived growth factor (PDGF) and transforming growth factor-β] (5,18,19,35,62).

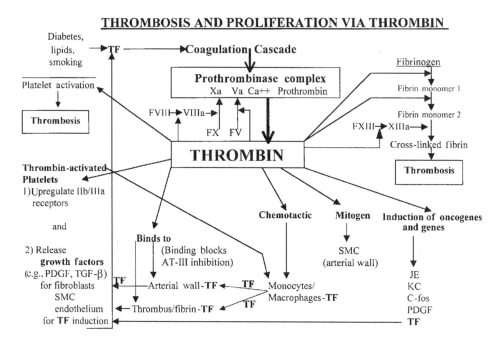

Figure 2 Thrombin activates coagulation and begets thrombin in the coagulation cascade by activating factors V to Va and VIII to VIIIa and via the induction of TF by several mechanisms. The other actions of thrombin stimulate neointimal proliferation, especially via platelet release of platelet-derived growth factor (PDGF), and transforming growth factor ß (TGG-ß). TF, tissue factor; AT-III, antithrombin III; GF, growth factors; SMC, smooth muscle cells.

V. CONCLUSIONS

The processes that lead to thrombosis are affected by the three major factors of rheology, arterial wall substrate, and blood. Favorably changing these factors can markedly reduce thrombosis. Lowering of LDL-C changes arterial wall substrate (decreased size of lipid pool) and reduces thrombogenicity of flowing blood, which reduces thrombus formation by 20%; this is comparable to the effect of adding clopidogrel to aspirin. Smoking cessation induces rheological changes via decreased vasoconstriction, reduces arterial wall tissue factor (substrate for thrombosis), and reduces catecholamine activation of platelets-rich thrombus (directly affecting blood). Improved control of diabetes improves rheology, substrate, and systemic factors such as impaired fibrinolysis, which occurs with hyperinsulinemia and glucose intolerance.

While current antithrombotic therapies have clearly improved cardiovascular outcomes in acute coronary syndromes, they are limited by lack of potency, narrow therapeutic windows, variable blood levels, and bleeding risk. New therapies are being developed as understanding of the pathophysiology of thrombosis increases. The central role of tissue factor in thrombosis and the connection of tissue factor with traditional cardiovascular risk factors such as lipids, diabetes, and smoking demonstrates an important mechanism by which risk factor reduction reduces thrombus in the arterial wall. Atherothrombosis leading to acute coronary syndromes is a great public health concern, and the aggressive treatment of risk factors can markedly reduce thromboembolic events and should continue to be a major focus of cardiovascular research.

REFERENCES

1. LaRosa JC. Future cardiovascular end point studies: where will the research take us? Am J Cardiol 1999; 84:454–458.
2. Davies MJ. The pathophysiology of acute coronary syndromes. Heart 2000; 83:361–366.
3. Chesebro JH, Rauch U, Fuster V, Badimon JJ. Pathogenesis of thrombosis in coronary artery disease. Haemostasis 1997; 27(suppl 1):12–18.
4. Falk E, Shah PK, Fuster V. Coronary plaque disruption. Circulation 1995; 92:657–671.
5. Badimon L, Badimon JJ. Mechanisms of arterial thrombosis in nonparallel streamlines: platelet thrombi grow on the apex of stenotic severely injured vessel wall. Experimental study in the pig model. J Clin Invest 1989; 84:1134–1144.
6. Badimon L, Badimon JJ, Galvez A, Chesebro JH, Fuster V. Influence of arterial wall damage and wall shear rate on platelet deposition: ex vivo study in a swine model. Arteriosclerosis 1986; 6:312–320.
7. Adams PC, Fuster V, Badimon L, Badimon JJ, Chesebro JH. Platelet/vessel wall interaction, rheologic factors, and thrombogenic substrate in acute coronary syndromes: preventative strategies. Am J Cardiol 1987; 60:9G-18G.
8. Lassila R, Badimon JJ, Vallabhajosula S, Badimon L. Dynamic monitoring of platelet deposition on severely damaged vessel wall in flowing blood: effects of different stenoses on thrombus growth. Arteriosclerosis 1990; 10:306–315.
9. Mailhac A, Badimon JJ, Fallon JT, Fernandez-Ortiz A, Meter B, Chesebro JH, Fuster V, Badimon L. Effect of eccentric stenosis on fibrin(ogen) deposition on severely damaged vessel wall in arterial thrombosis: relative contribution of fibrin(ogen) and platelets. Circulation 1994; 90:988–996.
10. Davies MJ, Thomas T. The pathologic basis and microanatomy of occlusive thrombus formation in human coronary arteries. Philos Trans R Soc Lond (Biol) 1981; 294:225–229.
11. Gertz SD, Roberts WC. Hemodynamic shear force in rupture of coronary arterial atherosclerotic plaques. Am J Cardil 1990; 66:1368–1372.

12. Ravn HB, Falk E. Histopathology of plaque rupture. Cardiol Clin 1999; 17:263–270.
13. Davies MJ. Stability and instability: two faces of coronary atherosclerosis. Circulation 1996; 94:2013–2020.
14. Loree HM, Kamm RD, Stringfellow RG, Lee RT. Effects of fibrous cap thickness on peak circumferential stress in model atherosclerotic vessels. Circ Res 1992; 71:850–858.
15. Lendon CL, Davies MJ, Born GVR, Richardson PD. Atherosclerotic plaque caps are locally weakened when macrophage density is increased. Atherosclerosis 1991; 87:87–90.
16. Moreno PR, Bernardi VH, Lopez-Cuellar JL, Alvaro MM, Igor FP, Gold HK, Mehran R, Sharma SK, Nemerson Y, Fuster V, Fallon JT. Macrophages, smooth muscle cells, and tissue factor in unstable angina: implications for cell-mediated thrombogenicity in acute coronary syndromes. Circulation 1996; 94:3090–3097.
17. Fernandez-Ortiz A, Badimon JJ, Falk E, Fuster V, Meyer B, Mailhac A, Weng D, Shah PK, Badimon L. Characterization of the relative thrombogenicity of atherosclerotic plaque components: implications for consequences of plaque rupture. J Am Coll Cardiol 1994; 23:1562–1569.
18. Toschi V, Gallo R, Lettino M, Fallon J, Gertz SD, Fernandez-Ortiz A, Chesebro JH, Badimon L, Nemerson Y, Fuster V, Badimon JJ. Tissue factor modulates the thrombogenicity of human atherosclerotic plaques. Circulation 1997; 95:594–599.
19. Chesebro JH, Toschi V, Lettino M, Gallo R, Badimon JJ, Fallon JT, Fuster V. Evolving concepts in the pathogenesis and treatment of arterial thrombosis. The Mount Sinai Journal of Medicine 1995; 62:275–286.
20. Giesen PL, Rauch U, Bohrmann B, Kling D, Roque M, Fallon JT, Badimon JJ, Himber J, Riederer MA, Nemerson Y. Blood-borne tissue factor: another view of thrombosis. Proc Natl Acad Sci USA 1999; 96(5):2311–2315.
21. Badimon L, Martinez-Gonzalez, Royo T, Lassila R, Badimon JJ. A sudden increase in plasma epinephrine levels transiently enhances platelet deposition on severely damaged arterial wall. Thromb Haemost 1999; 82:1736–1742.
22. Chesebro JH, Fuster V, Elveback LR, Frye RL. Strong family history and cigarette smoking as risk factors of coronary artery disease in young adults. Br Heart J 1982; 47:78–83.
23. Shepherd J, Cobbe SM, et al. Prevention of coronary heart disease with pravastatin in men with hypercholesterolemia. Engl J Med 1995; 333:1301–1307.
24. Scandinavian Simvastatin Survival Study Group. Randomized trial of cholesterol lowering in 4444 patients with coronary heart disease: the Scandinavian Simvastatin Survival Study Group (4S). Lancet 1994; 344:1383–1389.
25. The Long-Term Intervention with Pravastatin in Ischaemic Disease (LIPID) Study Group. Prevention of cardiovascular events and death with pravastatin in patients with coronary heart disease and a broad range of initial cholesterol levels. N Engl J Med 1998; 339:1349–1357.
26. Blankenhorn DH, Nessim SA, Johnson RL, SanMarco ME, Azen SP, Cachin-Hamphill L. Beneficial effects of colestipol niacin therapy on coronary atherosclerosis and coronary venous bypass grafts. JAMA 1987; 257:3233–3240.
27. Buchwald H, Varco RL, Matts JP, et al. Effect of partial ileal bypass on mortality and morbidity from coronary heart disease in patients with hypercholesterolemia. Report of the Program on Surgical Control of the Hyperlipidemias. N Engl J Med 1990; 323:946–955.
28. Watts GF, Lewis B, Brunt JNH, Lewis ES, Coltart DJ, Smith LDR, Mann JI, Swan AV: Effects on coronary artery disease of lipid-lowering diet, or diet plus cholestyramine, in the St. Thomas' Atherosclerosis Regression Study (STARS). Lancet 1992; 339:563–569.
29. Brown BG, Zhao XQ, Sacco DE, Albers JJ. Lipid lowering and plaque regression, new insights into prevention of plaque disruption and clinical events in coronary disease. Circulation 1993; 87:1781–1791.
30. Rauch U, Osende JI, Chesebro JH, Fuster V, Vorcheimer DA, Harris K, Harris P, Sandler DA, Fallon JT, Jayaraman S, Badimon JJ. Statins and cardiovascular diseases: the multiple effects of lipid-lowering therapy by statins. Atherosclerosis 2000; 153:181–189.
31. Fuster V. Lewis A Conner Memorial Lecture. Mechanisms leading to myocardial infarction: insights from studies of vascular biology. Circulation 1994; 90:2126–2146.

32. Davies MJ, Richardson PD, Woolf N, Katz DR, Mann J. Risk of thrombosis in human atherosclerotic plaques: role of extracellular lipid, macrophage, and smooth muscle cell content. Br Heart J 1993; 69:377–381.

33. Frick MH, Elo O, Haapa K, Heinonen OP, Heinsalmi P, Helo P, Huttunen JK, Kaitaniemi P, Koskinen P, Manninen V, et al. Helsinki Heart Study: primary-prevention trial with gemfibrozil in middle-aged men with dyslipidemia. Safety of treatment, changes in risk factors, and incidence of coronary heart disease. N Engl J Med 1987; 317:1237–1245.

34. Brown G, Alber JJ, Fisher LD, Schaefer SM, Lin JT, Kaplan C, Zhao XG, Bisson BD, Fitzpatrick VF, Dodge HT. Regression of coronary artery disease as a result of intensive lipid-lowering therapy in men with high levels of apolipoprotein B. N Engl J Med 1990; 323:1289–1298.

35. Fuster V, Badimon L, Badimon JJ, Chesebro JH. The pathogenesis of coronary artery disease and the acute coronary syndromes. N Engl J Med 1992; 326:310–318.

36. Brown BG, Zhao XQ, Chait A, Fisher LD, Cheung MC, Morse JS, Dowdy AA, Marino EK, Bolson EL, Alaupovic P, Frohlich, Albers JJ. Simvastatin and niacin, antioxidant vitamins, or the combination for the prevention of coronary disease. N Engl J Med 2001; 345:1583–1592.

37. Loscalzo J. Lipoprotein(a): a unique risk factor for atherothrombotic disease. Arteriosclerosis 1990; 10:672–679.

38. Loscalzo J. The relation between atherosclerosis and thrombosis. Circulation 1992; 86(suppl III):III-95–III-99.

39. Bozkurt E, Erol MK, Keles S, Acikel M, Mustafa Y, Gurlertop Y. Relation of plasma homocysteine levels to intracoronary thrombus in unstable angina pectoris and in non-q-wave acute myocardial infarction. Am J Card 2002; 90:413–415.

40. Al-Obaidi MK, Philippou H, Stubbs PJ, Adami A, Amersey R, Noble MM, Lane DA. Relationships between homocysteine, factor VIIa, and thrombin generation in acute coronary syndromes. Circulation 2000; 101:372–377.

41. Njolstad I, Arnesen E, Lund-Larsen PG. Smoking, serum lipids, blood pressure, and sex differences in myocardial infarction: a 12–year follow-up of the Finmark Study. Circulation 1996; 93:450–456.

42. Hung J, Lam JY, Lacoste L, Letchacovski G. Cigarette smoking acutely increases platelet thrombus formation in patients with coronary artery disease taking aspirin. Circulation 1995; 92:2432–2436.

43. Burke AP, Farb A, Malcom GT, Liang Y, Smialek J, Virmani R. Coronary risk factors and plaque morphology in men with coronary disease who died suddenly. N Engl J Med 1997; 336:1276–1282.

44. Matetzky S, Tani S, Kangavari S, Dimayuga P, Yano J, Xu H, Chyu KY, Fishbein M, Shah PK, Cercek B. Smoking increases tissue factor expression in atherosclerotic plaques: implications for plaque thrombogenicity.

45. Johnstone MT, Creager SJ, Scales KM, Cusco JA, Lee BK, Creager MA. Impaired endothelium-dependent vasodilation in patients with insulin-dependent diabetes mellitus. Circulation 1993; 88:2510–2516.

46. Moreno PR, Murcia AM, Palacios IF, Leon MN, Bernardi VH, Fuster V, Fallon JT. Coronary composition and macrophage infiltration in atherectomy specimens from patients with diabetes mellitus. Circulation 2000; 102:2180–2184.

47. Rao AK, Chouhan V, Chen X, Sun L, Boden G. Activation of the tissue factor pathway of blood coagulation during prolonged hyperglycemia in young healthy men. Diabetes 1999; 48:1156–1161.

48. McGill JB, Schneider DJ, Arfken CL, Lucore CL, Sobel BE. Factors responsible for impaired fibrinolysis in obese subjects and NIDDM patients. Diabetes. 1994; 43:104–109.

49. Juhan-Vague I, Alessi MC, Vague P. Increased plasma plasminogen activator inhibitor 1 levels. A possible link between insulin resistance and atherothrombosis. Diabetologia. 1991; 34:457–462.

50. Zuanetti G, Latini R, Maggioni AP, Santoro L, Franzosi MG. Influence of diabetes on mortality in acute myocardial infarction: data from the GISSI-2 study. J Am Coll Cardiol 1993; 22:1788–1794.

51. Gray RP, Yudkin JS, Patterson DL. Enzymatic evidence of impaired reperfusion in diabetic patients after thrombolytic therapy for acute myocardial infarction: a role for plasminogen activator inhibitor? Br Heart J 1993; 70:530–536

52. Rauch U, Crandall J, Osende JI, Fallon JT, Chesebro JH, Fuster V, et al. Increased thrombus formation relates to ambient blood glucose and leukocyte count in diabetes mellitus type 2. Am J Cardiol 2000; 86:246–249.

53. Rauch U, Schwippert B, Schultheiss HP, Tschoepe D. Platelet activation in diabetic microangiopathy. Platelets 1998; 9:237–240.

54. Becker RC, Bovill EG, et al. Pathobiology of thrombin in acute coronary syndromes. Am Heart J 1998; 136:S19–S31.

55. Chesebro JH, Webster MD, Zoldhelyi P, Roche PC, Badimon L, Badimon JJ. Antithrombotic therapy and progression of coronary artery disease. Antiplatelet versus antithrombins. Circulation 1992; 86(suppl III):III100–III110.

56. Heras M, Chesebro JH, Penny WJ, Bailey KR, Badimon L, Fuster V. Effects of thrombin inhibition on the development of acute platelet-thrombus deposition during angioplasty in pigs. Heparin versus recombinant hirudin, a specific thrombin inhibitor. Circulation 1989; 79:657–665.

57. Heras M, Chesebro JH, Webster MW, Mruk JS, Grill DE, Penny WJ, Bowie EJ, Badimon L, Fuster. Hirudin, heparin, and placebo during deep arterial injury in the pig. The in vivo role of thrombin in platelet-mediated thrombosis. Circulation 1990; 82:1476–1484.

58. Ardissino D, Merlini PA, Eisenberg PR, Kottke-Marchant K, Crenshaw BS, Granger CB. Coagulation markers and outcomes in acute coronary syndromes. Am Heart J 1998; 136:S7–S18.

59. Meade TW, Howarth DJ, Stirling Y, Welch TP, Crompton MR. Fibrinopeptide A and sudden coronary death. Lancet 1984; 2:607–609.

60. Ardissino D, Merlini PA, Gamba G, Barberis P, Demicheli G, Testa S, Colombi E, Poli A, Fetiveau R, Montemartini C. Thrombin Activity and early outcome in unstable angina pectoris. Circulation 1996; 93:1634–1639.

61. Merlini PA, Bauer KA, Oltrona L, Ardissino D, Cattaneo M, Belli C, Mannucci PM, Rosenberg RD. Persistent activation of coagulation mechanism in unstable angina and myocardial infarction. Circulation 1994; 90:61–68.

62. Rauch U, Osende JI, Fuster V, Badimon JJ, Fayad Z, Chesebro JH. Thrombus formation on atherosclerotic plaques: pathogenesis and clinical consequences. Ann Intern Med 2001; 134:224–238.

3-2

Atherosclerosis: A Lipid Disorder and a Chronic Inflammatory Disease

Scott Kinlay
Cardiovascular Division, Brigham Women's Hospital, Boston, Massachusetts, U.S.A.

Karen Moulton
Vascular Biology, Children's Hospital; Cardiovascular Division, Brigham Women's Hospital, Boston, Massachusetts, U.S.A.

I. INTRODUCTION

Atherosclerosis is a complex disease characterized by the accumulation of lipids, matrix, inflammatory cells, and smooth muscle cells in the walls of large arteries. This progressive chronic disease is the result of many insults. The natural history in humans typically progresses through a long clinically silent phase of atheroma formation, which is followed much later in life by the emergence of clinical syndromes, such as stroke and myocardial infarction, which are provoked by plaque disruption and thrombosis. In the last several decades our understanding of atherosclerosis has progressed rapidly because of advances in cell biology and molecular mechanisms of gene regulation, the development of experimental animal models amenable to genetic interventions, and numerous clinical studies identifying risk factors and improved therapies that modify the disease in humans. Pathological mechanisms are better characterized for some recognized clinical risk factors such as hypercholesterolemia, but remain incompletely understood for several other risk factors such as diabetes, smoking, hypertension and systemic inflammation.

This overview of atherosclerosis will discuss disease mechanisms that lead to the development of complex atheromas, which are capable of producing either acute vascular syndromes or more stable syndromes such as exertional angina related to inadequate blood flow to meet myocardial demands. This chapter outlines stages of atherosclerosis and describes important cellular, biochemical, and molecular events that are critical for lesion initiation, inflammatory cell recruitment, and foam cell generation in the artery wall, atheroma growth, and thrombosis. Recent excellent reviews provide more detailed descriptions of biological mechanisms and insights for future investigation (1–6).

II. RISK FACTORS FOR ATHEROSCLEROSIS

Epidemiological studies of large patient populations have identified major clinical risk factors that promote atherosclerosis. Conventional risk factors include nonmodifiable factors, such as age, gender, and family history. Modifiable risk factors include elevated levels of low-density lipoprotein (LDL) cholesterol, reduced levels of high-density lipoprotein (HDL) cholesterol, hypertension, diabetes, high-saturated-fat diets, smoking, obesity, and lack of exercise.

Many conventional risk factors are considered causal factors for the development of atherosclerosis because the risk is observed in different populations, it shows a dose-dependent response, and removal or reduction of the factor reduces clinical events. In the case of hypercholesterolemia, further proof of causality has been demonstrated by the development of atherosclerosis in experimental animals exposed to high cholesterol diets or engineered to have genetic deficiency of apolipoprotein E or LDL receptor genes that resemble genetic traits associated with atherosclerosis susceptibility in humans (7,8). Furthermore, gene-delivery treatments designed to reverse these genetic defects resulted in regression of atherosclerosis (9). Molecular analysis of cellular and biochemical changes activated by hypercholesterolemia have identified critical events required for the development of atherosclerosis that have helped explain the pathways linking many risk factors to atherosclerosis progression and clinical events.

A variety of novel risk markers are also under intense investigation, but their roles as causes of atherosclerosis are still uncertain. Serum markers of inflammation, including C-reactive protein, interleukin-6 (IL-6), and soluble intercellular adhesion molecule (ICAM), correlate with clinical risks for acute vascular syndromes such as myocardial infarction, unstable angina, and stroke. In comparison with hypercholesterolemia, our understanding of pathogenic mechanisms invoked by non–cholesterol-dependent risk factors remains incomplete, but unraveling these additional pathogenic mechanisms will likely reveal novel targets for new treatments.

III. CELLULAR AND BIOLOGIC EVENTS: PATHOGENIC MECHANISMS

Although the biological mechanisms that link the risk factors to the development of atherosclerosis and clinical events are known with variable detail, it is useful to understand how these risk factors target elements in the vascular wall and, in particular, the endothelium. By disturbing the normal homeostatic functions of the endothelium and vascular wall, risk factors promote the accumulation of lipid, activated inflammatory and smooth muscle cells, and other complex features within the arterial intima, which are characteristic features of atherosclerosis. Important stages in the development of atherosclerosis are identified in the following sections. Although these conceptual stages are presented as discrete steps, in reality they probably develop as a continuum. Even within the same individual, separate atheromas may represent various stages of disease development and atheromas may either regress or advance between stages over a chronic period of time. In pathological specimens, we see "snapshots" of various atheromas that resemble early, advanced, and complex atheromas associated with acute vascular complications, but we cannot predict the time course for transitions between phases. There is consensus about the sequence of events activated by hypercholesterolemia leading to the generation of the fatty streak type of lesion. However, in later phases of progression, the diversity of cells and factors in the plaque suggests that subsequent pathological events regulating the progression of atherosclerosis are complex and are not likely to proceed at a linear and predictable time course. The utility of these stages and diagrams are therefore to highlight important pathogenic mechanisms in atherosclerosis that may be affected by various known risk factors.

A. Lesion Initiation

1. Endothelial Dysfunction

The endothelium functions as a selective barrier between the blood and tissues. Disturbances of normal endothelial functions at this blood/tissue interface are important events that initiate early atherosclerotic lesions (Fig. 1). The response-to-injury hypothesis originally proposed that injury or disruption of the endothelium was an important early event that facilitated LDL entry and deposition in the artery wall. Although there is no physical break or denudation of the endothelium, there is evidence that functional properties of the endothelium, including the permeability of intercellular tight junctions to lipids and the production of nitric oxide, are altered in specific regions of lesion susceptibility even before lipid accumulation is observed. In regions of low shear stress, which are more susceptible to atherosclerosis, the endothelium has altered patterns of gene expression and endothelial cells have a different polygonal shape compared to endothelial cells from regions with laminar flow. The endothelial cells in these regions of atherosclerosis susceptibility express adhesion molecules that direct inflammatory cell rolling, firm adhesion, and then transmigration into these regions, which are required for early lesion generation (10–12). The perme-

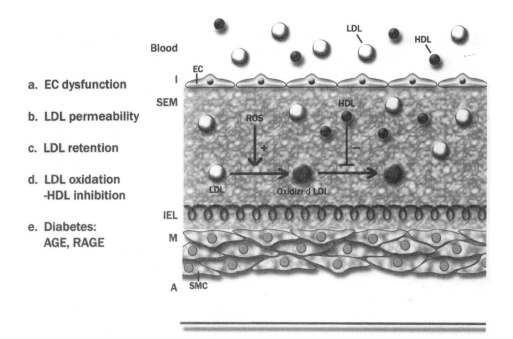

Figure 1 Lesion Initiation. (See text for discussion of critical events initiating early atherosclerotic lesions.) Early changes include endothelial cell (EC) dysfunction, permeability of LDL between endothelial cell junctions, and then retention of LDL to proteoglycans in the subendothelial cell matrix (SEM). Initial oxidation of LDL by reactive oxygen species (ROS) occurs after it leaves the circulation. Modified LDL and advanced glycosylated endproducts (AGE) may activate the overlying endothelium and facilitate inflammatory cell transmigration. Internal elastic lamina (IEL), media (M), and adventitia (A) layers in the blood vessel wall are shown. The intima layer over the internal elastic lamina is drawn in exaggerated size. (Illustration by S. Sonn.)

ability of the endothelium to macromolecules and lipid is similarly increased in these same regions (13).

2. LDL Permeability, Oxidation, and Retention

Most of the cholesterol in blood is carried in the native LDL particle, which is the principal form of cholesterol associated with increased risk for coronary artery disease (CAD) in epidemiological studies (14). Only a small fraction of LDL in the blood is modified by oxidation. A primary initiating event in atherosclerosis is the accumulation of LDL in the subendothelial matrix. The higher the levels of circulating LDL, the more that is delivered and retained in the artery wall (15). LDL is retained in the vessel wall because of binding interactions between apolipoprotein B proteins in the LDL particle and extracellular proteoglycans including biglycan and versican (16,17). Native LDL itself has few biological effects in the vessel wall, and uptake of unmodified LDL via the LDL receptor does not lead to intracellular lipid accumulation or foam cell generation because the receptor is downregulated (18,19). However, LDL trapped with proteoglycans can undergo oxidation and lipolysis to become modified LDL (20). Endogenous intracellular enzymes that contribute to LDL oxidation are the 12- and 15-lipoxygenases that insert oxygen molecules into unsaturated fatty acids, which can then diffuse into retained extracellular LDL. Additional aggregation and oxidation of modified LDL can be mediated by reactive oxygen species and the enzymes sphingomyelinase, phospholipase 2, and myeloperoxidase (21).

Modified lipoproteins have pro-inflammatory activities that stimulate the expression of cytokines growth factors and chemokines, recruit inflammatory cells, stimulate other vascular wall cells, induce adhesion molecules on the endothelium, and are taken up by scavenger receptors on macrophages and other vascular cells to generate foam cells in the vessel wall. Lipid accumulation continues as the deposition rate of lipids overwhelms the clearance rate, and the engorged foam cells cannot egress from the vessel wall or become apoptotic.

Oxidized LDL inhibits nitric oxide generation by the endothelium. Nitric oxide has multiple antiatherogenic effects, including arterial vasodilation, enhanced clearance of oxygen-derived free radicals, reduced expression of adhesion molecules and inflammatory chemokines, and inhibition of thrombus formation (22–24). The progressive depletion of nitric oxide in the vessel wall promotes paradoxical vasoconstriction instead of vasodilation to physiological stimuli. The resultant endothelial cell dysfunction is important during early stages of atherosclerosis, but also contributes to the propagation of atherosclerosis at advanced stages and promotes thrombotic complications (25,26).

3. High-Density Lipoprotein

A low plasma concentration of HDL is a significant risk factor for the development of atherosclerosis (27–29), but most current drug and diet treatments are only able to increase HDL modestly in free-living adults, limiting their role in preventing atherosclerosis. Some genetic factors such as apolipoprotein A deficiency, HDL-processing enzymes, and mutations in the ATP-binding cassette transporter A1 (ABCA1) responsible for Tangier disease, result in dramatically low levels of HDL and increased atherosclerosis (30). HDL has several antiatherogenic properties. These include reverse cholesterol transport and specific antioxidant functions.

Reverse cholesterol transport involving HDL occurs by passive diffusion or active transport (31). Phospholipids on the surface of HDL can reabsorb cholesterol from the plasma membrane of cells. Active transport of cholesterol from peripheral cells to HDL occurs by the interaction of HDL and with the ABCA1 transporters on peripheral tissues including macrophages. Cholesterol carried on HDL returns to the liver by direct and indirect pathways. Mature HDL that is laden with cholesterol may be removed from the circulation by the liver via the HDL specific scavenger receptor-B1 (SR-B1). There is also an exchange of cholesterol between HDL and very-low density lipoprotein (VLDL) facilitated by cholesterol ester transfer protein (CETP). Cholesterol that is transferred to VLDL may find its way back to the liver (or to peripheral tissues) via the LDL receptor. Abnormalities in some of these pathways have led to new pharmacological agents with greater effects on HDL. For example, rare genetic defects in CETP and HDL (Apo-A1 Milano) have led to the development of CETP inhibitors and recombinant HDL (Apo-A1 Milano) that increase HDL by 60–70% (32,33). These therapies may improve reverse cholesterol transport properties and are now being evaluated for atherosclerosis prevention in clinical trials (34).

HDL also contains the antioxidant paraoxonase and protects against atherosclerosis by inhibiting LDL oxidation (35). By these and other mechanisms, HDL can enhance endothelial cell function and activates production of nitric oxide (36).

4. Diabetes-Related Glycosylated Proteins

Diabetes and metabolic changes associated with insulin resistance lead to the formation of advanced glycation end products that interact with receptors on endothelial cells and inflammatory cells in the vessel wall to promote inflammation and oxidation. These changes combined with hypercholesterolemia accelerate the development of atherosclerosis (37).

B. Inflammatory Cell Recruitment and Foam Cell Generation

1. Endothelium-Dependent Recruitment

Monocyte recruitment and foam cell generation lead to the formation of fatty streak lesions as depicted in Figure 2. Initial changes in the endothelium direct the local recruitment of inflammatory cells through the endothelium into the subendothelial matrix. Retained oxidized lipoproteins, glycation products, and released growth factors induce endothelial cell expression of selectins and cellular adhesion molecules, most importantly vascular cell adhesion molecule (VCAM-1) (38). The recruitment of monocytes and T cells involves a highly ordered sequence of events on the luminal surface of endothelial cells (39,40). Leukocytes in the circulation are first slowed down by weak interactions with the selectin family of molecules that lead to rolling of the leukocytes on the endothelial cell surface. This allows more stable interactions with VCAM-1 and intercellular adhesion molecule (ICAM) that arrest the leukocytes and then permit the migration of these cells between endothelial cells into the arterial intima (39,40).

2. Monocyte Entry and Differentiation

Once monocytes have entered the subendothelial layer, these cells can amplify the recruitment process by the expression of chemokines monocyte chemoattractant protein MCP-1, its receptor CCR2, and cytokines M-CSF (41,42). These factors promote monocyte migration and the differentiation of monocytes into tissue macrophages. Modified lipoproteins augment the recruitment of inflammatory cells into the vascular wall by a number of mechanisms that act on both endothelial cells and inflammatory cells. The nuclear factor kappa B (NF-κB) signal transduction pathway is one particularly important mechanism that regulates the transcription of several pro-inflammatory genes including tumor necrosis factor

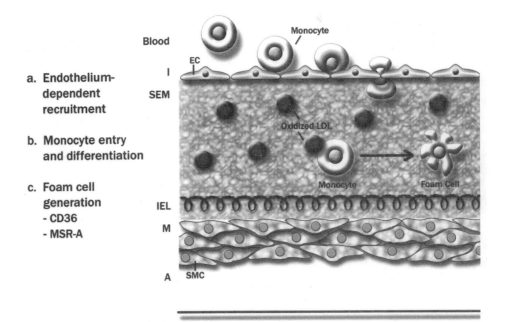

a. Endothelium-dependent recruitment

b. Monocyte entry and differentiation

c. Foam cell generation
 - CD36
 - MSR-A

Figure 2 Monocyte recruitment and foam cell generation. Expression of selectins and adhesion molecules ICAM-1 and VCAM-1 are cell surface receptors that engage ligands on inflammatory cells to mediate rolling and then firm adhesion that facilitates transmigration of inflammatory cells into the subendothelial space. Cytokines and chemokines enhance the recruitment of other inflammatory cells. Monocytes differentiate into macrophages in the artery wall and increase their expression of important receptors CD36 and the macrophage scavenger receptor A that are capable of clearing apoptotic bodies and modified lipoproteins. Unregulated uptake of modified lipids results in the formation of foam cells that comprise the fatty streak lesion. (Illustration by S. Sonn.)

-α (TNF-α). NF-κB is normally held in the cytoplasm as an inactive heterodimer complex with its inhibitory partner Iκ-Bα (43). Nitric oxide maintains this inhibitory complex, which may account for some of its anti-inflammatory effects (44,45). Oxidized LDL and oxygen-derived free radicals degrade the inhibitory Iκ-Bα (46,47), thereby activating NF-κB, which can then translocate to the nucleus to increase transcription of a number of pro-inflammatory genes.

3. Foam Cell Generation

Monocytes present in the arterial intima undergo changes in gene expression and mature into macrophages. Some of these developmental target genes include molecules such as matrix metalloproteinase-2 (gelatinase A), the macrophage scavenger receptor (MSR)-A, and CD-36, which play important roles in the pathogenesis of atherosclerosis (48,49). Experimental data have shown that MSR-A and CD36 are the principal receptors for the uptake of modified lipoproteins, since mice deficient in either or both receptors have incremental reductions in early lesion formation (50–53). This unregulated uptake of modified LDL cholesterol by macrophages and some vascular smooth muscle cells changes these cells into foam cells that comprise the fatty streak type of early atheroma. Foam cells express angiotensin II receptors and are capable of promoting further lipid oxidation (54,55). Angiotensin II increases the production of superoxide and stimulates NADPH oxidase on vascular smooth muscle cells. The accumulation of lipids in cells and tissues may also have direct effects on gene expression in macrophages. For instance, fatty acids are ligands for nuclear receptor transcription factors, including PPAR-α, PPAR-γ, and liver X receptor (LXR), which regulate macrophage and endothelial cell differentiation and alter expression of genes involved in fatty acid metabolism (56). These nuclear receptors also regulate inflammatory genes involved in TNF–α, interferon-γ (IFN-γ)–and lipopolysaccharide (LPS)–inducible responses of macrophages.

The macrophage response to oxidized LDL forms part of the rapidly responding innate immunity. Scavenger receptors CD36, MSR-A, and SR-B1 contribute to innate immunity through their recognition and clearance of diverse ligands associated with pathogens. During infections, oxidized phospholipids and apoptotic cells are generated, which may be cleared by these types of receptor. Specific antibodies recognizing oxidized LDL inhibit clearance of apoptotic bodies (57). Soluble factors of innate defense such as complement and C-reactive protein and IgM antibodies to oxidized LDL are also found in atherosclerotic plaques and may alter the progression of atherosclerosis (58). These observations link the response of macrophages during atherosclerosis to responses involved in innate immunity. Although these activities could provide survival benefits for host immune responses to pathogens, these activities could provide deleterious effects under environmental conditions associated with elevated serum lipoproteins and other clinical risk factors.

C. Growth of Fibroproliferative Atheroma

Several risk factors seem to contribute to the progression of atherosclerosis and the growth of fibrous lesions (Fig. 3). Some of the effects of systemic hypertension on atherosclerosis may be mediated by biomechanical forces and by humoral factors, including platelet-derived growth factor (PDGF) and components of the renin-angiotensin pathway. Angiotensin II activates smooth muscle cell proliferation and production of matrix.

1. Cytokines and Signal Amplification

The early arrival of monocytes within the artery wall sets the stage for the recruitment of other cell types including T lymphocytes, B lymphocytes, fibroblasts, and smooth muscle cells found in more complex atheromas. Myriad growth factors and cytokines are detected within atherosclerotic lesions, including fibroblast growth factors FGF-1 and FGF-2, PDGF, m-CSF, gm-CSF, vascular endothelial cell growth factor (VEGF), interleukins (IL-2, IL-6, and IL-10), insulin-like growth factor (IGF)-1, epidermal growth factor, TNF-α, and transforming growth factor (TGF-β)-β (59–61). Many of these mitogens affect several cell types in the atheroma. For example, FGF and PDGF promote the proliferation and migration of smooth muscle cells, endothelial cells, and fibroblasts (62). In turn, many of these factors act in concert to produce inflammatory mediators, vasoactive substances, matrix molecules, proteases, and protease inhibitors that have direct and indirect effects on several cell types also. This cascade of events creates complex networks of interactions between cells and biochemical and mechanical signals in the atheroma (63). Ultimately, these interactive networks converge to regulate important basic processes such as cell proliferation, apoptosis, matrix remodeling and inflammatory cell recruitment.

2. Smooth Muscle Cell and Fibroblast Recruitment

The proliferation of vascular smooth muscle cells (SMCs) is an important feature in the development of atherosclerotic lesions. The proliferation index of SMCs is relatively low at any given point in time but may continue over a chronic period (64). SMC pop-

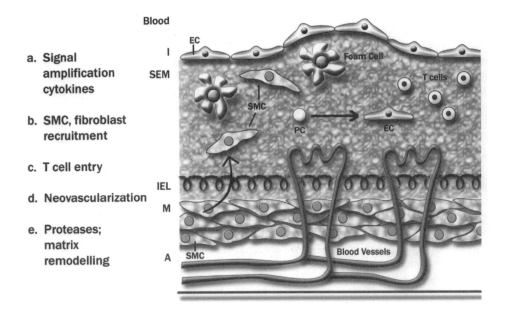

a. Signal
   amplification
   cytokines

b. SMC, fibroblast
   recruitment

c. T cell entry

d. Neovascularization

e. Proteases;
   matrix
   remodelling

Figure 3 Growth of fibroproliferative atheromas. Recruited macrophages in the plaque elaborate diverse mitogens, cytokines, and inflammatory mediators, all of which target many cell types including smooth muscle cells (SMC), fibroblasts, and T cells. Some advanced lesions develop neovascularization in the intimal layer that mostly arises as extensions from vasa vasorum in the outer blood vessel wall. Proteases released by inflammatory cells and invading capillary sprouts remodel the extracellular matrix. Positive remodeling or outward extension of the artery wall can preserve the caliber of the blood vessel lumen to optimize blood flow even in the presence of a large atheroma. Encroachment of the lumen due to negative remodeling or fibrous changes may restrict blood flow to levels that produce exertional angina.

ulations in atheromas are often monoclonal because they arise from preexisting clonal populations of vascular SMCs that form the vessel wall during embryological development (65). Animal studies and analysis of vascular lesions in transplanted organs have indicated that vascular SMCs may originate from subpopulations of bone marrow–derived cells or circulating precursor cells (66,67). SMCs are the main producers of extracellular matrix molecules such as collagen I and III, fibronectin, and proteoglycans. These matrix molecules provide biomechanical strength, interact with cell surface molecules such as integrins, and ultimately influence factors that determine plaque stability, which may explain why some lesion types with few SMCs, a thin fibrous cap, a necrotic lipid core, and increased numbers of macrophages are associated with acute ischemic complications (68–70). Given the diverse complex nature of cell mitogens found in the atheroma, instead of inhibiting individual growth factor pathways, several experimental strategies target common downstream regulators of the cell cycle (71,72). Pharmacological use of the cytostatic drugs rapamycin, sirolimus and paclitaxel, which were developed for use in cancer or immune suppression, have shown benefits in neointima growth of primary atherosclerosis and restenosis after angioplasty or stent placement (1,73,74).

3. T Cell Entry

The expression of cytokines, chemokines, and endothelial cellular adhesion molecules recruit T and B lymphocytes into the arterial wall, which form part of the acquired immune response in atherosclerosis (58). Macrophages activate T cells by presenting antigens to specific T cell receptors with co-stimulatory signals produced by interactions between CD40 ligand and CD40 on both cells. Oxidized LDL is one potential antigen that can activate T cells and B cells by this method (58). Production of antibodies to epitopes on oxidized lipoproteins can influence atherosclerotic progression (75,76).

Prior studies of atherosclerosis development in strains of mice that lack certain types of immune cells have previously shown that macrophages are critical cells for the development of early atherosclerotic lesions, but T cells and B cells contribute less to the extent of early and fibroproliferative plaques (77,78). These less abundant cell types in the plaque may not have substantial effects on the bulk of atheromas, but they may exert significant biological effects on local cells in the atheroma, which alter the gene expression patterns of macrophages, smooth muscle cells, and fibroblasts. For example, production of INF-γ by the Th1 subtype of T cells can regulate the expression of scavenger receptors by macrophages, inhibit the production of matrix by smooth muscle cells, and increase the expression of proteases such as metalloproteases that degrade extracellular matrix (79–82). Interferon-γ also induces CD40, which is widely expressed by many cells in the atheroma (83). Interruption of CD40 ligand receptor signaling by gene targeting or specific CD40 ligand antibodies reduce atherosclerosis at early and late stages of progression (83–86). The biological effects exerted by T cells on matrix turnover and diverse cells in lesions are consistent with major roles for lymphocytes in the progression of atherosclerosis.

4. Neovascularization

Neovascularization heralds the development of more complex plaques that are associated with clinical events. In normal large blood vessels, the vasa vasorum are confined to the outer layers of the vessel wall and have an organized pattern of first order longitudinal and second order circumferential branches (87). During early stages of lesion formation, the adventitial vasa vasorum proliferate and form a disordered vasa vasorum network that precedes the development of significant neointimal proliferation (88). At later stages of atherosclerosis, the vasa vasorum networks from the adventitia extend through the media into the intimal layer. In this location, neovascularization is associated with focal collections of inflammatory cells and may be a source of intraplaque hemorrhage.

Experimental evidence now suggests that neovascularization functions to promote the growth of atherosclerosis at advanced stages, but the functions of adventitial vasa vasorum proliferation at very early stages of atherosclerosis are still unclear. Some inhibitors of angiogenesis greatly reduced the growth of advanced atheromas but not early phases of plaque growth in mouse models of atherosclerosis. Conversely, endothelial cell growth factors promoted atherosclerosis (89–91). The observations that neovascularization is more frequently observed in large atheromas and interruption or compression of vasa vasorum induces medial necrosis in large thick-walled vessels suggests that neovascularization functions to perfuse the vessel wall (92). Although an additional source of perfusion beyond critical limits of diffusion from the main artery lumen may be a necessary condition for further growth, this does not mean that the extent of neovascularization has a linear dependence on plaque size. The correlations between vascular density of neovascularization and the sizes of atheromas are poor in both human and animal models (93,94). Not all advanced atheromas contain neovascularization, and like all forms of pathologic angiogenesis, neovascularization develops in focal regions, usually associated with inflammatory cells. During plaque regression, plaque blood flow and neovascularization dramatically declines, while only a modest reduction in plaque size is observed (95,96).

Intimal neovascularization is frequently observed in close proximity to areas within plaques that are rich in macrophages and T cells—cell types that are capable of stimulating angiogenesis (97,98). These vessels are also closely associated with cellular adhesion molecules and may provide a route for inflammatory cell recruitment into plaque (99). The vascular density of vasa vasorum networks show a strong linear correlation with the extent of adjacent inflammatory cell infiltrates. The spatial correlation could occur because these cells stimulate angiogenesis and/or the vasa vasorum networks are active conduits for the recruitment of inflammatory cells into the vessel wall. Once neovascularization is initiated, recruited inflammatory cells into sites of angiogenesis could further promote angiogenesis. Some agents that inhibit neovascularization may be able to interrupt this vicious cycle (94). Similarly, blocking antibodies against the VEGF receptor 1 on monocytes and endothelial cells inhibit both monocyte migration and angiogenesis (100). However, this approach has yet to be tested in humans.

The factors that regulate the formation of intimal neovascularization are not known. Several endothelial cell growth factors, including VEGF, FGF-1 and FGF-2, PDGF, and TGF-ß, are abundant within atherosclerotic lesions even at early stages, but their spatial patterns of expression do not correlate with the distribution of neovascularization. It is intriguing to ask why neovascular growth into the intimal layer occurs at much later stages than the appearance of endothelial cell growth factors. Several inhibitors of angiogenesis, including thrombospondin-1 and collagen XVIII, the parent molecule of endostatin, are present in the blood vessel wall and may oppose the actions of the endothelial cell growth factors expressed in early atheromas (101,102).

5. Proteases and Vascular Remodeling

Extracellular matrix and collagen in plaques is susceptible to several proteases, including members of the metalloproteinase family and cathepsins. Metalloproteinases are abundant in atherosclerotic plaque, especially in macrophages (103–105). Reactive oxygen species, cytokines, and CD40 stimulation of macrophages increase their production of metalloproteinases (79,106). Loss of nitric oxide and accumulation of its oxidized breakdown product peroxynitrite reduce the relative activity of tissue inhibitors of metalloproteinases TIMPs (107). Increased inflammatory cells and a relative reduced content of smooth muscle cells result in conditions in the plaque where the production of matrix proteins is exceeded by activities that degrade them. The relative loss of fibrous elements in the plaque may render these types of atheromas mechanically weak and more prone to rupture.

Although the activation of matrix proteases may result in pathological complications, these processes may be part of normal physiological responses of blood vessels to regulate their caliber according to changes in blood flow and perfusion. During blood vessel development, smaller vessels regress and coalesce to form dominant larger blood vessels that deliver blood through a hierarchical pattern of arteries, capillaries, and veins. During early stages of atheroma formation, the artery remodels as the lesion grows in an attempt to preserve the size of the arterial lumen. This compensatory enlargement, termed positive remodeling, was originally described from pathological studies of humans and animals, where the arterial segments with atheroma appeared to be larger than adjacent segments with less atheroma (108). In these cross-sectional studies, the lumen area was preserved until the area of plaque exceeded 40% of the total cross-sectional area of the artery. Specimens with greater proportions of plaque had a smaller lumen compared to adjacent segments with less atherosclerosis. Over a significant period of time, atheromas grow outward as cholesterol accumulates and proteases released by macrophages leads to medial thinning and cell apoptosis.

Remodeling also appears to occur in the opposite direction (negative remodeling). In these plaques, the cross-sectional area of the artery is smaller than adjacent segments and often accompanied by a narrower lumen area that might reduce blood flow. The mechanisms that drive positive and negative remodeling are poorly understood, but matrix metalloproteinases probably play an important role (109,110). Positive remodeling is associated with greater expression of metalloproteinases than artery regions that have negative or no remodeling (111–113). Disruption or inhibition of metalloproteinases prevents positive remodeling in atherosclerotic mice (114,115). Clinical studies suggest that negative remodeling is more common in smokers or those with insulin-dependent diabetes mellitus (116,117).

Local blood flow and biomechanical forces provide critical signals to regulate vascular remodeling. The presence of an atheroma can disturb laminar blood flow (118). Increased blood flow sensed by the endothelium stimulates endothelial cells to increase their production of nitric oxide (119) and decrease the expression of pro-atherogenic cellular adhesion molecules (120), endothelin (121), cytokines, and plasminogen activator inhibitor (122). These cellular responses favor positive remodeling and result in an increased lumen area and a compensatory reduction of elevated shear forces in the region near the atheroma.

Blood flow in the coronary arteries influences the development of restenosis after angioplasty. Areas of disturbed or low shear blood flow in coronary arteries tend to develop greater plaque accumulation detected by intravascular ultrasound over several months after percutaneous interventions (123,124). In contrast, regions with higher shear stress positively remodel without plaque accumulation to increase the lumen area—an effect that lowers blood flow velocity and shear stress to more physiological values and maintains vessel patency (124).

D. Advanced Lesions

The temporal onset for the development of advanced atheromas does not occur at a predictable time intervals in patients. Although ischemic symptoms during exertion are related to flow-limiting stenosis in coronary and peripheral arteries, unstable angina and acute thrombosis more often arise from plaques with only minimal narrowing of the artery lumen. Recent investigations are directed towards identifying biochemical and histological features that are associated with higher clinical risks for developing plaque rupture and thrombosis that result in stroke and myocardial infarctions. Many features found in advanced atheromas may render lesions more or less vulnerable to acute clinical complications (Fig. 4).

1. Lipid Pool

Over time, the unregulated accumulation of cholesterol by macrophages and smooth muscle cells leads to cell apoptosis and release of their contents into the extracellular space. Most acute coronary syndromes, including myocardial infarction, sudden cardiac death, or unstable angina, typically arise from disrupted complex plaques (68,125). Prior to disruption, these plaques typically cause only mild or no stenoses of the arterial lumen because of positive vascular remodeling. Autopsy studies of patients with sudden death have identified plaque morphologies in the culprit occluded coronary vessel that frequently have a thin fibrous cap overlying a large necrotic lipid-rich core. Abundant inflammatory

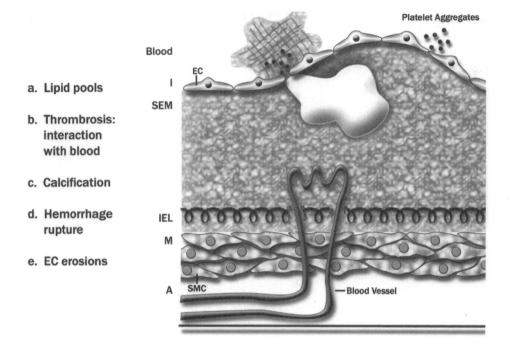

Figure 4 Advanced atheromas and complications. Lipid deposits and necrotic foam cells can result in the formation of lipid pools that are covered with a fibrous cap containing SMCs and matrix proteins. Inflammatory cells and neovascularization can invade the fibrous cap and provide a nidus for potential rupture. Exposure of the lipid core contents to blood may activate platelets and initiate plate aggregation and thrombus formation. Calcification and bone formation sometimes occur within vascular lesions, but it is not understood how this feature of atheromas relates to clinical complications.

cells infiltrate the edges or shoulders of the fibrous cap, and thrombosis is associated with the site of rupture into the artery lumen (4). Invasion of intimal neovascularization may also elaborate proteases and matrix remodeling in the shoulder regions of the plaque where biomechanical forces converge (126,127).

2. *Thrombosis and interaction with blood*

Exposure of subendothelial tissues to the blood is highly thrombogenic, but thrombosis in atheromas does not always cause complete vascular occlusion. Although local tissue conditions in a vulnerable atheroma may be critical substrates for the initiation of acute ischemic complications, hematological factors including platelets, fibrin, and other clotting factors may greatly influence the ability of the thrombus to propagate and cause vascular occlusion. Platelet activation, adhesion, and aggregation are important determinants in arterial thrombus formation. Platelets adhere to proteoglycans, collagens, nidogen, laminin, and fibulin in the basement membrane. Endothelial cells can modulate the balance between prothrombotic and antithrombotic interactions by the synthesis of prostacyclin PGI2 and nitric oxide that inhibit platelet activation, heparin sulfate that inactivates thrombin, and tissue plasminogen activator (t-PA) that generates plasmin and degrades fibrin. Thrombogenic substances produced by endothelial cells include von Willebrand factor (VWF), P-selectin, tissue factor, and plasminogen activator inhibitor. Genetic variations associated with increased levels of fibrinogen, plasminogen activator inhibitor type 1, and platelet reactivity promote the growth of thrombus and are associated with an increase the incidence of thrombotic complications (Table 1). Plasma levels of PAI-1 are increased in patients who have acute myocardial infarction compared to controls (128). Conversely, deficiency of vWF may provide some level of protection from atherosclerosis (129). Paradoxical vasoconstriction mediated by endothelial dysfunction can produce local vasospasm in association with a thrombus, which further limits blood flow and promotes thrombus growth (22,130,131).

3. Calcification

Calcification of the artery wall occurs more commonly in the elderly and is a feature of atherosclerosis. Artery calcification is an active process, more reminiscent of the active absorption and remodeling of calcium in bone (132). Calcification is associated with organizing thrombus and intraplaque hemorrhage (133), raising the possibility that intraplaque hemorrhage from rupture of intraplaque capillaries promotes calcification or facilitates the growth of chondrocyte-like cells in plaques. Diagnostic imaging modalities can quantify the extent of vascular calcification. Although extensive calcification may be associated with increase atherosclerotic burden, it is not known whether this feature predicts clinical risk for cardiovascular events. Arterial calcification may be more often associated with stable plaques compared to plaques with high inflammatory cell contents (126,134).

4. Hemorrhage, Rupture, and Erosions

Evidence for asymptomatic plaque rupture events, seen as intraplaque thrombosis or platelet aggregation on the endothelial surface, are often present at autopsy (125). Patients with sudden death due to an identified culprit lesion often show other active atheromas that were clinically silent (125). Thus, the incidence of atheromas with vulnerable features far exceeds the rate of acute tissue infarction associated with arterial occlusion.

Subclinical plaque rupture events may contribute to the progression of disease. For example, confined hemorrhage within the plaque could initiate an inflammatory response followed by wound healing cascades. The subsequent wound-healing from silent plaque ruptures may increase arterial stenosis by promoting plaque growth (135,136). In some cases superficial erosion of the intima without frank rupture leads to an acute syndrome (125,137,138). This type of vulnerable plaque morphology is rich with smooth muscle cells and proteoglycans and was more often observed in smokers who presented with sudden death (70). Inflammation also plays a role in superficial erosion by degrading collagens important in adhering endothelial cells to the subintimal matrix or by stimulating apoptosis of endothelial cells (4).

V. FUTURE DIRECTIONS

Over the last few decades our understanding of the progression and destabilization of atherosclerosis has increased exponentially. We now have a greater understanding of the mechanisms that link risk factors to advanced atherosclerosis and clinical events. This is particularly true for the role of LDL cholesterol as an important cause of atherosclerosis. Atherosclerosis is responsive to LDL cholesterol and the inflammation that is a consequence of exposure to this causative factor. This understanding has led to the concept of plaque stabilization as the main mechanism behind risk factor reduction and lowering the progression of atherosclerosis and the risk of clinical events. The increased use of invasive (e.g., intravascular ultrasound) and noninvasive imaging technologies makes these data increasingly obtainable, but further research is needed to validate these potential biological markers as reliable predictors of high clinical risk that can be modified therapeutically. An important goal is to develop ideally noninvasive tests or novel markers in addition to known clinical risk factors, which can stratify the large pool of patients at risk for sudden cardiac events at an early enough time interval to allow feasible interventions.

Since inflammation seems to be a key factor in the progression and destabilization of atherosclerosis, it seems logical that inhibitors of inflammatory pathways may offer new therapeutic options. The challenges for this approach include the importance of some immune regulators such as CD40 ligand for the maintenance of normal immune protection and the redundancy of molecular pathways. While future experimental studies may develop these new methods, current epidemiological, animal, and clinical studies strongly support the value of risk factor reduction as a primary method for preventing atherosclerosis progression and clinical events.

REFERENCES

1. Dzau VJ, Braun-Dullaeus RC, Sedding DG. Vascular proliferation and atherosclerosis: new perspectives and therapeutic strategies. Nat Med. 2002; 8:1249–1256.
2. Glass CK, Witztum JL. Atherosclerosis. the road ahead. Cell. 2001; 104:503–516.
3. Li AC, Glass CK. The macrophage foam cell as a target for therapeutic intervention. Nat Med. 2002; 8:1235–1242.
4. Libby P. Current concepts of the pathogenesis of the acute coronary syndromes. Circulation. 2001; 104:365–372.
5. Lusis AJ. Atherosclerosis. Nature. 2000; 407:233–241.
6. Steinberg D. Atherogenesis in perspective: hypercholesterolemia and inflammation as partners in crime. Nat Med. 2002; 8:1211–1217.
7. Plump AS, Smith JD, Hayek T, Aalto-Setala k, Walsh A, Verstuyft JG, Rubin EM, Breslow JL. Severe hypercholesterolemia and atherosclerosis in apolipoprotein E-deficient mice created by homologous recombination in ES cells. Cell. 1992; 71:343–353.
8. Ishibashi S, Goldstein JL, Brown MS, Herz J, Burns DK. Massive xanthomatosis and atherosclerosis in cholesterol-fed low density lipoprotein receptor-negative mice. J Clin Invest. 1994; 93:1885–1893.
9. Ishibashi S, Brown MS, Goldstein JL, Gerard RD, Hammer RE, Herz J. Hypercholesterolemia in low density lipoprotein receptor knockout mice and its reversal by adenovirus-mediated gene delivery. J Clin Invest. 1993; 92:883–893.
10. Cybulsky MI, Gimbrone MA, Jr. Endothelial expression of a mononuclear leukocyte adhesion molecule during atherogenesis. Science. 1991; 251:788–791.
11. Cybulsky MI, Iiyama K, Li H, Zhu S, Chen M, Iiyama M, Davis V, Gutierrez-Ramos JC, Connelly PW, Milstone DS. A major role for VCAM-1, but not ICAM-1, in early atherosclerosis. Journal of Clinical Investigation. 2001; 107:1255–1262.
12. Johnson RC, Chapman SM, Dong ZM, Ordovas JM, Mayadas TN, Herz J, Hynes RO, Schaefer EJ, Wagner DD. Absence of P-selectin delays fatty streak formation in mice. J Clin Invest. 1997; 99:1037–1043.
13. Richardson M, Gerrity RG, Alavi MZ, Moore S. Proteoglycan distribution in areas of differing permeability to Evans blue dye in the aortas of young pigs. An ultrastructural study. Arteriosclerosis. 1982; 2:369–379.
14. Kannel WB, Castelli WP, Gordon T. Cholesterol in the prediction of atherosclerotic disease. New perspectives based on the Framingham study. Ann Intern Med. 1979; 90:85–91.
15. Smith EB. Transport, interactions and retention of plasma proteins in the intima: the barrier function of the internal elastic lamina. Eur Heart J. 1990; 11 (suppl E):72–81.

16. Camejo G, Hurt-Camejo E, Wiklund O, Bondjers G. Association of apo B lipoproteins with arterial proteoglycans: pathological significance and molecular basis. Atherosclerosis. 1998; 139:205–222.

17. Skalen K, Gustafsson M, Rydberg EK, Hulten LM, Wiklund O, Innerarity TL, Boren J. Subendothelial retention of atherogenic lipoproteins in early atherosclerosis. Nature. 2002; 417:750–754.

18. Goldstein JL, Ho YK, Basu SK, Brown MS. Binding site on macrophages that mediates uptake and degradation of acetylated low density lipoprotein, producing massive cholesterol deposition. Proc Natl Acad Sci USA. 1979; 76:333–337.

19. Weinstein DB, Carew TE, Steinberg D. Uptake and degradation of low density lipoprotein by swine arterial smoot muscle cells with inhibition of cholesterol biosynthesis. Biochim Biophys Acta. 1976; 424:404–421.

20. Hurt-Camejo E, Camejo G, Rosengren B, Lopez F, Ahlstrom C, Fager G, Bondjers G. Effect of arterial proteoglycans and glycosaminoglycans on low density lipoprotein oxidation and its uptake by human macrophages and arterial smooth muscle cells. Arterioscler Thromb. 1992; 12:569–583.

21. Cyrus T, Witztum JL, Rader DJ, Tangirala R, Fazio S, Linton MF, Funk CD. Disruption of the 12/15–lipoxygenase gene diminishes atherosclerosis in apo E-deficient mice. Journal of Clinical Investigation. 1999; 103:1597–1604.

22. Kinlay S, Libby P, Ganz P. Endothelial function and coronary artery disease. Curr Opin Lipidol. 2001; 12:383–389.

23. Feron O, Dessy C, Moniotte S, Desager JP, Balligand JL. Hypercholesterolemia decreases nitric oxide production by promoting the interaction of caveolin and endothelial nitric oxide synthase. J Clin Invest. 1999; 103:897–905.

24. Harrison DG. Cellular and molecular mechanisms of endothelial cell dysfunction. J Clin Invest. 1997; 100:2153–2157.

25. Schachinger V, Britten MB, Zeiher AM. Prognostic impact of coronary vasodilator dysfunction on adverse long-term outcome of coronary heart disease. Circulation. 2000; 101:1899–1906.

26. Suwaidi JA, Hamasaki S, Higano ST, Nishimura RA, Holmes DR, Jr., Lerman A. Long-term follow-up of patients with mild coronary artery disease and endothelial dysfunction. Circulation. 2000; 101:948–594.

27. Gordon DJ, Probstfield JL, Garrison RJ, Neaton JD, Castelli WP, Knoke JD, Jacobs DR, Jr., Bangdiwala S, Tyroler HA. High-density lipoprotein cholesterol and cardiovascular disease. Four prospective American studies. Circulation. 1989; 79:8–15.

28. Yaari S, Goldbourt, Even-Zohar S, Neufeld HN. Associations of serum high density lipoprotein and total cholesterol with total, cardiovascular, and cancer mortality in a 7–year prospective study of 10 000 men. Lancet. 1981; 1:1011–1015.

29. Miller GJ, Miller NE. Plasma-high-density-lipoprotein concentration and development of ischaemic heart-disease. Lancet. 1975; 1:16–19.

30. Genest J. Lipoprotein disorders and cardiovascular risk. J Inherit Metab Dis. 2003; 26:267–287.

31. Oram JF, Yokoyama S. Apolipoprotein-mediated removal of cellular cholesterol and phospholipids. J Lipid Res. 1996; 37:2473–2491.

32. Barter PJ, Brewer HB, Jr., Chapman MJ, Hennekens CH, Rader DJ, Tall AR. Cholesteryl ester transfer protein: a novel target for raising HDL and inhibiting atherosclerosis. Arterioscler Thromb Vasc Biol. 2003; 23:160–167.

33. Chiesa G, Sirtori CR. Apolipoprotein A-I(Milano): current perspectives. Curr Opin Lipidol. 2003; 14:159–163.

34. Nissen SE, Tsunoda T, Tuzcu EM, Schoenhagen P, Cooper CJ, Yasin M, Eaton GM, Lauer MA, Sheldon WS, Grines CL, Halpern S, Crowe T, Blankenship JC, Kerensky R. Effect of recombinant ApoA-I Milano on coronary atherosclerosis in patients with acute coronary syndromes: a randomized controlled trial. JAMA. 2003; 290:2292–2300.

35. Mackness B, Durrington PN, Mackness MI. The paraoxonase gene family and coronary heart disease. Curr Opin Lipidol. 2002; 13:357–362.

36. Yuhanna IS, Zhu Y, Cox BE, Hahner LD, Osborne-Lawrence S, Lu P, Marcel YL, Anderson RG, Mendelsohn ME, Hobbs HH, Shaul PW. High-density lipoprotein binding to scavenger receptor-BI activates endothelial nitric oxide synthase. Nat Med. 2001; 7:853–857.

37. Libby P, Plutzky J. Diabetic macrovascular disease: the glucose paradox? Circulation. 2002; 106:2760–2763.

38. Li H, Cybulsky MI, Gimbrone MA, Jr., Libby P. An atherogenic diet rapidly induces VCAM-1, a cytokine-regulatable mononuclear leukocyte adhesion molecule, in rabbit aortic endothelium. Arterioscler Thromb. 1993; 13:197–204.

39. Luscinskas FW, Kansas GS, Ding H, Pizcueta P, Schleiffenbaum BE, Tedder TF, Gimbrone MA, Jr. Monocyte rolling, arrest and spreading on IL-4–activated vascular endothelium under flow is mediated via sequential action of L-selectin, beta 1–integrins, and beta 2–integrins. J Cell Biol. 1994; 125:1417–1427.

40. Springer TA. Traffic signals for lymphocyte recirculation and leukocyte emigration: the multistep paradigm. Cell. 1994; 76:301–314.

41. Cushing SD, Berliner JA, Valente AJ, Territo MC, Navab M, Parhami F, Gerrity R, Schwartz CJ, Fogelman AM. Minimally modified low density lipoprotein induces monocyte chemotactic protein 1 in human endothelial cells and smooth muscle cells. Proc Natl Acad Sci USA. 1990; 87:5134–5138.

42. Han KH, Han KO, Green SR, Quehenberger O. Expression of the monocyte chemoattractant protein-1 receptor CCR2 is increased in hypercholesterolemia. Differential effects of plasma lipoproteins on monocyte function. J Lipid Res. 1999; 40:1053–1063.

43. Barnes PJ, Karin M. Nuclear factor-kappaB: a pivotal transcription factor in chronic inflammatory diseases. N Engl J Med. 1997; 336:1066–1071.

44. Peng HB, Libby P, Liao JK. Induction and stabilization of I kappa B alpha by nitric oxide mediates inhibition of NF-kappa B. J Biol Chem. 1995; 270:14214–14219.

45. De Caterina R, Libby P, Peng HB, Thannickal VJ, Rajavashisth TB, Gimbrone MA, Jr., Shin WS, Liao JK. Nitric oxide decreases cytokine-induced endothelial activation. Nitric oxide selectively reduces endothelial expression of adhesion molecules and proinflammatory cytokines. J Clin Invest. 1995; 96:60–68.

46. Li D, Saldeen T, Romeo F, Mehta JL. Oxidized LDL upregulates angiotensin II type 1 receptor expression in cultured human coronary artery endothelial cells: the potential role of transcription factor NF-kappaB. Circulation. 2000; 102:1970–1976.

47. Cominacini L, Pasini AF, Garbin U, Davoli A, Tosetti ML, Campagnola M, Rigoni A, Pastorino AM, Lo Cascio V, Sawamura T. Oxidized low density lipoprotein (ox-LDL) binding to ox-LDL receptor-1 in endothelial cells induces the activation of NF-kappaB through an increased production of intracellular reactive oxygen species. J Biol Chem. 2000; 275:12633–12638.

48. Moulton KS, Semple K, Wu H, Glass CK. Cell-specific expression of the macrophage scavenger receptor gene is dependent on PU.1 and a composite AP-1/ets motif. Mol Cell Biol. 1994; 14:4408–4418.

49. Guidez F, Li AC, Horvai A, Welch JS, Glass CK. Differential utilization of Ras signaling pathways by macrophage colony-stimulating factor (CSF) and granulocyte-macrophage CSF receptors during macrophage differentiation. Mol Cell Biol. 1998; 18:3851–3861.

50. Suzuki OT, Sertie AL, Der Kaloustian VM, Kok F, Carpenter M, Murray J, Czeizel AE, Kliemann SE, Rosemberg S, Monteiro M, Olsen BR, Passos-Bueno MR. Molecular analysis of collagen XVIII reveals novel mutations, presence of a third isoform, and possible genetic heterogeneity in Knobloch syndrome. Am J Hum Genet. 2002; 71:1320–1329.

51. Febbraio M, Podrez EA, Smith JD, Hajjar DP, Hazen SL, Hoff HF, Sharma K, Silverstein RL. Targeted disruption of the class B scavenger receptor CD36 protects against atherosclerotic lesion development in mice. J Clin Invest. 2000; 105:1049–1056.

52. Endemann G, Stanton LW, Madden KS, Bryant CM, White RT, Protter AA. CD36 is a receptor for oxidized low density lipoprotein. J Biol Chem. 1993; 268:11811–6.

53. Kodama T, Reddy P, Kishimoto C, Krieger M. Purification and characterization of a bovine acetyl low density lipoprotein receptor. Proc Natl Acad Sci USA. 1988; 85:9238–9242.
54. Babior BM. Phagocytes and oxidative stress. Am J Med. 2000; 109:33–44.
55. Scheidegger KJ, Butler S, Witztum JL. Angiotensin II increases macrophage-mediated modification of low density lipoprotein via a lipoxygenase-dependent pathway. J Biol Chem. 1997; 272:21609–1615.
56. Welch JS, Ricote M, Akiyama TE, Gonzalez FJ, Glass CK. PPARgamma and PPARdelta negatively regulate specific subsets of lipopolysaccharide and IFN-gamma target genes in macrophages. Proc Nat Acad Sci USA. 2003; 100:6712–6717.
57. Boullier A, Bird DA, Chang MK, Dennis EA, Friedman P, Gillotre-Taylor K, Horkko S, Palinski W, Quehenberger O, Shaw P, Steinberg D, Terpstra V, Witztum JL. Scavenger receptors, oxidized LDL, and atherosclerosis. Ann N Y Acad Sci. 2001; 947:214–223.
58. Binder CJ, Chang MK, Shaw PX, Miller YI, Hartvigsen K, Dewan A, Witztum JL. Innate and acquired immunity in atherogenesis. Nat Med. 2002; 8:1218–1226.
59. Brogi E, Winkles JA, Underwood R, Clinton SK, Alberts GF, Libby P. Distinct patterns of expression of fibroblast growth factors and their receptors in human atheroma and nonatherosclerotic arteries. Association of acidic FGF with plaque microvessels and macrophages. J Clin Invest. 1993; 92:2408–2418.
60. Couffinhal T, Kearney M, Witzenbichler B, Chen D, Murohara T, Losordo DW, Symes J, Isner JM. Vascular endothelial growth factor/vascular permeability factor (VEGF/VPF) in normal and atherosclerotic human arteries. Am J Pathol. 1997; 150:1673–1685.
61. Smith JD, Bryant SR, Couper LL, Vary CP, Gotwals PJ, Koteliansky VE, Lindner V. Soluble transforming growth factor-beta type II receptor inhibits negative remodeling, fibroblast transdifferentiation, and intimal lesion formation but not endothelial growth. Circ Res. 1999; 84:1212–1222.
62. Nikol S, Isner JM, Pickering JG, Kearney M, Leclerc G, Weir L. Expression of transforming growth factor-beta 1 is increased in human vascular restenosis lesions. J Clin Invest. 1992; 90:1582–1592.
63. Ingber DE. Mechanical signaling and the cellular response to extracellular matrix in angiogenesis and cardiovascular physiology. Circ Res. 2002; 91:877–887.
64. Gordon D, Reidy MA, Benditt EP, Schwartz SM. Cell proliferation in human coronary arteries. Proc Nat Acad Sci USA. 1990; 87:4600–4460.
65. Chung IM, Schwartz SM, Murry CE. Clonal architecture of normal and atherosclerotic aorta: implications for atherogenesis and vascular development. Am J Pathol. 1998; 152:913–923.
66. Sata M, Saiura A, Kunisato A, Tojo A, Okada S, Tokuhisa T, Hirai H, Makuuchi M, Hirata Y, Nagai R. Hematopoietic stem cells differentiate into vascular cells that participate in the pathogenesis of atherosclerosis. Nat Med. 2002; 8:403–409.
67. Quaini F, Urbanek K, Beltrami AP, Finato N, Beltrami CA, Nadal-Ginard B, Kajstura J, Leri A, Anversa P. Chimerism of the transplanted heart. N Engl J Med. 2002; 346:5–15.
68. Falk E, Shah PK, Fuster V. Coronary plaque disruption. Circulation. 1995; 92:657–671.
69. Farb A, Tang AL, Burke AP, Sessums L, Liang Y, Virmani R. Sudden coronary death. Frequency of active coronary lesions, inactive coronary lesions, and myocardial infarction. Circulation. 1995; 92:1701–1709.
70. Burke AP, Farb A, Malcom GT, Liang YH, Smialek J, Virmani R. Coronary risk factors and plaque morphology in men with coronary disease who died suddenly [see comments]. N Engl J Med. 1997; 336:1276–1282.
71. Braun-Dullaeus RC, Mann MJ, Ziegler A, von der Leyen HE, Dzau VJ. A novel role for the cyclin-dependent kinase inhibitor p27(Kip1) in angiotensin II-stimulated vascular smooth muscle cell hypertrophy. J Clin Invest. 1999; 104:815–823.
72. Hiromura K, Pippin JW, Fero ML, Roberts JM, Shankland SJ. Modulation of apoptosis by the cyclin-dependent kinase inhibitor p27(Kip1). J Clin Invest. 1999; 103:597–604.
73. Morice MC, Serruys PW, Sousa JE, Fajadet J, Ban Hayashi E, Perin M, Colombo A, Schuler G, Barragan P, Guagliumi G, Molnar F, Falotico R. A randomized comparison of a sirolimus-

eluting stent with a standard stent for coronary revascularization. N Engl J Med. 2002; 346:1773–1780.

74. Moses JW, Leon MB, Popma JJ, Fitzgerald PJ, Holmes DR, O'Shaughnessy C, Caputo RP, Kereiakes DJ, Williams DO, Teirstein PS, Jaeger JL, Kuntz RE. Sirolimus-eluting stents versus standard stents in patients with stenosis in a native coronary artery. N Engl J Med. 2003; 349:1315–1323.

75. Palinski W, Ord VA, Plump AS, Breslow JL, Steinberg D, Witztum JL. ApoE-deficient mice are a model of lipoprotein oxidation in atherogenesis. Demonstration of oxidation-specific epitopes in lesions and high titers of autoantibodies to malondialdehyde-lysine in serum. Arterioscl Thrombosis. 1994; 14:605–616.

76. Palinski W, Tangirala RK, Miller E, Young SG, Witztum JL. Increased autoantibody titers against epitopes of oxidized LDL in LDL receptor-deficient mice with increased atherosclerosis. Arterioscl Thrombosis Vasc Biol. 1995; 15:1569–1576.

77. Smith JD, Trogan E, Ginsberg M, Grigaux C, Tian J, Miyata M. Decreased atherosclerosis in mice deficient in both macrophage colony-stimulating factor (op) and apolipoprotein E. Proc Nat Acad Sci USA. 1995; 92:8264–8268.

78. Dansky HM, Charlton SA, Harper MM, Smith JD. T and B lymphocytes play a minor role in atherosclerotic plaque formation in the apolipoprotein E-deficient mouse. Proc Nat Acad Sci USA. 1997; 94:4642–4646.

79. Galis ZS, Muszynski M, Sukhova GK, Simon-Morrissey E, Unemori EN, Lark MW, Amento E, Libby P. Cytokine-stimulated human vascular smooth muscle cells synthesize a complement of enzymes required for extracellular matrix digestion. Circ Res. 1994; 75:181–189.

80. Tontonoz P, Nagy L, Alvarez JG, Thomazy VA, Evans RM. PPARgamma promotes monocyte/macrophage differentiation and uptake of oxidized LDL. Cell. 1998; 93:241–252.

81. Gupta S, Pablo AM, Jiang X, Wang N, Tall AR, Schindler C. IFN-gamma potentiates atherosclerosis in ApoE knock-out mice. J Clin Invest 1997; 99:2752–2761.

82. Amento EP, Ehsani N, Palmer H, Libby P. Cytokines and growth factors positively and negatively regulate interstitial collagen gene expression in human vascular smooth muscle cells. Arterioscler Thromb. 1991; 11:1223–1230.

83. Mach F, Schonbeck U, Sukhova GK, Bourcier T, Bonnefoy JY, Pober JS, Libby P. Functional CD40 ligand is expressed on human vascular endothelial cells, smooth muscle cells, and macrophages: implications for CD40–CD40 ligand signaling in atherosclerosis. Proc Natl Acad Sci U S A. 1997; 94:1931–1936.

84. Lutgens E, Gorelik L, Daemen MJ, de Muinck ED, Grewal IS, Koteliansky VE, Flavell RA. Requirement for CD154 in the progression of atherosclerosis. Nat Med. 1999; 5:1313–1316.

85. Mach F, Schonbeck U, Sukhova GK, Atkinson E, Libby P. Reduction of atherosclerosis in mice by inhibition of CD40 signalling. Nature. 1998; 394:200–203.

86. Schonbeck U, Sukhova GK, Shimizu K, Mach F, Libby P. Inhibition of CD40 signaling limits evolution of established atherosclerosis in mice. Proc Natl Acad Sci U S A. 2000; 97:7458–463.

87. Kwon HM, Sangiorgi G, Ritman EL, McKenna C, Holmes DR, Jr., Schwartz RS, Lerman A. Enhanced coronary vasa vasorum neovascularization in experimental hypercholesterolemia. J Clin Invest. 1998; 101:1551–1556.

88. Herrmann J, Lerman LO, Rodriguez-Porcel M, Holmes DR, Jr., Richardson DM, Ritman EL, Lerman A. Coronary vasa vasorum neovascularization precedes epicardial endothelial dysfunction in experimental hypercholesterolemia. Cardiovascular Research. 2001; 51:762–766.

89. Moulton KS, Heller E, Konerding MA, Flynn E, Palinski W, Folkman J. Angiogenesis inhibitors endostatin or TNP-470 reduce intimal neovascularization and plaque growth in apolipoprotein E-deficient mice. Circulation. 1999; 99:1726–1732.

90. Celletti FL, Waugh JM, Amabile PG, Brendolan A, Hilfiker PR, Dake MD. Vascular endothelial growth factor enhances atherosclerotic plaque progression. Nature Medicine. 2001; 7:425–429.

91. Heeschen C, Jang JJ, Weis M, Pathak A, Kaji S, Hu RS, Tsao PS, Johnson FL, Cooke JP. Nicotine stimulates angiogenesis and promotes tumor growth and atherosclerosis. Nat Med. 2001; 7:833–839.

92. Williams JK, Armstrong ML, Heistad DD. Blood flow through new microvessels: factors that affect regrowth of vasa vasorum. Am J Physiol. 1988; 254:H126–132.

93. Kumamoto M, Nakashima Y, Sueishi K. Intimal neovascularization in human coronary atherosclerosis: its origin and pathophysiological significance. Hum Pathol. 1995; 26:450–456.

94. Moulton KS, Vakili K, Zurakowski D, Soliman M, Butterfield C, Sylvin E, Lo KM, Gillies S, Javaherian K, Folkman J. Inhibition of plaque neovascularization reduces macrophage accumulation and progression of advanced atherosclerosis. Proc Natl Acad Sci USA. 2003; 100:4736–4741.

95. Williams JK, Armstrong ML, Heistad DD. Vasa vasorum in atherosclerotic coronary arteries: responses to vasoactive stimuli and regression of atherosclerosis. Circ Res. 1988; 62:515–523.

96. Williams JK, Sukhova GK, Herrington DM, Libby P. Pravastatin has cholesterol-lowering independent effects on the artery wall of atherosclerotic monkeys. J Am Coll Cardiol. 1998; 31:684–691.

97. Polverini PJ, Cotran PS, Gimbrone MA, Jr., Unanue ER. Activated macrophages induce vascular proliferation. Nature. 1977; 269:804–806.

98. Auerbach R, Sidky YA. Nature of the stimulus leading to lymphocyte-induced angiogenesis. J Immunol. 1979; 123:751–754.

99. O'Brien ER, Garvin MR, Dev R, Stewart DK, Hinohara T, Simpson JB, Schwartz SM. Angiogenesis in human coronary atherosclerotic plaques. Am J Pathol. 1994; 145:883–894.

100. Luttun A, Tjwa M, Moons L, Wu Y, Angelillo-Scherrer A, Liao F, Nagy JA, Hooper A, Priller J, De Klerck B, Compernolle V, Daci E, Bohlen P, Dewerchin M, Herbert JM, Fava R, Matthys P, Carmeliet G, Collen D, Dvorak HF, Hicklin DJ, Carmeliet P. Revascularization of ischemic tissues by PlGF treatment, and inhibition of tumor angiogenesis, arthritis and atherosclerosis by anti-Flt1. Nat Med. 2002; 8:831–840.

101. Roth JJ, Gahtan V, Brown JL, Gerhard C, Swami VK, Rothman VL, Tulenko TN, Tuszynski GP. Thrombospondin-1 is elevated with both intimal hyperplasia and hypercholesterolemia. J Surg Res. 1998; 74:11–16.

102. Miosge N, Sasaki T, Timpl R. Angiogenesis inhibitor endostatin is a distinct component of elastic fibers in vessel walls. FASEB J. 1999; 13:1743–1750.

103. Galis ZS, Sukhova GK, Lark MW, Libby P. Increased expression of matrix metalloproteinases and matrix degrading activity in vulnerable regions of human atherosclerotic plaques. J Clin Invest. 1994; 94:2493–503.

104. Nikkari ST, O'Brien KD, Ferguson M, Hatsukami T, Welgus HG, Alpers CE, Clowes AW. Interstitial collagenase (MMP-1) expression in human carotid atherosclerosis. Circulation. 1995; 92:1393–1398.

105. Sukhova GK, Schonbeck U, Rabkin E, Schoen FJ, Poole AR, Billinghurst RC, Libby P. Evidence for increased collagenolysis by interstitial collagenases-1 and -3 in vulnerable human atheromatous plaques. Circulation. 1999; 99:2503–2509.

106. Rajagopalan S, Meng XP, Ramasamy S, Harrison DG, Galis ZS. Reactive oxygen species produced by macrophage-derived foam cells regulate the activity of vascular matrix metalloproteinases in vitro. Implications for atherosclerotic plaque stability. J Clin Invest. 1996; 98:2572–2579.

107. Frears ER, Zhang Z, Blake DR, O'Connell JP, Winyard PG. Inactivation of tissue inhibitor of metalloproteinase-1 by peroxynitrite. FEBS Lett. 1996; 381:21–24.

108. Glagov S, Weisenberg E, Zarins CK, Stankunavicius R, Kolettis GJ. Compensatory enlargement of human atherosclerotic coronary arteries. N Engl J Med. 1987; 316:1371–1375.

109. Galis ZS, Khatri JJ. Matrix metalloproteinases in vascular remodeling and atherogenesis: the good, the bad, and the ugly. Circ Res. 2002; 90:251–262.

110. Henney AM, Wakeley PR, Davies MJ, Foster K, Hembry R, Murphy G, Humphries S. Localization of stromelysin gene expression in atherosclerotic plaques by in situ hybridization. Proc Natl Acad Sci USA. 1991; 88:8154–1858.

111. Schoenhagen P, Vince DG, Ziada KM, Kapadia SR, Lauer MA, Crowe TD, Nissen SE, Tuzcu EM. Relation of matrix-metalloproteinase 3 found in coronary lesion samples retrieved by directional coronary atherectomy to intravascular ultrasound observations on coronary remodeling. Am J Cardiol. 2002; 89:1354–1359.

112. Pasterkamp G, Schoneveld AH, Hijnen DJ, de Kleijn DP, Teepen H, van der Wal AC, Borst C. Atherosclerotic arterial remodeling and the localization of macrophages and matrix metalloproteases 1, 2 and 9 in the human coronary artery. Atherosclerosis. 2000; 150:245–253.

113. Godin D, Ivan E, Johnson C, Magid R, Galis ZS. Remodeling of carotid artery is associated with increased expression of matrix metalloproteinases in mouse blood flow cessation model. Circulation. 2000; 102:2861–2866.

114. Kuzuya M, Kanda S, Sasaki T, Tamaya-Mori N, Cheng XW, Itoh T, Itohara S, Iguchi A. Deficiency of gelatinase a suppresses smooth muscle cell invasion and development of experimental intimal hyperplasia. Circulation. 2003.

115. Galis ZS, Johnson C, Godin D, Magid R, Shipley JM, Senior RM, Ivan E. Targeted disruption of the matrix metalloproteinase-9 gene impairs smooth muscle cell migration and geometrical arterial remodeling. Circ Res. 2002; 91:852–859.

116. Tauth J, Pinnow E, Sullebarger JT, Basta L, Gursoy S, Lindsay J, Jr., Matar F. Predictors of coronary arterial remodeling patterns in patients with myocardial ischemia. Am J Cardiol. 1997; 80:1352–1355.

117. Kornowski R, Lansky AJ, Mintz GS, Kent KM, Pichard AD, Satler LF, Bucher TA, Popma JJ, Leon MB. Comparison of men versus women in cross-sectional area luminal narrowing, quantity of plaque, presence of calcium in plaque, and lumen location in coronary arteries by intravascular ultrasound in patients with stable angina pectoris. Am J Cardiol. 1997; 79:1601–1605.

118. Gimbrone MA, Jr., Topper JN, Nagel T, Anderson KR, Garcia-Cardena G. Endothelial dysfunction, hemodynamic forces, and atherogenesis. Ann N Y Acad Sci. 2000; 902:230–240.

119. Uematsu M, Ohara Y, Navas JP, Nishida K, Murphy TJ, Alexander RW, Nerem RM, Harrison DG. Regulation of endothelial cell nitric oxide synthase mRNA expression by shear stress. Am J Physiol. 1995; 269:C1371–1378.

120. Tsao PS, Buitrago R, Chan JR, Cooke JP. Fluid flow inhibits endothelial adhesiveness. Nitric oxide and transcriptional regulation of VCAM-1. Circulation. 1996; 94:1682–1689.

121. Malek A, Izumo S. Physiological fluid shear stress causes downregulation of endothelin-1 mRNA in bovine aortic endothelium. Am J Physiol. 1992; 263:C389–296.

122. Ueba H, Kawakami M, Yaginuma T. Shear stress as an inhibitor of vascular smooth muscle cell proliferation. Role of transforming growth factor-beta 1 and tissue-type plasminogen activator. Arterioscler Thromb Vasc Biol. 1997; 17:1512–1516.

123. Kinlay S, Grewal J, Manuelin D, Fang JC, Selwyn AP, Bittl JA, Ganz P. Coronary flow velocity and disturbed flow predict adverse clinical outcome after coronary angioplasty. Arterioscler Thromb Vasc Biol. 2002; 22:1334–1340.

124. Stone PH, Coskun AU, Kinlay S, Clark ME, Sonka M, Wahle A, Ilegbusi OJ, Yeghiazarians Y, Popma JJ, Orav J, Kuntz RE, Feldman CL. Effect of endothelial shear stress on the progression of coronary artery disease, vascular remodeling, and in-stent restenosis in humans: in vivo 6–month follow-up study. Circulation. 2003; 108:438–444.

125. Davies MJ. Stability and instability: two faces of coronary atherosclerosis. The Paul Dudley White Lecture 1995. Circulation. 1996; 94:2013–2020.

126. Richardson PD, Davies MJ, Born GV. Influence of plaque configuration and stress distribution on fissuring of coronary atherosclerotic plaques. Lancet. 1989; 2:941–944.

127. Cheng GC, Loree HM, Kamm RD, Fishbein MC, Lee RT. Distribution of circumferential stress in ruptured and stable atherosclerotic lesions. A structural analysis with histopathological correlation. Circulation. 1993; 87:1179–1187.

128. Thogersen AM, Jansson JH, Boman K, Nilsson TK, Weinehall L, Huhtasaari F, Hallmans G. High plasminogen activator inhibitor and tissue plasminogen activator levels in plasma precede a first acute myocardial infarction in both men and women: evidence for the fibrinolytic system as an independent primary risk factor. Circulation. 1998; 98:2241–2247.

129. Methia N, Andre P, Denis CV, Economopoulos M, Wagner DD. Localized reduction of atherosclerosis in von Willebrand factor-deficient mice. Blood. 2001; 98:1424–1428.

130. Kinlay S, Behrendt D, Wainstein M, Beltrame J, Fang JC, Creager MA, Selwyn AP, Ganz P. Role of endothelin-1 in the active constriction of human atherosclerotic coronary arteries. Circulation. 2001; 104:1114–1118.

131. Ludmer PL, Selwyn AP, Shook TL, Wayne RR, Mudge GH, Alexander RW, Ganz P. Paradoxical vasoconstriction induced by acetylcholine in atherosclerotic coronary arteries. N Engl J Med. 1986; 315:1046–1051.

132. Bostrom K, Watson KE, Horn S, Wortham C, Herman IM, Demer LL. Bone morphogenetic protein expression in human atherosclerotic lesions. J Clin Invest. 1993; 91:1800–1809.

133. Bini A, Mann KG, Kudryk BJ, Schoen FJ. Noncollagenous bone matrix proteins, calcification, and thrombosis in carotid artery atherosclerosis. Arterioscler Thromb Vasc Biol. 1999; 19:1852–1861.

134. Beckman JA, Ganz J, Creager MA, Ganz P, Kinlay S. Relationship of clinical presentation and calcification of culprit coronary artery stenoses. Arterioscler Thromb Vasc Biol. 2001; 21:1618–1622.

135. Kolodgie FD, Gold HK, Burke AP, Fowler DR, Kruth HS, Weber DK, Farb A, Guerrero LJ, Hayase M, Kutys R, Narula J, Finn AV, Virmani R. Intraplaque hemorrhage and progression of coronary atheroma. N Engl J Med. 2003; 349:2316–2325.

136. Burke AP, Kolodgie FD, Farb A, Weber DK, Malcom GT, Smialek J, Virmani R. Healed plaque ruptures and sudden coronary death: evidence that subclinical rupture has a role in plaque progression. Circulation. 2001; 103:934–940.

137. van der Wal AC, Becker AE, van der Loos CM, Das PK. Site of intimal rupture or erosion of thrombosed coronary atherosclerotic plaques is characterized by an inflammatory process irrespective of the dominant plaque morphology. Circulation. 1994; 89:36–44.

138. Farb A, Burke AP, Tang AL, Liang TY, Mannan P, Smialek J, Virmani R. Coronary plaque erosion without rupture into a lipid core. A frequent cause of coronary thrombosis in sudden coronary death. Circulation. 1996; 93:1354–1363.

II. CLINICAL PHARMACOLOGY

4-1

Fundamental Concepts in Pharmacokinetics and Pharmacodynamics of Fibrinolytic Agents

Michael F. Caron and C. Michael White

Hartford Hospital, Hartford, Connecticut; and University of Connecticut School of Pharmacy, Storrs, Connecticut, U.S.A.

I. INTRODUCTION

Atherosclerotic plaque disruption with resultant coronary thrombosis is the predominant cause of acute myocardial infarction (AMI) (1). It is now evident that thrombolysis recanalizes the thrombotic occlusion associated with AMI, restores coronary flow improving myocardial function, and reduces mortality. Four thrombolytic agents are currently approved by the U.S. Food and Drug Administration (FDA) for intravenous (IV) use in patients with AMI (2,3). They are Class I interventions in the ACC/AHA Guidelines for the Management of Patients with Acute Myocardial Infarction (4). This indicates that there is evidence and/or general agreement that a given treatment is beneficial, useful, and effective.

Drug manufacturers have focused on developing thrombolytics with a rapid onset of action to establish artery patency, an adequate half-life for convenience of bolus administration and maintenance of coronary artery patency, and increased fibrin specificity resulting in less bleeding complications. When selecting an agent, clinicians should consider several pharmacokinetic (PK) and pharmacodynamic (PD) parameters such as these. This chapter will (a) assess the available efficacy trials performed in patients with acute myocardial infarction, (b) evaluate the PK and PD differences among the available thrombolytic agents, and (c) define how these agent-specific PK/PD features correlate to improved thrombolytic efficacy and safety.

II. EFFICACY TRIALS

Coronary artery patency trials have shown differences among streptokinase (STK; AstraZeneca, Wayne, PA), alteplase (rt-PA; Genentech Inc., South San Francisco, CA), reteplase (r-PA; Centocor Inc, Malvern, PA), and tenecteplase (TNK; Genentech Inc.). However, most of the landmark efficacy trials in AMI demonstrated similar survival benefit between thrombolytics.

The only survival trial that did show significant benefit of one agent over another was the first Global Use of Streptokinase and Tissue Plasminogen Activator for

Occluded Coronary Arteries (GUSTO I) trial (5). In this trial, rt-PA demonstrated a 6.3% 30-day mortality rate compared with 7.3% with STK ($p = 0.001$). This disparity was markedly reduced if the time to treatment was greater than 6 hours if it was not an anterior myocardial infarction (MI) and if the patient was greater than 75 years of age. In fact, the mortality was 10.4% in the rt-PA group compared with 8.3% in the STK group if the time to thrombolytic therapy was greater than 6 hours ($p =$ NS). Streptokinase also caused less hemorrhagic stroke overall than t-PA ($p = 0.03$) as well as in a subgroup of patients over the age of 75. The frequency of noncerebral systemic bleeding was more favorable with rt-PA. In another study, International Joint Efficacy Comparison of Thrombolytics (INJECT), 35-day mortality was 9.02% with r-PA and 9.53% with STK, a nonsignificant difference (6). In-hospital stroke rates were non-significantly higher in the r-PA group (1.23%) compared with the STK group (1.00%).

Why a significant benefit was found comparing rt-PA versus STK (GUSTO I trial) and not found comparing r-PA versus STK (INJECT trial) may be due to time to treatment. Earlier time to treatment with thrombolytic therapy corresponds to improved reductions in mortality, infarct size, and improved left ventricular (LV) function (7–9). Interestingly, thrombolytic therapy was administered more than 6 hours after symptom onset in approximately 20% of patients in the INJECT trial versus only 4% in the GUSTO trial.

The next two multicenter trials included subjects with infarct durations of less than 6 hours. The third Global Use of Strategies to Open Occluded Coronary Arteries (GUSTO III) trial demonstrated no difference in the 30-day mortality rate between r-PA and rt-PA (7.47% and 7.24%, respectively; $p = 0.54$)(10). Mortality was 9.7% in the r-PA group compared with 7.9% in the rt-PA group if treatment was greater than 4 hours after the onset of symptoms ($p = 0.07$). In addition, high-risk patients (age > 75 years, anterior MI) had slightly higher mortality with r-PA than with rt-PA ($p =$ NS). Similar bleeding risk for r-PA and rt-PA was demonstrated.

Finally, the second Assessment of the Safety of a New Thrombolytic (the ASSENT II) trial showed that TNK reduced 30-day mortality to a similar extent as rt-PA (6.18% vs. 6.15%, respectively)(11). However, mortality was significantly lower in the TNK group (7.0%) than the rt-PA group (9.2%) if the time to treatment was greater than 4 hours ($p = 0.018$). There were fewer noncerebral bleeding complications (26.43% vs. 28.95%; $p = 0.0003$) and less need for blood transfusion (4.25% vs. 5.49%; $p = 0.0002$) in the TNK group compared with the rt-PA group. No studies have been conducted comparing r-PA with TNK. Dosing of these agents in AMI trials are listed in Table 1.

Survival trials have established that STK, rt-PA, r-PA, and TNK are safe and effective agents for use in AMI. As of March 2001, the Average Wholesale Prices (AWP) of rt-PA, r-PA, and TNK were similar and priced at approximately $2,700 per agent(12). This is in sharp contrast to the AWP of STK, which is approximately $500. However, results of the GUSTO I trial provide us with clinical evidence that rt-PA is preferred over STK. The remaining thrombolytics have shown comparable clinical trial results and pricing, thus, agent selection should be based on other distinctive features of the drugs.

III. PHARMACOKINETIC PROPERTIES OF THROMBOLYTICS

The available thrombolytic agents differ markedly with respect to their PK profiles (Table 2). Notably, some thrombolytics have longer half-lives and lower plasma clearances that

Table 1 Dosing of IV Fribrinolytic Agents in Acute Myocardial Infarction

Drug	Patient weight (kg)	Recommended dosage	Ref.
STK	All weights	1.5 million U in 30–60 min	5,6
rt-PA	≤67	15 mg bolus, followed by 0.75 mg/kg infusion × 30 min; conclude with 0.50 mg/kg infusion × 60 min; not to exceed 100 mg	5,10
	≥67	15 mg bolus, followed by 50 mg infusion × 30 min; conclude with 35 mg infusion × 60 min; not to exceed 100 mg	
r-PA (*bolus doses administered 30 minutes apart over 2 minutes*)	All weights	10 U + 10 U	6, 10
TNK (*bolus dose administered over 5–10 seconds*)	< 60	30 mg	11
	60-69	35 mg	
	70-79	40 mg	
	80-89	45 mg	
	> 90	50 mg	

may influence dosage and administration. Thus, pharmacokinetics must be considered when comparing and evaluating these agents. However, very few thorough PK investigations of thrombolytic drugs have been conducted, and many of the available studies use different methodologies to assess PK profiles.

A. Absorption and Distribution

STK, rt-PA, r-PA, and TNK have large molecular sizes. This impedes diffusion across biological membranes, and they must be administered intravenously (13). Because they are given intravenously, bioavailability is considered to be 100%. Streptokinase and rt-PA require IV infusions to obtain adequate steady-state levels (13). Peak plasma concentration levels of r-PA and TNK are obtained in less than 10 minutes with IV double and single bolus doses, respectively (14,15).

Despite STK's longstanding use clinically, its PK profile is the least investigated in the thrombolytic class. In a PK study of STK, Grierson and Bjornsson determined plasma STK levels based on the amidolytic activity of the activator complex on a chromogenic substrate (16). When plasmin's activity on the chromogenic substrate is blocked by a protease inhibitor, the resulting rate of amidolysis has been shown to be a reflection of the activator complex activity present. This assay demonstrated that over the range of plasma STK concentrations from 12.5 to 800 U/mL, a linear relationship existed between the amount of STK added to plasma and the rate of amidolysis of chromogenic substrate.

More recent PK studies of thrombolytics have investigated both the activity and antigen concentration to determine the relevant parameter for pharmacological action.

Table 2 Fribrinolytic Parameters of Fibrinolytic Agents in Patients with Acute Myocardial Infarction

Agent	Dose	C_{max} (mg/mL)	Cl (mL/min)	V_{ss} (L)	$T_{1/2\alpha}$ (min)	$T_{1/2\beta}$ (min)	AUC_a (%)	Ref
STK	1.5×10^6 IU[a]	3.85 ± 1.18	118 ± 48.5	5.68 ± 2.29	N/A[b]	36.6 ± 14.4	N/A[b]	53
rt-PA	100 mg[c]	4 ± 1	572 ± 132	8.4 ± 5	3.5 ± 1.4	72 ± 68	85	17
r-PA	10 U + 10 U	3.38	283 ± 101	39.3 ± 18.8	14.4 ± 6.6	97.8 ± 39	>80	24
TNK	30 mg	10.0 ± 7.3	98.5 ± 42	6.34 ± 3.3	21.5 ± 8.2	116 ± 63	72	24
	40 mg	10.9 ± 11	119 ± 49	8.01 ± 5.9	23.8 ± 5.5	129 ± 87	75	
	50 mg	15.2 ± 12	99.9 ± 32	6.12 ± 2.4	20.1 ± 10	90.4 ± 35	66	

C_{max}, maximum plasma concentration; Cl, plasma clearance; V_{ss}, steady-state volume of distribution; $T_{1/2\beta}$, initial half-life; $T_{1/2\beta}$, terminal half-life; AUC_a, area under the curve associated with the initial half-life: N/A, not available.

[a]Infused intravenously over 60 minutes.

[b]Postpeak decline in concentration was mono-exponential.

[c]15 mg was infused in 2 min, followed by 50 mg in 30 min and 35 mg in 60 min.

When measuring plasma levels, activity reflects only functionally active molecules, whereas antigen concentrations represent active and inactive molecules (14). One study with rt-PA demonstrated that steady-state plasma concentrations based on rt-PA functional activity were approximately 30% lower than antigen concentrations, and therefore the clearance calculated from functional activity was correspondingly higher (17).

The PK behavior of rt-PA provides a good correlation between the dose and serum concentration. An accelerated infusion of rt-PA (given over a period of 90 minutes) demonstrated that the antigen concentrations in plasma reached a maximum of 4 mg/mL after the 15 mg bolus injection, maintained an initial steady state value of 3.2 mg/mL during the first infusion of 50 mg over 30 minutes, and decreased to a second steady state of 1.08 mg/mL during the subsequent infusion of 35 mg over 60 minutes (17). The initial steady-state value during the accelerated infusion was 45% higher in terms of the antigen concentration than during the standard 3-hour infusion regimen. This may explain the results found in the GISSI-2 trial that found no difference in mortality between the use of STK and rt-PA administered over 3 hours (18). The authors of this study theorized that the elevated initial plasma concentration of rt-PA is the primary determinant of high early coronary artery patency and that the principal function of the maintenance infusions is the prevention of reocclusion.

Reteplase's pharmacokinetics are well defined, but much of the primary PK litera-ture describing its PK profile consist of data on file at Centocor, Inc. and was not made available to the authors. Since there is not a steady-state concentration after bolus injec-tion, the AUC of r-PA activity was used as a correlate for its effectiveness in terms of thrombolytic effect. Animal models have demonstrated the that the AUC increases linearly with increasing doses of r-PA (19,20). In addition, the AUC and maximum plasma con-centration increased in a reasonably linear manner with dose in both healthy volunteers and patients with AMI unpublished, Steven J. Mack, Pharm.D., Centocor, Inc.)

Because rt-PA is a fibrin-specific agent, it was used to define the equieffective dose of r-PA. An animal model of coronary artery thrombosis demonstrated that a bolus dose of r-PA would achieve similar clinical effects (a patency rate of about 70% at 90 minutes and an acceptably low bleeding risk) as a conventionally infused dose of rt-PA (3-hour infusion regimen) (14). The study also found that the AUC for r-PA after doses equieffective to rt-PA was about 30% lower than that of rt-PA. It has been hypothesized that some of the rt-PA dose is lost after bolus injection because of its short half-life and that high peak drug concentrations have to be achieved in order to have thrombolytically active plasma rt-PA concentrations. Another explanation is that r-PA easily penetrates into the clot, whereas rt-PA is tightly bound to the fibrin matrix and primarily accumu-lates at the surface of the clot. A dose-ranging study found that the target AUC for reteplase activity to achieve about a 70% patency rate was calculated to be 700 mUΣh/L (21). This and previous PK studies were the foundation for the single IV bolus injection of 10 units for a clinical starting dose. However, the GRECO study (22) demonstrated that the predefined minimal 90-minute patency of 70% required by the protocol was not achieved. In addition, the RAPID study (23) showed superior patency rates with a double bolus regimen of 10 + 10 units compared to a single bolus of 15 units and a double bolus of 10 + 5 units. Hence, the 10 + 10 unit strategy was established and is cur-rently recommended clinically.

With regard to TNK, mean observed peak plasma concentration escalated with increasing dose in the 30–50 mg dose range (24). The initial plasma concentration using antigen concentrations for doses of 30, 40, and 50 mg were 10, 10.9, and 15.2 mg/mL respectively. However, a study evaluating the dose of TNK and the AUC showed a trend towards nonlinear pharmacokinetics (15). When comparing rt-PA (accelerated dose regimen) to TNK (single bolus of 30, 40, or 50 mg over 5–10 seconds), plasma concentrations after a single bolus dose of TNK were initially higher but the AUC approximates that of rt-PA (25).

B. Metabolism and Elimination

Alteplase, r-PA, and TNK plasma concentrations decrease in a biphasic manner, with a more prominent initial a-phase half-life compared with the slower terminal b-phase half-life (13). The initial phase is dominant, accounting for up to 85, > 80, and 69% of the total AUC for rt-PA, r-PA, and TNK, respectively (13,15,17). STK activity is characterized by a monoexponential decline (16).

The half-life of STK was not related to the doses administered. The average half-life was 82 minutes but ranged from 34 to 116 minutes in one study (16). The clearance averaged 10.8 mL/min (ranging from 2.75 to 29.3 mL/min), and the apparent volume of distribution averaged 1.10 L (ranging from 0.265 to 2.81 L). The clearance and apparent volume of distribution demonstrated high interpatient variability, with an approximate 10-fold variation for both parameters.

Drug resistance is a result of the production of neutralizing antibodies that reduces a drug's effectiveness. A positive correlation between STK resistance and the apparent volume of distribution ($p = 0.028$) and STK resistance and clearance ($p = 0.047$) was found (16). Low STK plasma levels were associated with high STK resistance, small AUC, high clearance, and a large apparent volume of distribution. Conversely, higher plasma STK levels had low STK resistance, large AUC, low clearance, and a small apparent volume of distribution. High STK resistance was associated with decreased fibrinolytic activity as well.

Among fibrin-specific thrombolytic agents, r-PA and TNK's longer half-lives allow them to be administered as IV boluses as opposed to rt-PA's IV infusion. A PK study of 30 mg of TNK (15) revealed a fourfold slower plasma clearance (143 mL/min) than that obtained in a PK evaluation of accelerated doses of rt-PA (17) (572 mL/min) in patients with AMI. The clearance for r-PA is somewhat in between that of rt-PA and TNK. Following a 10 unit dose of r-PA, the clearance was 283 mL/min (26). The slower plasma clearance of TNK compared to rt-PA and r-PA is a result of its longer initial a-phase half-life (18 ± 8, 3.5 ± 1.4, and 14.4 ± 6.6, respectively) (15,17,26). This effect is also partially explained by TNK's smaller percentage of drug cleared during the initial half-life (69, 85, and > 80% for TNK, rt-PA, and r-PA, respectively) (13,15,17).

Bolus dosing of r-PA and TNK may correspond to improved clinical outcomes. In the GUSTO-trial, for patients treated with infusions of STK and rt-PA, 13.5% and 11.5% had medication errors, respectively (27). Medication errors were defined as an incorrect dose or infusion length. The most troublesome finding was that mortality was higher (40% and 77% for rt-PA and STK, respectively) in patients with a medication error compared with patients who received the correct dose ($p < 0.001$). In contrast, the InTIME-II trial found that single bolus lanoteplase (not FDA approved) demonstrated fewer doing errors compared to an infusion of rt-PA (5.7% vs 7.3%; $p < 0.001$) (27). Therefore, preliminary investigation demonstrates that bolus administration of thrombolytics is less complicated and can decrease medications errors. Whether this translates into improved clinical outcomes has yet to be established.

Liver metabolism is the major clearance mechanism for STK, rt-PA, and TNK, and no active metabolites have been identified for these agents (13,28–30). Decreased plasma clearance with increasing doses occurs and may be related to a saturation of hepatic receptors responsible for the clearance of these agents (15,16). A study of TNK pharmacokinetics found that women, lighter patients, and older patients had lower plasma clearance (15). In fact, patients who were older than 65 years had a mean plasma clearance of 97 mL/min compared to 143 mL/min for patients younger than 45 years of age. The authors suggested that older patients, who also tend to weigh less, might have a larger exposure to thrombolytic agents compared to younger patients. Reteplase has both renal and hepatic elimination pathways, and no active metabolites have been identified (13,31). Animal studies of renal and hepatic failure have shown that r-PA continued to be inactivated in plasma, indicating the possibility of compensatory mechanisms of elimination (unpublished Steven J. Mack, Pharm.D., Centocor, Inc.)

Despite their respective routes of elimination, none of the manufacturers of STK, rt-PA, r-PA, and TNK recommend dosage adjustment for hepatic and renal impairment in their prescribing information. They do, however, provide precautionary statements. The prescribing information recommends using (a) streptokinase with caution in patients with liver and/or kidney disease, (b) alteplase with caution in patients with significant liver dysfunction and/or advanced age (older than 75 years), (c) reteplase with caution in patients with severe renal and/or hepatic dysfunction, and (d) tenecteplase with caution in patients with severe hepatic dysfunction and/or advanced age.

Because of the potentially life-threatening bleeding complications, including intracranial hemorrhage (ICH), associated with thrombolytics, sound clinical judgment makes us exercise extreme caution when using these agents in patients with significant hepatic or renal dysfunction or advanced age. If r-PA can show appreciable compensatory elimination, it may have a clinical advantage in these select populations but more data are needed.

Aside from decreased elimination and advanced age, other studies have attempted to identify patients at risk for ICH when using thrombolytics. A retrospective cohort found the following characteristics to be independent predictors of ICH in patients receiving thrombolytic therapy (32): >75 years of age, female, black race, prior stroke, systolic blood pressure ≥160 mmHg, treatment with rt-PA versus other thrombolytic agents, excessive anticoagulation (INR > 4 or PT > 24), and below median body weight (£65 kg for women and £80 kg for men). Gurwitz and colleagues also found that older age (≥65 years of age), female sex, black ethnicity, systolic blood pressure of 140 mmHg or more, diastolic blood pressure of 100 mmHg or more, history of stroke, rt-PA dose of more than 1.5 mg/kg, and lower body weight (£70.3 kg) were all significantly associated with intracranial hemorrhage AMI patients receiving rt-PA (33). Similarly, Gore et al. found that in AMI patients taking thrombolytics, advanced age, lower weight, prior cerebrovascular disease or hypertension, systolic and diastolic blood pressures, randomization to tissue plasminogen activator, and an interaction between age and hypertension were significant predictors of ICH (34). Therefore, recognizing patient subgroups at high risk for bleeding complications is an important factor when choosing therapeutic regimens in patients with AMI.

IV. PHARMACODYNAMIC PROPERTIES OF THROMBOLYTICS

Pharmacodynamics refer to the relationship between drug concentrations at the site of action and pharmacological response (35). The various thrombolytics differ considerably with respect to their PD characteristics. The PD parameters most commonly discussed for thrombolytic therapy are mechanism of action, fibrin specificity, plasminogen activator inhibitor (PAI-1) resistance, and drug interactions.

Table 3 Pharmacodynamic Properties of Thrombolytic Agents

Drug	Fibrin specificity	PAI-1 resistance	Potency	Ref.
STK	Negligible	+	N/A	37,40,54
rt-PA	++	++	+	25,37,40,54,55
rt-PA	+	++	++	38,55
TNK	+++	+++	+++	25,56

+, lowest intensity; ++, intermediate intensity; +++, highest intensity. PAI, plasminogen activator inhibitor. N/A, not available.

A. Mechanism of Action

STK, rt-PA, r-PA, and TNK achieve thrombolysis by acting upon plasminogen to elicit the breakdown of fibrin and, ultimately, the occlusive thrombus that prevents or severely impedes coronary artery blood flow. Fibrin-specific thrombolytic agents (rt-PA, r-PA, and TNK) preferentially bind to fibrin in a thrombus and enzymatically cleave plasminogen to plasmin (3). They produce limited conversion of plasminogen in the absence of fibrin and initiate local fibrinolysis at the site of a thrombus. Streptokinase produces an "activator complex," exposing the plasminogen-activating site and indirectly triggering the breakdown of fibrin (3,28). It degrades fibrin clots as well as fibrinogen and other plasma proteins.

B. Fibrin Specificity

As fibrin specificity decreases, circulating plasminogen becomes more prone to convert to plasmin, increasing the likelihood of degrading plasma proteins other than fibrin systemically (13). These plasma proteins include fibrinogen, factor V, albumin, and factors VIII, IX, and X (36). Also, as levels of plasmin in the circulating plasma increase, available supplies of a-antiplasmin (endogenous neutralizer of plasmin) are depleted and the risk of a systemic fibrinolytic state increases (13). If bleeding complications develop during thrombolytic therapy, the patient's ability to regain normal hemostatic function will be dictated by the fibrin specificity of the thrombolytic utilized. This may be of clinical value for subsequent invasive procedures, such as percutaneous coronary intervention (PCI) or coronary artery bypass grafting (CABG). Streptokinase has weak fibrin specificity and can induce bleeding complications. Consequently, agents that convert only fibrin-complexed plasminogen to plasmin were developed with the hope that they would induce local fibrinolysis and reduce bleeding caused by systemic fibrinolysis. Rt-PA, r-PA, and TNK possess fibrin specificity to varying degrees (Table 3), as measured by decreases in systemic plasminogen and fibrinogen levels.

Fibrin specificity was assessed in an investigation comparing STK to rt-PA in 254 patients with AMI (37). The study demonstrated that posttreatment plasma fibrinogen levels declined significantly more in STK-treated patients (57, 58, and 21%) compared to rt-PA–treated patients (26, 33, and 11%) at 3, 5, and 27 hours, respectively ($p < 0.001$ at 3 and 5 hours and $p < 0.01$ at 27 hours). At these same time points the decreases in the plasma plasminogen levels were significantly greater in STK-treated patients (83, 82, 54%) compared to rt-PA–treated patients (63, 57, and 38%) ($p < 0.001$). At all three time points, the circulating fibrin(ogen) degradation products levels were significantly higher in the STK-treated patients ($p < 0.001$). In both treatment groups, the frequency of hemorrhagic events was higher in patients with greater changes in fibrinogen, plasminogen, and circulating fibrin(ogen) degradation products. Plasma levels of fibrin(ogen) degradation products correlated most with hemorrhage (correlation coefficient 0.282 and 0.272 for rt-PA and STK, respectively, $p < 0.005$). Increased rt-PA fibrin specificity is a plausible reason for the decreased noncerebral bleeding observed in the rt-PA group compared to the STK group in the GUSTO I trial(5).

In a study comparing r-PA and rt-PA in 50 patients with AMI, fibrin specificity was lower for r-PA ($p < 0.05$), as shown by a faster and more pronounced decrease in fibrinogen (38). In fact, at 3 hours r-PA reduced fibrinogen to about half the level compared to patients who received rt-PA (122 ± 27 vs. 224 ± 28 mg/dL; $p < 0.01$ and $p < 0.05$ vs controls, respectively).

The TIMI 10B trial showed a 5–10% drop in fibrinogen over the first 6 hours at the 30–50 mg doses of TNK compared with a 40% drop after rt-PA(25). There was a 10–15% decrease in plasminogen after TNK compared with a 50% decrease in plasminogen for rt-PA. In addition, the consumption of a-antiplasmin was four to five times greater with rt-PA than with TNK at any of the three doses. These findings are supported by the lower frequency of noncerebral bleeding complications and the need for blood transfusions found in the TNK group compared to the rt-PA in ASSENT II(11).

C. PAI-1 Resistance

PAI-1 is a natural substance released at the site of vessel injury or thrombus formation by endothelial and muscle cells. It is an inhibitor of both endogenous and exogenous fibrinolysis and can contribute to thrombolytic resistance(13). Thrombolytic resistance may increase the risk of reinfarction and can delay reperfusion. In fact, failure of STK therapy (i.e., reinfarction) was found to be significantly associated with pretreatment PAI-1 levels in 60 patients with AMI ($p < 0.05$) (9). Paganelli and colleagues investigated the relationships between PAI-1 levels before and after STK and rt-PA and the patency of infarct-related arteries in 55 patients with AMI (40). PAI-1 levels increased significantly with both STK ($p < 0.001$ at 12 and 18 hours) and rt-PA ($p < 0.05$ at 3 hours) compared to a control group. However, the increase was greater in the STK group as compared to rt-PA group ($p < 0.01$) and the PAI-1 levels peaked later with STK than with rt-PA (18 vs. 3 hours, respectively). Although PAI-1 peaked earlier in the rt-PA group, PAI-1 concentrations in the rt-PA group were approximately 1.6-fold higher than the control group at 3 hours compared to approximately 2.1-fold higher than the control group at 18 hours in the STK group. In addition, PAI-1 levels in the rt-PA equated those of the control group at 12 hours and were lower than the control group from 12 to 48 hours. PAI-1 levels 6 and 18 hours after STK therapy and the area under the PAI-1 curve were significantly higher in patients with occluded arteries, suggesting a relationship between increased PAI-1 levels after thrombolytic therapy and poor patency. Although increased PAI-1 levels are not directly correlated with inferior patency rates, the lower total systemic exposure of PAI-1 found with rt-PA relative to STK may be the reason for the significant mortality benefit found in the rt-PA group compared to the STK group in the GUSTO I trial (5).

In contrast, a study by Genser et al. found no difference in PAI-1 concentrations among 50 AMI patients treated with STK, rt-PA, and urokinase (41). The contrasting results observed in these two studies may be attributed to different study design (40,41). Paganelli et al. (40) investigated an accelerated infusion of rt-PA compared to Genser and colleagues' 3-hour infusion. In addition, the study by Paganelli and coinvestigators had higher patient numbers to use to detect a difference ($n = 28$ and $n = 27$ in the rt-PA and

STK groups, respectively) than the study by Genser et al. ($n = 23$, $n = 17$, and $n = 10$ in the STK, urokinase, and rt-PA groups, respectively).

In a study by Nordt and colleagues, PAI-1 levels were determined in 31 patients with AMI receiving rt-PA or r-PA (42). Although PAI-1 concentrations increased in comparison with baseline values ($p < 0.001$), this observation was independent of the thrombolytic agent used.

TNK, most likely due to amino acid substitutions on the tissue plasminogen activator molecule, has improved resistance to inactivation by PAI-1 (43). The results of the TIMI 10B trial demonstrated lower PAI-1 levels in all doses utilized (30, 40, and 50 mg) in the TNK group compared to a front-loaded rt-PA regimen (25). Comparative PAI-1 resistance and thrombolytic potency for these agents are summarized in Table 3.

D. Drug Interactions

Anticoagulants (coumarin derivatives and unfractionated/low molecular weight heparin) and inhibitors of platelet function (aspirin, nonsteroidal anti-inflammatory drugs, clopidogrel, ticlopidine, dipyridamole, and glycoprotein IIb/IIIa receptor antagonists) may increase bleeding complications when given prior to, during, or after thrombolytic therapy (3). Therefore, careful monitoring is advised. Despite this, most thrombolytic trials coadministered both aspirin and unfractionated heparin (UH) with beneficial results and are recommended treatment modalities in AMI (4). However, it is prudent to achieve therapeutic aPTTs when utilizing UH. Large multicenter studies of patients with AMI receiving thrombolytics and UH have demonstrated progressively increased risk of major bleeding as the aPTT exceeded 75 seconds (44). For this reason, current ACC/AHA Guidelines for the Management of Patients with Acute Myocardial Infarction recommend UH at an initial IV bolus of 60 U/kg and an infusion of 12 U/kg/h (with a maximum of 4000 U bolus and 1000 U/kg/h for patients weighing >70 kg), adjusted to maintain aPTT at 1.5–2.0 times control (50–70 s) (4).

Despite their potential to increase bleeding complications when coadministered with a thrombolytic, glycoprotein IIb/IIIa receptor antagonists are currently being studied in combination with reduced doses of thrombolytics. Small clinical trials have shown increased reperfusion rates without increasing bleeding risk (45,46), but larger clinical trials are underway (ASSENT-3 and GUSTO-IV) and may produce more concrete conclusions.

Other than these obvious drug interactions, which may potentiate bleeding complications, investigation of drug interactions with thrombolytics has been limited. Nitroglycerin has been observed to have a pharmacodynamic interaction with rt-PA. In a canine model, when rt-PA was given with nitroglycerin, the time to reperfusion was increased by 70%, and the time to reocclusion was 74% shorter compared with rt-PA alone (47). The plasma rt-PA antigen concentration was 3.4 times lower when rt-PA and nitroglycerin were combined. In human studies, reperfusion occurs less often and is slower, and the risk of coronary reocclusion is higher when rt-PA is given concurrently with IV nitroglycerin (48,49). In these human studies, rt-PA was administered over 3 hours and its plasma concentrations were significantly decreased. Whether this outcome will occur during a 60-minute infusion is yet to be investigated. The investigators (48,49) speculated that increased hepatic blood flow occurs and results in increased rt-PA metabolism. However, pharmacological studies have shown that hepatic blood flow does not change after nitrate administration (50,51). In another study, when rt-PA and supraphysiological concentrations of nitroglycerin are combined, degradation of alteplase in plasma is enhanced (52). Therapeutic concentrations of nitroglycerin also increased the degradation of rt-PA by 45% versus alteplase alone, but this was not statistically significant. Although the exact mechanism is not known, degradation of rt-PA in plasma is enhanced when rt-PA and nitroglycerin are combined. A secondary outcome in the TIMI 10A trial found that TNK plasma clearance did not differ in a group of patients that received nitrates ($p = 0.09$) (15). It is not known if this interaction occurs with STK and r-PA.

V. CONCLUSION

The INJECT, GUSTO III, and ASSENT II trials have demonstrated similar mortality benefit with rt-PA, r-PA, and TNK in AMI patients. The GUSTO I trial demonstrated that rt-PA provided a 14.6% relative risk reduction in 30-day mortality compared with STK. Despite similarities in clinical trial results, the four available agents possess several unique characteristics. Structural modifications have led to agents with a more favorable PK profile, higher degrees of fibrin specificity, and enhanced resistance to PAI-1. Reteplase and TNK's longer half-lives and slower plasma clearances allow for IV bolus administration. The convenience of bolus dosing may make drug administration less cumbersome for clinicians and may improve clinical outcomes compared to infusions of STK and rt-PA. Tenecteplase's single bolus over 5–10 seconds is more convenient than r-PA's bolus doses over 2 minutes given 30 minutes apart. However, r-PA's 10 unit dose is the same regardless of the weight of the patient, which is less ambiguous than TNK's weight-based dosing regimen. Dosage adjustment is not mandated in patients with compromised hepatic or renal function for any thrombolytic. However, caution should be taken when using these agents in this patient population, since drug clearance may be reduced. Reteplase may not have altered clearance in hepatic or renal dysfunction, but further studies are needed to verify this. Thrombolytic agents with higher degrees of fibrin specificity and improved resistance to inactivation by PAI-1 have theoretical advantages such as decreased bleeding and reducing rethrombosis. The results of the survival trials strengthen these theories, but further investigation will provide additional insight. Finally, a pharmacodynamic interaction between rt-PA and nitroglycerin exists, which enhances rt-PA degradation. Nitroglycerin does not appear to decrease TNK levels, and it is not known if this interaction occurs with STK or r-PA.

REFERENCES

1. Pasternak RC, Braunwald E, Sobel BE. Acute myocardial infarction. In: Braunwald E, ed. *Heart Disease: A Textbook of Cardiovascular Medicine*. 4th ed. Philadelphia, W. B. Saunders Company; 1992: 1200–1291.
2. The GUSTO Angiographic Investigators. The comparative effects of tissue plasminogen activator, streptokinase, or both on coronary artery patency, ventricular function, and survival after acute myocardial infarction. N Engl J Med 1993; 329: 1615–1622.
3. Burnham TH, Short RM, Bell WL, Schweain SL, Snitker J, eds. *Drug Facts and Comparisons*. St. Louis, MO: Facts and Comparisons; 2000.
4. American College of Cardiology/American Heart Association Task Force on Practice Guidelines (Committee on Management of Acute Myocardial Infarction). 1999 Update: ACC/AHA guidelines for the management of patients with acute myocardial infarction: executive summary and recommendations. Circulation 1999; 100: 1016–1030.
5. The GUSTO Investigators. An international randomized trial comparing four thrombolytic strategies for acute myocardial infarction. N Engl J Med 1993; 329: 673–682.

6. The INJECT Investigators. Randomized, double blind comparison of reteplase double-bolus administration with streptokinase in acute myocardial infarction. Lancet 1995; 346: 329–336.

7. Weaver WD, Cerqueira M, Hallstrom AP, et al. Prehospital-initiated vs hospital-initiated thrombolytic therapy: the Myocardial Infarction Triage and Intervention Trial. JAMA 1993; 270: 1211–1216.

8. Koren G, Weiss AT, Hasin Y, et al. Prevention of myocardial damage in acute myocardial ischemia by early treatment with intravenous streptokinase. N Engl J Med 1985; 313: 1384–1389.

9. Hermens WT, Willems GM, Nijssen KM, Simoons ML. Effect of thrombolytic treatment delay on myocardial infarct size. Lancet 1992; 340: 1297.

10. The GUSTO III Investigators. A comparison of reteplase with alteplase for acute myocardial infarction. N Engl J Med 1997; 337: 1118–1123.

11. The ASSENT-2 Investigators. Single-bolus tenecteplase compared with front-loaded alteplase in acute myocardial infarction: the ASSENT-2 double blind randomised trial. Lancet 1999; 354: 716–722.

12. Cardinale V, Chi JC, eds. *Red Book*. Montvale, NJ: Medical Economics Company, Inc., 2000.

13. Tsikouris JP, Tsikouris AP. A Review of available fibrin-specific thrombolytic agents used in acute myocardial infarction. Pharmacotherapy 2001; 21: 207–217.

14. Martin U, Kaufmannn B, Neugebauer. Current clinical use of reteplase for thrombolysis: a pharmacokinetic-pharmacodynamic perspective. Clin Pharmacokinet 1999; 36: 265-276.

15. Modi NB, Eppler S, Breed J, Cannon CP, Braunwald E, Love TW. Pharmacokinetics of a slower clearing tissue plasminogen activator variant, TNK-tPA, in patients with acute myocardial infarction. Thromb Haemost 1998; 79: 134–139.

16. Grierson DS, Bjornsson TD. Pharmacokinetics of streptokinase in patients based on amidolytic activator complex activity. Clin Pharmacol Ther 1987; 41: 304–313.

17. Tanswell P, Tebbe U, Neuhaus KL, Glasle-Schwarz L, Wojcik J, Seifried E. Pharmacokinetics and fibrin specificity of alteplase during accelerated infusions in acute myocardial infarction. J Am Coll Cardio 1992; 19: 1071–1075.

18. Gruppo Italiano per lo Studio della Sopravvivencza nell'Infarto Miocardico. GISSI-2: a factorial randomized trial of alteplase versus streptokinase and heparin versus no heparin among 12, 490 patients with acute myocardial infarction. Lancet 1990; 336: 65–71.

19. Martin U, Fischer S, Kohnert U, et al. Thrombolysis with an Excherichica coli-produced recombinant plasminogen activator (BM 06.022) in the rabbit model of jugular vein thrombosis. Thromb Haemost 1991; 65: 560–564.

20. Martin U, Fischer S, Kohnert U, et al. Coronary thrombolytic properties of a novel recombinant plasminogen activator (BM 06.022) in a canine model. J Cardiovasc Pharmacol 1991; 18: 111–119.

21. Martin U, von Moellendorf E, Akpan W, et al. Dose-ranging study of the novel recombinant plasminogen activator BM 06.022 in healthy volunteers. Clin Pharmacol Ther 1991; 50: 429–436.

22. Neuhaus KL, von Essen R, Vogt A, et al. Dose finding with a novel recombinant plasminogen activator (BM 06.022) in patients with acute myocardial infarction: results of the German recombinant plasminogen activator study. J Am Coll Cardiol 1994; 24: 55–60.

23. Smalling RW, Bose C, Kalbfleisch J, et al. More rapid, complete, and stable coronary thrombolysis with bolus administration of reteplase compared with alteplase infusion in acute myocardial infarction. Circulation 1995; 91: 2725–2732.

24. Modi NB, Fox NL, Clow FW, et al. Pharmacokinetics and pharmacodynamics of tenecteplase: results from a phase II study in patients with acute myocardial infarction. J Clin Pharmacol 2000; 40: 508–515.

25. Cannon CP, Gibson CM, McCabe CH, et al. TNK-tissue plasminogen activator compared with front-loaded alteplase in acute myocardial infarction: results of the Thrombolysis in Myocardial Infarction (TIMI) 10B Trial. Circulation 1998; 98: 2805–2814.

26. Boehringer Mannheim GmbH. Open randomized monocenter pilot study of the effect of various dosages of reteplase (r-PA; BM 06.022) in patients with actue myocardial infarction (MF 4292). Boehringer Mannheim Unpublished Report, 1994.

27. Cannon CP. Thrombolysis medication errors: benefits of bolus thrombolytic agents. Am J Cardiol 2000; 85: 17C–22C.
28. Streptase [package insert]. Wayne, PA: September, 1998.
29. Activase [package insert]. South San Francisco, CA: April, 1999.
30. TNKase [package insert]. South San Francisco, CA: June, 2000.
31. Retavase [package insert]. Malvern, PA: February, 2000.
32. Brass LM, Lichtman JH, Wang Y, Gurwitz JH, Radford MJ, Krumholz HM. Intracranial hemorrhage associated with thrombolytic therapy for elderly patients with acute myocardial infarction: results from the Cooperative Cardiovascular Project. Stroke 2000; 31: 1802–1811.
33. Gurwitz JH, Gore JM, Goldberg RJ, et al. Risk for intracranial hemorrhage after tissue plasminogen activator treatment for acute myocardial infarction. Ann Intern Med 1998; 129: 597–604.
34. Gore JM, Granger CB, Simoons ML, et al. Stroke after thrombolysis. Mortality and functional outcomes in the GUSTO-1 trial. Global use of strategies to open occluded coronary arteries. Circulation 1995; 92: 2811–2818.
35. Shargel L, Yu ABC. *Applied Biopharmaceutics and Pharmacokinetics*. 3rd ed. Norwalk, CT: Appleton & Lange, Inc., 1993.
36. Bell Jr WR. Evaluation of thrombolytic agents. Drugs 1997; 54 (suppl 3): 11–17.
37. Koneti Rao A, Pratt C, Berke A, et al. Thrombolysis in myocardial infarction (TIMI) trial-phase I: hemorrhagic manifestations and changes in plasma fibrinogen and the fibrinolytic system in patients treated with recombinant tissue plasminogen activator and streptokinase. J Am Coll Cardiol 1988; 11: 1–11.
38. Hoffmeister HM, Kastner C, Szabo S, et al. Fibrin specificity and procoagulant effect related to the kallikrein-contact phase system and to plasmin generation with double-bolus reteplase and front-loaded alteplase thrombolysis in acute myocardial infarction. Am J Cardiol 2000; 86: 263–268.
39. Sinkovic A. Pretreatment plasminogen activator inhibitor-1 (PAI-1) levels and the outcome of thrombolysis with streptokinase in patients with acute myocardial infarction. Am Heart J 1998; 136: 406–411.
40. Paganelli F, Alessi MC, Morange P, Maixent JM, Levy S, Vague IJ. Relationship of plasminogen activator inhibitor-1 levels following thrombolytic therapy with rt-PA as compared to streptokinase and patency of infarct related coronary artery. Thromb Haemost 1999; 82: 104–108.
41. Genser N, Lechleitner P, Maier J, et al. Rebound increase of plasminogen activator inhibitor type I after cessation of thrombolytic treatment for acute myocardial infarction is independent of type of plasminogen activator used. Clin Chem 1998; 44: 209–214.
42. Nordt TK, Moser M, Kohler B, et al. Augmented platelet aggregation as predictor of reocclusion after thrombolysis in acute myocardial infarction. Thromb Haemost 1998; 80: 881–886.
43. Keyt BA, Paoni NF, Refino CJ, et al. A faster-acting and more potent form of tissue plasminogen activator. Proc Natl Acad Sci USA 1994; 91: 3670–3674.
44. Hirsh J, Warkentin TE, Raschke R, Ohman EM, Dalen JE. Heparin and low molecular weight heparin. Chest 1998; 114: 489s–510s.
45. Antman Em, Giugliano RP, Gibson CM, et al. Abciximab facilitates the rate and extent of thrombolysis: results of the Thrombolysis in Myocardial Infarction (TIMI) 14 trial. Circulation 1999; 99: 2720–2732.
46. Strategies for Patency Enhancement in the Emergency Department (SPEED) Group. Trial of abciximab with and without low-dose reteplase for acute myocardial infarction. Circulation 2000; 101: 2788–2794.
47. Mehta JL, Nicoline FA, Nichols WW, et al. Concurrent nitroglycerin administration decreases thrombolytic potential of tissue-type plasminogen activator. J Am Coll Cardiol 1991; 17: 805–811.
48. Nicoline FA, Ferrini D, Ottani F, et al. Concurrent nitroglycerin therapy impairs tissue-type plasminogen activator-induced thrombolysis in patients with acute myocardial infarction. Am J Cardiol 1994; 74: 662–666.

49. Romeo F, Rosano GMC, Martuscelli E, et al. Concurrent nitroglycerin administration reduces the efficacy of recombinant tissue-type plasminogen activator in patients with acute anterior wall myocardial infarction. Am Heart J 1995; 130: 692–697.

50. Leier CV, Magorien RD, Desch CE, Thompson MJ, Univerferth DV. Hydralazine and isosorbide dinitrate: comparative central and regional hemodynamic effects when administered alone or in combination. Circulation 1981; 63: 102–109.

51. Leier CV, Bambach D, Thompson MJ, et al. Central and regional hemodynamic effects of intravenous isosobide dinitrate, nitroglycerin and nitroprusside in patients with congestive heart failure. Am J Cardiol 1981; 48: 1115–1123.

52. White CM, Fan C, Chen BP, Kluger J, Chow MSS. Assessment of the drug interaction between alteplase and nitroglycerin: an in vitro study. Pharmacotherapy 2000; 20: 380–382.

53. Gemmill JD, Hogg KJ, Burns, et al. A comparison of the pharmacokinetic properties of streptokinase and anistreplase in acute myocardial infarction. Br J Clin Pharmacol 1991; 31: 143–147.

54. Collen D. Coronary thrombolysis: streptokinase or recombinant tissue-type plasminogen activator? Ann Intern Med 1990; 112: 529–538.

55. Fischer S, Kohnert U. Major mechanistic differences explain the higher clot lysis potency of reteplase over alteplase: lack of fibrin binding is an advantage for bolus application of fibrin-specific thrombolytics. Fibrinolysis Proteolysis 1997; 11: 129–135.

56. Benedict CR, Refino CJ, Keyt BA et al. New variant of human tissue plasminogen activator (TPA) with enhanced efficacy and lower incidence of bleeding compared with recombinant human TPA. Circulation 1995; 92: 3032–3040.

4-2

Fundamental Concepts in the Pharmacokinetics and Pharmacodynamics of Antithrombotic Agents

Michael F. Caron, James S. Kalus, Brian McBride, and C. Michael White
Hartford Hospital, Hartford, Connecticut; and University of Connecticut School of Pharmacy, Storrs, Connecticut, U.S.A.

I. INTRODUCTION

Antithrombotics have been used for decades and have vastly improved outcomes for patients with acute coronary syndromes, percutaneous coronary interventions, deep venous thrombosis, pulmonary embolus, and thrombus formation due to atrial fibrillation. The traditional antithrombotics warfarin and heparin have complex pharmacokinetics and pharmacodynamics, which need to be appreciated for optimal pharmacotherapy to occur. Over the past several years, new antithrombotics have given us new treatment choices with pharmacokinetic and pharmacodynamic advantages over traditional agents.

This chapter will review the pharmacokinetic and pharmacodynamic aspects of warfarin, unfractionated heparin (UFH), low molecular weight heparins (LMWHs), danaparoid, fondaparinux, and the direct thrombin inhibitors. Clinical implications germane to these aspects will be highlighted.

II. WARFARIN

A. History

Bishydroxycoumarin (dicoumarol) is a natural anticoagulant derived from Dakota sweet clover and served as the prototype substance from which the synthetic hydroxycoumarin warfarin sodium was derived (1). While several coumarin-type oral anticoagulants are available for therapeutic use, warfarin sodium remains the most popular agent, with over 1 million patients receiving the drug annually in the United States alone (2). Warfarin sodium was initially used as a rodent poison until the therapeutic potential of the drug was determined.

B. Pharmacodynamics

1. Mechanism of Action

The synthesis of clotting factors VII, IX, X, and II (i.e., the SNOT factors) and anticlotting proteins C and S takes place almost entirely in the liver. Following RNA-to-protein translation of these clotting factor precursors, gamma carboxylation is required to enter their inactive clotting factor form. From this point, only calcium is needed to induce the final conformational change required to enhance binding to cofactors on phospholipid surfaces within in the body (activation). Hence, without the gamma carboxylation, the clotting factor precursors and proteins C and S cannot exhibit biological activity. The carboxylation reaction requires the reduced form of vitamin K (vitamin KH_2), oxygen, and carbon dioxide. In order to produce vitamin KH_2, the dietary form of vitamin K accepts hydrogen molecules from the NADH cofactor responsible for the carboxylation reaction. The reaction is accelerated by vitamin KH_2 reductase. When vitamin KH_2 is utilized in the gamma carboxylation of the clotting factor precursors, it is converted into the epoxide form of vitamin K (vitamin KO). Vitamin KO is then converted back to the dietary form of vitamin K via vitamin KO reductase to repeat the cycle.

Warfarin sodium primarily inhibits vitamin KO reductase and to a lesser extent blocks vitamin K reductase. This gradually reduces the amount of reduced vitamin K available to the reaction synthesizing the inactive clotting factors and proteins C and S. Vitamin KO reductase inhibition is reversible at therapeutic doses but can become an irreversible inhibition at fatal concentrations. Since warfarin only modestly inhibits antithrombotic effect is closer to the half-lives of factor II and X. In an animal model, the protective effect of warfarin was overcome with the infusion of factor II and, to a lesser extent, to factor X. In contrast, infusions of factor VII and IX had no effect. This has important clinical implications. Patients deplete the natural anticoagulants protein C and S early in therapy but do not experience appreciable antithrombotic effects for several days after therapy initiation (see below). This underscores the need to overlap warfarin with heparin or another antithrombotic until the INR is therapeutic for several days. In addition, using an initial warfarin-loading dose (e.g. 10 mg) is generally not desirable, as this does not appreciably enhance the depletion of factor II over a standard 5 mg dose but does increase the rate of protein C and factor X depletion. Loading doses also ultimately increase the risk of undesirable hemorrhagic effects several days after therapy initiation (3–5).

2. Adverse Drug Reactions

Hemorrhage and minor bleeding are the principal pharmacodynamic adverse effects of warfarin. The extent and severity of the bleeding is dependent upon the intensity of the overanticoagulation and the risk factors particular to the patient. Such risk factors include age greater than 65 years, history of a cerebrovascular accident, gastrointestinal bleeding, heart disease, concomitant use of aspirin, hypertension, and an extended duration of warfarin therapy.

Patients can also possess a genetic mutation causing deficiencies in factor IX. In response to warfarin administration, the concentrations of factor IX are reduced to 1–3% from baseline. In comparison, other coagulation factors are reduced to 30–40% of their normal activity. Patients who do not have this mutation experience a 30–40% reduction in all four of the vitamin K–dependent factors when warfarin is administered (1).

Elevations of the INR above the indicated therapeutic range without any bleeding can usually be managed safely by withholding the administration of warfarin for 1–2 days. In the presence of active bleeding, the administration of vitamin K (phytonidione) is essential to control the severity of the overdose (dosing described in detail later in the chapter). For serious bleeding, the administration of fresh frozen plasma (FFP) is essential. FFP contain clotting factors with gamma carboxylation.

Among the first factors inhibited by the administration of warfarin are protein C and protein S, the endogenous anticoagulants. Until other pro-coagulant proteins are cleared, there is a transient hypercoagulable state associated with the use of warfarin. The pharmacodynamic effect manifests as a gangrenous dermatological disorder of the extremities secondary to the formation of microemboli occluding peripheral capillaries (3).

The use of warfarin to treat thromboembolic disorders in the pregnant patient is contraindicated due to the effects on the formation of the fetal bone structures. In the bone there are vitamin K–dependent proteins responsible for the carboxylation of 1,25-dihydroxyvitamin D3. In the fetus, this can result in osteomalacia. The process is selective only for the formation of new bone and is not seen in adults (1).

3. Drug Interactions

Pharmacodynamic drug interactions are those that accentuate or diminish the effects of a drug without changing the drug's therapeutic concentration. For warfarin, this is generally manifested as increased bleeding risk or elevation of the INR unrelated to warfarin concentrations. Drug interactions with warfarin have been summarized in Table 1.

The antiplatelet effects of aspirin have been shown to be beneficial in patients with coronary artery disease, diabetes mellitus, and other risk factors for cardiovascular morbidity. However, irreversible inhibition of platelet thromboxane A_2 (TXA2) by aspirin decreases platelet aggregation and predisposes a patient to additive bleeding risks when combined with warfarin. In studies of patients with atrial fibrillation, the use of 81 mg of aspirin in combination with adjusted-dose warfarin (INR 2–3) showed an insignificant increase in minor bleeding with no difference in the rates of major bleeding (6, 7). Patients should be advised of the increased risk for bleeding, which can persist for up to 7 days following discontinuation of aspirin therapy.

Patients who are co-prescribed acetylated nonsteroidal anti-inflammatory agents (NSAIDs) must also be advised of excessive bleeding. The increased risk of bleeding is due to the acetylated NSAIDs exhibiting a reversible obstruction of prostaglandin G/H synthetase (also known as cyclooxygenase-1) enzyme. Acetylated NSAIDs decrease the amount of TXA2 available for platelet aggregation, and this effect on the platelets is dependent on the half-life of the agent; e.g., the effects of naproxen ($t_? =$ 12 hours) on platelets last 24 hours (8). Ibuprofen ($t_? = 2$ hours) sustains maximal prostaglandin G/H synthetase obstruction for 4–6 hours with a single dose (9). Like those using aspirin, patients using acetylated NSAIDs should be advised of the additional bleeding risks that can extend for up to 24 hours, depending upon the half-life of the product. Nonacetylated NSAIDs (trilisate, disalcid) do not exhibit antiplatelet activity. Therefore, they do not have an additive effect on bleeding when administered with warfarin.

The cyclooxygenase-2 (COX-2) inhibitors were thought to offer an alternative to the acetylated NSAIDs because they do not inhibit platelet aggregation. However, all of the agents have a pharmacokinetic drug interaction with warfarin, which is described below (14).

Thienopyridines (ticlopidine, clopidogrel) prevent the aggregation of platelets by binding to two ADP receptors (PDX1 and $P2Y_{12}$) on the platelet. Both agents form an irreversible disulfide bridge on platelet ADP receptors. Therefore, an increased risk of bleeding when administered with warfarin can persist for up to 7 days.

Table 1 Warfarin Drug Interaction Severity Guide

Mechanism	Drug/drug class	Severity[a]
Increased coagulation factor production	Estrogens	1
	Vitamin K	1
	Glucocorticoids	1
Decreased coagulation factors	Propylthiouracil	4
CYP 450 enzyme induction-increased warfarin metabolism	Barbiturates	1
	Carbamazepine	2
	Chronic ethanol use	4
	Dicloxacillin	2
	Griseofulvin	2
	Nafcillin	2
	Phenytoin	1
	Primodone	2
	Rifampin	1
Gastrointestinal binding	Cholestyramine	2
	Colesevelam	2
	Colestipol	2
Unknown	Azathioprine	4
	Cyclosporin A	2
Increased catabolism of clotting factors	Thyroid hormones	1
Decreased synthesis of clotting factors	Cephalosporins	2
	Vitamin E	1
Impaired vitamin KH_2 secretion by GI organisms	Cephalosporins	2
	Tetracyclines	4
	Fluroquinolones	4
	Azithromycin	1
Inhibition of warfarin metabolism	Acute alcohol use	2
	Amiodarone	1
	Fluconazole	1
	Fluvoxamine	1
	Propafenone	2
	HMG CoA reductase inhibitors (except pravastatin)	4
	Selective serotoin reuptake inhibitors (SSRs)[b]	4
Unknown/Other	Orlistat	4
	Acetaminophen (>2225 mg/week)	3
	Androgens (gemfibrozil)	
Increased bleeding risk not associated with warfarin metabolism	Aspirin	1
	Nonacetylated salicylates	1

[a] 1 = highest; 5 = lowest.
[b] Citalopram is metabolized by CYP 2C19, and sertraline is metabolized by CYP 3A4.
Source: Refs. 11–14.

Dipyridamole, an agent that indirectly inhibits the release of platelet TXA_2, does not exhibit an additive effect when given with warfarin. A combination product of aspirin and dipyridamole (Aggrenox®) does have an additive effect secondary to the aspirin component.

Several herbal products, including *Ginkgo biloba*, chondroitin, Danshen, tocotrienols (Evolve, Cardiem), coenzyme Q10, and high-dose vitamin E, have antiplatelet effects. These products are not well studied, so the time course of antiplatelet effects is not well known. Avoidance is therefore the best policy.

The heparin family of anticoagulants expresses overlapping inhibition of clotting factors, including thrombin (factor II), factor X, and factor IX. UFH also inhibits the conversion of factor VII by blocking chemokine release in the intrinsic pathway. Additive effects of bleeding are seen when patients are cross-covered with UFH/LMWH while warfarin therapy is being titrated. These effects are dose dependent and less likely to cause excessive bleeding when dosed for the prophylaxis of deep vein thrombosis (DVT). The risk of bleeding can certainly be managed, and overlap may be needed for optimal pharmacotherapy (see above)

Synthetic or dietary forms of vitamin K do not need to be activated in vivo to offset the anticoagulant effects of warfarin. Dietary vitamin K intake remains a problem for clinicians and creates a type of resistance to warfarin secondary to hepatic accumulation of vitamin K (15) (see below)

Bacterial flora in the gastrointestinal tract produce vitamin KH_2, and the use of broad-spectrum antibiotic therapy can elevate the INR by destroying the bacterial flora in the gastrointestinal tract. These antibiotics include tetracyclines, chloramphenicol, azithromycin, aminoglycosides, third-generation cephaolosporins, and aminopenicillins (ampicillin and amoxicillin). The greatest elevations in the INR are seen when the aforementioned antibiotics are administered by the oral route. Additionally, antibiotics may also inhibit the metabolism of warfarin via the cytochrome P450 enzyme pathways. (see below)

Glucocorticoids, estrogen, and progestins induce the hepatic biosynthesis of precursor proteins in the liver. Coagulation factor precursors can then be gamma carboxylated to inactive coagulation factors using reductase enzymes other than vitamin KH_2 reductase. These secondary reductase enzymes are not inhibited by warfarin therapy. The clinical significance of these drug interactions is minor.

C. Pharmacokinetics

1. Absorption and Distribution

Warfarin sodium is rapidly and completely absorbed from the gastrointestinal tract with no difference in absorption between the oral and intravenous forms. Complete absorption is attained in about 90 minutes.

Maximum concentrations are obtained within 2–8 hours following oral administration. Warfarin binds extensively to plasma proteins, mainly albumin, at a rate of 99%. As a result, the volume of distribution of warfarin closely approximates the volume of distribution of albumin (0.14 L/kg).

2. Metabolism and Elimination

Metabolism of the enantiomers of warfarin (R and S) takes place through two microsomal pathways. R warfarin is metabolized by the cytochrome P 450 (CYP) 1A2 enzyme system. S warfarin, a more potent anticoagulant, is metabolized by CYP 2C9. The elimination half-life of the racemic mixture is approximately 40 hours, with a range of 25–60 hours. The overall duration of anticoagulant effect lasts from 2 to 5 days. It should also be noted that the R isomer has a longer half-life than the S isomer. The difference in the half-life contributes to the long duration of anticoagulation, which can present a difficulty to the clinician in terms of drug interactions and overanticoagulation (1,3).

3. Drug Interactions

Pharmacokinetic drug interactions alter the concentration of drug available to exert an anti-coagulant effect. Decreases in protein binding or serum albumin lead to an elevated free fraction of the drug, which leads to a transient elevated INR with the same serum concentration. Protein-binding alteration interactions are transient because the excess free form of the drug increases metabolism that ultimately leads to similar free concentrations. However, the inhibition or induction of CYP 450 3A4, 2C9, and 1A2 are more significant, with CYP2C9 being the most important.

Cyclooxygenase inhibitors cause additive antithrombotic effects not by inhibiting platelet aggregation, but by altering warfarin metabolism. With the exception of celecoxib, all COX-2 inhibitors reduce cytochrome P450 (CYP 450)3A4 metabolism of both R and S warfarin. Celecoxib has a higher affinity for the CYP 450 2C9 enzyme, thus inhibiting metabolism of S warfarin (14). These pharmacokinetic interactions do not have a large amount of clinical application.

Amiodarone, an inhibitor of 2C9, 1A2, and 3A4, is frequently employed to manage several rhythm disorders that concomitantly increase the risk of thromboemolism. Amiodarone is the only agent studied to provide dosing for concomitant warfarin administration. In a retrospective analysis of 43 patients, amiodarone was added to a stable dose of warfarin (mean 5.2 ± 2.6 mg). At 4 and 7 weeks, warfarin dosage was reduced by 37 and 45%, respectively. By the end of the 12-month study, the total reduction in warfarin dose from baseline was 20%. The extent of empiric warfarin reduction is dependent upon the maintenance dose of amiodarone used (Table 2) (16).

D. Clinical Application

1. Reversal of Anticoagulation

Patients presenting with an INR outside of the therapeutic range of 2–3 (2.5–3.5 for mechanical bioprosthetic heart valves) are at an increased risk of bleeding. The risk increases proportionally with the INR level. Three modalities are used to reverse over anti-coagulation: FFP, temporary discontinuation of warfarin, and administration of vitamin KH_2. The use of FFP is only recommended for patients with serious bleeding and/or an INR of >20 (3). Temporary discontinuation of warfarin administration reduces the level of anticoagulation with no risk of developing resistance to warfarin. In a retrospective analysis, withholding warfarin and adjusting the dose was shown to be effective for asymptomatic patients with an INR of <10 (2).

Whether to administer vitamin KH_2 via the subcutaneous, intravenous, or oral route has been a topic of debate over the past decade. In a randomized evaluation of

Table 2   Recommended Warfarin Dosage Reduction with Concomitant Amiodarone

Amiodarone maintenance dose (mg)	Reduction in warfarin dose (%)
400	38 ±1.7
300	36 ± 4.4
200	31 ± 1.9
100	25 ± 4.4

Source: Ref. 16.

patients receiving either intravenous or subcutaneous vitamin KH_2, 95% of patients who received the IV form of vitamin KH_2 had an INR of 5.0 at 24 hours. This was compared with only 45% of those receiving subcutaneous vitamin KH_2. The rate of overcorrection was the same in both groups (2). Intravenous therapy is currently recommended for patients with an INR of >20 because studies have shown that high doses of vitamin KH_2 can produce overcorrection and warfarin resistance that lasts for up to 7 days. Lower doses rapidly reversed the INR without causing warfarin resistance. Furthermore, lower doses of intravenous vitamin KH_2 have a lower risk of developing anaphylaxis compared to high-dose (10 mg) therapy. Oral therapy was evaluated in a prospective study of patients with asymptomatic elevations in their INR. Seventy-three percent of patients receiving 2.5 mg experienced a reduction in PT to <35 seconds at 12 hours. In patients who received 5 mg of vitamin KH_2, 90% had a PT of <35 seconds at 12 hours. There were no episodes of overanticoagulation (2). The American College of Chest Physicians (ACCP) now recommends the use of oral vitamin KH_2 in patients with an INR of >10 (but <20) or in patients undergoing a surgical procedure. For more information on the reversal of anticoagulation, the reader is referred to the ACCP Guidelines on Anticoagulation. Finally, oral vitamin KH_2 was compared to temporary discontinuation of warfarin in patients with an INR of <10. The withholding of warfarin was found to be safe and effective in patients who were not actively bleeding. For patients with an INR of <10, withholding warfarin therapy is the recommended treatment to reverse over-anticoagulation and prevent resistance to warfarin therapy (3).

2. *Warfarin Resistance*

Resistance to oral anticoagulation is defined as the inability of a therapeutic concentration of warfarin to cause therapeutic elevations in the INR. Resistance can occur in two forms: acquired resistance and hereditary resistance.

Acquired resistance gradually develops over time as a result of decreased patient compliance, interacting drugs, increased clearance of warfarin, decreased absorption, or the administration of exogenous vitamin KH_2. Following administration of vitamin KH_2, it accumulates in the liver, attenuating the effects of warfarin. The administration of large doses of vitamin KH_2 for overanticoagulation can antagonize the effects of warfarin for up to 7 days (see above). Additionally, there are case reports of decreased warfarin efficacy in patients consuming high amounts of Ensure® for dietary supplementation. Following these case reports, the manufacturer of Ensure® has reduced the amount of vitamin K to 20 μg per 8-ounce can. Patients receiving warfarin therapy who partake in a weight reduction diet may also decrease their INR if they consume large amounts of leafy green vegetables (which are rich in vitamin KH_2). Therefore, patients taking warfarin therapy should be advised to maintain a constant intake of vitamin KH_2 (5). Clearly the beginning and end of the growing season for home gardeners are temporally higher risk times as the innate consumption of green leafy vegetables are altered and increased monitoring is needed for patients at risk.

Hereditary resistance to warfarin therapy is defined as the presence of an abnormal enzyme or receptor that has decreased affinity for warfarin or an increased affinity for vitamin KH_2 (15). To date, there have been only three case reports of warfarin resistance. In order to diagnose warfarin resistance, pharmacokinetic and pharmacodynamic studies can be performed, such as area under the curve (AUC), total body clearance, and clotting factor assays.

III. HEPARIN

A. History

Endogenous heparin was initially discovered by a medical student in 1916. Complete understanding of its mechanism of action was not known until 1939 when antithrombin (AT, formerly known as antithrombin III) was discovered. The name heparin results from the high concentration of endogenous heparin in hepatic tissue. Clinically, exogenous heparin (UFH) is the most widely used anticoagulant in that it serves as the treatment of choice for many acute thromboembolic disorders and as a bridge to oral anticoagulant treatment with warfarin.

B. Pharmacodynamics

UFH is a member of the family of glycosaminoglycans. Glycosaminoglycans are polymer chains of 200–300 monosaccharides that attach to a protein core. Up to 15 of these polymer chains attach to a single protein core (1). UFH indirectly inhibits the clotting cascade by enhancing the effect of AT. To accomplish this, the pentasaccharide sequence of heparin binds to AT, which catalyzes the exposure of the arginine-reactive site on the AT molecule. Free circulating thrombin, other clotting factors (XII, XI, X, IX), and kallikrien bind to the arginine-reactive site of AT through a covalent bond. As such, these factors are not available to be activated. Thrombin inhibition by the UFH/AT complex prevents the activation of factors VIII and V, which interrupts a positive feedback mechanism that causes enhanced thrombin generation. Thrombin already bound to a clot is not able to bind to AT. Thus, UFH is ineffective against clot-bound thrombin.

To inhibit conversion of prothrombin to its active form, thrombin, UFH molecules must not only have the pentasaccharide structure bound to AT, but the remainder of the sequence bound to thrombin itself. This effect is not possible with chains less than 18 saccharides in length. However, the other coagulation factors inhibited by UFH only require the binding of the pentasaccharide sequence to AT (1). Exploitation of this mechanism led to the development of LMWHs and selective factor Xa inhibitors, which are discussed in detail later in this chapter. In addition to anticoagulant effects, UFH inhibits platelet aggregation by platelet surface binding, which prolongs the bleeding time independent of the effects of UFH on the clotting factors (1).

The pharmacodynamic response of UFH can be measured in two ways. Clinicians monitor therapy by examining the coagulation cascade as a whole or by examining the plasma levels of specific clotting factors. Activated partial thromboplastin time (aPTT) and activated clotting time (ACT) are two global measures of anticoagulation for monitoring heparin therapy. Although aPTT has a stronger correlation to the concentration of UFH, ACT is often used in situations where a rapid turnaround time is essential, such as in operating suites and critical care units. While aPTT and ACT are measures of the pharmacodynamic effects of UFH therapy, they can also be used to predict or diagnose certain pharmacokinetic abnormalities associated with UFH therapy. Due to interlaboratory variations, the normal therapeutic range of the aPTT is defined as 1.5–2.0 times the laboratory control value. For the ACT, the normal level is 70–120 seconds. A therapeutic level of anticoagulation is defined as 150–190 seconds when measured by the ACT (17,18).

C. Pharmacokinetics

1. Absorption and Distribution

Due to the lipophilic nature of the gastrointestinal mucosa, UFH cannot be administered orally but has a 100% bioavailability by the intravenous route. When the drug is administered subcutaneously to provide low-intensity anticoagulation for thromboprophylaxis, absorption is delayed due to a low blood flow to the injection site. This is known as the depot effect, and it provides a persistent low level of anticoagulation for up to 12 hours. With standard dosing, the anticoagulant effect is very small secondary to the amount of unbound UFH reaching the plasma.

Although the ability of UFH to bind to substances other than AT is present at any dose, the effects become less significant when UFH is administered intravenously at higher doses for the treatment of thromboembolic disorders such as pulmonary embolism or acute coronary syndromes (ACS) (19). Intravenous dosing is usually initiated with a bolus dose (60 U/kg for ACS; 70–80 U/kg for venous thrombosis) to reduce the time to reach therapeutic aPTT levels (1.5–2.0 times standard laboratory control).

Due to the electrostatic charge of the UFH molecule, it has a great affinity for cationic plasma proteins such as AT and albumin. Because of this high affinity, the volume of distribution closely approximates the volume of plasma (0.7 L/kg) (20). However, the volume of distribution is variable due to the binding of the UFH molecules to endothelial cells and macrophages. This binding alters the interpatient pharmacodynamic response and varies the volume of distribution between patients as well. Excessive binding also contributes the clinical syndrome of heparin resistance in some patients (see below).

2. Metabolism and Elimination

The principal route of UFH elimination is via the reticuloendotheial system. In this system, macrophages depolymerize the molecule, eliminating its biological activity. Since the reticuloendotheial system can be saturated, UFH can exhibit nonlinear pharmacokinetics at high doses. The hallmark of nonlinear pharmacokinetics is that a small change in the dose of UFH affords a huge and disproportionate change in the serum level of UFH.

Table 3 Approximate Pharmacokinetic Parameters of LMWHs in Healthy Subjectsa

Agent	C_{max} (U/mL)	T_{max} (h)	$T_{1/2}$ (h)
Preventive doses			
Ardeparin	0.2	2.7	3.1
Dalteparin	0.2	2.8	2.8
Enoxaparin	0.3–0.6	2.4–3.0	2.9-4.4
Tinzaparin	0.3–0.4	3.7	3.4
Treatment doses			
Ardeparin	0.3	3.0	3.3
Dalteparin	0.82	4.0	2.1–2.3
Enoxaparin	1.0–1.1	3.0–5.0	4.5
Tinzaparin	0.9	4.4–5.0	3.3–4.4

C_{max} = maximum anti-factor Xa activity; LMWH = low-molecular weight heparins; T_{max} = time maximum anti-factor Xa activity was achieved; $T_{1/2}$ = half-life of anti-factor Xa elimination.
a 70 kg patient is assumed when parameters were reported per kg.
Source: Refs. 36–46.

Clinically, a small increase in an already high dose of UFH (as in pulmonary embolism) can predispose a patient to excessive bleeding. Additionally, when the system becomes saturated, the duration of anticoagulant effect is also prolonged. Saturation of the reticuloendotheial system occurs at a faster rate in patients with hepatic cirrhosis secondary to a decreased production and availability of reticuloendotheial cells in the diseased liver. Renal elimination of UFH is a secondary zero order process that operates at a slow rate. In patients with end-stage renal disease, including peritoneal dialysis or hemodialysis, the renal pathway is blocked and can contribute to a rapid saturation of the primary pathway. The overall rate of elimination by both systems is quantified by the half-life of UFH, which is approximately 90 minutes (20). This half-life is important to the clinician when reversal of UFH therapy is needed (see below).

3. Drug Interactions

Most drug interactions with UFH are clinically insignificant and have conflicting results when examined in clinical trials. Despite the conflicting reports of significant interactions with most of the agents, it is advisable to monitor all patients receiving one of the agents discussed below since there is a large interpatient variability in the response to UFH administration.

Penicillins and cephalosporins are proposed to increase bleeding by inhibiting platelet aggregation and decreasing bacteria that produce vitamin KH_2 in the gastrointestinal tract. As discussed in the warfarin section, depletion of vitamin KH_2 causes a reduction in the carboxylation of the coagulation factors precursors of factors VII, IX, X, and II needed for biological activity. A decline in inactive coagulation factors can lead to excessive bleeding because there are fewer coagulation factors for the UFH/AT complex to inhibit. Combining UFH with warfarin, a LMWH, or a direct thrombin inhibitor represents a pharmacodynamic interaction that can also increase the risk of bleeding.

The concurrent administration of intravenous nitroglycerin with UFH is common in clinical practice for the treatment of ACS. However, there have been conflicting reports that nitroglycerin causes a reduction in aPTT. Subsequent studies have shown that the interaction is minimal and only occurs with supratherapeutic doses of intravenous nitroglycerin (>40 µg/min) and is unaffected by the excipients used in the manufacturing of the product. Whether this is a pharmacokinetic or pharmacodynamic interaction is not known.

Acetylated NSAIDs have been shown to moderately increase the risk for bleeding with UFH therapy. The interaction is due to a reversible obstruction of the active site responsible for TXA2 production by prostaglandin G/H synthetase (commonly known as the cycloxygenase-1 enzyme) (9). Aspirin represents the only member of the NSAID family that can significantly increase the rate of bleeding, which is the result of an irreversible acetylation of prostaglandin G/H synthetase that can persist for up to 7 days. The use of aspirin and UFH concomitantly require monitoring for the signs and symptoms of bleeding. Finally, the use of streptokinase with UFH has been demonstrated in vivo to produce a mild resistance to UFH therapy due to an unknown reaction. However, patients who receive both UFH and streptokinase have a higher risk of intracranial hemorrhage compared with the use of UFH with synthetic plasminogen activators.

4. Adverse Drug Reactions

The principal adverse drug reaction of UFH is hemorrhage. The bleeding risk with UFH is increased with an aPTT greater than 2.0 times the normal laboratory control value. The bleeding episode can usually be controlled by a discontinuation of UFH therapy. With significant, life-threatening bleeding the administration of protamine, a basic substance that binds UFH, is necessary to reduce morbidity. Since protamine has been shown to cause an independent anticoagulant effect by inhibition of platelets and fibrinogen, dosage for UFH overdose must be conservative. The general clinical practice is to administer 1 mg of protamine for every 100 units of UFH that was infused in the preceding 90 minutes.

Prolonged infusions of UFH (>3 months) can contribute to osteoporosis. UFH binds to osteoblasts causing the release of chemical mediators that stimulate the activity of osteoclasts. Osteoclasts are responsible for decreases in bone mineral density.

In rare instances, hypersensitivity to UFH administration occurs with symptoms such as fever, chills, or urticaria. However, the production of antiheparin antibodies can lead to a serious immune reaction known as heparin-induced thrombocytopenia (HIT) or the more severe heparin-induced thrombocytopenia with thrombotic syndrome (HITTS).

HIT develops as macrophages digest and clear the UFH molecules. An epitope of the UFH molecule is presented by the macrophage to T-helper 2 (TH2) cells. A TH2 cell ultimately induces the generation of antiheparin antibodies. The crystallizeable unit of the antibody (Fc) binds to a receptor on the platelet while the antigen-binding fragment binds to a UFH molecule. This process eventually causes the formation of a complex of platelets causing a precipitous drop in the platelet count over several days. The thrombotic syndrome, HITTS, associated with HIT occurs when a complex of UFH, platelets, and antibodies occlude a vessel and produce ischemia. Further use of UFH therapy once HIT or HITTS occurs is contraindicated and necessitates the use of a direct thrombin inhibitor. HIT is generally diagnosed when the platelet count falls to <100,000 cells/μL or a 50% decrease from a baseline value, there is the presence of an unexplained thrombosis, and the patient has marked resistance to heparin therapy (21). HIT is more likely to develop when UFH is administered for 7–10 days (as with venous thromboembolism) because the immune reaction described above takes several days to develop. However, if a prior exposure of HIT was undetected, HIT can reoccur in as little 48 hours upon reexposure due to the presence of the memory cells of the immune system. Memory cells speed the immune response to antigens that previously caused a hypersensitivity reaction by reducing the number of steps needed to generate antiheparin antibodies.

5. Heparin Resistance

Patients are defined as being resistant to UFH therapy when they receive more than 35,000 units of UFH in a given 24-hour period. Common etiologies of UFH resistance include, AT deficiency, increased UFH clearance, increased heparin-binding proteins, and elevations in factor VIII, fibrinogen, or platelet factor 4 (19). As factor VIII levels rise, the antithrombotic effect is not correlated with the aPTT. As such, the pharmacodynamic effects of UFH therapy must be measured by a specific test such as the factor Xa assay. Measurement by this test provides an appropriate antithrombotic effect with a lower risk of bleeding (19). For patients who experience UFH resistance or a dose of >35,000 units in 24 hours, an anti-factor Xa level should be 0.35–0.7 IU/mL.

IV. LOW MOLECULAR WEIGHT HEPARIN

As discussed in detail above, unfractionated heparin has poor bioavailability, protein-binding interactions, and dose-dependent clearance that is both rapid and unpredictable. These limitations of UFH have led to the development of the LMWHs. The LMWHs currently available in the United States include ardeparin (Normiflo®), dalteparin (Fragmin®), enoxaparin (Lovenox®), and tinzaparin (Innohep®). Depending on the specific agent and dose used, LMWHs are similar or superior to UFH in the prevention or treatment of venous or pulmonary thromboembolism (22,23), management of acute coronary syndromes (24–27), and the treatment of MI (28).

LMWHs are produced by cleaving UFH through either chemical or enzymatic means. Each LMWH product is a heterogeneous mixture of oligosaccharides of varying chain lengths and range from 2 to 7 kDa in molecular weight (19,29). Differences in length and weight have some impact on the pharmacodynamic and pharmacokinetic profiles of the individual LMWHs.

A. Pharmacodynamics

Similar to UFH, LMWHs produce anticoagulation by interacting with and enhancing the activity of AT. LMWH chains will interact with AT if the length of the chain is at least five saccharides (i.e., a pentasaccharide) (19). Approximately 15–25% of the chains in LMWH preparations contain this critical pentasaccharide chain length (29). The chain must be at least 18 saccharides long for the formation of a ternary complex between the heparin, AT, and activated thrombin (Factor IIa), which subsequently causes deactivation of thrombin. Few chains are long enough to form this ternary complex in any LMWH preparation. In contrast, the pentasaccharide/AT complex alone is adequate to effectively deactivate activated factor X (factor Xa), which inhibits the formation of thrombin. As a result, LMWHs appear to derive their anticoagulant benefit primarily from their effect on factor Xa and have minimal direct antithrombin effects (19).

Interaction with tissue factor pathway inhibitor (TFPI) may also contribute to the mechanism of action of the LMWHs. TFPI is a protease inhibitor, which plays a role in the physiological anticoagulation process (30). TFPI is bound to the endothelium, lipoproteins, and platelets and acts as an anticoagulant by complexing with and inactivating factor Xa. Additionally, the TFPI/factor Xa complex inactivates the factor VIIa/tissue factor complex, which plays a central role in the initiation of the coagulation cascade (19,31). Limited data suggest that release of both free and total TFPI after administration of enoxaparin or ardeparin is similar to that observed after UFH administration (30,31). Effects on TFPI appear to have some role in producing the physiological effects observed with the LMWHs.

Interaction of the LMWHs with other biological substrates may account for some of the pharmacological properties of the LMWHs. Many of the pharmacokinetic advantages of the LMWHs (discussed below) over UFH are directly related to a lower binding affinity of the LMWHs for plasma proteins (histidine-rich glycoproteins, vitronectin, fibronectin, platelet factor 4, and multimers of von Willebrand factor), endothelium, and reticuloendothelial cells including macrophages. Less binding to these superfluous materials allows for more LMWH to interact at the site of action and allows for a more predictable, longer lasting anticoagulant response (32,33).

Less binding to extraneous substances may also have safety implications. It has been suggested that heparin-induced thrombocytopenia (HIT) occurs as a result of the formation of antibodies to the complex of a heparin chain and platelet factor 4 (PF4). Since only a few chains in a LMWH preparation are long enough to form this complex (>12 saccharides), the risk of HIT is reduced but not absent (19). LMWHs may also be associated with a lower incidence of osteopenia. This could be due to less interaction of the LMWHs with osteoblasts, resulting in less osteoclast activation and subsequently less bone resorption (19).

B. Pharmacokinetics

As with UFH, it is not possible to determine pharmacokinetic parameters by simply measuring LMWH blood concentrations. Instead, anti-factor Xa activity is used as a surrogate measure of the drug's pharmacokinetic behavior.

UFH possesses the ability to inactivate factor Xa and IIa (thrombin) to a similar degree (i.e., Xa to IIa inhibiting ratio = 1), while the shorter-chain LMWHs preferentially inactivate factor Xa. Consequently, the LMWHs are described in terms of the agents' in vitro factor Xa to IIa inhibiting ratio. These ratios range from 1.9 to 3.8, with enoxaparin possessing the highest ratio (32,34). The international standard for LMWH possesses a Xa to IIa inhibiting ratio of approximately 2.5 (35). Since anti-factor Xa activity is commonly used to describe the pharmacokinetic parameters of LMWHs, the pharmacokinetic section refers to parameters derived from factor Xa activity unless otherwise stated. Approximate values of important pharmacokinetic parameters are summarized in Table 3 (36–46).

1. Absorption and Distribution

Subcutaneous (SC) administration of a LMWH results in a predictable rate and extent of absorption. SC bioavailability based on anti-factor Xa activity is approximately 90%, while bioavailability based on antithrombin activity is lower (~60%). This may explain why in vivo anti-factor Xa:IIa ratios are reportedly larger than those measured in vitro. Absorption and bioavailability of the LMWHs is superior to that observed with SC UFH (~30%) (29,32). Peak anti-Xa activity is achieved approximately 4 hours after the SC LMWH dose.

Reduced binding to plasma proteins, endothelium, and macrophages accounts for greater LMWH bioavailability and could explain the smaller volume of distribution of the LMWHs as compared to UFH (32). LMWH volume of distribution approximates plasma volume, suggesting that the drugs remain primarily in the central compartment (29,47).

Certain patient conditions and characteristics can alter the absorption and distribution of the LMWHs. In a study investigating the effect of pregnancy on enoxaparin pharmacokinetics, volume of distribution was greater during the first trimester than the postpartum period. As such, this study reported a smaller peak anti-Xa activity and area under the plasma activity-versus-time curve (AUC) during the first trimester as well (48). Given the larger volume of distribution in pregnant women, higher doses of LMWH may be necessary to achieve an optimal response. A warning against the use of enoxaparin in pregnant women for prophylaxis of valve thrombosis has recently been added to its package insert. This is secondary to reports of enoxaparin failure and a study in which approximately 30% of women treated with enoxaparin (1 mg/kg) developed valve thrombosis (46).

The pharmacokinetic properties of the LMWHs may also be altered in obestity. In patients treated with dalteparin for deep vein thrombosis or pulmonary embolism, volume of distribution in patients with a body mass index (BMI) of >30 was 1.63 times larger than volume of distribution in nonobese patients (BMI 20–29). Although this difference was not statistically significant, the study was not adequately powered. There was a modest correlation between volume of distribution and total body weight ($r = 0.52$) in this study (36).

Results from other studies in obese subjects have differed. In a study investigating the pharmacokinetic properties of prophylactic and treatment doses of tinzaparin, there was no difference in peak anti-Xa activity or AUC when obese subjects (100–160 kg) were compared to historical controls. If volume of distribution were larger in the obese subjects, peak anti-Xa activity and AUC should have been lower (37). Another study found that patients who did and did not experience a thromboembolic event while being treated with enoxaparin (30 mg twice daily) after knee or hip surgery were of similar body weight and had similar mean anti-factor Xa activity on treatment (49). Additionally, body weight was not well correlated with anti-factor Xa levels. The true effect of obesity on the pharmacokinetics of the LMWHs remains unclear. The conflicting results observed in obese patients could be due to differences in study designs or to differences in the pharmacokinetic behavior of individual LMWHs. Given the currently available data, it is prudent to use the LMWHs cautiously and to consider periodic monitoring of anti-factor Xa levels in obese patients. Alternatively, a different antithrombotic agent could be chosen in lieu of the LMWHs in these patients.

Altered LMWH pharmacokinetics have been reported in critically ill patients on vasopressor agents such as dopamine or norepinephrine. In a small study of postoperative patients, the anti-factor Xa levels for intensive care unit (ICU) patients receiving vasopressors were compared to those without such therapy and patients who were not in the ICU. Mean anti-factor Xa levels in patients treated with vasopressor agents were lower as compared to the other two groups. The mean peak anti-factor Xa level in patients receiving vasopressors (0.09 IU/mL) was lower than the usual "therapeutic range" for prophylaxis of venous thromboembolism (0.25–0.37 IU/mL), which suggests that critically ill patients on vasopressor agents could be at risk of developing thromboembolic complications (50). The reduction in bioavailability when the LMWHs were given via the subcutaneous route in this study is likely due to a reduction in absorption caused by vasopressor-induced peripheral vasoconstriction.

2. Metabolism and Elimination

Negligible binding of LMWHs to macrophages, endothelial cells, and reticulocytes limit alternate clearance routes (29,32,33,47). As such, LMWHs are predominantly renally eliminated and have a half-life of approximately 4 hours, which allows for once- or twice-daily dosing (32,51–53). The elimination rate is linear, following first-order pharmacokinetics. Since elimination is not saturable, as with UFH, the elimination rate is independent of the dose of LMWH administered (33,52,53).

Clearance of antithrombin activity is faster than clearance of anti-factor Xa activity with administration of the LMWHs. This is likely because LMWH chains large enough to interact with thrombin are also more likely to undergo the saturable metabolic pathways described above (32).

Metabolism and elimination may also be affected by patient disease states or characteristics. In the study discussed previously (48), clearance of enoxaparin was greater in pregnant women during the first trimester compared to postpartum women and women in later stages of pregnancy.

Since renal mechanisms primarily account for LMWH clearance, renal insufficiency may impact elimination (33,52). The effect of renal insufficiency [creatinine clearance (CrCl) < 50 mL/min] on the pharmacokinetics of the LMWHs has not been adequately studied (38,47,54–57).

Most studies report a reduction in clearance and an increase in half-life directly proportional to the patient's level of renal dysfunction (38,54,55). In fact, one study reported that anti-factor Xa clearance was reduced by nearly 50% and half-life was doubled in hemodialysis patients (CrCl = 5–21 mL/min) (38). Reduction in clearance apparently results in drug accumulation, as the degree of renal impairment has been associated with degree of bleeding complications (54). Conversely, three studies found no relationship between renal dysfunction and altered pharmacokinetics and recommend no dosage adjustment in this popultion (47,56,57). In two of these studies, pharmacokinetic parameters measured in hemodialysis patients receiving a single dose of enoxaparin were compared to the parameters measured in historical control patients (56,57). A third study prospectively compared anti-factor Xa activity in patients with renal impairment (CrCl < 15 mL/min) to a control group with normal renal function (58). However, the first two studies have a flawed study design (56,57), and the last one cannot be fully evaluated because it has not been published (58). Well-designed clinical studies have demonstrated that cautious use of the LMWHs in patients with renal insufficiency is warranted because pharmacokinetic parameters are altered with varying degrees of renal dysfunction (57,58).

Delayed LMWH elimination may also occur in elderly patients. In one investigation, pharmacokinetic parameters in otherwise healthy elderly subjects (65 ± 3 years) receiving treatment doses of nadroparin (a LMWH not available in the United States) were compared to measurements obtained from healthy young volunteers (25 ± 4 years) and elderly patients being treated for deep vein thrombosis (65 ± 11 years) (59). LMWH was administered for 6–10 days and pharmacokinetic parameters were measured on the first and last days of therapy. At the end of therapy, peak anti-Xa activity and AUC were increased from day 1 levels in elderly subjects, and these parameters were also greater in elderly subjects than in healthy subjects. Accumulation of the LMWH occurred in elderly patients treated for DVT as well. There was a modest but significant correlation between CrCl and anti-factor Xa clearance ($r = 0.49$; $p < 0.002$), therefore, the findings of this study may be due to differences in renal function among the study groups, as renal function was normal in young subjects (CrCl = 114 ± 15 mL/min) and was somewhat impaired in elderly subjects (CrCl = 62 ± 6) and the treatment group (71 ± 24).

Although monitoring of anti-factor Xa activity does not enhance LMWH efficacy or safety in most cases, the pharmacokinetic properties of these agents suggest that anti-factor Xa levels should be monitored in some individuals (19,60). The pharmacokinetics of the LMWHs appear to be less predictable in pregnant patients, obese patients, or patients with impaired renal function (CrCl < 50 mL/min). Periodic monitoring of anti-factor Xa levels may be prudent in these patients (19).

If monitoring is to be preformed, timing of the blood draw should be approximately 3–4 hours after the dose. This ensures that anti-factor Xa measurements will approximate peak activity, as these peaks have been associated with more frequent bleeding complications (61–64). The most accurate assessment of steady-state anti-factor Xa activity would be obtained by measuring after the second or third dose, as the half-life for the LMWHs ranges from 3 to 4 hours and steady state will have been achieved by this time (65).

The therapeutic range for peak anti-factor Xa level is dependent on the indication for LMWH and whether dosing is once or twice daily. If treating an established thromboembolism with once- or twice-daily dosing, the therapeutic range is 1–2 or 0.6–1 IU/mL, respectively. For prevention of thromboembolism in moderate- and high-risk patients, target peak anti-factor Xa levels of 0.1–0.25 and 0.2–0.5 IU/mL, respectively, are suggested (19,66,67). Target anti-factor Xa levels are less apparent when treating unstable angina with a LMWH. However, in a study demonstrating the efficacy of enoxaparin (1 mg/kg/12 h) in patients with unstable angina, peak anti-factor Xa measurements were within the typical therapeutic range for treatment of thromboembolism (68). Consequently, anti-factor Xa levels of 0.5–1.2 IU/mL could be a reasonable choice in these patients as well. Alternatively, UFH could be used for patients with risk factors for altered pharmacokinetic behavior of the LMWHs.

Limited data are available to guide dosage adjustment in patients with anti-factor Xa activity outside of the "therapeutic range." In most cases, empiric dosing and clinical judgment are the only tools available to assist in treating these patients with LMWH. One study that may provide some guidance in patients being treated with twice-daily enoxaparin for unstable angina has reported that patients with CrCl of <30 mL/min, 30–60 mL/min, and >60 mL/min achieved reasonably safe and effective anti-factor Xa levels (0.95–1.01 IU/mL) with doses of 0.64, 0.84, and 0.92 mg/kg/12 h (69). However, when no dosing recommendations are available, it should be noted that the linear dose-response relationship of the LMWHs allow for a change in dose to produce a change in anti-factor Xa activity of a similar magnitude and direction (i.e., decreasing the dose of LMWH by 40% would produce an approximate 40% reduction in steady-state anti-factor Xa levels). Once steady-state concentrations have been measured and deemed acceptable, further monitoring is unnecessary unless a change in patient condition warrants it (19,65).

3. Drug Interactions

Drug interactions with the LMWHs are generally similar to those described above with UFH. In particular, additive pharmacodynamic effect interactions are possible when LMWHs are administered with other antithrombotic, antiplatelet, or thrombolytic agents (13). However, it should be noted that in many situations coadministration of a LMWH with one of these agents is appropriate and safe (28).

V. DANAPAROID

Danaparoid is a heparinoid composed of heparan sulfate, dermatan sulfate, and condroitin sulfate. With a pharmacodynamic profile similar to the LMWHs, danaparoid primarily acts on factor Xa, but the degree of factor Xa inhibition is considerably less than is seen with the LMWHs (64). Danaparoid is not likely to cause HIT on its own, but cross-reactivity of HIT antibodies is possible in approximately 10% of patients who have established HIT and are treated with danaparoid (64). Absorption of danaparoid when administered subcutaneously is nearly complete, and as with the LMWHs, the drug appears to be renally eliminated. Elimination may be delayed in the patient with renal insufficiency (70–72).

VI. FONDAPARINUX

Fondaparinux is the first antithrombotic agent of the pentasaccharide class, which has been studied for the prevention of postoperative deep vein thrombosis (73–75). This drug could be considered a very low molecular weight heparin, as it is only made up of the five-saccharide chain necessary for binding ATIII. Similar to the LMWHs, the interaction of ATIII with fondaparinux causes a conformational change favoring the deactivation of factor Xa. The drug does not appear to have any effect on thrombin, nor does it appear to interact with PF4 (75,76). The latter suggests that thrombocytopenia should not occur with this agent. This hypothesis has thus far been supported by published clinical trials, as none have reported significant thrombocytopenia (73–75,77–79).

   The bioavailability of fondaparinux is nearly complete, and absorption occurs in 2–3 hours. Similar to the LMWHs, fondaparinux exhibits a linear relationship between dose and anticoagulant response. The volume of distribution is similar to plasma volume, suggesting that the pentasaccharide remains within the central compartment. Fondaparinux appears to be principally eliminated unchanged in the urine and the half-life is approximately 15 hours, allowing for once daily dosing (80).

Limited data are available regarding drug interactions with fondaparinux. However, two studies have been performed (81,82) in which the pharmacokinetic parameters of fondaparinux were not altered by coadministration of either warfarin (81) or aspirin (82).

VII. DIRECT THROMBIN INHIBITORS

The center of the clotting cascade is the generation of thrombin, which plays a pivotal role in fibrin deposition and platelet activation (83). Because of the complex thrombotic processes in vivo (discussed above) and the limitations of traditional indirect thrombin inhibitors such as UFH and LMWH (e.g., the potential for varied anticoagulant response and resistance to clot-bound thrombin), direct thrombin inhibitors were developed.

The direct thrombin inhibitors currently available in the United States include argatroban (Argatroban®), bivalirudin (Angiomax®), and lepirudin (Refludan®). Interestingly, these agents differ considerably with respect to pharmacodynamics and pharmacokinetics. They also have dissimilar indications, with bivalirudin being the only agent approved for use in patients with unstable angina undergoing percutaneous coronary intervention (PCI) (84). Argatroban is approved for use as an anticoagulant for prophylaxis or treatment of thrombosis in HIT, including patients undergoing PCI (85). Lepirudin is approved for use as an anticoagulant in patients with HIT and associated thromboembolic disease (86). Lepirudin has limited clinical trial data in the interventional cardiology arena, but argatroban may have unacceptable efficacy in this population (87).

A. Pharmacodynamics

UFH and LMWH require a specific pentasaccharide sequence allowing them to bind to AT, disrupting the activation of free circulating thrombin (1). Thrombin already bound to a clot is not able to bind to AT. This limits indirect thrombin inhibitors' effectiveness since bound thrombin remains enzymatically active and amplifies thrombus growth by activating coagulation factors V, VIII, and XI and activating platelets (83). In contrast, direct thrombin inhibitors do not require the cofactor AT and inhibit both soluble and fibrin-bound thrombin. Further, platelet factor 4 (PF4), a protein released from activated platelets, binds heparin with high affinity, potentially eliminating heparin activity (88). More importantly, this can generate heparin antibodies leading to HIT or HITTS. Direct thrombin inhibitors do not interact with PF4 and are not associated with HIT (89).

The major mechanistic differences between the direct thrombin inhibitors are whether they have reversible or irreversible thrombin binding and if they exhibit bivalent or univalent thrombin binding. Argatroban is a univalent, synthetic small molecule that binds reversibly to the thrombin active site (89,90). It is highly selective for thrombin and exerts its effects by inhibiting thrombin-catalyzed or -induced reactions.

Lepirudin is a bivalent, recombinant form of hirudin (most potent natural and specific thrombin inhibitor) that demonstrates a highly specific, irreversible (one molecule of lepirudin binds to one molecule of thrombin) binding to thrombin at the active site (89,91). Unlike argatroban, it additionally competes with fibrin for the exosite 1 (ensures that substrates are bound in the proper orientation and mediates binding to fibrin) (89).

Bivalirudin is a bivalent, 20-amino-acid polypeptide and is modeled after the hirudin molecule (92). It demonstrates a specific binding to thrombin at the active site (one molecule of bivalirudin binds to one molecule of thrombin) and, like lepirudin, competes with fibrin for the exosite 1 (89,93). What makes bivalirudin pharmacologically distinct is that the binding is reversible. Once bound, bivalirudin is cleaved by thrombin at the active site, thus restoring active site functions (93).

Theoretically, the aPTT, ACT, PT, INR, and thrombin time (TT) are affected by direct thrombin inhibitors and could be utilized to measure pharmacodynamic response. However, the recommendations for monitoring each direct thrombin inhibitor differ considerably. For argatroban, the recommended monitoring test is the aPTT (90). Argatroban displays linear dose- and concentration-dependent anticoagulant activity at infusion doses up to 40 µg/kg/min (85,90). An aPTT should be performed at baseline, 2 hours following initiation of therapy, and until the steady-state (usually within 1–3 hours after initiation) aPTT is 1.5–3 times the initial baseline value (not to exceed 100 seconds) (85).

The aPTT ratio (a patient's aPTT at a given time over an aPTT reference value, usually median of the laboratory normal range for aPTT) is recommended to monitor lepirudin therapy (86,94). Increases in aPTT were observed with increased plasma concentrations of lepirudin, with no saturable effect up to the highest tested dose (0.5 mg/kg) (86). However, the pharmacodynamic response is dependent on renal function. Lepirudin should not be started in patients with a baseline aPTT ratio ≥ 2.5 and the target ratio during treatment should be 1.5–2.5 (86). The first aPTT should be performed 4 hours following initiation of therapy and 4 hours after every dosage change and daily as long as therapy continues (86,91). Patients with renal insufficiency require more frequent monitoring.

Given its use in PCI, the ACT has been evaluated predominantly for bivalirudin monitoring (93). When given IV, bivalirudin exhibits linear dose- and concentration dependent anticoagulant activity as demonstrated by ACT prolongation (92). However, the ACT is not predictive of the efficacy and safety of bivalirudin for most patient subtypes and should therefore be reserved for specific patient populations (i.e., those with renal impairment and bleeding complications) (93).

1.   Drug Interactions

As mentioned above, additive pharmacodynamic effect interactions are possible when direct thrombin inhibitors are administered with other antithrombotic, antiplatelet, or thrombolytic agents. However, few pharmacokinetic drug interactions with direct thrombin inhibitors are known.

Studies have demonstrated that argatroban can be administered safely in combination with digoxin and acetaminophen (90). The combination of these agents with argatroban did not alter the pharmacokinetics or pharmacodynamics of either agent. The combination of argatroban with aspirin did prolong bleeding times but had no effect on APTT, TT, and PT (90). Because argatroban and lidocaine both bind to a_1-acid glycoprotein, the potential interaction was assessed in a drug interaction study. Argatroban plasma concentrations were decreased by 20% and aPTT values were lowered when argatroban was administered to 12 normal volunteers (90). However, the effect was considered clinically insignificant and dosage adjustment is not recommended. There were no alterations in the pharmacokinetics of either argatroban or erythromycin with coadministration. (see below) The combination of argatroban and warfarin increases PT/INR measurements (90). When initiating warfarin therapy in patients receiving argatroban at doses ≤2 µg/kg/min, argatroban can be safely discontinued once the PT/INR is 4.0. When measured with PT reagents with international sensitivity index (ISI) values of up to 1.78, an INR of 4.0 is approximately equivalent to an INR of 2–3 with warfarin therapy alone. Because the INR relationship is more variable when argatroban doses are >2 µg/kg/min, the dose should be reduced to 2 µg/kg/min and the PT/INR should be reassessed within 4–6 hours when initiating warfarin (90).

Limited drug interaction data exist for lepirudin. Like argatroban, the combination of lepirudin with aspirin does have the potential to prolong bleeding time (91). Lepirudin administered to patients also receiving fibrinolytics may prolong the aPTT and increase bleeding risk (91), however, no studies have been performed assessing the combination of lepirudin with glycoprotein IIb/IIIa antagonists, clopidogrel or ticlopidine, LMWH, or UFH. The manufacturer does recommend a gradual dosage reduction in order to reach an aPTT ratio just above 1.5 before initiating warfarin therapy. Lepirudin should then be discontinued when an INR of 2.0 is reached (86).

Since bivalirudin is not metabolized by the cytochrome P450 enzyme system and does not bind to plasma proteins other than thrombin, the potential for drug-drug interactions is low. Studies have demonstrated that bivalirudin did not have a pharmacodynamic interaction with the thienopyridine ticlopidine, glycoprotein IIb/IIIa antagonists, LMWH, or UFH (93). In addition, bivalirudin has been administered safely concomitantly with aspirin. These data are important since the aforementioned antiplatelet or antithrombotic agents may be administered during PCI, when bivalirudin would most commonly be employed.

2. Adverse Drug Reactions

As with the aforementioned antithrombotic agents, hemorrhage and minor bleeding are the most significant adverse effects of direct thrombin inhibitors. The extent and severity of the bleeding is dependent upon the intensity of the overanticoagulation and the patient-specific risk factors (e.g., coadministration with other drugs that increase bleeding risk, renal or hepatic impairment, duration of treatment, and underlying disease). In addition, no specific antidote is available to reverse the anticoagulant effect of direct thrombin inhibitors and should be used in caution in these patient populations. With this in mind, a direct thrombin inhibitor with a shorter half-life may be more advantageous since faster reversal of effect will occur upon drug discontinuation (see below).

There have been no reports of antibody formation to argatroban or bivalirudin; therefore, reexposure to the drug would not increase the risk of adverse effects or decrease efficacy. In contrast, lepirudin does have immunogenic properties. In a study of 198 individuals with HIT, 45% developed antihirudin antibodies when treated with lepirudin for ≥5 days (95). The antibodies were thought to produce an enhanced effect in 2–3% of patients, requiring a 60% dosage reduction to maintain the aPTT within the target range. Reduced renal clearance of lepirudin immune complexes may be responsible for this effect (96). The clinical relevance of lepirudin antibody formation has yet to be determined.

B. Pharmacokinetics

1. Absorption and Distribution

Argatroban's onset of action is approximately 30 minutes (90). Its peak plasma concentrations occur approximately 2 hours following initiation of therapy (90). Also, argatroban's steady-state levels and anticoagulant effect occur in approximately 1–3 hours (85). It distributes mainly in the extracellular fluid as demonstrated by an apparent steady-state volume of distribution of 174 mL/kg. Argatroban is 54% bound to human serum proteins, with binding to albumin and a_1-acid glycoprotein being 20 and 34%, respectively (90).

Lepirudin also is mainly distributed to extracellular fluid with volume of distribution of 200 mL/kg, with less than 10% bound to plasma proteins (94). Maximum serum concentrations occur in 0.08–0.29 hours.

Bivalirudin's peak plasma concentration after a 15-minute IV bolus infusion of 0.05–0.6 mg/kg was directly related to the dose and occurred within 5 minutes of completion of the infusion (84,92). Peak concentrations occurred within 2 minutes after a bolus injection of 0.3 mg/kg. A mean steady-state concentration of 12.3 μg/mL was observed following an IV bolus of 1 mg/kg and a 2.5 mg/kg/h infusion over 4 hours. Bivalirudin is distributed mainly in the intravascular space as demonstrated by a volume of distribution of 240 mL/kg (93). It does not bind to plasma proteins other than thrombin.

2. Metabolism and Elimination

The principal route of argatroban elimination is by hydroxylation and aromatization the liver, forming four metabolites catalyzed in vitro by cytochrome P450 3A4/5 enzymes (85). The primary metabolite has an approximate fourfold weaker anticoagulant activity compared to argatroban. Sixty-five percent of argatroban elimination is in the feces via biliary secretion (90). Despite this cytochrome P450 3A4/5 metabolism, the pharmacokinetics of argatroban and erythromycin (a cytochrome P450 3A4/5 inhibitor) were not altered in 14 healthy patients when the drugs were coadministered, suggesting that this is not clinically relevant in vivo (97). A pharmacokinetic study of argatroban showed that clearance was decreased was decreased fourfold, AUC was increased threefold, and elimination half-life was increased twofold in hepatically impaired individuals, suggesting that dosing reduction and careful monitoring are necessary (98). The same study demonstrated that argatroban's pharmacokinetics are not affected by age, gender, or renal failure. Steady-state clearance and half-life ranged from 3.8 to 5.4 mL/min/kg and 39 to 51 minutes, respectively.

Lepirudin is eliminated principally via the kidney and to some extent by proteolytic cleavage (86). Up to 90% of the administered dose is recovered in the urine, which consists of 38–65% unchanged lepirudin and 30% active catabolic metabolites (94). Thus, lepirudin clearance is decreased considerably in patients with renal impairment and the potential for increased risk of bleeding is enhanced. The half-life is 0.8–2 hours in normal volunteers but is prolonged up to 2 days in individuals with severe renal impairment (CrCl < 15 mL/min) and on hemodialysis (86,94). As a result, dosage reductions are necessitated in patients with CrCl < 60 mL/min and frequency of dosing should be guided by aPTT results.

Similarly to lepirudin, bivalirudin elimination occurs via a combination of renal excretion and proteolytic cleavage, with renal elimination being the primary route (93). Urinary excretion data showed that 21%, 28%, and 35% of unchanged bivalirudin was cleared renally in patients with normal renal function (CrCl ≥ 90 mL/min), mild renal impairment (CrCl = 60–89 mL/min), and moderate renal impairment (CrCl = 30–59 mL/min), respectively (99). The lack of total urinary recovery of bivalirudin may result from tubular reabsorption and subsequent metabolism. Pharmacokinetic studies of bivalirudin have demonstrated that plasma clearance [3.4 mL/min/kg in normal renal function (CrCl ≥ 90 mL/min)] is reduced by approximately 20% in patients with moderate (CrCl = 30–59 mL/min) or severe (CrCl = 10–29 mL/min) renal impairment (99,100). Also, the half-life of bivalirudin in patients with moderate and severe renal impairment was increased to 34 minutes and 57 minutes, respectively, compared to 25 minutes in patients with normal renal function (99). Therefore, a 20% and 60% reduction in the infusion dose of bivalirudin is warranted in patients with moderate and severe renal impairment, respectively (99).

REFERENCES

1. Majerus PW, Broze GJ, Miletich JP, Tollefsen DM. Anticoagulant, thrombolytic and antiplatelet drugs. In: Hardman JG, and Limbird LE, eds. Goodman and Gilman's The Pharmacological Basis of Therapeutics. 10th ed. New York: McGraw-Hill, 2002:1341–1359.
2. Taylor CT, Chester EA, Byrd DC, Stephens MA. Vitamin K to reverse excessive anticoagulation: a review of the literature. Pharmacotherapy 1999;19:1415–1425.
3. Hirsh J, Dalen JE, Anderson DR, Poller L, Bussey H, Ansell J, et al. Oral anticoagulants: mechanism of action, clinical effectiveness, and optimal therapeutic range. Chest 2001;119:8S–21S
4. Harrison L, Johnston M, Massicote PM, Crowther M, Moffat K, and Hirsh J. Comparison of 5 mg and 10 mg loading doses in initiation of warfarin therapy. Ann Intern Med 1997;126:133–135.
5. O'Connell MB, Kowal PR, Allivato CJ, Repka TL. Evaluation of warfarin initiation regimens in elderly patients. Pharmacotherapy 2000;20:923–930.
6. Gullov AL, Koefoed BG, Petersen P, Padersen TS, Andersen ED, Godtfredsen J, et al. Fixed minidose warfarin and aspirin alone and in combination vs adjusted-dose warfarin for stroke prevention in atrial fibrillation. Arch Intern Med 1998;158:1513–1521.
7. Stroke Prevention in Atrial Fibrillation Investigators. Adjusted-dose warfarin versus low-intensity, fixed dose warfarin plus aspirin for high risk patients with atrial fibrillation: stroke prevention in atrial fibrillation III randomised clinical trial. Lancet. 1996:348;633–638.
8. Watson DJ, Rhodes T, Cai B, and Guess HA. Lower risk of thromboembolic cardiovascular complications with naproxen among patients with rheumatoid arthritis. Arch Intern Med 2002:162;1105–1110.
9. Catella-Lawson F, Reilly MP, Kapoor SC, Cucchiara AJ, Demarco S, Tournier B, Vyas SN, and FitzGerald GA. Cyclooxygenase inhibitors and the antiplatelet effects of aspirin. N Engl J Med 2001;345:1809–1817.
10. Wittkowsky AK. Drug interactions update: drugs herbs, and oral anticoagulation. J Thromb Thrombolysis 2001;12:67–71
11. Wittkowsky AK. Thrombosis. In Koda-Kimble MA and Young LL. Applied Therapeutics: The Clinical Use of Drugs. 2001 Philadelphia. W.B. Saunders
12. Cytochrome P450 Drug Interactions. Available at: http://medicine.iupui.edu/flockhart. Accessed July 12, 2002.
13. MICROMEDEX (database online). Greenwood Village, CO: Thompson Healthcare. Updated June 2002.
14. Tatro DS (ed). Drug Interaction Facts. St. Louis: Facts and Comparisons 2002.
15. Sanoski CA, and Bauman JL. Clinical observations with the amiodarone/warfarin interaction. Chest 2002;121:19–23.
16. Hulse ML. Warfarin resistance: diagnosis and therapeutic alternatives. Pharmacotherapy 1996;16:1009–1017.
17. Corbett JV. Laboratory Tests and Diagnostic Procedures. 4th ed. Stamford, CT: Appelton and Lange. 1996.
18. Smythe MA, Koerber JM, Nowak SN, Mattson JC, Begle RL, Westley SJ, et al. Correlation between activated clotting time and Activated Partial Thromboplastin Times. Ann Pharmacother. 2002;36:7–11.
19. Hirsh J, Warkentin TE, Shaughnessy SG, Anand SS, Halperin JL, Raschke R, et al. Heparin and low-molecular-weight-heparin. Mechanisms of action, pharmacokinetics, dosing, monitoring, efficacy, and safety. Chest 2001;119(suppl):64S–94S.
20. Estes JW. Clinical pharmacokinetics of heparin. Clin Pharmacokinet 1980;5:204–220.
21. Januzzi JL, Jang IK. Heparin induced thrombocytopenia: diagnosis and contemporary management. J Thromb Thrombolysis 1999; 7:259–264.
22. Samama MM, Cohen AT, Darmon JY, Desjardins L, Eldor A, Janbon C, et al. A comparison of enoxaparin with placebo for the prevention of venous thromboembolism in acutely ill medical patients. N Engl J Med 1999;341:793–800.

23. The Columbus Investigators. Low-molecular-weight heparin in the treatment of patients with venous thromboembolism. N Engl J Med 1997;337:657–662.
24. Klein W, Buchwald A, Hillis SE, Monrad S, Sanz G, Turpie GG, et al. Comparison of low-molecular-weight heparin with unfractionated heparin acutely and with placebo for 6 weeks in the management of unstable coronary artery disease. Fragmin in unstable coronary artery disease study (FRIC). Circulation 1997;96:61–68.
25. Fragmin during instability in coronary artery disease (FRISC) study group. Low-molecular-weight heparin during instability in coronary artery disease. Lancet 1996;347:561–568.
26. Cohen M, Demers C, Gurfinkel EP, Turpie AGG, Fromell GJ, Goodman S, et al. A comparison of low-molecular-weight heparin with unfractionated heparin for unstable coronary artery disease. N Engl J Med 1997;337:447–452.
27. Gurfinkel EP, Manos EJ, Mejail RI, Cerda MA, Duronto EA, Garcia CN, et al. Low molecular weight heparin versus regular heparin or aspirin in the treatment of unstable angina and silent ischemia. J Am Coll Cardiol 1995;26:313–318.
28. The Assessment of the Safety and Efficacy of a New Thrombolytic Regimen (ASSENT)-3 Investigators. Efficacy and safety of tenecteplase in combination with enoxaparin, abciximab, or unfractionated heparin: the ASSENT-3 randomised trial in acute myocardial infarction. Lancet 2001;385:605–613.
29. Andrassy K, Eschenfelder V. Are the pharmacokinetic parameters of low molecular weight heparins predictive of their clinical efficacy. Thromb Res 1996;81(suppl 2):S29–38.
30. Alban S, Gastpar R. Plasma levels of total and free tissue factor pathway inhibitor (TFPI) as individual pharmacologic parameters of various heparins. Thromb Haemost 2001;85:824–829.
31. Hoppensteadt DA, Walenga JM, Fasanella A, Jeske W, Fareed J. TFPI antigen levels in normal human volunteers after intravenous and subcutaneous administration of unfractionated heparin and low molecular weight heparin. Thromb Res 1995;77:175–185.
32. Weitz JI. Low-molecular-weight heparins. N Engl J Med 1997;337:688–698.
33. Howard PA. Dalteparin: a low-molecular-weight heparin. Ann Pharmacother 1997;31:192–203.
34. KesslerCM. Low molecular weight heparins: practical considerations. Semin Haematol 1997;34:35–42.
35. Barrowcliffe TW, Curtis AD, Johnson EA, Thomas DP. An international standard for low molecular weight heparin. Thromb Haemost 1988;60:1–7.
36. Yee JYV, Duffull SB. The effect of body weight on dalteparin pharmacokinetics. A preliminary study. Eur J Clin Pharmacol 2000;56:293–297.
37. Hainer JW, Barrett JS, Assaid CA, Fossler MJ, Cox DS, Leathers T, et al. Dosing in heavy-weight/obese patients with the LMWH, tinzaparin: a pharmacodynamic study. Thromb Haemost 2002;87:817–823.
38. Cadroy Y, Pourrat J, Baladre MF, Saivin S, Houin G, Montastruc JL, et al. Delayed elimination of enoxaparine in patients with chronic renal insufficiency. Thromb Res 1991;63:385–390.
39. Cambus JP, Saivin S, Heilmann JJ, Caplain H, Boneu B, Houin G. The pharmacodynamics of tinzaparin in healthy volunteers. Br J Haematol 2002;116:649–652.
40. Barrett JS, Hainer JW, Kornhauser DM, Gaskill JL, Hua TA, Sprogel P, et al. anticoagulant pharmacodynamics of tinzaparin following 175 IU/kg subcutaneous administration to healthy volunteers. Thromb Res 2001;101:243–254.
41. Fossler MJ, Barrett JS, Hainer JW, Riddle JG, Ostergaard P, Van Der Elst E, et al. Pharmacodynamics of intravenous and subcutaneous tinzaparin and heparin in healthy volunteers. AJHP 2001;58:1614–1621.
42. Collignon F, Frydman A, Caplain H, Ozoux ML, Le Roux Y, Bouthier J, et al. Comparison of the pharmacokinetic profiles of three low molecular mass heparins—dalteparin, enoxaparin and nadroparin—administered subcutaneously in healthy volunteers (doses for prevention of thromboembolism). Thromb Haemost 1995;73:630–640.
43. Troy S, Fruncillo R, Ozawa T, Mammen E, Holloway S, Chiang S. The dose proportionality of the pharmacokinetics of ardeparin, a low molecular weight heparin, in healthy volunteers.
44. Bara L, Planes A, Samama MM. Occurrence of thrombosis and haemorrhage, relationship with anti-Xa, anti-IIa activities, and D-dimer plasma levels in patients receiving a low molecular

weight heparin, enoxaparin or tinzaparin, to prevent deep vein thrombosis after hip surgery. Br J Haematol 1999; 104:230–240.

45. Fragmin [package insert]. Kalamazoo, MI: Pharmacia and Upjohn Corp.;2002.

46. Lovenox [package insert]. Bridgewater, NJ: Aventis Pharmaceuticals Products Inc.; 2001.

47. Frydman A. Low-molecular-weight heparins: an overview of their pharmacodynamics, pharmacokinetics and metabolism in humans. Haemostasis 1996;26(suppl 2):24–38.

48. Casele HL, Laifer SA, Woelkers DA, Venkataramanan R. Changes in the pharmacokinetics of the low-molecular-weight heparin enoxaparin sodium during pregnancy. Am J Obstet Gynec 1999;181:1113–1117.

49. Kovacs MJ, Weir K, MacKinnon K, Keeney M, Brien WF, Cruickshank MK. Body weight does not predict for anti-Xa levels after fixed dose prophylaxis with enoxaparin after orthopedic surgery. Thromb Res 1998;91:137–142.

50. Dorffler-Melly J, de Jonge E, de Pont AC, Meijers J, Vroom MB, Buller HR. Bioavailability of subcutaneous low-molecular-weight heparin to patients on vasopressors. Lancet 2002;359:849–850.

51. Verstraete M. Pharmacotherapeutic aspects of unfractionated and low molecular weight heparins. Drugs 1990;40:498–530.

52. Buckley MM, Sorkin EM. Enoxaparin. A review of its pharmacology and clinical applications in the prevention and treatment of thromboembolic disorders. Drugs 1992;44:465–497.

53. Freedman MD. Pharmacodynamics, clinical indications, and adverse effects of heparin. J Clin Pharmacol 1992;32:584–596.

54. Becker RC, Spencer FA, Gibson M, Rush JE, Sanderink G, Murphy SA, et al. Influence of patients characteristics and renal function on factor Xa inhibition pharmacokinetics and pharmacodynamics after enoxaparin administration in non-ST-segment elevation acute coronary syndromes. Am Heart J 2002;143:753–759.

55. Sanderink GCM, Guimart CG, Ozoux ML, Jariwala NU, Shukla UA, Boutouyrie BX. Pharmacokinetics and pharmacodynamics of the prophylactic dose of enoxaparin once daily over 4 days in patients with renal impairment. Thromb Res 2002;105:225–231.

56. Brophy DF, Wazny LD, Geher TWB, Comstock TJ, Venitz J. The pharmacokinetics of subcutaneous enoxaparin in end-stage renal disease. Pharmacotherapy 2001;21:169–174.

57. Follea G, laville M, Pozet N, Dechavanne M. Pharmacokinetic studies of standard heparin and low molecular weight heparin in patients with chronic renal failure. Haemostasis 1986;16:147–151.

58. Busby LT, Weyman A, Rodgers GM. Excessive anticoagulation in patients with mild renal insufficiency receiving long-term therapeutic enoxaparin. Am J Hematol 2001;67:54–56.

59. Mismetti P, Laporte-Simitsidis S, Navarro C, Sie P, d'Azemar P, Necciari J, et al. Aging and venous thromboembolism influence the phramacodynamics of the anti-factor Xa and antithrombin activities of a low molecular weight heparin (nadroparin). Thromb Haemost 1998;79:1162–1165.

60. Alhenc-Gelas M, Jestin-Le Guernic C, Vitoux JF, Kher A, Aiach M, Fiessinger JN. Adjusted versus fixed doses of the low molecular weight heparin Fragmin in the treatment of deep venous thrombosis. Thromb Haemost 1994;71:698–702.

61. STA®-Rotachrom® HBPM/LMWH 4 [package insert] Asnieres-Sur-Seine, France: Diagnostica Stago; 1997.

62. Boneu B, de Moerloose P. How and when to monitor a patient treated with low molecular weight heparin. Semin Thromb Hemost 2001;27:519–522.

63. Nieuwenhuis HK, Albada J, Banga JD, Sixma JJ. Identification of risk factors for bleeding during treatment of acute venous thromboembolism with heparin or low molecular weight heparin. Blood 1991;78:2337–2343.

64. Laposata M, Green D, Van Cott EM, Barrowcliffe TW, Goodnight SH, Sosolik RC. College of American Pathologists Conference XXXI on laboratory monitoring of anticoagulant therapy. The clinical use and laboratory monitoring of low-molecular-weight heparin, danaparoid, hirudin and related compounds, and argatroban. Arch Pathol Lab Med 1998;122:799–807.

65. Winter ME. Basic Clinical Pharmacokinetics. 3rd ed. Vancouver, WA: Applied Therapeutics, Inc; 1994.
66. Samama MM. Contemporary laboratory monitoring of low molecular weight heparins. Clin Lab Med 1995;15:119–123.
67. Handeland GF, Abildgaard U, Holm HA, Arnesen KE. Dose adjusted heparin treatment of deep venous thrombosis: a comparison of unfractionated and low molecular weight heparin. Eur J Clin Pharmacol 1990;39:107–112.
68. The thrombolysis in myocardial infarction (TIMI) 11A trial investigators. Dose-ranging trial of enoxaparin for unstable angina: Results of TIMI 11A. J Am Coll Cardiol 1997;29:1474–1482.
69. Collet JP, Montalescot G, Choussat R, Lison L, Ankri A. Enoxaparin in unstable angina patients with renal failure. Int J Cardiol 2001;80:81–82.
70. Danhof M, de Boer A, Magnani HN, Stiekema JC. Pharmacokinetic considerations on orgaran (Org 10172) therapy. Haemostasis 1992;22:73–84.
71. Stiekema JC, Wijnand HP, Van Dinther TG, et al. Safety and pharmacokinetics of the low molecular weight heparinoid Org 10172 administered to healthy elderly volunteers. Br J Clin Pharmacol. 1989;27:39–48.
72. ten Cate H, Henny CP, ten Cate JW, et al. Anticoagulant effects of a low molecular weight heparinoid (Org 10172) in human volunteers and haemodialysis patients. Thromb Res 1985;29:211–222.
73. Bauer KA, Eriksson BI, Lassen MR, Turpie AGG for the Steering Committee of the Pentasaccharide in Major Knee Surgery Study. Fondaparinux compared with enoxaparin for the prevention of venous thromboembolism after elective major knee surgery. N Engl J Med 2001;345:1305–1310.
74. Eriksson BI, Bauer KA, Lassen MR, Turpie AGG for the steering committee of the pentasaccharide in hip-fracture surgery study. Fondaparinux compared with enoxaparin for the prevention of venous thromboembolism after hip-fracture surgery. N Engl J Med 2001;345:1298–1304.
75. Turpie AGG, Gallus AS, Hoek JA for the Pentasaccharide Investigators. A synthetic pentasaccharide for the prevention of deep-vein thrombosis after total hip replacement. N Engl J Med 2001;344:619–625.
76. Walenga JM, Jeske WP, Bara L, Samama MM, Fareed J. Biochemical and pharmacological rationale for the development of a synthetic heparin pentasaccharide. Thromb Res 1997;86:1–36.
77. Lassen MR. The Epheseus Study: Comparison of the first synthetic factor Xa Inhibitor with low molecular weight heparin in the prevention of venous thromboembolism after elective hip replacement surgery (abstr). Blood 2000;96:490a.
78. The Pentathalon 2000 Study: Comparison of the first synthetic factor Xa Inhibitor with low molecular weight heparin in the prevention of venous thromboembolism after elective hip replacement surgery (abstr). Blood 2000;96:491a.
79. Coussement PK, Bassand JP, Convens C, Vrolix M, Boland J, Grollier G, et al. A synthetic factor-Xa inhibitor (ORG31540/SR9017A) as an adjunct to fibrinolysis in acute myocardial infarct. The PENTALYSE study. Eur Heart J 2001;22:1716–1724.
80. Boneu B, Necciari J, Cariou R, Sie P, Gabaig AM, Kieffer G, et al. Pharmacokinetics and tolerance of the natural pentasaccharide (SR90107/ORG31540) with high affinity to antithrombin III in man. Thromb Haemost 1995;74:1468–1473.
81. Faaij RA, Burggraaf J, Cohen AF. Lack of pharmacokinetic (PK) and pharmacodynamic (PD) interaction between the first synthetic factor Xa inhibitor and warfarin in human volunteers (abstr). Blood 2000;96:56a.
82. Donat F, Ollier C, Santoni A, Duvauchelle T. Safety and pharmacokinetics (PK) of co-administration of the first synthetic factor Xa inhibitor and aspirin in human volunteers (abstr). Blood 2000;96:54a.
83. Nappi J. Heparin, bivalirudin, and reduction of complications during percutaneous coronary intervention. Pharmacotherapy 2002;22:89S–96S.

84. Product information. Angiomax (bivalirudin). Cambridge, MA: The Medicines Company, December 2000.

85. Product information. Argatroban (Argatroban). Philadelphia: SmithKline Beecham Pharmaceuticals, August 2000.

86. Product information. Refludan (lepirudin). Wayne, NJ: Berlex Laboratories, September 2001.

87. Yusuf S, for the Direct Thrombin Inhibitor Trialists' Collaborators Group. Direct thrombin inhibitors in acute coronary syndromes: principal results of a meta-analysis based on individual patients' data. Lancet 2002;359:294–302.

88. Kelton J, Smith J, Warkentin T, et al. Immunoglobulin G from patients with heparin-induced thrombocytopenia binds to a complex of heparin and platelet factor 4. Blood 1994;83:3232–3239.

89. Wittkowsky AK. The role of thrombin inhibition during percutaneous coronary intervention. Pharmacotherapy 2002;22:97S–104S.

90. Kondo LM, Wittkowsky AK, Wiggins BS. Argatroban for prevention and treatment of thromboembolism in heparin-induced thrombocytopenia. Ann Pharmacother 2001;35:440–451.

91. Greinacher A, Lubenow N. Recombinant hirudin in clinical practice: focus on lepirudin. Circulation 2001;103:1479–1484.

92. Sciulli TM, Mauro VF. Pharmacology and clinical use of bivalirudin. Ann Pharmacother 2002;36:1028–1041.

93. Reed MD, Bell D. Clinical pharmacology of bivalirudin. Pharmacotherapy 2002;22:105S–111S.

94. Wittkowsky AK, Kondo LM. Lepirudin dosing in dialysis-dependent renal failure. Pharmacotherapy 2002;20:1123–1128.

95. Song X, Huhle G, Wang L, et al. Generation of anti-hirudin antibodies in heparin-induced thrombocytopenia patients treated with r-hirudin. Circulation 1999;100:1528–1532.

96. Eichler P, Friesen H-J, Lubenow N, et al. Anti-hirudin antibodies in patients with heparin-induced thrombocytopenia treated with lepirudin: incidence, effects on aPTT, and clinical relevance. Blood 2000;96:2373–2378.

97. Tran JQ, Di Cicco RA, Sheth SB, et al. Assessment of the potential pharmacokinetic and pharmacodynamic interaction between erythromycin and argatroban. ZJZ Clin Pharmacol 1999;39:513–519.

98. Swan SK, Hursting MJ. The pharmacokinetics and pharmacodynamics of argatroban: effects of age, gender, and hepatic or renal dysfunction. Pharmacotherapy 2000;20:318–329.

99. Robson R, White H, Aylward P, Frampton C. Bivalirudin pharmacokinetics and pharmacodynamics: effect of renal function, dose, and gender. Clin Pharmcol Ther 2002;71:433–439.

100. Fox I, Dawson A, Loynds P, et al. Anticoagulant activity of hirulog, a direct thrombin inhibitor, in humans. Thromb Haemost 1993;69:157–163.

5-1

In-Hospital Cardiology Clinical Pharmacy Services

William Brennan, Jr. and Alisha Dunn
*Massachusetts College of Pharmacy and Health Sciences, Boston; Massachusetts, U.S.A.
Hartford Hospital, Hartford, Connecticut; and University of Connecticut School of
Pharmacy, Storrs, Connecticut, U.S.A.*

Paralleling the advancements in the practice of cardiovascular medicine and thrombocardiology, in-hospital clinical pharmacy services have also evolved. The increasing utilization of these services by cardiologists has resulted in the development of a number of multidisciplinary patient care models that include a clinical pharmacy component. It is useful to briefly examine the changes within the pharmacy profession that have contributed to the development of cardiology clinical pharmacy services. Some of the roots of this movement can be found in three distinct, yet overlapping entities: early clinical pharmacy efforts, pharmacy education governing bodies, and federal government initiatives.

I. EVOLUTION OF CLINICAL PHARMACY SERVICES

Until the mid to late twentieth century, the practice of pharmacy was focused almost entirely on preparing and dispensing drug products. Early efforts by pharmacists to define and provide clinical pharmacy services have been reported (1–4). Implemented to demonstrate enhanced pharmacy services, the underlying goal of these undertakings was improved pharmacy patient care. These ventures utilized the expertise of the pharmacist to review medication use, gather information regarding medication side effects, and provide medication counseling upon discharge. While not designed to produce definitive results, these initial works sought to highlight the therapeutic and cognitive aspects of pharmacy services. Hence, a profession that had trained rigorously to assume only an apothecary role was now beginning to integrate an additional component into the delivery of patient care (Fig. 1).

The clarion call to the pharmacy profession to deepen and expand these initial clinic pharmacy services can be found within the oft-cited article of Hepler and Strand (5). In this visionary article, the now-common concept of pharmaceutical care was discussed, as the authors envisioned the pharmacist as a working member of a multidisciplinary health care team. In particular, Hepler and Strand called for the pharmacist to work with other health care providers to "design, implement and monitor a drug therapy plan that will produce specific therapeutic outcomes for the patient."

Perhaps in response to some of the pioneering efforts of clinical pharmacists, pharmacy education organizations initiated a resetting of the course of study for all pharma-

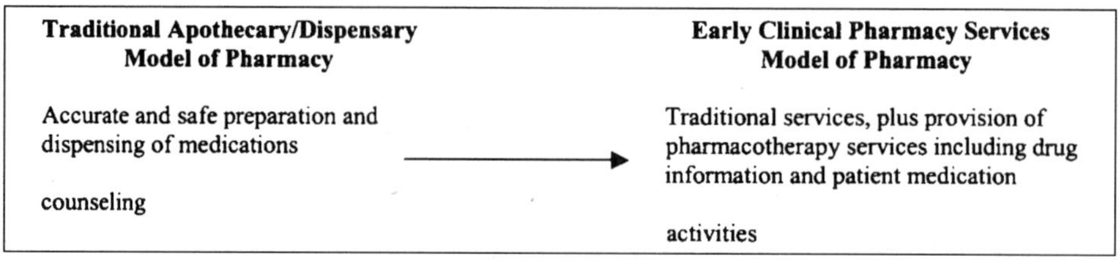

Traditional Apothecary/Dispensary Model of Pharmacy	Early Clinical Pharmacy Services Model of Pharmacy
Accurate and safe preparation and dispensing of medications counseling	Traditional services, plus provision of pharmacotherapy services including drug information and patient medication activities

Figure 1 Evolution of clinical pharmacy services.

cists (6). The academic training of pharmacists was lengthened to a 6-year Doctor of Pharmacy (Pharm.D.) program, which offered expanded and intensive coursework in pharmacokinetics, therapeutics, and additional areas of professional study. However, it is the increase in post-Pharm.D. residency training that arguably has had the greatest impact on the development of a pharmacist's clinical skills. In the United States, pharmacy practice residency provides a graduate with an additional year of clinical training in the acute/ambulatory setting. The increased demand for clinical training has resulted in a doubling in the number of accredited general and specialty residencies nationwide in the past 10 years (7). Fellowship training is also available to pharmacists seeking to develop independent research skills for use in academic careers.

The ambulatory care setting provided the venue for a third component in the development of contemporary clinical pharmacy. The Omnibus Budget Reconciliation Act of 1990 (OBRA '90) mandated the implementation of drug utilization review (DUR) for all ambulatory patients enrolled in Medicaid-related programs (8). OBRA '90, in calling for retrospective and prospective drug utilization review by pharmacists, served to further hasten the development of clinical pharmacy programs. The proactive premise underlying OBRA '90 has been firmly embraced by health care providers practicing in the cardiology setting of acute and ambulatory services.

The task of accurate preparation and dispensing of drug product remains a central part of the pharmacy profession. However, due in part to the initiatives and clinical training described above, the professional role of the pharmacist has evolved to include cognitive services with direct application at the in-hospital and ambulatory level of patient care (9–13).

II. IMPLEMENTING CLINICAL PHARMACY IN THE ACUTE CARE SETTING

During the period in which clinical pharmacy services was emerging, an increasing number of reports identified problem areas in the medication-delivery process (14). A number of studies examined the cost of medication noncompliance or nonadherence, incidence of adverse drug reactions, and medical errors in hospitalized patients (15–18). Attempts to measure medication-related morbidity and morality have also been described (19). These and numerous other data served to sharpen the desire of researchers to determine if clinical pharmacy services could demonstrate benefit in the acute care setting.

Three recent studies evaluated the impact of clinical pharmacy services in patient care. One study examined the impact on adverse drug events (ADEs) of having a senior pharmacist present during physician rounds in an ICU setting (20). Another study utilized a clinical pharmacist on a heart failure management team and sought to assess differences in patient outcomes as a result of adding a pharmacist to the team (21). A third study examined the cost impact of clinical pharmacist activities in the acute care setting (22). Decreased ADEs, a decrease in all-cause mortality and heart failure events, and a decrease in drug costs, respectively, were reported. As a result of these and other reports, the benefit of in-hospital clinical pharmacy services has become more broadly recognized. The interest in clinical pharmacy services has increased to such a degree that a pharmacist scope of practice was the focus of a 2002 Position Paper of the American College of Physicians–American Society of Internal Medicine (ACP-ASIM) (23). The ACP-ASIM paper calls upon the medical community to "proactively respond to the pharmacy movement" and proposes suggestions for "how the medical profession can work with pharmacists to enhance patient safety and quality of care" (23).

While the establishment of clinical pharmacy services has occurred in a number of medical specialties, none has appeared to integrate these services more than cardiology. From amiodarone to warfarin, angina to Wolff-Parkinson-White syndrome, the dynamic nature of cardiovascular disease (CVD) creates the necessity for frequent initiation, monitoring, assessment, and titration of medication. As a result, cardiology and thrombocardiology have been at the forefront in seeking to optimize clinical pharmacy services.

III. CARDIOLOGY AND CLINICAL PHARMACY SERVICES

The morbidity and mortality of CVD along with its staggering direct and indirect costs have been reported previously (24). While nonpharmacological treatments of CVD are a vital component of patient care (e.g., nutrition, lifestyle), the role of medication in the treatment of cardiovascular disease and thromboembolic disorders is fundamental. As a result, the cardiologist places an extraordinary reliance on the accurate delivery of, and continued patient adherence to, the prescribed cardiovascular medication regimen.

Despite the rational use of cardiovascular medications and their ubiquitous presence in a patient's treatment, the number of hospital readmissions and recurrent cardiovascular events—is still of great concern. In one attempt to address this situation, cardiology has seized on a natural extension of the activities of early clinical pharmacy. The specialty of cardiology has sought to leverage clinical pharmacy services not only to identify and reduce medication adverse effects, but also to minimize avoidable *therapeutic failure* (25). Recognizing that presumptions are made in the void between medication-prescribing and patient medication adherence, cardiology has supported the innovative use of clinical pharmacists within various models of multidisciplinary care.

The following are descriptions of in-hospital and transitional care clinical pharmacy cardiology services. The models of clinical pharmacy services and the type of involvement of a clinical pharmacist in the cardiology service will vary by size and type of health care system. Additionally, the amount of resources allocated to clinical pharmacy activities by hospital administration, the commitment to multidisciplinary care, and an affiliation with a school of pharmacy are all contributors to a model's design.

IV. CLINICAL PHARMACY IN THE CARDIOLOGY
ACUTE CARE SETTING

Regardless of the model details, there is a basic set of activities and patient-care duties that a well-trained clinical pharmacist will bring to an acute care setting (Table 1). One of the most important aspects of these activities is the delivery of a pharmacist's specialized knowledge at the point of medication ordering or decision making by the medical team

(20). When implemented, these duties may include consultation with team members regarding dosage adjustments for renal/hepatic dysfunction, including for noncardiac medications (e.g., antibiotics, benzodiazepines, and phenytoin). A more subtle, focused activity of the in-patient clinical pharmacist involves vigilance for any signs or symptoms of drug-induced disease(s) among the cardiology unit's patients. Academic detailing for the cardiology team members of newly released or heavily marketed medications is also a service offered by the well-trained clinical pharmacy specialist. Other specific clinical pharmacy activities may include sedation medication management utilizing sedation scales with frequent patient assessment, information to the team in response to dosage form questions regarding tablet-splitting and transdermal dosing, and dosage equivalency information for patients admitted with nonformulary medications (e.g., fosinopril-for-lisinopril interchange). A few examples of broader activities and interventions a clinical pharmacist might perform in the acute care setting include conversion of a patient's medication from intravenous (IV) to an oral formulation, consideration of a less expensive yet efficacious agent, or discontinuation of an unnecessary medication(s) (26–28).

From the perspective of a coronary care unit (CCU) medical team, the patient may transfer from the CCU having received an accurate diagnosis, superb intervention procedures where necessary, and appropriately prescribed pharmacotherapy for continued recovery and treatment. However, from the perspective of the patient, the importance of the newly prescribed medication regimen in the management of CVD may not be fully appreciated. Therefore, the patient's transfer from the CCU to transitional care unit (TCU) setting presents another opportunity for delivery of care by a multidisciplinary team (29,30), including the involvement of clinical pharmacy services.

V. CLINICAL PHARMACY IN THE CARDIOLOGY TRANSITIONAL CARE SETTING

A CCU patient diagnosed with acute coronary syndrome or myocardial infarction will likely have a number of newly prescribed medications at the onset of transitional care. In today's health care environment of pharmacy benefits provider networks, the patient may additionally be faced with formulary-driven therapeutic interchanges. There are a number of medication-related cognitive services that may be beneficial to the patient at this transition in care. The following is a description of three specific clinical pharmacy activities that can be performed in the post-CCU setting: patient medication education, information-gathering from the patient and family members for the assessment of potential obstacles to

Table 1 Sample Daily Activities of a Clinical Pharmacy Specialist in the Cardiology Acute Care Setting

- Preround and walk-around services, including drug-drug interaction monitoring, recommendations to the medical team for any pharmacokinetic- or pharmacodynamic-related dosing adjustments, laboratory monitoring of drug serum concentration levels, adverse drug reaction monitoring
- In-unit drug information consultations for medical and nursing teams, including indication and dosing of agents; safety, efficacy and cost of available alternative agents
- Delivery of pharmacotherapy teaching to medical residents and health care providers in the acute care unit
- Intermediary between unit nursing staff and pharmacy vis-à-vis patient's prescribed medication regimen, e.g., medication availability, dosing, and administration instructions, including any nutrient or food-drug interactions

medication adherence, and recommendations to the patient's cardiologist and primary care physician for the titration and optimization of pharmacotherapy.

During transfer from the acute care setting, the clinical pharmacist has an excellent opportunity to provide the patient/family members with detailed medication information (Table 2). In one study within a cardiology clinic setting, a CHF multidisciplinary team utilized the clinical pharmacist member to ask the patient a series of 10 open-ended questions related to the patient's prescribed regimen (21). Implementing this effective interviewing technique, a trained clinical pharmacist can assist the patient in the early identification of medication-related patient concerns that may hinder adherence to a prescribed regimen. An additional benefit of such an interview approach is a review with the patient of the place in therapy of each medication and its role in treating CVD. In the absence of this clinical pharmacy service, a patient experiencing side effects may subsequently decide to self-adjust or discontinue medications without informing the physician or medical team. This nonadherence can further jeopardize the patient's treatment and result in ill-informed dosing titrations by the physician. Therefore, if performed repeatedly and properly at various stages of a patient's care, a medication education/counseling session may garner useful information for the patient's cardiology team.

The desire to optimize guideline-derived medication regimens has produced another role for the clinical pharmacist in the treatment of CVD patients. Utilizing a previously agreed-upon heart failure management protocol, one study examined the impact on hospitalizations of heart failure and related costs when a clinical pharmacist participated in medication dosage optimization (31).

Working as a member of a multidisciplinary team, the clinical pharmacist conducted chart review and monitoring of medication-pertinent laboratory values (e.g., serum creatinine, serum potassium, and blood pressure). If subsequent to monitoring, an optimization of angiotensin-converting enzyme inhibitor (ACE-I) dosing was deemed warranted, the clinical pharmacist forwarded dosing recommendations to the patient's attending physician for review and possible action (31). An improvement in heart failure outcomes was reported in two studies in which a clinical pharmacist conducted this type of dose-optimization activity (21,31).

Table 2 Medication Counseling and Information-Gathering Activities of a Clinical Pharmacist in the Cardiology Acute Care–Transitional Care Setting[a]

- Gather a complete medication history from patient, including prescriptions written by outside providers, over-the-counter, alternative, and herbal therapies. This includes gathering any pre-hospitalization reports of medication-induced adverse effects.
- Assess possible obstacles to patient adherence to newly prescribed medications. This includes any cultural, financial, social, or religious concerns of the patient or any educational obstacles that could preclude adherence.
- Perform a thorough medication review with the patient, including the place in therapy, administration instructions, and common side effects of the patient's medication regimen. Imperative in this and any subsequent reviews is the utilization of open-ended assessment questions to maximize information sharing and instruction (21).
- Assess any special drug-drug, drug-food/nutrient interactions that may diminish efficacy, and work with providers and patient to minimize or avoid these concerns.
- Offer the patient written medication information, medication organizational supplies, and a telephone contact for any subsequent questions and concerns regarding administration, side effects, or the newly prescribed medications after TCU discharge.

---

[a]All information gathered by the clinical pharmacist in the TCU setting should be conveyed in writing to the other members of the patient's cardiology/primary care team for future prescribing considerations.

In addition to the delivery of patient medication education and dosage optimization of cardiovascular medications, the clinical pharmacist may be responsible for performing telephone follow-up with the patient (21). Combining pharmacotherapy knowledge with practiced listening skills, the clinical pharmacist may again be able to identify nascent, yet manageable, medication side effects reported by the patient. The telephone encounter can also be used to determine if obstacles to medication adherence have developed in the period since hospital discharge. Strategies for mitigating any admitted medication nonadherence can then be formulated with the patient as an active participant. Operating within the context of a multidisciplinary team, any medication-related patient information that is gathered in telephone follow-up would be conveyed, along with recommendations, to the team and attending physician (21,31).

VI. INTEGRATING CLINICAL PHARMACY SERVICES ACROSS PATIENT CARE SETTINGS

The multidisciplinary team approach to managing coronary artery disease (CAD) patients also has included the innovative use of clinical pharmacy services. For instance, the goal of optimizing lipid-lowering medication in CAD patients in order to decrease the risk of adverse ischemic events (32) is one in which a clinical pharmacist can play an active role (33–36). Employing the expertise of each of its multidisciplinary team members, one such model initiates its team care at the point of hospital admission (37). In this model, patients with confirmed coronary artery disease are identified during an in-hospital stay and then, based on a number of criteria, stratified to one of four clinical pathways. The use of nurses, dieticians, physical therapists, psychologists, clinical pharmacists, and physicians is included in the pathway. In one part of the clinical pharmacy pathway, the clinical pharmacist performs close monitoring of pertinent laboratory values, dose titrations of antihyperlipidemic medications, and patient follow-up. All of these lipid-management activities are conducted under physician oversight and previously agreed-upon dosing protocols (37). The proactive nature of this model, initiated in the inpatient setting and continued after discharge, is a clear attempt at acknowledging the continuum of treatment that is important in the treatment of the cardiovascular patient. This type of comprehensive patient management is identified by some as continuity of patient care (38,39). Regardless of the label, the provision of clinical pharmacy services across the patient care setting would naturally seem to follow the pharmacotherapy that remains an integral part of a cardiovascular disease patient's treatment. The wide variety of health care systems and the varying degree to which multidisciplinary care is adopted will impact the actual configuration of clinical pharmacy services that span patient care settings.

VII. CONCLUSION

The cardiologist, keenly aware of the complex nature of cardiovascular disease, has gathered together a number of health care specialties to assist in the provision of care to the CVD patient. The inclusion of clinical pharmacy services in this multidisciplinary effort is indeed rational, given the prominent role of pharmacotherapy in the treatment of CVD.

From proactive pharmacodynamic and pharmacokinetic monitoring in the CCU to the ongoing need to assess obstacles to medication adherence in the transitional care setting, the goal of the clinical pharmacist is the efficacious and safe use of medication. Knowing the consideration the cardiologist takes in prescribing CVD medication and the reliance placed on its efficacy by the entire team, the well-trained clinical pharmacist fully realizes the responsibility to act thoroughly to ensure therapeutic success. Observant and attentive to patient response *after* the delivery of medication, the clinical pharmacist is capable of providing valuable feedback information to the cardiologist, primary care physician, and, indeed, the patient vis-à-vis a prescribed regimen. Ideally, this information gathering and feedback would be provided along the continuum of the cardiology patient's care.

One of the goals in delivering a continuum of clinical pharmacy services is the accurate collection of the patient's medication regimen and his or her response and adherence to it. The value of these data is magnified when it is thoughtfully and repeatedly gathered, reassessed, and resubmitted to the patient's cardiologist, primary care physician, and medical team. Hopefully, as a result, the patient's CVD pharmacotherapy may become as dynamic as the cardiovascular disease itself. Any resulting improvement in clinical outcome of the patient is one in which all members of the multidisciplinary team can take satisfaction.

REFERENCES

1. McKenney JM, Slining JM, Henderson HR, Devins D, Barr M. The effect of clinical pharmacy services on patients with essential hypertension. Circulation 1973;48:1104–1111.
2. Sczupak CA, Conrad WF. Relationship between patient-oriented pharmaceutical services and therapeutic outcomes of ambulatory patients with diabetes mellitus. Am J Hosp Pharm 1977;34:1238–1242
3. Hoffmann RP, Sveska KJ. A clinical pharmacy program for cardiac patients. Hosp Pharm 1982;17:17–24.
4. Hawkins DW. Fiedler FP. Douglas HL. Eschbach RC. Evaluation of a clinical pharmacist in caring for hypertensive and diabetic patients. Am J Hosp Pharm 1979;36:1321–1325.
5. Hepler CD, Strand LM. Opportunities and responsibilities in pharmaceutical care. Am J Hosp Pharm. 1990;47:533–542.
6. ACCP. Pharmaceutical education. A commentary from the American College of Clinical Pharmacy. Pharmacotherapy. 1992;12(5):419–427
7. Residency Accreditation Service Database. American Society of Health-System Pharmacy. 2002.
8. Omnibus Budget Reconciliation Act, 1990. Section 1927 GH of the Social Security Act (Public Law 101508), Washington, DC.
9. Lipton HL, Byrns PJ, Soumerai SB, Chrischilles EA. Pharmacists as agents of change for rational drug therapy. Int J Tech Assess Health Care. 1995;11(3):485–508.
10. American College of Clinical Pharmacy. Establishing and Evaluating Clinical Pharmacy Services in Primary Care. Pharmacotherapy 1994;14(6):743–758
11. Winslade NE, Strand LM, Pugsley JA, Perrier DG. Practice functions necessary for the delivery of pharmaceutical care. Pharmacotherapy 1996;1616(5)889–898.
12. Kirk JK, Michael KA, Markowsky SJ, Restino MR, Zarowitz BJ. Critical pathways: the time is here for pharmacist involvement. Pharmacotherapy 1996;16(4)723–733.
13. Carmichael JM, O'Connell MB, Devine B, Kelly HW, Ereshefsky L, Linn WD, Stimmel GL. Collaborative drug therapy management by pharmacists. Pharmacotherapy 1997;17(5):1050–1061.
14. Phillips DP, Christenfeld N, Glynn LM. Increase in US medication-error deaths between 1983–1993. Lancet 1998;351:643–644.

15. Sullivan SD, Kreling DH, Hazlet TK. Noncompliance with medication regimens and subsequent hospitalization: a literature analysis and cost of hospitalization estimate. J Res Pharm Econ. 1990;2:19–33.

16. Noncompliance with Medications: An Economic Tragedy with Important Implications for Health Care Reform. Baltimore, MD:The Task Force for Noncompliance, 1993.

17. Lazarou J, Pomeranz BH, Corey PN. Incidence of adverse drug reactions in hospitalized patient. JAMA. 1998;279(15):1200–1205

18. Kohn LT, Corrigan JM, Donaldson MS. To Err is Human:Building a Safer Health System. Committee on Quality of Health Care in America. Institute of Medicine. 2000

19. Johnson JA, Bootman L. Drug-related morbidity and mortality. Arch Intern Med 1995;155:1949–1956

20. Leape LL, Cullen DJ, Clapp MD, Burdick E, Demonaco HJ, Erickson JI, Bates DW. Pharmacist participation on physician rounds and adverse drug events in the intensive care unit. JAMA 1999;281(3):267–270.

21. Gattis WA, Hasselblad V, Whellan DJ, O'Connor CM. Reduction in heart failure events by the addition of a clinical pharmacist to the heart failure management team. Arch Intern Med 1999;159:1939–1945.

22. McMullin ST, Hennenfent JA, Ritchie DJ, Huey WY, Lonergan TP, Schaiff RA, et al. A prospective, randomized trial to assess the cost impact of pharmacist initiated interventions. Arch Intern Med 1999;159:2306–2309.

23. American College of Physicians–American Society of Internal Medicine. Pharmacist scope of practice. Ann Intern Med. 2002;136:79–85

24. American Heart Association. Heart Disease and Stroke Statistics—2003 Update. Dallas, TX:American Heart Association, 2002.

25. Talley CR. Continuity of care. Am J Hosp Pharm. 1994;51:1423.

26. Gandhi PJ, Smith BS, Tataronis GR, Maas B. Impact of a pharmacist on drug costs in a coronary care unit. Am J Health-Syst Pharm. 2001;58:497–503.

27. Montazeri M, Cook DJ. Impact of a clinical pharmacist in a multidisciplinary intensive care unit. Crit Care Med. 1994;22:1044–1048.

28. Herfindal ET, Bernstein LR, Kishi DT. Impact of clinical pharmacy services on prescribing on a cardiothoracic/vascular surgical unit. Drug Intell Clin Pharm. 1985;19:440–444.

29. Stewart S, Marley JE, Horowitz JD. Effects of multidisciplinary, home-based intervention on unplanned readmissions and survival among patients with chronic congestive heart failure: a randomised controlled study. Lancet. 1999;354:1077–1083.

30. Rich MW, Gray DB, Beckham V, Wittenberg C, Luther P. Effect of multidisciplinary intervention on medication compliance in elderly patients with congestive heart failure. Am J Med. 1996;101:270–276.

31. Luzier AB, Forrest A, Feurstein SG, Schentag J, Izzo JL. Containment of heart failure hospitalizations and cost by angiotensin-converting enzyme inhibitor dosage optimization. Am J Cardiol 2000;86:519–523.

32. Scandinavian Simvastatin Survivial Study Group. Randomised trial of cholesterol lowering in 4444 patients with coronary heart disease: the Scandinavian Simvastatin Survival Study (4S). Lancet. 1994;344:1383–1389.

33. Marciniak TA, Ellerbeck EF, Radfrod MJ, et al. Improving the quality of care for Medicare patients with acute myocardial infarction. Results from the cooperative cardiovascular project. JAMA 1998;279:1351–1357.

34. Krumholz HM, Radford MJ, Wang Y, Chen J, Heiat A, Marciniak TA. National use and effectiveness of beta-blockers for the treatment of elderly patients after acute myocardial infarction. National cooperative cardiovascular project. JAMA 1998;280:623–629.

35. Stringer KA, Lopez L, Talbert RL. A call for pharmacists to improve the care of patients with myocardial infarction. Pharmacotherapy 2001;21(11):1317–1319.

36. Faulkner MA, Wadibiea EC, Lucas BD, Hilleman DE. Impact of pharmacy counseling on compliance and effectiveness of combination lipid-lowering therapy in patients undergoing coro-

nary artery revascularization: a randomized, control trial. Pharmacotherapy. 2000;20(4):410–416.

37. Merenich JA, Lousberg TR, Brennan SH, Calonge NB. Optimizing treatment of dyslipidemia in patients with coronary artery disease in the managed-care environment. Am J Cardiol. 2000;85:36A–42A.

38. Cameron B. The impact on pharmacy discharge planning on continuity of care. Can J Hosp Pharm. 1994;47:101–109.

39. Rogers J, Curtis P. The concept and measurement of continuity in primary care. Am J Public Health 1980;70:122–127.

5-2

Clinical Pharmacy Services in the Outpatient Cardiology Setting

Mary Amato
Massachusetts College of Pharmacy and Health Sciences, Boston, Massachusetts, U.S.A.

I. INTRODUCTION

The Institute of Medicine (IOM) issued a national call in 2001 for the rebuilding of the healthcare delivery system in the United States. This initiative sought the implementation of safer, more effective, patient-centered healthcare. The IOM specifically advocated for interdisciplinary collaboration, evidence-based practice, and quality improvement initiatives as a means toward improved patient outcomes (1). In practice, cardiology is one medical specialty that has continually demonstrated a desire to collaborate with other healthcare providers in the acute care and ambulatory setting. Clinical pharmacy services represent one healthcare discipline that has been invited to participate as a member of the interdisciplinary team in the outpatient cardiology setting. Several roles of the clinical pharmacist in the outpatient cardiology clinic will be highlighted in this chapter. Prior to a discussion of specific cardiology clinics in which clinical pharmacists participate, a brief discussion of clinical pharmacist training will be presented.

Recent surveys have revealed an increase in medication-related clinical functions of pharmacists in the ambulatory setting (2). This increase in clinical pharmacy services reflects a major shift in the education and training of pharmacists in the United States. Today's graduating pharmacists obtain more clinical experience in direct patient care settings than their predecessors. Additionally, they complete courses in physical assessment and patient communication and receive extensive training in pathophysiology and pharmacotherapy. Upon successful completion of the nationally mandated 6-year doctor of pharmacy degree (Pharm.D.) and state pharmacy board examination, some licensed pharmacists (R.Ph.) pursue postgraduate residency, fellowship programs, or disease state–management training programs in areas such as anticoagulation, heart failure, and hyperlipidemia (Fig. 1).

Those clinical pharmacists with more extensive experience and/or training may sit for rigorous certification exams, including the pharmacotherapy specialist examinations provided by the board of pharmaceutical specialties (BPS). The designation board-certified pharmacotherapy specialist (BCPS) is given to those who pass an examination assessing advanced pharmacotherapy knowledge. The BPS offers exams in a number of specialty areas (Fig. 1).

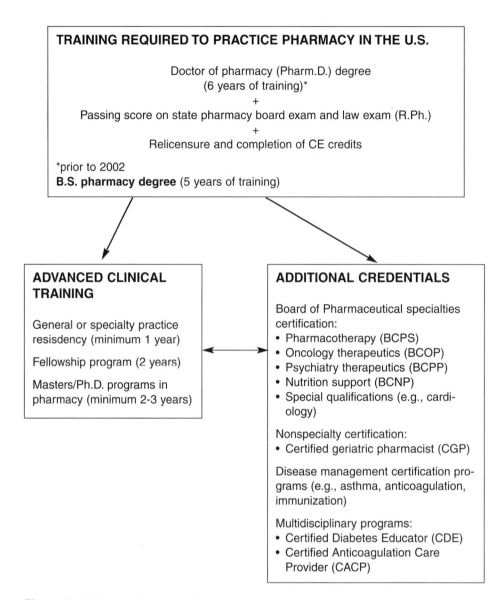

Figure 1   Pharmacist education and credentials.

Other organizations offer specialty certification in areas such as geriatrics (Certified Geriatric Pharmacist offered by the Commission for Certification in Geriatric Pharmacy), diabetes (Certified Diabetes Educator offered by the National Certification Board for Diabetes Educators), and anticoagulation (Certified Anticoagulation Provider offered by the National Board of Anticoagulation Providers). Well-trained pharmacists working in the ambulatory clinic setting are able to work closely with cardiologists, primary care physicians, and other health care professionals in promoting optimal pharmacotherapy. Potential clinical roles of pharmacists in outpatient settings are listed in Table 1.

The increasing shift of healthcare delivery from acute care to the ambulatory setting has resulted in more outpatients receiving complex drug therapy regimens requiring close monitoring (3). In light of this trend, it is disturbing to realize that inappropriate patient manage-

Table 1 Direct Patient Care Roles of Pharmacists in the Cardiology Outpatient Setting

- Provide patient education about medications and treatment goals
- Implement strategies to improve compliance
- Provide patient education for drug therapy devices such as home blood pressure monitors
- Monitor and adjust therapy to achieve therapeutic goals on referral by physician (e.g., collaborative drug therapy management in general and specialty pharmacotherapy clinics including anticoagulation, hypertension, hyperlipidemia, heart failure, and cardiac risk reduction)
- Provide recommendations to physicians as to selection and adjustment of drug therapy

ment of drug therapy in the ambulatory setting is reported to be a significant problem, with preventable drug-related hospital admissions comprising an estimated 3–9% of overall admissions (4). The National Committee for Quality Assurance's (NCQA) health plan employer data and information set (HEDIS) is one tool used to evaluate healthcare providers and systems. One HEDIS data set includes cardiology-related measures such as blood pressure control, beta-blocker use after admission for myocardial infarction, cholesterol management after acute cardiovascular events, and whether Medicare patients admitted with heart failure receive beta-blockers within 90 days of hospital discharge (5). These medication-related indicators, coupled with the desire of cardiologists to optimize prescribed pharmacotherapy in the setting of the cardiology clinic, serve as the basis for a number of interdisciplinary endeavors between cardiologists, clinical pharmacists, and other healthcare providers.

II. MODELS OF PHARMACEUTICAL CARE IN THE OUTPATIENT CARDIOLOGY SETTING

In the cardiology setting, clinical pharmacists may work directly with cardiologists in identifying and resolving drug-related problems. They also may meet with patients referred by cardiologists with whom they have collaborative drug therapy agreements in specialized drug-monitoring clinics.

A. Generalized Pharmacotherapy Clinics

Outcome of several cardiac conditions improves significantly with appropriate pharmacotherapy. It is well documented that achievement of treatment goals improves outcomes with interventions such as aggressive cholesterol lowering, hypertension control, intense glucose control in patients with diabetes, antiplatelet therapy and beta-blockers for patients with ischemic heart disease, and adequate angiotensin-converting enzyme (ACE) inhibitor doses in patients with chronic heart failure (6–13). However, due to fragmented healthcare systems with gaps in care, patients often do not receive therapy or reach treatment goals for these conditions (14).

Pharmacists in generalized pharmacotherapy clinics follow patients in whom pharmacotherapy is indicated and must be monitored and/or adjusted to reach and maintain treatment goals. Pharmacist activities, including patient education, assessment of efficacy and compliance, monitoring for adverse drug reactions, and providing drug therapy recommendations, assist in achieving improved disease control and freeing up physician time. In a typical pharmacotherapy monitoring clinic, the physician initiates and determines duration of therapy, then authorizes the clinical pharmacist to follow the patient at shorter intervals between physician visits in order to monitor and adjust therapy. Pharmacists performing these activities have been shown to improve measures of disease control and reduce costs of therapy (15,16). Services provided by pharmacists providing direct patient care outlined in Table 2. Since pharmacist training does not provide expertise in diagnosis, patients who are referred for drug therapy monitoring should have previously been evaluated and assigned a diagnosis by the referring physician. Clinical pharmacists learn enough about the significance of various patient-reported symptomatology and physical findings to report concerning findings to physicians for further assessment. Benefits of outpatient pharmacotherapy services include improvements in patient safety, improved disease control, and reduction of overall costs (17–19).

B. Physician–Pharmacist Collaborative Agreements

Collaborative drug therapy management describes the collaboration of pharmacists with physicians in the overall prescribing process (20,21). Pharmacists who have collaborative practice agreements with physicians are authorized to implement drug therapy protocols upon initiation or referral by the physician. A majority of states in the United States have passed some type collaborative drug therapy management legislation allowing pharmacists to initiate, continue, modify, administer, and monitor and assess response to drug therapy. State pharmacy boards in these states have worked with credentialing committees, physicians, and pharmacy and therapeutics committees to develop protocols and guidelines for managing patients. Physicians who enter collaborative practice agreements with pharmacists may specify a disease state(s) or classes of medications such as anticoagulants or hyperlipidemia therapy that a pharmacist may manage for patients they refer. Collaborative drug therapy management is more extensively practiced in the Department of Veterans Affairs, academic settings, and selected areas of the country where ambulatory care clinical pharmacy practice is well established.

Certification of competence is important before allowing pharmacists to assume direct patient care roles. Approval for clinical privileges or scope of practice by a credentialing committee in a health system or insurance plan, completing disease certification programs, or earning specialty board certification are various mechanisms to document pharmacist competence in performing clinical activities.

C. Specialized Pharmacotherapy Clinics

1. Anticoagulation Services

Many clinical pharmacists are involved in outpatient anticoagulation monitoring programs and clinics. Warfarin therapy requires intensive monitoring due to its complex pharma-

Table 2 Clinical Functions of the Pharmacist in Direct Patient Care Clinics

- Obtain patient histories
- Perform physical assessment necessary to monitor and adjust drug therapy
- Collect other objective information, including laboratory and results of other tests
- Develop medication-related problem lists
- Provide an assessment and plan for each problem
- Communicate goals of therapy and monitoring for each plan
- Provide patient education regarding disease state and drug therapy
- Recommend and implement pharmacotherapy plan
- Follow patient to monitor for outcomes of therapy

cokinetic and pharmacodynamic properties, its interaction with multiple drugs, and its narrow therapeutic index. Frequent monitoring is required to reduce the risk of bleeding and thrombotic episodes in patients taking chronic warfarin. Outpatient therapy with low molecular weight heparins for anticoagulation initiation or bridge therapy also requires close monitoring. Studies have documented that pharmacists with expertise in this area are able to optimally manage therapy with anticoagulants and prevent complications (22–24). Patients followed in one clinical pharmacist-managed anticoagulation clinic maintained their therapeutic INR more often, had lower bleeding and clotting complications, and had fewer hospitalizations and emergency room visits compared to patients receiving usual medical care (23). Bleeding was reduced from 35% to 8%, major to fatal bleeding from 3.9% to 1.6%, and mortality from 2.9% to 0%. Hospitalizations were reduced from 19% to 5%, and emergency room visits were reduced from 22% to 6%, resulting in $162,058 saved per 100 patients managed in the clinic per year. Other studies have also documented reduced bleeding and thrombotic rates in pharmacist-managed anticoagulation clinics (22,24).

2. Heart Failure Specialty Clinics and Programs

Pharmacists can promote optimal drug therapy in heart failure patients by providing drug therapy recommendations to physicians, participating in a heart failure interdisciplinary team, or developing pharmacotherapy clinics for heart failure patients. Key functions of pharmacists in this setting are to verify that patients have been treated with agents known to reduce mortality, such as ACE inhibitors and beta-adrenergic blockers, to titrate therapy in order to improve symptoms without causing toxicity, and to monitor response to therapy. Studies have that shown when pharmacists are involved in the overall care of patients with heart failure, outcomes are improved. In one study, 181 outpatients with heart failure caused by left ventricular dysfunction were randomized to receive either pharmacist interventions (making evidence-based therapy recommendations, performing patient drug therapy education, and providing follow-up telephone care) or standard care with no pharmacist intervention (25). The patients who received pharmacist intervention had a significantly lower all-cause mortality, fewer heart failure events, and more compliance with clinical practice guidelines regarding ACE inhibitor use than the control group. This study highlights the benefits of interdisciplinary patient care and the benefits of having a pharmacist as a member of an interdisciplinary team.

3. Hyperlipidemia Clinics

Despite the well-documented risk of hyperlipidemia and ischemic heart disease and evidence that treating hyperlipidemia reduces cardiovascular risk, a majority of patients do not reach lipid-treatment goals (26). Lack of screening and insufficient education and motivation of patients to follow lifestyle modification and comply with pharmacotherapy regimens contribute to this problem. Pharmacists can contribute to achievement of lipid goals by patients by assisting in screening, promoting a healthy diet, exercise, and smoking cessation, and monitoring and adjusting pharmacotherapy regimens.

In the community setting, pharmacists have demonstrated success in assisting hyperlipidemic patients to achieve therapeutic goals. Providing disease-management services in 26 community-based pharmacies to 397 patients with increased cholesterol levels, pharmacists were able to help patients comply with their medication regimens more than 90% of the time (27). Goal cholesterol levels were maintained at the end of the 2-year study in 62% of patients, which is well over the national average of about 30% (26,28). Pharmacist participation in other multidisciplinary lipid clinics has also been associated with positive outcomes (29,30).

4. *Cardiovascular Risk-Reduction Clinics*

Pharmacists may participate in cardiovascular clinics by promoting rational preventive therapies in patients with known cardiovascular disease and in those at risk, such as those with metabolic syndrome. Activities of pharmacists in this setting include providing patient education, promoting compliance, recommending appropriate therapy such as antiplatelet therapy or beta-blockers, titrating medications to achieve treatment goals for blood pressure, lipid levels, and promoting lifestyle changes such as exercise, healthy diet, and smoking cessation. Clinical pharmacists in a large managed care group managed drug therapy of patients with known heart disease and were able to achieve treatment goals for secondary prevention by screening and initiating treatment to lower cholesterol and recommending use of antiplatelet therapy and beta-blocker therapy. Their study showed a positive impact on patient satisfaction with pharmaceutical care (31).

5. *Hypertension Clinics*

Data show that blood pressure is still uncontrolled in a significant proportion of the population (32). Hypertension is a significant cardiovascular risk factor that often requires pharmacotherapy in addition to lifestyle changes. Hypertension management requires adequate knowledge of pharmacotherapy and familiarity with outcome studies and national treatment guidelines in order to tailor therapeutic regimens to achieve optimal outcomes. In addition, knowledge of interactions of therapy with comorbid disease states and other drugs, as well as the ability to monitor for patient compliance and adverse effects of therapy, is essential. Studies have shown that when clinical pharmacists participate in the detection, monitoring, and management of patients with hypertension that more patients achieve their blood pressure goals (33–37).

D. Additional Functions of Clinical Pharmacists in the Cardiology Setting

In addition to direct patient care roles of clinical pharmacists, there are many activities pharmacists can perform as a healthcare team member in order to increase efficiency, improve patient outcomes and satisfaction, and decrease healthcare costs (Table 3). These include participating in the development of clinical practice guidelines, critical pathways and disease-management programs for patients in healthcare systems (38). Pharmacists can also be available for drug therapy consultation and information provision, reducing the physician time required to answer clinical questions that require extensive searches of drug therapy databases and the primary literature.

E. Barriers to Pharmacists in Providing Pharmaceutical Care

The greatest limitation for pharmacists in providing direct patient care is the current Medicare reimbursement system overseen by the Centers for Medicare and Medicaid Services (CMS), which does not recognize clinical pharmacists as eligible providers of care. Since pharmacists are not reimbursed as providers, their only source of reimbursement is through an overall facility fee billed in hospital outpatient clinics, or through a minimal incident-to-physician fee billed in private physicians' offices. Some private insur-

Table 3 Health System Support Roles of Clinical Pharmacy Services

- Coordinate adverse drug event–monitoring programs
- Participate in interdisciplinary quality improvement programs
- Develop medication assistance programs for indigent patients
- Conduct medication utilization evaluation programs
- Direct medication safety issues
- Participate in formulary management and drug policy issues
- Clinical research involvement
- Collect and report data on prescribing and clinical outcomes to physicians
- Assist in education of medical students, residents, and fellows regarding pharmacotherapy
- Provide drug information consultative services
- Participate on a CPR team

ance companies and managed care programs do reimburse pharmacists for clinical functions, but in general these organizations follow similar guidelines to CMS for reimbursement. Some clinics employ pharmacists after documenting that their services are cost-effective or for risk-management purposes. For example, hiring a pharmacist to provide anticoagulation services can be justified by reduced admissions for bleeding and thrombosis in anticoagulated patients.

III. SUMMARY

Clinical pharmacists are now more prepared than ever to participate as an important part of a cardiovascular patient care team. They embrace evidence-based pharmacotherapy and understand the complexity of therapeutic regimens. The importance of adequate monitoring and titration of medication regimens is foremost in the activity of a clinical pharmacist, and they are trained to work with other professionals in optimizing drug therapy in patients. Whether utilized as a drug information source, a developer and implementer of drug use policies, or a direct patient care provider, most clinically trained pharmacists have the desire and the ability to positively affect patient care outcomes.

REFERENCES

1. Institute of Medicine. Crossing the quality chasm: a new health system for the 21st century. Washington, DC: National Academy Press; 2001. (available at http://www.nap.edu/books/0309072808/html/
2. Knapp KK. Blalock S, O'Malley C. ASHP survey of ambulatory care of pharmacists in managed care and integrated health systems-1999. Am J Health-Syst Pharm 1999;56:2431–2423.
3. American Heart Association. Heart disease and stroke statistics: 2003 update. Available at www.americanheart.org/downloadable/heart/1040391091015HDS_stats_03.pdf, assessed February 13, 2003.
4. Winterstein AG, Sauer BC, Hepler CD, Poole C. Preventable drug-related hospital admissions. Ann Pharmacother 2002;36:1236–1248.
5. Available at: www.ncqa.org/Programs/HEDIS/HEDIS2004/publiccomment.htm
6. Expert Panel on Detection, Evaluation, and Treatment of High Blood Cholesterol in Adults. Executive summary of the third report of the National Cholesterol Education Program (NCEP). Expert Panel on Detection, Evaluation and Treatment of High Blood Cholesterol in Adults (Adult Treatment Panel III). JAMA 2001;285:2486–2497.

7. The Joint National Committee on Detection, Evaluation, and Treatment of High Blood Pressure. The Sixth Report of the Joint National Committee on Detection, Evaluation, and Treatment of High Blood Pressure (JNC-VI). Arch Intern Med 1997;157:2412–2446.

8. UK Prospective Diabetes Study Group. Intensive blood-glucose control with sulphonylureas or insulin compared with conventional treatment and risk of complications in patients with type 2 diabetes (UKPDS 33). Lancet 1998;352:837–853.

9. Diabetes Control and Complications Trial Research Group. The effect of intensive treatment of diabetes on the development and progression of long-term complications in insulin-dependent diabetes mellitus. N Engl J Med 1993;329:977–986.

10. Smith SC, Blair SN, Bonow RO, et al. AHA/ACC guidelines for preventing heart attack and death in patients with atherosclerotic cardiovascular disease: 2001 update. Circulation 2001;104:1577–1579.

11. Gottlieb SS, McCarter RJ, Vogel RA. Effect of beta-blockade in mortality among high-risk and low-risk patients after myocardial infarction. N Engl J Med 1998;339:489–497.

12. Cairns JA, Theroux P, Lewis HD, et al. Antithrombotic agents in coronary artery disease. Chest 2001;119:228S–252S.

13. Hunt SA, Baker DW, Chin MH, et al. ACC/AHA guidelines for the evaluation and management of chronic heart failure in the adult: executive summary: a report of the American College of Cardiology/American Heart Association Task Force on Practice Guidelines (Committee to Revise the 1995 Guidelines for the Evaluation and Management of Heart Failure) J Am Coll Cardiol 2001;38:2101–2113.

14. Presidential Address: Quality of Cardiovascular care in the U.S. Beller GA. J Am Coll Cardiol 2001;38:587–594

15. Galt KA. Cost avoidance, acceptance, and outcomes associated with a pharmacotherapy consult clinic in a veterans affairs medical center. Pharmacotherapy 1998;18:1103–1111.

16. Geber J, Parra D, Beckey NP, Korman L. Optimizing drug therapy in patients with cardiovascular disease: the impact of pharmacist-managed pharmacotherapy clinics in a primary care setting. Pharmacotherapy 2002;22:738–747.

17. Schumock GT, Butler MG, Meek PD, Vermeulen LC, Arondekar BV, Bauman J. Evidence of the economic benefit of clinical pharmacy services: 1996–2000. Pharmacotherapy 2003;23:113–132.

18. Schumock GST, Meek PD, Ploetz PA, Vermeulen LC. Economic evaluations of clinical pharmacy servicers—1988–1995. Pharmacotherapy 1996;16:1188–1208.

19. Hatoum HT, Akhras K. A 32-year literature review on the value and acceptance of ambulatory care provided by clinical pharmacists. Ann Pharmacother 1993;27:1108–1119.

20. Carmichael JM, O'Connell MB, Devine B, et al. ACCP Position Statement. Collaborative drug therapy management by pharmacists. Pharmacotherapy 1997;17(5):1050–1061.

21. Koch KE. Trends in collaborative drug therapy management. Drug Benefit Trends; 21:45–54.

22. Wilt VM, Gums JG, Ahmed OI, Moore LM. Outcome analysis of a pharmacist-managed anticoagulation service. Pharmacotherapy 1995;15:732–739.

23. Chiquette E, Amato MG, Bussey HL. Comparison of an anticoagulation clinic with usual medical care: anticoagulation control, patient outcomes, and health care costs. Arch Intern Med 1998;158:1641–1647.

24. Gray DR, Garabedian-Ruffalo SM, Chretieu SD. Cost justification of a clinical pharmacist managed anticoagulation clinic. Drug Intell Clin Pharmacy 1985;19:575–580.

25. Gattis WA, Hasselblad V, Whellan DJ, O'Connor CM. Reduction in heart failure events by the addition of a clinical pharmacist to the heart failure management team: results of the pharmacist in heart failure assessment recommendation and monitoring (PHARM) study. Arch Intern Med 1999;159:1939–1945.

26. Pearson TA, Laurora I, Chu H, Kafonek S. The lipid treatment assessment project (L-TAP): a multicenter survey to evaluate the percentages of dyslipidemic patients receiving lipid-lowering therapy and achieving low-density lipoprotein cholesterol goals. Arch Intern Med 2000;160:459–467.

27. Bluml BM, McKenney JM, Czirsky. Pharmaceutical care services and results in ImPACT: hyperlipidemia. J Am Pharm Assoc 2000;40:157–165.
28. Hoerger TJ, Bala MV, Bray J, Wilcosky TC, LaRosa J. Treatment patterns and distribution of low-density lipoprotein cholesterol levels in treatment-eligible United States adults. Am J Cardiol 1998;82:61–65.
29. Shaffer J, Wexler LF. Reducing low-density lipoprotein cholesterol levels in an ambcare system. Results of a multidisciplinary collaborative practice lipid clinic compared with traditional physician-based care. Arch Intern Med 1995;155:2330–2335.
30. Harris DE, Record NB, Gibson GW et al. Lipid lowering in a multidisciplinary clinic compared with primary physician involvement. Am J Cardiol 1998;81:929–933.
31. Merenich JA, Lousberg TR, Brennan SH, Calonge NB. Optimizing treatment of dyslipidemia in patients with coronary artery disease in the managed-care environment (the Rocky Mountain Kaiser Permanente experience). Am J Cardiol 2000;85(3A):36A–42A.
32. Joint National Committee on the Detection Evaluation and Treatment of High Blood Pressure. The sixth report of the Joint National Committee on Detection, Evaluation and Management of High Blood Pressure (JNC-VI). Arch Intern Med 1997;157:2413–2446.
33. McGhan WF, Stimmel GL, Hall TG, Gilman TM. A comparison of pharmacists and physicians on the quality of prescribing for ambulatory hypertensive patients. Med Care 1983;21:435–444.
34. McKenney JM, Slining JM, Henderson GR, Devins D, Barr M. The effect of clinical services on patients with essential hypertension. Circulation 1973;48:1104–1111.
35. Solomon DK, Portner TS, Bass GE, Gourley DR, Gourley GA, Holt JM et al. Part 2. Clinical and economic outcomes in the hypertension and COPD arms of a multicenter outcomes study. J Am Pharm Assoc 1998;38:574–585.
36. Carter BL, Elliott WJ. The role of pharmacists in the detection, management, and control of hypertension: a national call to action. Pharmacotherapy 2000;20:119–122.
37. Erickson SR, Slaughter R, Halapy G. Pharmacists' ability to influence outcomes of hypertension therapy. Pharmacotherapy 1997;17:140–147.
38. Ellrodt G, Cook DJ, Lee J. Cho M, Hunt D. Evidence-based disease management. JAMA 1997;278:1687-1692.

6-1

Cost-Effective Drug Selection

Gordon J. Vanscoy
University Pharmacotherapy Associates, LLC, Pittsburgh Veterans Affairs Health System, and University of Pittsburgh School of Pharmacy, Pittsburgh, Pennsylvania, U.S.A.

When patients are hospitalized, the primary interventions targeted to enhance health are surgery and medications. Appropriate medication selection and monitoring can make the difference between a chemical being a toxin or a life-saving/prolonging tool. Efficacy and safety must be of utmost consideration when selecting medications. However, within drug classes we frequently do not have the benefit of head-to-head trials, which define superiority or equivalence. If a superiority trial produces negative results, equivalence cannot be ruled out. Likewise, if equivalence trial results are found to be positive, superiority cannot be excluded.

Without documented differentiation between products, how does one choose? Today's cost-conscience health care environment has added a third criterion to enable more informed drug selection, namely pharmacoeconomics. This type of analysis provides insight into value for prescribers and drug policy makers. Value in this setting can be described as optimizing outcomes for the least overall health care costs.

When assessing the combined impact on outcomes and costs, understanding a study's perspectives is essential to determine the applicability of the results to your situation. Patients desire "high-tech" medicine provided in a service-oriented fashion. Society is demanding less spending on health care. Providers want to deliver the best possible care and be partners in profit. Payers want control of costs and want providers to demonstrate that their services are appropriate, high quality, and cost-effective. It is feasible that a pharmacoeconomic study can demonstrate significant value for society but could be too costly for a particular health care system.

There are many types of pharmacoeconomic analysis including, but not limited to, cost analysis, cost benefit, cost-of-illness, cost utility, number-needed-to-treat, pharmacoepidemiological, and decision-analysis modeling. Cost-minimization studies require equivalent impact on outcomes and only compare the effect on costs. Cost-effectiveness analyzes the relationship between costs and differing outcomes. In a basic form, cost-benefit analysis results in a ratio of the difference in costs to the difference in benefits. Cost utility requires additional data such as assessments on quality of life.

Questions posed by Lawrence Lehman enable a framework for a practical analysis of a pharmacoeconomic study (1). Can the issue or problem be analyzed? Does the selected analysis make sense? Is the analysis appropriate? Is the analysis thorough, complete, and accurate? Are the variables, assumptions, estimates, and computations correct? Does the construct address the most probable outcomes, costs, comorbidities, and benefits? Can the analysis address expected and unexpected changes? Is the analysis an accepted one for the specified indication? Is the chosen analysis the best one for the issue at hand? Is the pharmacoeconomic analysis usable?

In summary, cost-effective thrombo-cardiology drug selection requires a thorough efficacy-and-safety analysis. Appropriate assessment of a drug's value impact and definition of economic perspective provide decision makers additional tools for rationalizing drug selection. The next three chapters focus on cost-effective selection of fibrinolytics, injectable anticoagulants, and antiplatelet agents. Advances in new drug development will necessitate an ongoing assessment of current agents of choice based on efficacy, safety, and value.

REFERENCE

1. Lehman LB. P&T. 2001;26:312–315. 3832

6-2

Cost-Effective Drug Selection: Antiplatelet Agents

Paul Dobesh

St. Louis College of Pharmacy, St. Louis; and St. Luke's Hospital, Chesterfield, Missouri, U.S.A.

Although others may be used on an occasional basis, the main antiplatelet classes utilized to prevent and treat cardiovascular disease are aspirin, ADP antagonists, and glycoprotein (GP) IIb/IIIa receptor inhibitors. These agents have shown their clinical benefits in a wide variety of well-designed clinical trials. As health care advances into the new millennium, the clinical benefits of medical therapies need to be accompanied by an economic analysis of this benefit. For clinicians to make cost-effective selection of antiplatelet agents, the efficacy, safety and pharmacoeconomic data all need to be considered.

I. ORAL ANTIPLATELET AGENTS

Aspirin has been shown to be safe and effective for the acute treatment of myocardial infarction (MI), as well as secondary and primary prevention of MI (1–4). Due to aspirin being readily available, inexpensive, and very effective, few contest the attractive pharmacoeconomic impact of aspirin therapy. For treatment of MI, a 30 day course of treatment costs about $0.30, which calculates into a cost of about $13 per life saved (5). Long-term use for secondary prevention of MI is also inexpensive. Treating 1000 patients for 2–3 years would prevent 12 deaths and 32 nonfatal vascular events. This translates into a cost of $830 per life saved and $310 per nonfatal vascular event prevented (2,6). Primary prevention of MI with aspirin is the least impressive economically but, with appropriate patient selection, still cost-effective. Five years of aspirin therapy for primary prevention of MI in 1000 patients would not significantly affect mortality but would prevent 5 nonfatal MI. This translates into a cost of $3,650 per MI prevented (2,6).

The currently available ADP antagonists—clopidogrel (Plavix; Bristol-Myers Squibb/Sanofi Pharmaceuticals, New York, NY) and ticlopidine (Ticlid; Roche Laboratories Inc, Nutley, NJ)—have been shown to be clinically effective in preventing in-stent thrombosis when added to aspirin for 2–6 weeks. The efficacy of the two agents seems to be similar from the clinical trials (7). Clopidogrel has for the most part replaced ticlopidine as the ADP antagonist of choice for several reasons. First, clopidogrel has a better safety profile, with significantly less neutropenia and thrombotic thrombocytopenic purpura (TTP). Second, clopidogrel has similar clinical efficacy and its loading doses are better tolerated. Finally, clopidogrel costs less (one month of clopidogrel is approximately

$95 vs. $135 for ticlopidine). Not only is the acquisition cost less, but the cost difference is even greater when the need for less hematological monitoring is considered.

One of the more difficult pharmacoeconomic questions is: Should clopidogrel be used instead of aspirin for secondary prevention of ischemic complications? This question comes from the CAPRIE (Clopidogrel versus Aspirin in Patients at Risk of Ischemic Events) trial 9). This trial evaluated the ability of either clopidogrel or aspirin to prevent secondary ischemic complications in over 15,000 patients who recently were diagnosed with either stroke, MI, of peripheral vascular disease. Clopidogrel proved to be significantly better than aspirin at preventing ischemic complications, but the benefit was not impressive. The absolute reduction was only 0.5%, which calculates into a number needed to treat (NNT) to prevent one ischemic complication of 200. Due to the higher cost of clopidogrel (approximately $456,000 to prevent one event) compared to aspirin, this marginal benefit does not seem to justify its use.

The other difficult pharmacoeconomic question is: Should clopidogrel be added to aspirin for all patients with acute coronary syndromes (ACS)? This question comes from the CURE (Clopidogrel in Unstable Angina to Prevent Recurrent Ischemic Events) trial (9,10). This trial evaluated aspirin versus aspirin plus clopidogrel for a year to prevent ischemic complications in patients with ACS. The combination arm was proven to be more effective. The main benefit came from a 2% absolute reduction in MI, which calculates into a NNT of 50 patients to prevent one MI. Based on the acquisition cost of clopidogrel, this roughly calculates to $42,750 to prevent one MI. This does not take into consideration the 1% absolute increases in major bleeding seen with the combination arm. Formal cost-effective analysis for the CURE trial has been completed (11). The use of clopidogrel in substitution for the 5% of patients not eligible for aspirin therapy has a favorable cost-effective ratio of $31,000 per quality-adjusted life-year gained. The routine addition of clopidogrel to aspirin therapy has a much less favorable cost-effective ratio of about $130,000 per quality-adjusted life-year gained.

II.   INJECTABLE GP IIb/IIIA INHIBITORS

GP IIb/IIIa inhibitors are the most potent platelet inhibitors in our arsenal to treat patients suffering from an ACS. There are currently three FDA-approved agents available for use in the United States. These agents are abciximab (ReoPro; Centocor/Eli Lilly & Co., Indianapolis, IN), tirofiban (Aggrastat; Merck, West Point, PA), and eptifibatide (Integrilin; Cor/Schering-Key, Kenilworth, NJ). All block GP IIb/IIIa receptors, but there are some pharmacological differences (12). Abciximab is a monoclonal antibody, while the other "small-molecule" agents are either a nonpeptide (tirofiban) or a peptide (eptifibatide) molecule. Both tirofiban and eptifibatide inhibit the platelet for about 4–8 hours and are GP IIb/IIIa–specific inhibitors (12). Abciximab inhibits the platelet for at least 24 hours and also blocks the vitronectin and MAC-1 receptors (12). The clinical relevance of these differences has not been fully clarified.

These agents have been evaluated in a few different settings. The agents have mainly been evaluated in patients undergoing immediate percutaneous coronary intervention (PCI) or in the medical stabilization of patients with ACS may or may not be undergoing PCI in the near future. The benefits seen with the use of GP IIb/IIIa inhibitors in clinical trials are usually a significant reduction in the composite endpoint of death, nonfatal MI, and the need for repeat coronary intervention (PCI or CABG). Since prevention of repeat coronary interventions may be considered a "soft" endpoint by some, the composite of death and nonfatal MI is also commonly reported. The major safety concern with the use of these agents is bleeding. Aside from the EPIC (Evaluation of 7E3 for the Prevention of Ischemic Complications) trial (13), which was the first large experience with abciximab, major bleeding is not significantly increased with the use of GP IIb/IIIa inhibitors.

GP IIb/IIIa inhibitors have had a large impact on pharmacy budgets. The acquisition cost for the agents differs between agents and treatment strategy. When the agents are used in the setting of PCI, the acquisition costs are about $1,350 for abciximab, $740 for tirofiban, and $600 for eptifibatide. For patients who are to receive the agents upstream for medical stabilization (with or without PCI), the acquisition costs are $1,800 for abciximab, $1,100 for tirofiban, and $1,630 for eptifibatide. As many practitioners know, the longer these agents are infused, the higher the cost. This is especially true for the small molecules (tirofiban and eptifibatide), since most of the dose is given during the infusion, whereas most of the dose of abciximab is given during the bolus. These acquisition costs are based on the average infusion times from clinical trials in the published literature (13–21). An example of this would be the >70-hour infusions of tirofiban and eptifibatide utilized in the PRISM-PLUS (Platelet Receptor Inhibition in Ischemic Syndrome-Management in Patients Limited by Unstable Signs and Symptoms) and PURSUIT (Platelet Glycoprotein IIb/IIIa in Unstable Angina: Receptor Suppression Using Integrilin Therapy) trials, respectively (18,20). While some may advocate shorter infusion times to reduce costs, it is critical to remember that the benefits from utilizing the agents from these trials are based on specific infusion times, and the outcomes with shorter infusion times are not known and may not result in clinical benefit.

For most institutions that treat patients with ACS, especially those that perform PCI, this group of agents is usually in the top 10 for pharmacy expenditures. The ability to utilize these agents has also increased over the last several years with the increasing number of PCIs in this country. In 1998 an estimated 550,000 PCIs were completed in the United States alone (22). While these agents have contributed to greatly increasing hospital pharmacy budgets, the reimbursement to hospitals for treating patients with ACS has not increased to the same degree. Therefore, despite the clinical benefits seen with these agents, there can be a disincentive to utilize these agents from the payer perspective. But as increasing numbers of clinical trials have shown the benefits utilizing GP IIb/IIIa inhibitors, refraining from utilizing these agents becomes less and less appealing. This has led many clinicians to become more familiar with the available pharmacoeconomic data on the use of these agents. While the acquisition cost to institutions may be high, this must be combined with the clinical benefits seen in patients with ACS, and related to the total economic impact from the payer, patient, and societal perspectives. It is unfortunate when economic discussions regarding the use of GP IIb/IIIa inhibitors begin and end with the comparison of acquisition costs. The pharmacoeconomic evaluation of these agents must go beyond the acquisition cost and include more important considerations such as the effectiveness of the agent, total hospital costs, and the overall cost-effectiveness of using each specific agent.

The most common driving forces of in-hospital costs for patients undergoing PCI have been determined. The largest contributor to total hospital cost is the occurrence of unplanned ischemic complications (23–27). Different ischemic complications have different impacts on hospital cost 24,27,28). By decreasing the occurrence of ischemic complications, therapeutic interventions can have a dramatic impact on the total hospital costs associated with patients receiving PCI. Because of the beneficial reduction in ischemic complications observed with the use of GP IIb/IIIa inhibitors, these agents have the ability reduce the cost of care and possibly recover some of their own cost through their effectiveness.

III. TRIAL COMPARISONS (NUMBER NEEDED TO TREAT)

When clinicians decide which GP IIb/IIIa inhibitor to utilize, the outcomes the agents provide must be part of the discussion of cost-effective drug selection. The prevention of ischemic complications represents the driving force for the economics rather than the acquisition cost of the different agents. The utility of the GP IIb/IIIa inhibitors has been evaluated in a number of clinical trials with patients going to PCI. Most of these trials have evaluated patients who present with ACS. The use of abciximab has been evaluated in the EPIC, EPILOG (Evaluation in PTCA to Improve Long-Term Outcome with Abciximab GP IIb/IIIa Blockade), and EPISTENT (Evaluation of Platelet IIb/IIIa Inhibitor for Stenting) trials (13–15). Tirofiban has been evaluated in the RESTORE (Randomized Efficacy Study of Tirofiban for Outcomes and REstenosis) trial, and eptifibatide has been evaluated in the IMPACT II (Integrilin to Minimize Platelet Aggregation and Coronary Thrombosis II) trial (17,19). Eptifibatide has also been evaluated in the more recent ESPRIT (Enhanced Suppression of Platelet IIb/IIIa Receptor with Integrilin Therapy) trial, but this trial evaluated eptifibatide in patients undergoing elective procedures, and not in patients currently experiencing an ACS (21). It can be difficult to make direct comparisons between these trials because of some differences in the definition of endpoints used, known and unknown differences in the study populations, and different utilization of intracoronary stents. However, one may combine the data and make comparisons such as outcomes and economic impact of the agents. This can be accomplished by determined the number of patients that need to be treated (NNT) in order to prevent one ischemic event (29–31).

As previously discussed, these trials generally share a common combined triple endpoint of death, MI, and urgent revascularization, usually evaluated at 30 days and 6 months. The NNT to prevent one of these ischemic complications at these time points is shown in Table 1. The data suggest that approximately 20 patients need to be treated with abciximab in order to prevent one of these ischemic event at 30 days and out to 6 months. The trials with small molecules each produce a NNT that is approximately twice that of abciximab in the short term and up to five times that of abciximab with "harder" endpoints (death or MI) at 6 months.

Utilizing NNT one can then calculate how much it costs to prevent one ischemic event. The overall cost to prevent one death or MI at 30 days from the abciximab trial data is approximately $20,000 compared to >$30,000 for either of the of the small molecules (Table 1). Using this method of analyzing cost spent to prevent ischemic events shows that less money is spent when using abciximab as compared to one of the other agents. When examining the data regarding the use of the GP IIb/IIIa receptor inhibitors for medical stabilization, the NNT can also be calculated (Table 1). The PURSUIT data seem to be an outlier compared to similar trials. However, subgroup analysis of the North American (NA) patients in this trial showed a NNT of 30, which is very consistent with data from PRISM PLUS. These findings support the cost of about $30,000 to prevent one death or MI when using one of the small molecules. This concept of viewing abciximab as less costly is counterintuitive for most individuals because the acquisition cost is higher than that for the small molecules. This type of analysis emphasizes the importance of evaluating the clinical benefit as part of the overall economic impact of the agents and looking beyond acquisition costs. If the ESPRIT data are included, the cost to prevent one death or MI with eptifibatide is similar to that of the abciximab ACS trials. The NNT are slightly higher for the ESPRIT trial, but the acquisition cost for eptifibatide is less than for abciximab (21).

It is important to remember the limitations of these cross-trial comparisons discussed earlier. A better understanding of the economic impact an agent may have requires

Table 1 Number Needed to Treat for the Prevention of Ischemic Events for PCI Trials with GP IIb/IIIa Inhibitors

Trial (Ref.)	Agent	NNT to prevent 1 D/MI/UR at 30 days	NNT to prevent 1 D/MI at 30 days	Cost to prevent 1 D/MI at 30 days	NNT to prevent 1 D/MI/UR at 6 months	NNT to prevent 1 D/MI at 6 months
EPIC (12)	Abciximab	22	11	$15,477	13	17
EPILOG (13)	Abciximab	16	16	$22,512	16	19
EPISTENT (14)	Abciximab	19	10	$13,500	18	18
RESTORE (16)	Tirofiban	40	53	$37,100	34	111
IMPACT II (18)	Eptifibatide	39	67	$29,212	N/A	91
CAPTURE (15)	Abciximab		24	$43,200		
PRISIM-PLUS (17)	Tirofiban		31	$32,550		
PURSUIT (19)	Eptifibatide		67	$81,941		
PURSUIT NA (19)	Eptifibatide		30	$36,690		
ESPRIT (20)	Eptifibatide		28	$16,800		25

NNT = numbers needed to treat; D = death; MI = myocardial infarction; UR = urgent revascularization; N/A = not available; NA = North American patients.

more formal pharmacoeconomic analysis. Some of these data come from different sources. Some of the analysis is collected as substudies from large clinical trials. This type of data has the strengths of randomization and maybe even blinding of study groups. The limitation that can exist with this type of pharmacoeconomic analysis is that it is not "real world." There are several aspects of care in a clinical trial that may not reflect real-world treatment and expenses due to the well-structured environment created by the clinical trial. To balance this, there are real-world pharmacoeconomic studies available for review, where health centers or systems have collected clinical outcome and economic data. These have the strength of being more comparable to other institutions for how patients are cared for, but these data are not randomized or blinded.

IV. PHARMACOECONOMIC ANALYSES: CLINICAL TRIALS

Formal pharmacoeconomic substudies have been performed for some of the large clinical trial that have been already mentioned. One of these is the economic analysis of the EPIC trial (27,32). Even with the increase in bleeding events, at 6 months the overall hospital costs for patients treated with abciximab were only $145 more than those in the placebo arm. In other words, the drug was able to recover the majority of its cost through sustained prevention of adverse ischemic outcomes at 6 months. Since the clinical outcomes with abciximab were better and it appeared to be relatively cost-neutral, it can be said that the therapy was cost-beneficial. A cost-effectiveness analysis was also done on the EPIC trial. At 6 months the cost to keep a patient free from ischemic complications in the placebo arm was $27,700 compared to $25,400 in the abciximab arm. This represents a $3,000 savings at 6 months in patients treated with abciximab. From the hospital prospective, the cost of GP IIb/IIIa therapy often cannot be passed on to the payer, particularly with fixed diagnostic-related groups (DRGs) or capitated reimbursement. In this situation, the institution absorbs these costs. This is why the acquisition cost is focused on rather than the overall cost-effectiveness of the therapeutic intervention. This assessment of the long-term benefits allows institutions to look past acquisition cost, act in the best interest of patients, and continue to implement cost-effective strategies.

Formal economic analysis of the EPILOG trial allows for a better representation of abciximab data because of the improvement in heparin dosing that resulted in decrease bleeding complications (33). The in-hospital costs for abciximab-treated patients was $800 less than placebo-treated patients ($p =0.004$). This reduction in cost was due to decreased ischemic events in the abciximab-treated patients. When the cost of the drug is factored into this equation, the net cost of abciximab therapy upon discharge was determined to be $544. Therefore, the agent is able to recover about 65% of its cost by the time the patient completes the initial hospitalization. At 6 months the cost of abciximab therapy had increased to $1,180.

This ability of abciximab to recuperate much of its expense by the time the patient leaves the hospital has also been evaluated outside of the well-controlled clinical trial environment. A retrospective evaluation of abciximab therapy at a University Medical Center was able to reproduce similar findings in data collected between 1/1/96 and 6/30/98 (31). An assessment of approximately 1150 patients and 1350 interventions found the adjusted cost for abciximab upon discharge to be about $600, similar to the EPILOG trial. It would seem that whether in a controlled clinical environment of a study protocol or the real-world setting, the agent was able to recover about 65% of its cost before the patient left the hospital.

Economic analysis of the RESTORE trial, in which tirofiban was administered to patients undergoing PCI, has also been completed (34). The cost difference between tirofiban and placebo patients was $438 ($p$ = NS). When the cost of tirofiban is added in, the total costs are increased by $262. The reason costs are not reduced before adding in acquisition cost as much as with abciximab is due to less clinical benefit seen in the trials with abciximab than with tirofiban (13,14,17). This example emphasizes the importance of evaluating clinical efficacy along with cost to create a complete economic picture. It is also important to put these economic analyses into perspective. The analyses discussed so far utilized little intracoronary stenting ≤10% of patients) compared to practice today (~80%).

Another formal pharmacoeconomic analysis of a clinical trial was conducted on the PURSUIT trial (35), which trial assessed the efficacy of an average 72-hour infusion of eptifibatide in patients with a non–ST segment elevation ACS. The economic assessment demonstrated no difference in the total hospital costs at 6 months, excluding drug cost ($18,456 eptifibatide vs. 18,828 placebo; p = NS). The cost of the agent must be factored into this equation—approximately $1200 for a 72-hour infusion into the eptifibatide arm.

V. PHARMACOECONOMIC ANALYSES: CLINICAL PRACTICE EXPERIENCES

There have been several nonrandomized analyses of the economic impact of GP IIb/IIIa inhibitors on individual hospitals and health systems (36–43). It is thought that these analyses give a real world look at the economic impact of these agents. A fairly common measure that is evaluated is the impact the agents have on length of hospitalization (LOH). LOH can be an important indirect measure of ischemic complications and cost. If ischemic complications are increased, so will be LOH. If LOH is increased, so will be hospital cost. This allows hospitals and health systems to evaluate the impact of these agents beyond acquisition costs. Even though the pharmacy budget may be heavily impacted by the use of these agents, other areas of the hospital or health system may see benefits. Consequently, these agents may not be as much of an economic burden when considering the entire expense of care to the patient. This should be helpful from the payer perspective, since most formal pharmacoeconomic analyses are based more on a societal perspective.

Ohio Heart Christ Hospital collected information on unstable angina patients undergoing PCI in 1995 and 1997 (36). Between these time periods, they witnessed a dramatic increase in the use of abciximab (15% to 70%) and stents (20% to 60%). This increased utilization led to a substantial reduced in LOH in 1997 (1.8 days) compared to 1995 (2.8 days), along with a 28% reduction in hospital costs, despite the increase utilization of these new technologies.

The Hospital Corporation Information Association (HCIA) has a database of patients from over 1500 hospitals across the country. They found a statistically significant reduction in LOH of 0.89 days ($p < 0.05$) in patients who received abciximab compared to those undergoing PCI without the use of abciximab (37). There was also a consistent reduction in LOH of 0.54 days ($p < 0.05$) in the subgroup of patients diagnosed with MI. The HCIA has also collected similar data comparing all three GP IIb/IIIa inhibitors (38–40). The LOH was statistically increased by almost a full day in patients given either of the small molecules when compared to patients given abciximab (0.91 more days with eptifibatide, $p = 0.002$; and 0.98 more days with tirofiban, $p < 0.001$). This increased LOH contributes to the increase in the hospitalization costs of $1,336 in the patients given eptifibatide ($p < 0.001$) and $2,671 in patients given tirofiban ($p < 0.001$) when compared to the patients given abciximab in this evaluation.

An economic evaluation of elective patients undergoing PCI who could have received either tirofiban or abciximab in an unrandomized fashion has been conducted in the community hospital setting (41). In this analysis, patients who received abciximab had a significantly shorter LOH than patients who received tirofiban (2.4 days vs. 3.0 days; $p < 0.01$). This did not correlate to a reduction in sin-hospital cost with the use of abciximab compared to tirofiban as in the HCIA evaluation. Another small economic evaluation of GP IIb/IIIa inhibitor therapy was conducted by the PRICE investigators (42). This was a relatively small trial ($n = 320$) of low-risk patients undergoing elective PCI who were to randomly receive abciximab or eptifibatide. The adverse clinical outcomes at hospital discharge (4.9% abciximab and 5.1% eptifibatide) and at 30 days (5.6% abciximab and 6.3% eptifibatide) were statistically similar, although an assessment of clinical differences would be difficult with this low number of patients. Due to the assumption of similar clinical outcomes between the agents and the lower acquisition cost of eptifibatide, there was a cost benefit to using eptifibatide over abciximab in these elective PCI patients.

VI. PHARMACOECONOMIC ANALYSES: COST PER LIFE-YEAR SAVED

Cost-effective analysis is a common method to help determine if the added cost of a therapy represents a good value, especially in regard to improved survival or life expectancy. This type of analysis creates a ratio that the health-care system then needs to determine if it is economically attractive. A commonly held benchmark for cost-effectiveness has been <$50,000 per life-year gained (44). Therapies that have ratios less than this may be economically attractive, while those that are higher may not be. In the pure sense of this analysis, the therapy needs to show a reduction in mortality in order for such an analysis to be appropriate. The only clinical trial to show a statistically significant reduction in mortality at one year with GP IIb/IIIa inhibitor therapy has been the EPISTENT Trial (1.0% stent with abciximab vs. 2.4% stent without abciximab; $p = 0.037$) (45). Based on the results of this trial, adding abciximab to intracoronary stenting would give a cost-effectiveness ratio of $6,213 for an additional life-year saved. This would be classified as highly cost-effective therapy (44). This ratio is in line with or even more attractive than other cost-effective therapies, such as ACE inhibitor therapy post-MI, t-PA over streptokinase for MI, or secondary prevention of MI with HMG-CoA reductase inhibitors (44). This impressive cost-effective ratio may change the question from, "Can we afford to use this therapy?" to "Can we afford not to use this therapy?" It is important to remember that this type of analysis is from a societal prospective, and the payer may not share the same perspective.

Kereiakes and associates have completed a similar analysis at their institutions (46). The data were presented as a real-world evaluation of a high-volume interventional practice. In their evaluation of 1472 patients they found a significant reduction in mortality with the use of abciximab compared to no abciximab. Based on this reduction in mortality they were able to calculate a cost-effective ratio of $2,875 per life-year saved with the use of abciximab. While this evaluation carries the limitations of small size and lack of randomization, it still confirms an attractive cost-effective ratio for the use of abciximab in the reduction in mortality.

Another formal cost-effective analysis was performed in the PURSUIT Trial (34). This analysis calculated a cost-effective ratio of $16,491 per life-year saved. There are a couple of important limitations to this calculation. First, this ratio is based only on the U.S. cohort of patients from the trial, which is the half of the patients who had the best outcomes. When the entire PURSUIT population is analyzed, the ratio increases to $33,619. Second, and most important, mortality was not reduced in the PURSUIT trial. Mortality for patients in both groups was 6.2%. Therefore, cost of life-years saved is calculated without the saving of lives. This is done by assumptions of lives saved by reductions in myocardial infarction. In comparison, the EPISTENT cost-effective ratio is calculated on the mortality benefit, and myocardial infarction reductions are not added into the equation. The cost-effectiveness of eptifibatide from the EPRINT trial has also been presented (47). This analysis concluded the one-year cost of eptifibatide to be $291 per patient with a cost per life-year gained of $1,407—highly cost-effective. As in the PURSUIT trial, mortality was not significantly reduced with the use of eptifibatide in the ESPRIT trial and assumptions from the incidence of reduction in MI are made.

VII. CONCLUSIONS

The efficacy and safety of GP IIb/IIIa receptor inhibitors is well known and accepted. This leaves cost as the leading barrier to more widespread use of these agents. Pharmacoeconomic data from the relevant prospective become critically important when making cost-effective drug selection. Economic substudies are becoming more common and soon may become standard. When considering the use of high-cost agents such as GP IIb/IIIa inhibitors, this type of analysis can be very helpful tool. These analyses evaluate this issue in terms of cost to prevent ischemic events, in-hospital costs, follow-up costs, LOH, and cost-effectiveness for added years of life. Currently most of the available data exist with the use of abciximab. This may be attributed to the higher acquisition cost of the agent compared to the small molecule agents, and therefore a greater need to prove its worth. Arguably, the data reveal that the higher acquisition cost of abciximab is offset by the resultant prevention in ischemic complications. The acquisition costs of eptifibatide and tirofiban are less than that of abciximab, and these agents are not as economically prohibitive, but, fewer economic data exist an these agents. Currently the only head-to-head large clinical trial has been the TARGET (Do Tirofiban and ReoPro Give Similar Efficacy) trial (48), which showed a significant benefit of abciximab over tirofiban at 30 days. Pharmacoeconomic analysis of this trial is needed. The current comparison pharmacoeconomic data may favor abciximab, but some analyses report a benefit for either of the small molecules. In today's health-care environment, clinicians are required to learn and utilize more pharmacoeconomic data than ever before in an attempt to make cost-effective drug selection. If more head-to-head data become available, agent selection may become easierr.

REFERENCES

1. ISIS-2 Collaborative Group. Randomized trial of intravenous streptokinase, oral aspirin, both, of neither among 17,187 cases of suspected acute myocardial infarction: ISIS-2. Lancet 1988; ii:349–360.
2. Antiplatelet Trialists' Collaboration. Collaborative overview of randomized trials of antiplatelet therapy-1: prevention of death, myocardial infarction, and stroke by prolonged antiplatelet therapy in various categories of patients. Br Med J 1994; 308:81–106.
3. Steering Committee of the Physicians' Health Study Research Group. Final report on the aspirin component of the ongoing Physicians' Health Study. N Engl J Med 1989; 321:129–135.

4. Peto R, Gray R, Collins R, et al. Randomized trial of prophylactic daily aspirin in British male doctors. Br Med J 1988; 296:313–316.

5. Hennekens CH, Jonas MA, Buring JE. The benefits of aspirin in acute myocardial infarction. Still a well kept secret in the United States. Arch Intern Med 1994; 154:37–39.

6. Gaziano JM, Skerrett PJ, Buring JE. Aspirin in the treatment and prevention of cardiovascular disease. Haemostasis 2000; 30(suppl 3):1–13.

7. Calver AL, Blows LJ, Harmer S. Clopidogrel for prevention of major cardiac events after coronary stent implantation: 30-day and 6-month results in patients with smaller stents. Am Heart J 2000; 140:483–491.

8. CAPRIE Steering Committee. A randomized, blinded, trial of clopidogrel versus aspirin in patients at risk of ischemic events (CAPPRIE). Lancet 1996; 348:1329–1339.

9. The CURE Trial Investigators. Effects of clopidogrel in addition to aspirin in patients with acute coronary syndromes without ST-segment elevation. N Engl J Med 2001; 345:494–502.

10. Mehta SR, Yusuf S, Peters RJG, et al. Effects of pretreatment with clopidogrel and aspirin followed by long-term therapy in patients undergoing percutaneous coronary intervention: the PCI-CURE study. Lancet 2001; 358:527–533.

11. Gaspoz JM, Coxson PG, Goldman PA, et al. Cost-effectiveness of aspirin, clopidogrel, or both for secondary prevention of coronary heart disease. N Engl J Med 2002; 346:1800–1806.

12. Dobesh PP, Latham KA. Advancing the battle against acute ischemic syndromes: a focus on the GP IIb/IIIa inhibitors. Pharmacotherapy 1998; 18:663–685.

13. The EPIC Investigators. Use of a monoclonal antibody directed against the platelet glycoprotein IIb/IIIa receptor in high-risk coronary angioplasty. N Engl J Med 1994; 330:956–961.

14. The EPILOG Investigators. Platelet glycoprotein IIb/IIIa receptor blockade and low-dose heparin during percutaneous coronary revascularization. N Engl J Med 1997; 336:1689–1696.

15. The EPISTENT Investigators. Randomized placebo-controlled and balloon-angioplasty-controlled trial to assess safety of coronary stenting with use of platelet glycoprotein IIb/IIIa blockade. Lancet 1998; 352:87–92.

16. The CAPTURE Investigators. Randomized placebo-controlled trial of abciximab before and during coronary intervention in refractory unstable angina: the CAPTURE study. Lancet 1997; 349:1429–1435.

17. The RESTORE Investigators. Effects of platelet glycoprotein IIb/IIIa blockade with tirofiban on adverse cardiac events in patients with unstable angina or acute myocardial infarction undergoing coronary angioplasty. Circulation 1997; 96:1445–1453.

18. The PRISM-PLUS Study Investigators. Inhibition of the platelet glycoprotein IIb/IIIa receptor with tirofiban in unstable angina and non-Q-wave myocardial infarction. N Engl J Med 1998; 338:1488–1497.

19. The IMPACT II Investigators. Randomized placebo-controlled trial of effects of eptifibatide on complications of percutaneous coronary intervention: IMPACT II. Lancet 1997; 349:1422–1428.

20. The PURSUIT Trial Investigators. Inhibition of platelet glycoprotein IIb/IIIa with eptifibatide in patients with acute coronary syndromes. N Engl J Med 1998; 339:436–443.

21. The ESPRIT Investigators. Novel dosing regimen of eptifibatide in planned coronary stent implantation (ESPRIT): a randomized, placebo-controlled trial. Lancet 2000; 356:2037–2044.

22. 2001 Heart and Stroke Facts: Statistical supplement. American Heart Association.

23. Hlatky MA, Boothroyd DB, Brooks BB, et al. Clinical correlates of the initial and long-term cost of coronary bypass surgery and coronary angioplasty. Am Heart J 1999; 138:376–383.

24. Vaitkus PT, Witmer WT, Brandenburg RG, et al. Economic impact of angioplasty salvage techniques with an empasis on coronary stents: a method incorporating cost, revenues, clinical effectiveness and payer mix. J Am Coll Cardiol 1997; 4:894–900.

25. Mark DB, O'Neil WW, Brodie B, et al. Baseline and 6-month cost of primary angioplasty therapy for acute myocardial infarction: results from the Primary Angioplasty Registry. J Am Coll Cardiol 1995; 26:688–695.

26. Adele C, Vaitkus PT, Wells SK, et al. Cost advantages of an as hoc angioplasty strategy. J Am Coll Cardiol 1998; 31:321–325.

27. Hillegass WB. The economics of IIb/IIIa therapy. J Invasive Cardiol 1996; 8(suppl B):30B–33B.

28. Popma JJ, Redwood SR, Chuang YC, et al. Procedure-related complications are the major contributors of incremental in-hospital cost after angioplasty (abstr). Circulation 1995; 92(suppl I):I–662.

29. Hillegass WB, Newman AR, Raco DL. Economic issues in glycoprotein IIb/IIIa receptor therapy. Am Heart J 1999; 136:S24–S32.

30. Bell DM. Analysis of number needed to treat and cost of platelet glycoprotein IIb/IIIa inhibitors in percutaneous coronary interventions in acute coronary syndromes. Pharmacotherapy 1999; 19:1086–1093.

31. Hillegass WB, Newman AR, Raco DL. Glycoprotein IIb/IIIa receptor therapy in percutaneous coronary intervention and non-ST-segment elevation acute coronary syndromes. Pharmacoeconomics 2001; 19:41–55.

32. Mark DB, Talley JD, Topol EJ, et al. Economic assessment of platelet glycoprotein IIb/IIIa inhibition for prevention of ischemic complications of high-risk coronary angioplasty. Circulation 1996; 94:629–635.

33. Lincoff AM, Mark DB, Tcheng JE, et al. Economic assessment of platelet glycoprotein IIb/IIIa receptor blockade with abciximab and low-dose heparin during percutaneous coronary revascularization. Circulation 2000; 102:2923–2929.

34. Weintraub WS, Culler S, Boccuzzi SJ, et al. Economic impact of GP IIb/IIIa blockade after high-risk angioplasty. J Am Coll Cardiol 1999; 34:1061–1066.

35. Mark DB, Harrington RA, Lincoff AM, et al. Cost-effectiveness of platelet glycoprotein IIb/IIIa inhibition with eptifibatide in patients with non-ST-elevation acute coronary syndromes. Circulation 2000; 101:366–371.

36. Kereiakes DJ. Preferential benefit of platelet glycoprotein IIb/IIIa receptor blocker: specific considerations by device and disease state. Am J Cardiol 1998; 81:49E–54E.

37. Lage MJ, Barber BL, Bowman L, Ball DE, Bala M. Shorter hospital stays for angioplasty patients who receive abciximab. J Invas Cardiol 2000; 12:179–186.

38. Lage MJ, Barber BL, Scherer J, McCollam P. Shorter hospital length of stay for coronary angioplasty patients who receive abciximab versus eptifibatide or tirofiban (abstr). Value Health 2000; 3:57.

39. Lage MJ, Barber BL, McCollam P, Bala M, Scherer. Impact of abciximab versus eptifibatide on length of hospital stay for PCI patients. Cathet Cardiovasc Intervent 2001; 53:296–303.

40. Lage MJ, Barber BL, McCollam P, Bala M, Scherer. Impact of abciximab versus tirofiban on length of hospital stay for PCI patients. Cathet Cardiovasc Intervent 2001; 52:298–305.

41. Lucore CL, Mishkel GJ, Ligon RW, Rocha-Singh K. Economic implications of coronary stenting with adjunctive IIb/IIIa receptor antagonist in a community hospital. J Invas Cardiol 1999; 11:14C–20C.

42. The PRICE Investigators. Comparative 30-day economic and clinical outcomes of platelet glycoprotein IIb/IIIa inhibitor use during elective percutaneous coronary intervention: Prairie ReoPro Versus Integrilin Cost Evaluation (PRICE) Trial. Am Heart J 2001; 141:402–409.

43. Dobesh PP, Lanfear SL, Abu-Shanab JR, Lakamp JE, Gowda G, Haikal M. Outcomes associated with a change in prescribing of glycoprotein IIb/IIIa inhibitors in percutaneous intervention in a community hospital setting. Ann Pharmacother 2003; 37:1375–1380.

44. Goldman, L, Garber, AM, Grover SA, Hlatky MA. Task force 6. Cost-effectiveness of assessment and management of risk factors. J Am Coll Cardiol 1996; 27:1020–1030.

45. Topol EJ, Mark DB, Lincoff AM, et al. Outcomes at 1 year and economic implications of platelet glycoprotein IIb/IIIa blockade in patients undergoing coronary stenting: results from a multicentre randomized trial. Lancet 1999; 354:2019–2024.

46. Kereiakes DJ, Obenchain RL, Barber BL, et al. Abciximab provides cost-effective survival advantage in high-volume interventional practice. Am Heart J 2000; 140:603–610.

47. Cohen DJ. Cost-effectiveness of eptifibatide in patients undergoing planned coronary stenting: results from the EPRIT trail. Presented at the American Heart Association Scientific Sessions, November 12, 2001, Anaheim, CA.

48. Topol EJ, Moliterno DJ, Herrmann HC, et al. Comparison of two platelet glycoprotein IIb/IIIa inhibitors, tirofiban and abciximab, for prevention of ischemic events with percutaneous coronary revascularization. N Engl J Med 2001; 344:1888–1894.

6-3

Cost-Effective Drug Selection: Fibrinolytics

Thomas L. Rihn
University Pharmacotherapy Associates, LLC, and Duquesne University School of Pharmacy, Pittsburgh, Pennsylvania, U.S.A.

Nearly one in every two Americans dies of cardiovascular disease. The 1.1 million acute myocardial infarctions (AMIs) each year in the United States are an important component of cardiovascular disease. Acute myocardial infarction represents a high-cost DRG ($10,428 per Medicare discharge for AMI), which contributes significantly to total cardiovascular expenditures (1). Approximately 400,000 infarct patients are admitted to hospitals each year with ST-segment elevation myocardial infarction (STEMI).

DeWood et al. observed that occlusive intracoronary thrombi were present in the majority of AMI patients, establishing thrombosis as the primary pathophysiological mechanism of acute infarct (2). Thus, it is critical to initiate early reperfusion therapy in the form of fibrinolytic therapy or primary angioplasty [percutaneous coronary intervention (PCI)] to minimize infarct size and reduce mortality. The time-to-treatment goal for administration of a fibrinolytic in STEMI is within 30 minutes of the patient presenting to the door of the hospital.

Double-blind, placebo-controlled, randomized trials of fibrinolytic therapy for AMI have established fibrinolytics as a pharmacological standard of care in patients with STEMI presenting within 12 hours of onset of chest pain (3–12). Considering the number of STEMI patients, the time to presentation, potential contraindications to fibrinolytic therapy, and the number of patients treated today with primary angioplasty/stenting, ~100,000–150,000 patients per year are actual candidates for fibrinolytic therapy. The acquisition cost of commonly used next-generation fibrinolytics is in the range of $2,200 although the cost may vary depending on specific group purchasing agreements. This cost is appreciable when considering total hospital costs and current reimbursement patterns for AMI admissions.

I. PHARMACOLOGICAL DIFFERENTIATION

Common fibrinolytics currently FDA approved for the treatment of AMI include streptokinase, or SK (Streptase™, AstraZeneca), reteplase or r-PA (Retavase™, Centocor, Inc.), alteplase, or t-PA (Activase™, Genentech, Inc.), and tenecteplase, or TNK (TNKase™, Genentech, Inc.). The key criteria for fibrinolytic selection in AMI are the comparative pharmacological characteristics, clinical efficacy/safety, and economics.

SK is antigenic, is an indirect plasminogen activator, and is not fibrin specific. It has been associated with significant allergic manifestations including hypotension. As a result, SK is not generally considered optimal in drug selection in the United States today, even though the acquisition cost of the drug is significantly lower than that of the other fibrinolytics. The other three fibrinolytics are not antigenic. r-PA possesses a low degree of fibrin specificity. t-PA is much more fibrin specific than r-PA, but, TNK possesses fibrin specificity (selectivity) 14-fold greater than that of wild-type t-PA (13). A high level of fibrin specificity is desirable in a fibrinolytic agent because it permits targeting of the clot in the infarct-related artery while conserving fibrinogen and minimizing systemic plasminogen activation. The pharmacokinetics of the fibrinolytics, including the elimination half-life, are important in determining the preferred mode and ease of administration. The elimination half-lives of r-PA, t-PA, and TNK are 18, 5, and 20 minutes, respectively (13). TNK exhibits a biphasic disposition from the plasma and is cleared from the plasma more than four times more slowly than native t-PA. Although the initial elimination half-life of TNK is approximately 20 minutes, the terminal phase half-life of the drug is 90–130 minutes. This permits the drug to be administered as a single weight-adjusted bolus dose. r-PA is administered as a double bolus (30 minutes apart), and t-PA is given as a weight-based bolus plus infusion over 90 minutes. TNK-tPA is relatively resistant to inactivation by plasminogen activator inhibitor-1 (PAI-1) (13). PAI-1 is a primary regulator of the fibrinolytic system and a major inhibitor of t-PA. The lytic action of plasminogen activators affects primarily the fibrin portion of coronary thrombi, exposing the large pool of clot-bound thrombin. Because thrombin is a potent activator of platelets, this partial lysis stimulates further platelet aggregation, thereby increasing the concentration of PAI-1 near the site of lytic activity. Therefore, enhanced resistance to PAI-1 is a desirable characteristic for a fibrinolytic agent.

Although no single fibrinolytic agent is ideal in terms of pharmacological characteristics, recently bioengineered agents such as TNK offer potential safety advantages and greater ease of use.

II. ANALYSIS OF CLINICAL EVIDENCE

Double-blind, placebo-controlled, randomized trials of fibrinolytic therapy for AMI began to appear in the literature in the mid-1980s (3–5). Multicenter clinical trials have evaluated the clinical efficacy and safety profiles of various fibrinolytic drugs. The evaluation of efficacy has focused on 30-day mortality rates because AMI had been associated with death rates of 20–30% at 30 days. Numerous early trials (6–8). failed to show a significant difference between streptokinase and t-PA, and the less expensive streptokinase had a lower risk of stroke. Thus, the decisions faced by initial Pharmacy and Therapeutics (P&T) committees were relatively straightforward. Because no difference in mortality rates were found between these agents, the preferred agent could then be chosen on the basis of cost minimization with the lowest acquisition cost. Because streptokinase was a fraction of the cost of t-PA, it became the preferred agent, although t-PA had to be available on formularies for patients with contraindications to streptokinase, which included significant allergic reactions to the drug.

In 1993, the Global Utilization of Streptokinase and Tissue Plasminogen Activator to Open Occluded Coronary Arteries (GUSTO) trial was the first major study to demonstrate a statistically significant improvement in survival when patients were given "frontloaded" or accelerated t-PA followed by intravenous heparin for STEMI (9). The study found an absolute decrease of 1% in the 30-day mortality rate with t-PA compared with streptokinase, slightly offset by a 0.1% increase in the risk of intracerebral hemorrhage for patients treated within 4 hours of the onset of chest pain.

For a large integrated health care system with 2 million covered lives, this decrease in mortality could translate into 10–20 additional lives saved annually. Based on these results, the use of t-PA was reevaluated in a timely manner. Because of the agent's improved efficacy, P&T guidelines had to reflect this data. The GUSTO Economic Substudy was not published until 2 years later in 1995 (14). This substudy currently provides the best cost analysis of fibrinolytic therapy in STEMI.

Other key mortality trials included the INJECT trial, an equivalence trial that demonstrated that r-PA was equivalent to SK in lowering 30-day mortality (10). The GUSTO III trial was a superiority trial that failed to demonstrate that r-PA was superior to t-PA (11). In addition, 30-day mortality equivalence between r-PA and t-PA could not be concluded from the GUSTO III trial.

ASSENT-2, a phase III equivalence trial, compared weight-based single-bolus TNK and weight-based front-loaded t-PA in myocardial infarction (12). The reduction in 30-day mortality was shown to be equivalent except in patients presenting later than 4 hours, in which case TNK was more effective. In terms of safety, ASSENT-2 revealed a significant difference in total bleeding and need for transfusion in favor of TNK. The incidence of noncerebral major bleeding was also significantly lower in TNK-treated patients. In addition, it produced fewer noncerebral major bleeds in high-risk patients such as elderly females with lower body weight. As discussed, neither the GUSTO III (r-PA) nor the ASSENT-2 (TNK) trial demonstrated greater overall efficacy in reducing 30-day mortality rates compared with t-PA. Thus, detailed economic analysis of these trials has not yet emerged.

III. ECONOMIC ASSESSMENT IN PERSPECTIVE

Cost-effectiveness analysis is a widely used method for determining the value of any health intervention. It serves as an aid in selecting a clinical intervention that leads to the greatest health improvement for a given expenditure. The cost-effectiveness ratio is defined as the difference in total health costs between two interventions divided by the difference in effectiveness, defined as life-years saved (LYS) or quality-adjusted life-years (QALY). In cost-effectiveness analysis, the costs are expressed in monetary terms, whereas the effectiveness is expressed as a health benefit. For example, in assessing the cost-effectiveness of fibrinolytics in AMI, it is usually expressed as the cost (in dollars) per life-year saved. Because interventions rarely save both costs and lives, the relative benefit achieved from one intervention can be compared with what would be expected from another intervention.

Because a cost-effectiveness ratio is determined by dividing the change in total cost by the change in total effectiveness, the same ratio may be obtained for interventions with markedly different total costs and effectiveness. It is important to understand not only the relative cost-effectiveness of an intervention, but also the total investment that would be required if it were to be applied across the target population.

In cost-effectiveness analysis, costs and benefits in the future are not as highly valued as costs or benefits that may be realized immediately. Thus, to adjust for the diminished value of future costs (cash flow) and benefits, analyses use the principle of discounting. Generally, future costs and benefits are discounted by 3–5% per year.

All cost-effectiveness analyses of fibrinolytic agents in AMI generally include any direct medical costs related to the diagnosis and treatment of AMI as well as any disease-specific costs that may be induced or averted. Such analyses are intended to improve clinical practice and aid in the development of clinical guidelines by providing information about the value of different fibrinolytics in AMI patients.

An accepted benchmark for overall cost-effectiveness for medical interventions in the United States is $50,000 per year of life saved. A stratification for medical interventions relative to cost-effectiveness has been described by Goldman et al. and Kupersmith et al. (15,16) as follows:

Highly cost-effective: <$20,000 LYS
Relatively cost-effective: $20,000–$40,000/LYS
Borderline cost-effective: $40,000–$$60,000/LYS
Expensive: >$60,000/LYS

As the clinical value of fibrinolysis in STEMI was established, a number of economic questions emerged regarding its value or cost-effectiveness compared to other treatments. A relatively small number of studies have evaluated the economics or cost-effectiveness of fibrinolytic therapy in STEMI. They have assessed the value of fibrinolytic therapy versus no-fibrinolytic therapy and have compared the value of various fibrinolytic agents. As discussed, the earliest trials of fibrinolytic therapy employed streptokinase. Thus, early economic evaluations focused on this agent.

Krumholtz et al. focused on the use of steptokinase for the treatment of elderly patients with AMI, where there had been some debate regarding the use of fibrinolytic therapy (17). Based on data from the GISSI-1 and ISIS-2 trials, the relative benefit of fibrinolytic therapy was assumed by some to be lower in elderly patients. The risk of fibrinolytic therapy for elderly patients was also assumed to be higher in elderly patients; however, the absolute risk of an AMI was much higher for this population compared with younger patients. Considering the costs of treatment, complications, and long-term health care of survivors, Krumholtz et al. estimated that the cost-effectiveness ratio of streptokinase compared with conventional therapy (without fibrinolytic) was $21,000 per life-year saved for an 80-year-old patient. The authors calculated similar estimates for younger patients. Other early cost-effectiveness analyses also found streptokinase to be cost-effective relative to other commonly used medical interventions (18,19).

The final results of the GUSTO trial were published in September 1993. Despite the 1% absolute decrease in 30-day mortality with t-PA versus SK, some concern about the accuracy of the predictions of 1-year mortality made investigators cautious about submitting the GUSTO Economic Substudy publication on cost-effectiveness. The substudy was finally published in May 1995 (14).

The analysis of cost-effectiveness in the GUSTO Economic Substudy used life expectancy projected on the basis of the records of survivors of myocardial infarction in the Duke Cardiovascular Disease Database. In the primary analysis it was assumed that there were no additional treatment costs due to the use of t-PA after the first year and that the comparative survival benefit of t-PA was still evident one year after enrollment. Effectiveness was measured in terms of additional life expectancy, and the effects of the treatments on the patients' quality of life were assessed in a sensitivity analysis. Cost-effectiveness ratios were expressed as the additional total lifetime costs required to add one extra year of life with t-PA treatment as compared with SK therapy. For the primary analysis, incremental costs included cumulative hospital and physician costs for the first year after treatment. All costs were expressed in 1993 dollars.

Both treatment groups were similar in their use of resources in the year after admission for a STEMI. Also, both groups had a mean length of stay of 8 days, including an average of 3.5 days in the intensive care unit. Overall, the 1-year health costs, excluding the difference in the cost of the fibrinolytic agent, were $24,990 per patient treated with t-PA versus $24,575 per patient treated with SK. The major difference in the cost of the therapies was the cost of the drug: $2,750 for t-PA and $320 for SK. One year after enrollment, patients who received t-PA had a total incremental cost of $2,845 and a higher survival rate (an increase of 1.1%, or 11 per 1000 patients treated). This incremental cost is similar to that estimated by Kalish et al. (20) by modeling the costs.

The effectiveness of t-PA over SK was expressed as the years of life saved. This number was calculated by taking the number of lives saved and multiplying it by an estimate of the patients' life expectancy. The addition in life expectancy per patient treated with t-PA was 0.14 years. On the basis of the projected life expectancy of each treatment group, the final published incremental cost-effectiveness ratio, with both future costs and benefits discounted at 5% a year, was $32,678 per year of life saved. Thus, according to the cost-effectiveness stratification of Goldman and Kupersmith (15,16), the cost-effectiveness of treatment with accelerated t-PA rather than SK compares favorably with that of other therapies whose added medical benefit for dollars spent is judged by society to be worthwhile. Thus, t-PA was found to be cost-effective in the treatment of STEMI. The cost-effectiveness ratio varied considerably among eight different groups based on the infarction site and the age of the patient. In general, the younger patients at lower risk had higher cost-effectiveness ratios. For example, the cost-effectiveness ratio for t-PA in the rare patient 40 years of age or younger with an inferior infarction was $203,071 per year of life saved compared with $13,410 per year of life saved for a patient 75 years or older with an anterior wall infarction.

Deciding which fibrinolytic agent to recommend in a treatment protocol or pathway should include an assessment of efficacy and safety, cost-effectiveness, and net clinical benefit (NCB) (9,14). NCB simultaneously considers issues of efficacy and safety. It is an excellent tool for clinical evaluation in that it includes mortality (or survival) and morbidity considerations. The GUSTO trial's measure of 30-day NCB was defined by survival without a disabling stroke (or mortality due to any cause and all nonfatal disabling strokes). A patient was classified as disabled if at discharge he or she had a moderate deficit, as defined by substantial limitation of activity or capability, or as severe deficit, as defined by inability to live independently or work.

The 30-day absolute results of the combined endpoint of death plus non-fatal disabling (ND) strokes were 7.8% for SK vs. 6.9% for accelerated t-PA (9). Thus, t-PA produced a net increase of one nonfatal disabling stroke per 1000 patients treated. If nonfatal disabling stroke is considered an endpoint equivalent to death in the hospital, then the increase in life expectancy estimated for t-PA in the substudy model is reduced to 0.13 years per patient, and the primary cost-effectiveness ratio increased to $35,538 per life-year saved. Thus, cost-effectiveness was maintained even after considering the incidence of nonfatal disabling stroke and NCB with t-PA.

As mentioned, new fibrinolytics agents such as TNK, have been approved by the FDA for the treatment of STEMI. Ideally, new fibrinolytic agents would be evaluated for FDA approval with available clinical and pharmacoeconomic data. However, TNK was shown to be equivalent to t-PA in terms of mortality reduction in the ASSENT-2 trial. Because increased overall efficacy with newer drugs like r-PA and TNK has not been evaluated, detailed economic analyses of these agents have not been performed.

It should also be noted that clinical evidence evolves rapidly in cardiovascular medicine. Novel combination antithrombotic therapy in STEMI patients is being evaluated. The ASSENT-3 trial demonstrated that the combination of TNK plus the low molecular weight heparin (LMWH) enoxaparin in STEMI patients had a better efficacy and safety profile than combinations employing reduced-dose fibrinolytics plus a glycoprotein IIb/IIIa inhibitor or full-dose fibrinolytic plus standard unfractionated heparin (21). Even though an economic analysis of TNK in STEMI has not been performed, clinicians and health systems may feel that the drug provides greater value than a drug like t-PA because of the overall efficacy and safety profile of the drug, and thus it is adopted in clinical practice.

Many studies attempt to provide timely data on the cost-effectiveness of a drug or therapy, but most fall short of intended goals. Data are often not available for years after studies demonstrate efficacy such as in the GUSTO trial. This lapse is due partly to the complexities inherent in analyzing and processing financial information from multiple hospital systems, complexities such as those that arise in obtaining uniform billing data, interpreting fee-for-service versus prepaid plan data, and justifying costs versus charges.

Pharmacoeconomic studies may not be useful and can even be misleading if their results are not applicable to a specific population served by a health system. Patients enrolled in research protocols may not be representative of the general patient population within that system. From an institution's perspective it is critical that data from Pharmacoeconomic studies apply to the patient populations served at their institutions, and that the P&T committee understands the limitations of Pharmacoeconomic analyses and their underlying assumptions. The advent of multiway sensitivity analysis was useful in providing perspective on the impact of underlying assumptions and potential costs when a therapy is applied in a variety of environments.

A number of trials have examined the role of primary angioplasty stenting for the management of AMI (22). These procedures have significant ramifications on health care systems in terms of the allocations and availability of resources. Pharmacoeconomic data prospectively collected and comparing the cost-effectiveness of fibrinolytic therapy (often followed by later PCI or surgery) versus primary angioplasty (including the cost development of resources to provide these services 24 hours a day) would be extremely useful to an integrated health care system. Such data would assist a system not only in organizing its resources, but also in making decisions about the expenditure of financial resources.

The GUSTO Economic Substudy remains a model for future fibrinolytic investigations of cost-effectiveness. The study was prospectively designed at the inception of the main clinical trial and was analyzed and authored by an independent academic group. Complex modeling was used to estimate the effects of the acute benefit on long-term outcome. The GUSTO Economic Substudy demonstrated that the incremental cost-effectiveness of t-PA was within the accepted range for medical interventions. Unfortunately, this type of Pharmacoeconomic information for most therapies is rarely available at the time P&T committees evaluate agents for inclusion on the formulary. Placing the benefit of a drug like t-PA within the cost-effectiveness framework provided a rationale for its clinical use even in financially constrained health systems.

IV. CONCLUSION

Although pharmacoeconomic data are an important component in the assessment of new or recent therapies, their current utility in large integrated health care systems is somewhat limited by a number of factors. The timing of available data is the most critical factor, and currently these data lag behind by 2–3 years. Consideration should be given to incorporating a Pharmacoeconomic assessment prospectively into the initial clinical trial design and developing guidelines to help investigators report financial information that may facilitate and improve the data obtained. Until better and more timely Pharmacoeconomic data become available, health systems will continue to evaluate fibrinolytic agents based on clinical efficacy and safety data, and equivalent therapies will primarily be differentiated on the basis of acquisition costs alone. In the United States, as financial pressures have increased in health systems, the market share of fibrinolytic agents in STEMI is split between r-PA, t-PA, and TNK. The cost-effectiveness demonstrated with t-PA has been extrapolated to r-PA and TNK because of their somewhat similar efficacy and safety profiles. Thus, the pricing structure for each agent has become a critical determinant in health systems when selecting a fibrinolytic agent for the treatment of STEMI patients.

REFERENCES

1. Heart Disease and Stroke Statistics—2003 Update. American Heart Association, 2003.
2. DeWood MA, Spores J, Notske R, et al. Prevalence of total coronary occlusion during the early hours of transmural myocardial infarction. N Engl J Med 1980; 303:897–902.
3. Gruppo Italiono per lo Studio della Streptochinasi nell' Infarto Miocardico (GISSI). Effectiveness of intravenous thrombolytic treatment in acute myocardial infarction. Lancet 1986; 1:397–402.
4. ISIS-2 (Second International Study of Infarct Survival) Collaborative Group. Randomized trial of intravenous streptokinase, oral aspirin, both, or neither among 17,187 cases of suspected myocardial infarction: ISIS-2. Lancet 1988; 2:349–360.
5. Chesebro J, Knatterud G, Roberts R, et al. Thrombolysis in Myocardial Infarction (TIMI) trial, phase 1: a comparison between intravenous tissue plasminogen activator and intravenous streptokinase. Clinical findings through hospital discharge. Circulation 1987; 76:142–514.
6. Gruppo Italiono per lo Studio della Streptochinasi nell' Infarto Miocardico (GISSI). GISSI-2: a factorial randomized trial of alteplase versus streptokinase and heparin versus no heparin among 12,490 patients with acute myocardial infarction. Lancet 1990; 336:65–71.
7. International Study Group. In-hospital mortality and clinical course of 20,819 patients with suspected acute myocardial infarction randomized between alteplase and streptokinase with or without heparin. Lancet 1990:336; 71–75.
8. International Study of Infarct Survival (ISIS) Collaborative Group. ISIS-3: a randomized comparison of streptokinase vs tissue plasminogen activator and of aspirin plus heparin vs aspirin alone among 41,299 cases of suspected acute myocardial infarction. Lancet 1992; 339:753–770.
9. GUSTO Investigators. An international randomized trial comparing four thrombolytic strategies for acute myocardial infarction. N Engl J Med 1993; 329:673–682.
10. International Joint Efficacy Comparison of Thrombolytics. Randomised, double-blind comparison of reteplase double-bolus administration with streptokinase in acute myocardial infarction (INJECT) trial to investigate equivalence. Lancet 1995; 346:329–336.
11. GUSTO III Investigators. A comparison of reteplase with alteplase for acute myocardial infarction. The global use of strategies to open occluded coronary arteries. N Engl J Med 1997; 337:1118–1123.
12. The ASSENT-2 Investigators. Single-bolus tenecteplase compared with front-loaded alteplase in acute myocardial infarction: The ASSENT-2 double-blind randomized trial. Lancet 1999; 354:716–722.
13. Ross AM. New plasminogen activators: a clinical review. Clin Cardiol 1999; 22:165–171.
14. Mark D, Hlatky M, Califf R, et al. Cost effectiveness of thrombolytic therapy with tissue plasminogen activator as compared to streptokinase for acute myocardial infarction. N Engl J Med 1995:332; 1418–1424.
15. Goldman L, Garber AM, Grover SA, et al. Task Force 6. Cost effectiveness of assessment and management of risk factors. J Am Coll Cardiol 1996; 27:1020
16. Kupersmith J, Holmes-Rovner M, Hogan A, et al. Cost-effectiveness analysis in heart disease. Part I: general principles. Prog Cardiovasc Dis 1994; 34:161–181.
17. Krumholtz HM, Pasternak RC, Weinstein MC, et al. Cost effectiveness of thrombolytic with streptokinase in elderly patients with suspected acute myocardial infarction. N Engl J Med 1992; 327:7–13.

18. Herve C, Cstiel D, Gaillard M, et al. Cost-benefit analysis of thrombolytic therapy. Eur Heart J 1990; 11:1006–1010.
19. Naylor CD, Bronskill S, Goel V. Cost-effectiveness of intravenous thrombolytic drugs for acute myocardial infarction. Can J Cardiol 1993; 9:553–558.
20. Kalish SC, Gurwitz JH, Krumholtz HM, et al. A cost-effectiveness model of thrombolytic therapy for acute myocardial infarction. J Gen Intern Med 1995; 10:321–330.
21. The ASSENT-3 Investigators. Efficacy and safety of tenecteplase in combination with enoxaparin, abciximab, or unfractionated heparin: the ASSENT-3 randomised trial in acute myocardial infarction. Lancet 2001; 358:605–613.
22. Weaver D. Comparison of primary coronary angioplasty and intravenous thrombolytic therapy for acute myocardial infarction: a quantitative review. JAMA 1998; 278:2093–2098.

6-4

Cost-Effective Drug Selection: Injectable Anticoagulants

Sarah Spinler
Philadelphia College of Pharmacy, University of the Sciences in Philadelphia, Philadelphia, Pennsylvania, U.S.A.

Compared to other antithrombotic classes for treatment of acute coronary syndromes (ACS), anticoagulants are relatively inexpensive. Available injectable anticoagulants for treating patients with ACS include unfractionated heparin (UFH), the low molecular weight heparins (LMWHs) enoxaparin and dalteparin, and the direct thrombin inhibitor lepirudin (1–5). Currently, either the LMWHs or UFH are acceptable agents for treating patients with non–ST segment elevation (NSTE) ACS based upon the 2002 American Heart Association (AHA)/American College of Cardiology (ACC) practice guidelines, while enoxaparin is the preferred agent (6). While UFH is the preferred agent for patients with ST segment elevation (STE) ACS, AHA/ACC data suggests that enoxaparin may be a preferred alternative (7,8). Lepirudin, due to its expense (approximately \$500–\$750 per day), marginal superiority to UFH in clinical trials, and high rate of bleeding complications, is reserved for patients with heparin-induced thrombocytopenia (2,4).

I. UFH VS. LMWHs

The pharmacological profile of LMWHs makes them an attractive alternative anticoagulant to UFH. In contrast to UFH, the LMWHs have excellent bioavailability when given by subcutaneous injection. Also, the half-life of LMWHs is approximately 3–4 hours while that of UFH is approximately 60–90 minutes. Therefore, LMWHs may be administered as weight-based subcutaneous injections twice daily, therefore avoiding the need for intravenous (iv) infusion pumps and potentially additional iv access lines. When compared to UFH, which requires frequent monitoring of the activated partial thromboplastin time (aPTT), LMWHs require no special monitoring of coagulation activity. The reason that UFH requires frequent aPTT monitoring is primarily because it is highly bound to plasma proteins, which, during times of acute stress, change dramatically in plasma concentration. In addition, UFH is bound and cleared by the endothelium. Therefore, the amount of "free" UFH available to inactivate clotting factors changes frequently during the course of the patient's hospitalization, making frequently aPTT monitoring necessary. It is currently recommended that the aPTT be monitored with UFH within 4–6 hours of initiation and every 6 hours thereafter until the target range of 50–70 seconds is achieved. In contrast to UFH, which is cleared primarily non-renally as described previously, LMWHs are cleared primarily through glomerular filtration. Currently, no prospective ACS clinical trials have specifically addressed LMWH efficacy and safety in patients with creatinine clearance values of less than 30 mL/min. However, retrospective analysis of the ESSENCE/TIMI 11B data suggests that patients with renal insufficiency have a higher rate of major bleeding than patients without renal insufficiency, but this increase is observed in patients receiving either UFH or enoxaparin (9). Recent dosing recommendations for patients with creatinine clearance less than 30 mL/min that have been added to the product label recommend a 50% dose reduction for enoxaparin (1 mg/kg every 24 hours). Therefore, at this time, ACS patients with renal insufficiency may be treated with either enoxaparin or UFH. However, patients receiving renal replacement therapy should probably still be treated with UFH due to lack of clinical trials in this patient group. Also, LMWHs are theoretically more difficult to reverse should bleeding occur. However, there are no case reports documenting a relevant clinical disadvantage. Unfractionated heparin is reversible with protamine, while LMWHs, which primarily inhibit factor Xa, are partially reversible with protamine and have a longer half-life, making clearance from the circulation longer after drug discontinuation (9,10). At this time there is no drug available clinically for reversal of bleeding associated with direct thrombin inhibitors such as lepirudin.

II. DIFFERENTIATION OF EFFICACY

Enoxaparin has proven superior to UFH in two large clinical NSTE ACS trials—Efficacy and Safety of Enoxaparin in Non-Q-Wave Coronary Events (ESSENCE) (1) and Thrombolysis in Myocardial Infarction (TIMI) 11B (2)—while dalteparin has demonstrated equivalency to UFH in one study, FRIC (4). In ESSENCE, a randomized, double-blind trial of 3171 patients with NSTE ACS, enoxaparin reduced the primary endpoint of death, myocardial infarction (MI), or recurrent angina by 20% ($p = 0.0019$) (1). In TIMI 11B, a randomized, double-blind trial of 3910 patients with NSTE ACS, enoxaparin reduced the primary endpoint of death, myocardial infarction (MI) or urgent revascularization at 8 days by 17% ($p = 0.048$) (2). Extended outpatient therapy with low-dose enoxaparin did not result in a further reduction in clinical events. In meta-analysis of the combined trials with more than 7000 NSTE ACS patients, enoxaparin also demonstrated a statistically significant reduction in the combined endpoint of death or MI at days 8 (23%), 14 (21%), and 43 (18%) ($p = 0.02$) (3). These benefits were apparent with approximately 2.5–4 days of treatment or 5–8 doses of enoxaparin, but benefit was observed within the first 48 hours after therapy was initiated (2,3).

   In the Fragmin in Unstable Coronary Artery Disease (FRIC) study, dalteparin and UFH were equivalent in terms of rates of death, MI, or recurrent angina at 6 days (7.6% in the UFH group and 9.3%) in the dalteparin group (3). Various reasons have been proposed for the lack of superiority of dalteparin to UFH in the FRIC trial when compared to enoxaparin's superiority in the ESSENCE and TIMI 11B trials, including low study sample size ($n = 1482$), differing pharmacological characteristics between dalteparin and enoxaparin (9,10), and a potential dose-ceiling effect. When administering enoxaparin, a patient receives a full mg/kg dose no matter how much the patient weights, whereas the dose of dalteparin is capped at 10,000 U (3).

   The efficacy of extended duration of treatment with dalteparin at a lower daily dose of either 5000 or 7500 IU subcutaneously twice daily compared to placebo was studied in the Fragmin and Fast Revascularization During Instability in Coronary Artery Disease (FRISC) II trial of patients with NSTE ACS (11). In FRISC II, all patients were treated with higher-dose dalteparin during the first several days after admission and then randomized to placebo or lower-dose extended treatment with dalteparin for 3 months. As with extended low-dose treatment of enoxaparin in TIMI 11B, there was no significant benefit with dalteparin compared to placebo, with no reduction in the composite endpoint of death or MI at 3 months (11). Results from a smaller clinical trial comparing enoxaparin and UFH in patients with NSTE ACS receiving eptifibatide suggest a lower rate of clinical events (secondary endpoint the composite of death or MI) in patients receiving enoxaparin (12).

All NSTE ACS studies evaluating LMWHs compared to UFH in NSTE ACS have been criticized for the poor performance of UFH in terms of rates of patients achieving the target aPTT. This is not a valid criticism for the following reasons: a clinical trial scenario with set monitoring likely achieves a higher rate of time in therapeutic range of UFH than does "real-world" experience, and it has never been demonstrated that achieving a target aPTT range for UFH in NSTE ACS is associated with benefit or harm.

In the Assessment of the Safety and Efficacy of a New Thrombolytic Regimen (ASSENT) trial, 3, utilization of either enoxaparin with full-dose tenecteplase or abciximab, UFH, plus half-dose tenecteplase was associated with a lower rate of 30-day death, in-hospital reinfarction or in-hospital refractory ischemia than the combination of UFH and full-dose tenecteplase in 6095 STE ACS patients (16% reduction for enoxaparin and 18% with abciximab; $p < 0.0001$) (7). The abciximab, UFH, plus half-dose tenecteplase group had a significantly higher rate of bleeding than the UFH-treated patients, while enoxaparin did not. Therefore, the authors suggested that the preferred treatment regimen was enoxaparin plus full-dose tenecteplase (7). Enoxaparin has also been studied for STE ACS in combination with alteplase and demonstrated marginal benefit in TIMI flow (13). A meta-analysis of studies of enoxaparin din STE ACS demonstrate a reduction in the composite endpoint of death or MI compared to UFH (14).

III. SAFETY CONSIDERATIONS

In most major clinical ACS LMWH trials, the rates of major bleeding have been similar to those reported with UFH (1–3,7,14). In INTERACT, the rate of major bleeding with enoxaparin was lower than UFH in patients with NSTE ACS receiving eptifibatide (12). The rates of minor bleeding are increased with LMWHs compared to UFH, but this is primarily due to subcutaneous hematomas occurring when giving a subcutaneous injectable anticoagulant compared to an intravenous infusion (1–3,7). The rate of total mortality has not been reduced in any clinical ACS trials of LMWHs (1-3,7,12,14).

IV. ECONOMICS

Economic evaluations of anticoagulants should include comparisons of efficacy, safety, and administration concerns. There are no published trials evaluating dalteparin or lepirudin in acute treatment of patients with ACS. Dalteparin, although more convenient to administer than UFH, is much more expensive than UFH while providing equivalent clinical results in patients with NSTE ACS; therefore, dalteparin would not be economically advantageous. Economic analysis of extended low-dose dalteparin treatment in NSTE ACS patients suggests an incremental one-month cost-effectiveness ratio of approximately $3750 (15). A secondary endpoint of the FRISC II trial was a 47% reduction in the rate of death or MI (11). This clinical benefit was not durable as there was no difference, and therefore no pharmacoeconomic benefit, of 3-month treatment (11). This analysis may be more relevant in Europe, where NSTE ACS patients may not necessarily undergo angiography and revascularization during the index hospitalization where clinicians could consider outpatient therapy as a short-term bridge to revascularization.

Lepirudin, the most expensive anticoagulant for patients with NSTE ACS, increases bleeding, offers no clinical or administration advantages when compared to UFH, and therefore would not be economically advantageous as primary therapy. Because it is not associated with heparin-induced thrombocytopenia, lepirudin is reserved for this special population patient group.

Enoxaparin has been evaluated in several pharmacoeconomic studies based upon the short-term results of the ESSENCE trial (16,17). In one study evaluating prospective data collected from hospital billing records of 655 U.S. patients enrolled in ESSENCE, a cumulative 30-day cost-savings of $1172 per patient was estimated ($p = 0.04$). In this model, the drug costs of enoxaparin were estimated at $155 per patient, and average UFH costs were estimated to be $80, which included hospital pharmacy acquisition costs, infusion pump costs for UFH, pharmacy preparation costs, and monitoring costs for UFH. Personnel costs for running the infusion pumps and changing UFH infusion rates were not utilized in the calculation (17). In a similar analysis of 1259 Canadian ESSENCE patients (40% of the total ESSENCE Canadian population), use of enoxaparin during the initial hospitalization was associated with a one-year cumulative savings of $1485 (Canadian dollars) ($p = 0.06$) (16). Both of these studies have drawn some criticism because the primary benefits and cost-savings demonstrated for enoxaparin have involved a reduction in re-hospitalization and revascularization. In the original ESSENCE study, less than 35% of patients underwent revascularization with either percutaneous coronary intervention (PCI) or coronary artery bypass graft (CABG) surgery (3). Currently, it is estimated that more than 85% of ACS patients undergo revascularization (18). Cost savings in terms of monitoring, especially personnel costs, may be more important today than in the past. Additional short-term pharmacoeconomic analyses of the ESSENCE data demonstrating cost savings with enoxaparin over UFH have been published from the perspective of the United Kingdom and French health care systems, as well as one using the entire worldwide population (19). Additional U.S. and Canadian pharmacoeconomic analyses using the long-term data from ESSENCE demonstrate durability of the cost-savings out to one year population (19). There are no published pharmacoeconomic evaluations of LMWHs in STE ACS.

V. CONCLUSIONS

While total mortality is not reduced with use of anticoagulants in ACS, they are a mainstay of therapy. LMWHs offer pharmacological benefits without the need for therapeutic monitoring. Limited pharmacoeconomic data suggests cost benefit with the use of enoxaparin. The utilization of LMWHs continues to increase in the United States, and additional pharmacoeconomic trials in patients with ACS are warranted.

REFERENCES

1. Cohen M, Demers C, Gurfinkel EP, Turpie AGG, Frommell GJ, Goodman S, et al. A comparison of low-molecular-weight heparin with unfractionated heparin for unstable coronary artery disease. N Engl J Med 1997; 337:447–452.
2. Antman EM, McCabe CH, Gurfinkel EP, Turpie AGG, Bernink PJLM, Salein D, et al. Enoxaparin prevents death and cardiac ischemic events in unstable angina/non-Q-wave

myocardial infarction. Results of the Thrombolysis in Myocardial Infarction (TIMI) 11B Trial. Circulation 1999; 100:1593–1601.

3. Antman EM, Cohen M, Radley D, McCabe C, Rush J, Premmereur J, et al. Assessment of the treatment effect of enoxaparin for unstable angina/non-Q-wave myocardial infarction . TIMI 11B-ESSENCE meta-analysis. Circulation 1999; 100:1602–1608.

4. Klein W, Buchwald A, Hillis SE, Monrad S, Sanz G, Turpie AGG, et al. Comparison of a low-molecular-weight heparin with unfractionated heparin acutely and with placebo for 6 weeks in the management of unstable coronary artery disease. Fragmin in Unstable Coronary Artery Disease Study (FRIC). Circulation 1997; 96:61–68.

5. Organisation to Assess Strategies for Ischemic Syndromes (OASIS-2) Investigators. Effects of recombinant hirudin (lepirudin) compared with heparin on death, myocardial infarction, refractory angina, and revascularization procedure sin patients with acute myocardial ischemia without ST elevation: a randomized trial. Lancet 1999; 353:429–438.

6. Braunwald E, Antman EM, Beasley JW, et al. American College of Cardiology (ACC)/American Heart Association (AHA) 2002 guideline update for the management of patients with unstable angina and non-ST-segment elevation myocardial infarction: a report of the ACC/AHA Task Force on Practice Guidelines (Committee on the Management of Patients with Unstable Angina). J Am Coll Cardiol 2002; 40:1366–1374.

7. The Assessment of the Safety and Efficacy of a New Thrombolytic Regimen (ASSENT)-3 Investigators. Efficacy and safety of tenecteplase in combination with enoxaparin, abciximab, or unfractionated heparin: the ASSENT-3 randomised trial in acute myocardial infarction. Lancet 2001; 358:605–613.

8. Spinler SA, Inverso SM. Update in strategies to improve thrombolysis for acute myocardial infarction. Pharmacotherapy 2001; 21:691–716.

9. Spinler SA, Inverso SM, Cohen M, Goodman SG, Stringer KA, Antman EM for the ESSENCE and TIMI 11B Investigators. Safety and Efficacy of Unfractionated Heparin versus Enoxaparin in Obese Patients and Patients with Severe Renal Impairment: Analysis from the ESSENCE and TIMI 11B Studies. Am Heart J 2003; 146:33–41.

10. Hirsh J, Warkentin TE, Shaughnessy SG, Anand S, Halperin JL, Raschke R, et al. Heparin and low-molecular-weight heparin: mechanisms of action, pharmacokinetics, dosing , monitoring, efficacy and safety. Chest 2001; 119:64S–94S.

11. FRISC II Investigators. Long-term low molecular mass heparin in unstable coronary artery disease: FRISC II prospective randomised multicetre study. Lancet 1999; 354:701–707.

12. Goodman S. Randomized evaluation of the safety and efficacy of enoxaparin versus unfractionated heparin in high-risk patients with non-ST-segment elevation acute coronary syndromes receiving the glycoprotein IIb/IIIa inhibitor eptifibatide. Circulation 2003; 107(2):238–244.

13. Ross AM, Molhoek P, Lundergan C, et al. Randomized comparison of enoxaparin, a low-molecular-weight heparin, with unfractionated heparin adjunctive to recombinant tissue plasminogen activator thrombolysis and aspirin: second trial of Heparin and Aspirin Reperfusion Therapy (HART II). Circulation 2001; 104:648–652.

14. Theroux P, Welsh RC. Meta-analysis of randomized trials comparing enoxaparin versus unfractionated heparin as adjunctive therapy to fibrinolysis in ST-elevation acute myocardial infarction. Am J Cardiol 2003; 91:860–864.

15. Janzon M, Levin LA, Swahn E, et al. Cost effectiveness of extended treatment with low molecular weight heparin (dalteparin) in unstable coronary artery disease: results from the FRISC II trial. Heart 2003; 89:287–292.

16. Smith SC, Dove JT, Kern MJ, Jacobs AK, Kuntz RE, Kennedy JW, et al. ACC/AHA guidelines for percutaneous coronary intervention (revision of the 1993 PTCA guidelines). J Am Coll Cardiol 2001; 37:1–66.

17. Mark DB, Cowper PA, Berkowitz SD, Davidson-Ray L, DeLong ER, Turpie AGG, et al. Economic assessment of low-molecular-weight heparin, enoxaparin, versus unfractionated heparin in acute coronary syndrome patients. Results from the ESSENCE randomized trial. Circulation 1998; 97:1702–1707.

18. O'Brien BJ, Willian A, Blackhouse G, Coeree R, Cohen M, Goodman S. Will the use of low-molecular-weight heparin (enoxaparin) in patients with acute coronary syndrome save costs in Canada? Am heart J 2000; 139:423–429.

19. Bosanquet N, Jonsson B, Fox KAA. Costs and cost effectiveness of low molecular weight heparins and platelet glycoprotein IIb/IIIa inhibitors in the management of acute coronary syndromes. Pharmacoeconomics 2003; 21:1135–1152.

7-1

The Pathobiology of Acute Coronary Syndromes: Mechanisms and Implications for Therapy

David A. Morrow and Elliott M. Antman
Brigham & Women's Hospital, Boston, Massachusetts, U.S.A.

I. INTRODUCTION

The acute management of patients with acute coronary syndromes (ACS) proceeds from and has evolved with our understanding of the pathobiology of this complex syndrome and its complications. The spectrum of patients with ACS is heterogeneous, ranging from those with complete coronary occlusion resulting in ST segment elevation on the electrocardiogram and myocardial infarction that is typically transmural to patients presenting with severe, but not occlusive, coronary obstruction resulting in myocardial ischemia with or without myocyte necrosis. The varied risk of complications in this population demands a careful prognostic assessment as a guide to triage and individualized therapeutic decision making. Nevertheless, consistent pathobiological contributors across the entire spectrum of ACS support a common foundation of therapy, including anticoagulant and antiplatelet therapy, as well as agents to reduce myocardial oxygen demand. In addition, over the past decade substantial advances in vascular biology have shed new light on the complex processes that promote atherothrombosis. In particular, experimental, pathologic and clinical data have implicated inflammatory contributions at every stage of atherogenesis (1–3). Such observations have provided new directions for therapy designed to target specific steps in the inflammatory cascade believed to mediate atherothrombosis. A deeper understanding of the underlying mechanisms of atherogenesis and ACS is important to the clinician as this insight will continue to guide the contemporary and future management of patients with acute coronary ischemia.

II. PRINCIPAL MECHANISMS OF ACS

Ultimately, an imbalance between oxygen supply and demand is always the fundamental cause of myocardial ischemia, which if severe and persistent culminates in irreversible myocardial injury. Five major mechanisms that contribute to the genesis of this imbalance have been identified and may be used as a framework to understand the heterogeneous presentations of patients with ACS (Fig. 1) (4). It is rare that any of these contributors exist in isolation; for example, it has become apparent that inflammatory processes play an impor-

Mechanisms of Acute Coronary Ischemia
- **Progressive mechanical obstruction**
- **Acute thrombosis on pre-existing plaque**
- **Dynamic obstruction (coronary spasm or vasoconstriction)**
- **Inflammation and/or infection**
- **Secondary unstable angina**

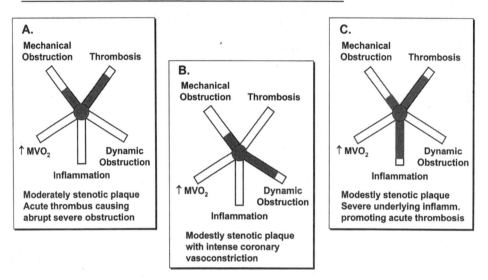

Figure 1   Principal mechanisms of acute coronary ischemia. MVO_2 = myocardial oxygen demand; inflamm. = inflammation. (Adapted from Ref. 4.)

tant role in the progression of atherosclerosis (mechanical obstruction), promotion of thrombosis, and, perhaps, initiation of coronary vasospasm (2,4). Each of these principal mechanisms will be reviewed individually while highlighting areas of overlap.

A.   Mechanical Obstruction and Acute Plaque Rupture

Most patients who develop unstable angina have significant obstructive coronary atherosclerosis, and until the 1990s the prevailing view of the pathogenesis of ACS was strongly influenced by the angiographic visualization of high-grade "culprit" stenoses. However, pathological and clinical data have demonstrated discordance between the degree of fixed coronary stenosis and the probability of acute symptomatic thrombosis (Fig. 2) (5). Angiographic studies performed before or at the time of acute MI have documented that the culprit stenosis is frequently not "critical" by standard angiographic criteria (6–9). Moreover, clinical studies assessing the degree of regression of luminal narrowing in response to interventions such as lipid lowering have shown minimal change in the degree of stenosis despite clinically important reductions in the risk of acute coronary events (10). Concurrently, pathological and clinical data have indicated the importance of plaque rupture or erosion in provoking the development of superimposed flow-limiting thrombus (5,11–16).

1.   Fixed Obstructive Stenoses

These observations do not obviate severely obstructive coronary lesions as an important cause of ACS. Such lesions remain substrate for acute thrombosis (12). Furthermore, rapid

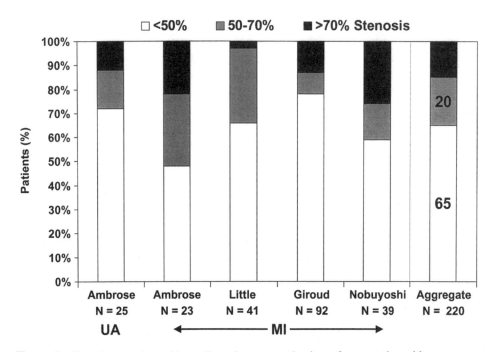

Figure 2   Data from angiographic studies prior to or at the time of presentation with acute coronary syndrome. UA = unstable angina; MI = myocardial infarction. (Adapted from Ref. 5.)

progression of coronary disease, especially complex stenoses, has been documented in angiographic studies (17,18). Acute coronary ischemia may also be precipitated by a fixed advanced stenosis with a superimposed increase in myocardial oxygen demand, such as that due to sustained tachycardia or uncontrolled hypertension. The severity of obstruction from coronary stenoses and the number of severely diseased vessels is thus an established predictor of cardiovascular morbidity and mortality (19).

2. Vulnerable Plaque

Nevertheless, for the majority of patients with ACS, the underlying culprit atheroma is responsible for only a modest reduction (<50%) in the diameter of the coronary lumen, but is a nidus for acute plaque compromise that provokes formation of intracoronary thrombus (8, 9, 20). As such, attention has shifted from an emphasis on the degree of stenosis of the coronary lumen to the properties of the underlying atheroma that influence its propensity to rupture (21). Pathologic data have highlighted the importance of the structural integrity of the fibrous cap as the primary characteristic that determines the "vulnerability" of the plaque to acute rupture (22). Lesions with thin, friable caps are most likely to rupture and expose the highly procoagulant contents of the atheroma core (13, 23, 24). Morphological characterization from pathological and imaging studies demonstrate consistent presence of a large lipid pool with compensatory eccentric enlargement resulting in typically modest stenosis by angiography (25–28) Both focal shear stress forces and dynamic coronary artery constriction at the site of the plaque may precipitate plaque rupture (29). The area of compromise is most frequently found at the edge or "shoulder" region of the atheroma (22,30). It is in this region that inflammatory cells accumulate, with a predominance of macrophages and T lymphocytes (31–33). Sensitive thermal catheters have also demonstrated higher temperatures in atherosclerotic regions compared to healthy arterial wall and an increased frequency of thermal hetero-geneity in plaques with high macrophage content as well as among patients with ACS (34,35). Together, these observations characterize the "vulnerable" plaque as one with a thin fibrous cap, a large lipid core, and a prominent inflammatory infiltrate and as one that may be literally "hot."

3. Implications for Therapy

The central role of inflammatory cells and the cytokines that they elaborate, as well as therapies aimed at stabilizing the vulnerable plaque, will be discussed in detail later in this chapter. It is worth noting, however, in this context that while invasive treatment of the apparent acute culprit lesion reduces the short-term risk of death and recurrent ischemic events (36), preventive interventions aimed at the diffuse, mildly to moderately stenotic plaques that are prone to rupture is likely necessary to achieve optimal long-term reduc-tion in the risk of future events. Data based on sampling of inflammatory indicators from the coronary sinus underscore the concept that it is probably not only the culprit lesion that is vulnerable, but rather that there is diffuse inflammatory involvement of the coronary tree in patients presenting with ACS (37). Contemporary therapy as well as future advances in treatment for patients with ACS should take into account the diffuse nature of the under-lying pathology.

B. Acute Thrombosis

Triggered by exposure of the highly pro-coagulant materials within the core of the rup-tured coronary atheroma, concomitant activation of platelets and the coagulation cascade culminates in the rapid formation of coronary thrombus in patients with ACS. Probable or definite intracoronary thrombus is suggested angiographically in up to 75% of patients with non-ST elevation ACS and nearly 100% of patients with STEMI (38). Angioscopy and pathological examination have also directly confirmed the presence of coronary thrombi in many patients with ACS (13,39,40). Patients presenting with ACS also have ele-vated circulating biomarkers indicating activation of the coagulation cascade, fibrin for-mation, and platelet activation (41,42), which may persist for several months after presentation (43). Variability in the propensity to form thrombus may relate to patient-spe-cific factors, such as underlying abnormalities of the coagulation cascade, platelet func-tion, or other contributors to a prothrombotic state (44–46).

1. The Coagulation Cascade

Tissue factor has now been recognized to be the principal determinant of coagulation in vivo (47). Tissue factor is expressed by activated endothelial cells, is an integral membrane protein on the surface of smooth muscle cells and fibroblasts exposed during arterial intimal injury, and is also produced in large quantities by inflammatory monocytes (47,48). When exposed to circulating blood, tissue factor within the atheroma binds to factor VII to initiate the extrinsic coagulation pathway and generate activated factor X (Xa) (Fig. 3) (49). Factor Xa converts pro-thrombin to thrombin (factor IIa), the key enzyme that gen-erates fibrin from fibrinogen. Both factors Xa and IIa exert feedback interactions that enhance production of additional factor Xa, as well as promote platelet activation and aggregation (50). Thrombin also activates factor XIII, which stabilizes the forming clot by cross-linking the fibrin strands. In addition, thrombin stimulates the release of multiple vasoactive mediators that may adversely influence vascular reactivity resulting in further compromise of coronary blood flow (51,52). At each branch in this pathway, one molecule

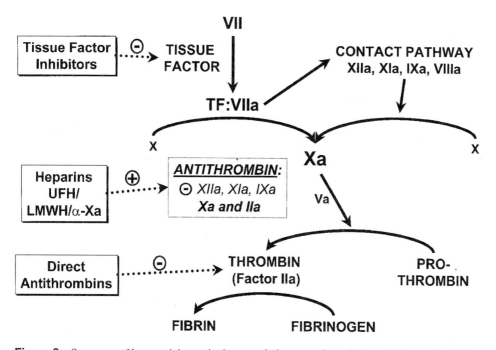

Figure 3 Summary of key participants in the coagulation cascade, and its regulation, as targets for therapy. TF = tissue factor; TF:VIIa = tissue factor:VIIa complex; TFPI = tissue factor pathway inhibitor; UFH = unfractionated heparin; αXa = anti-factor Xa; FDPs = fibrin degradation products.

of activated enzyme is able to activate many molecules of its substrate protein, thereby amplifying each step in the coagulation cascade. This cascade of sequential proteolytic interactions is most efficient when supported on the surface of activated endothelial cells and platelets that bring the enzymes into contact through membrane phospholipids (53). This interaction is just one example of the many levels of interdependence of platelet activation and the coagulation cascade.

In Vivo Control of Coagulation. This cascade of proteins is restrained by several mechanisms, including the protein C system, tissue factor pathway inhibitor, and the serine protease inhibitor, antithrombin (50). Antithrombin exerts its inhibitory effect by binding to each of the serine proteases except VIIa (i.e., factors XIIa, XIa, IXa, Xa, and thrombin) to form highly stable, 1:1 complexes that are no longer capable of proteolysis. This interaction between antithrombin and key proteases in the coagulation cascade is enhanced substantially by endothelial cell proteoglycans. The final product of the cascade, fibrin, is endogenously cleaved by plasmin, which is generated from plasminogen by the action of endothelial cell–derived plasminogen activators (54). Two naturally occurring plasminogen activators [tissue-type (t-PA), and urokinase-type (u-PA] convert plasminogen to plasmin via cleavage of a single peptide bond. The efficiency of this proteolytic action of t-PA is increased several hundred–fold upon binding to fibrin, providing its relative "fibrin specificity." The by-products of fibrin degradation also exert some antithrombotic effect by competing with fibrin monomer for fibrin polymer-binding sites.

Implications for Therapy. Given the critical role of the coagulation cascade in the pathogenesis of acute atherothrombosis, interventions aimed at achieving anticoagulant effects are a fundamental element of treatment for patients with suspected ACS (55,56). This complex system of multiple interacting proteases and controls presents several targets for therapeutic intervention in patients with acute arterial thrombosis (Fig. 3) (57). Clinicians have long exploited the ability to mimic the catalytic action of endothelial proteoglycans on antithrombin with heparins. Specifically, both unfractionated heparin (UFH), a complex mixture of mucopolysaccharide chains of widely varying length and molecular weight (3,000–30,000 daltons), and low molecular weight heparins (LMWH), a more homogeneous mixture of smaller chains (1000–10,000 daltons), interact with antithrombin by binding of a unique pentasaccharide sequence on the heparin molecule (58,59). Recently, a synthetic analog of this unique pentasaccharide has also become available (60,61). Binding of any of these agents induces a conformational change in antithrombin that promotes a nearly 1000-fold increase in the affinity of antithrombin for factors Xa and IIa (59,62).

By virtue of a greater relative activity against factor Xa compared with UFH, the LMWHs have the advantage of interrupting the coagulation system at a higher point in the cascade and acting to inhibit both thrombin activity and thrombin generation (63). Moreover, LMWHs, may have less propensity to stimulate, and may even act to suppress, platelet activation and aggregation (64). LMWHs also appear to restrain coagulation through inhibition of the tissue factor–VIIa complex (65,66). Specifically, while both UFH and LMWHs stimulate the release of tissue factor pathway inhibitor (TFPI), UFH appears to deplete blood levels of TFPI compared with LMWHs (65–68). The possibility of interrupting the multiplier effect earlier in the coagulation cascade, thus providing even more potent inhibition of thrombin generation than LMWH, has also stimulated interest in inhibiting the activity of tissue factor. Agents targeted at blocking either the binding of tissue factor to factor VIIa or the binding of the tissue factor–VIIa complex to factor X have been developed and are in clinical testing in patients with coronary disease (69,70).

Inhibition of thrombin may also be accomplished with agents that bind to and inhibit factor IIa directly without requiring the participation of antithrombin (57,71). Because the heparin-binding domain of clot-bound thrombin is less accessible to heparin, unfractionated heparin has relatively diminished effect against clot-bound thrombin (72). The so-called direct antithrombins have a theoretical advantage over UFH because of their greater ability to block both fluid-phase and clot-bound thrombin (72,73). Another advantage is the availability of oral formulations, which may achieve dose-dependent reliable levels of chronic anticoagulation without the need for frequent monitoring of the prothrombin time, such as is necessary for warfarin (74). These agents have now been studied in intravenous and oral forms for anticoagulation in a number of clinical settings including medical and interventional management of ACS (75–81). Similar advantages may also be achieved with direct inhibitors of Xa (82).

Such agents also provide hope for a convenient option for extended anticoagulation for secondary prevention among patients stabilized after ACS. Given the prolonged activation of thrombin and persistently increased risk of recurrent atherothrombotic events among patients with ACS, researchers have maintained an intense interest in long-term anticoagulation as a means for modifying risk beyond the acute presentation. Indeed, anticoagulation with coumadin after acute MI may reduce the risk of recurrent events. However, chronic treatment with LMWHs appears to increase the risk of bleeding without detectable reductions in ischemic events. Additional research with potent and practical antithrombins may prove the value of such agents in secondary prevention (82,83).

2. *Platelet Activation and Aggregation*

Concurrent with the activation of the coagulation cascade by tissue factor, circulating platelets adhere to subendothelial matrix exposed by compromise of the atheroma's protective fibrous cap. Adhesion of platelets to the disrupted endothelial surface via interaction of the platelet surface glycoprotein Ib with endothelial von Willebrand factor and via the collagen Ia/IIa receptor triggers the activation of adherent and surrounding platelets through direct contact and the release of multiple chemical agonists such as thromboxane A_2, adenosine diphosphate (ADP), and serotonin (Fig. 4). Activated platelets undergo a morphological change that substantially increases the surface area on which thrombin generation may occur. In addition, activated platelets express the glycoprotein IIb/IIIa inhibitor in an active form that is capable of binding to fibrinogen and thus cross-linking

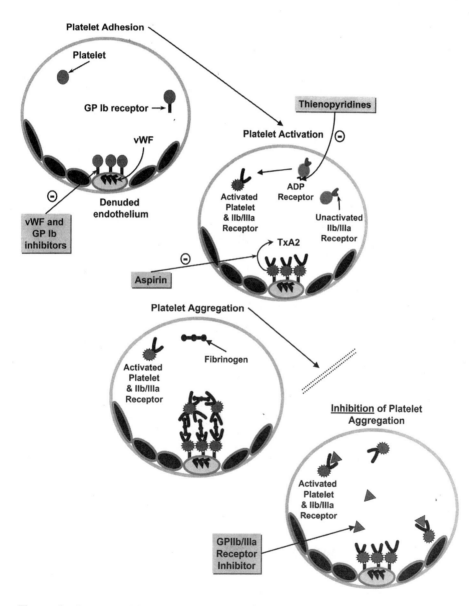

Figure 4 Summary of key participants platelet adhesion, activation and aggregation as targets for therapeutic intervention. ADP = adenosine diphosphate; vWF = won Willebrand factor; TxA2 = thromboxane A2. (Adapted from Guiglian RP. Antiplatelet therapy. In Antman EM (ed). Cardiovascular Therapeutics: A Companion to Braunwald's Heart Disease, 2nd ed. Philadelphia, WB Saunders, 2002.)

to other platelets. The ensuing process of platelet aggregation culminates in formation of the platelet plug. Studies using a variety of indices of platelet activation and aggregation have provided consistent evidence for the importance of these steps in the onset of ACS (84–86). In parallel with the coagulation cascade, the key participants in the process of platelet adhesion, activation, and aggregation are targets for therapy.

Platelets and a Possible Role in Inflammation.   Recent evidence also implicates platelets in contributing to the inflammation that occurs in ACS (87). Specifically, activated platelets appear to interact with endothelial and inflammatory cells via CD40-ligand on the platelet surface. The interaction with activated platelets stimulates endothelial cells to express adhesion molecules and chemokines, resulting in additional recruitment of inflammatory monocytes to areas of vascular injury (88,89). This interaction may also promote additional elaboration of tissue factor (90). The presence of platelet-monocyte aggregates has been documented in patients with stable coronary artery disease and was reported to be increased after coronary angioplasty and at presentation with unstable angina (91–95).

Implications for Therapy.   The progressive evolution in our understanding of platelet biology has directed us toward multiple effective forms of antiplatelet therapy (Fig. 4). Inhibition of platelet aggregation may be achieved by blocking the production of thromboxane A_2, the key chemokine promoting platelet aggregation and vasoconstriction. As such, the irreversible inhibition of platelet cycloxygenase by aspirin has proved to be one of the most effective interventions in the acute and long-term management of patients presenting with ACS (96). Although aspirin effectively inhibits thromboxane A_2 production, it only partially inhibits platelet aggregation induced by ADP, collagen, and thrombin (97). Inhibitors of the glycoprotein IIb/IIIa receptor, which functions in the final common step in platelet aggregation, have a theoretical advantage over other agents that may antagonize only one of the myriad of pathways for platelet activation and recruitment (Fig. 4B). Platelet inhibition may also be achieved through antagonism of one or more of the many receptors that mediate platelet activation. For example, thienopyridines which bind irreversibly to the ADP receptor have been proven to complement aspirin with respect to clinical benefit in patients with non–ST elevation acute coronary syndromes (98).

The intriguing observations regarding the importance of platelets in the inflammatory pathobiology of ACS suggest that platelet inhibition may confer additional anti-inflammatory actions that may contribute to the clinical benefit of these agents. For example, clopidogrel decreases the expression of both CD40 ligand and P-selectin (99,100), and may have a greater impact on reducing ischemic events after PCI in patients with elevated markers of inflammation (101). In addition, novel strategies that aim at interrupting platelet-monocyte interactions directly at the level of the involved receptors are also under study (102–104). Other agents that have targeted pathways for platelet inhibition include phosphodiesterase inhibitors, thromboxane receptor antagonists, serotonin receptor blockers, von Willebrand factor inhibitors, and agents that interfere with the GP Ib receptor (105–108).

C.   Inflammation and Infection

Substantial data indicate that inflammatory processes participate at every stage of atherothrombosis, from initiation of the earliest progenitor of the mature atheroma to plaque destabilization and acute thrombosis (1,109). Epidemiological and pathological data have also pointed toward infectious agents as one of the potential triggers for the inflammation that drives atherogenesis (110). The tremendous progress in our understanding of the specific inflammatory pathways involved in atherothrombosis has created opportunities to translate these findings into novel tools for detection of asymptomatic atherosclerosis and risk assessment as well as development of new therapies targeting inflammation and infection.

1. Inflammation in Atherothrombosis

Endothelial Dysfunction and Atherogenesis. The vascular endothelium is a complex organ capable of many functions, including regulation of vasomotor tone, modification of lipoproteins, and orchestration of cellular traffic through generation of an array of intercellular messengers (111). This organ may be injured by a number of varied insults, including but not limited to oxidative stress (112,113), hemodynamic forces (114,115), modified lipoproteins (116), infectious agents (110,117,118), and other cytotoxic elements, such as advanced glycosylation end products (119) and homocysteine (120). In addition, other traditional risk factors for atherosclerosis, such as obesity, are associated with inflammatory processes that may contribute to endothelial dysfunction (121,122). Regardless of the inciting injury, the resulting endothelial cell dysfunction triggers a largely stereotyped response (Fig. 5) (1,109).

The activation of endothelial cells is first marked by upregulation of intercellular adhesion molecules and the elaboration of chemokines that stimulate increased adhesion and migration of mononuclear leukocytes. Vascular cell adhesion molecule 1 (VCAM-1),

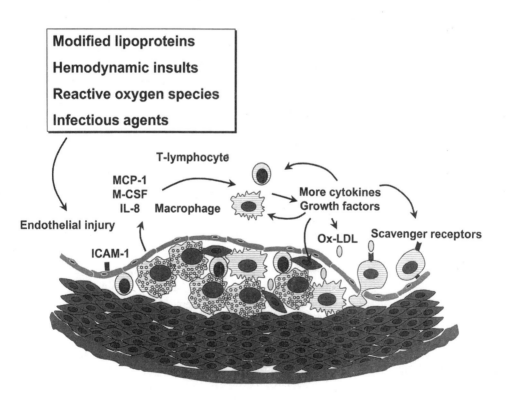

Figure 5 Inflammatory pathobiology of atherogenesis. See text for details. ICAM-1 = intercellular adhesion molecule-1; MCP-1 = monocyte chemotactic protein-1; M-CSF = macrophoge colony stimulating factor; IL-8 = interleukin-8; Ox-LDL = oxidized LDL. (From Ref. 2.)

E-selectin, and intercellular adhesion molecule 1 (ICAM-1) are among the adhesion molecules expressed in response to endothelial dysfunction caused by oxidatively modified low-density lipoprotein (LDL) and hemodynamic shear stress (123–129). VCAM-1, in particular, is exposed on the surface of vascular endothelial cells in response to an atherogenic diet in rabbits, as well as to angiotensin II in rats and has been shown to be an important component of atherogenesis in mice (130–132). These adhesion molecules interact with proteins on the surface of leukocytes to facilitate migration of inflammatory cells into the subendothelial space (127,133). In addition, endothelial cells, smooth muscle cells, and arriving monocytes secrete a number of chemoattractant molecules, such as monocyte chemotactic protein 1 (MCP-1), interleukin-6 (IL-6), IL-8, tumor necrosis factor alpha (TNF-α), and macrophage colony-stimulating factor (M-CSF), that further enhance the recruitment of inflammatory cells (134–138). Importantly, experimental absence of MCP-1 has been shown to slow atherogenesis in a mouse model, and to correlate with vascular risk factors and adverse prognosis in patients with ACS (139–141). As such, in response to any of a varied group of insults to the vascular endothelium, an inflammatory infiltrate dominated by monocyte-derived macrophages and T lymphocytes is established in the arterial intima (142–144). Notably, mechanisms that restrain the expression of adhesion molecules and establishment of the inflammatory infiltrate appear to be impaired at branch points in arteries, where endothelial cells are subjected to disturbed flow (124,145,146).

Uptake of LDL by inflammatory macrophages transforms them into lipid-laden foam cells, the defining constituent of the fatty streak, the first progenitor of the advanced atheroma (147–150). The continued generation of inflammatory cytokines by arriving monocytes promotes further expression of adhesion molecules, cellular recruitment, and the oxidation and uptake of LDL, as well as the production of reactive oxygen species that perpetuate the endothelial injury (126,149,151–155). Simultaneously released mitogens, including platelet-derived growth factor, and fibroblast growth factor, along with IL-1 and IL-6, trigger the proliferation of smooth muscle cells that contribute to maturation of the fatty streak into an intermediate atheroma (156–159). Both macrophages as well as T lymphocytes appear to elaborate the inflammatory cytokines and mitogens that promote progression of the atheroma (109). Concurrently, a resilient fibrous cap forms over the admixture of inflammatory monocytes, smooth muscle cells, intra- and extracellular lipid, and necrotic cellular debris that form the core of the advanced complex atherosclerotic lesion.

Inflammation and Plaque Rupture. As the critical barrier between the procoagulant contents of the atheroma core and blood within the coronary lumen, the structure of the fibrous cap and the balance of forces that maintain its integrity have become a focus of intense investigation (Fig. 6) (22). The fibrous cap is composed of an extracellular matrix reinforced primarily by types I and III collagen as well as elastin synthesized by vascular smooth muscle cells (21,158). Smooth muscle cells within the matrix contribute to maintaining this barrier by ongoing synthesis of collagen and elastin. This synthetic activity is counterbalanced by collagenases, elastases, and proteases released by foam cells within the atheroma (160,161). In addition, interferon-γ (IFN-γ) produced by T lymphocytes exerts an inhibitory effect on the ability of smooth muscle cells to synthesize collagen (21). As such, focal thinning of the fibrous cap is observed to occur most frequently in the shoulder regions of the atheroma, where macrophages and T lymphocytes tend to accumulate (11,23,30–32). Indeed, these inflammatory cells predominate at the site of plaque rupture or erosion in ACS regardless of the overall plaque morphology (31–33).

Researchers have identified specific cytokines and proteolytic enzymes that appear to play important roles in compromise of the atheroma plaque (Fig. 6) (3). Detection of

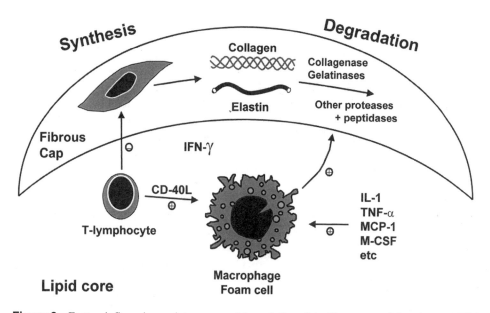

Figure 6 Factors influencing maintenance and degradation of the fibrous cap of the atheroma. IFN = interferon; CD40L = CD40 ligand; IL = interleukin; TNF = tumor necrosis factor; MCP = monocyte chemotactic protein; M-CSF = macrophage colony-stimulating factor. (Adapted from Ref. 21.)

high levels of the tranplant antigen HLA-DRα, a protein that appears to be induced only by IFN-γ, on the surface of smooth muscle cells at the site of rupture or erosion supports a role for this cytokine in plaque vulnerability (21). In addition, several members of the family of matrix metalloproteinases (MMPs) have been implicated in compromise of the protective fibrous cap (162–165). These proteolytic enzymes act extracellularly to degrade both collagen and elastin and are produced by smooth muscle cells and macrophages under the influence of IL-1 and TNF as well as cell-cell interactions with T lymphocytes. Immunostain preparations of materials from human atheroma demonstrate the presence of metalloproteinases in macrophages, T lymphocytes, and vascular endothelial cells, with the highest enzyme activity observed in the "shoulder" region of the plaque (161,162).

Thrombosis and Vascular Reactivity

In addition to a probable role in determining the vulnerability of the atheromatous plaque, inflammatory cells and messengers may also promote a pro-coagulant state and abnormal vasomotor function. Activated macrophages produce large quantities of tissue factor which activates the extrinsic coagulation pathway and plays an important role in the formation of thrombus in ACS (48,49,166,167). Although the stimuli for tissue factor expression are not fully characterized, T lymphocytes are known to induce tissue factor production through interaction of cell surface proteins mediated by cell-cell contact rather than via circulating cytokines (49,165).

Vascular inflammation has been postulated to influence arterial vasomotor function through several possible mechanisms. Endothelin-1 is a potent modulator of vasoconstriction that can be produced by leukocytes. IL-1 is also released by activated inflammatory cells and can increase smooth muscle cell reactivity (168). In addition, inflammatory infiltrates have been documented in the arterial adventitia with vascular nerve involvement and therefore have been hypothesized to stimulate coronary vasospasm (169).

Implications for Therapy. Advances in our insight into the details of inflammatory participation in atherothrombosis has directed investigators toward specific targets for novel therapeutic intervention. Moreover, laboratory and clinical studies have provided evidence for anti-inflammatory effects of established treatments aimed at other risk factors for atherogenesis (e.g., aspirin, statins, and angiotensin-converting enzyme (ACE) inhibitors), effects that may contribute, at least in part, to the proven clinical efficacy of these therapies (170). These advances have also guided the investigation of new biological markers and application of imaging techniques to identify patients with evidence of systemic inflammation who are at higher risk of future cardiovascular events and to detect arterial plaques that may be particularly vulnerable to rupture.

Inflammatory Biomarkers. Elevated levels of inflammatory biomarkers such as C-reactive protein (CRP), serum amyloid A, and IL-6 are detectable in a substantial proportion of patients presenting with ACS, including those without evidence of myocyte necrosis using our most sensitive biological markers (171–174). A consistent body of evidence indicates that elevated levels of at least several of these markers portend poor short- and long-term prognosis (171–178). In particular, high-sensitivity testing for CRP appears to add to traditional tools for risk assessment in ACS (172,176).

It is plausible that elevation of circulating markers of inflammation during ACS are manifestations of intensification of the focal inflammatory processes that contribute to destabilization of vulnerable plaque. Nevertheless, the precise pathophysiological basis for the relationship between inflammatory markers and risk in ACS has not been conclusively established. Studies that demonstrate elevation of CRP and IL-6 in the absence of myocyte necrosis refute the position that the rise in inflammatory markers is solely a response to cellular necrosis (171,172). Growing evidence implicates CRP as a potential direct participant in atherothrombosis rather than merely a measurable epiphenomenon. CRP promotes uptake of LDL cholesterol by monocytes (179), induces the production of tissue factor (180,181), activates complement within arterial plaque (182), stimulates the expression of multiple adhesion molecules (183), and may also directly aid in monocyte recruitment through a monocyte-CRP receptor (184).

Treatments Targeting Inflammation. Whether direct mediators of risk or markers of underlying processes contributing to plaque rupture, CRP and other biomarkers of inflammation have the potential to become valuable tools for targeting therapy among patients with ACS (109,185,186). Strong support for this paradigm comes from the compelling evidence for an interaction between CRP and the efficacy of certain therapeutic and preventive interventions.

ASPIRIN. Aspirin was the first agent to be studied with respect to its interaction with inflammatory markers in cardiovascular disease. Observations from the Physician's Health Study demonstrated a 55% reduction in risk of first MI attributable to aspirin among men in the highest quartile of hs-CRP, compared with a 13% risk reduction in the lowest quartile of hs-CRP (187). Although the mechanism underlying these observations is not defined, these data raised the possibility that the anti-inflammatory actions of aspirin as well as its antiplatelet effects may contribute to the efficacy of this drug in cardiovascular disease prevention. It is also possible that, as suggested for clopidogrel (101), there are anti-inflammatory consequences of effective platelet inhibition. Subsequent studies exploring the interaction of aspirin and inflammatory markers have provided mixed results. A study of patients with ischemia on Holter monitoring who were randomized to aspirin (300 mg orally each day) or placebo showed a reduction in levels of hs-CRP, IL-6, and macrophage colony stimulating factor after 3 weeks of treatment (188). However, in a trial of lower-dose aspirin in healthy volunteers, neither 81 mg every day nor 325 mg every 3 days was associated with a detectable decrease in levels of hs-CRP (189). Similarly, 325 mg of aspirin administered for 7 days does not appear to lower levels of hs-CRP in apparently healthy volunteers (190). It is possible that higher doses of aspirin or longer periods of treatment are necessary to reduce vascular inflammation. It is also possible that low-dose aspirin impacts vascular inflammation without measurable effects on hs-CRP (189).

Few data are available on the interaction of aspirin and inflammatory biomarkers in patients with ACS. In an observational study of 304 patients with non–ST elevation ACS, aspirin used prior to hospitalization appeared to modify the risk associated with increased levels of hs-CRP. Patients who were not previously on aspirin had a two- to threefold higher risk of death or MI for each standard deviation higher peak CRP, whereas a relationship between CRP and the risk of recurrent events was not detectable among those previously taking aspirin (191).

HMG-CoA REDUCTASE INHIBITORS.   Outcome data demonstrating an interaction between the effects of HMG-CoA reductase inhibitors (statins) and hs-CRP now support the clinical relevance of substantial experimental evidence indicating that statins attenuate inflammation and influence stability of atheromatous plaque (Fig. 7). Again, the clinical data derive primarily from studies of primary or secondary prevention among stable patients rather than in the acute management of ACS. In a nested case-control analysis of patients enrolled in the Cholesterol and Recurrent Events (CARE) trial of pravastatin or placebo for secondary prevention after prior MI, the magnitude of risk reduction with pravastatin was greater among patients with evidence of inflammation (risk reduction attributable to pravastatin 54%) compared to those without evidence of inflammation (risk reduction 25%) (192). Moreover, the risk associated with elevated hs-CRP was significant among those receiving placebo (RR 3.2; $p = 0.048$) but was attenuated among those treated with pravastatin (RR 1.29; $p = 0.5$). A substudy from the Air Force/Texas Coronary Athersoclerosis Prevention Study (AFCAPS/TexCAPS) trial provided additional evidence for an interaction between evidence of low-level systemic inflammation and the clinical benefit of statins (Fig. 7b) (193). In this study of lovastatin for primary prevention among patients with low to moderate risk of cardiovascular events, an overall 37% reduction in the risk of acute coronary events was observed in the active treatment group. As expected, lovastatin was highly effective in patients with elevated LDL cholesterol. In addition, treatment with lovastatin provided a significant reduction in the risk of future coronary events among patients with elevated levels of hs-CRP and baseline LDL below the median for the trial. Notably, the number needed to treat to prevent one coronary event in the group with elevated CRP and low LDL was similar to that for patients with elevated LDL but low CRP (48 vs. 38) (193). There was no detectable benefit of lovastatin in patients with below-average LDL and CRP.

Together the data from CARE and AFCAPS/TexCAPS, as well as numerous studies that demonstrate lowering of circulating levels of hs-CRP after treatment with statins (Fig. 7a), lend strong support to the hypothesis that statins are effective in modifying the risk associated with evidence of systemic inflammation (194–197). Statins have been suggested to have particular benefit in patients with elevated CRP undergoing PCI (198,199), and there has been substantial interest in statins as a component of the early management of ACS. At least one small study has suggested a marked reduction in short-term recurrent events with early statin therapy after presentation with non-STE ACS (200). The Myocardial Ischemia Reduction with Aggressive Cholesterol Lowering (MIRACL) trial showed only a modest reduction in the risk of the composite of death, MI, cardiac arrest, or recurrent ischemia (14.8% vs. 17.4%; $p = 0.048$) during 16 weeks of follow-up among 3086 patients with ACS (201). Over that same period of time aggressive treatment with atorvastatin (80 mg) was associated with a 34% greater decline in levels of hs-CRP compared with placebo (202). Two other trials of early aggressive statin therapy for patients with ACS have been completed and shown both clinical benefit and greater reductions in

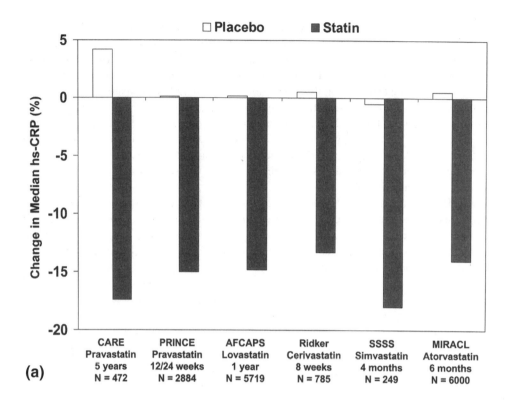

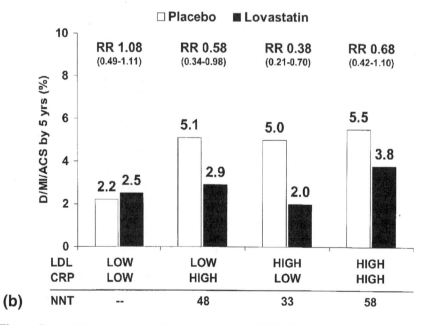

Figure 7 **(a)** Median change in C-reactive protein (CRP) during statin therapy in patients with atherosclerotic vascular disease. **(b)** Effect of lovastatin for primary prevention of atherothrombosis among patients with and without elevated hs-CRP and LDL cholesterol. NNT = number needed to treat to avoid one event.

CRP with more intensive statin therapy (203,204). In the PROVE-IT Trial, the benefit of more aggressive statin therapy could be attributed largely to changes in CRP (204b).

The precise pathophysiological mechanisms for the impact of statins on inflammatory measures and their associated risk are not yet clear. However, laboratory and animal studies have revealed a broad spectrum of nonlipid effects of statins, including modulation of immune function, antiproliferative effects on vascular smooth muscle cells, amelioration of endothelial dysfunction, as well as antithrombotic properties (205–212). Treatment of hypercholesterolemic rabbits with statins reduces the accumulation of macrophages and expression of metalloproteinases and tissue factor (213,214). However, dietary lipid lowering has also been shown to alter the morphology of atherosclerotic plaque, reducing macrophage accumulation, matrix metalloproteinase expression, tissue factor production, and endothelial and smooth muscle cell activation, as well as increasing interstitial collagen (215–217). Thus, it remains unclear to what degree the apparent anti-inflammatory effects of statins reside with their effect on lipids compared with nonlipid actions (170,218).

OTHER INTERVENTIONS. Other established preventive interventions as well as novel therapeutic strategies may also have anti-inflammatory effects that could prove beneficial in the management of patients with ACS. For example, the reduction in cardiovascular risk achieved with ACE inhibitors is greater than that expected from observed levels of blood pressure lowering (219,220). In vitro experiments show that angiotensin induces inflammatory changes in human vascular smooth muscle cells (115) and treatment with ACE inhibitors can reduce signs of inflammation in animal models of atherosclerosis (221). Fibric acid derivatives act through a molecular target, PPAR-α, which has been the object of mounting evidence demonstrating anti-inflammatory effects. Specifically, PPAR-α agonists can reduce the expression of VCAM-1 on endothelial cells, inhibit T-lymphocyte function, improve vascular reactivity, and reduce tissue factor production (222–226). Likewise, the family of insulin-sensitizing thiazolidinediones, which act through PPAR-γ are now appreciated to exert anti-inflammatory actions, reduce atherogenesis in animal models, and reduce CRP as well as MMPs in patients with diabetes (227–230). To date, more potent anti-inflammatory therapies, such as intravenous administration of steroids, have undergone very limited evaluation without fruitful results (231).

Other novel therapies are likely to result from specific targets revealed by recent advances in vascular biology. For example, interruption of key intercellular adhesion molecules might inhibit atherogenesis at its earliest stage—the response to endothelial injury. Antagonism of other cytokine and receptor signaling pathways might also serve to stabilize the vulnerable plaque. As one example, inhibition of CD40-ligand signaling reduces lesion size and favorably shifts the balance of collagen production and proteolysis in mice (232). Alternatively, pharmacological interventions targeted at reducing smooth muscle proliferation might slow or prevent progression of the fatty streak to the intermediate atheromatous plaque. Nevertheless, interruption of the complex inflammatory and immunological pathways that mediate response to injury and infection could also have important detrimental effects. The action of cyclooxygenase inhibitors is a good example of the complexities involved, as data suggest that anti-inflammatory effects of these inhibitors may be outweighed by an imbalance in the relative inhibition of prostacyclin vs. thromboxane resulting in a prothrombotic state (233–236). Carefully designed studies will be critical to evaluate the consequences of the multiple effects of agents that target inflammatory pathways.

2. Infection

Animal and epidemiological studies have suggested associations between atherothrombotic vascular disease and evidence of prior or ongoing infection. Specifically, evidence has arisen from detection of organisms within human atheroma, ascertainment of serological measures of infection in those with established and incident vascular disease, and demonstration in animal models that infection with specific pathogens is associated with more extensive or progressive atherosclerosis. Systemic or local infections may contribute to endothelial injury through autoimmune or inflammatory responses (237–239). These data have raised the possibility that infectious pathogens are one, if not the major, stimulus for inflammation as a byproduct or mediator of cardiovascular risk.

Pathological and Experimental Evidence. Pathological data have revealed evidence for the presence of viral and bacterial pathogens within arterial plaque (240–242). The frequency of evidence of the presence of *Chlamydia pneumoniae* (chlamydial DNA, antigens, or elementary bodies) varies widely with technique but has been found in up to 86% of specimens of human atherosclerotic plaque taken either at the time of coronary atherectomy or autopsy (243–247), whereas the organism is rarely seen in nonatheromatous arterial sections (244). It has also been possible to culture *C. pneumoniae* from atherosclerotic arteries (246). In addition, animal studies have indicated that infection with certain viral and bacterial pathogens can induce the genesis of arterial lesions similar to the early fatty streak. Such observations date back to the 1970s when Fabricant demonstrated that chickens infected with an avian herpes virus developed vascular lesions comparable to human atherosclerosis (248). More recent studies have shown that Cytomegalovirus (CMV) may induce endothelial cell proliferation and intimal thickening in animal models of transplantation (118), and that cholesterol-fed rabbits infected with *C. pneumoniae* show significant acceleration of aortic atherosclerosis compared with controls (249). Furthermore, in an apo-E knockout mouse model that develops atherosclerosis spontaneously, investigators have demonstrated persistence of *C. pneumoniae* in aortic atheroma >20 weeks after intranasal innoculation and that lesion area is significantly greater among animals infected with *C. pneumoniae* (250,251). Such studies also suggest possible synergism between the infection and hypercholesterolemia in atherogenesis (252).

Serological Evidence.   There is also evidence of a higher frequency of serological evidence of exposure to cytomegalovirus (253), *C. pneumoniae* (254,255), and *Helicobacter pylori* (256,257), among patients with documented atherosclerotic vascular disease. Early studies indicated a possible association between *C. pneumoniae* and prevalent coronary heart disease (254). A subsequent meta-analysis of 20 epidemiological studies including 2700 total subjects with coronary or cerebrovascular disease reported a greater than twofold higher prevalence of coronary heart disease among patients with elevated titers of antibodies to *C. pneumoniae* (258). There has, however, been doubt as to whether the observed associations between infection and atherosclerosis in cross-sectional and case-control studies reflect a true pathophysiological relationship or a manifestation of confounding relationships with other factors such as age, smoking patterns, and socioeconomic status (259–261). Such studies are also limited by available methods for establishing evidence of infection. The multiple prospective studies that are able to account for the effects of such confounders have shown either substantially more modest risk relationships or no evidence of an independent relationship between infection and incident atherothrombosis (262–267). It is possible that the interaction between infection and atherogensis requires cumulative effects from multiple pathogens or interaction with other risk factors (268–271), and that independent relationships are difficult to detect because of the complex contributions of multiple factors to atherothrombosis (272). Moreover, antibody titers against CMV have been shown to exhibit a graded relationship between subsequent development of subclinical atherosclerosis measured by carotid intimal-medial thickening (273). In addition, higher rates of restenosis and transplant graft atherosclerosis have been observed among patients with serological evidence of prior infection with CMV (274,275).

Proposed Mechanisms. On the basis of the collective experimental and clinical evidence it has been hypothesized that the activation of vessel-associated leukocytes or transformation of vascular smooth muscle and endothelial cells by infectious pathogens may establish a pathophysiological link between infection, inflammation, and atherogenesis (Fig. 8) (110,276). Indirect evidence to support this hypothesis is provided by studies showing an association between serologic evidence of exposure to several infectious pathogens and levels of inflammatory markers such as hs-CRP (277–279) In vitro studies have shown that *C. pneumoniae* can multiply within human macrophages, endothelial cells, and smooth muscle cells and that macrophages infected with *C. pneumoniae* accumulate lipid to a greater extent than those not infected (280). Endothelial cells infected with *C. pneumoniae* elaborate inflammatory cytokines and express leukocyte adhesion molecules stimulating transendothelial migration of inflammatory monocytes (281). The possible induction of autoimmune responses to proteins such as heat shock protein through molecular mimicry may also promote arterial inflammation and stimulate release of TNF-α or MMPs (282–284). These findings suggest that, in addition to contributing to the initiation and progression of atherosclerosis, new endovascular infection of a previously stable plaque could trigger local inflammation, plaque rupture, and a consequent acute coronary syndrome. Similarly, reactivation of latent endovascular infection could produce a similar local inflammatory response. Finally, it is possible that an immune response to a distant (extravascular) infection could lead to generalized cytokine release, which could provoke plaque instability.

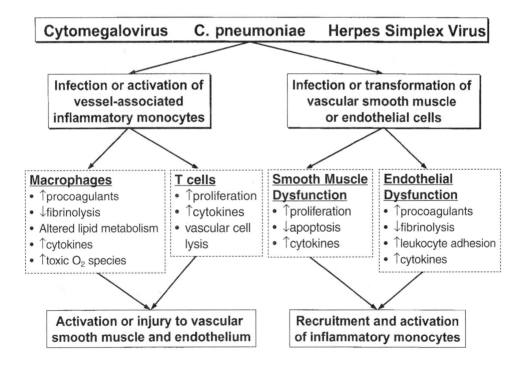

Figure 8 Proposed mechanisms mediating the cardiovascular risk associated with infection. Sm Muscle = smooth muscle. (Adapted from Ref. 110.)

Implications for Therapy. If systemic or local infection within the arterial wall accelerates or provokes atherothrombosis, it is plausible that therapy directed at the inflammatory response or at specific pathogens may be effective for primary or secondary prevention. However, the results from randomized trials completed to date are mixed.

The pilot experience with trials of macrolide antibiotics supported the possibility of substantial benefit from antimicrobial therapy in patients with coronary artery disease (CAD) (285,286). For example, in a randomized trial of roxithromycin vs. placebo for 30 days in patients with non–ST elevation MI ($n = 202$), the ROXIS investigators observed a statistically significant reduction in recurrent cardiac events at 30-days among patients treated with the antibiotic (2% vs. 9%; $p = 0.032$) (285). Several trials have reinforced these preliminary but promising clinical results with results showing improvements in surrogate endpoints such as inflammatory markers. In the Azithromycin in Coronary Artery Disease: Elimination of Myocardial Infarction with Chlamydia (ACADEMIC) study, treatment with azithromycin, administered daily for 3 days and then weekly for 3 months, was associated with reductions in hs-CRP and IL-6 among 302 patients with CAD and *Chlamydia* antibody IgG titers ≥ 1:16 (287). Similar effects on fibrinogen were observed in patients with ischemic heart disease treated with clarithromycin (288). Others have shown improvement in measures of endothelial function, such as endothelium-dependent nitric oxide vasodilation and levels of E-selectin, among patients with CAD treated with azithromycin compared with placebo (289).

Despite the encouraging results of mechanistic and pilot outcomes studies, the first large randomized, placebo-controlled trial to test antibiotic treatment for patients with CAD failed to show an advantage. In the Weekly Intervention with Zithromax for Atherosclerosis and its Related Disorders (WIZARD) trial, investigators randomly allocated 7747 seropositive (IgG titers ≥ 1:16) patients with stable CAD to placebo or azithromycin (600 mg QD × 3 days followed by 600 mg once weekly × 11 weeks) (290). After a mean follow-up of 2.1 years, treatment with azithromycin was associated with a nonsignificant trend toward a lower rate of death, nonfatal MI, hospitalization for angina, or revascularization (7% relative reduction; $p = 0.23$) (290). Exploratory analyses suggested a possible benefit of azithromycin during the phase of active treatment and in specific subgroups such as those with diabetes.

Several trials of antibiotic therapy among patient with acute coronary syndromes are ongoing or recently completed. The Clarithromycin in Acute Coronary Syndrome patients in Finland (CLARIFY) trial showed a weak trend toward decreased death, MI, or unstable angina at 3 months in patients treated with clarithromycin daily for 85 days or matching placebo (291). Similarly, among 1400 patients with ACS allocated to azithromycin for 5 days or placebo in the Zithromycin in Acute Coronary Syndromes (AZACS) trial, antibiotic therapy had no demonstrable effect on the endpoint of death, MI, or recurrent ischemia requiring revascularization at 6 months (290). The Pravastatin or Atorvastatin Evaluation and Infection Therapy (PROVE-IT) trial enrolled ~4000 patients with ACS and showed no advantage of quinilone antibiotic gatifloxicin administered 10 days monthly for 2 years compared with placebo in patients treated either with atorvastatin or pravastatin. Moreover, the NHLBI-sponsored ACES study involving 4000 patients with stable CAD compared with azithromycin (600 mg/week for one year) or placebo through 3–4 years of follow-up and showed no effect of long-term antibiotic therapy.

The aggregate data to date regarding antibiotic therapy for prevention of atherothrombosis have been disappointing in light of the strong mechanistic evidence for a role of infection. At this time there is not sufficient evidence to support antibiotic therapy directed at secondary prevention in patients with CAD. Additional studies are ongoing, and it remains possible that chronic therapy may be necessary, that multiple pathogens must be targeted, or that only specific groups of patients will derive benefit from antibiotics for CAD. Although at least one study suggests that treatment with statins may ameliorate the inflammatory response to infection with *Chlamydia*, the clinical relevance is uncertain (292).

D. Dynamic Obstruction

Dynamic coronary obstruction due to coronary vasoconstriction occurs most commonly on the substrate of underlying coronary atherosclerosis. Increased release of endothelin-1 with concurrent impaired production of the potent vasodilator nitric oxide in the setting of endothelial dysfunction is a common underpinning. In addition, a number of vasoactive substances produced during thrombosis, such as thromboxane A_2 and serotonin from platelets and thrombin, may contribute to local vasoconstriction (84,86,293,294). In patients with Prinzmetal variant angina intense focal epicardial coronary vasospasm may occur in the absence of atherosclerosis (295). Constriction of small intramural coronary resistance vessels may also slow epicardial flow in the absence of epicardial stenoses (296). Such abnormal vasomotor function in the coronary "microvasculature" may be an important complication of acute coronary thrombosis and distal embolization for some patients (297,298). Clinically significant coronary vasoconstriction may also occur during exposure to potent adrenergic stimuli, such as cold immersion, cocaine, or mental stress (299–302).

E. Increased Oxygen Demand

A sustained increase in myocardial oxygen demand is an important contributor to the onset of unstable angina in some cases. Examples of conditions that may precipitate unstable angina through this mechanism include sustained supraventricular tachyarrhythmias, fever, thyrotoxicosis, hyperadrenergic states, and severe elevation of left ventricular diastolic pressure due to aortic stenosis or uncontrolled hypertension. The treatment of ACS due to increased myocardial oxygen demand is usually targeted at the specific etiology of the increase.

III. SUMMARY

The clinician's options for treating patients with ACS continue to expand. Recapitulating history, the next line of strategies for management of these patients is likely to derive from advances in our understanding of the coagulation cascade, platelet biology, and, in particular, the inflammatory mediators that participate in atherothrombosis. Moreover, noninvasive tools, such as cardiac biomarkers, that may aid in characterizing the dominant mechanisms (e.g., inflammatory vs. hypercoaguable) for the individual patient may make personalized therapy for ACS possible in the foreseeable future. Prospective randomized studies testing specific interventions among patients with elevated inflammatory markers will provide critical evidence toward establishing the validity of the promising preliminary findings to date. Lastly, advanced biomarker, imaging, and invasive techniques may allow clinicians to identify vulnerable patients prior to onset of acute atherothrombosis and intervene with preventive measures.

REFERENCES

1. Ross R. Atherosclerosis—an inflammatory disease. N Engl J Med 1999; 340:115–126.
2. Morrow DA, Ridker PM. Inflammation in cardiovascular disease. In: Topol E, ed. Textbook of Cardiovascular Medicine Updates. Cedar Knolls: Lippincott Williams & Wilkins; 1999. p. 1–12.
3. Libby P. Inflammation in atherosclerosis. Nature 2002; 420:868–874.
4. Braunwald E. Unstable angina: an etiologic approach to management. Circulation 1998; 98:2219–2222.
5. Fuster V. Lewis A. Conner Memorial Lecture. Mechanisms leading to myocardial infarction: insights from studies of vascular biology. Circulation 1994; 90:2126–246.
6. Serruys PW, Wijns W, van den Brand M, et al. Is transluminal coronary angioplasty mandatory after successful thrombolysis? Quantitative coronary angiographic study. Br Heart J 1983; 50:257–265.
7. Hackett D, Davies G, Maseri A. Pre-existing coronary stenoses in patients with first myocardial infarction are not necessarily severe. Eur Heart J 1988; 9:1317–1323.
8. Little WC, Constantinescu M, Applegate RJ, et al. Can coronary angiography predict the site of a subsequent myocardial infarction in patients with mild-to-moderate coronary artery disease? Circulation 1988; 78:1157–1166.
9. Ambrose JA, Tannenbaum MA, Alexopoulos D, et al. Angiographic progression of coronary artery disease and the development of myocardial infarction. J Am Coll Cardiol 1988; 12:56–62.
10. Brown B, Zhao X, Sacco E, Albers J. Lipid lowering and plaque regression: new insights into prevention of plaque disruption and clinical events in coronary disease. Circulation 1993; 87:1781–1791.
11. Constantinides P. Plaque fissuring in human coronary thrombosis. J Atheroscler Res 1966; 6:1–17.
12. Falk E. Plaque rupture with severe pre-existing stenosis precipitating coronary thrombosis. Characteristics of coronary atherosclerotic plaques underlying fatal occlusive thrombi. Br Heart J 1983; 50:127–134.
13. Davies MJ, Thomas AC. Plaque fissuring—the cause of acute myocardial infarction, sudden ischaemic death, and crescendo angina. Br Heart J 1985; 53:363–373.
14. Ambrose JA, Winters SL, Stern A, et al. Angiographic morphology and the pathogenesis of unstable angina pectoris. J Am Coll Cardiol 1985; 5:609–616.
15. Farb A, Burke AP, Tang AL, et al. Coronary plaque erosion without rupture into a lipid core. A frequent cause of coronary thrombosis in sudden coronary death. Circulation 1996; 93:1354–1363.
16. Lee RT, Libby P. The unstable atheroma. Arterioscler Thromb Vasc Biol 1997; 17:1859–1867.
17. Moise A, Theroux P, Taeymans Y, et al. Unstable angina and progression of coronary atherosclerosis. N Engl J Med 1983; 309:685–689.
18. Kaski JC, Chester MR, Chen L, Katritsis D. Rapid angiographic progression of coronary artery disease in patients with angina pectoris. The role of complex stenosis morphology. Circulation 1995; 92:2058–2065.
19. Moise A, Lesperance J, Theroux P, et al. Clinical and angiographic predictors of new total coronary occlusion in coronary artery disease: analysis of 313 nonoperated patients. Am J Cardiol 1984; 54:1176–1181.
20. Mann JM, Davies MJ. Vulnerable plaque. Relation of characteristics to degree of stenosis in human coronary arteries. Circulation 1996; 94:928–931.
21. Libby P. Molecular bases of the acute coronary syndromes. Circulation 1995; 91:2844–2850.
22. Falk E. Why do plaques rupture? Circulation 1992; 86:III30–42.
23. Davies MJ. A macro and micro view of coronary vascular insult in ischemic heart disease. Circulation 1990; 82:II38–46.
24. Loree HM, Kamm RD, Stringfellow RG, Lee RT. Effects of fibrous cap thickness on peak circumferential stress in model atherosclerotic vessels. Circ Res 1992; 71:850–858.

25. Glagov S, Weisenberg E, Zarins CK, et al. Compensatory enlargement of human atherosclerotic coronary arteries. N Engl J Med 1987; 316:1371–1375.
26. Thieme T, Wernecke KD, Meyer R, et al. Angioscopic evaluation of atherosclerotic plaques: validation by histomorphologic analysis and association with stable and unstable coronary syndromes. J Am Coll Cardiol 1996; 28:1–6.
27. Yamagishi M, Terashima M, Awano K, et al. Morphology of vulnerable coronary plaque: insights from follow-up of patients examined by intravascular ultrasound before an acute coronary syndrome. J Am Coll Cardiol 2000; 35:106–111.
28. Takano M, Mizuno K, Okamatsu K, et al. Mechanical and structural characteristics of vulnerable plaques: analysis by coronary angioscopy and intravascular ultrasound. J Am Coll Cardiol 2001; 38:99–104.
29. Lee RT, Grodzinsky AJ, Frank EH, et al. Structure-dependent dynamic mechanical behavior of fibrous caps from human atherosclerotic plaques. Circulation 1991; 83:1764–1770.
30. Richardson PD, Davies MJ, Born GV. Influence of plaque configuration and stress distribution on fissuring of coronary atherosclerotic plaques. Lancet 1989; 2:941–944.
31. van der Wal AC, Becker AE, van der Loos CM, Das PK. Site of intimal rupture or erosion of thrombosed coronary atherosclerotic plaques is characterized by an inflammatory process irrespective of the dominant plaque morphology. Circulation 1994; 89:36–44.
32. Moreno PR, Falk E, Palacios IF, et al. Macrophage infiltration in acute coronary syndromes. Implications for plaque rupture. Circulation 1994; 90:775–778.
33. Boyle JJ. Association of coronary plaque rupture and atherosclerotic inflammation. J Pathol 1997; 181:93–99.
34. Stefanadis C, Diamantopoulos L, Vlachopoulos C, et al. Thermal heterogeneity within human atherosclerotic coronary arteries detected in vivo: a new method of detection by application of a special thermography catheter. Circulation 1999; 99:1965–1971.
35. Verheye S, De Meyer GR, Van Langenhove G, et al. In vivo temperature heterogeneity of atherosclerotic plaques is determined by plaque composition. Circulation 2002; 105:1596–1601.
36. Cannon CP, Weintraub WS, Demopoulos LA, et al. Comparison of early invasive and conservative strategies in patients with unstable coronary syndromes treated with the glycoprotein IIb/IIIa inhibitor tirofiban. N Engl J Med 2001; 344:1879–1887.
37. Buffon A, Biasucci LM, Liuzzo G, et al. Widespread coronary inflammation in unstable angina. N Engl J Med 2002; 347:5–12.
38. TIMI IIIA Investigators. Early effects of tissue-type plasminogen activator added to conventional therapy on the culprit coronary lesion in patients presenting with ischemic cardiac pain at rest. Results of the Thrombolysis in Myocardial Ischemia (TIMI IIIA) Trial. Circulation 1993; 87:38–52.
39. Sherman CT, Litvack F, Grundfest W, et al. Coronary angioscopy in patients with unstable angina pectoris. N Engl J Med 1986; 315:913–919.
40. de Feyter PJ, Ozaki Y, Baptista J, et al. Ischemia-related lesion characteristics in patients with stable or unstable angina. A study with intracoronary angioscopy and ultrasound. Circulation 1995; 92:1408–1413.
41. Theroux P, Latour JG, Leger-Gauthier C, De Lara J. Fibrinopeptide A and platelet factor levels in unstable angina pectoris. Circulation 1987; 75:156–162.
42. Hamm CW, Lorenz RL, Bleifeld W, et al. Biochemical evidence of platelet activation in patients with persistent unstable angina. J Am Coll Cardiol 1987; 10:998–1006.
43. Merlini PA, Bauer KA, Oltrona L, et al. Persistent activation of coagulation mechanism in unstable angina and myocardial infarction. Circulation 1994; 90:61–68.
44. Weiss EJ, Bray PF, Tayback M, et al. A polymorphism of a platelet glycoprotein receptor as an inherited risk factor for coronary thrombosis. N Engl J Med 1996; 334:1090–1094.
45. Ault KA, Cannon CP, Mitchell J, et al. Platelet activation in patients after an acute coronary syndrome: results from the TIMI-12 trial. Thrombolysis in Myocardial Infarction. J Am Coll Cardiol 1999; 33:634–639.
46. Rosenberg RD, Aird WC. Vascular-bed—specific hemostasis and hypercoagulable states. N Engl J Med 1999; 340:1555–1564.

47. Taubman MB, Giesen PL, Schecter AD, Nemerson Y. Regulation of the procoagulant response to arterial injury. Thromb Haemost 1999; 82:801–805.

48. Moreno PR, Bernardi VH, Lopez-Cuellar J, et al. Macrophages, smooth muscle cells, and tissue factor in unstable angina. Implications for cell-mediated thrombogenicity in acute coronary syndromes. Circulation 1996; 94:3090–3097.

49. Camerer E, Kolsto AB, Prydz H, Kolst AB. Cell biology of tissue factor, the principal initiator of blood coagulation. Thromb Res 1996; 81:1–41.

50. Dahlback B. Blood coagulation. Lancet 2000; 355:1627–1632.

51. Harker LA, Hanson SR, Runge MS. Thrombin hypothesis of thrombus generation and vascular lesion formation. Am J Cardiol 1995; 75:12B-17B.

52. Antman EM, Handin R. Low-molecular-weight heparins: an intriguing new twist with profound implications. Circulation 1998; 98:287–289.

53. Zwaal RF, Comfurius P, Bevers EM. Lipid-protein interactions in blood coagulation. Biochim Biophys Acta 1998; 1376:433–453.

54. Collen D, Lijnen HR. Basic and clinical aspects of fibrinolysis and thrombolysis. Blood 1991; 78:3114–3124.

55. Ryan TJ, Antman EM, Brooks NH, et al. 1999 update: ACC/AHA guidelines for the management of patients with acute myocardial infarction. A report of the American College of Cardiology/American Heart Association Task Force on Practice Guidelines (Committee on Management of Acute Myocardial Infarction). J Am Coll Cardiol 1999; 34:890–911.

56. Braunwald E, Antman EM, Beasley JW, et al. ACC/AHA 2002 guideline update for the management of patients with unstable angina and non-ST-segment elevation myocardial infarction— summary article: a report of the American College of Cardiology/American Heart Association task force on practice guidelines (Committee on the Management of Patients With Unstable Angina). J Am Coll Cardiol 2002; 40:1366–1374.

57. Antman EM. The search for replacements for unfractionated heparin. Circulation 2001; 103:2310–2314.

58. Hirsh J, Warkentin TE, Raschke R, et al. Heparin and low-molecular-weight heparin: mechanisms of action, pharmacokinetics, dosing considerations, monitoring, efficacy, and safety. Chest 1998; 114:489S-510S.

59. Weitz JI. Low-molecular-weight heparins. N Engl J Med 1997; 337:688–698.

60. Walenga JM, Bara L, Petitou M, et al. The inhibition of the generation of thrombin and the antithrombotic effect of a pentasaccharide with sole anti-factor Xa activity. Thromb Res 1988; 51:23–33.

61. Turpie AG, Gallus AS, Hoek JA. A synthetic pentasaccharide for the prevention of deep-vein thrombosis after total hip replacement. N Engl J Med 2001; 344:619–625.

62. Danielsson A, Raub E, Lindahl U, Bjork I. Role of ternary complexes, in which heparin binds both antithrombin and proteinase, in the acceleration of the reactions between antithrombin and thrombin or factor Xa. J Biol Chem 1986; 261:15467–15473.

63. Wong GC, Giugliano RP, Antman EM. Use of low-molecular-weight heparins in the management of acute coronary artery syndromes and percutaneous coronary intervention. JAMA 2003; 289:331–342.

64. Serra A, Esteve J, Reverter JC, et al. Differential effect of a low-molecular-weight heparin (dalteparin) and unfractionated heparin on platelet interaction with the subendothelium under flow conditions. Thromb Res 1997; 87:405–410.

65. Hansen JB, Sandset PM. Differential effects of low molecular weight heparin and unfractionated heparin on circulating levels of antithrombin and tissue factor pathway inhibitor (TFPI): a possible mechanism for difference in therapeutic efficacy. Thromb Res 1998; 91:177–181.

66. Hansen JB, Naalsund T, Sandset PM, Svensson B. Rebound activation of coagulation after treatment with unfractionated heparin and not with low molecular weight heparin is associated with partial depletion of tissue factor pathway inhibitor and antithrombin. Thromb Res 2000; 100:413–417.

67. Sandset PM, Bendz B, Hansen JB. Physiological function of tissue factor pathway inhibitor and interaction with heparins. Haemostasis 2000; 30:48–56.
68. Lupu C, Poulsen E, Roquefeuil S, et al. Cellular effects of heparin on the production and release of tissue factor pathway inhibitor in human endothelial cells in culture. Arterioscler Thromb Vasc Biol 1999; 19:2251–2262.
69. Broze GJ, Jr. Tissue factor pathway inhibitor and the revised theory of coagulation. Annu Rev Med 1995; 46:103–112.
70. Lee A, Agnelli G, Buller H, et al. Dose-response study of recombinant factor VIIa/tissue factor inhibitor recombinant nematode anticoagulant protein c2 in prevention of postoperative venous thromboembolism in patients undergoing total knee replacement. Circulation 2001; 104:74–78.
71. Weitz JI, Buller HR. Direct thrombin inhibitors in acute coronary syndromes: present and future. Circulation 2002; 105:1004–1011.
72. Weitz JI, Hudoba M, Massel D, et al. Clot-bound thrombin is protected from inhibition by heparin-antithrombin III but is susceptible to inactivation by antithrombin III- independent inhibitors. J Clin Invest 1990; 86:385–391.
73. Fox I, Dawson A, Loynds P, et al. Anticoagulant activity of Hirulog, a direct thrombin inhibitor, in humans. Thromb Haemost 1993; 69:157–163.
74. Gustafsson D, Nystrom J, Carlsson S, et al. The direct thrombin inhibitor melagatran and its oral prodrug H 376/95: intestinal absorption properties, biochemical and pharmacodynamic effects. Thromb Res 2001; 101:171–181.
75. Antman EM. Hirudin in acute myocardial infarction. Thrombolysis and Thrombin Inhibition in Myocardial Infarction (TIMI) 9B trial. Circulation 1996; 94:911–921.
76. GUSTO IIb Investigators. A comparison of recombinant hirudin with heparin for the treatment of acute coronary syndromes. Global Use of Strategies to Open Occluded Coronary Arteries (GUSTO) IIb. N Engl J Med 1996; 335:775–782.
77. Neuhaus KL, Molhoek GP, Zeymer U, et al. Recombinant hirudin (lepirudin) for the improvement of thrombolysis with streptokinase in patients with acute myocardial infarction: results of the HIT-4 trial. J Am Coll Cardiol 1999; 34:966–973.
78. Kong DF, Topol EJ, Bittl JA, et al. Clinical outcomes of bivalirudin for ischemic heart disease. Circulation 1999; 100:2049–2053.
79. Antman EM, McCabe CH, Braunwald E. Bivalirudin as a replacement for unfractionated heparin in unstable angina/non-ST-elevation myocardial infarction: observations from the TIMI 8 trial. The Thrombolysis in Myocardial Infarction Investigators. Am Heart J 2002; 143:229–234.
80. Eriksson BI, Bergqvist D, Kalebo P, et al. Ximelagatran and melagatran compared with dalteparin for prevention of venous thromboembolism after total hip or knee replacement: the METHRO II randomised trial. Lancet 2002; 360:1441–1447.
81. Eriksson BI, Arfwidsson AC, Frison L, et al. A dose-ranging study of the oral direct thrombin inhibitor, ximelagatran, and its subcutaneous form, melagatran, compared with dalteparin in the prophylaxis of thromboembolism after hip or knee replacement: METHRO I. MElagatran for THRombin inhibition in Orthopaedic surgery. Thromb Haemost 2002; 87:231–237.
82. Dyke CK, Becker RC, Kleiman NS, et al. First experience with direct factor Xa inhibition in patients with stable coronary disease: a pharmacokinetic and pharmacodynamic evaluation. Circulation 2002; 105:2385–2391.
83. Becker RC. Antithrombotic therapy after myocardial infarction. N Engl J Med 2002; 347:1019–1022.
84. Hirsh PD, Hillis LD, Campbell WB, et al. Release of prostaglandins and thromboxane into the coronary circulation in patients with ischemic heart disease. N Engl J Med 1981; 304:685–691.
85. Fitzgerald DJ, Roy L, Catella F, FitzGerald GA. Platelet activation in unstable coronary disease. N Engl J Med 1986; 315:983–989.
86. Willerson JT, Golino P, Eidt J, et al. Specific platelet mediators and unstable coronary artery lesions. Experimental evidence and potential clinical implications. Circulation 1989; 80:198–205.

87. Freedman JE, Loscalzo J. Platelet-monocyte aggregates: bridging thrombosis and inflammation. Circulation 2002; 105:2130–2132.

88. Henn V, Slupsky JR, Grafe M, et al. CD40 ligand on activated platelets triggers an inflammatory reaction of endothelial cells. Nature 1998; 391:591–594.

89. Phipps RP. Atherosclerosis: the emerging role of inflammation and the CD40–CD40 ligand system. Proc Natl Acad Sci USA 2000; 97:6930–6932.

90. Slupsky JR, Kalbas M, Willuweit A, et al. Activated platelets induce tissue factor expression on human umbilical vein endothelial cells by ligation of CD40. Thromb Haemost 1998; 80:1008–1014.

91. Ott I, Neumann FJ, Gawaz M, et al. Increased neutrophil-platelet adhesion in patients with unstable angina. Circulation 1996; 94:1239–1246.

92. Neumann FJ, Ott I, Gawaz M, et al. Neutrophil and platelet activation at balloon-injured coronary artery plaque in patients undergoing angioplasty. J Am Coll Cardiol 1996; 27:819–824.

93. Furman MI, Benoit SE, Barnard MR, et al. Increased platelet reactivity and circulating monocyte-platelet aggregates in patients with stable coronary artery disease. J Am Coll Cardiol 1998; 31:352–358.

94. Furman MI, Barnard MR, Krueger LA, et al. Circulating monocyte-platelet aggregates are an early marker of acute myocardial infarction. J Am Coll Cardiol 2001; 38:1002–1006.

95. Sarma J, Laan CA, Alam S, et al. Increased platelet binding to circulating monocytes in acute coronary syndromes. Circulation 2002; 105:2166–2171.

96. Antiplatelet Trialists' Collaboration. Collaborative overview of randomised trials of antiplatelet therapy—I: Prevention of death, myocardial infarction, and stroke by prolonged antiplatelet therapy in various categories of patients. BMJ 1994; 308:81–106.

97. Patrono C. Aspirin as an antiplatelet drug. N Engl J Med 1994; 330:1287–1294.

98. Yusuf S, Zhao F, Mehta SR, et al. Effects of clopidogrel in addition to aspirin in patients with acute coronary syndromes without ST-segment elevation. N Engl J Med 2001; 345:494–502.

99. Hermann A, Rauch BH, Braun M, et al. Platelet CD40 ligand (CD40L)—subcellular localization, regulation of expression, and inhibition by clopidogrel. Platelets 2001; 12:74–82.

100. Moshfegh K, Redondo M, Julmy F, et al. Antiplatelet effects of clopidogrel compared with aspirin after myocardial infarction: enhanced inhibitory effects of combination therapy. J Am Coll Cardiol 2000; 36:699–705.

101. Chew DP, Bhatt DL, Robbins MA, et al. Effect of clopidogrel added to aspirin before percutaneous coronary intervention on the risk associated with C-reactive protein. Am J Cardiol 2001; 88:672–674.

102. Theoret JF, Bienvenu JG, Kumar A, Merhi Y. P-selectin antagonism with recombinant P-selectin glycoprotein ligand-1 (rPSGL-Ig) inhibits circulating activated platelet binding to neutrophils induced by damaged arterial surfaces. J Pharmacol Exp Ther 2001; 298:658–664.

103. Bienvenu JG, Tanguay JF, Theoret JF, et al. Recombinant soluble P-selectin glycoprotein ligand-1-Ig reduces restenosis through inhibition of platelet-neutrophil adhesion after double angioplasty in swine. Circulation 2001; 103:1128–1134.

104. Simon DI, Chen Z, Xu H, et al. Platelet glycoprotein ibalpha is a counterreceptor for the leukocyte integrin Mac-1 (CD11b/CD18). J Exp Med 2000; 192:193–204.

105. Gralnick HR, Williams S, McKeown L, et al. A monomeric von Willebrand factor fragment, Leu-504–Lys-728, inhibits von Willebrand factor interaction with glycoprotein Ib-IX. Proc Natl Acad Sci USA 1992; 89:7880–7884.

106. Kawasaki T, Kaku S, Kohinata T, et al. Inhibition by aurintricarboxylic acid of von Willebrand factor binding to platelet GPIb, platelet retention, and thrombus formation in vivo. Am J Hematol 1994; 47:6–15.

107. Katayama T, Ikeda Y, Handa M, et al. Immunoneutralization of glycoprotein Ibalpha attenuates endotoxin-induced interactions of platelets and leukocytes with rat venular endothelium in vivo. Circ Res 2000; 86:1031–1037.

108. Miller JL, Thiam-Cisse M, Drouet LO. Reduction in thrombus formation by PG-1 F(ab')2, an anti-guinea pig platelet glycoprotein Ib monoclonal antibody. Arterioscler Thromb 1991; 11:1231–1236.

109. Libby P, Ridker PM, Maseri A. Inflammation and atherosclerosis. Circulation 2002; 105:1135–1143.

110. Libby P, Egan D, Skarlatos S. Roles of infectious agents in atherosclerosis and restenosis: an assessment of the evidence and need for future research. Circulation 1997; 96:4095–4103.

111. Gimbrone MA, Jr. Culture of vascular endothelium. Prog Hemost Thromb 1976; 3:1–28.

112. Liao F, Andalibi A, Qiao JH, et al. Genetic evidence for a common pathway mediating oxidative stress, inflammatory gene induction, and aortic fatty streak formation in mice. J Clin Invest 1994; 94:877–884.

113. Gong KW, Zhu GY, Wang LH, Tang CS. Effect of active oxygen species on intimal proliferation in rat aorta after arterial injury. J Vasc Res 1996; 33:42–46.

114. Glagov S, Zarins C, Giddens DP, Ku DN. Hemodynamics and atherosclerosis. Insights and perspectives gained from studies of human arteries. Arch Pathol Lab Med 1988; 112:1018–1031.

115. Kranzhofer R, Schmidt J, Pfeiffer CA, et al. Angiotensin induces inflammatory activation of human vascular smooth muscle cells. Arterioscler Thromb Vasc Biol 1999; 19:1623–1629.

116. Steinberg D. Antioxidants and atherosclerosis. A current assessment. Circulation 1991; 84:1420–1425.

117. Benditt EP, Barrett T, McDougall JK. Viruses in the etiology of atherosclerosis. Proc Natl Acad Sci USA 1983; 80:6386–6389.

118. Lemstrom K, Koskinen P, Krogerus L, et al. Cytomegalovirus antigen expression, endothelial cell proliferation, and intimal thickening in rat cardiac allografts after cytomegalovirus infection. Circulation 1995; 92:2594–2604.

119. Schmidt AM, Yan SD, Wautier JL, Stern D. Activation of receptor for advanced glycation end products: a mechanism for chronic vascular dysfunction in diabetic vasculopathy and atherosclerosis. Circ Res 1999; 84:489–497.

120. Harker LA, Ross R, Slichter SJ, Scott CR. Homocystine-induced arteriosclerosis. The role of endothelial cell injury and platelet response in its genesis. J Clin Invest 1976; 58:731–741.

121. Yudkin JS, Stehouwer CD, Emeis JJ, Coppack SW. C-reactive protein in healthy subjects: associations with obesity, insulin resistance, and endothelial dysfunction: a potential role for cytokines originating from adipose tissue? Arterioscler Thromb Vasc Biol 1999; 19:972–978.

122. Yudkin JS, Yajnik CS, Mohamed-Ali V, Bulmer K. High levels of circulating proinflammatory cytokines and leptin in urban, but not rural, Indians. A potential explanation for increased risk of diabetes and coronary heart disease. Diabetes Care 1999; 22:363–364.

123. Quinn MT, Parthasarathy S, Fong LG, Steinberg D. Oxidatively modified low density lipoproteins: a potential role in recruitment and retention of monocyte/macrophages during atherogenesis. Proc Natl Acad Sci USA 1987; 84:2995–2998.

124. Nagel T, Resnick N, Atkinson WJ, et al. Shear stress selectively upregulates intercellular adhesion molecule-1 expression in cultured human vascular endothelial cells. J Clin Invest 1994; 94:885–891.

125. Cybulsky MI, Gimbrone MA, Jr. Endothelial expression of a mononuclear leukocyte adhesion molecule during atherogenesis. Science 1991; 251:788–791.

126. Osborne L, Hession C, Tizard R, et al. Direct expression cloning of vascular cell adhesion molecule 1, a cytokine-induced protein that binds to lymphocytes. Cell 1989; 59:1203–1211.

127. Osborne L. Leukocyte adhesion to endothelium in inflammation. Cell 1990; 62:3–6.

128. Poston RN, Haskard DO, Coucher JR, et al. Expression of intercellular adhesion molecule-1 in atherosclerotic plaques. Am J Pathol 1992; 140:665–673.

129. Nakashima Y, Raines E, Plump A, et al. Upregulation of VCAM-1 and ICAM-1 at atherosclerosis-prone sites on the endothelium in the ApoE-deficient mouse. Arterioscler Thromb Vasc Biol 1998; 18:842–851.

130. Li H, Cybulsky MI, Gimbrone MA, Jr., Libby P. An atherogenic diet rapidly induces VCAM-1, a cytokine-regulatable mononuclear leukocyte adhesion molecule, in rabbit aortic endothelium. Arterioscler Thromb 1993; 13:197–204.

131. Tummala PE, Chen XL, Sundell CL, et al. Angiotensin II induces vascular cell adhesion molecule-1 expression in rat vasculature: A potential link between the renin-angiotensin system and atherosclerosis. Circulation 1999; 100:1223–1229.

132. Cybulsky MI, Iiyama K, Li H, et al. A major role for VCAM-1, but not ICAM-1, in early atherosclerosis. J Clin Invest 2001; 107:1255–1262.

133. Navab M, Hama SY, Nguyen TB, Fogelman AM. Monocyte adhesion and transmigration in atherosclerosis. Coron Artery Dis 1994; 5:198–204.

134. Valente AJ, Rozek MM, Sprague EA, Schwartz CJ. Mechanisms in intimal monocyte-macrophage recruitment. A special role for monocyte chemotactic protein-1. Circulation 1992; 86:III20–25.

135. Nelken NA, Coughlin SR, Gordon D, Wilcox JN. Monocyte chemoattractant protein-1 in human atheromatous plaques. J Clin Invest 1991; 88:1121–1127.

136. Wang JM, Sica A, Peri G, et al. Expression of monocyte chemotactic protein and interleukin-8 by cytokine-activated human vascular smooth muscle cells. Arterioscler Thromb 1991; 11:1166–1174.

137. Cushing SD, Berliner JA, Valente AJ, et al. Minimally modified low density lipoprotein induces monocyte chemotactic protein 1 in human endothelial cells and smooth muscle cells. Proc Natl Acad Sci USA 1990; 87:5134–5138.

138. Rajavashisth TB, Andalibi A, Territo MC, et al. Induction of endothelial cell expression of granulocyte and macrophage colony-stimulating factors by modified low-density lipoproteins. Nature 1990; 344:254–257.

139. Gu L, Okada Y, Clinton SK, et al. Absence of monocyte chemoattractant protein-1 reduces atherosclerosis in low density lipoprotein receptor-deficient mice. Mol Cell 1998; 2:275–281.

140. Boring L, Gosling J, Cleary M, Charo IF. Decreased lesion formation in CCR2–/- mice reveals a role for chemokines in the initiation of atherosclerosis. Nature 1998; 394:894–897.

141. de Lemos JA, Morrow DA, Sabatine MS, et al. Plasma levels of monocyte chemoattractant protein (MCP)-1 in patients with acute coronary syndromes. Circulation 2003; 107:690–695.

142. Mitchinson MJ, Ball RY. Macrophages and atherogenesis. Lancet 1987; 2:146–148.

143. Jonasson L, Holm J, Skalli O, et al. Regional accumulations of T cells, macrophages, and smooth muscle cells in the human atherosclerotic plaque. Arteriosclerosis 1986; 6:131–138.

144. Yla-Herttuala S, Lipton BA, Rosenfeld ME, et al. Expression of monocyte chemoattractant protein 1 in macrophage-rich areas of human and rabbit atherosclerotic lesions. Proc Natl Acad Sci USA 1991; 88:5252–5256.

145. Topper JN, Cai J, Falb D, Gimbrone MA, Jr. Identification of vascular endothelial genes differentially responsive to fluid mechanical stimuli: cyclooxygenase-2, manganese superoxide dismutase, and endothelial cell nitric oxide synthase are selectively up-regulated by steady laminar shear stress. Proc Natl Acad Sci USA 1996; 93:10417–10422.

146. Lee RT, Yamamoto C, Feng Y, et al. Mechanical strain induces specific changes in the synthesis and organization of proteoglycans by vascular smooth muscle cells. J Biol Chem 2001; 276:13847–13851.

147. Aqel NM, Ball RY, Waldmann H, Mitchinson MJ. Monocytic origin of foam cells in human atherosclerotic plaques. Atherosclerosis 1984; 53:265–271.

148. Yla-Herttuala S, Palinski W, Rosenfeld ME, et al. Evidence for the presence of oxidatively modified low density lipoprotein in atherosclerotic lesions of rabbit and man. J Clin Invest 1989; 84:1086–1095.

149. Steinberg D, Parthasarathy S, Carew TE, et al. Beyond cholesterol. Modifications of low-density lipoprotein that increase its atherogenicity. N Engl J Med 1989; 320:915–924.

150. Stary HC. Evolution and progression of atherosclerotic lesions in coronary arteries of children and young adults. Arteriosclerosis 1989; 9:I19–32.

151. Mantovani A, Bussolino F, Dejana E. Cytokine regulation of endothelial cell function. Faseb J 1992; 6:2591–2599.

152. Raines EW, Dower SK, Ross R. Interleukin-1 mitogenic activity for fibroblasts and smooth muscle cells is due to PDGF-AA. Science 1989; 243:393–396.

153. Seino Y, Ikeda U, Ikeda M, et al. Interleukin 6 gene transcripts are expressed in human atherosclerotic lesions. Cytokine 1994; 6:87–91.

154. Rus HG, Vlaicu R, Niculescu F. Interleukin-6 and interleukin-8 protein and gene expression in human arterial atherosclerotic wall. Atherosclerosis 1996; 127:263–271.

155. Libby P, Ordovas JM, Auger KR, et al. Endotoxin and tumor necrosis factor induce interleukin-1 gene expression in adult human vascular endothelial cells. Am J Pathol 1986; 124:179–185.

156. Schwartz SM, Reidy MA. Common mechanisms of proliferation of smooth muscle in atherosclerosis and hypertension. Hum Pathol 1987; 18:240–247.

157. Libby P, Warner SJ, Salomon RN, Birinyi LK. Production of platelet-derived growth factor-like mitogen by smooth-muscle cells from human atheroma. N Engl J Med 1988; 318:1493–1498.

158. Ip JH, Fuster V, Badimon L, et al. Syndromes of accelerated atherosclerosis: role of vascular injury and smooth muscle cell proliferation. J Am Coll Cardiol 1990; 15:1667–1687.

159. Ikeda U, Ikeda M, Oohara T, et al. Interleukin 6 stimulates growth of vascular smooth muscle cells in a PDGF-dependent manner. Am J Physiol 1991; 260:H1713–1717.

160. Lendon CL, Davies MJ, Born GV, Richardson PD. Atherosclerotic plaque caps are locally weakened when macrophages density is increased. Atherosclerosis 1991; 87:87–90.

161. Henney AM, Wakeley PR, Davies MJ, et al. Localization of stromelysin gene expression in atherosclerotic plaques by in situ hybridization. Proc Natl Acad Sci USA 1991; 88:8154–8158.

162. Galis ZS, Sukhova GK, Lark MW, Libby P. Increased expression of matrix metalloproteinases and matrix degrading activity in vulnerable regions of human atherosclerotic plaques. J Clin Invest 1994; 94:2493–2503.

163. Galis ZS, Muszynski M, Sukhova GK, et al. Cytokine-stimulated human vascular smooth muscle cells synthesize a complement of enzymes required for extracellular matrix digestion. Circ Res 1994; 75:181–189.

164. Saren P, Welgus HG, Kovanen PT. TNF-alpha and IL-1beta selectively induce expression of 92–kDa gelatinase by human macrophages. J Immunol 1996; 157:4159–4165.

165. Mach F, Schonbeck U, Bonnefoy JY, et al. Activation of monocyte/macrophage functions related to acute atheroma complication by ligation of CD40: induction of collagenase, stromelysin, and tissue factor. Circulation 1997; 96:396–399.

166. Wilcox JN, Smith KM, Schwartz SM, Gordon D. Localization of tissue factor in the normal vessel wall and in the atherosclerotic plaque. Proc Natl Acad Sci USA 1989; 86:2839–2843.

167. Neri Serneri G, Abbate R, Gori A, et al. Transient intermittent lymphocyte activation is responsible for the instability of angina. Circulation 1992; 86:790–797.

168. Shimokawa H, Ito A, Fukumoto Y, et al. Chronic treatment with interleukin-1 beta induces coronary intimal lesions and vasospastic responses in pigs in vivo. The role of platelet-derived growth factor. J Clin Invest 1996; 97:769–776.

169. Kohchi K, Takebayashi S, Hiroki T, Nobuyoshi M. Significance of adventitial inflammation of the coronary artery in patients with unstable angina: results at autopsy. Circulation 1985; 71:709–716.

170. Libby P, Aikawa M. Stabilization of atherosclerotic plaques: new mechanisms and clinical targets. Nat Med 2002; 8:1257–1262.

171. Liuzzo G, Biasucci LM, Gallimore JR, et al. The prognostic value of C-reactive protein and serum amyloid a protein in severe unstable angina. N Engl J Med 1994; 331:417–424.

172. Morrow DA, Rifai N, Antman EM, et al. C-Reactive protein is a potent predictor of mortality independently and in combination with troponin T in acute coronary syndromes. J Am Coll Cardiol 1998; 31:1460–1465.

173. Biasucci LM, Vitelli A, Liuzzo G, et al. Elevated levels of interleukin-6 in unstable angina. Circulation 1996; 94:874–877.

174. Morrow DA, Rifai N, Antman EM, et al. Serum amyloid A predicts early mortality in acute coronary syndromes: a TIMI 11A substudy. J Am Coll Cardiol 2000; 35:358–362.

175. Toss H, Lindahl B, Siegbahn A, Wallentin L. Prognostic influence of increased fibrinogen and C-reactive protein levels in unstable coronary artery disease. FRISC Study Group. Fragmin during Instability in Coronary Artery Disease. Circulation 1997; 96:4204–4210.

176. Ferreiros ER, Boissonnet CP, Pizarro R, et al. Independent prognostic value of elevated C-reactive protein in unstable angina. Circulation 1999; 100:1958–1963.

177. Heeschen C, Hamm CW, Bruemmer J, Simoons ML. Predictive value of C-reactive protein and troponin T in patients with unstable angina: a comparative analysis. CAPTURE Investigators. Chimeric c7E3 AntiPlatelet Therapy in Unstable angina REfractory to standard treatment trial. J Am Coll Cardiol 2000; 35:1535–1542.

178. Lindahl B, Toss H, Siegbahn A, et al. Markers of myocardial damage and inflammation in relation to long-term mortality in unstable coronary artery disease. FRISC Study Group. Fragmin during Instability in Coronary Artery Disease. N Engl J Med 2000; 343:1139–1147.

179. Zwaka TP, Hombach V, Torzewski J. C-reactive protein-mediated low density lipoprotein uptake by macrophages: implications for atherosclerosis. Circulation 2001; 103:1194–1197.

180. Nakagomi A, Freedman SB, Geczy CL. Interferon-gamma and lipopolysaccharide potentiate monocyte tissue factor induction by C-reactive protein: relationship with age, sex, and hormone replacement treatment. Circulation 2000; 101:1785–1791.

181. Penn MS, Topol EJ. Tissue factor, the emerging link between inflammation, thrombosis, and vascular remodeling. Circ Res 2001; 89:1–2.

182. Yasojima K, Schwab C, McGeer EG, McGeer PL. Generation of C-reactive protein and complement components in atherosclerotic plaques. Am J Pathol 2001; 158:1039–1051.

183. Pasceri V, Willerson JT, Yeh ET. Direct proinflammatory effect of C-reactive protein on human endothelial cells. Circulation 2000; 102:2165–2168.

184. Torzewski M, Rist C, Mortensen RF, et al. C-reactive protein in the arterial intima: role of C-reactive protein receptor-dependent monocyte recruitment in atherogenesis. Arterioscler Thromb Vasc Biol 2000; 20:2094–2099.

185. Bhatt DL, Topol EJ. Need to test the arterial inflammation hypothesis. Circulation 2002; 106:136–140.

186. Pearson TA, Mensah GA, Alexander RW, et al. Markers of inflammation and cardiovascular disease: application to clinical and public health practice: a statement for healthcare professionals from the Centers for Disease Control and Prevention and the American Heart Association. Circulation 2003; 107:499–511.

187. Ridker PM, Cushman M, Stampfer MJ, et al. Inflammation, aspirin, and the risk of cardiovascular disease in apparently healthy men. N Engl J Med 1997; 336:973–979.

188. Ikonomidis I, Andreotti F, Economou E, et al. Increased proinflammatory cytokines in patients with chronic stable angina and their reduction by aspirin. Circulation 1999; 100:793–798.

189. Feldman M, Jialal I, Devaraj S, Cryer B. Effects of low-dose aspirin on serum C-reactive protein and thromboxane B2 concentrations: a placebo-controlled study using a highly sensitive C-reactive protein assay. J Am Coll Cardiol 2001; 37:2036–2041.

190. Feng D, Tracy RP, Lipinska I, et al. Effect of short-term aspirin use on C-reactive protein. J Thromb Thrombolysis 2000; 9:37–41.

191. Kennon S, Price CP, Mills PG, et al. The effect of aspirin on C-reactive protein as a marker of risk in unstable angina. J Am Coll Cardiol 2001; 37:1266–1270.

192. Ridker PM, Rifai N, Pfeffer MA, et al. Inflammation, pravastatin, and the risk of coronary events after myocardial infarction in patients with average cholesterol levels. Cholesterol and Recurrent Events (CARE) Investigators. Circulation 1998; 98:839–844.

193. Ridker PM, Rifai N, Clearfield M, et al. Measurement of C-reactive protein for the targeting of statin therapy in the primary prevention of acute coronary events. N Engl J Med 2001; 344:1959–1965.

194. Ridker PM, Rifai N, Pfeffer MA, et al. Long-term effects of pravastatin on plasma concentration of C-reactive protein. Circulation 1999; 100:230–235.

195. Ridker PM, Rifai N, Lowenthal SP. Rapid reduction in C-reactive protein with cerivastatin among 785 patients with primary hypercholesterolemia. Circulation 2001; 103:1191–1193.

196. Albert MA, Danielson E, Rifai N, Ridker PM. Effect of statin therapy on C-reactive protein levels: the pravastatin inflammation/CRP evaluation (PRINCE): a randomized trial and cohort study. JAMA 2001; 286:64–70.

197. Jialal I, Stein D, Balis D, et al. Effect of hydroxymethyl glutaryl coenzyme a reductase inhibitor therapy on high sensitive C-reactive protein levels. Circulation 2001; 103:1933–1935.

198. Horne BD, Muhlestein JB, Carlquist JF, et al. Statin therapy, lipid levels, C-reactive protein and the survival of patients with angiographically severe coronary artery disease. J Am Coll Cardiol 2000; 36:1774–1780.

199. Walter DH, Fichtlscherer S, Britten MB, et al. Statin therapy, inflammation and recurrent coronary events in patients following coronary stent implantation. J Am Coll Cardiol 2001; 38:2006–2012.

200. Kayikcioglu M, Turkoglu C, Kultursay H, et al. The short term results of combined use of pravastatin with thrombolytic therapy in acute myocardial infarction (abstr). Circulation 1999; 100:I-303.

201. Schwartz GG, Olsson AG, Ezekowitz MD, et al. Effects of atorvastatin on early recurrent ischemic events in acute coronary syndromes: the MIRACL study: a randomized controlled trial. JAMA 2001; 285:1711–1718.

202. Kinlay S, Rifai N, Libby P, Ganz P. Effect of atorvastatin on c-reactive protein in patients with acute coronary syndromes: a substudy of the MIRACL trial (abstr). J Am Coll Cardiol 2002; 39:304A.

203. de Lemos Aj, Blazing MA, Wivitt SD, et al. Early intensive vs. a delayed conservative simvastatin strategy in patients with acute coronary syndrome: Phase Z of the A to Z trial. JAMA 2004; 292(11):307

204. Cannon CP, Braunwald E, McCabe CH, et al. Comparison of intensive and moderate lipid lowering with statins after acute coronary syndromes. New Engl J Med (abst.) 2004, 350.

205. Treasure CB, Klein JL, Weintraub WS, et al. Beneficial effects of cholesterol-lowering therapy on the coronary endothelium in patients with coronary artery disease. N Engl J Med 1995; 332:481–487.

206. Williams JK, Sukhova GK, Herrington DM, Libby P. Pravastatin has cholesterol-lowering independent effects on the artery wall of atherosclerotic monkeys. J Am Coll Cardiol 1998; 31:684–691.

207. Wilson SH, Simari RD, Best PJ, et al. Simvastatin preserves coronary endothelial function in hypercholesterolemia in the absence of lipid lowering. Arterioscler Thromb Vasc Biol 2001; 21:122–128.

208. Sparrow CP, Burton CA, Hernandez M, et al. Simvastatin has anti-inflammatory and antiatherosclerotic activities independent of plasma cholesterol lowering. Arterioscler Thromb Vasc Biol 2001; 21:115–121.

209. Bourcier T, Libby P. HMG CoA reductase inhibitors reduce plasminogen activator inhibitor-1 expression by human vascular smooth muscle and endothelial cells. Arterioscler Thromb Vasc Biol 2000; 20:556–562.

210. Lopez S, Peiretti F, Bonardo B, et al. Effect of atorvastatin and fluvastatin on the expression of plasminogen activator inhibitor type-1 in cultured human endothelial cells. Atherosclerosis 2000; 152:359–366.

211. Dangas G, Smith DA, Unger AH, et al. Pravastatin: an antithrombotic effect independent of the cholesterol- lowering effect. Thromb Haemost 2000; 83:688–692.

212. Dangas G, Badimon JJ, Smith DA, et al. Pravastatin therapy in hyperlipidemia: effects on thrombus formation and the systemic hemostatic profile. J Am Coll Cardiol 1999; 33:1294–1304.

213. Bustos C, Hernandez-Presa MA, Ortego M, et al. HMG-CoA reductase inhibition by atorvastatin reduces neointimal inflammation in a rabbit model of atherosclerosis. J Am Coll Cardiol 1998; 32:2057–2064.

214. Aikawa M, Rabkin E, Sugiyama S, et al. An HMG-CoA Reductase inhibitor, cerivastatin, suppresses growth of macrophages expressing matrix metalloproteinases and tissue factor in vivo and in vitro. Circulation 2001; 103:276–283.

215. Aikawa M, Rabkin E, Okada Y, et al. Lipid lowering by diet reduces matrix metalloproteinase activity and increases collagen content of rabbit atheroma: a potential mechanism of lesion stabilization. Circulation 1998; 97:2433–2444.

216. Aikawa M, Sugiyama S, Hill CC, et al. Lipid lowering reduces oxidative stress and endothelial cell activation in rabbit atheroma. Circulation 2002; 106:1390–1396.

217. Aikawa M, Voglic SJ, Sugiyama S, et al. Dietary lipid lowering reduces tissue factor expression in rabbit atheroma. Circulation 1999; 100:1215–1222.

218. Sukhova GK, Williams JK, Libby P. Statins reduce inflammation in atheroma of nonhuman primates independent of effects on serum cholesterol. Arterioscler Thromb Vasc Biol 2002; 22:1452–1458.

219. Yusuf S, Sleight P, Pogue J, et al. Effects of an angiotensin-converting-enzyme inhibitor, ramipril, on cardiovascular events in high-risk patients. The Heart Outcomes Prevention Evaluation Study Investigators. N Engl J Med 2000; 342:145–153.

220. Sleight P, Yusuf S, Pogue J, et al. Blood-pressure reduction and cardiovascular risk in HOPE study. Lancet 2001; 358:2130–2131.

221. Hernandez-Presa M, Bustos C, Ortego M, et al. Angiotensin-converting enzyme inhibition prevents arterial nuclear factor-kappa B activation, monocyte chemoattractant protein-1 expression, and macrophage infiltration in a rabbit model of early accelerated atherosclerosis. Circulation 1997; 95:1532–1541.

222. Neve BP, Corseaux D, Chinetti G, et al. PPARalpha agonists inhibit tissue factor expression in human monocytes and macrophages. Circulation 2001; 103:207–212.

223. Marx N, Sukhova GK, Collins T, et al. PPARalpha activators inhibit cytokine-induced vascular cell adhesion molecule-1 expression in human endothelial cells. Circulation 1999; 99:3125–3131.

224. Marx N, Mackman N, Schonbeck U, et al. PPARalpha activators inhibit tissue factor expression and activity in human monocytes. Circulation 2001; 103:213–219.

225. Malik J, Melenovsky V, Wichterle D, et al. Both fenofibrate and atorvastatin improve vascular reactivity in combined hyperlipidaemia (fenofibrate versus atorvastatin trial—FAT). Cardiovasc Res 2001; 52:290–298.

226. Marx N, Kehrle B, Kohlhammer K, et al. PPAR activators as antiinflammatory mediators in human T lymphocytes: implications for atherosclerosis and transplantation-associated arteriosclerosis. Circ Res 2002; 90:703–710.

227. Pasceri V, Wu HD, Willerson JT, Yeh ET. Modulation of vascular inflammation in vitro and in vivo by peroxisome proliferator-activated receptor-gamma activators. Circulation 2000; 101:235–238.

228. Li AC, Brown KK, Silvestre MJ, et al. Peroxisome proliferator-activated receptor gamma ligands inhibit development of atherosclerosis in LDL receptor-deficient mice. J Clin Invest 2000; 106:523–531.

229. Collins AR, Meehan WP, Kintscher U, et al. Troglitazone inhibits formation of early atherosclerotic lesions in diabetic and nondiabetic low density lipoprotein receptor-deficient mice. Arterioscler Thromb Vasc Biol 2001; 21:365–371.

230. Haffner SM, Greenberg AS, Weston WM, et al. Effect of rosiglitazone treatment on nontraditional markers of cardiovascular disease in patients with type 2 diabetes mellitus. Circulation 2002; 106:679–684.

231. Azar RR, Rinfret S, Theroux P, et al. A randomized placebo-controlled trial to assess the efficacy of antiinflammatory therapy with methylprednisolone in unstable angina (MUNA trial). Eur Heart J 2000; 21:2026–2032.

232. Schonbeck U, Sukhova GK, Shimizu K, et al. Inhibition of CD40 signaling limits evolution of established atherosclerosis in mice. Proc Natl Acad Sci USA 2000; 97:7458–7463.

233. Mukherjee D, Nissen SE, Topol EJ. Risk of cardiovascular events associated with selective COX-2 inhibitors. JAMA 2001; 286:954–959.

234. Ray WA, Stein CM, Daugherty JR, et al. COX-2 selective non-steroidal anti-inflammatory drugs and risk of serious coronary heart disease. Lancet 2002; 360:1071–1073.

235. Ray WA, Stein CM, Hall K, et al. Non-steroidal anti-inflammatory drugs and risk of serious coronary heart disease: an observational cohort study. Lancet 2002; 359:118–123.

236. Hennan JK, Huang J, Barrett TD, et al. Effects of selective cyclooxygenase-2 inhibition on vascular responses and thrombosis in canine coronary arteries. Circulation 2001; 104:820–825.

237. Zhou YF, Shou M, Guetta E, et al. Cytomegalovirus infection of rats increases the neointimal response to vascular injury without consistent evidence of direct infection of the vascular wall. Circulation 1999; 100:1569–1575.

238. Mayr M, Metzler B, Kiechl S, et al. Endothelial cytotoxicity mediated by serum antibodies to heat shock proteins of Escherichia coli and *Chlamydia pneumoniae:* immune reactions to heat shock proteins as a possible link between infection and atherosclerosis. Circulation 1999; 99:1560–1566.

239. Epstein SE, Zhou YF, Zhu J. Infection and atherosclerosis: emerging mechanistic paradigms. Circulation 1999; 100:e20–28.

240. Hendrix MG, Dormans PH, Kitslaar P, et al. The presence of cytomegalovirus nucleic acids in arterial walls of atherosclerotic and nonatherosclerotic patients. Am J Pathol 1989; 134:1151–1157.

241. Hendrix MG, Salimans MM, van Boven CP, Bruggeman CA. High prevalence of latently present cytomegalovirus in arterial walls of patients suffering from grade III atherosclerosis. Am J Pathol 1990; 136:23–28.

242. Grayston JT, Kuo CC, Coulson AS, et al. *Chlamydia pneumoniae* (TWAR) in atherosclerosis of the carotid artery. Circulation 1995; 92:3397–3400.

243. Kuo CC, Shor A, Campbell LA, et al. Demonstration of *Chlamydia pneumoniae* in atherosclerotic lesions of coronary arteries. J Infect Dis 1993; 167:841–849.

244. Kuo CC, Grayston JT, Campbell LA, et al. *Chlamydia pneumoniae* (TWAR) in coronary arteries of young adults (15–34 years old). Proc Natl Acad Sci U S A 1995; 92:6911–6914.

245. Muhlestein JB, Hammond EH, Carlquist JF, et al. Increased incidence of *Chlamydia* species within the coronary arteries of patients with symptomatic atherosclerotic versus other forms of cardiovascular disease. J Am Coll Cardiol 1996; 27:1555–1561.

246. Maass M, Bartels C, Engel PM, et al. Endovascular presence of viable *Chlamydia pneumoniae* is a common phenomenon in coronary artery disease. J Am Coll Cardiol 1998; 31:827–832.

247. Ericson K, Saldeen TG, Lindquist O, et al. Relationship of *Chlamydia pneumoniae* infection to severity of human coronary atherosclerosis. Circulation 2000; 101:2568–2571.

248. Fabricant CG, Fabricant J, Litrenta MM, Minick CR. Virus-induced atherosclerosis. J Exp Med 1978; 148:335–340.

249. Muhlestein JB, Anderson JL, Hammond EH, et al. Infection with *Chlamydia pneumoniae* accelerates the development of atherosclerosis and treatment with azithromycin prevents it in a rabbit model. Circulation 1998; 97:633–636.

250. Moazed TC, Kuo C, Grayston JT, Campbell LA. Murine models of *Chlamydia pneumoniae* infection and atherosclerosis. J Infect Dis 1997; 175:883–890.

251. Moazed TC, Campbell LA, Rosenfeld ME, et al. *Chlamydia pneumoniae* infection accelerates the progression of atherosclerosis in apolipoprotein E-deficient mice. J Infect Dis 1999; 180:238–241.

252. Hu H, Pierce GN, Zhong G. The atherogenic effects of chlamydia are dependent on serum cholesterol and specific to *Chlamydia pneumoniae.* J Clin Invest 1999; 103:747–753.

253. Melnick JL, Adam E, DeBakey ME. Possible role of cytomegalovirus in atherogenesis. JAMA 1990; 263:2204–2207.

254. Saikku P, Leinonen M, Mattila K, et al. Serological evidence of an association of a novel *Chlamydia,* TWAR, with chronic coronary heart disease and acute myocardial infarction. Lancet 1988; 2:983–986.

255. Thom DH, Grayston JT, Siscovick DS, et al. Association of prior infection with *Chlamydia pneumoniae* and angiographically demonstrated coronary artery disease. JAMA 1992; 268:68–72.

256. Patel P, Mendall MA, Carrington D, et al. Association of *Helicobacter pylori* and *Chlamydia pneumoniae* infections with coronary heart disease and cardiovascular risk factors [published erratum appears in BMJ 1995 Oct 14; 311(7011):985]. BMJ 1995; 311:711–4.

257. Mendall MA, Goggin PM, Molineaux N, et al. Relation of *Helicobacter pylori* infection and coronary heart disease. Br Heart J 1994; 71:437–439.

258. Danesh J, Collins R, Peto R. Chronic infections and coronary heart disease: is there a link? Lancet 1997; 350:430–436.

259. Hahn DL, Golubjatnikov R. Smoking is a potential confounder of the *Chlamydia pneumoniae*-coronary artery disease association. Arterioscler Thromb 1992; 12:945–947.

260. Mendall MA, Carrington D, Strachan D, et al. *Chlamydia pneumoniae:* risk factors for seropositivity and association with coronary heart disease. J Infect 1995; 30:121–128.

261. Ridker P. Are associations between infection and coronary risk causal or due to confounding? Am J Med 1999; 106:376–377

262. Whincup PH, Mendall MA, Perry IJ, et al. Prospective relations between *Helicobacter pylori* infection, coronary heart disease, and stroke in middle aged men. Heart 1996; 75:568–572.

263. Wald NJ, Law MR, Morris JK, Bagnall AM. *Helicobacter pylori* infection and mortality from ischaemic heart disease: negative result from a large, prospective study. BMJ 1997; 315:1199–1201.

264. Ridker P, Hennekens C, Stampfer M, Wang F. Prospective study of herpes simplex virus, cytomegalovirus, and the risk of future myocardial infarction and stroke. Circulation 1998; 98:2796–2799.

265. Ridker P, Kundsin R, Stampfer M, et al. Prospective study of *Chlamydia pneumoniae* IgG seropositivity and risks of future myocardial infarction. Circulation 1999; 99:1161–1164.

266. Danesh J, Whincup P, Walker M, et al. *Chlamydia pneumoniae* IgG titres and coronary heart disease: prospective study and meta-analysis. BMJ 2000; 321:208–213.

267. Danesh J, Whincup P, Lewington S, et al. Chlamydia pneumoniae IgA titres and coronary heart disease; prospective study and meta-analysis. Eur Heart J 2002; 23:371–375.

268. Muhlestein JB, Horne BD, Carlquist JF, et al. Cytomegalovirus seropositivity and C-reactive protein have independent and combined predictive value for mortality in patients with angiographically demonstrated coronary artery disease. Circulation 2000; 102:1917–1923.

269. Zhu J, Nieto FJ, Horne BD, et al. Prospective study of pathogen burden and risk of myocardial infarction or death. Circulation 2001; 103:45–51.

270. Rupprecht HJ, Blankenberg S, Bickel C, et al. Impact of viral and bacterial infectious burden on long-term prognosis in patients with coronary artery disease. Circulation 2001; 104:25–31.

271. Espinola-Klein C, Rupprecht HJ, Blankenberg S, et al. Impact of infectious burden on extent and long-term prognosis of atherosclerosis. Circulation 2002; 105:15–21.

272. Buja LM. Does atherosclerosis have an infectious etiology? Circulation 1996; 94:872–873.

273. Nieto FJ, Adam E, Sorlie P, et al. Cohort study of cytomegalovirus infection as a risk factor for carotid intimal-medial thickening, a measure of subclinical atherosclerosis. Circulation 1996; 94:922–927.

274. Zhou YF, Leon MB, Waclawiw MA, et al. Association between prior cytomegalovirus infection and the risk of restenosis after coronary atherectomy. N Engl J Med 1996; 335:624–630.

275. Grattan MT, Moreno-Cabral CE, Starnes VA, et al. Cytomegalovirus infection is associated with cardiac allograft rejection and atherosclerosis. JAMA 1989; 261:3561–3566.

276. Vallance P, Collier J, Bhagat K. Infection, inflammation, and infarction: does acute endothelial dysfunction provide a link? Lancet 1997; 349:1391–1392.

277. Mendall MA, Patel P, Ballam L, et al. C reactive protein and its relation to cardiovascular risk factors: a population based cross sectional study. BMJ 1996; 312:1061–1065.

278. Anderson JL, Carlquist JF, Muhlestein JB, et al. Evaluation of C-reactive protein, an inflammatory marker, and infectious serology as risk factors for coronary artery disease and myocardial infarction. J Am Coll Cardiol 1998; 32:35–41.

279. Zhu J, Quyyumi AA, Norman JE, et al. Cytomegalovirus in the pathogenesis of atherosclerosis: the role of inflammation as reflected by elevated C-reactive protein levels. J Am Coll Cardiol 1999; 34:1738–1743.

280. Kalayoglu MV, Byrne GI. Induction of macrophage foam cell formation by Chlamydia pneumoniae. J Infect Dis 1998; 177:725–729.

281. Molestina RE, Miller RD, Ramirez JA, Summersgill JT. Infection of human endothelial cells with Chlamydia pneumoniae stimulates transendothelial migration of neutrophils and monocytes. Infect Immun 1999; 67:1323–1330.

282. Kol A, Sukhova GK, Lichtman AH, Libby P. Chlamydial heat shock protein 60 localizes in human atheroma and regulates macrophage tumor necrosis factor-alpha and matrix metalloproteinase expression. Circulation 1998; 98:300–307.

283. Epstein SE, Zhu J, Burnett MS, et al. Infection and atherosclerosis: potential roles of pathogen burden and molecular mimicry. Arterioscler Thromb Vasc Biol 2000; 20:1417–1420.

284. Fong IW, Chiu B, Viira E, et al. Chlamydial heat-shock protein-60 antibody and correlation with Chlamydia pneumoniae in atherosclerotic plaques. J Infect Dis 2002; 186:1469–1473.

285. Gurfinkel E, Bozovich G, Daroca A, et al. Randomised trial of roxithromycin in non-Q-wave coronary syndromes: ROXIS Pilot Study. ROXIS Study Group. Lancet 1997; 350:404–7.

286. Gupta S, Leatham EW, Carrington D, et al. Elevated Chlamydia pneumoniae antibodies, cardiovascular events, and azithromycin in male survivors of myocardial infarction. Circulation 1997; 96:404–407.

287. Anderson JL, Muhlestein JB, Carlquist J, et al. Randomized secondary prevention trial of azithromycin in patients with coronary artery disease and serological evidence for Chlamydia pneumoniae infection: The Azithromycin in Coronary Artery Disease: Elimination of Myocardial Infection with Chlamydia (ACADEMIC) study. Circulation 1999; 99:1540–1547.

288. Torgano G, Cosentini R, Mandelli C, et al. Treatment of Helicobacter pylori and Chlamydia pneumoniae infections decreases fibrinogen plasma level in patients with ischemic heart disease. Circulation 1999; 99:1555–1559.

289. Parchure N, Zouridakis EG, Kaski JC. Effect of azithromycin treatment on endothelial function in patients with coronary artery disease and evidence of Chlamydia pneumoniae infection. Circulation 2002; 105:1298–1303.

290. Ferguson JJ. Meeting highlights: highlights of the 51st annual scientific sessions of the American College of Cardiology. Atlanta, Georgia, USA. March 17– 20, 2002. Circulation 2002; 106:E24–30.

291. Sinisalo J, Mattila K, Valtonen V, et al. Effect of 3 months of antimicrobial treatment with clarithromycin in acute non-q-wave coronary syndrome. Circulation 2002; 105:1555–1560.

292. Kothe H, Dalhoff K, Rupp J, et al. Hydroxymethylglutaryl coenzyme A reductase inhibitors modify the inflammatory response of human macrophages and endothelial cells infected with Chlamydia pneumoniae. Circulation 2000; 101:1760–1763.

293. McFadden EP, Clarke JG, Davies GJ, et al. Effect of intracoronary serotonin on coronary vessels in patients with stable angina and patients with variant angina. N Engl J Med 1991; 324:648–654.

294. Eisenberg PR, Kenzora JL, Sobel BE, et al. Relation between ST segment shifts during ischemia and thrombin activity in patients with unstable angina. J Am Coll Cardiol 1991; 18:898–903.

295. Prinzmetal M, Kennamer R, Merliss R. A variant form of angina pectoris. Am J Med 1959; 27:375.

296. Epstein SE, Cannon RO, 3rd. Site of increased resistance to coronary flow in patients with angina pectoris and normal epicardial coronary arteries. J Am Coll Cardiol 1986; 8:459–461.

297. Topol EJ, Yadav JS. Recognition of the importance of embolization in atherosclerotic vascular disease. Circulation 2000; 101:570–580.

298. de Lemos JA, Braunwald E. ST segment resolution as a tool for assessing the efficacy of reperfusion therapy. J Am Coll Cardiol 2001; 38:1283–1294.

299. Nabel EG, Ganz P, Gordon JB, et al. Dilation of normal and constriction of atherosclerotic coronary arteries caused by the cold pressor test. Circulation 1988; 77:43–52.

300. Pitts WR, Lange RA, Cigarroa JE, Hillis LD. Cocaine-induced myocardial ischemia and infarction: pathophysiology, recognition, and management. Prog Cardiovasc Dis 1997; 40:65–76.

301. Ganz P, Weidinger FF, Yeung AC, et al. Coronary vasospasm in humans: the role of atherosclerosis and of impaired endothelial vasodilator function. Basic Res Cardiol 1991; 86:215–222.

302. Yeung AC, Vekshtein VI, Krantz DS, et al. The effect of atherosclerosis on the vasomotor response of coronary arteries to mental stress. N Engl J Med 1991; 325:1551–1556.

8-1

Risk Assessment in Acute Coronary Syndromes

Cheuk–Kit Wong and Harvey D. White
Green Lane Hospital, Auckland, New Zealand

I. INTRODUCTION

Risk assessment is an important part of the clinical evaluation of patients with acute coronary syndromes (ACS). It can determine the prognosis and the response to medical and interventional therapies, guide clinical decisions as to which therapeutic approach is most appropriate, indicate the likely duration of the hospital stay, and provide information for patients and relatives.

Before an evidence-based approach was developed, clinical experience and opinion-guided risk assessment dominated this area of medicine. In the past two decades, data from clinical trials and registries have provided an evidence base for assessing the relative importance of individual risk factors, leading to the development of risk models. Due to the patient selection process for clinical trials, risk models derived from specific trial populations may not accurately represent patients encountered in routine clinical practice (1,2). Registry data may better evaluate how co-morbidities such as renal disease, pulmonary disease, cerebrovascular disease and malignancy may influence risk—an increasingly relevant issue as the demographic profile of ACS patients moves more towards elderly subjects with multiple medical problems. Unlike risk factors identified in ACS trials, these co-morbidities are often pathologically unrelated to the ACS.

The concept of "risk" is usually thought of as the risk of death, but composite end-points such as death/nonfatal myocardial infarction (MI)/revascularization are often used in clinical trials. Revascularization is a "softer" endpoint than death and may be influenced by factors unrelated to the risk of death. Whether or not an individual risk factor predicts the benefit of treatment depends upon whether that risk factor is pathophysiologically related to the development and severity of the ACS and whether it is reversible (see Chapter 7-1). Qualitative clinical observations (e.g., "the patient looks sick and is pale and sweating") have been omitted from risk models, possibly because of the likelihood of interobserver variability.

II. CLASSIFICATION OF ACS

ACS is classified according to the presence or absence of ST-segment elevation on the presenting electrocardiogram (ECG). Patients with ST-elevation ACS have a high early mortality rate (3) due to a rapid wavefront of myocardial necrosis resulting from total or near-total coronary artery occlusion, requiring emergency reperfusion therapy with either fibrinolysis or primary percutaneous coronary intervention (PCI). Non–ST-elevation ACS is usually due to subtotal coronary occlusion, which causes less myocardial necrosis. These patients have a lower early mortality rate than those with ST-elevation ACS (4), and there is a longer time window for administration of antiplatelet and antithrombotic treatments to maintain coronary flow and to passivate the plaque prior to a revascularization procedure (4–6).

The prognostic difference between ST-elevation ACS and non–ST-elevation ACS changes over time. In the Global Use of Strategies to Open Occluded Coronary Arteries (GUSTO) IIB study, the 30-day mortality rate was higher in patients with ST-elevation ACS ($n = 4125$) than in those with non–ST-elevation ACS ($n = 8001$, 6.1% vs. 3.8%; $p < 0.001$), but the difference in mortality was no longer significant at 1 year (9.6% vs. 8.8%) (7). Among patients with non–ST-elevation ACS in GUSTO IIB, those with enzymatic evidence of MI at baseline ($n = 3513$) had higher rates of reinfarction (9.8% vs. 6.2% at 6 months; $p < 0.001$) and mortality (8.8% vs. 5.0% at 6 months; $p < 0.001$; and 11.1% vs. 7.0% at 1 year; $p < 0.001$) than those without MI at baseline ($n = 4488$) (7). A recent report from the same trial showed that creatine kinase levels at baseline independently predicted 6-month outcomes across the whole spectrum of ACS (8), irrespective of the patient's ST-segment changes. In a registry study from Minnesota (1), patients were followed up for 6.3 years, and there was no difference in death/reinfarction rates between those with and those without ST elevation on their initial ECGs.

III. ACUTE RISK ASSESSMENT IN NON–ST-ELEVATION ACS

The major risk factors identified in patients with non–ST-elevation ACS include age (9), severity of ST-segment depression (10–13), elevated cardiac protein levels (particularly the troponins) (9,12–17), heart failure (9,18), diabetes (13,19), coronary artery disease (9), and renal disease (1,2,13,20,21).

Elevated troponin levels in the blood signify necrosis of cardiac myocytes, and numerous studies (16,17,22–28) have shown that elevated troponin levels are associated with increased risk. This risk is additional to that conferred by elevated creatine kinase-MB levels and the presence of ST-segment depression (Table 1). For example, in the Thrombolysis in Myocardial Infarction (TIMI) IIIB trial of patients with unstable angina or non–Q-wave MI, those with elevated troponin I levels within 6 hours after symptom onset had almost double the mortality rate at 42 days compared those without elevated troponin levels (3.1% vs 1.7%) (29). Meta-analysis has shown that patients with elevated troponin levels have a fourfold risk of death/MI within 30 days (30).

The prognostic value of elevated troponin levels is greater than the extent of myocardial damage and left ventricular dysfunction might suggest. Elevated troponin levels have

Table 1 Predictors of Death/MI Within 30 Days ($n = 773$)

Predictors	Patients with positive status		Patients with negative status		Odds ratio	
	n	Death/MI	n	Death/MI	(95% CI)	p value
Troponin T	123	27 (22%)	650	7 (1.1%)	25.8 (9.6–48.6)	<0.001
Troponin I	171	32 (19%)	602	2 (0.3%)	61.4 (14.9–511.7)	<0.001
Creatine kinase-MB	86	12 (14%)	687	N/A	3.5 (1.4–8.9)	0.008
ST depression	158	14 (8.9%)	615	N/A	2.9 (1.47–5.9)	0.003

CI = confidence interval; N/A = not available.
Source: Modified from Ref. 28.

been shown to be associated with complex plaques and the presence of visible thrombus at angiography (31,32), and hence may signify plaque instability and platelet embolism downstream from the culprit lesion, causing further minor myocyte necrosis (33). Antithrombotic treatments (e.g., platelet glycoprotein IIb/IIIa inhibitors and low molecular weight heparins) (34) and early revascularization have been shown to be more beneficial in patients with elevated troponin levels (Fig. 1) (4,16,34–36). It should be borne in mind, however, that ischemia resulting from plaque fissuring or rupture is not the only possible cause of myocardial necrosis. Furthermore, a normal troponin test result does not guarantee that the patient is at low risk because troponin elevations cannot be detected for least 6 hours after the onset of myocyte necrosis, and so patients presenting very early after symptom onset may initially not have elevated troponin levels. For this reason it is important that troponin tests are performed 6–8 hours after symptom onset.

A. Acute Risk Models for Non–ST-Elevation ACS

A number of acute risk models have been developed for patients presenting acutely with non–ST-elevation ACS. The Platelet IIb/IIIa in Unstable Angina Receptor Suppression Using

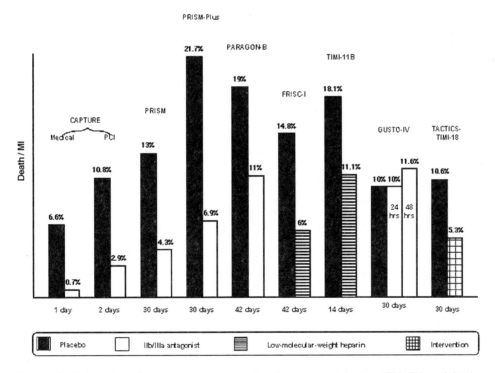

Figure 1 Interaction of elevated troponin levels with treatment in the c7E3 Fal-Antiplatelet Therapy in Unstable Refactory Anagina (CAPTURE) study of abciximab with PCI (22), the Platelat Receptor Inhibitor in Ischamic Syndrome Management (PRISM) (23) and PRISM-Plus (Patients Limited by Unstable Signs and Symptoms (24) studies of tirofiban, the Platelet IIb/IIIa Antagonism for the Reduction of Acute Coronary Syndrome Events in a Global Organization Network (PARAGON-B) trial of lamifiban (36), the Fragmin During Instability in Coronary Artery Disease (FRISC I) study of dalteparin (26), the TIMI 11B trial of enoxaparin (27), the GUSTO IV trial of abciximab (which was administered for 24 or 48 hours, as indicated) (17), and the Treat Angana With Aggrastat and Determine Cost of Therapy with an Invasive or Conservative Strategy (TACTICS)-TIMI-18 trial with intervention. (From Ref. 4)

Table 2 Factors Included in Risk Stratification Models for Patients with Non–ST-Elevation Acute Coronary Syndromes

Factor	PURSUIT	TIMI 11B	GUSTO IIB	GUSTO IV
Age	√	√	√	√
Cardiac markers	√	√	√	√
ST-segment deviation	√	√	√	√
Congestive heart failure	√		√	√
Previous coronary artery disease or MI	√	√	√	√
Risk factors	√	√	√	
Prior beta-blocker therapy	√			
Prior aspirin therapy	√	√		
Previous coronary artery bypass surgery	√	√	√	
Renal insufficiency			√	
Severe chronic obstructive pulmonary disease			√	

Source: Modified from Ref. 127.

Integrilin Therapy (PURSUIT) investigators developed a risk model including 33 variables identified as predictors of death/MI within 30 days (Table 2) (9). Most of the prognostic information is contained in seven variables: age, gender, Canadian Cardiovascular Society (CCS) angina class (37), heart rate, blood pressure, the presence of rales, and the presence of ST depression (Fig. 2). The model varies according to the presence or absence of MI on admission (Fig. 3) and gives separate risk scores for the endpoints of death or death/MI.

Using data from patients randomized to receive unfractionated heparin in the TIMI 11B trial (27), the TIMI investigators devised a simple risk score incorporating variables predictive of death/MI/severe ischemia requiring revascularization within 14 days (Table 3) (13). This

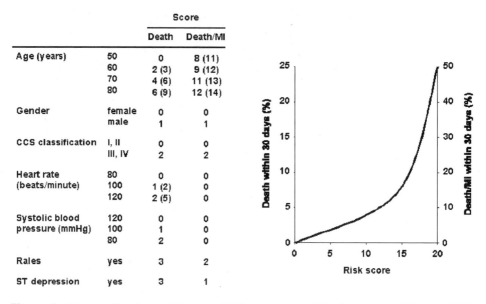

Figure 2 Risk stratification model for the 30-day endpoints of death and death/MI in the PURSUIT trial. Points were given for each predictive factor. With respect to age and heart rate, separate points were given for the enrollment diagnoses of unstable angina and MI (indicated in parentheses). CCS = Canadian Cardiovascular Society. (Modified from Ref. 9.)

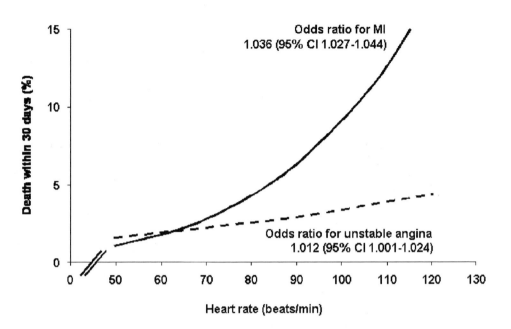

Figure 3 Univariate association between heart rates and 30-day mortality in patients with MI or unstable angina in the PURSUIT trial. (Modified from Ref. 9.)

user-friendly score includes seven baseline characteristics—some of which differ from those in the PURSUIT risk model (Table 2)—and can be easily calculated at the patient's bedside. However, some variables identified as being important prognosticators in other studies are not included in the TIMI risk score. For example, heart rate, blood pressure, and presence of heart failure are not included as risk factors, perhaps because patients considered to require revascularization were excluded from enrollment and so few patients with heart failure were enrolled in the TIMI 11B trial (38), which consequently included few patients with heart failure. Cardiac markers such as creatine kinase or creatine kinase-MB levels are included in the TIMI risk score, but troponin levels are not specifically included because troponin testing was not routinely performed in TIMI 11B.

The TIMI risk score has been validated in a number of populations including patients randomized to receive enoxaparin in the TIMI 11B trial (27), patients randomized to receive either unfractionated heparin or enoxaparin in the Efficacy and Safety of Subcutaneous Enoxaparin in Non–Q-Wave Coronary Events (ESSENCE) trial (39), and patients in the Platelet Receptor Inhibition in Ischemic Syndrome Management in Patients

Table 3 Baseline Characteristics Included in the TIMI Risk Score for Unstable Angina/Non–ST-Elevation ACS

Age ≥ 65 years
≥3 risk factors for coronary artery disease
Known coronary stenosis of ≥50%
ST-segment deviation
≥2 anginal events within previous 24 hours
Aspirin therapy within previous 7 days
Elevated cardiac markers

Source: Modified from Ref. 13.

Limited by Unstable Signs and Symptoms (PRISM-Plus) study (40), a placebo-controlled trial of the IIb/IIIa inhibitor, tirofiban, in patients receiving background aspirin and heparin therapy (24). The TIMI risk score has also been shown to maintain its predictive value in a registry of "real-world" patients with unstable angina and non–ST-elevation MI (41).

The TIMI risk score has also been used to predict the effectiveness of therapy. In the TIMI 11B and ESSENCE trials, the advantage of enoxaparin over unfractionated heparin increased in a graded fashion with higher TIMI risk scores (13). In the Treat Angina with Aggrastat and Determine Cost of Therapy with an Invasive or Conservative Strategy (TAC-TICS) TIMI 18 trial (4), invasive management was more beneficial than medical management in patients with higher TIMI risk scores. In the PRISM-Plus study, tirofiban was more effective in patients scoring ≥4 points than in those with lower TIMI risk scores (40).

The predictive value of a model is measured by its C-statistic (i.e., the area under the receiver-operator characteristic curve). In general, a C-statistic of >0.8 is generally considered useful and a C-statistic of <0.7 is considered limited. The TIMI 11B and PURSUIT risk models have good predictive value for death, with C-statistics of 0.74 (13) and 0.819, respectively, but have lower predictive value for death/MI, with C-statistics of 0.63 and 0.67, respectively.

B. Diabetes

Diabetes is an independent risk factor for 30-day mortality in patients with non–ST-elevation ACS (4,24,42) This higher mortality risk may be due to a greater degree of platelet activation in diabetics (43–46). In a meta-analysis of six large-scale IIb/IIIa inhibitor trials involving a total of 6458 diabetic patients (22% of the total cohort), diabetes was associated with a twofold increase in 30-day mortality (adjusted odds ratio 2.05; $p < 0.0001$). The use of IIb/IIIa inhibitors was associated with a significant 30-day mortality reduction from 6.2%

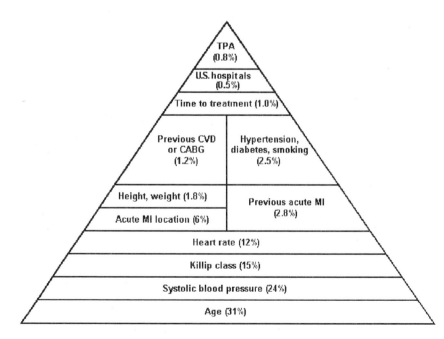

Figure 4   Influence of clinical characteristics on 30-day mortality after MI in patients treated with fibrinolytic agents in the GUSTO I trial. The numbers in brackets represent the percentage of the total 30-day mortality risk associated with that particular characteristic CABG = artary bypass surgery; CVD = cardiovascular disease; TPA = tissue plasminogen activator (alteplasa). (Adapted from Ref. 47)

to 4.6% ($p = 0.007$) in diabetic patients (42). In the TACTICS TIMI 18 trial (4), invasive treatment was found to reduce the relative risk of death/MI/rehospitalization with ACS by 27% (from 27.7% to 16.4%) in diabetic patients, who made up 28% of the trial population.

IV. ACUTE RISK ASSESSMENT IN ST-ELEVATION ACS

The major risk factors in patients presenting with ST-elevation ACS are traditionally considered to be age, systolic blood pressure, pulse rate, and Killip class. In the GUSTO I database of 41,021 patients randomized to one of four fibrinolytic regimes, a regression model was developed to illustrate the relative influence of clinical characteristics on 30-day mortality (47). The resulting mortality pyramid (Fig. 4) shows that the traditional baseline risk factors (age, blood pressure, heart rate, Killip class) had a greater combined influence on the outcome than modifiable or semi-modifiable factors such as the fibrinolytic agent used and the time to treatment.

The GUSTO risk score is computed by summing points for the Killip class (stratified according to age because age and Killip class interacted in the mortality model), heart rate, systolic blood pressure, prior MI, and infarct location (Fig. 5) (48). From this score, the likelihood of mortality with streptokinase or alteplase treatment can be estimated.

1. Find points for each marker

Killip class	I	II	III	IV	Heart rate		Systolic BP	Points
Age	Points	Points	Points	Points	Beats/minute	Points	40	34
30	19	35	48	53	0	12	60	25
40	28	42	53	59	10	10	80	17
50	38	49	59	65	20	7	100	8
60	47	56	64	70	30	5	120+	0
70	57	63	70	76	40	2		
80	66	70	75	82	50	0		
90	75	77	81	88	70	4	Prior MI	Points
100	85	84	86	94	90	8	Yes	5
110	94	91	92	100	110	13	No	0
					130	17		
					150	21		
					170	25	MI location	Points
					190	30	Anterior	6
					210	34	Inferior	0
					230	38	Other	3

2. Sum points for all risk factors

Age/Killip class _____
Heart rate _____
Systolic BP _____
Prior MI _____
MI location _____
Points total _____

3. Look up risk corresponding to points total

Points	SK mortality	TPA mortality	TPA mortality reduction
20	0.1%	0.1%	-
30	0.4%	0.4%	-
40	0.8%	0.8%	0.01%
50	1.7%	1.4%	0.3%
60	3.5%	2.8%	0.8%
70	10%	8.3%	1.7%
80	20%	17%	3%
90	40%	35%	5%

Figure 5 Nomogram to determine the estimated 30-day mortality risk with streptokinase (SK) treatment in patients with given characteristics and the absolute mortality reduction that would result from substitution of accelerated alteplase treatment. The point scores for each variable (1) are added to produce an overall points total (2), which corresponds to the mortality risk at the bottom of the figure (3). Note: because age interacts with Killip class, the age score that corresponds to the patient's Killip class should be used. BP = blood pressure. (Modified from Ref. 48.)

A TIMI risk score for 30-day mortality in patients with ST-elevation ACS has recently been developed using data from patients in the Intravenous NPA for the Treatment of Infarcting Myocardium Early (InTIME II) trial, which randomised patients to receive either alteplase or lanoteplase (Fig. 6) (49). Unlike the GUSTO risk score, the TIMI risk score rates each variable in a dichotomous fashion (e.g., heart rate > 100 or ≤ 100 beats/min, systolic pressure > 100 or ≤ 100 mmHg) with heavy weighting for age, blood pressure, pulse, and Killip class. Patients with the minimum score of 0 have a 0.8% risk of death, while those with the maximum score of >8 have a 35.9% risk of death. This risk score has been validated externally using patient data derived from the TIMI 9 trial, which randomized patients to receive either unfractionated heparin or hirudin as adjunctive therapy with either alteplase or streptokinase.

When applied to the InTIME II dataset, the TIMI risk score had a C-statistic of 0.779 for 30-day mortality, and the GUSTO risk score had a C-statistic of 0.803. From the InTIME II dataset, a risk index was developed to predict 30-day mortality using the three key parameters of age, heart rate, and systolic blood pressure as continuous variables in the equation: (heart rate × $[age/10]^2$)/systolic blood pressure (50). This algorithm has been shown to have C-statistics of 0.81 for 24-hour mortality and 0.78 for 30-day mortality, and has been validated externally in the TIMI 9 database. Unlike the simple dichotomous classification of variables in the TIMI risk score, the algorithm maximizes the information obtained from the three key baseline parameters.

A. Predictive Value of ECG Parameters in ST-Elevation ACS

The baseline ECG provides measures of potential infarct size and outcome. The European Cooperative Study Group observed that patients with a large ST-segment shift (i.e., initial ST elevation and reciprocal ST depression) on their baseline ECG had larger

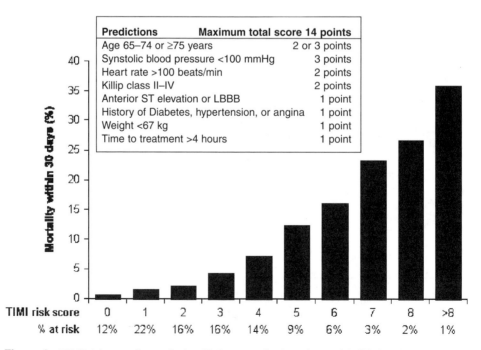

Predictions	Maximum total score 14 points
Age 65–74 or ≥75 years	2 or 3 points
Synstolic blood pressure <100 mmHg	3 points
Heart rate >100 beats/min	2 points
Killip class II–IV	2 points
Anterior ST elevation or LBBB	1 point
History of Diabetes, hypertension, or angina	1 point
Weight <67 kg	1 point
Time to treatment >4 hours	1 point

TIMI risk score	0	1	2	3	4	5	6	7	8	>8
% at risk	12%	22%	16%	16%	14%	9%	6%	3%	2%	1%

Figure 6 TIMI risk score for predicting 30-day mortality in patients with ST-elevation acute coronary syndromes. LBBB = left brundle branch block (Modified from Ref. 49.)

infarcts and a higher mortality rate, and that these patients benefited more than most from alteplase (51). In the Gruppo Italiano per lo Studio della Streptochinasi nell'Infarto Miocardico (GISSI-1) study, streptokinase was most beneficial in patients with ST elevation in multiple ECG leads (52). The addition of baseline ECG features to demographic and hemodynamic factors has been shown to improve risk assessment. After excluding ECGs that showed left bundle branch block or ventricular/paced rhythms, the GUSTO I investigators used their remaining dataset of 34,166 ECGs to identify independent ECG predictors of 30-day mortality (53). These predictors included a prolonged QRS duration, a large summed absolute ST-segment deviation, evidence of prior MI, and current anterior MI. The addition of these factors to the risk model improved its C-statistic to 0.83 (Table 4).

Right-sided ST elevation is the major diagnostic criterion for right ventricular MI. In a recent meta-analysis totaling almost 4000 patients, right ventricular MI occurred in nearly half of the patients with inferior wall MI, and these patients had triple the rates of early mortality, cardiogenic shock, ventricular tachyarrhythmia, and advanced heart block when compared with patients who had only inferior AMI without right ventricular involvement (54). The association between right ventricular MI and early mortality has been shown to be independent of the left ventricular ejection fraction (54–56).

Table 4 Independent Multivariate ECG and Clinical Predictors of 30-Day Mortality in the GUSTO I Trial

Predictors[a]	χ^2 test[b]	Degrees of freedom	p value
Age	540	1	<0.001
Systolic blood pressure	292	1	<0.001
Killip class	189	3	<0.001
Sum of absolute ST-segment deviation	*64*	*2*	*<0.001*
Pulse	60	2	<0.001
QRS duration	*58*	*2*	*<0.001*
Previous MI on admission ECG	*31*	*2*	*<0.001*
Previous coronary artery bypass surgery	28	1	<0.001
History of diabetes	27	1	<0.001
Height	23	1	<0.001
Acute anterior MI on ECG	*21*	*2*	*<0.001*
QRS duration × acute anterior MI	*21*	*1*	*<0.001*
Sum of ST-segment depression	*17*	*1*	*<0.001*
Acute inferior MI on ECG	*16*	*2*	*<0.001*
Previous MI × acute inferior MI	*16*	*1*	*<0.001*
History of hypertension	16	1	<0.001
Current smoking	14	1	<0.001
History of cerebrovascular disease	14	1	<0.001
Sum of inferior ST-segment elevation[c]	*14*	*1*	*<0.001*
Time to treatment	12	1	<0.001
Accelerated alteplase therapy	11	3	0.001
ECG heart rate	*8*	*1*	*<0.005*
Previous smoking	7	1	0.007
Weight	7	1	0.01

[a]ECG variables are shown in italics and were derived from the admission ECG.
[b]Wald χ^2 values with corresponding p values represent the statistical significance of each factor after adjustment for all others.
[c]ST-segment elevation includes leads II, III, and aVF.
Source: From Ref. 53.

The TIMI risk score, with its dichotomous categorization of pulse rate and systolic blood pressure, may fail to stratify risk in patients with right ventricular MI, as they typically have low systolic blood pressure and reflex tachycardia due to acute right ventricular dilatation, which bulges the septum towards the left ventricle and restricts diastolic filling (57). Further studies are required to assess the value of right-sided ECG readings in order to establish whether risk scores should incorporate points for right-sided ECG changes.

B. Predictive Value of Early Angiography in ST-Elevation ACS

Angiography provides a direct assessment of "angiographic" epicardial coronary disease in both culprit and nonculprit arteries, and is required when planning revascularization. Some angiographic findings have a major impact on treatment decisions (e.g., a finding of severe left main coronary artery disease), but there is little information available regarding the value of angiographic findings in risk assessment. The presence of visible thrombus on angiography has been shown to denote higher risk in patients with non–ST-elevation ACS (58), but there are few data in patients with ST-elevation ACS to indicate how angiographic findings before and after primary PCI should be integrated into risk assessment algorithms. In the four Primary Angioplasty in Myocardial Infarction (PAMI) trials, the presence of TIMI grade 3 (i.e., normal) coronary artery flow (59) prior to PCI was associated with a higher 6-month survival rate ($p = 0.04$, Fig. 7) (60). Successful PCI has been shown to be associated with better patient outcomes than unsuccessful PCI, and institutions performing high volumes of procedures tend to produce better patient outcomes (61). In additional to quantitation of epicardial infarct artery flow by TIMI flow grading or corrected TIMI frame counting, assessment of the myocardial blush grade has been shown to be an independent predictor of survival after primary PCI (62).

Multifocal plaque instability involving both the infarct artery and non–infarct-related coronary arteries can occur in patients with ST-elevation ACS and is detectable at angiog-

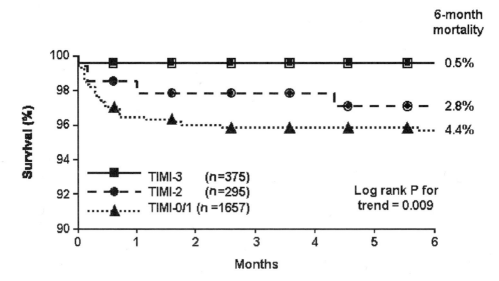

Figure 7 Six-month mortality rates according to TIMI flow grades prior to PCI in the PAMI trials. The presence of TIMI grade 3 flow prior to PCI was an independent predictor of survival ($p = 0.04$). (Modified from Ref. 60.)

raphy (63). A three-vessel intravascular ultrasound study performed in 24 patients with ACS (9 with and 15 without ST elevation) found multiple atherosclerotic plaque ruptures in addition to the culprit lesion in 19 patients (79%) (64). Whether or not patients with multiple plaque ruptures fare worse remains to be determined in future studies.

C. Prediction of Early Mortality Risk in ST-Elevation ACS

The mortality rate from ST-elevation ACS is typically high in the first 24–48 hours. In the Fibrinolytic Therapy Trialists' (FTT) overview, 4.0% of patients receiving fibrinolytics died on days 0–1 and 5.9% died during days 2–35 (65). In GUSTO I, 40% of deaths occurred in the first 24 hours, and most were from left ventricular pump failure. High early mortality rates were also noted in the recent GUSTO V (66) and Hirulog and Early Reperfusion or Occlusion (HERO)-2 trials. The GUSTO I trial showed that sinus tachycardia (>100 beats/min) and hypotension (<100 mmHg) were the most potent predictors of early mortality (3). The InTIME II risk index, (heart rate × $[age/10]^2$)/systolic blood pressure, is also highly predictive of 24-hour mortality (50).

Left ventricular dysfunction usually occurs early in patients with ST-elevation ACS and is due either to myocyte necrosis or to myocardial stunning, which may recover with time. Cardiogenic shock is common within the first 24 hours, occurring in 74% of patients in the Should We Emergently Revascularize Occluded Coronaries for Cardiogenic Shock (SHOCK) trial registry (68). About 5% of patients in the registry had nonhypotensive shock (i.e., peripheral hypoperfusion in conjunction with a systolic blood pressure of >90 mmHg), and these patients had a 43% in-hospital mortality rate (69). Thus the occurrence of peripheral vasconstriction with cold, clammy extremities is a bad sign even when the systolic blood pressure is maintained. These features are not included in any risk assessment algorithm.

V. ONGOING RISK ASSESSMENT

Patients presenting initially with a non–ST-elevation ACS can subsequently develop an ST-elevation ACS. Similarly, some patients with ST-elevation ACS develop postinfarction angina with a non–ST-elevation ACS. Although patients presenting with ACS are classified primarily according to the presence or absence of ST elevation, the two categories do partly overlap. It is important that the risk assessment process is continued right through until discharge, as the patient's risk may change over time depending on whether complications of MI or continuing ischemia occur.

A. The First 24–48 Hours

1. Serial ECG Changes in Non–ST-Elevation ACS

The presence of ST changes on continuous monitoring signifies an increased risk of death/MI (70), as does rebound ischemia occurring after the cessation of unfractionated heparin (71). In the Fast Assessment of Thoracic Pain (FAST) study, the presence of transient ST elevation or depression of ≥1mm was a predictor of death/MI within 30 days (72).

The presence of dynamic ST depression on a resting ECG has been shown to be an important risk marker (73). In a meta-analysis of continuous monitoring data obtained in the c7E3 Fab Antiplatelet Therapy in Unstable Refractory Angina (CAPTURE) trial (74), the PURSUIT trial (75), and the Fibrinogen Receptor Occupancy (FROST) trial (76), the

30-day rates of death/MI were 5.7% in patients with no ischemic events, 9.5% in those with 1–2 events, 12.7% in those with 3–5 events, and 19.7% in those with ≥5 events (77).

Other important risk factors include prolonged or accelerating angina (78,79), marked T-wave inversion (79), hemodynamic instability (79), major arrhythmias (79), previous coronary artery bypass surgery (79), postinfarction angina (79), and the presence of visible coronary artery thrombus at angiography (58).

2. Serial ECG Changes in ST-Elevation ACS

An important part of risk assessment is the evaluation of myocyte reperfusion by analysis of ST-segment resolution after fibrinolysis or PCI. Studies in patients treated with fibrinolysis have reported correlations between ST resolution and infarct artery patency (80), ventricular wall motion (81) and survival (82–91).

ST resolution of >25% within 3 hours in the lead showing the greatest magnitude of ST elevation has been shown to predict both coronary artery patency and improvement in left ventricular function (92). Resolution of the sum of ST elevation in all ECG leads within 1 hour has been shown to correlate with patency of the infarct artery at 72 hours, smaller infarcts (as indicated by cardiac enzyme testing), better left ventricular function, and lower mortality (82). Investigators from the Gruppo Italiano per lo Studio della Sopravvivenza nell'Infarto Miocardico (GISSI-2) study (83) showed that the greater the magnitude of ST resolution at 4 hours, the better the outcome. Dissmann et al. proposed three categories for resolution of ST elevation (<30%, 30–70%, >70%) and demonstrated an association between increasing ST resolution, smaller infarct size, and better ventricular function at follow-up (93). Schröder verified these cut-points in the Intravenous Streptokinase in Acute Myocardial Infarction (ISAM) trial (84), and prospectively confirmed the value of the magnitude of ST resolution at 180 minutes in predicting outcomes at 35 days in the International Joint Efficacy Comparison of Thrombolytics (INJECT) trial (85). In the Hirudin for the Improvement of Thrombolysis (HIT) 4 trial, which used streptokinase as the fibrinolytic agent, >70% ST resolution was observed in 25% of patients by 90 minutes and in 50% of patients by 180 minutes, and the presence of ST resolution at either time point predicted a low risk of mortality (86,87).

The speed of ST resolution depends on the efficacy of the fibrinolytic agent being used. In the GUSTO III trial, which compared reteplase with alteplase, complete ST resolution was observed in 44.2% of patients by 90 minutes and in 56.5% by 180 minutes (88), and the presence of ST resolution at either time point predicted a low risk of 30-day mortality. The InTIME II investigators recently found that 33% of patients treated with alteplase or lanoteplase achieved ST resolution within 60 minutes and that these patients had a low 30-day mortality rate of 1.7% (94).

Failure of ST resolution in the presence of a patent infarct artery is thought to be due to impairment of myocyte reperfusion by microvascular dysfunction. The presence of ST resolution in patients with an early creatine kinase peak after fibrinolytic therapy has been used to distinguish between those with and those without myocardial perfusion (95). A small angiographic trial by the TIMI investigators found that complete ST resolution predicted infarct artery patency, but that failed ST resolution did not necessarily predict vessel occlusion (96). In the HERO-1 trial, the presence of a patent infarct artery at 90 minutes and earlier ST resolution on continuous monitoring each predicted greater preservation of wall motion in the infarct zone (81). In 258 patients from the Thrombolysis and Angioplasty in Myocardial Infarction (TAMI) 7 and GUSTO I trials, ST resolution was found to be the only independent predictor of the combined endpoint of in-hospital mortality and congestive heart failure (89).

Primary PCI studies have provided further insights. In the Zwolle trial, the 15% of patients with no ST resolution at 1 hour after successful PCI had a 8.7-fold risk of death (95% CI 3.7–20.1), and the 34% of patients with partial ST resolution had a 3.6-fold risk of death (95% CI 1.6–8.3) compared with the remaining 51% of patients who had complete ST resolution (90). In another study of patients with successful PCI, those who did not achieve ST resolution had lower ejection fractions and higher rates of heart failure and short- and long-term mortality than those who did achieve ST resolution (91). Taken together, these findings illustrate that early ST resolution can be considered a marker of myocyte reperfusion.

ST-segment analysis after the first 24–36 hours may be a better indicator of the overall success of reperfusion. The Assessment of the Safety and Efficacy of a New Thrombolytic Agent (ASSENT)-2 investigators reported that the presence of ST resolution at 24–36 hours after fibrinolysis was a predictor of survival at 1 year (Fig. 8) (97). It should be noted that 23% of patients did not undergo ST-segment monitoring, and these patients had a higher mortality rate than those who were monitored. Further studies are needed to evaluate the prognostic significance and utility of ST resolution measured at this later timepoint.

B. After 24–48 Hours

1. Non–ST-Elevation ACS

When patients with non–ST-elevation ACS have been relatively free of ischemia for 24–48 hours, they should be assessed for inducible ischemia if an early invasive strategy is not part of the overall management plan (4–6). If the exercise test is negative for ischemia, the likelihood of 5-year survival is 95% (98), whereas the occurrence of ischemia at < 6 mets is associated with a poor prognosis (98,99). Predischarge exercise testing has been shown to add to the prognostic information obtained from troponin testing (5). In the Fragmin During Instability in Coronary Artery Disease (FRISC I) study, patients with a troponin T level of < 0.06 mg/L and a low-risk exercise test result had a 1% risk of death/MI within

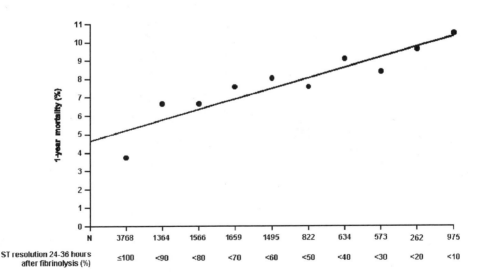

Figure 8 ST resolution at 24–36 hours after fibrinolysis, partitioned into 10% intervals, and its relation to 1-year mortality ($r = -0.963$; $p < 0.001$) in the ASSENT-2 trial. (Modified from Ref. 97.)

5 months, whereas the risk in those with a troponin T level of > 0.2 mg/L and a positive exercise test was 34% (Fig. 9) (15).

2. ST-Elevation ACS

Postinfarction Angina or Recurrent Ischemia. Postinfarction ischemia has been shown in several studies to be a major risk factor for death and MI (7,100). Recurrent ischemia was diagnosed in 23% of the 4125 patients who had ST-elevation ACS in the GUSTO IIB trial (7), and 22% of these cases were considered refractory to medical therapy (defined as having ischemic symptoms associated with ECG changes persisting for > 10 minutes despite the use of nitrates and either beta-blockers or calcium-channel antagonists). The 30-day reinfarction rates were 2.7% in patients without recurrent ischemia, 10.7% in those with nonrefractory ischemia, and 28.0% in those with refractory ischemia. The 30-day mortality rates were 5.4%, 7.2%, and 11.8%, respectively.

In the Danish Trial in Acute Myocardial Infarction (DANAMI) trial (100), 1008 patients who had spontaneous angina >36 hours after ST-elevation MI or who experienced angina or silent ST changes during their predischarge exercise stress test were randomized to undergo either conservative treatment or invasive treatment 2–10 weeks after MI. After 2.4 years of follow-up there was no significant reduction in mortality (3.6% with invasive treatment vs 4.4% with conservative treatment; p = NS), but invasive treatment was associated with lower rates of reinfarction (5.6% vs 10.5%; p = 0.0038) and admission for recurrent unstable angina (17.9% vs. 29.5%; p <0.00001) Fig. 10).

Left Ventricular Function. Contrast left ventriculography performed 4–8 weeks after acute MI showed that the presence of a low left ventricular ejection fraction or larger end-systolic volume had prognostic significance, with end-systolic volume being the most important prognostic factor (101). A recent study of over 1000 patients compared the rel-

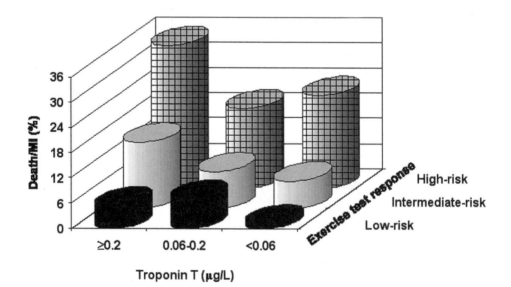

Figure 9 Five-month risk of cardiac death/MI according to exercise test response and maximal troponin T levels during the first 24 hours after MI in the FRISC I study. With respect to the exercise test response: high-risk = both low maximal workload (<90 W for men and <70 W for women) and presence of ≥1 mm of ST depression in 3 or more ECG leads; intermediate risk = either low workload or ST depression present; low risk = both absent. (Modified from Ref. 15.)

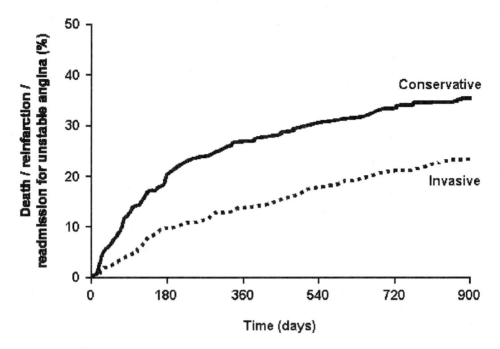

Figure 10 Risk of first occurrence of the combined primary endpoint of death/reinfarction/admission for unstable angina pectoris in the DANAMI trial. (Modified from Ref. 100.)

ative prognostic values of the left ventricular ejection fraction, end-systolic volume, and infarct size as assessed by radionuclide imaging 1–2 weeks after ST-elevation MI treated with fibrinolysis (102). While each of these parameters was a predictor of 6-month mortality, on univariate analysis, the ejection fraction was the only independent predictor on multivariate analysis.

Infarct Artery Patency. A patent infarct artery not only salvages cardiac myocytes, but is also associated with less ventricular dilatation and improved electrical stability and provides the capacity to supply collateral circulation to another infarct zone in the event of subsequent reinfarction (103). A 3-year follow-up study of patients treated with fibrinolysis showed that in those with an ejection fraction of ≥50%, infarct artery patency was a predictor of survival only if the occluded artery supplied >25% of the left ventricle, whereas in those with an ejection fraction of <50%, infarct artery patency predicted survival even if the occluded artery supplied <25% of the left ventricle (104). In a 2-year follow-up study of the 2431 patients who underwent early angiography in the GUSTO I trial, those who had early TIMI grade 3 flow and a preserved ejection fraction had an incremental survival advantage after the first 30 days (105). In another 10-year follow-up study, the degree of infarct artery patency 3 weeks after MI (measured either by TIMI flow grading or by corrected TIMI frame counting) independently predicted 5- but not 10-year survival (106).

Ventricular Arrhythmias. In a 1-year follow-up study of 3178 patients recruited into the Canadian Assessment of Myocardial Infarction (CAMI) study in the early 1990s, 9.9% of patients died in hospital and 7.1% died within 1 year. Only 1.9% of patients died from a presumed arrhythmic caused (107). Risk factors for ventricular arrhythmia include severe left ventricular dysfunction, recurrent ischemia, a positive electrophysiological ventricular extra-stimulation test, frequent ventricular ectopic beats, presence of late potential, and reduced heart rate variability. Despite intensive efforts over the decades, no pharmacological antiarrhythmic therapies have been found to improve the outcome of patients at high risk of arrhythmias after ST-elevation ACS. In contrast, implantation of artificial defibrillators is an established therapy (108) that improves survival rates in patients with impaired left ventricular function after acute MI. Effectively, this makes routine screening for arrhythmias less relevant.

VI. RISK ASSESSMENT ALGORITHMS FROM REGISTRIES

There are several reasons why cardiovascular risk algorithms derived from clinical trial populations may differ from those derived from patients treated in routine clinical practice. First, elderly patients and those with comorbidities are often underrepresented in clinical trial populations. In addition, patients treated in trials may receive different treatments than patients treated routinely, such as different reperfusion strategies, higher rates of revascularization procedures and higher usage rates of other evidence-based therapies.

In 103,164 patients (mean age 76.8 years) with MI in the Cooperative Cardiovascular Project (CCP) database, the following eight factors were found to have the strongest association with 1-year mortality: older age, urinary incontinence, assisted mobility, heart failure or cardiomegaly, peripheral vascular disease, body mass index of <20 kg/m^2, renal dysfunction, and ejection fraction of <40%.

The Predicting Risk of Death in Cardiac Disease Tool (PREDICT) risk score is based on information routinely collected for the Minnesota Heart Survey from admissions to community hospitals in 1985 and 1990 (21). The score takes into account cardiac parameters, comorbidities and renal function, and was validated in a 6.3-year follow-up study of 717 patients admitted with non–ST-elevation MI to Olmsted County hospitals between 1993 and 1994. The discriminatory accuracy of the community PREDICT risk score was found to be consistently superior to that of the TIMI risk score for patients with non–ST-elevation ACS. However, the difference between the two scores' C-statistics was narrowed when measurement of comorbidities was added to the TIMI risk score (1).

Variations in clinical management may influence the accuracy of risk scores derived from trials using specific protocols. In a study of 84,039 patients with ST-elevation MI listed in the National Registry of Myocardial Infarction (NRMI)-3 between the years 1998 and 2000 (48% of whom received reperfusion therapy), the TIMI risk score was a good predictor of in-hospital mortality in patients reperfused by fibrinolysis ($n = 23,960$, C-statistic 0.79) or by primary PCI ($n = 15,348$, C-statistic 0.80). However, in those not receiving any reperfusion therapy, a TIMI risk score in the low or middle ranges consistently underestimated the mortality risk, with an overall C-statistic of only 0.65 (109). Risk estimates in these patients were enhanced by inclusion of the bleeding risk, uncertainty regarding the diagnosis of MI, major organ failure, and chronic renal insufficiency as variables in the model (109).

Registry-derived risk scores may better predict risk by including broader groups of older patients with comorbidities. However, many of these risk factors are nonmodifiable and extraneous to the pathophysiology of ACS. Treatments for ACS would not be expected to have a greater effect in patients whose higher-risk status is due to extraneous factors, whereas risk factors that are related to the pathophysiology of ACS (such as elevated troponin levels) may predict the likelihood of benefit from antithrombotic (16) or revascularization therapies (4).

VII. VARIATIONS IN MEDICAL PRACTICE IN DIFFERENT COMMUNITIES

The InTIME II investigators evaluated the association between availability of on-site catheterization and clinical outcomes in a study of 15,078 patients treated in 855 hospitals in 35 countries. On-site catheterization facilities were available 24 hours a day in 31% of hospitals, during the daytime only in 25% of hospitals, and not at all in 44% of hospitals. Although the usage of procedures varied considerably according to the availability of on-site catheterization facilities (cardiac angiography being performed in 57%, 38%, and 26% of hospitals, respectively, and revascularization procedures being performed in 37%, 21%, and 17%, respectively), the 1-year mortality rates did not vary (Fig. 11) (110). The duration of hospitalization and the risk of ischemic events might be reduced if *all* patients (not just those experiencing recurrent symptoms) were to undergo routine angiography 24 hours after fibrinolysis with PCI provided their anatomy was suitable (111). While it is possible that longer-term follow-up studies will reveal longer-term benefits from the use of revascularization procedures during the index hospitalization, the data available to date do not suggest that more routine use of angiography would reduce mortality rates.

VIII. ASSESSMENT OF LONG-TERM RISK

The GISSI-Prevenzione investigators recently devised a risk algorithm from their widely inclusive trial conducted in the mid-1990s, which included 11,324 patients enrolled within 3 months after acute MI (50% of whom were recruited within 16 days) and followed-up for 4 years (112). The dataset represented a low-risk patient group with a 4-year mortality rate of 9.5%. The average age was 59 years, and 16% of patients were over the age of 70. Only

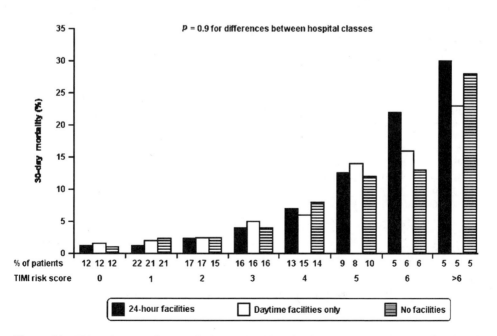

Figure 11 Thirty-day mortality rates in the InTIME II study, shown according to the availability of on-site catheterization facilities and stratified by the TIMI risk score. (Modified from Ref. 110.)

15% of patients were women, and only 12% had an ejection fraction of <40%. A mortality model was generated, which incorporated different categories of risk factors such as age and gender; postinfarction complications including residual ischemia (present in ~50%), electrical instability (~24%) and left ventricular dysfunction (~21%); and cardiovascular risk factors including current smoking (13%), diabetes (15%), history of hypertension (36%) and history of claudication (4%). Other variables including blood pressure, lipid levels, fibrinogen levels and white blood cell count were also monitored during the trial period. The rate of revascularization procedures over the 4-year study period was low (19%).

In this study (112), age was found to be the most powerful prognostic factor. While women were at lower risk than men up to the age of 60, they were at higher risk after that age. Diabetes and a history of claudication were important prognostic factors. While total cholesterol and triglyceride levels were not prognostic factors, a low high-density lipoprotein (HDL) cholesterol level was an independent positive predictor of mortality. In this population, residual ischemia was a prognostic factor but was much less important than left ventricular dysfunction.

The GISSI-Prevenzione risk algorithm may not be applicable to other higher-risk populations or to populations with higher rates of revascularization, but it represents one of the few attempts to integrate multiple risk factors that are present after acute MI into a risk model. The Long-Term Intervention with Pravastatin in Ischemic Disease (LIPID) study investigators constructed a risk model using data from 8557 patients who were enrolled in the LIPID study 3–36 months after MI or unstable angina and followed up for 6 years (Table 5). The summed risk points predicted the combined 5-year risk of cardiac death and nonfatal MI (113).

IX. NEWER CARDIAC MARKERS

A number of new markers may soon be included in risk models (Table 6). High-sensitivity C-reactive protein (CRP) is the most likely of these to enter routine clinical practice. CRP is an inflammatory marker that correlates with long-term risk, both in patients with no known heart disease (114,115) and in those with non–ST-elevation ACS (116). Inflammation has been shown to play an important role in the pathophysiology of

Table 5 Factors Included in the LIPID Risk Score

	Score
Total cholesterol level ≥ 5.5 mmol/L	1
HDL cholesterol level ≤ 1.0 mmol/L	2
Age 60–64 years	1
Age 65–69 years	2
Age ≥ 70 years	3
Male sex	2
Current smoking	3
Single previous MI	1
Multiple previous MIs	6
Revascularization since the acute coronary event qualifying for trial entry	4
Previous stroke	3
Diabetes	3
History of hypertension	1

Source: Modified from Ref. 113.

Table 6   Future Candidate Markers of Coronary Risk

Markers of endothelial injury	Markers of inflammation
Human neutrophil elastase	Antibodies to heat shock protein
Inducible nitric oxide synthase	CRP
Matrix metalloproteinases	Endothelial selectin
Thrombomodulin	Infectious agents
Markers of hemostasis	Intracellular adhesion molecule-1
Anti-IIa	Interleukin-6
Anti-Xa	Neopterin
D-dimer	Oxidized low-density lipoprotein
Fibrinogen	Platelet selectin
Fibrinopeptide-A	Serum amyloid-A
Platelet-derived growth factor	Tumor necrosis factor α
Thromboglobulin	Vascular cell adhesion molecule-1
Tissue factor	CD40 ligand
von Willebrand factor	Markers of necrosis
Markers of platelet activation	Creatine kinase-MB and its isoforms
Glycoprotein IIb/IIIb receptor occupancy	Fatty acid binding proteins
Monocyte-platelet conjugates	Myoglobin
PAC-1	Troponin I
P-selectin	Troponin T
Soluble fibrinogen binding	Markers of hemodynamic stress
	B-type natriuretic peptide

Source: Modified from Ref. 127.

atherosclerosis (117), and it is possible that CRP itself may promote plaque rupture, the proximate cause of ACS (see Chapter 7-1) (118). Various treatments such as aspirin (115), statins (119), and revascularization (4) have been shown to be more effective in patients with elevated CRP levels. When myocardial necrosis has occurred, elevated CRP levels may be due more to inflammation from necrosis of cardiac myocytes than to inflammation associated with atherosclerosis.

The presence of elevated von Willebrand factor levels in the acute stage of non–ST-elevation ACS has been shown to predict adverse outcomes independently of CRP levels (120). It has also been shown that different antithrombotic regimens may have differing effects on the release of von Willebrand factor (121). B-type natriuretic peptide (BNP) levels become elevated when left ventricular afterload and left ventricular wall stress are increased (122). BNP levels have been shown to be elevated in patients with non–ST-elevation ACS even when there is no evidence of MI (123). Increasing BNP levels may therefore reflect the extent of left ventricular global ischemia.

Point-of-care testing is now available for a number of the new biomarkers. The use of multiple markers has been shown to increase the accuracy of risk assessment (Table 7) (124). The TIMI investigators have recently shown that troponins T and I, high-sensitivity CRP (Fig.12), and BNP each provide unique and complementary prognostic information (125,126). In the Orbofiban in Patients with Unstable Coronary Syndromes (OPUS) TIMI 16 trial (126), the mortality risk almost doubled for each additional biomarker that was elevated ($p = 0.01$). These findings were validated in a TACTICS TIMI 18 risk model adjusted for age, diabetes, previous MI, prior congestive heart failure and ST elevation, where the combined incidence of death/MI/heart failure within 6 months increased by 2.1 times in patients with one risk factor, 3.1 times in those with two risk factors, and 3.7 times in those with three risk factors (126).

Table 7 30-Day Mortality Rates in the CHECKMATE Study, According to Cardiac Marker
Test Results

Multimarker testing[a]			Single marker testing[b]		
Positive ($n = 149$)	Negative ($n = 641$)	p value	Positive ($n = 44$)	Negative ($n = 807$)	p value
3 (2.0%)	0	0.007	0	4 (0.5%)	1.000

CHECKMATE = Chest Pain Evaluation by Creatine Kinase-MB, Myoglobin, and Troponin I.
[a]Myoglobin, creatine kinase-MB, and troponin I.
[b]Creatine kinase-MB if available, otherwise troponin I or T.
Source: Modified from Ref. 124.

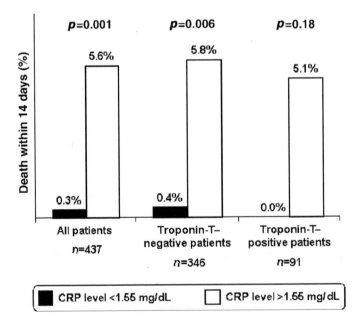

Figure 12 Mortality rate at 14 days according to CRP concentrations in all patients and in patients
with negative or positive troponin T tests in the TIMI 11A study. (Modified from Ref. 125.).

X. THE FUTURE

There is growing evidence from mega-trials and registry studies to support the adoption of risk assessment into routine clinical practice. Further work is required to compare the utility of the various risk models. The usage of evidence-based therapies has varied widely among different trials and registries. Future risk-assessment algorithms should be derived from populations receiving appropriate contemporary evidence-based treatments such as aspirin, clopidogrel, beta-blockers, angiotensin-converting-enzyme (ACE) inhibitors and/or angiotensin II antagonists, aldosterone antagonists, lipid-lowering agents, revascularization procedures, and lifestyle modification measures such as smoking cessation, weight management, and regular exercise.

Genomic testing is on the horizon as a tool to detect the likely benefit and risk of adverse events with any given therapy, and in the near future handheld computers may be used to individualize risk assessment and treatment selection.

REFERENCES

1. Singh M, Reeder GS, Jacobsen SJ, et al. Scores for post-myocardial infarction risk stratification in the community. Circulation 2002; 106:2309–2314.
2. Krumholz HM, Chen J, Chen YT, et al. Predicting one-year mortality among elderly survivors of hospitalization for an acute myocardial infarction: results from the Cooperative Cardiovascular Project. J Am Coll Cardiol 2001; 38:453–459.
3. Kleiman NS, White HD, Ohman EM, et al. Mortality within 24 hours of thrombolysis for myocardial infarction: the importance of early reperfusion. Circulation 1994; 90:2658–2665.
4. Cannon CP, Weintraub WS, Demopoulos LA, et al. Comparison of early invasive and conservative strategies in patients with unstable coronary syndromes treated with the glycoprotein IIb/IIIa inhibitor tirofiban. N Engl J Med 2001; 344:1879–1887.
5. Fragmin and Fast Revascularisation During Instability in Coronary Artery Disease (FRISC II) Investigators. Invasive compared with non-invasive treatment in unstable coronary-artery disease: FRISC II prospective randomised multicentre study. Lancet 1999; 354:708–715.
6. Fox K, Poole-Wilson P, Henderson R, et al. Interventional versus conservative treatment for patients with unstable angina or non-ST-elevation myocardial infarction: the British Heart Foundation RITA 3 randomised trial. Lancet 2002; 360:743–751.
7. Armstrong PW, Fu Y, Chang W-C, et al. Acute coronary syndromes in the GUSTO-IIb trial: prognostic insights and impact of recurrent ischemia. Circulation 1998; 98:1860–1868.
8. Savonitto S, Granger CB, Ardissino D, et al. The prognostic value of creatine kinase elevations extends across the whole spectrum of acute coronary syndromes. J Am Coll Cardiol 2002; 39:22–29.
9. Boersma E, Pieper KS, Steyerberg EW, et al. Predictors of outcome in patients with acute coronary syndromes without persistent ST-segment elevation: results from an international trial of 9461 patients. Circulation 2000; 101:2557–2567.
10. Cannon CP, Thompson B, McCabe CH, et al. Predictors of non-Q-wave acute myocardial infarction in patients with acute ischemic syndromes: an analysis from the Thrombolysis in Myocardial Ischemia (TIMI) III trials. Am J Cardiol 1995; 75:977–981.
11. Hyde TA, French JK, Wong CK, et al. Four-year survival of patients with acute coronary syndromes without ST-segment elevation and prognostic significance of 0.5–mm ST-segment depression. Am J Cardiol 1999; 84:379–385.
12. The Global Use of Strategies to Open Occluded Coronary Arteries (GUSTO) IIB Investigators. A comparison of recombinant hirudin with heparin for the treatment of acute coronary syndromes. N Engl J Med 1996; 335:775–782.

13. Antman EM, Cohen M, Bernink PJLM, et al. The TIMI risk score for unstable angina/non-ST elevation MI: a method for prognostication and therapeutic decision making. JAMA 2000; 284:835–482.

14. Hamm CW, Ravkilde J, Gerhardt W, et al. The prognostic value of serum troponin T in unstable angina. N Engl J Med 1992; 327:146–150.

15. Lindahl B, Andrén B, Ohlsson J, et al. Risk stratification in unstable coronary artery disease: additive value of troponin T determinations and pre-discharge exercise tests. Eur Heart J 1997; 18:762–770.

16. Heeschen C, Hamm CW, Goldmann B, et al. Troponin concentrations for stratification of patients with acute coronary syndromes in relation to therapeutic efficacy of tirofiban. Lancet 1999; 354:1757–1762.

17. The GUSTO IV-ACS Investigators. Effects of glycoprotein IIb/IIIa receptor blocker abciximab on outcome in patients with acute coronary syndromes without early coronary revascularisation: the GUSTO IV-ACS randomized trial. Lancet 2001; 357:1915–1924.

18. Bahit MC, Shah M, Granger C, et al. Prognostic significance of manifestations of acute congestive heart failure: results from GUSTO IIb [abstract]. J Am Coll Cardiol 2000; 35 (suppl A): 213A.

19. McGuire DK, Emanuelsson H, Granger CB, et al. Influence of diabetes mellitus on clinical outcomes across the spectrum of acute coronary syndromes: findings from the GUSTO-IIb study. Eur Heart J 2000; 21:1750–1758.

20. The Global Use of Strategies to Open Occluded Coronary Arteries (GUSTO) IIa Investigators. Randomized trial of intravenous heparin versus recombinant hirudin for acute coronary syndromes. Circulation 1994; 90:1631–1637.

21. Jacobs DR Jr, Kroenke C, Crow R, et al. PREDICT: a simple risk score for clinical severity and long-term prognosis after hospitalization for acute myocardial infarction or unstable angina: the Minnesota Heart Survey. Circulation 1999; 100:599–607.

22. The CAPTURE Investigators. Randomised placebo-controlled trial of abciximab before and during coronary intervention in refractory unstable angina: the CAPTURE study. Lancet 1997; 349:1429–1435.

23. The Platelet Receptor Inhibition in Ischemic Syndrome Management (PRISM) Study Investigators. A comparison of aspirin plus tirofiban with aspirin plus heparin for unstable angina. N Engl J Med 1998; 338:1498–1505.

24. The Platelet Receptor Inhibition in Ischemic Syndrome Management in Patients Limited by Unstable Signs and Symptoms (PRISM-Plus) Study Investigators. Inhibition of the platelet glycoprotein IIb/IIIa receptor with tirofiban in unstable angina and non-Q-wave myocardial infarction. N Engl J Med 1998; 338:1488–1497.

25. The Platelet IIb/IIIa Antagonist for the Reduction of Acute Coronary Syndrome Events in a Global Organization Network (PARAGON)-B Investigators. Randomized, placebo-controlled trial of titrated intravenous lamifiban for acute coronary syndromes. Circulation 2002; 105:316–321.

26. Fragmin During Instability in Coronary Artery Disease (FRISC) Study Group. Low-molecular-weight heparin during instability in coronary artery disease. Lancet 1996; 347:561–568.

27. Antman EM, McCabe CH, Gurfinkel EP, et al. Enoxaparin prevents death and cardiac ischemic events in unstable angina/non-Q-wave myocardial infarction: results of the Thrombolysis in Myocardial Infarction (TIMI) 11B trial. Circulation 1999; 100:1593–1601.

28. Hamm CW, Goldmann BU, Heeschen C, et al. Emergency room triage of patients with acute chest pain by means of rapid testing for cardiac troponin T or troponin I. N Engl J Med 1997; 337:1648–1653.

29. The TIMI IIIB Investigators. Effects of tissue plasminogen activator and a comparison of early invasive and conservative strategies in unstable angina and non-Q-wave myocardial infarction: results of the TIMI IIIB trial. Circulation 1994; 89:1545–1556.

30. Ottani F, Galvani M, Nicolini FA, et al. Elevated cardiac troponin levels predict the risk of adverse outcome in patients with acute coronary syndromes. Am Heart J 2000; 140:917–927.

31. Heeschen C, van den Brand MJ, Hamm CW, et al. Angiographic findings in patients with refractory unstable angina according to troponin T status. Circulation 1999; 104:1509–1514.

32. deFilippi CR, Tocchi M, Parmar RJ, et al. Cardiac troponin T in chest pain unit patients without ischemic electrocardiographic changes: angiographic correlates and long-term clinical outcomes. J Am Coll Cardiol 2000; 35:1827–1834.

33. Goldmann BU, Christenson RH, Hamm CW, et al. Implications of troponin testing in clinical medicine. Curr Control Trials Cardiovasc Med 2001; 2:75–84.

34. Fragmin and Fast Revascularisation During Instability in Coronary Artery Disease (FRISC II) Investigators. Long-term low-molecular-mass heparin in unstable coronary-artery disease: FRISC II prospective randomised multicentre study [published erratum appears in Lancet 1999; 354:1478]. Lancet 1999; 354:701–707.

35. Morrow DA, Cannon CP, Rifai N, et al. Ability of minor elevations of troponins I or T to predict benefit from an early invasive strategy in patients with unstable angina and non-ST elevation myocardial infarction. JAMA 2001; 286:2405–2412.

36. Newby LK, Ohman EM, Christenson RH, et al. Benefit of glycoprotein IIb/IIIa inhibition in patients with acute coronary syndromes and troponin T-positive status: the PARAGON-B troponin T substudy. Circulation 2001; 103:2891–2896.

37. Campeau L. Grading of angina pectoris [letter]. Circulation 1976; 54:522–523.

38. Ohman EM, Granger CB, Harrington RA, et al. Risk stratification and therapeutic decision making in acute coronary syndromes [commentary]. JAMA 2000; 284:876–878.

39. Cohen M, Demers C, Gurfinkel EP, et al. A comparison of low-molecular-weight heparin with unfractionated heparin for unstable coronary artery disease. N Engl J Med 1997; 337:447–452.

40. Morrow DA, Antman EM, Snapinn SM, et al. An integrated clinical approach to predicting the benefit of tirofiban in non-ST elevation acute coronary syndromes: application of the TIMI risk score for UA/NSTEMI in PRISM-Plus. Eur Heart J 2002; 23:223–229.

41. Scirica BM, Cannon CP, Antman EM, et al. Validation of the Thrombolysis in Myocardial Infarction (TIMI) risk score for unstable angina pectoris and non-ST-elevation myocardial infarction in the TIMI III registry. Am J Cardiol 2002; 90:303–305.

42. Roffi M, Chew DP, Mukherjee D, et al. Platelet glycoprotein IIb/IIIa inhibitors reduce mortality in diabetic patients with non-ST-segment elevation acute coronary syndromes. Circulation 2001; 104:2767–2771.

43. Tschoepe D, Roesen P, Kaufmann L, et al. Evidence for abnormal platelet glycoprotein expression in diabetes mellitus. Eur J Clin Invest 1990; 20:166–170.

44. Shukla SD, Paul A, Klachko DM. Hypersensitivity of diabetic human platelets to platelet activating factor. Thromb Res 1992; 66:239–246.

45. Jilma B, Fasching P, Ruthner C, et al. Elevated circulating P-selectin in insulin dependent diabetes mellitus. Thromb Haemost 1996; 76:328–332.

46. Davi G, Gresele P, Violi F, et al. Diabetes mellitus, hypercholesterolemia, and hypertension but not vascular disease per se are associated with persistent platelet activation in vivo: evidence derived from the study of peripheral arterial disease. Circulation 1997; 96:69–75.

47. Lee KL, Woodlief LH, Topol EJ, et al. Predictors of 30–day mortality in the era of reperfusion for acute myocardial infarction: results from an international trial of 41,021 patients. Circulation 1995; 91:1659–1668.

48. Califf RM, Woodlief LH, Harrell FE Jr, et al. Selection of thrombolytic therapy for individual patients: development of a clinical model. Am Heart J 1997; 133:630–639.

49. Morrow DA, Antman EM, Charlesworth A, et al. TIMI risk score for ST-elevation myocardial infarction: a convenient, bedside, clinical score for risk assessment at presentation: an Intravenous nPA for Treatment of Infarcting Myocardium Early II trial substudy. Circulation 2000; 102:2031–2037.

50. Morrow DA, Antman EM, Giugliano RP, et al. A simple risk index for rapid initial triage of patients with ST-elevation myocardial infarction: an InTIME II substudy. Lancet 2001; 358:1571–1575.

51. Willems JL, Willems RJ, Willems GM, et al. Significance of initial ST segment elevation and depression for the management of thrombolytic therapy in acute myocardial infarction.

European Cooperative Study Group for Recombinant Tissue-Type Plasminogen Activator. Circulation 1990; 82:1147–1158.

52. Mauri F, Gasparini M, Barbonaglia L, et al. Prognostic significance of the extent of myocardial injury in acute myocardial infarction treated by streptokinase (the GISSI trial). Am J Cardiol 1989; 63:1291–1295.

53. Hathaway WR, Peterson ED, Wagner GS, et al. Prognostic significance of the initial electrocardiogram in patients with acute myocardial infarction. JAMA 1998; 279:387–391.

54. Mehta SR, Eikelboom JW, Natarajan MK, et al. Impact of right ventricular involvement on mortality and morbidity in patients with inferior myocardial infarction. J Am Coll Cardiol 2001; 37:37–43.

55. Bueno H, Lopez-Palop R, Bermejo J, et al. In-hospital outcome of elderly patients with acute inferior myocardial infarction and right ventricular involvement. Circulation 1997; 96:436–441.

56. Bueno H, Lopez-Palop R, Perez-David E, et al. Combined effect of age and right ventricular involvement on acute inferior myocardial infarction prognosis. Circulation 1998; 98:1714–1720.

57. Wong CK, White HD. Risk stratification of patients with right ventricular infarction: is there a need for a specific risk score? [editorial]. Eur Heart J 2002; 23:1642–1645.

58. Zhao XQ, Théroux P, Snapinn SM, et al. Intracoronary thrombus and platelet glycoprotein IIb/IIIa receptor blockade with tirofiban in unstable angina or non-Q-wave myocardial infarction: angiographic results from the PRISM-Plus trial (Platelet Receptor Inhibition for Ischemic Syndrome Management in Patients Limited by Unstable Signs and Symptoms). Circulation 1999; 100:1609–1615.

59. Chesebro JH, Knatterud G, Roberts R, et al. Thrombolysis in Myocardial Infarction (TIMI) trial, phase I: a comparison between intravenous tissue plasminogen activator and intravenous streptokinase: clinical findings through hospital discharge. Circulation 1987; 76:142–154.

60. Stone GW, Cox D, Garcia E, et al. Normal flow (TIMI-3) before mechanical reperfusion therapy is an independent determinant of survival in acute myocardial infarction: analysis from the Primary Angioplasty in Myocardial Infarction trials. Circulation 2001; 104:636–641.

61. Canto JG, Every NR, Magid DJ, et al. The volume of primary angioplasty procedures and survival after acute myocardial infarction. N Engl J Med 2000; 342:1573–1580.

62. van't Hof AWJ, Liem A, Suryapranata H, et al. Angiographic assessment of myocardial reperfusion in patients treated with primary angioplasty for acute MI: myocardial blush grade. Circulation 1998; 97:2302–2306.

63. Goldstein JA, Demetriou D, Grines CL, et al. Multiple complex coronary plaques in patients with acute myocardial infarction. N Engl J Med 2000; 343:915–922.

64. Rioufol G, Finet G, Ginon I, et al. Mulitple atherosclerotic plaque rupture in acute coronary syndrome: a three-vessel intravascular ultrasound study. Circulation 2002; 106:804–808.

65. Fibrinolytic Therapy Trialists' (FTT) Collaborative Group. Indications for fibrinolytic therapy in suspected acute myocardial infarction: collaborative overview of early mortality and major morbidity results from all randomised trials of more than 1000 patients. Lancet 1994; 343:311–322.

66. The GUSTO V Investigators. Reperfusion therapy for acute myocardial infarction with fibrinolytic therapy or combination reduced fibrinolytic therapy and platelet glycoprotein IIb/IIIa inhibition: the GUSTO V randomized trial. Lancet 2001; 357:1905–1914.

67. The Hirulog and Early Reperfusion or Occlusion (HERO)-2 Trial Investigators. Thrombin-specific anticoagulation with bivalirudin versus heparin in patients receiving fibrinolytic therapy for acute myocardial infarction: the HERO-2 randomised trial. Lancet 2001; 358:1855–1863.

68. Webb JG, Sleeper LA, Buller CE, et al. Implications of the timing of onset of cardiogenic shock after acute myocardial infarction: a report from the SHOCK trial registry. J Am Coll Cardiol 2000; 36:1084–1090.

69. Menon V, Slater JN, White HD, et al. Acute myocardial infarction complicated by systemic hypoperfusion without hypotension: report of the SHOCK trial registry. Am J Med 2000; 108:374–380.

70. Langer A, Freeman MR, Armstrong PW. ST segment shift in unstable angina: pathophysiology and association with coronary anatomy and hospital outcome. J Am Coll Cardiol 1989; 13:1495–1502.

71. Goodman SG, Barr A, Sobtchouk A, et al. Low molecular weight heparin decreases rebound ischemia in unstable angina or non-Q-wave myocardial infarction: the Canadian ESSENCE ST segment monitoring substudy. J Am Coll Cardiol 2000; 36:1507–1513.

72. Jernberg T, Lindahl B, Wallentin L. The combination of a continuous 12–lead ECG and troponin T; a valuable tool for risk stratification during the first 6 hours in patients with chest pain and a non-diagnostic ECG. Eur Heart J 2000; 21:1464–1472.

73. Kaul P, Fu Y, Chang WC, et al. Prognostic value of ST segment depression in acute coronary syndromes: insights from PARAGON-A applied to GUSTO-IIb. J Am Coll Cardiol 2001; 38:64–71.

74. Klootwijk P, Meij S, Melkert R, et al. Reduction of recurrent ischemia with abciximab during continuous ECG-ischemia monitoring in patients with unstable angina refractory to standard treatment (CAPTURE). Circulation 1998; 98:1358–1364.

75. The PURSUIT Trial Investigators. Inhibition of platelet glycoprotein IIb/IIIa with eptifibatide in patients with acute coronary syndromes. N Engl J Med 1998; 339:436–443.

76. Akkerhuis KM, Neuhaus KL, Wilcox RG, et al. Safety and preliminary efficacy of one month glycoprotein IIb/IIIa inhibition with lefradafiban in patients with acute coronary syndromes without ST-elevation: a phase II study. Eur Heart J 2000; 21:2042–2055.

77. Akkerhuis M, Klootwijk PAJ, Lindeboom WK, et al. The risk of adverse outcome in patients with acute coronary syndromes is directly proportional to the number of episodes of recurrent ischemia detected by multilead ST-segment monitoring: meta-analysis of three studies involving 995 patients [abstract]. Circulation 2000:102 (suppl II): II-589.

78. Bertrand ME, Simoons ML, Fox KAA, et al. Management of acute coronary syndromes: acute coronary syndromes *without* persistent ST segment elevation: recommendations of the Task Force of the European Society of Cardiology. Eur Heart J 2000; 21:1406–1432.

79. Braunwald E, Antman EM, Beasley JW, et al. ACC/AHA guidelines for the management of patients with unstable angina and non-ST-segment elevation myocardial infarction: a report of the American College of Cardiology/American Heart Association Task Force on Practice Guidelines (Committee on the Management of Patients with Unstable Angina). J Am Coll Cardiol 2000; 36:970–1062.

80. Krucoff MW, Croll MA, Pope JE, et al. Continuous 12–lead ST-segment recovery analysis in the TAMI 7 study: performance of a noninvasive method for real-time detection of failed myocardial reperfusion. Circulation 1993; 88:437–446.

81. Andrews J, Straznicky IT, French JK, et al. ST-segment recovery adds to the assessment of TIMI 2 and 3 flow in predicting infarct wall motion after thrombolytic therapy. Circulation 2000; 101:2138–2143.

82. Barbash GI, Roth A, Hod H, et al. Rapid resolution of ST elevation and prediction of clinical outcome in patients undergoing thrombolysis with alteplase (recombinant tissue-type plasminogen activator): results of the Israeli Study of Early Intervention in Myocardial Infarction. Br Heart J 1990; 64:241–247.

83. Mauri F, Maggioni AP, Franzosi MG, et al. A simple electrocardiographic predictor of the outcome of patients with acute myocardial infarction treated with a thrombolytic agent: a Gruppo Italiano per lo Studio della Sopravvivenza nell'Infarto Miocardico (GISSI-2)-derived analysis [published erratum appears in J Am Coll Cardiol 1995; 25:805]. J Am Coll Cardiol 1994; 24:600–607.

84. Schröder R, Dissmann R, Bruggemann T, et al. Extent of early ST segment elevation resolution: a simple but strong predictor of outcome in patients with acute myocardial infarction. J Am Coll Cardiol 1994; 24:384–391.

85. Schroder R, Wegscheider K, Schroder K, et al. Extent of early ST segment elevation resolution: a strong predictor of outcome in patients with acute myocardial infarction and a sensi-

tive measure to compare thrombolytic regimens: a substudy of the International Joint Efficacy Comparison of Thrombolytics (INJECT) trial. J Am Coll Cardiol 1995; 26:1657–1664.

86. Neuhaus KL, Molhoek GP, Zeymer U, et al. Recombinant hirudin (lepirudin) for the improvement of thrombolysis with streptokinase in patients with acute myocardial infarction: results of the HIT-4 trial. J Am Coll Cardiol 1999; 34:966–973.

87. Schroder R, Zeymer U, Wegscheider K, et al. Comparison of the predictive value of ST segment elevation resolution at 90 and 180 min after start of streptokinase in acute myocardial infarction: a substudy of the Hirudin for Improvement of Thrombolysis (HIT)-4 study. Eur Heart J 1999; 20:1563–1571.

88. Anderson RD, White HD, Ohman EM, et al. Predicting outcome after thrombolysis in acute myocardial infarction according to ST-segment resolution at 90 minutes: a substudy of the GUSTO-III trial. Am Heart J 2002; 144:81–88.

89. Shah A, Wagner GS, Granger CB, et al. Prognostic implications of TIMI flow grade in the infarct related artery compared with continuous 12–lead ST-segment resolution analysis: reexamining the "gold standard" for myocardial reperfusion assessment. J Am Coll Cardiol 2000; 35:666–672.

90. van't Hof AWJ, Liem A, de Boer M-J, et al. Clinical value of 12–lead electrocardiogram after successful reperfusion therapy for acute myocardial infarction. Lancet 1997; 350:615–619.

91. Matetzky S, Novikov M, Gruberg L, et al. The significance of persistent ST elevation versus early resolution of ST segment elevation after primary PTCA. J Am Coll Cardiol 1999; 34:1932–1938.

92. Saran RK, Been M, Furniss SS, et al. Reduction in ST segment elevation after thrombolysis predicts either coronary reperfusion or preservation of left ventricular function. Br Heart J 1990; 64:113–117.

93. Dissmann R, Schroder R, Busse U, et al. Early assessment of outcome by ST-segment analysis after thrombolytic therapy in acute myocardial infarction. Am Heart J 1994; 128:851–857.

94. de Lemos JA, Antman EM, Giugliano RP, et al. Comparison of a 60– versus 90–minute determination of ST-segment resolution after thrombolytic therapy for acute myocardial infarction. Am J Cardiol 2000; 86:1235–1237.

95. Matetzky S, Freimark D, Chouraqui P, et al. The distinction between coronary and myocardial reperfusion after thrombolytic therapy by clinical markers of reperfusion. J Am Coll Cardiol 1998; 32:1326–1330.

96. de Lemos JA, Antman EM, Giugliano RP, et al. ST-segment resolution and infarct-related artery patency and flow after thrombolytic therapy. Am J Cardiol 2000; 85:299–304.

97. Fu Y, Goodman S, Chang WC, et al. Time to treatment influences the impact of ST-segment resolution on one-year prognosis: insights from the Assessment of the Safety and Efficacy of a New Thrombolytic (ASSENT-2) trial. Circulation 2001; 104:2653–2659.

98. Severi S, Orsini E, Marraccini P, et al. The basal electrocardiogram and the exercise stress test in assessing prognosis in patients with unstable angina. Eur Heart J 1988; 9:441–446.

99. Swahn E, Areskog M, Berglund U, et al. Predictive importance of clinical findings and a predischarge exercise test in patients with suspected unstable coronary artery disease. Am J Cardiol 1987; 59:208–214.

100. Madsen JK, Grande P, Saunamäki K, et al. Danish multicenter randomized study of invasive versus conservative treatment in patients with inducible ischemia after thrombolysis in acute myocardial infarction (DANAMI). Circulation 1997; 96:748–755.

101. White HD, Norris RM, Brown MA, et al. Left ventricular end-systolic volume as the major determinant of survival after recovery from myocardial infarction. Circulation 1987; 76:44–51.

102. Burns RJ, Gibbons RJ, Yi Q, et al. The relationships of left ventricular ejection fraction, end-systolic volume index and infarct size to six-month mortality after hospital discharge following myocardial infarction treated by thrombolysis. J Am Coll Cardiol 2002; 39:30–36.

103. White HD. Should all occluded infarct-related arteries be opened? [editorial]. Eur Heart J 1997; 18:1207–1209.

104. White HD, Cross DB, Elliott JM, et al. Long-term prognostic importance of patency of the infarct-related coronary artery after thrombolytic therapy for acute myocardial infarction. Circulation 1994; 89:61–67.

105. Ross AM, Coyne KS, Moreyra E, et al. Extended mortality benefit of early postinfarction reperfusion. Circulation 1998; 97:1549–1556.

106. French JK, Hyde TA, Straznicky IT, et al. Relationship between corrected TIMI frame counts at three weeks and late survival after myocardial infarction. J Am Coll Cardiol 2000; 35:1516–1524.

107. Rouleau JL, Talajic M, Sussex B, et al. Myocardial infarction patients in the 1990s—their risk factors, stratification and survival in Canada: the Canadian Assessment of Myocardial Infarction (CAMI) study. J Am Coll Cardiol 1996; 27:1119–1127.

108. Moss AJ, Zareba W, Hall WJ, et al. Prophylactic implantation of a defibrillator in patients with myocardial infarction and reduced ejection fraction. N Engl J Med 2002; 346:877–883.

109. Morrow DA, Antman EM, Parsons L, et al. Application of the TIMI risk score for ST-elevation MI in the National Registry of Myocardial Infarction 3. JAMA 2001; 286:1356–1359.

110. Llevadot J, Giugliano RP, Antman EM, et al. Availability of on-site catheterization and clinical outcomes in patients receiving fibrinolysis for ST-elevation myocardial infarction. Eur Heart J 2001; 22:2104–2115.

111. Williams SB, Ferguson JJ. Meeting highlights: highlights of the 24th Congress of the European Society of Cardiology. Circulation 2002; 106:e211–e219.

112. Marchioli R, Avanzini F, Barzi F, et al. Assessment of absolute risk of death after myocardial infarction by use of multiple-risk-factor assessment equations: GISSI-Prevenzione mortality risk chart. Eur Heart J 2001; 22:2085–2103.

113. Marschner IC, Colquhoun D, Simes RJ, et al. Long-term risk stratification for survivors of acute coronary syndromes: results from the Long-Term Intervention with Pravastatin in Ischemic Disease (LIPID) study. J Am Coll Cardiol 2001; 38:56–63.

114. Ridker PM, Cushman M, Stampfer MJ, et al. Inflammation, aspirin, and the risk of cardiovascular disease in apparently healthy men. N Engl J Med 1997; 336:973–979.

115. Ridker PM, Hennekens CH, Buring JE, et al. C-reactive protein and other markers of inflammation in the prediction of cardiovascular disease in women. N Engl J Med 2000; 342:836–843.

116. Heeschen C, Hamm CW, Bruemmer J, et al. Predictive value of C-reactive protein and troponin T in patients with unstable angina: a comparative analysis. J Am Coll Cardiol 2000; 35:1535–1542.

117. Ross R. Atherosclerosis—an inflammatory disease. N Engl J Med 1999; 340:115–126.

118. Lagrand WK, Visser CA, Hermens WT, et al. C-reactive protein as a cardiovascular risk factor. Circulation 1999; 100:96–102.

119. Ridker PM. High-sensitivity C-reactive protein: potential adjunct for global risk assessment in the primary prevention of cardiovascular disease. Circulation 2001; 103:1813–1818.

120. Montalescot G, Philippe F, Ankri A, et al. Early increase of von Willebrand factor predicts adverse outcome in unstable coronary artery disease: beneficial effects of enoxaparin. Circulation 1998; 98:294–299.

121. Montalescot G, Collet JP, Lison L, et al. Effects of various anticoagulant treatments on von Willebrand factor release in unstable angina. J Am Coll Cardiol 2000; 36:110–114.

122. Levin ER, Gardner DG, Samson WK. Mechanisms of disease—natriuretic peptides. N Engl J Med 1998; 339:321–328.

123. de Lemos JA, Morrow DA, Bentley JH, et al. The prognostic value of B-type natriuretic peptide in patients with acute coronary syndromes. N Engl J Med 2001; 345:1014–1021.

124. Newby LK, Storrow AB, Gibler WB, et al. Bedside multimarker testing for risk stratification in chest pain units: the Chest Pain Evaluation by Creatine Kinase-MB, Myoglobin, and Troponin I (CHECKMATE) study. Circulation 2001; 103:1832–1837.

125. Morrow DA, Rifai N, Antman EM, et al. C-reactive protein is a potent predictor of mortality independently of and in combination with troponin T in acute coronary syndromes: a TIMI 11A substudy. J Am Coll Cardiol 1998; 31:1460–1465.

126. Sabatine MS, Morrow DA, de Lemos JA, et al. Multimarker approach to risk stratification in non-ST elevation acute coronary syndromes: simultaneous assessment of troponin I, C-reactive protein, and B-type natriuretic peptide. Circulation 2002; 105:1760–1763.

9-1

Monitoring Anticoagulants in the Catheterization Laboratory and in the ICU When Using Combination Therapies

Debabrata Mukherjee and David J. Moliterno
Division of Cardiovascular Medicine, Gill Heart Institute, University of Kentucky, Lexington, Kentucky, U.S.A.

I. BACKGROUND AND RATIONALE FOR MONITORING

The availability of potent antiplatelet, antithrombin, and fibrinolytic therapies for the treatment of acute coronary syndromes (ACS) and during percutaneous coronary interventions (PCI) has made monitoring these therapies an important issue. The use of these agents in combination has led to improved antithrombotic efficacy, albeit at the cost of higher bleeding in some situations. Current and evolving technologies to monitor the extent of inhibition of platelet aggregation and activity of antithrombotic agents when used as combination therapy will be covered in this overview. Table 1 lists various scenarios in which the monitoring of combination therapies may be useful. The clinically important question to be considered is whether the results generated from monitoring will effect a change that will improve efficacy (prevent thrombotic events) or reduce adverse events (bleeding) from these therapies. Since novel and increasingly potent agents continue to be developed, monitoring anticoagulation will continue to be of special interest.

II. UNFRACTIONATED HEPARIN

Unfractionated heparin (UFH) remains the leading antithrombotic therapy used in the catheterization laboratory and in the intensive care unit (ICU) setting. The clinical value of anticoagulation monitoring has been well studied with UFH. Several trials including GUSTO I (1) and GUSTO IIa (2) have demonstrated a linear relationship between increasing activated partial thromboplastin time (aPTT) and risk of hemorrhage in the setting of fibrinolytic therapy. Each 10% increase in aPTT was associated with a 1% absolute increase in moderate or severe hemorrhage (1). The current ACC/AHA guidelines recommend that in the setting of fibrinolytic therapy heparin be administered at the lower weight-adjusted dose of 60 U/kg bolus followed by 12 U/kg/h with a target aPTT of 50–70 seconds (3).

Table 1 Scenarios in which Monitoring Would Be Clinically Useful When Using Combination Therapies

---

Patient
  Confirm adequate anticoagulation and platelet inhibition
Prior to PCI
    In patients with refractory ischemia on IIb/IIIa inhibitors
    Abnormal platelet count
    Renal insufficiency
    High or low body weight
Clinical
  Bleeding
    Confirm excess inhibition
    Guidance during reversal of therapy
  Emergent surgery
    Confirm 50% aggregation inhibition
    Guidance to reverse therapy if needed
Other
  Drug-specific
    Switching among agents
    Transition from intravenous to oral agents

There are at present no large randomized trials of different levels of anticoagulation with UFH during PCI, but a number of observational studies have suggested that the degree of anticoagulation as measured by the ACT correlates with risk of thrombotic events (4–8).

A. Tests

The standard method for measuring the degree of anticoagulation with UFH is the aPTT, which primarily reflects the effect of UFH on thrombin (factor IIa), factor Xa, and factor IXa. Technologies that enable rapid determination of the degree of anticoagulation with UFH in the form of whole blood activated clotting time (ACT) have evolved for use in the catheterization laboratory. The two commonly used systems for ACT measurement include the Hemochron® device (International Technidyne Corporation) and the Hemotec Device (Medtronic Hemotec, Englewood, CO).

1. Hemochron® ACT

The Hemochron system has two separate platforms for monitoring ACT. The tube-based technology was first developed decades ago and is still commonly used during percutaneous and surgical coronary revascularization procedures. The Hemochron Response is a tube-based machine (Fig. 1a), which uses a magnet inside glass specimen tubes that hold celite, kaolin, or glass particles. After blood is placed into the tube, coagulation becomes activated, and the tubes are rotated inside the machine's prewarmed cylinder. As the blood clots, the magnet is displaced from the bottom of the tube, thereby activating a proximity switch within the cylinder. The clotting time is the interval taken for the activated blood to clot and displace the magnet.

More recently a cuvette-based microsample technology has been developed and is more commonly used on the hospital ward or outpatient setting where portability of

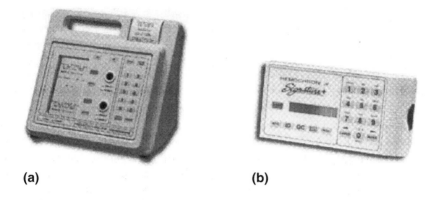

(a)   (b)

Figure 1   (a) The HEMOCHRON Response is a whole blood coagulation monitoring instrument designed to be used at the point-of-care. It includes an easy-to-read screen and data management features, including patient and operator ID options. (b) The HEMOCHRON microcoagulation system rapidly and accurately monitors low to moderate levels of heparin (0–2.5 units/mL), reporting results as Celite® equivalent values useful in dialysis, extracorporeal membrane oxygenation (ECMO), and catheterization laboratory procedures.

this smaller device needed. The Hemochron microcoagulation system (Fig. 1b) utilizes a mechanical endpoint clotting mechanism in which testing occurs within the disposable ACT cuvette (9). Following whole blood sample introduction, the instrument precisely measures 15 mL of blood and automatically moves it into the test channel within the cuvette. After mixing with the reagent (silica, kaolin, and phospholipid), the sample is then moved back and forth within the test channel and monitored by the analyzer for clot formation. The clot detection mechanism consists of two light-emitting diode (LED) optical detectors aligned with the test channel of the cuvette. The speed at which the blood sample moves between the two detectors is measured. As clot formation begins, blood flow is impeded and the movement slows. The instrument recognizes that a clot endpoint has been achieved when the movement decreases below a predetermined rate. Electronic optical detection of a fibrin clot in the blood sample automatically terminates the test. The instrument's digital timer then displays the ACT value in seconds.

2.   Hemotec ACT

This technique uses a double-well reagent cartridge containing kaolin as activator (10). A whole blood sample is dispensed into a prewarmed reagent cartridge inserted into the instrument. When the testing cycle is initiated, plungers in the cartridge move up and down, mixing the reagent and blood together. These plungers continue to move until fibrin is formed. As fibrin strands adhere to the plunger, the reduced movement of the plunger is detected optically and the resultant time is displayed in seconds as the ACT.

B.   Clinical Utility and Relevance

Narins et al. (6) demonstrated procedural ACT during PCI to be inversely related to the likelihood of abrupt vessel closure but could not identify a minimum target ACT. Chew et al. pooled data from six randomized PCI trials and analyzed the rates of ischemic and bleeding events stratified by ACT (8). Using ACT results divided into 25-second intervals, they demonstrated that there was a near-linear decrease in the 7-day composite of death, myocardial infarction, and revascularization with increasing levels of ACT from heparin alone (Fig. 2a). A U-shaped distribution was noted for major and minor bleeding stratified by ACT (Fig. 2b). The lowest rate of bleeding events corresponded to an ACT of 300–350 seconds. The authors also analyzed ACT values among patients who received concomitant IIb/IIIa inhibitors. There was no significant difference in the rates of ischemic events over a range of ACT values, but there was an increase in bleeding episodes with higher ACT levels, particularly if the ACT was greater that 300 seconds. The authors concluded that a target ACT for patients not receiving a glycoprotein IIb/IIIa inhibitor should be approximately 350 seconds and ≥200 seconds for patients being treated with concomitant IIb/IIIa inhibitors (8). Data from the EPILOG trial, had demonstrated that a reduction in the dose of heparin from 100 to 70 U/kg with adjunctive abciximab resulted in a significant reduction in major bleeding from 3.5 to 2.0% with no reduction in benefit (11). Thus, a lower target ACT is recommended with use of adjunctive glycoprotein (GP) IIb/IIIa inhibitors.

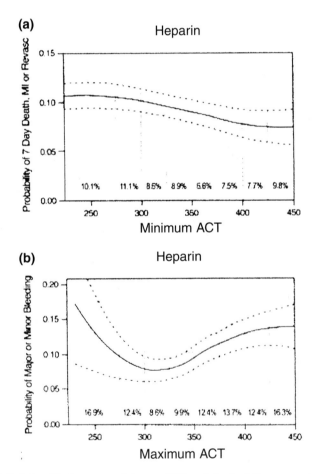

Figure 2 (a) Relationship between minimum ACT and death, MI, or urgent revascularization (Revasc) at 7 days. (b) Relationship between maximum ACT and major or minor bleeding events at 7 days. Lowess smoothing estimate and 95% confidence intervals are indicated by solid and dotted lines, respectively. Percentages represent actual event rates observed. (Adapted from Ref. 8.)

The ACC/AHA currently recommends that in patients who do not receive GP IIb/IIIa inhibitors, sufficient UFH should be given during coronary angioplasty to achieve an ACT of 250–300 seconds with the Hemotec device and 300–350 seconds with the Hemochron device (12). Typically the Hemochron device gives ACT values 30–50 seconds higher than the Hemotec at all UFH concentrations (13). Weight-adjusted bolus heparin (≤70–100 IU/kg) can be used to avoid excess anticoagulation. If the target value for ACT is not achieved after an initial bolus of heparin, additional smaller heparin boluses (1000–2000 IU) should be given. Early sheath removal when the ACT falls to less than 150–180 seconds is recommended to reduce access site bleeding complications. The UFH bolus should be reduced to ≤50–70 IU/kg when GP IIb/IIIa inhibitors are given in order to achieve a target ACT of ≥200 seconds using either the Hemotec or Hemochron device. Monitoring of the degree of anticoagulation with aPTT and ACT may translate into improved clinical outcomes or improved safety when using UFH (14).

III. LOW MOLECULAR WEIGHT HEPARINS

Because unfractionated heparin (UFH) has a number of important limitations related to its pharmacokinetic properties, low molecular weight heparins (LMWHs) have been produced. Compared with UFH, LMWHs have better subcutaneous absorption and bioavailability, longer half-life, and a lower likelihood of inducing heparin-associated platelet antibodies. Other distinctions between UFH and LMWH include the fact that low molecular weight fractions of heparin do not prolong standard measures of anticoagulation such as aPTT and ACT. Whereas a standard dose of UFH in a setting of PCI would prolong the activated clotting time to 300–350 seconds, a similarly appropriate dose of LMWH would have minimal effect on the ACT (15). Rabah et al. (16) randomized 60 patients to receive intravenous enoxaparin (1 mg/kg bolus dose) or UFH at the time of PCI. Thirty percent of patients who received unfractionated heparin required a second bolus of intravenous heparin to achieve the target-activated clotting time of 300 seconds before PCI. Enoxaparin showed antithrombotic properties comparable to that of unfractionated heparin as measured by anti-Xa levels, with less inhibition of thrombin (factor IIa) at all time points measured ($p < 0.0001$). Angioplasty success rates, in-hospital ischemia, bleeding, and vascular complications were similar in both groups (16). Thus, intravenous enoxaparin has predictable and effective antithrombotic effects during elective PCI. LMWHs have become more commonplace in the treatment of ACS and are becoming more frequently seen in cardiac catheterization laboratories. A desire to monitor the extent of anticoagulant effect of LMWH has emerged in some situations. LMWHs are also currently being tested in combination with fibrinolytic agents, and the adequacy of the antithrombotic effect in this setting may also be clinically important.

Henry et al. (15) demonstrated that ACTs are not helpful in the management of anticoagulation with subcutaneous enoxaparin during PCI. The investigators obtained peak (mean 4.3 hours after enoxaparin) and trough (mean 11.5 hours after enoxaparin) anti-Xa levels and ACTs for 26 patients in the Thrombolysis In Myocardial Infarction (TIMI) 11A trial. Despite doses of enoxaparin in the range of 89 ± 19 mg every 12 hours and significant increases in anti-Xa levels even at trough, there was no change in the ACT measured by HemoTec and only a small increase with Hemochron. The correlation of peak Hemochron ACT with peak anti-Xa levels was poor (R = 0.5; $p = 0.08$). The authors concluded that in contrast to UFH, ACTs are not useful for assessment of anticoagulation with subcutaneous enoxaparin and should not be relied on in patients receiving enoxaparin who require acute PCI.

Prospective studies to determine the optimal dose, safety, and efficacy of enoxaparin in patients undergoing PCI are underway. Anti-Xa levels or tissue factor pathway inhibitor (TFPI) levels may also be helpful to monitor anticoagulation levels with LMWH in the cardiac catheterization laboratory. One assay has the potential to monitor a combination of antithrombotic and antiplatelet effect but has not been tested thoroughly in a clinical setting (17). Holmes et al. developed this assay based on initiation of clotting by tissue factor in minimally altered whole blood. Blood samples were obtained from healthy subjects, and the contact pathway of coagulation was inhibited with corn trypsin inhibitor (a specific factor XIIa inhibitor without effect on other coagulation factors). Clotting was initiated with relipidated tissue factor and detected with a Hemochron ACT instrument. Results were reproducible with samples from 25 healthy volunteers (mean time to clot 125 ± 17 s). Blood was also exposed to pharmacological concentrations of antithrombotic and antiplatelet agents in vitro. Heparin (0.25 anti-IIa/Xa U/mL) prolonged the time to clot by 2.4-fold (172 s; $p < 0.05$); hirudin (1.0 anti-IIa U/mL) by 3-fold (250 s; $p < 0.05$); and enoxaparin (0.6 anti-Xa U/mL) by 2-fold (123 s; $p < 0.05$). Additive effects of antiplatelet agents were readily detectable with both heparin and hirudin. Thus, addition of 3 mg/mL abciximab to 1.0 anti-IIa/Xa U/mL heparin and to 1.0 anti-IIa U/mL hirudin further prolonged the times to clot by 140 and 67 seconds, respectively ($p < 0.05$ for each). Addition of abciximab to enoxaparin did not further prolong the time to clot (increment, 13 s; $p =$ NS) (17). The assay, if validated, may facilitate improved dose selection, titration, and monitoring of combination antithrombotic and antiplatelet treatment regimens in the future. Interassay variability in anti-Xa monitoring exists as for the ACT (18) and will require standardization prior to widespread acceptance.

A. Tests

1. RapidPoint™

Pharmanetics, Inc. (Cardiovascular Diagnostics) has developed a point-of-care device for measuring the extent of anticoagulation provided by enoxaparin based on the Thrombolytic Assessment System (Fig. 3). In the Rapidpoint ENOX test, factor X is rapidly converted to factor Xa by a specific activator, initiating the clotting process. Enoxaparin from the patient's blood complexes with antithrombin (AT) to inhibit factor Xa and proportionally lengthen the clotting time. The reported clotting time is related to the enoxaparin concentration present in the sample. The results generated by the ENOX test are thus indicative of the anticoagulant effect produced by enoxaparin in whole blood.

Because each LMWH has a specific ratio of effect against factors Xa and IIa, it is not possible to create a generic LMWH test card. Rather, the card-based technology must be modified to optimize measuring the effect of each agent. The Rapidpoint system has been tested and shown to correlate well with several available LMWHs (Fig. 4). The current test card is optimized for use with enoxaparin and will not provide reliable results if used to monitor other LMWHs.

B. Clinical Utility/Relevance

Several studies have evaluated the safety of LMWHs during PCI (19). The National Investigators Collaborating on Enoxaparin (NICE)-1 pilot was a phase I study of 60 patients undergoing PCI and compared the antithrombotic properties of enoxaparin (1.0 mg/kg) to UFH (procedural ACT > 300 s) (16). The primary observation of the study was equivalent immediate anti-factor Xa activity of enoxaparin and UFH. This protocol was

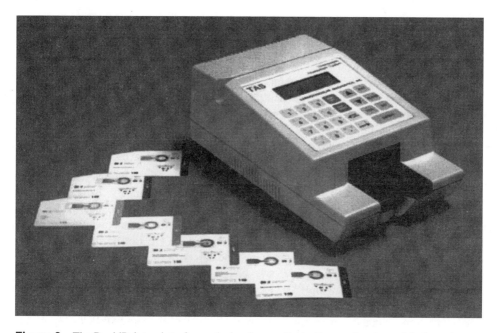

Figure 3 The RapidPoint point-of-care device for monitoring low molecular weight heparin.

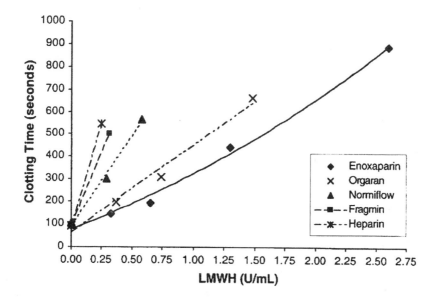

Figure 4 With the RapidPoint system, the effect of various low molecular weight heparins can be observed. To accurately discern the therapeutic effect for each low molecular weight heparin, a specific monitoring card must be used. (Adapted from Ref. 45.)

subsequently expanded to the NICE-1 registry, in which 828 patients received enoxaparin (1.0 mg/kg) intravenously immediately prior to PCI. The registry evaluated major and minor bleeding following PCI and demonstrated that the major bleeding rate of 0.5% and minor bleeding rate of 5.6% with enoxaparin at 30 days compared favorably with bleeding rates reported with UFH in the literature (20). In an observational cohort study of 451 patients with ACS, Collet et al. evaluated the feasibility of PCI after enoxaparin injection and demonstrated that PCI can be performed within 8 hours of the last injection of enoxaparin (21). The Clinical Revascularization Using Integrilin Simultaneously with Enoxaparin (CRUISE) trial designed to evaluate the potential utility of eptifibatide combined with either UFH or enoxaparin, a LMWH, demonstrated similar safety and efficacy outcomes for both treatment groups in 261 patients undergoing intracoronary stenting. The primary endpoint of the CRUISE study, the bleeding index (change in hemoglobin corrected for blood transfusions), was 0.8 in the patients randomized to enoxaparin and 1.1 in patients randomized to UFH, ($p = 0.15$) (22). The NICE-4 study was an open-label registry of 800 patients with combined LMWH (enoxaparin) and a GP IIb/IIIa blockade (abciximab) during PCI. This registry demonstrated the safety of this combination with a low incidence of major (0.5%) and minor (5.6%) bleeding at 30 days and infrequent major cardiac events at 30-day follow-up (23). Kereiakes et al. demonstrated that dalteparin 60 IU/kg IV appears to be safe and effective when administered in conjunction with abciximab for percutaneous coronary intervention in 107 patients undergoing PCI (24). As the use of LMWH increases in the catheterization laboratory, appropriate monitoring will become an important issue.

The Evaluation of ENOX Clotting Times (ELECT) study prospectively evaluated the predictive value of the Rapidpoint assay to assess the ischemic and hemorrhagic events associated and PCI and determine the optimal therapeutic reference range for PCI and sheath removal. This study confirmed the safety of PCI among patients receiving enoxaparin with a 30-day composite death, myocardial infarction, and revascularization rate of 5.4%. This incidence of major adverse cardiac events compares favorably with large contemporary PCI trials. The major bleeding rate of <1% was also low with enoxaparin. The optimal clotting time for PCI appears to be an ENOX Rapidpoint clotting time of 250–450 seconds, which corresponds to an anti-Xa activity of 0.8–2.2 IU/mL. Arterial sheaths can be safely pulled with an ENOX clotting time of <200–250 seconds depending on concomitant use of GP IIb/IIIa agents.

IV. DIRECT THROMBIN INHIBITORS

Direct thrombin inhibitors have the theoretical advantage over heparin of inhibiting clot-bound thrombin and not being inhibited by circulating plasma proteins and platelet factor 4. A number of studies have evaluated direct thrombin inhibitors for PCI. Bittl et al. compared bivalirudin with high-dose heparin during coronary angioplasty for unstable angina and assessed differences in rates of death, myocardial infarction, or repeat revascularization at 7, 90, and 180 days (25,26). The combined end point occurred in 135 of 2161 patients (6.2%) in the bivalirudin group and in 169 of 2151 patients (7.9%) in the heparin group at 7 days ($p = 0.039$). Differences persisted between the groups at 90 days ($p = 0.012$) and 180 days ($p = 0.153$). Bleeding occurred in 76 patients (3.5%) in the bivalirudin group versus 199 (9.3%) in the heparin group ($p < 0.001$) (25). The authors concluded that bivalirudin reduces ischemic complications and bleeding after angioplasty. The Comparison of Abciximab Complications with Hirulog for Ischemic Events Trial (CACHET) randomized 268 patients who underwent coronary intervention in three sequential phases to treatment with bivalirudin (with or without abciximab) or the control regimen of low-dose weight-adjusted heparin with abciximab. Patients in the bivalirudin arms received bivalirudin (1.0 mg/kg bolus, infusion of 2.5 mg/kg/h for 4 h) plus abciximab in phase A, bivalirudin (0.5 mg/kg bolus, infusion of 1.75 mg/kg/h for the procedure duration) plus provisional ("rescue") abciximab in phase B, or bivalirudin (0.75 mg/kg bolus, infusion of 1.75 mg/kg/h for the procedure duration) plus provisional abciximab in phase C (27). Abciximab was required on a provisional basis in 24% of the patients in the bivalirudin arms of phases B and C. A composite clinical endpoint of death, myocardial infarction, repeat revascularization, or major bleeding by 7 days occurred in 3.3, 5.9, 0, and 10.6% of the patients in the bivalirudin phase A, bivalirudin phase B, bivalirudin phase C, and heparin plus planned abciximab arms, respectively ($p = 0.018$ for the pooled bivalirudin groups vs. the heparin group). The authors concluded that bivalirudin with planned or provisional abciximab may be at least as safe and effective as low-dose heparin plus abciximab during percutaneous coronary intervention (27).

The efficacy and safety of bivalirudin for PCI has generated questions regarding monitoring of the degree of anticoagulation with bivalirudin. Direct thrombin inhibitors affect aPTT and the ACT, although the effects vary among agents. Fenyvesi et al. tested plasma samples of six healthy donors treated with lepirudin and argatroban to 3000 ng/mL and UFH up to 0.48 IU/mL, (28). Partial thromboplastin times (aPTT) and ecarin clotting times (ECT) were measured. At 3000 ng/mL ECT values were 339.1 ± 25.0 seconds with lepirudin and 457.5 ± 29.5 seconds with argatroban. ECT was more sensitive to therapeutic drug concentration ranges than aPTT and could therefore be suitable for monitoring anticoagulation with direct thrombin inhibitors (28). Cho et al. assessed point-of-care clotting times among 64 consecutive patients undergoing PCI on bivalrudin (29). Anti-factor IIa activity was measured with two different ACT assays and a rapid ecarin clotting time (ECT) assay. Following bivalirudin bolus, the correlations between bivalirudin concentrations and the Hemochron and Pro/DM ACT assays were weak ($r = 0.15$ and 0.42, respectively), whereas the bivalirudin concentration was strongly correlated with ECT results ($r = 0.72$) (29). The clinical relevance of these measurements remains to be determined, and measurement of the degree of anticoagulation may be less crucial with direct thrombin inhibitors.

A. Tests

1. Ecarin Clotting Time

The Rapidpoint ECT is a one-stage, two-step test that measures the clotting time of whole blood. The test utilizes the ability of venom from the snake *Echis carinatus* to directly activate prothrombin to meizothrombin, which converts fibrinogen to fibrin. The fibrin clot is detected by the analyzer as integrated iron particle movement becomes restricted. Meizothrombin is rapidly inhibited by direct thrombin inhibitors. The longer the ECT, the greater the concentration of the thrombin inhibitor. This assay also has the advantage of being relatively specific for the effect of direct thrombin inhibitors, as heparin is a poor inhibitor of meizothrombin. Therefore, ECT may be a more accurate and reliable measurement of direct thrombin inhibitor activity (30).

B. Clinical Utility/Relevance

A number of studies have now considered the efficacy and safety of direct thrombin inhibitors in PCI (25,27) and as an adjunct to fibrinolysis. Bivalirudin is currently approved for use during PCI and for patients with heparin-induced thrombocytopenia

(HIT). As use of these agents increase in the catheterization laboratory and in the ICU, appropriate monitoring will become clinically important. The ACT has not been found to be fully useful to monitor the degree of anticoagulation with these agents, and monitoring may be especially important in patients with renal insufficiency. The ECT may be more reliable.

V. PLATELET INHIBITORS

The goal of platelet function testing in the catheterization laboratory or intensive care unit is to provide information about platelet contributions to the risk of thrombotic or hemorrhagic events and optimization of antiplatelet therapy for PCI or ACS. Important clinical questions before PCI include whether an antiplatelet agent is achieving the desired effect on platelet inhibition and whether the patient has sufficient residual platelet function to avoid bleeding. The role of aspirin and thienopyridines has been well established in the management of coronary artery disease, and intravenously adminis-tered platelet glycoprotein (GP) IIb/IIIa antagonists have become the standard of care in several scenarios.

The 35–55% reduction in early ischemic events after PCI among patients receiving abciximab is predicated on a targeted >80% inhibition of platelet aggregation to 20 mmol/L adenosine disphosphate (ADP). Likewise, the empiric treatment (i.e., not neces-sarily associated with PCI) with eptifibatide or tirofiban for unstable angina or non–Q-wave MI has been shown to reduce death or MI by 10–35%, and the beneficial effects persist at 6 months. Here, too, the extent of platelet inhibition is believed central to the drugs' efficacy. Data from the Assessing Ultegra (Au - GOLD) (31) study suggest the per-cent inhibition of platelet aggregation (%IPA) as measured by the Ultegra rapid platelet function assay (RPFA') should be 95% at 10 minutes after platelet GPIIb/IIIa inhibitor bolus and >70% at 8 hours later during drug infusion to achieve optimal clinical outcomes (reduction in death, myocardial infarction, or requirement for repeat revascularization). This is separately supported by clinical trial observations of better outcome when more potent therapies are used (32–35).

A.   Tests

1. PFA-100 Analyzer

The Dade Behring platelet function analyzer (PFA-100) evaluates primary hemostasis through platelet-platelet interaction as whole blood flows under shear stress conditions through an aperture (36). This assay evaluates multiple factors involved in primary hemostasis similar to the template bleeding time without the incisional variability. It uses whole blood, is simple to perform, and is quick and automatic. The normal closure time is 100 seconds, and the instrument can detect a closure times up to 300 seconds, so this assay has a limited range. Its usefulness in monitoring GPIIb/IIIa therapy is hindered because the closure times are increased beyond 300 seconds with currently used GP IIb/IIIa antagonists.

2.   Flow Cytometry

Flow cytometry can rapidly measure specific characteristics of a large number of indi-vidual platelets. In response to agonists such as thrombin, collagen, or ADP, a spectrum of specific activation-dependent modifications of platelet surface antigens can be detected. This process leads to an intracellular signal transduction cascade involving ion fluxes and activation of the cytoskeleton. The end result is secretion of endosomes, which causes reorganization and conformational changes of surface receptor expression through inside-out signaling. Platelet activation also leads to an altered expression of already constitutively expressed surface glycoproteins. Thus, measuring the expression of these antigens on circulating platelets reflects not only the activation state of the platelets, but also the extent to which secretion has occurred. In addition to the benefits of whole blood analysis and a small amount of blood required, the minimal handling of samples needed prevents artifactual in vitro platelet activation. Also, with this assay both the activation state and the reactivity of platelets can be considered. Flow cytometry is helpful in assessing specific platelet functions, activity, and hyperreactivity. Thus, this test can be used to monitor the inhibition of the GP IIb/IIIa receptor by specific antagonists (33,34).

3. Clot Signature Analyzer

The Clot Signature Analyzer (Xylum Corporation, Scarsdale, NY) (Fig. 5a) has a collagen channel to simulate the exposure of blood to thrombogenic subendothelial tissue and measures several aspects of platelet function and clotting properties.. Blood is perfused over the collagen fiber at a high shear rate (approximately 6200/s). Platelets activated by collagen adhere and aggregate to form a thrombus. The clot signature analyzer (CSA) has a punch channel that provides information on platelet function. While blood flows through the channel, the channel is punched by a 0.15 mm needle, resulting in two fine holes. A high shear rate at the punch point promotes platelet adhesion to the injury site and recruitment of activated platelets and resultant aggregation at the site. A growing fibrin clot gradually occludes the pathway, resulting in reduction of the flow as evidenced by decrease in the pressure. Pressure (mmHg) is plotted against time for both channels to produce a clot signature (Fig. 5b). This automated assay uses whole blood under conditions of physiological flow and temperature and evaluates both platelet activation and aggregation. These ideal features are, however, somewhat offset since the current instrument is rather large for routine use and interpretation of the results is complex.

B. Clinical Utility/Relevance

Several clinical studies have considered platelet function assays and optimal GPIIb/IIIa blockade (31,37–39). These include the GOLD (31) and the PARADISE (39) studies. The PARADISE study involved 100 patients and demonstrated substantial interpatient variability in response to standard, weight-adjusted abciximab. Almost all patients achieved >80% of platelet inhibition after an abciximab bolus, but ~13% of patients did not maintain this level of inhibition during the infusion.

Even a wider range of variability was noted after the termination of the infusion. Although this study was not designed to evaluate clinical outcomes, systematic measuring of postprocedural myocardial enzymes was carried out. Of the 13 patients with platelet function inhibited by <80% at 8 hours, 6 (46%) had an adverse cardiac event. This is in comparison with only 5 (7%) events among 75 patients with more than 80% inhibition at 8 hours ($p < 0.001$). Although not a predefined objective of the study, these results are consistent with the hypothesis that a specific level of platelet inhibition must be maintained to prevent thrombotic complications associated with PCI.

The GOLD study (31) prospectively enrolled 469 patients undergoing elective PCI with adjunctive GPIIb/IIIa therapy. The RPFA device was used to assess %IPA at base-

(a)

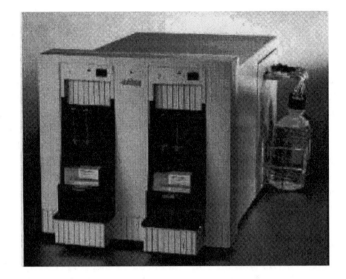

(b)

CSA PUNCH CHANNEL

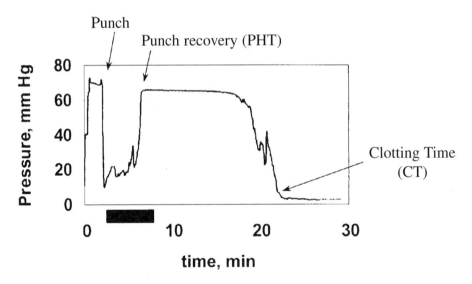

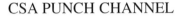

Figure 5 (a) Clot signature analyzer (CSA) instrument. (b) A growing fibrin clot gradually occludes the punched pathway, resulting in reduction of the flow as evidenced by decrease in the pressure. Pressure is plotted against time for both channels to produce a clot signature and generate a clotting time.

line, during PCI, and serially after PCI. The occurrence of death, myocardial infarction, or urgent target revascularization was correlated to the extent of %IPA during the procedure. Specifically, the incidence of this composite ischemic outcome occurred in 14.4% of patients whose platelets were <95% inhibited versus 6.4% for those whose platelets were >95% inhibited ($p = 0.006$). A multivariable model was performed on this data set and showed that the extent of percent IPA was strongly and independently correlated to the ischemic endpoint composite with an odds ratio of 0.44 for those achieving greater than 95% IPA ($p = 0.019$). In the Do Tirofiban And Reopro Give similar Efficacy outcome Trial (TARGET), a lower 30-day incidence of the combined endpoint of death, myocardial infarction, and urgent target vessel revascularization was seen in patients treated with abciximab compared with those who received tirofiban. Kabbani et al. studied whether the difference observed reflected suboptimal inhibition of platelet aggregation during the first 2 hours after initiation of treatment with tirofiban (33). The inhibition of maximal aggregation was greater 15–60 minutes after onset of treatment with abciximab than with tirofiban when aggregation was induced by 20 M adenosine diphosphate. The average inhibition of maximal aggregation ranged from 94 to 94% from 15 to 45 minutes after initiation of treatment with abciximab and from 61 to 66% after initiation of tirofiban ($p < 0.001$ at 15, 30, and 45 min) (33). Similarly, Herrmann et al. demonstrated that that the dose of tirofiban used in TARGET may not have fully inhibited platelet aggregation at the key time point near the initial balloon inflation (35). These findings may potentially explain improved clinical outcomes at 30 days with abciximab compared to tirofiban in the TARGET trial. The pharmacology of higher-dose eptifibatide in percutaneous coronary intervention (the PRIDE study) revealed that a double bolus of eptifibatide at 180 g/kg followed by a 2.0 g/kg/min infusion at steady state achieved >80% inhibition of platelet aggregation (40). With the single-bolus regimen, however, there was an early loss of inhibition of platelet aggregation before steady state was reached. The double-bolus regimen was associated with improved clinical outcomes (41).

Mukherjee et al. reported several illustrative cases in which platelet monitoring with the Ultegra Rapid Platelet Function Assay was used to guide dosing of a GP IIb/IIIa inhibitor for coronary and peripheral intervention among patients at increased bleeding risk (42). While GP IIb/IIIa inhibitors are not currently indicated for patients with thrombocytopenia or those on oral anticoagulants, the case series demonstrated that these agents may be used safely and effectively in some of these patients with reduction of GP IIb/IIIa dosage and monitoring of IPA% (42).

In summary, GP IIb/IIIa antagonists are becoming the standard of care for patients undergoing PCI and those with ACS. As such, there are many scenarios related to the patient, clinical situation, or other phenomenon whereby monitoring the extent of platelet aggregation inhibition would be useful. Outcome data are becoming available, suggesting that a specific extent of %IPA may be optimal. With evolution of monitoring techniques, the hope is that this class of drug can be extended to more patients without increasing bleeding rates. Among those currently receiving therapy, monitoring may not only improve efficacy but also reduce adverse events.

VI. ASPIRIN RESISTANCE

Despite proven benefit of aspirin in patients with coronary artery disease, there is evidence that a subset of patients may not benefit from aspirin therapy. There are no drugs that are 100% effective, but there appears an identifiable subset of patients in whom aspirin is less efficacious, and these individuals are considered aspirin resistant. Gum et al. (43) demonstrated that among patients with cardiac disease, 5–9% are aspirin resistant and an additional 23% are aspirin semiresponders. Previous studies have demonstrated a significantly higher vascular event rate in aspirin nonresponders (44). The availability of safe and effective alternate antiplatelet therapy makes the identification of these individuals with aspirin resistance clinically relevant.

VII. COMBINATION THERAPIES

The use of combination antithrombotic and antiplatelet therapies in the treatment of cardiovascular diseases has significantly increased in the last few years. The most commonly used combination is glycoprotein IIb/IIIa inhibitor and UFH. To investigate the possible influence of platelet IIb/IIIa antagonism on procedural ACT, Moliterno et al. analyzed data from the Evaluation of c7E3 Fab in the Prevention of Ischemic Complications (EPIC) trial. In the EPIC trial, 2099 patients undergoing PCI were randomized to receive placebo ($n =$ 696) or the IIb/IIIa platelet receptor antagonist abciximab ($n = 1403$). Despite receiving less procedural heparin and fewer patients receiving very high heparin doses (>14,000 U) than the placebo group, those receiving abciximab had a higher mean (401 vs. 367 s; $p < 0.001$) ACT when corrected for body weight. The ACT was increased approximately 35 seconds by abciximab. Subsequent studies using lower doses of heparin have not found a significant prolongation of the ACT by abciximab. The dose of heparin used in the EPIC trial (100 U/kg) resulted in significantly higher bleeding complications compared to placebo. In the EPILOG trial, a reduction in the dose of heparin from 100 to 70 U/kg with adjunctive abciximab resulted in a significant reduction in major bleeding from 3.5 to 2.0% with no reduction in benefit (11). Thus, it is apparent that dose adjustment is indicated when using potent therapies in combination. There are evolving data on the combination of bivalirudin and enoxaparin with glycoprotein IIb/IIIa inhibitors. Several studies are also evaluating more effective adjunctive therapy with fibrinolytics in the form of LMWH such as enoxaparin, abciximab (a glycoprotein IIb/IIIa inhibitor), and bivalirudin (a direct thrombin inhibitor). The combination of two long-acting agents such as tenecteplase and enoxaparin raises questions about adequacy/excessive anticoagulation if the patient needs catheterization and PCI. Streptokinase is probably best avoided as a fibrinolytic therapy in combination with LMWH or glycoprotein IIb/IIIa inhibitors as fibrinogen can no longer be used as a parameter to measure anticoagulation. Monitoring of these potent combinations may be especially important in patients with renal insufficiency and individuals with high or low body weight.

VIII. FUTURE DIRECTIONS

Several antithrombotic and antiplatelet agents have been separately shown to reduce the risk of adverse events during PCI and in the medical management of patients. These therapies are now being used in combination in a significant proportion of patients. In attempts to improve efficacy and safety while broadening the population receiving these drugs, rapid point-of-care devices have been developed. Although no monitoring device has clearly been shown to improve clinical outcome, data are emerging that show the ability to correlate the extent of anticoagulation/antiplatelet effect with outcome. At the same time, evolution of device technology has improved, such that correlation with central laboratory monitoring has a very high correlation coefficient. For the future a therapeutic window will continue to be defined for each of these newer agents when used either as monotherapy or, more likely, as part of combination therapy.

REFERENCES

1. Granger CB, Hirsch J, Califf RM, et al. Activated partial thromboplastin time and outcome after thrombolytic therapy for acute myocardial infarction: results from the GUSTO-I trial. Circulation 1996; 93:870–878.

2. Randomized trial of intravenous heparin versus recombinant hirudin for acute coronary syndromes. The Global Use of Strategies to Open Occluded Coronary Arteries (GUSTO) IIa Investigators. Circulation 1994; 90:1631–1637.

3. Ryan TJ, Antman EM, Brooks NH, et al. 1999 update: ACC/AHA guidelines for the management of patients with acute myocardial infarction. A report of the American College of Cardiology/American Heart Association Task Force on Practice Guidelines (Committee on Management of Acute Myocardial Infarction). J Am Coll Cardiol 1999; 34:890–911.

4. McGarry TF, Jr., Gottlieb RS, Morganroth J, et al. The relationship of anticoagulation level and complications after successful percutaneous transluminal coronary angioplasty. Am Heart J 1992; 123:1445–1451.

5. Ferguson JJ, Dougherty KG, Gaos CM, et al. Relation between procedural activated coagulation time and outcome after percutaneous transluminal coronary angioplasty. J Am Coll Cardiol 1994; 23:1061–1065.

6. Narins CR, Hillegass WB, Jr., Nelson CL, et al. Relation between activated clotting time during angioplasty and abrupt closure. Circulation 1996; 93:667–671.

7. Bittl JA, Ahmed WH. Relation between abrupt vessel closure and the anticoagulant response to heparin or bivalirudin during coronary angioplasty. Am J Cardiol 1998; 82:50P–56P.

8. Chew DP, Bhatt DL, Lincoff AM, et al. Defining the optimal activated clotting time during percutaneous coronary intervention: aggregate results from 6 randomized, controlled trials. Circulation 2001; 103:961–966.

9. Giavarina D, Carta M, Fabbri A, et al. Monitoring high-dose heparin levels by ACT and HMT during extracorporeal circulation: diagnostic accuracy of three compact monitors. Perfusion 2002; 17:23–26.

10. Gravlee GP, Haddon WS, Rothberger HK, et al. Heparin dosing and monitoring for cardiopulmonary bypass. A comparison of techniques with measurement of subclinical plasma coagulation. J Thorac Cardiovasc Surg 1990; 99:518–527.

11. Platelet glycoprotein IIb/IIIa receptor blockade and low-dose heparin during percutaneous coronary revascularization. The EPILOG Investigators. N Engl J Med 1997; 336:1689–1696.

12. Smith SC, Jr., Dove JT, Jacobs AK, et al. ACC/AHA guidelines of percutaneous coronary interventions (revision of the 1993 PTCA guidelines)—executive summary. A report of the American College of Cardiology/American Heart Association Task Force on Practice Guidelines (committee to revise the 1993 guidelines for percutaneous transluminal coronary angioplasty). J Am Coll Cardiol 2001; 37:2215–2239.

13. Avendano A, Ferguson JJ. Comparison of Hemochron and HemoTec activated coagulation time target values during percutaneous transluminal coronary angioplasty. J Am Coll Cardiol 1994; 23:907–910.

14. Boccara A, Benamer H, Juliard JM, et al. A randomized trial of a fixed high dose vs a weight-adjusted low dose of intravenous heparin during coronary angioplasty. Eur Heart J 1997; 18:631–635.

15. Henry TD, Satran D, Knox LL, et al. Are activated clotting times helpful in the management of anticoagulation with subcutaneous low-molecular-weight heparin? Am Heart J 2001; 142:590–593.

16. Rabah MM, Premmereur J, Graham M, et al. Usefulness of intravenous enoxaparin for percutaneous coronary intervention in stable angina pectoris. Am J Cardiol 1999; 84:1391–1395.

17. Holmes MB, Schneider DJ, Hayes MG, et al. Novel, bedside, tissue factor-dependent clotting assay permits improved assessment of combination antithrombotic and antiplatelet therapy. Circulation 2000; 102:2051–2057.

18. Kitchen S, Iampietro R, Woolley AM, et al. Anti Xa monitoring during treatment with low molecular weight heparin or danaparoid: inter-assay variability. Thromb Haemost 1999; 82:1289–1293.

19. Kereiakes DJ, Montalescot G, Antman EM, et al. Low-molecular-weight heparin therapy for non-ST-elevation acute coronary syndromes and during percutaneous coronary intervention: an expert consensus. Am Heart J 2002; 144:615–624.

20. Kereiakes DJ, Grines C, Fry E, et al. Enoxaparin and abciximab adjunctive pharmacotherapy during percutaneous coronary intervention. J Invasive Cardiol 2001; 13:272–278.

21. Collet JP, Montalescot G, Lison L, et al. Percutaneous coronary intervention after subcutaneous enoxaparin pretreatment in patients with unstable angina pectoris. Circulation 2001; 103:658–663.

22. Bhatt D, Lee B, Casterella P, et al. Safety of concomitant therapy with eptifibatide and enoxaparin in patients undergoing percutaneous coronary intervention: Results of the coronary revascularization using integrilin and single bolus enoxaparin study. J Am Coll Cardiol 2003; 41:20–25.

23. Kereiakes DJ, Fry E, Matthai W, et al. Combination enoxaparin and abciximab therapy during percutaneous coronary intervention: "NICE guys finish first." J Invasive Cardiol 2000; 12(suppl A):1A–5A.

24. Kereiakes DJ, Kleiman NS, Fry E, et al. Dalteparin in combination with abciximab during percutaneous coronary intervention. Am Heart J 2001; 141:348–352.

25. Bittl JA, Chaitman BR, Feit F, et al. Bivalirudin versus heparin during coronary angioplasty for unstable or postinfarction angina: final report reanalysis of the Bivalirudin Angioplasty Study. Am Heart J 2001; 142:952–959.

26. Bittl JA, Strony J, Brinker JA, et al. Treatment with bivalirudin (Hirulog) as compared with heparin during coronary angioplasty for unstable or postinfarction angina. Hirulog Angioplasty Study Investigators. N Engl J Med 1995; 333:764–769.

27. Lincoff AM, Kleiman NS, Kottke-Marchant K, et al. Bivalirudin with planned or provisional abciximab versus low-dose heparin and abciximab during percutaneous coronary revascularization: results of the Comparison of Abciximab Complications with Hirulog for Ischemic Events Trial (CACHET). Am Heart J 2002; 143:847–853.

28. Fenyvesi T, Jorg I, Harenberg J. Monitoring of anticoagulant effects of direct thrombin inhibitors. Semin Thromb Hemost 2002; 28:361–368.

29. Cho L, Kottke-Marchant K, Roffi M, et al. A new rapid ecarin clotting time assay but not activated clotting time strongly correlates with bivalirudin cocentration: a percutaneous coronary intervention study. J Am Coll Cardiol 2002; in press.

30. Nowak G, Bucha E. Quantitative determination of hirudin in blood and body fluids. Semin Thromb Hemost 1996; 22:197–202.

31. Steinhubl SR, Talley JD, Braden GA, et al. Point-of-care measured platelet inhibition correlates with a reduced risk of an adverse cardiac event after percutaneous coronary intervention: results of the GOLD (AU-Assessing Ultegra) multicenter study. Circulation 2001; 103:2572–2578.

32. Chew DP, Moliterno DJ. A critical appraisal of platelet glycoprotein IIb/IIIa inhibition. J Am Coll Cardiol 2000; 36:2028–2035.

33. Kabbani SS, Aggarwal A, Terrien EF, et al. Suboptimal early inhibition of platelets by treatment with tirofiban and implications for coronary interventions. Am J Cardiol 2002; 89:647–650.

34. Kabbani SS, Watkins MW, Ashikaga T, et al. Platelet reactivity characterized prospectively: a determinant of outcome 90 days after percutaneous coronary intervention. Circulation 2001; 104:181–186.

35. Herrmann HC, Swierkosz TA, Kapoor S, et al. Comparison of degree of platelet inhibition by abciximab versus tirofiban in patients with unstable angina pectoris and non-Q-wave myocardial infarction undergoing percutaneous coronary intervention. Am J Cardiol 2002; 89:1293–1297.

36. Mammen EF, Comp PC, Gosselin R, et al. PFA-100 system: a new method for assessment of platelet dysfunction. Semin Thromb Hemost 1998; 24:195–202.

37. Kereiakes DJ, Mueller M, Howard W, et al. Efficacy of abciximab induced platelet blockade using a rapid point of care assay. J Thromb Thrombolysis 1999; 7:265–276.

38. Kereiakes DJ, Broderick TM, Roth EM, et al. Time course, magnitude, and consistency of platelet inhibition by abciximab, tirofiban, or eptifibatide in patients with unstable angina pectoris undergoing percutaneous coronary intervention. Am J Cardiol 1999; 84:391–395.

39. Steinhubl SR, Kottke-Marchant K, Moliterno DJ, et al. Attainment and maintenance of platelet inhibition through standard dosing of abciximab in diabetic and nondiabetic patients undergoing percutaneous coronary intervention. Circulation 1999; 100:1977–1982.

40. Tcheng JE, Talley JD, O'Shea JC, et al. Clinical pharmacology of higher dose eptifibatide in percutaneous coronary intervention (the PRIDE study). Am J Cardiol 2001; 88:1097–1102.

41. O'Shea JC, Hafley GE, Greenberg S, et al. Platelet glycoprotein IIb/IIIa integrin blockade with eptifibatide in coronary stent intervention: the ESPRIT trial: a randomized controlled trial. JAMA 2001; 285:2468–2473.

42. Mukherjee D, Chew DP, Robbins M, et al. Clinical application of procedural platelet monitoring during percutaneous coronary intervention among patients at increased bleeding risk. J Thromb Thrombolysis 2001; 11:151–154.

43. Gum PA, Kottke-Marchant K, Poggio ED, et al. Profile and prevalence of aspirin resistance in patients with cardiovascular disease. Am J Cardiol 2001; 88:230–235.

44. Grotemeyer KH, Scharafinski HW, Husstedt IW. Two-year follow-up of aspirin responder and aspirin non responder. A pilot-study including 180 post-stroke patients. Thromb Res 1993; 71:397–403.

45. Moliterno DJ, Mukherjee D. Applications of monitoring platelet glycoprotein IIb/IIIa antagonism and low molecular weight heparins in cardiovascular medicine. Am Heart J 2000; 140:S136–142.

9-2

Clinical Trials of Combination Pharmacotherapy for ST-Elevation Acute Myocardial Infarction

Craig R. Narins
University of Rochester School of Medicine and Dentistry,
Rochester, New York, U.S.A.

In acute myocardial infarction, regardless of the reperfusion strategy employed, survival is a direct function of the rapidity and reliability with which patency of the infarct-related artery can be restored. While numerous clinical trials have established the efficacy of both mechanical (primary percutaneous coronary intervention [PCI]) and pharmacological (fibrinolytic therapy) approaches to achieve reperfusion, both of these therapeutic modalities possess limitations in clinical practice. Primary PCI, while generally regarded as the treatment of choice for acute ST elevation myocardial infarction (MI), is available in less than 20% of hospitals in the United States, limiting its widespread applicability (1). Fibrinolytic therapy, although universally available, is hampered by lower rates of reperfusion and higher incidences of infarct artery reocclusion and major bleeding events relative to catheter-based strategies.

These shortcomings have led to attempts to improve the effectiveness and safety of medical reperfusion therapy, and "combination therapy" consisting of the conjoint administration of a fibrinolytic agent at a reduced dose and a platelet glycoprotein (GP) IIb/IIIa receptor antagonist has emerged as a possible alternative to stand-alone fibrinolytic therapy. The use of GP IIb/IIIa antagonists as an adjunct to fibrinolytics in acute ST segment MI is based on (a) the proven effectiveness of these agents in the setting of both percutaneous coronary intervention (PCI) and non–ST elevation acute coronary syndromes (2–4), (b) expanding observations that have highlighted the importance of platelet activation and aggregation in the pathogenesis of both acute coronary syndromes and of fibrinolytic failure (5,6), (c) the well-established safety profile of GP IIb/IIIa antagonists (7–9), and (d) a theoretic perspective of the enhanced compatibility of this regimen with the practice of early coronary angiography and percutaneous revascularization as commonly employed in the United States (10). Over the past several years combination therapy has been examined in a series of clinical trials, and this chapter will critically review the results of these studies and outline areas of ongoing investigation aimed at better clarifying the role of combination therapy in clinical practice.

I. SHORTCOMINGS OF FIBRINOLYTIC THERAPY

The primary shortcoming of stand-alone fibrinolytic therapy is its failure, among a substantial proportion of patients with acute MI, to bring about timely restoration of normal flow within the infarct-related artery. In the Global Utilization of Streptokinase and Tissue Plasminogen Activator of Occluded Coronary Arteries (GUSTO) I angiographic substudy, TIMI-3 flow was present 90 minutes after initiation of fibrinolytics in only 32% of individuals randomized to streptokinase plus intravenous heparin and in 54% treated with t-PA and heparin (11–13). The speed and completeness of reperfusion correlate strongly with preservation of left ventricular function and the likelihood of adverse clinical events including death. As elegantly demonstrated by the GUSTO I investigators, failure to achieve TIMI-3 flow by 90 minutes was associated with an approximate doubling of the 30-day mortality rate (Fig. 1). While newer fibrin-selective fibrinolytic agents have emerged over the past decade, these drugs have not been associated with further improvements in reperfusion rates or survival benefits beyond those of t-PA (14–16).

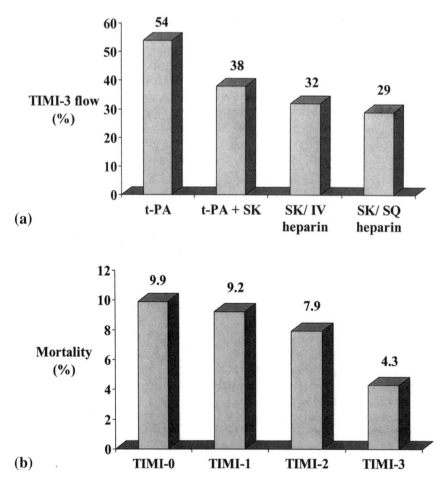

Figure 1   (a) TIMI-3 flow at 90 minutes by treatment arm in the GUSTO I trial; (b) The relationship between completeness of revascularizton at 90-minutes and 30-day survival in the GUSTO I angiographic substudy.

Early infarct artery reocclusion following initial restoration of patency, an event that occurs in 15–30% of fibrinolytic-treated patients, represents a second major deficiency of fibrinolytic therapy. Reocclusion, when it does occur, is associated with a two- to threefold increase in mortality (17). A third drawback relates to the increased potential for major bleeding complications among patients who receive fibrinolytic agents, relative to placebo-treated patients or individuals who undergo primary PCI for treatment of acute MI. Intracranial hemorrhage, the most feared of such events, is observed with frequencies of approximately 0.4% following streptokinase administration and 0.5–1.0% after t-PA. Fourth, among patients treated with full-dose fibrinolytic therapy who require immediate percutaneous revascularization, most often in the setting of persistent or recurrent culprit vessel occlusion, the failure and complication rates of angioplasty are increased (relative to patients undergoing direct primary angioplasty) (18,19). Whether this is due to a selection bias or an adverse effect of the fibrinolytic agent is not certain.

II. THEORETICAL RATIONALE FOR COMBINATION THERAPY

Fibrinolytic agents, via activation of endogenous plaminogen, promote dissolution of the fibrin-rich component of the occlusive thrombus but are not directly capable of producing degeneration of the platelet aggregates that are also integral to the structure of the clot. In fact, fibrinolysis results in the liberation and enhanced production of thrombin, which is among the most potent of known platelet agonists (20,21). Consequently, the byproducts of fibrinolysis can engender a pro-platelet aggregatory response within the microenvironment of the clot undergoing dissolution which may, paradoxically, favor persistent or recurrent vessel occlusion (22,23). Some controversy exists regarding this issue, as other investigators have found that plasmin and various fibrinolytic agents may actually promote platelet disaggregation (24). From a clinical perspective, however, the synergism that exists between fibrinolytic and antiplatelet agents in the treatment of acute MI is exemplified by the additive survival benefits and reduced likelihood of coronary reocclusion and recurrent ischemia when aspirin is co-administered with fibrinolytic therapy (25,26).

The robust clinical benefits of aspirin therapy during thrombolysis likely relate at least in part to the drug's ability to modulate the pro-platelet aggregatory effects of fibrinolytics. Aspirin exerts its anti-platelet properties by inhibition of thromboxane A_2–induced platelet activation, and concentrations of thromboxane A_2 metabolites and other platelet agonists have been shown to increase during fibrinolysis (22,27). Despite the clinical benefits of aspirin administration during acute MI, aspirin is a relatively weak platelet antagonist, and it has been postulated that some patients who fail to achieve reperfusion after fibrinolytic administration may do so as a result of inadequate platelet inhibition rather than inadequate fibrinolysis. Because thromboxane A_2 represents only one of possibly more than 100 promoters of platelet activation, aspirin monotherapy may be insufficient in instances to overcome the pro-platelet triggers present in the highly prothrombotic milieu of a clot undergoing lysis. In addition, a growing body of evidence suggests that a certain percentage of individuals may be "resistant" to the antiplatelet effects of aspirin (28,29). Depending upon the measurement technique used and the population under study, between 5 and 55% of individuals treated with aspirin fail to demonstrate the expected degree of platelet inhibition and have been termed aspirin "nonresponders" or "partial responders" (Table 1) (30–36). Two small clinical follow-up studies have shown an association between aspirin nonresponsiveness and an increased likelihood of future

Table 1 Prevalence of Aspirin Resistance Among Patients with Cardiovascular Disease

n	Aspirin-resistant (%)	Method	Ref.
40	42.5	Bleeding Time	31
289	54.7	Bleeding time	32
180	33	Platelet reactivity test	34
Not stated	55	Flow cytometry and aggregometry	69
326	5.2	Optical aggregometry	36

adverse cardiac events among patients with stable cardiovascular disease (30,34). The potential relationship between aspirin resistance and lytic failure, while intriguing, remains to be studied.

Given the potential link between inadequate or incomplete platelet inhibition following aspirin therapy and failed reperfusion or vessel reocclusion following fibrinolysis, GP IIb/IIIa antagonist therapy was proposed as a potentially more effective adjunct to fibrinolytic therapy. While aspirin therapy results in modest (well below 50%) relative reductions in platelet aggregation, the GP IIb/IIIa antagonists, by occupying the IIb/IIIa receptor and thereby disabling the final common pathway of platelet aggregation, have the ability to result in dose-dependent 80–100% relative reductions in platelet aggregatory capacity. The clinical benefits of combined GP IIb/IIIa antagonist plus aspirin therapy (versus aspirin monotherapy) have been well demonstrated among patients presenting with non–ST segment elevation acute coronary syndromes and those undergoing elective or urgent percutaneous coronary revascularization (2,4). The safety of the GP IIb/IIIa antagonist therapy has also been established in these patient populations (8,9). For example, among the 10,948 patients enrolled in the randomized PURSUIT trial of eptifibitide versus placebo for treatment of acute coronary syndromes, primary hemorrhagic stroke occurred with an incidence of only 0.1% among those who received GP IIb/IIIa antagonist therapy, which was identical to the occurrence rate in the placebo control arm (9).

III. CLINICAL TRIALS OF COMBINATION THERAPY: PILOT STUDIES

After exploratory work in the canine model of coronary thrombosis was performed (37,38), a series of eight small to medium-sized dose-ranging clinical studies were undertaken to evaluate the safety and derive preliminary insights regarding the efficacy of combinations of various fibrinolytic agents and GP IIb/IIIa antagonists administered in the setting of acute MI (39–46). In all trials, patients were treated with either combination therapy or stand-alone fibrinolytic therapy. Aspirin and heparin therapy were routinely administered to all patients. While not adequately powered to evaluate clinical endpoints, most of these phase II trials employed early (60–90 min) angiography as a surrogate endpoint to assess the speed and completeness of reperfusion associated with various combinations of agents (Table 2). Based on the generally encouraging findings of these pilot studies, two larger multicenter randomized trials, GUSTO V and Assessment the Safety and Effficacy of a New Thrombolytic Regimen 3 (ASSENT-3), were performed (47,48).

1. Trials of Full-Dose Fibrinolytic Administration

The first clinical study to evaluate combination pharmacotherapy for acute MI was the non-randomized Thrombolytic and Angioplasty in Myocardial Infarction (TAMI-8) trial

Table 2 Angiographic and Bleeding Complication Data from Phase II Trials of Combination Pharmacotherapy

Study	n	Therapy	60- to 90-Minute TIMI-3 flow (%)		Vessel patency (TIMI-2 or -3 flow, %)		Major bleeding (%)	
			Combination arm	Lytic control arm	Combination arm	Lytic control arm	Combination arm	Lytic control arm
Full-Dose Lytic								
TAMI-8	70	rt-PA, abciximab	—	—	92	56[a]	25	50
IMPACT-AMI	180	Alteplase, eptifibitaide	66	39[a]	87	69[a]	4	5
Ronner et al.	181	Streptokinase, eptifibitide	44	31	61	78[a]	14	0*
Half-Dose Lytic								
SPEED	419	Reteplase, abciximab	54	47	77	77	9.8	3.7[a]
TIMI-14	888	Streptokinase or alteplase, abciximab[b]	76	62[a]	94	75[a]	6	7
INTEGRETI	438	TNK, eptifibitide	59	49	85	77	7.6	2.5
ENTIRE-TIMI 23	483	TNK, abciximab	51	50	76	75	6.6	2.1[a]

[a] $p < 0.05$.
[b] Angiographic data presented are for alteplase plus abciximab versus alteplase alone.

(39), in which 60 patients with acute ST elevation MI within 6 hours of symptom onset were treated with standard full-dose recombinant tissue-type plasminogen activator (rt-PA) and one of four doses (0.1, 0.15, 0.20, or 0.25 mg/kg) of monoclonal antibody 7E3 Fab (abciximab). Abciximab was administered as three sequential boluses given at 3, 6, and 15 hours after initiation of rt-PA. Ten patients who received standard dose rt-PA without abciximab therapy served as the control group. Patients were observed for bleeding complications and clinical events. With this "delayed IIb/IIIa" dosing strategy, only patients who received the highest abciximab dose (0.25 mg/kg) demonstrated consistent blockade of ≥ 80% of platelet GP IIb/IIIa receptors. Major bleeding, defined as a ≥ 15% drop in hematocrit with or without need for blood transfusion, was common among both the abciximab and control groups (incidences of 25 and 50%, respectively), although half of the bleeding events in the abciximab group were related to subsequent coronary artery bypass surgery. Routine coronary angiography was not performed, but 61% of patients did undergo angiography an average of 5 days following rt-PA administration. Infarct artery patency (TIMI grade 2 or 3 flow) was more common among patients who received rt-PA and abciximab compared to those treated with rt-PA alone (92 vs. 56%). Clinical ischemic events were uncommon and similar in frequency among the treatment and control arms.

The Integrelin to Manage Platelet Aggregation to Prevent Coronary Thrombosis in Acute MI (IMPACT-AMI) trial was a placebo-controlled trial of eptifibitide administered with accelerated full-dose alteplase during ST elevation MI. In the dose-ranging phase of this trial, 132 patients were treated with one of six ascending doses of eptifibitide (bolus plus a 24-hour infusion) begun concomitantly with the alteplase (40). The group that received the highest eptifibitide dose (180 μg bolus and 0.75 μg/kg/min infusion, $n = 16$) achieved ≥70% inhibition in platelet aggregation relative to baseline that persisted for 24 hours, experienced no deaths or reinfarctions, and demonstrated a 6% incidence of severe bleeding. In the second (randomized, placebo-controlled) phase, 48 additional patients were randomized to receive combination therapy (alteplase plus the highest eptifibatide dose from phase 1) or alteplase alone. Patients who received combination therapy demonstrated evidence of more rapid reperfusion than control patients as measured by faster time to ST segment recovery on continuous ECG monitoring (65 vs. 116 minutes; $p = 0.05$) and higher likelihood of TIMI grade 3 flow at 90-minute angiography (66 vs. 39%; $p = 0.006$). Severe bleeding events were infrequent in both the study groups (4 vs. 5%).

Ronner et al. performed a phase II multicenter, randomized, double-blind dose-escalating study of eptifibatide (180 μg/kg bolus plus 72-hr infusion at 0.75, 1.33, or 2.0 μg/kg/min) plus full-dose streptokinase versus streptokinase without GP IIb/IIIa antagonist therapy (41). Enrollment in the highest dose eptifibatide group was terminated early due to excess bleeding complications (54% incidence of major or minor bleeding). Patients randomized to eptifibatide (all dose groups combined) demonstrated a strong trend toward greater likelihood of TIMI grade 3 flow at 90-minute angiography than did control patients (44 vs. 31%, p=0.07) and a significant improvement in combined TIMI-2/3 flow (78 vs. 61%; $p = 0.02$). Vessel patency rates were similar among the three eptifibitide dosing groups. Major bleeding events occurred more commonly among patients who received eptifibatide rather than placebo (14 vs. 0%).

In the Platelet Aggregation Receptor Antagonist Dose Investigation and Reperfusion Gain in Myocardial Infarction (PARADIGM) Trial, 252 patients with acute MI were treated with combinations of the nonpeptide GP IIb/IIIa antagonist lamifiban and either accelerated t-PA or standard-dose streptokinase (42). In the dose-escalating phase of the trial, lamifiban was found to result in dose-dependent inhibition of adenosine diphosphate (ADP) and thrombin receptor agonist peptide (TRAP)-induced platelet aggregation, with the highest doses yielding >85% inhibition. Including all patients enrolled in the dose-finding and randomized phases of the trial, time to resolution of ST elevation on continuous ECG monitoring was significantly shorter among patients receiving combination lamifiban and fibrinolytic treatment compared to those who received fibrinolytic therapy alone (88 vs. 122 minutes, $p = 0.003$). Bleeding events requiring transfusion were, however, more frequent among patients assigned to combined lytic and GP IIb/IIIa antagonist therapy (16.1 vs. 10.3%).

2. Trials of Reduced-Dose Fibrinolytic Administration

In aggregate, the initial four phase II trials described above highlighted the potential for more frequent and more rapid restoration of infarct artery patency when fibrinolytic therapy was administered with an adjuvant GP IIb/IIIa antagonist, at the cost of a heightened risk of bleeding events in some but not all of the studies. Four subsequent studies— Strategies for Patency Enhancement in the Emergency Department (SPEED), Thrombolysis in Myocardial Infarction 14 (TIMI 14), Enoxaparin and TNK-tPA with or without GP IIb/IIIa Inhibitor as Reperfusion Strategy in ST Elevation MI (ENTIRE-TIMI 23), and Integrelin and Tenecteplase in Acute Myocardial Infarction (INTEGRETI)— sought to determine whether a strategy of combining reduced dosages of fibrinolytics with GP IIb/IIIa antagonists could result in a reduction of bleeding risk without a sacrifice in thrombolytic efficacy.

The SPEED trial was a two-phase study that included a total of 419 patients with acute ST elevation MI who presented within 12 hours of symptom onset (43). In the initial (dose-finding) phase, patients were randomized to receive abciximab (0.25 mg/kg bolus and 0.125 µg/kg/min infusion for 12 hr) alone or concomitantly with one of five escalating dosage regimens of reteplase (ranging from 25 to 50% of the standard dose in various bolus combinations). All patients also received aspirin and heparin therapy. Angiography was routinely performed 60–90 minutes following drug initiation (Figure 2). Percutaneous revascularization could be performed at this time at the discretion of the treating physician. Interestingly, 27% of patients treated with abciximab alone demonstrated normalization of flow in the infarct vessel on early angiography. Among patients assigned to combined abciximab and reteplase, those who received half-standard dose

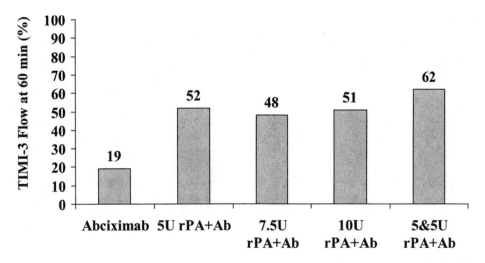

Figure 2 Rates of TIMI-3 flow at 60 minutes by treatment assignment in the SPEED study. RPA = reteplase; Ab = abciximab.

dual-bolus reteplase (serial 5 mg boluses 30 min apart) demonstrated the highest rates of early TIMI-3 flow. The incidences of major bleeding and need for transfusion were similar among individuals treated with the abciximab and 5 & 5 U reteplase regimen and those treated with abciximab alone (5.3 vs. 3.3% for major bleeding, 9.3 vs. 9.8% for transfusion for reteplase + abciximab vs. abciximab-alone groups).

In the second phase of the SPEED trial, patients were randomized to receive either the abciximab plus half-dose reteplase regimen that was most effective in the dose-finding phase of the study or standard-dose reteplase without GP IIb/IIIa antagonist therapy. Patients in the combination therapy arm received either a standard (60 U/kg) or low-dose (40 U/kg) heparin bolus, while reteplase-treated patients were treated with a 70 U/kg bolus. Angiography at 60–90 minutes (mean 62 min) demonstrated no significant difference between the treatment groups with respect to TIMI-3 flow in the infarct artery (54 vs. 47%; $p = 0.39$). On a post hoc analysis, which was limited to combination therapy patients who received the 60 U/kg heparin bolus, a borderline significant improvement in TIMI-3 flow rates was observed relative to reteplase-only treated patients (61 vs. 47%; $p = 0.05$). A nonsignificant trend toward increased major bleeding events was also noted in the combination therapy arm (9.8 vs. 3.7%).

The TIMI 14 trial was likewise a multiphase exploratory study that in total included 888 patients with acute MI who were randomized to standard-dose alteplase monotherapy or abciximab (same dose as used in SPEED) alone or in combination with one of several reduced doses of alteplase (20–65 mg) or reduced-to-full doses of streptokinase (0.5–1.5 million units) (44,49,50). Patients underwent 60- and 90-minute angiograms (Fig. 3) and were followed for clinical bleeding events. Consistent with observations from the SPEED trial, 32% of patients with acute MI who received treated with abciximab alone demonstrated TIMI-3 flow by 90 minutes posttreatment (similar to the rate of TIMI-3 flow noted with stand-alone streptokinase therapy in the GUSTO I study). Alteplase monotherapy, comparable to prior reports, was associated with a 57% rate of TIMI-3 flow at 90 minutes. Interestingly, 90-minute TIMI-3 rates for patients assigned to combination abciximab plus streptokinase therapy (all doses combined) were inferior to those observed for patients treated with alteplase alone (42 vs. 57%). The most effective regimen based on the 90-minute angiogram consisted of half-dose alteplase (15 mg bolus and 35 mg infusion over 60 min) plus abciximab, which was associated with a 76% rate of TIMI-3 flow ($p = 0.08$ compared to alteplase alone).

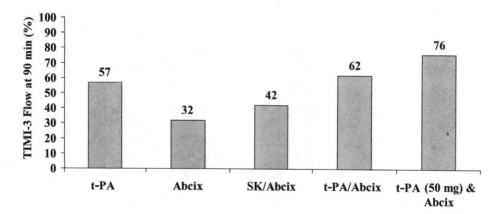

Figure 3 Relationship between various pharmacological regimens and TIMI-3 flow at 90 minutes in the TIMI 14 study. Abcix = abciximab; SK = streptokinase.

In the dose-confirmation phase of the study, additional patients were randomized to the abciximab + half-dose alteplase regimen or to full-dose alteplase without abciximab. Pooled data from both phases of the study revealed a significant improvement in the rate of TIMI-3 flow at 60 minutes (72% vs. 43%; $p = 0.0009$) and 90 minutes (77 vs. 62%; $p = 0.01$) for patients treated with combination therapy (and low-dose heparin) rather than fibrinolytic therapy and heparin, respectively. Major bleeding events occurred among 6% of patients treated with alteplase alone, 7% who received any abciximab/alteplase combination, and 10% of streptokinase/abciximab-treated individuals.

The INTEGRETI trial explored the safety and efficacy of combined therapy with eptifibatide and tenecteplase among patients with acute MI (46). In the dose-finding phase of the trial ($n = 189$), various regimens of epitifibitide combined with half-dose tenecteplase yielded similar rates of TIMI-3 flow (ranging from 64 to 68%) at 60 minutes, but the eptifibitide dose of sequential 180 µg/kg boluses 10 minutes apart in conjunction with a 2 µg/kg/min infusion produced the highest rate of arterial patency at 60 minutes (96%) and was chosen for the dose-confirmation phase of the trial. In this latter phase, 249 patients with acute MI were randomized to either combined eptifibitide and half-dose tenecteplase or full-dose tenecteplase. Nonsignificant trends toward improved angiographic outcomes at 60 minutes were observed in the combination arm, including increased incidences of TIMI-3 flow (59 vs. 49%; $p = 0.015$) and arterial patency (85 vs. 77%; $p = 0.17$). A significant decrease in the combined clinical endpoint of death, reinfarction, or urgent target vessel revascularization was noted at 48 hours (3.4 vs. 11.0%; $p = 0.02$), but this difference was no longer observed at 30 days. No difference in the rate of intracranial hemorrhage was observed between the groups, but the rate of transfusion and major noncerebral bleeding events was significantly greater in the combination therapy arm.

The ENTIRE-TIMI 23 trial was an open-label phase 2 study that examined the safety of various doses of enoxaparin in comparison to unfractionated heparin as an adjunct to either full-dose tenecteplase (TNK) or half-dose TNK plus abciximab (45). The trial enrolled 483 patients and demonstrated a significantly reduced incidence of clinical events (defined as the composite of death, reinfarction, or major hemorrhage at 30 days) among patients treated with enoxaparin rather than unfractionated heparin in conjunction with either full-dose TNK or half-dose TNK and abciximab (Table 3). Patients assigned to full-dose TNK plus enoxaparin demonstrated a reduced rate of major hemorrhage compared to patients treated with combination GP IIb/IIIa antagonist and half-dose TNK therapy.

In summary, SPEED and TIMI 14 expanded the observations of the earlier small phase II trials by demonstrating that (a) that reduced (half-standard) doses of fibrin-specific fibrinolytic agents administered simultaneously with abciximab are associated with similar or perhaps improved rates of early reperfusion compared to those achieved when full doses of fibrinolytics are used in conjunction with GP IIb/IIIa antagonists, (b) while maintaining therapeutic efficacy, reduced doses of fibrinolytics as part of combination therapy are associated with a rates of bleeding events that appear to be only slightly in excess of those observed with full-dose fibrinolytic monotherapy, (c) as part of a combination regimen, selective fibrinolytic agents are associated with more rapid and more consistent restoration of infarct vessel patency than is streptokinase, and (d) lower-dose heparin (40–60 U/kg bolus) regimens are probably best from the standpoint of safety when combination therapy is being employed. In addition, the ENTIRE-TIMI 23 study provided preliminary evidence that the low molecular weight heparin (LMWH) enoxaparin may have a safety and efficacy profile that is superior to that of unfractionated heparin when used as an adjunct to either combination therapy or stand-alone fibrinolytic therapy (45,51).

Table 3 Clinical Results of the ENTIRE TIMI 23 Study

Endpoint	Full-dose TNK and unfractionated heparin	Full-dose TNK and enoxaparin	Half-dose TNK, abciximab, and unfractionated heparin	Half-dose TNK, abciximab, and enoxaparin
Complete resolution of ST elevation at 180 minutes (%)	38	4	52	55
30-day death or nonfatal MI (%)	15.9	4.4	6.5	5.5
Major hemorrhage (%)	2.4	1.9	5.2	8.5

IV. CLINICAL ENDPOINT STUDIES

A. GUSTO V

As a whole, phase II trials suggested that combination therapy could be administered with a modestly increased but hopefully acceptable risk of bleeding complications and a modest, statistically significant benefit in terms of the speed and reliability of reperfusion. The GUSTO V trial was designed and statistically powered to determine if the improvements in angiographic endpoints observed with combination therapy in these smaller trials would translate into improvements in clinical outcomes including mortality (52). In this trial, 16588 patients with acute ST elevation MI within 6 hours of symptom onset were randomly assigned to receive half-dose reteplase (5 + 5 u boluses, 30 min apart) and abciximab (0.25 mg/kg bolus and 0.125 µg/kg/min infusion, maximum of 10 µg/min, for 12 hr) or full-dose reteplase (10 + 10 u boluses 30 min apart) and placebo. The dosing strategy selected for the combination therapy group represented the regimen associated with the most favorable results in the dose-ranging phase of the SPEED study. All patients received aspirin and heparin with a goal-activated partial thromboplastin time of 50–70 seconds.

The incidence of 30-day mortality, the prespecified primary endpoint of the study, was lower than anticipated in both the experimental and control groups and disappointingly did not differ significantly based on treatment assignment (5.6 vs. 5.9% for combination therapy vs. reteplase alone, $p = 0.43$), (see Table 4). Among several prespecified characteristic subgroups, including gender, age, diabetes, anterior location of the MI, and time from symptom onset to treatment, no mortality differences emerged between the treatment arms. Small but statistically significant reductions in the frequency of several secondary clinical endpoints were noted, however, at 30-day follow-up among patients randomized to the combination therapy arm, including reinfarction (2.3 vs. 3.5%; $p < 0.0001$), recurrent myocardial ischemia (11.3 vs. 12.8%; $p = 0.004$) and ventricular arrhythmias. The composite endpoint of death, reinfarction, or urgent percutaneous revascularization until hospital discharge or day 7 (whichever came first) was also significantly reduced among patients treated with combination therapy (16.2 vs. 20.6%; $p < 0.0001$).

Severe and moderate nonintracranial bleeding complications were uncommon, but were twice as likely to occur in the half-dose reteplase plus abciximab group than in the full-dose reteplase group (4.6 vs. 2.3%; $p < 0.0001$). The need for transfusions was also slightly but significantly greater among patients assigned to the combination therapy arm (5.7 vs. 4.0%; $p < 0.0001$). The incidence of intracranial hemorrhage did not differ based on treatment assignment (1.0 vs. 0.9% for combination vs. monotherapy). Among those

Table 4 Major Clinical Endpoints in the GUSTO V Trial

Endpoint	Reteplase ($n = 8260$)	Reteplase and abciximab ($n = 8328$)	Odds ratio (95% CI)	p value
30-day death (%)	5.9	5.6	0.95 (0.84, 1.08)	0.43
30-day death or reinfarction (%)	8.8	7.4	0.83 (0.74, 0.93)	0.0011
7-day death, MI, or urgent PCI (%)	20.6	16.2	0.75 (0.69, 0.81)	<0.0001
Use of PCI within 6- hours (%)	8.6	5.6	0.64 (0.56, 0.72)	<0.0001
Use of PCI within 7 days (%)	27.9	25.4	0.88 (0.82, 0.94)	<0.0001
Severe or moderate bleeding (%)[a]	2.3	4.6	2.03 (1.70, 2.42)	<0.0001
Intracranial hemorrhage (%)	0.6	0.6	1.05 (0.71, 1.56)	0.79

[a]Nonintracranial bleeding.

treated with combination therapy, the youngest group of patients (those <57 years old) did demonstrate a relative decrease in the incidence of intracranial hemorrhage compared to those treated with full-dose reteplase, while combination therapy was associated with an excess of this feared complication among the oldest (>83 years old) patients.

In summary, combination therapy was not associated with a survival advantage compared to standard fibrinolytic therapy at 30 days. No subgroup was identified that fared better in terms of mortality at 30 days, although nonsignificant trends toward better survival were observed in higher-risk patients: those with anterior MI, and those treated late, i.e., > 6 hours, after symptom onset. The incidence of several nonfatal adverse events, including reinfarction and recurrent ischemia, was lower in the combination therapy group, but this came at the cost of a two-fold excess in moderate or major bleeding in this group. The authors postulated that the lack of mortality benefit might have resulted from the generalized low-risk nature of the patients enrolled in this study, as reflected by a lower than anticipated overall mortality rate of 5.7%. Indeed, many investigators may have opted not to enroll certain higher-risk patients in GUSTO V, but rather treat them with primary PCI. At the time GUSTO V was published, the authors also speculated that, although no mortality differences were present at 30 days, the reduced incidence of early reinfarction in the combination therapy arm might ultimately translate into a survival advantage on longer-term follow-up. At one-year follow-up, however, identical all-cause mortality rates (8.4%) were observed among the combination therapy and full-dose fibrinolytic arms (53) Subgroup analysis at one year did suggest a trend toward benefit among younger patients with anterior MI.

B. ASSENT-3

The ASSENT-3 trial was an open-label randomized study in which a total of 6095 patients with acute MI were assigned to one of three treatment groups: (a) full-dose TNK plus the low molecular weight heparin enoxaparin (30 mg iv bolus, followed by 1 mg/kg subcutaneously every 12 hours until hospital discharge for a maximum of 7 days), (b) half-dose TNK plus abciximab (same dose as in GUSTO V) with low-dose unfractionated heparin, or (c) full-dose TNK plus unfractionated heparin (48). The primary endpoint was the composite of death, in-hospital reinfarction, or refractory ischemia at 30 days, which occurred less often ($p = 0.0001$) among patients in the TNK plus enoxaparin (11.4%) and TNK plus abciximab (11.1%) arms compared to those treated with TNK plus unfractionated heparin (15.4%) (Table 5; Fig. 4). The trial was not sufficiently powered to detect significant mortality differences based on treatment assignment, but a trend toward decreased mortality in the TNK-plus-enoxaparin group was observed relative to the other treatment strategies. As in GUSTO V, the incidence of intracranial hemorrhage was identical (at 0.9%) among all three arms, and a modest but statistically significant excess in bleeding complications occurred in the abciximab and enoxaparin arms compared to the TNK-plus-unfractionated heparin controls.

While not performed in a double-blinded manner and not sized to detect mortality benefits, the findings of ASSENT-3 echo those of the larger GUSTO V trial. Combination therapy with half-dose fibrinolytic-plus-abciximab therapy was associated with a small but significant reduction in reinfarction and recurrent ischemia, but carried an increased risk of nonintracranial major bleeding events. In addition, and concordant with the findings of the smaller ENTIRE-TIMI 23 study, the combination of full-dose TNK and enoxaparin (administered for up to 7 days) appeared equivalent or perhaps slightly superior to combined TNK and abciximab in terms of efficacy and safety. The findings of this exploratory trial await confirmation in larger studies.

Table 5 Major Clinical Endpoints in the ASSENT-3 Trial

Endpoint	Enoxaparin ($n = 2040$)	Abciximab ($n = 2017$)	Unfractionated heparin ($n = 2038$)	p value
30-day death (%)	5.4	6.6	6.0	0.25
30-day death, or in-hospital reinfarction or refractory Ischemia(%)	11.4	11.1	15.4	0.0001
30-day death, or in-hospital reinfarction, refractory ischemia, or major bleeding (%)	13.8	14.2	17.0	0.0081
In-hospital urgent PCI (%)	11.9	9.1	14.4	<0.0001
Major (nonintracranial) bleeding (%)	3.0	4.3	2.2	0.0005
Intracranial hemorrhage (%)	0.9	0.9	0.9	0.98

Patients in the abciximab arm received half-dose TNK (15–25 mg, based on body weight), while patients in the other arms received full-dose TNK (30–50 mg).

V. DIRECT THROMBIN INHIBITORS IN COMBINATION WITH FIBRINOLYSIS

The procoagulant effects of thrombin, liberated during fibrinolysis, likely contribute to the occurrence of both fibrinolytic failure and early vessel reocclusion. Whereas heparin is limited in that the heparin/antithrombin-III complex is unable to inactivate thrombin once the thrombin molecule has become bound to fibrin, the direct thrombin inhibitors, a group of small- to-medium length peptide molecules that interact directly with the active site on thrombin, do possess the capability of inhibiting clot-bound thrombin. In addition, because the direct thrombin inhibitors do not bind to plasma proteins and are not neutralized by

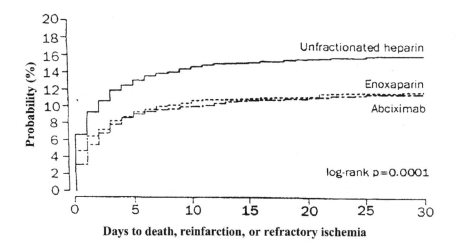

Figure 4 Kaplan-Meier curves for the primary efficacy endpoint (death, MI, or refractory ischemia) by treatment arm in the ASSENT-3 trial. The unfractionated heparin and enoxaparin groups received full-dose TNK, whereas the abciximab patients received half-dose TNK.

platelet factor-4, these agents also provide a more predictable level of anticoagulation than unfractionated heparin. Because of these attributes, a variety of direct thrombin inhibitors have been studied as possible adjuncts to fibrinolytics in lieu of unfractionated heparin (54,55).

Following a series of safety and feasibility studies of combined fibrinolytic and direct thrombin inhibitor therapy, several small randomized dose-ranging trials were performed (56–60) The Promotion of Reperfusion in Myocardial Infarction Evolution (PRIME) trial randomized 336 patients with acute ST elevation MI to receive one of five doses of the direct thrombin inhibitor efegatran sulfate or heparin infusion for 72–96 hours in addition to accelerated alteplase and aspirin (56). A shorter median time to ST segment recovery was observed among individuals assigned to efegatran (107 vs. 154 min; $p = 0.025$), but the primary composite endpoint of 30-day death or reinfarction, or less than TIMI-3 flow at 90-minute angiography was similar in efegatran and heparin-treated patients (53.8 vs. 53.0%, respectively; $p = 0.90$). Major bleeding complications did not differ based on treatment assignment. In the Myocardial Infarction with Novastatin (argatroban) and t-PA (MINT) Study, 125 patients with ST elevation MI were treated with t-PA and randomized to receive heparin versus low- or high-dose argatroban (58) A nonsignificant trend toward more frequent TIMI 3 flow on early angiography was observed among patients who received argatroban.

Three initial phase III trials, TIMI 9a, GUSTO IIa, and, Hirudin for improvement of thrombolysis (HIT)-3, compared recombinant hirudin (at moderate to high doses) versus unfractionated heparin (with moderately high aPTT ranges, up to 85 s) combined with fibriniolytic therapy for acute ST elevation MI. All three of these trials, however, were terminated early as a result of an excess of bleeding complications in both the hirudin and heparin arms. The subsequent large randomized TIMI 9b, GUSTO IIb, and HIT-4 trials employed more modest doses of anticoagulants, resulting in reduced bleeding events. GUSTO IIb included 3289 patients with ST elevation MI who were treated with t-PA or steptokinase and randomized to a 72-hour infusion of hirudin or heparin (61,62). Among all enrolled patients, a nonsignificant trend toward a reduced incidence of death or recurrent MI at 30 days was observed among individuals randomized to hirudin. Interestingly, among the subgroup of patients treated with streptokinase, randomization to hirudin was associated with a significant reduction in the incidence of 30-day death or nonfatal MI [8.6 vs. 14.4%; OR 1.78, 95% confidence interval (CI) 1.20 to 2.66; $p = 0.004$]), whereas patients treated with t-PA displayed no added benefit from hirudin over heparin in relation to 30-day events (10.3% vs.10.9%, respectively; OR 1.06, 95% CI 0.81–1.38; $p = 0.68$).

In the similarly designed TIMI-9b study, 3,002 patients with acute ST elevation MI treated with streptokinase or t-PA were randomized to heparin or hirudin administration for 96 hours (63). The results of this trial were less encouraging than those of GUSTO IIb, as the primary composite end- point (death, recurrent MI, or development of severe congestive heart failure or cardiogenic shock by 30 days) occurred in 11.9% of patients in the heparin group and 12.9% of patients in the hirudin group ($p = $ NS). Subgroup analysis did not identify any group that derived greater benefit from direct antithrombin than heparin therapy. When combined, data from the GUSTO IIb and TIMI 9b trials did not demonstrate a mortality advantage of hirudin over heparin at 30 days, but a borderline significant reduction in 30-day recurrent MI was observed (4.7% for hirudin vs. 5.8% for heparin, 19% relative reduction; $p = 0.55$). No significant differences in the incidence of bleeding events were noted among patients treated with heparin or hirudin. In the HIT-4 study, which randomized 1208 streptokinase-treated patients to either hirudin or heparin, treatment assignment was not associated with significant differences 30-day reinfarction rate or mortality (64).

The Hirulog and Early Reperfusion/Occlusion (HERO)-2 trial, which randomized 17,073 patients with acute ST elevation myocardial infarction to either an intravenous bolus and 48-hour infusion of either bivalirudin or heparin, together with standard-dose streptokinase, represents the largest trial comparing a direct thrombin inhibitor to unfractionated heparin (65). Despite a significant 30% relative reduction in the incidence of early reinfarction at 96 hours among bivalirudin-treated patients, no significant difference in 30-day mortality was observed (10.8% for heparin vs. 10.9% for bivalirudin; $p = 0.85$). Severe bleeding complications were slightly more prevalent among bivalirudin-treated patients in this trial.

In aggregate, the trials of combined fibrinolytic and direct thrombin inhibitor therapy, involving a total of >25,000 patients, suggest a small (but inconsistent among the trials) absolute reduction in the incidence of early reinfarction among patients treated with direct thrombin inhibiters rather than unfractionated heparin. Unfortunately, no benefit in 30-day mortality has been recognized in any trial (Table 6). Data from the GUSTO IIb trial suggested that direct thrombin inhibitors may provide preferential benefit over heparin among individuals treated with streptokinase rather than t-PA, but this relationship was not confirmed in the TIMI 9b, HIT-4, or HERO-2 trials. Although higher doses of hirudin and efegatran were associated with an excess of bleeding risk in earlier studies, moderation of dosing strategies resulted in increased safety of direct thrombin inhibitor therapy in subsequent trials.

VI. SUMMARY: CURRENT STATUS AND FUTURE DIRECTIONS

The clinical studies presented above have provided a great deal of information regarding combination pharmacotherapy during the treatment of acute MI. Based upon the results of several phase II studies that employed early angiograpy, certain fibrinolytic plus GP IIb/IIIa antagonist combinations have proven capable of effecting more rapid and reliable reperfusion than traditional fribrinolytic regimens. These advantages, however, did not translate into a hoped-for mortality benefit in the large randomized GUSTO V trial, rendering the ultimate role that combination therapy will play in daily clinical practice still uncertain. Among the most fascinating of several issues to be addressed in future trials are the following:

1. Are there certain patient subsets that will preferentially benefit from combination therapy? As previously mentioned, the overall population studied in GUSTO-V was a "low-risk" group, but there was a trend toward benefit from combination therapy among higher-risk subgroups within this cohort. Likewise, a trend toward reduced incidence of intracranial hemorrhage was noted among younger individuals.

2. What is the role of LMWH combined either with full-dose fibrinolytic therapy or with a reduced-dose fibrinolytic and a GP IIb/IIIa antagonist? Nonblinded studies, both ENTIRE-TIMI 23 and ASSENT-3, suggested that addition of the LMWH enoxaparin to a full-dose fibrinolytic agent may be equally or perhaps more effective than combination therapy with a half-dose fibrinolytic and a GP IIb/IIIa antagonist.

3. Will combination therapy lend itself to a strategy of "facilitated angioplasty," whereby the most favorable attributes of both medical and catheter-based reperfusion therapies are integrated with the hope of restoring arterial patency as quickly and reliably as possible? This strategy will be examined in detail in the

Table 6 Results of Randomized Trials of Direct Thrombin Inhibitor Versus Heparin Therapy in Conjunction with Fibrinolysis for Acute ST Elevation MI

Trial	(Ref.)	n	Incidence of primary endpoint			Primary endpoint	Medications used	
			Direct thrombin inhibitor (%)	Heparin (%)	p value		Direct thrombin inhibitor	Lytic agent
HERO-2	(65)	17,073	10.9	10.8	NS[b]	30-day death	Bivalirudin	SK
GUSTO-IIb	(61)	4,131[a]	9.9	11.3	NS[c]	30-day death or MI	Hirudin	t-PA or SK
TIMI-9b	(63)	3,002	12.9	11.9	NS	30-day death, MI, or severe CHF	Hirudin	t-PA or SK
HIT-4	(64)	1,208	22.7	24.3	NS	30-day death, MI, stroke, urgent PCI, or refractory angina	Hirudin	SK
HERO	(66)	412	47	35	0.023	90–120 min TIMI-3 flow	Bivalirudin	SK
PRIME	(56)	336	53.8	53.0	NS	30-day death, MI or <TIMI-3 flow	Efegatran	t-PA
TIMI-5	(67)	246	38.2	50.6	NS[c]	36-hr death or MI, or <TIMI-3 flow at 90 min	Hirudin	t-PA
ESCALAT	(57)	245	40	53	NS	90-min TIMI-3 flow	Efegatran	t-PA
TIMI-6	(68)	175	35.0	32.3	NS	Death, MI, CHF, or LVEF < 0.40 at hospital discharge	Hirudin	SK
ARGAMI	(59)	127	76	82	NS	90-min TIMI 2 or 3 flow	Artgatroban	t-PA
MINT	(58)	125	57	42	NS	90-min TIMI-3 flow	Argatroban	t-PA

SK, streptokinase; t-PA, tissue plasminogen activator.
[a] Subset of patients with acute ST-elevation MI
[b] $p = 0.13$
[c] $p = 0.07$

ongoing Facilitated Intervention with Enhanced Reperfusion Speed to Stop Events (FINESSE) trial, in which patients with acute MI will undergo primary PCI after pretreatment with one of the following regimens: (a) combination therapy with half-dose reteplase plus abciximab, started in the emergency department; (b) abciximab alone, started in the emergency department; or (c) abciximab alone, started in the cath lab immediately prior to undergoing primary PCI.

REFERENCES

1. Weaver WD, Simes RJ, Betriu A, et al. Comparison of primary coronary angioplasty and intravenous thrombolytic therapy for acute myocardial infarction: a quantitative review. Jama. 1997; 278:2093–8.
2. The EPISTENT Investigators. Randomised placebo-controlled and balloon-angioplasty-controlled trial to assess safety of coronary stenting with use of platelet glycoprotein-IIb/IIIa blockade. The EPISTENT Investigators. Evaluation of Platelet IIb/IIIa Inhibitor for Stenting. Lancet. 1998; 352:87–92.
3. Montalescot G, Barragan P, Wittenberg O, et al. Platelet glycoprotein IIb/IIIa inhibition with coronary stenting for acute myocardial infarction. N Eng J Med. 2001; 344:1895–1903.
4. Bhatt DL, Topol EJ. Current role of platelet glycoprotein IIb/IIIa inhibitors in acute coronary syndromes. Jama. 2000; 284:1549–1558.
5. Ault KA, Cannon CP, Mitchell J, et al. Platelet activation in patients after an acute coronary syndrome: results from the TIMI-12 trial. Thrombolysis in Myocardial Infarction. J the Am Coll Cardiol. 1999; 33:634–639.
6. Cannon CP. Combination therapy for acute myocardial infarction: glycoprotein IIb/IIIa inhibitors plus thrombolysis. Clin Cardiol. 1999; 22:IV37–43.
7. The EPILOG Investigators. Platelet glycoprotein IIb/IIIa receptor blockade and low-dose heparin during percutaneous coronary revascularization. New England Journal of Medicine. 1997; 336:1689–1696.
8. Akkerhuis KM, Deckers JW, Lincoff AM, et al. Risk of stroke associated with abciximab among patients undergoing percutaneous coronary intervention. Jama. 2001; 286:78–82.
9. Mahaffey KW, Harrington RA, Simoons ML, et al. Stroke in patients with acute coronary syndromes: incidence and outcomes in the platelet glycoprotein IIb/IIIa in unstable angina. Receptor suppression using integrilin therapy (PURSUIT) trial. The PURSUIT Investigators. Circulation. 1999; 99:2371–2377.
10. Li RH, Herrmann HC. Facilitated percutaneous coronary intervention: a novel concept in expediting and improving acute myocardial infarction care. Am Heart J. 2000; 140:S125–135.
11. The GUSTO Angiographic Investigators. The effects of tissue plasminogen activator, streptokinase, or both on coronary-artery patency, ventricular function, and survival after acute myocardial infarction. N Engl J Med. 1993; 329:1615–1622.
12. Lundergan CF, Ross AM, McCarthy WF, et al. Predictors of left ventricular function after acute myocardial infarction: effects of time to treatment, patency, and body mass index: the GUSTO-I angiographic experience. Am Heart J. 2001; 142:43–50.
13. Simes RJ, Topol EJ, Holmes DR, Jr., et al. Link between the angiographic substudy and mortality outcomes in a large randomized trial of myocardial reperfusion. Importance of early and complete infarct artery reperfusion. GUSTO-I Investigators. Circulation. 1995; 91:1923–1938.
14. The ASSENT-2 Investigators. Single-bolus tenecteplase compared with front-loaded alteplase in acute myocardial infarction: the ASSENT-2 double-blind randomised trial. Assessment of the Safety and Efficacy of a New Thrombolytic Investigators. Lancet. 1999; 354:716–722.
15. The Global Use of Strategies to Open Occluded Coronary Arteries (GUSTO III) Investigators. A comparison of reteplase with alteplase for acute myocardial infarction. N Engl J Med. 1997; 337:1118–1123.

16. Llevadot J, Giugliano RP, Antman EM. Bolus fibrinolytic therapy in acute myocardial infarction. Jama. 2001; 286:442–449.

17. Brouwer MA, Bohncke JR, Veen G, et al. Adverse long-term effects of reocclusion after coronary thrombolysis. J Am Coll Cardiol. 1995; 26:1440–1444.

18. Jong P, Cohen EA, Batchelor W, et al. Bleeding risks with abciximab after full-dose thrombolysis in rescue or urgent angioplasty for acute myocardial infarction. Am Heart J. 2001; 141:218–225.

19. Ellis SG, Da Silva ER, Spaulding CM, et al. Review of immediate angioplasty after fibrinolytic therapy for acute myocardial infarction: insights from the RESCUE I, RESCUE II, and other contemporary clinical experiences. Am Heart J. 2000; 139:1046–1053.

20. Eisenberg PR, Sobel BE, Jaffe AS. Activation of prothrombin accompanying thrombolysis with recombinant tissue-type plasminogen activator. J American Coll Cardiol. 1992; 19:1065–1069.

21. Moser M, Nordt T, Peter K, et al. Platelet function during and after thrombolytic therapy for acute myocardial infarction with reteplase, alteplase, or streptokinase. Circulation. 1999; 100:1858–1864.

22. Fitzgerald DJ, Catella F, Roy L, et al. Marked platelet activation in vivo after intravenous streptokinase in patients with acute myocardial infarction. Circulation. 1988; 77:142–150.

23. Terres W, Umnus S, Mathey DG, et al. Effects of streptokinase, urokinase, and recombinant tissue plasminogen activator on platelet aggregability and stability of platelet aggregates. Cardiovasc Res. 1990; 24:471–477.

24. Loscalzo J, Vaughan DE. Tissue plasminogen activator promotes platelet disaggregation in plasma. J Clin Invest. 1987; 79:1749–1755.

25. ISIS-2 Collaborative Group. Randomised trial of intravenous streptokinase, oral aspirin, both, or neither among 17,187 cases of suspected acute myocardial infarction: ISIS-2. Lancet. 1988; 2:349–360.

26. Roux S, Christeller S, Ludin E. Effects of aspirin on coronary reocclusion and recurrent ischemia after thrombolysis: a meta-analysis. J Am Coll Cardiol. 1992; 19:671–677.

27. Kerins DM, Roy L, FitzGerald GA, et al. Platelet and vascular function during coronary thrombolysis with tissue-type plasminogen activator. Circulation. 1989; 80:1718–1725.

28. Halushka MK, Halushka PV. Why are some individuals resistant to the cardioprotective effects of aspirin? Could it be thromboxane A2? Circulation. 2002; 105:1620–1622.

29. Eikelboom JW, Hirsh J, Weitz JI, et al. Aspirin-resistant thromboxane biosynthesis and the risk of myocardial infarction, stroke, or cardiovascular death in patients at high risk for cardiovascular events. Circulation. 2002; 105:1650–1655.

30. Gum PA, Kottke-Marchant K, Welsh PA, et al. A prospective, blinded determination of the natural history of aspirin resistance among stable patients with cardiovascular disease.[comment]. J Am Coll Cardiol. 2003; 41:961–965.

31. Buchanan MR, Brister SJ. Individual variation in the effects of ASA on platelet function: implications for the use of ASA clinically. Can J Cardiol. 1995; 11:221–227.

32. Buchanan MR, Schwartz L, Bourassa M, et al. Results of the BRAT study—a pilot study investigating the possible significance of ASA nonresponsiveness on the benefits and risks of ASA on thrombosis in patients undergoing coronary artery bypass surgery. Can J Cardiol. 2000; 16:1385–1390.

33. Grotemeyer KH. Effects of acetylsalicylic acid in stroke patients. Evidence of nonresponders in a subpopulation of treated patients. Thromb Res. 1991; 63:587–593.

34. Grotemeyer KH, Scharafinski HW, Husstedt IW. Two-year follow-up of aspirin responder and aspirin non responder. A pilot-study including 180 post-stroke patients. Thromb Research. 1993; 71:397–403.

35. Helgason CM, Tortorice KL, Winkler SR, et al. Aspirin response and failure in cerebral infarction. Stroke. 1993; 24:345–350.

36. Gum PA, Kottke-Marchant K, Poggio ED, et al. Profile and prevalence of aspirin resistance in patients with cardiovascular disease. Am J Cardiol. 2001; 88:230–235.

37. Gold HK, Coller BS, Yasuda T, et al. Rapid and sustained coronary artery recanalization with combined bolus injection of recombinant tissue-type plasminogen activator and monoclonal antiplatelet GPIIb/IIIa antibody in a canine preparation. Circulation. 1988; 77:670–677.

38. Nicolini FA, Lee P, Rios G, et al. Combination of platelet fibrinogen receptor antagonist and direct thrombin inhibitor at low doses markedly improves thrombolysis. Circulation. 1994; 89:1802–1809.

39. Kleiman NS, Ohman EM, Califf RM, et al. Profound inhibition of platelet aggregation with monoclonal antibody 7E3 Fab after thrombolytic therapy. Results of the Thrombolysis and Angioplasty in Myocardial Infarction (TAMI) 8 Pilot Study. J Am Coll Cardiol. 1993; 22:381–389.

40. Ohman EM, Kleiman NS, Gacioch G, et al. Combined accelerated tissue-plasminogen activator and platelet glycoprotein IIb/IIIa integrin receptor blockade with Integrilin in acute myocardial infarction. Results of a randomized, placebo-controlled, dose-ranging trial. IMPACT-AMI Investigators. Circulation. 1997; 95:846–854.

41. Ronner E, van Kesteren HA, Zijnen P, et al. Safety and efficacy of eptifibatide vs placebo in patients receiving thrombolytic therapy with streptokinase for acute myocardial infarction; a phase II dose escalation, randomized, double-blind study. Eur Heart J. 2000; 21:1530–1536.

42. The PARADIGM Investigators. Combining thrombolysis with the platelet glycoprotein IIb/IIIa inhibitor lamifiban: results of the Platelet Aggregation Receptor Antagonist Dose Investigation and Reperfusion Gain in Myocardial Infarction (PARADIGM) trial. J Am Coll Cardiol. 1998; 32:2003–2010.

43. Strategies for Patency Enhancement in the Emergency Department (SPEED) Group. Trial of abciximab with and without low-dose reteplase for acute myocardial infarction. Circulation. 2000; 101:2788–2794.

44. Antman EM, Giugliano RP, Gibson CM, et al. Abciximab facilitates the rate and extent of thrombolysis: results of the thrombolysis in myocardial infarction (TIMI) 14 trial. The TIMI 14 Investigators. Circulation. 1999; 99:2720–2732.

45. Antman EM, Louwerenburg HW, Baars HF, et al. Enoxaparin as Adjunctive Antithrombin Therapy for ST-Elevation Myocardial Infarction: results of the ENTIRE-Thrombolysis in Myocardial Infarction (TIMI) 23 Trial. Circulation. 2002; 105:1642–1649.

46. Giugliano RP, Roe MT, Harrington RA, et al. Combination reperfusion therapy with eptifibatide and reduced-dose tenecteplase for ST-elevation myocardial infarction: results of the integrilin and tenecteplase in acute myocardial infarction (INTEGRITI) Phase II Angiographic Trial. J Am Coll Cardiol. 2003; 41:1251–1260.

47. The Gusto V. Investigators. Reperfusion therapy for acute myocardial infarction with fibrinolytic therapy or combination reduced fibrinolytic therapy and platelet glycoprotein IIb/IIIa inhibition: the GUSTO V randomised trial. Lancet. 2001; 357:1905–1194.

48. The Assessment of the S, Efficacy of a New Thrombolytic Regimen I. Efficacy and safety of tenecteplase in combination with enoxaparin, abciximab, or unfractionated heparin: the ASSENT-3 randomised trial in acute myocardial infarction. Lancet. 2001; 358:605–613.

49. de Lemos JA, Antman EM, Gibson CM, et al. Abciximab improves both epicardial flow and myocardial reperfusion in ST-elevation myocardial infarction. Observations from the TIMI 14 trial. Circulation. 2000; 101:239–243.

50. de Lemos JA, Gibson CM, Antman EM, et al. Abciximab and early adjunctive percutaneous coronary intervention are associated with improved ST-segment resolution after thrombolysis: Observations from the TIMI 14 Trial. Am Heart J. 2001; 141:592–598.

51. Ross AM, Molhoek P, Lundergan C, et al. Randomized comparison of enoxaparin, a low-molecular-weight heparin, with unfractionated heparin adjunctive to recombinant tissue plasminogen activator thrombolysis and aspirin: second trial of Heparin and Aspirin Reperfusion Therapy (HART II). Circulation. 2001; 104:648–652.

52. The GUSTO-V Investigators. Reperfusion therapy for acute myocardial infarction with fibrinolytic therapy or combination reduced fibrinolytic therapy and platelet glycoprotein IIb/IIIa inhibition: the GUSTO V randomised trial. Lancet. 2001; 357:1905–1914.

53. Lincoff AM, Califf RM, Van de Werf F, et al. Mortality at 1 year with combination platelet glycoprotein IIb/IIIa inhibition and reduced-dose fibrinolytic therapy vs conventional fibrinolytic therapy for acute myocardial infarction: GUSTO V randomized trial. JAMA. 2002; 288:2130–2135.

54. Weitz JI, Buller HR. Direct thrombin inhibitors in acute coronary syndromes: present and future. Circulation. 2002; 105:1004–1011.

55. Moliterno DJ. Anticoagulants and their use in acute coronary syndromes and In: In Topol EJ, ed. coronary intervention. Textbook of Interventional Cardiology. 4th ed.: Philadelphia: WB Saunders, 2003

56. The Prime Investigators. Multicenter, dose-ranging study of efegatran sulfate versus heparin with thrombolysis for acute myocardial infarction: The Promotion of Reperfusion in Myocardial Infarction Evolution (PRIME) trial. Am Heart J. 2002; 143:95–105.

57. Fung AY, Lorch G, Cambier PA, et al. Efegatran sulfate as an adjunct to streptokinase versus heparin as an adjunct to tissue plasminogen activator in patients with acute myocardial infarction. ESCALAT Investigators. Am Heart J. 1999; 138:696–704.

58. Jang IK, Brown DF, Giugliano RP, et al. A multicenter, randomized study of argatroban versus heparin as adjunct to tissue plasminogen activator (TPA) in acute myocardial infarction: myocardial infarction with novastan and TPA (MINT) study. J Am Coll Cardiol. 1999; 33:1879–1885.

59. Vermeer F, Vahanian A, Fels PW, et al. Argatroban and alteplase in patients with acute myocardial infarction: the ARGAMI Study. J Thromb Thrombolysis. 2000; 10:233–240.

60. Rott D, Behar S, Hod H, et al. Improved survival of patients with acute myocardial infarction with significant left ventricular dysfunction undergoing invasive coronary procedures. American Heart Journal. 2001; 141:267–276.

61. The GUSTO IIb investigators. A comparison of recombinant hirudin with heparin for the treatment of acute coronary syndromes. N Engl J Med. 1996; 335:775–782.

62. Metz BK, White HD, Granger CB, et al. Randomized comparison of direct thrombin inhibition versus heparin in conjunction with fibrinolytic therapy for acute myocardial infarction: results from the GUSTO-IIb Trial. Global Use of Strategies to Open Occluded Coronary Arteries in Acute Coronary Syndromes (GUSTO-IIb) Investigators. J Am Coll Cardiol. 1998; 31:1493–1498.

63. Antman EM. Hirudin in acute myocardial infarction. Thrombolysis and Thrombin Inhibition in Myocardial Infarction (TIMI) 9B trial. Circulation. 1996; 94:911–921.

64. Neuhaus KL, Molhoek GP, Zeymer U, et al. Recombinant hirudin (lepirudin) for the improvement of thrombolysis with streptokinase in patients with acute myocardial infarction: results of the HIT-4 trial. J Am Coll Cardiol. 1999; 34:966–973.

65. White H, The H, Early Reperfusion or Occlusion -2 Trial I. Thrombin-specific anticoagulation with bivalirudin versus heparin in patients receiving fibrinolytic therapy for acute myocardial infarction: the HERO-2 randomised trial. Lancet. 2001; 358:1855–1863.

66. White HD, Aylward PE, Frey MJ, et al. Randomized, double-blind comparison of hirulog versus heparin in patients receiving streptokinase and aspirin for acute myocardial infarction (HERO). Hirulog Early Reperfusion/Occlusion (HERO) Trial Investigators. Circulation. 1997; 96:2155–2161.

67. Cannon CP, McCabe CH, Henry TD, et al. A pilot trial of recombinant desulfatohirudin compared with heparin in conjunction with tissue-type plasminogen activator and aspirin for acute myocardial infarction: results of the Thrombolysis in Myocardial Infarction (TIMI) 5 trial. J Am Coll Cardiol. 1994; 23:993–1003.

68. Lee LV. Initial experience with hirudin and streptokinase in acute myocardial infarction: results of the Thrombolysis in Myocardial Infarction (TIMI) 6 trial. Am J Cardiol. 1995; 75:7–13.

69. Farrell TP, Hayes KB, Sobel BE, et al. The lack of augmentation by aspirin of inhibition of platelet reactivity by ticlopidine. Am J Cardiol 1999; 83:770–774.

10-1

Acute Coronary Syndromes: Electrocardiographic Diagnosis

Aaron Satran and Robert C. Hendel
*Rush-Presbyterian-St. Luke's Medical Center,
Chicago, Illinois, U.S.A.*

The 12-lead electrocardiogram (ECG) is the one of the most well-established diagnostic tools in cardiology. It was brought into widespread clinical use by Willem Einthoven in the early 1900s and today, despite dramatic advances in the detection of acute coronary syndrome (ACS), the ECG remains invaluable. During ACS, evidence of myocardial ischemia can be identified by characteristic changes in the T wave and ST segment, as well as by the appearance of Q waves. Frequently, these changes permit localization and quantification of myocardial injury, but their interpretation and subsequent therapeutic interventions may be confounded by normal variants. Thus, it is critical to establish and maintain proficiency in proper ECG interpretation.

I. UNSTABLE ANGINA AND NON–ST SEGMENT ELEVATION MYOCARDIAL INFARCTION

ACS is a clinical spectrum with unstable angina/non–ST segment elevation MI (UA/NSTEMI) at one end, and acute myocardial infarction (AMI) associated with electrocardiographic ST segment elevation MI (STEMI) on the other. In approximately 50% of patients presenting with UA/NSTEMI, the earliest and most consistent ECG finding is dynamic ST segment deviation (1,2).

Transient ST segment depression of ≥1 mm on ECG has long been recognized as a marker of adverse outcome among patients presenting with UA (3–8). However, reviews of several large clinical trials have demonstrated that ≥ 0.05 mV of ST segment deviation is also a high-risk marker (9–12). Investigators from the TIMI III registry reported that the 1-year incidence of death or MI was 16.3% among patients with this finding at presentation, compared with 6.8% of patients with isolated T-wave changes and 8.2% of those with no ECG changes (1). Similarly, Lloyd-Jones et al. showed that NSTEMI was three to four times more likely among patients with chest pain and three or more ECG leads showing ST segment depression and/or isolated ST segment depression of ≥0.2 mV (13).

Patients with UA/NSTEMI may also present with abnormal T-wave inversion (TWI), which is classically sharp, symmetrical, and preceded by an isoelectric ST segment that bows upward. An important subgroup of patients will demonstrate deep (>0.2 mV), symmetrical, and occasionally biphasic TWI in the anterior precordial leads (14), termed

Wellen's syndrome, after the group who first described the ECG findings associated with significant stenosis of the left anterior descending coronary artery (LAD) (15–18) (Fig. 1). Interestingly, Wellen's syndrome is generally not accompanied by chest pain, but it is nonetheless a high-risk marker for acute ischemia and should be treated in a similar manner to dynamic ST segment depression or elevation (10). In contrast, nonspecific ST-T wave changes, defined as ST segment deviation of <0.05 mV or TWI of <0.2 mV, are less helpful clinically. Similarly, although established pathological Q waves may not be helpful in diagnosing UA/NSTEMI, their presence suggests prior MI, and thus a high likelihood of coronary artery disease (CAD).

A single ECG provides a transient view of an ongoing process. A normal ECG in a patient with chest pain does not exclude the possibility of ACS, as 1–6% of such patients will eventually progress to NSTEMI, and more than 4% are subsequently diagnosed with UA (19–22). Continuous 12-lead ECG monitoring to detect ST segment shifts can detect ischemic episodes that are not evident upon presentation and also predict future death, MI, or the need for urgent revascularization (23–25), especially when combined with elevated serum troponin levels (26). At present, however, the utility of continuous ST segment monitoring for initial risk stratification is still inconclusive.

II. ST SEGMENT ELEVATION MYOCARDIAL INFARCTION

Transmural ischemia is caused by interruption of blood supply to the myocardium via occlusion of one of the three epicardial coronary arteries or their branches, which shifts the overall ST vector in the direction of the epicardium and results in ST segment elevation (STE). The earliest ECG finding of STEMI is a prominent "hyperacute" T wave, which occurs as early as 30 minutes after coronary artery occlusion and can be either upright or inverted (27). The origin of the hyperacute T wave is uncertain, but it is presumably caused by the same mechanisms that precipitate a current-of-injury pattern (28,29). Morphologically, hyperacute T waves are often asymmetrical with a broad base

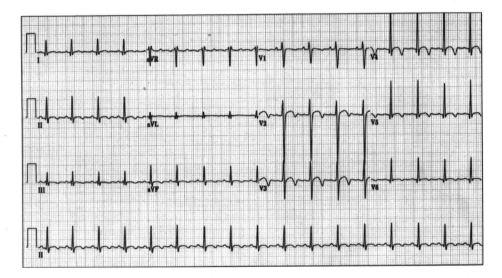

Figure 1   Wellen's syndrome, with biphasic T-wave inversion in the anterior precordial leads.

and are not infrequently associated with reciprocal ST segment depression (STD). During STEMI, rapid progression to STE in the leads facing the area of injury is the rule, with an upsloping portion that is generally convex or flat. STE is reflected by reciprocal STD in approximately 75% of inferior wall STEMIs, but less frequently in anterior wall STEMI (~30%) (30).

Hyperacute T waves and STE are typically followed by evolving T-wave inversion and associated QT prolongation over the next hours to days. These changes can resolve over days to weeks, but they may persist indefinitely depending on the amount of myocardial damage. Complete normalization of the ECG after STEMI is uncommon but can occur with smaller infarcts, spontaneous recanalization, or good collateral circulation.

Although classically ascribed to transmural infarction, Q waves do not reliably differentiate STEMI from NSTEMI (31,32). Any infarction of significant size results in necrotic myocardium and subsequent loss of depolarization forces, which leads to a redirection of electrical activity away from that area. The main component of this redirection occurs during early ventricular depolarization, so if there is a large area of necrosis, a Q wave is seen on the surface ECG. A smaller infarction, on the other hand, may be insufficient to produce a Q wave, but it can reduce the magnitude of the normal anterior forces, resulting in diminished R-wave voltage (33). Small, nonpathological Q waves are commonly seen in leads I, aVF, and V_4–V_6. Significant (pathological) Q waves are abnormally wide ($\geq$0.04 s) and deep (25% of the height of the R wave), with the exception of isolated Q waves in either lead III or aVL (33). Pathologic Q alwaves usually develop within 8–12 hours after STEMI but can occasionally be seen within 1–2 hours of complete coronary occlusion (30) and as such should not preclude reperfusion therapy with thrombolysis when otherwise clinically indicated.

As with UA/NSTEMI, the initial ECG findings during STEMI may be unremarkable; in fact, they are diagnostic in only 50% of cases. Multiple studies have demonstrated that more than 20% of patients with AMI present with normal or nondiagnostic ECG findings, including hyperacute T waves (34–37). Regardless, the ECG diagnosis of STEMI in the absence of a bundle branch block is immediately confirmed by presentation with typical angina and STE of $\geq$1 mm in two contiguous leads.

A. Acute Anterior STEMI

Anterior wall STEM is most often caused by an acute occlusion of the LAD, and is usually seen in consecutive anterior precordial leads, particularly V_2 (sensitivity, 99%) and V_3 (38,39). Diffuse anterior STE (leads V_1–V_6) with concurrent lateral STE (leads I and AVL) is especially concerning, because it suggests proximal LAD occlusion at or before the first septal perforator (Fig. 2). Complications, such as cardiogenic shock or various degrees of bundle branch block due to compromised perfusion of the His-Purkinje system, are common in this cohort, as is increased mortality. In the GUSTO-1 study, a subgroup of patients with angiographically documented proximal LAD occlusion had 30-day and 1-year mortality rates of 19.6% and 25.6%, respectively, compared with 9.2% and 12.4 % for mid-LAD occlusion and 6.8 and 10.2% for distal LAD or diagonal occlusion (40).

B. Acute Inferior and Right Ventricular STEMI

Patients with inferior STEMI comprise a diverse subgroup, with variable presentations and outcomes depending on the degree of myocardial involvement. A proximal, dominant right coronary artery (less commonly the circumflex coronary artery) is responsible for sup-

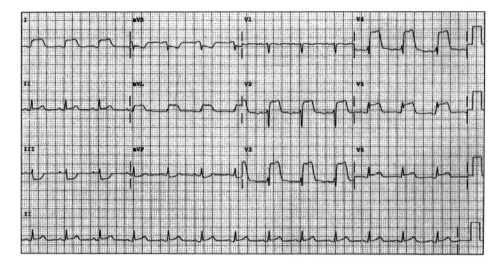

Figure 2 Acute anterolateral MI secondary to proximal LAD occlusion. Note the reciprocal ST segment depression in lead IIII. (Courtesy of K. Wang, M.D.)

plying the inferior portion of the left ventricle. The ECG leads demonstrating acute inferior STEMI most commonly include II, II, AVF (inferior leads, in 50% of patients) (38), with additional STE possible in V_5 and V_6 (lateral leads), V_1 and V_3R or V_4R (right ventricular leads, see below), or an R/S ratio >1 in V_1 and V_2 with or without ST depression in the anterior precordial leads (posterior infarction with reciprocal change). Inferior STEMI with precordial ST segment depression indicates a large area of infarction (41–45), and is associated with significant short- and long-term complications and mortality, even with the appropriate utilization of reperfusion therapy (41,44–50). Ten to 20% of patients with inferior MI have isolated circumflex coronary artery lesions and may also present with STE in V_5 and V_6, or STD in V_2 (38,51). In contrast to anterior STEMI, the conduction disturbances associated with inferior STEMI are usually benign and transient; frequently, they require no specific therapy.

Inferior STEMI in combination with right precordial STE (including the standard V1 lead) suggests right ventricular involvement (Fig. 3). RV infarction is usually a complication of inferior wall STEMI and is an independent risk factor for increased morbidity and mortality (52). Right-sided leads are much more sensitive and specific for detecting the changes of RV infarction, particularly in lead V_4R, where ≥1 mm of STE has both sensitivity and predictive accuracy of more than 90% (53). Isolated right ventricular infarction is rare and occurs mainly in patients with right ventricular hypertrophy (54).

C. Acute Lateral STEMI

In contrast to anterior STEMI with lateral involvement, the ECG is often electrically silent in the setting of isolated circumflex coronary artery occlusion. When these patients undergo angioplasty, STE in the lateral leads (I, AVL, V_5, or V_6) is seen only 50% of the time (55), possibly because of the smaller ventricular area supplied by the circumflex coronary artery or the anatomical position of the lateral wall of the left ventricle within the mediastinum. One helpful sign may be the presence of STE in V_5 and V_6, combined with prominent U waves in leads V_1 to V_3, which in two studies had a positive predictive value of more than 80% for circumflex occlusion (56,57)

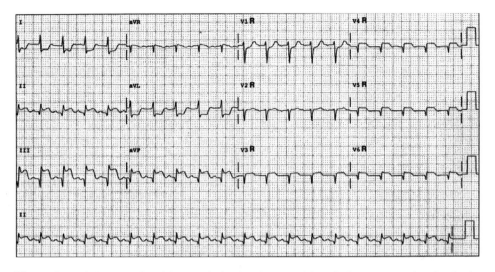

Figure 3 Inferior MI with right ventricular involvement. There is ST segment elevation in the inferior leads and in the right-sided precordial leads, as well as reciprocal ST segment depression in leads I and AVL. (Courtesy of K. Wang, M.D.)

D. Acute Posterior STEMI

Posterior wall STEMI, although rare in isolation, occurs in up to 20% of all STEMI, usually in conjunction with an inferior wall or lateral wall MI involving either the right coronary artery or circumflex coronary artery (58,59). As the standard ECG does not have posterior leads, posterior STEMI is most commonly reflected by STD in the anterior leads V_1–V_3, which are opposite the site of injury. Additional findings include tall, upright T waves, tall, broad R waves, and an R/S ratio of >1 (Fig. 4). The dominant R wave is actually an evolving Q wave and is thus not often seen on the initial ECG. If posterior leads

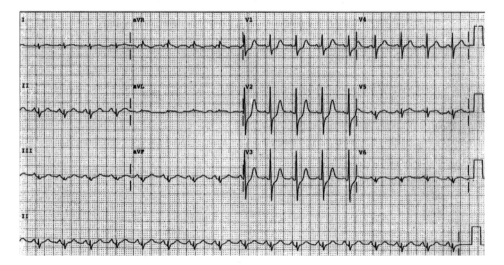

Figure 4 Posterior MI, demonstrated by tall R waves in leads V_1 to V_3 with concurrent ST segment depression. (Courtesy of K. Wang, M.D.)

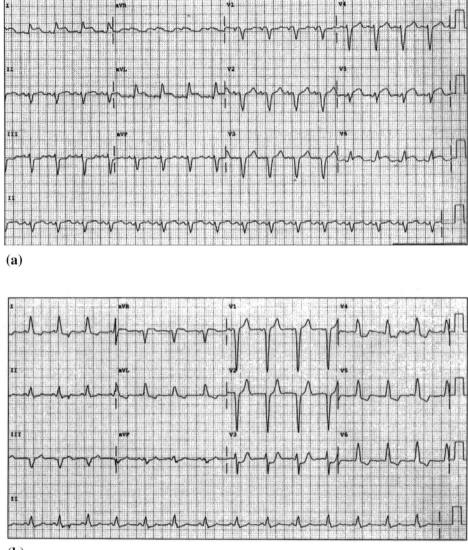

(a)

(b)

Figure 5 **(a)** LBBB with acute anterolateral MI. There is concordant ST segment elevation in leads I, AVL, and V$_6$. **(b)** LBBB with acute posterior MI. There is concordant ST segment depression in lead V$_6$, representing reciprocal posterior wall ST segment elevation. (c) (*Facing page*) LBBB with acute inferior MI. There is concordant ST segment elevation in lead III. (Courtesy of K. Wang, M.D.

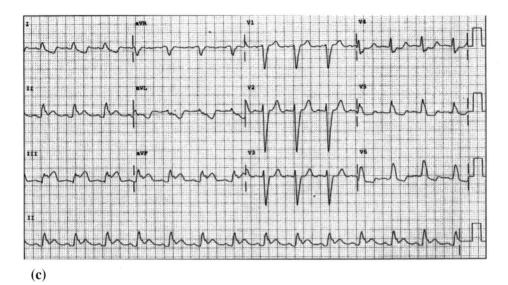

(c)

Figure 5 (*Continued*)

are used, they can show STE in leads V_7–V_9. Such a finding suggests occlusion of the right coronary artery rather than of the circumflex coronary artery (56).

III. CONFOUNDING PATTERNS

There are multiple nonischemic conditions that suggest the ECG diagnosis of ACS. These syndromes are commonly misdiagnosed, reinforcing the point that STE is an insensitive marker for AMI (60). The ECG abnormalities most commonly mistaken for STE include various forms of intraventricular conduction delay, LVH, and early repolarization.

Bundle branch block may be present at the time of AMI or develop as a complication of the infarction. Regardless, the diagnosis of AMI is usually not affected by the presence of right bundle brance block (RBBB), which primarily affects the terminal phase of ventricular depolarization. Preexisting left bundle brance block (LBBB), in contrast, may mask or mimic the diagnosis of AMI because of abnormalities in both the early and late phases of ventricular depolarization. Still, the electrocardiographic diagnosis of AMI in the presence of LBBB can still be made using several simple criteria devised by Sgarbossa et al (61), who compared the baseline ECGs of patients enrolled in GUSTO-1 with LBBB and AMI (confirmed by elevated serum CK-MB) to a control group with chronic CAD and LBBB. Three electrocardiographic criteria independently suggestive of AMI were (a) STE of ≥ 1 mm concordant with the QRS complex (most suggestive), 2) STD of ≥1 mm in leads V_1, V_2, or V_3, and (c) STE of ≥ 5 mm discordant from the QRS complex (Table 1; Fig. 5). In a separate study, Sgarbossa et al. showed that similar criteria are useful for diagnosing AMI in the presence of a ventricular paced rhythm: (a) discordant STE ≥ 5 mm, (b) concordant STE ≥ 1 mm, and (c) STD ≥ 1 mm in leads V_1, V_2, or V_3 (62).

Left ventricular hypertrophy (LVH) is frequently associated with ST-T wave abnormalities secondary to altered repolarization (Fig. 6). As with LBBB, these changes can mask or mimic the findings consistent with ACS. Generally speaking, LVH is associated with poor R wave progression and a precordial QS pattern in leads V_1–V_3. Up to 5 mm of

Table 1 ECG Findings in Acute Coronary Syndrome

ECG finding	Diagnosis	Sensitivity	Specificity
STD, giant TWI, or transient STE	Unstable angina	+++	++
	NSTEMI, if elevated biomarkers		
STE in V₁–V₆, I, and/or aVL	Anterior infarction	++++	+++
STE in II, III, aVF	Inferior infarction	++++	+++
STE in V₁, V₃R, V₄R	RV infarction	++++	+++
STE in V₅, V₆ and/or I, aVR, aVL	Lateral infarction	+	+++
Tall R-waves and STD in V₁–V₃	Posterior infarction	+++	+++

STE, ST segment elevation; STD, ST segment depression; NSTEMI, non–ST segment elevation myocardial infarction.

STE can be seen in this distribution, along with prominent T waves. A "strain" pattern, characterized by downsloping STD with abnormal, asymmetrical T waves (gradually downsloping and rapidly returning to baseline) in leads with prominent R waves (I, aVL, V₄–V₆) is common and is frequently misinterpreted as ischemia. Other specific criteria for abnormal repolarization in the setting of LVH include J point depression, terminal positivity of the T wave, TWI > 3 mm in V₆, and TWI greater in lead V₆ than lead V₄ (63). ST segment elevation in the setting of LVH has a morphologically flattened or convex pattern as opposed to the concave pattern that is seen with LVH and ACS.

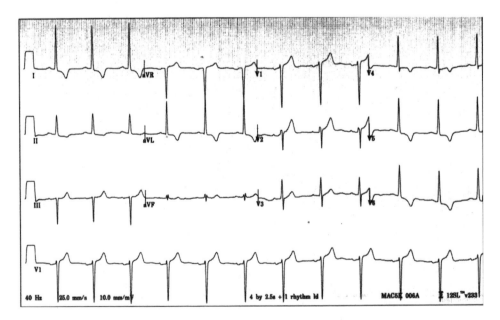

Figure 6 LVH, with "strain" pattern ST segment depression, prominent lateral R wave voltage, and left atrial enlargement.

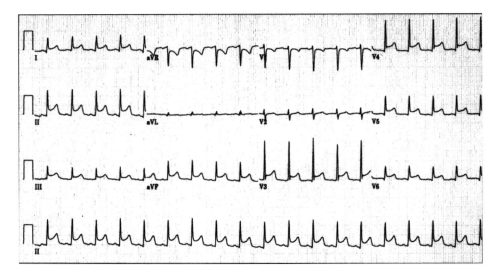

Figure 7 Acute pericarditis, with diffuse ST segment elevation involving more than one coronary vascular territory and PR segment depression.

ECG abnormalities during acute pericarditis include widespread STE (usually <5 mm) with upright T waves (Fig. 7). Diffuse STE is seen because the inflamed myocardium is only partially depolarized, resulting in the development of new ST vectors directed away from the ventricular cavity and toward the apical epicardium. As a result, STE can be seen in all leads except for AVR (and sometimes V_1), where STD is seen. Additionally, concurrent PR segment depression is often noted, except in leads AVR and V_1 (64). Acute pericarditis usually persists for 3–4 weeks, at which time the ST segments normalize and the T waves become inverted.

The correlation between serum potassium levels and ECG changes is poor, but the first ECG manifestations of hyperkalemia are tall, peaked T waves similar to the hyperacute T waves of acute infarction. Progressive severity of hyperkalemia results in decreased P wave amplitude, PR prolongation, widening of the QRS complex (which may resemble RBBB, RBBB, or STE), and, if untreated, ultimately AV block and ventricular fibrillation.

Table 2 Diagnosis of ST Segment Elevation Myocardial Infarction in the Presence of Left Bundle-Branch Block

ECG finding	Sensitivity %	Specificity %
ST segment elevation ≥ 1mm (concordant with QRS complex)	73	92
ST segment elevation ≥ 5 mm (discordant with QRS complex)	31	92
ST segment depression ≥ 1mm in lead V_1, V_2, or V_3	25	96
Positive T wave in lead V_5 or V_6	26	92
Left axis deviation	72	48

Source: Adapted from Ref. 61.

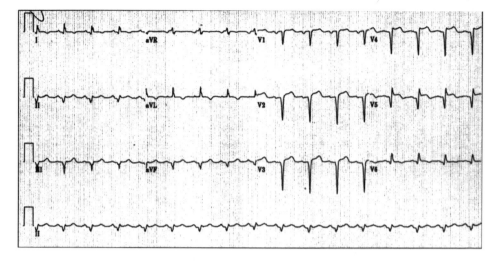

Figure 8 Left ventricular aneurysm. There is a QS pattern in leads V_1 to V_4, with diffuse, persistent ST segment elevation.

Early repolarization is a normal variant. The STE of early repolarization, as in pericarditis, is diffuse. It is usually <2 mm in the precordial leads and <0.5 mm in the limb leads. Morphologically, early repolarization is characterized by an upward concavity of the initial ST segment, notching or slurring of the terminal QRS complex, and relative temporal stability. The ST segment should appear to have been evenly lifted upwards from the J point (65). STE associated with early repolarization solely in the limb leads is uncommon without concurrent precordial STE; such a finding should prompt consideration of other precipitants of STE.

Left ventricular aneurysm (LVA) is a localized, dyskinetic area of infarction. Usually LVAs occur after transmural anterior MI, but they can also occur after blunt chest trauma,

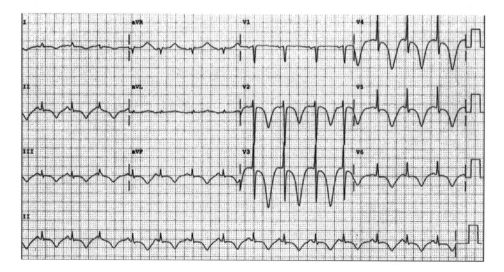

Figure 9 Neurogenic T-wave changes. The T waves are deeply inverted and symmetrical, with a prolonged QT interval. (Courtesy of K. Wang, M.D.)

Chagas' disease, and sarcoidosis (66). Electrocardiographically, LVA is characterized by persistent STE of variable magnitude and morphology observed weeks after AMI. The mechanism responsible for persistent STE is unknown, but is postulated to arise from mechanical stress on viable perianeurysmal myocardium (15) (Fig. 8).

ECG manifestations of central nervous system disease can also resemble myocardial ischemia (Fig. 9). The underlying mechanism is unknown, but it is probably mediated by the sympathetic nervous system. Deep, symmetrical T wave inversion and QT prolongation can occur during subarachnoid hemorrhage, ischemic stroke, and various other noncardiac illnesses (67–71).

IV. CONCLUSION

Despite the rapid, ongoing development of costly and sophisticated diagnostic modalities, the ECG is still critically important in the diagnosis and treatment of ACS. It can provide independent prognostic information even after adjustment for elevated cardiac biomarkers and clinical findings, and it may be the only abnormal finding among patients with ACS and transient symptoms. To that end, all patients with suspected ACS should be placed in an environment where continuous cardiac monitoring is available. A 12-lead ECG should be obtained and definitively interpreted within 10 minutes (10) in order to quickly deliver appropriate therapy or recognize other causes of chest pain. If possible, previous tracings should be obtained for comparison, especially when STE is noted. Serial tracings are invaluable and should be obtained expeditiously, especially when symptoms are intermittent or recurrent. As with all patients suspected of having ACS, the ECG should not be interpreted in isolation, but should be integrated with other clinical and laboratory findings. Thus, as it passes its 100th year of clinical use, the ECG remains an invaluable tool in the armamentarium of all physicians, and will it continue to be useful for diagnosing ischemic heart disease and arrhythmias in the future.

REFERENCES

1. Cannon CP, McCabe CH, Stone PH, Rogers WJ, Schactman M, Thompson BW, Pearce KJ, Diver DJ, Kells C, Feldman T, Williams M, Gibson RS, Kronenberg MW, Ganz LI, Anderson HV, Braunwald E. The electrocardiogram predicts one-year outcome of patients with unstable angina and non-Q-wave myocardial infarction: Results of the TIMI III Registry ECG Ancillary Study. Thrombolysis in Myocardial Ischemia. J Am Coll Cardiol 1997; 30:133–140.
2. Gazes PC, Mobley EM, Faris HM, Duncan RC, Humphries GB. Preinfarctional (unstable) angina—a prospective study—ten year follow-up: prognostic significance of electrocardiographic changes. Circulation 1973; 48:331–337.
3. Stenton RE, Flamm MD Jr, Zaret BL, McGowan RL. Transient ST-segment elevation with postmyocardial infarction angina: prognostic significance. Am Heart J 1975; 89:449–454.
4. Plotnick GD, Conti CR. Transient S-T segment deviation in unstable angina: prognostic significance. Am J Med 1979; 67:800–803.
5. Sclarovsky S, Davidson E, Lewin RF, Strasberg B, Arditti A, Agmon J. Unstable angina pectoris evolving to acute myocardial infarction: significance of ECG changes during chest pain. Am Heart J 1986; 112:459–462.
6. Scarovsky S, Davidson E, Strasberg B, Lewin RF, Arditti A, Wurtzel M, Agmon J. Unstable angina: the significance of ST segment elevation or depression in patients without evidence of increased myocardial oxygen demand. Am Heart J 1986; 112:463–467.

7. Cohen M, Hawkins L, Greenberg S, Fuster V. Usefulness of ST-segment changes in greater than or equal to 2 leads on the emergency room electrocardiogram in either unstable angina or non-Q-wave myocardial infarction in predicting outcome. Am J Cardiol 1991; 67:1368–137

8. Savonitto S, Ardissino D, Granger CB, Morando G, Prando MD, Mafrici A, Cavallini C, Melandri G, Thompson TD, Vahanian A, Ohman EM, Califf RM, Van de Werf F, Topol EJ. Prognostic value of the admission electrocardiogram in acute coronary syndromes. JAMA 1999; 281:707–713.

9. Hyde TA, French JK, Wong CK, Straznicky IT, Whitlock M, White HD. Four-year survival of patients with acute coronary syndromes without ST-segment elevation and prognostic significance of 0.5 mm ST-segment depression. Am J Cardiol 1999; 84:379–385.

10. Braunwald E, Antman EM, Beasley JW, Califf RM, Cheitlin MD, Hochman JS, Jones RH, Kereiakes D, Kupersmith J, Levin TN, Pepine CJ, Schaeffer JW, Smith EE III, Steward DE, Théroux P. ACC/AHA 2002 guideline update for the management of patients with unstable angina/non-ST segment elevation myocardial infarction: A report of the American College of Cardiology/American Heart Association task force on practice guidelines (Committee on the Management of Patients with Unstable Angina). 2002.

11. Inhibition of platelet glycoprotein IIb/IIIa with eptifibatide in patients with acute coronary syndromes. PURSUIT Trial Investigators. Platelet glycoprotein IIb/IIIa in unstable angina: receptor suppression using integrilin therapy. N Engl J Med 1998; 339:436–443.

12. Cohen M, Stinnett S, Weatherley BD, Gurfinkel EP, Fromelli GJ, Goodman SG, Fox KA, Califf RM. Predictors of recurrent ischemic events and death in unstable coronary artery disease after treatment with combination antithrombotic therapy. Am Heart J 2000; 139:962–970.

13. Lloyd-Jones DM, Camargo CAJ, Lapuerta P, Giugliano RP, O'Donnell, CJ. Electrocardiographic and clinical predictors of acute myocardial infarction in patients with unstable angina pectoris. Am J Cardiol 1998; 81:1182–1186.

14. Hayden GE, Brady WJ, Perron AD, Somers MP, Mattu A. Electrocardiographic T-wave inversion: differential diagnosis in the chest pain patient. Am J Emerg Med 2002; 20:252–262.

15. Goldberger AL. Myocardial Infarction: Electrocardiographic Differential Diagnosis. 4th ed. St. Louis: Mosby-Year Book, 1991.

16. de Zwaan C, Bär FWHM, Wellens HJJ. Characteristic electrocardiographic pattern indicating a critical stenosis high in the left anterior descending coronary artery in patients admitted because of impending acute myocardial infarction. Am Heart J 1982; 103:730–736.

17. de Zwaan C, Bär FWHM, Janssen JH, De Swart HB, Vermeer F, Wellens HJJ. Effects of thrombolytic therapy in unstable angina: clinical and angiographic results. J Am Coll Cardiol 1988; 12:301–309.

18. Renkin J, Wijns W, Ladha Z, Col J. Reversal of segmental hypokinesis by coronary angioplasty in patients with unstable angina, persistent T wave inversion, and left anterior descending coronary stenosis: additional evidence for myocardial stunning in humans. Circulation 1990; 82:913–919.

19. Rouan GW, Lee TH, Cook EF, Brand DA, Weisberg MC, Goldman L. Clinical characteristics and outcome of acute myocardial infarction in patients with initially normal or nonspecific electrocardiograms (a report from the Multicenter Chest Pain Study). Am J Cardiol 1999; 33:107–118.

20. McCarthy BD, Wong JB, Selker HP. Detecting acute cardiac ischemia in the emergency department: a review of the literature. J Gen Intern Med 1990; 5:365–373.

21. Slater DK, Hlatky MA, Mark DB, Harrell FEJ, Pryor DB, Califf RM. Outcome in suspected acute myocardial infarction with normal or minimally abnormal admission electrocardiographic findings. Am J Cardiol 1987; 60:766–770.

22. Langer A, Freeman MR, Armstrong PW. ST segment shift in unstable angina: pathophysiology and association with coronary anatomy and hospital outcome. J Am Coll Cardiol 1989; 13:1495–1502.

23. Langer A, Freeman MR, Armstrong PW. Relation of angiographic detected intracoronary thrombus and silent myocardial ischemia in unstable angina pectoris. Am J Cardiol 1990; 66:1381–1382.

24. Patel DJ, Knight CJ, Holdright DR, Mulcahy D, Clarice D, Wright C, Purcell H, Fox KM. Long-term prognosis in unstable angina: the importance of early risk stratification using continuous ST segment monitoring. Eur Heart J 1998; 19:240–249.

25. Jernberg T, Lindhal B, Wallentin L. ST-segment monitoring with continuous 12-lead ECG improves early risk stratification in patients with chest pain and ECG nondiagnostic of acute myocardial infarction. J Am Coll Cardiol 1999; 34:1413–1419.

26. Aguiar C, Ferreria J, Seabra-Gomes R. Prognostic value of continuous ST-segment monitoring in patients with non–ST-segment elevation acute coronary syndromes. Ann Nonivas Electrocardiol 2002; 7:29–39.

27. Madias JE. The earliest electrocardiographic signs of acute transmural myocardial infarction. J Electrocardiol 1977; 10:193.

28. Rosen, P. Emergency Medicine: Concepts and Clinical Practice. 4th ed. St. Louis: Mosby-Year Book, 1998.

29. Kondo T, Kubota I, Tachibana H, Yamaki M, Tomoike H. Glibenclamide attenuates peaked T wave in early phase of myocardial ischemia. Cardiovasc Res 1996; 31:683–687.

30. Brady WJ, Aufderheide TP, Chan T, Perron AD. Electrocardiographic diagnosis of acute myocardial infarction. Emerg Med Clin North Am 2001; 19:295–319.

31. Phibbs B, Marcus F, Marriott HJ, Moss A, Spodick DH. Q-wave versus non-Q-wave myocardial infarction: a meaningless distinction. J Am Coll Cardiol 1999; 33:576–582.

32. Mirvis DM, Ingram LA, Ramanathan KB, Wilson JL. R and S wave changes produced by experimental nontransmural and transmural myocardial infarction. J Am Coll Cardiol 1986; 8:675–681.

33. Goldschlager N, Goldman MJ. Principles of Clinical Electrocardiography. East Norwalk: Appleton and Lange, 1989.

34. Brady WJ, Roberts D, Morris F. The nondiagnostic ECG in the chest pain patient: normal and nonspecific initial ECG presentations of acute MI. Am J Emerg Med 1999; 17:394–397.

35. Rouan GW, Lee TH, Cook EF, Brand DA, Weisberg MC, Goldman L. Clinical characteristics and outcome of patients with acute myocardial infarction and initially normal or nonspecific electrocardiograms. Am J Cardiol 1989; 64:1087–1092.

36. Lee T, Cook F, Weisberg M, Sargent RK, Wilson C, Goldman L. Acute chest pain in the emergency room: identification and examination of low risk patients. Arch Intern Med 1985; 145:65–69.

37. Fesmire FM, Percy RF, Wears RL, MacMath TL. Initial ECG in Q wave and non-Q wave myocardial infarction. Ann Emerg Med 1989; 18:741–746.

38. Blanke H, Cohen M, Schlueter GU, Karsch KR, Rentrop KP. Electrocardiographic and coronary correlations during acute myocardial infarction. Am J Cardiol 1984; 54:249–255.

39. Aldrich HR, Hindman NB, Hinoara T, Jones MG, Boswick J, Lee KL, Bride W, Califf RM. Identification of optimal electrocardiographic leads for detecting acute epicardial injury in acute myocardial infarction. Am J Cardiol 1987; 59:20–23.

40. Topol EJ, Van de Werf FJ. Acute myocardial infarction: early diagnosis and management. In: Topol EJ, ed. Textbook of Cardiovascular Medicine. Philadelphia: Lippincott-Raven,1998:403–404.

41. Gelman JS, Saltrups A. Precordial ST depression in patients with inferior infarctions: clinical implications. Br Heart J 1982; 48:560–565.

42. Shah PK, Pichler M, Berman DS, Maddahi J, Peter T, Singh BN, Swan HJ. Noninvasive identification of a high-risk subset of patients with acute inferior myocardial infarction. Am J Cardiol 1980; 46:915–921.

43. Goldberg HL, Borer JS, Jacobstein JG, Kluger J, Scheidt SS, Alonso DR. Anterior ST-segment depression in acute inferior myocardial infarction: indicator of posterolateral infarction. Am J Cardiol 1981; 48:1009–1015.

44. Ong L, Valdellon B, Coromilas J, Brody R, Reiser P, Morrison J. Precordial S-T segment depression in acute inferior myocardial infarction: evaluation by quantitative thallium-201 scintigraphy and technetium-99m ventriculography.

45. Gibson RS, Crampton RS, Watson DD, et al. Precordial ST-segment depression during acute inferior myocardial infarction: clinical, scintigraphic, and angiographic correlations. Circulation 1982; 66:732–741.

46. Roubin GS, Shen WF, Nicholson M, Dunn RF, Kelly DT, Harris PJ. Anterolateral ST segment depression in acute inferior myocardial infarction: angiographic and clinical implications. Am Heart J 1984; 107:1177–1182.

47. Hlatky MA, Califf RM, Lee KL, Pryor DB, Wagner GS, Rosati RA. Prognostic significance of precordial ST-segment depression during inferior myocardial infarction. Am J Cardiol 1985; 55:325–329.

48. Nasmith J, Marpole D, Rahal D, Homan J, Stewart S, Sniderman A. Clinical outcomes after inferior infarction. Ann Intern Med 1982; 96:22–26.

49. Krone RJ, Greenberg H, Dwyer EM, Kleiger RE, Boden WE. Long-term prognostic significance of ST segment depression during acute myocardial infarction. The Multicenter Diltiazem Postinfarction Trial Research Group. J Am Coll Cardiol 1993; 22:361–367.

50. Birnbaum Y, Herz I, Sclarovsky S, Zlotikamien B, Chetrit A, Olmer L, Barbash G. Prognostic significance of precordial ST segment depression on admission electrocardiogram in patients with inferior wall myocardial infarction. J Am Coll Cardiol 1996; 28:313–318.

51. Kontos MC, Desai PV, Jesse RL, Ornato JP. Usefulness of the admission electrocardiogram for identifying the infarct-related artery in inferior wall myocardial infarction. Am J Cardiol 1997; 79:182–184.

52. Zehender M, Kasper W, Kauder E, Schönthaler M, Geibel M, Olschewski M, Just H. Right ventricular infarction as an independent predictor of prognosis after acute inferior myocardial infarction. N Engl J Med 1993; 328:981–988.

53. Braat SH, Brugada P, den Dulk K, van Ommen V, Wellens HJJ. Value of lead V4R for recognition of the infarct coronary artery in acute inferior myocardial infarction. Am J Cardiol 1984; 53:1538–1541.

54. Kopelman HA, Forman MB, Wilson H, Kolodgie FD, Smith RF, Friesinger GC, Virmani R. Right ventricular myocardial infarction in patients with chronic lung disease: possible role of right ventricular hypertrophy. J Am Coll Cardiol 1985; 5:1302–1307.

55. Huey BL, Beller GA, Kaiser DL, Gibson RS. A comprehensive analysis of myocardial infarction due to left circumflex artery occlusion: comparison with infarction due to right coronary artery and left posterior descending artery occlusion. J Am Coll Cardiol 1988; 12:1156–1166.

56. Kulkarni AU, Brown R, Ayoubi M, Banka VS. Clinical use of posterior electrocardiographic leads: a prospective electrocardiographic analysis during coronary occlusion. Am Heart J 1996; 131:736–741.

57. Blanke H, Cohen M, Schlueter GU, et al. Electrocardiographic and coronary correlations during acute myocardial infarction. Am J Cardiol 1984; 54:249–255.

58. Boden WE, Kleiger RE, Gibson RS, Schwartz DJ, Schechtman KB, Capone RJ, Roberts R, and the diltiazem reinfarction study group. Electrocardiographic evolution of posterior acute myocardial infarction: Importance of early precordial ST-segment depression. Am J Cardiol 1987; 59:782–792.

59. Brady WJ, Hwang V, Sullivan R, Chang N, Beagle C, Carter CT, Martin ML, Aufderheide TP. A comparison of the 12 lead ECG to the 15–lead ECG in emergency department chest pain patients: impact on diagnosis, therapy, and disposition. Am J Emerg Med 2000; 18:239–243.

60. Rude RE, Poole WK, Muller JE, Zoltan T, Rutherford J, Parker C, Roberts R, Raabe DS Jr, Gold HK, Stone PH, Willerson JT, Braunwald E and the MILIS Study Group. Electrocardiographic and clinical criteria for recognition of acute myocardial infarction based on analysis of 3697 patients. Am J Cardiol 1983; 52:936–942.

61. Sgarbossa EB, Pinski SL, Barbagelata A, Underwood DA, Gates KB, Topol EJ, Califf RM, Wagner GS. Electrocardiographic diagnosis of evolving acute myocardial infarction in the presence of left bundle-branch block. GUSTO-1 (Global Utilization of Streptokinase and Tissue Plasminogen Activator for Occluded Coronary Arteries) investigators. N Engl J Med 1996; 334:481–487.

62. Sgarbossa EB, Pinski SL, Gates KB, Wagner GS. Early electrocardiographic diagnosis of acute myocardial infarction in the presence of ventricular paced rhythm. GUSTO-1 (Global Utilization of Streptokinase and Tissue Plasminogen Activator for Occluded Coronary Arteries) investigators. Am J Cardiol 1996; 77:423–424.

63. Beach C, Kenmure CF, Short D. Electrocardiogram of pure left ventricular hypertrophy and its differentiation from lateral ischemia. Br Heart J 1981; 46:285–289.
64. Spodik DH. Differential characteristics of the electrocardiogram in early repolarization and acute pericarditis. N Engl J Med 1976; 295:523–526.
65. Wasserburger RM, Alt WJ, Lloyd C. The normal RS-T segment evolution variant. Am J Cardiol 1961; 8:184–192.
66. Engel J, Brady WJ, Mattu A, Perron AD. Electrocardiographic ST segment elevation: left ventricular aneurysm. Am J Emerg Med 2002; 20:238–242.
67. Yamour BJ, Sridharan MR, Rice JF, Flowers NC. Electrocardiographic changes in cerebrovascular hemorrhage. Am Heart J 1980; 99:294–300.
68. Hugenholtz PG. Electrocardiographic changes typical for central nervous system after right radical neck dissection. Am Heart J 1967; 74:438–441.
69. Gould L, Gopalaswami C, Chandy F, Kim B. Electroconvulsive therapy-induced ECG changes simulating a myocardial infarction. Arch Intern Med 1983; 143:1786–1787.
70. Koepp M, Schmidt D, Kern A. Electrocardiographic changes in patients with brain tumors. Arch Neurol 1995; 52:152–155.
71. Sharkey SW, Shear W, Hodges M, Herzog CA. Myocardial contraction abnormalities in patients with an acute noncardiac illness. Chest 1998; 114:98–105.

10-2

Acute Coronary Syndromes: Serum Biomarkers

Aaron Satran and Robert C. Hendel
Rush-Presbyterian–St. Luke's Medical Center, Chicago, Illinois, U.S.A.

Accurate identification and prompt, appropriate treatment of acute coronary syndrome (ACS) is essential. However, recognizing patients with unstable angina (UA) or acute myocardial infarction (AMI) can often be difficult. The baseline ECG and a history of ischemic-type chest pain remain primary screening methods for ACS, but they are imperfect modalities at best. A significant number (at least 50%) of patients who are ultimately shown to have AMI present with nondiagnostic ECGs, and atypical chest pain is common. Thus, in the majority of patients, clinicians require additional information such as that obtained with serial biochemical cardiac markers in order to exclude or establish the diagnosis of AMI.

Following severe ischemic injury, myocytes become necrotic and lose membrane integrity. Intracellular macromolecules then diffuse into the cardiac interstitium and ultimately into the lymphatics and microvasculature (1). Depending on several factors, they eventually become detectible in the peripheral circulation. These markers of myocardial damage should be specific for cardiac tissue and absent from the periphery (2,3) to ensure a high level of diagnostic accuracy. For optimal sensitivity, they should be rapidly released into the blood in direct proportion to the degree of myocardial injury. The ideal markers should persist long enough to allow for a convenient diagnostic time frame and fall rapidly enough not to mask reinjury. Finally, they should be easily, inexpensively, and rapidly assayed. At present, no single biochemical cardiac marker satisfies all of these requirements. When clinically integrated, however, each one can provide potentially valuable diagnostic and prognostic information in the management of ACS.

I. CREATINE KINASE

Creatine kinase (CK) is a large enzyme (molecular weight 86,000 d) that is ubiquitous in cardiac and skeletal muscle. Functionally, it catalyzes the transfer of phosphate groups in tissues with high metabolic rates requiring large amounts of energy (4). On the molecular level, CK is too large to enter the capillaries; it must be transported by lymphatics prior to release into the serum. Thus, there is a delay between tissue release and serum elevation. Elevated serum CK is a sensitive indicator of AMI. It is detectible within 3–8 hours and peaks between 12 and 24 hours; a return to baseline values occurs within 3–4 days (5). However, peak levels occur earlier in patients who receive thrombolytic therapy, undergo percutaneous recanalization, or experience spontaneous thrombolysis, all of which limit the ability of CK to detect infarct size (1,6). Also, the specificity of CK is limited, as multiple conditions can result in elevated serum values (Table 1). Because of these limitations, total CK assays are now performed primarily as screening tests prior to ordering a specific, more expensive isozyme assay such as CK-MB.

II. CK ISOENZYMES

There are two subunits of CK, B (named for brain tissue), and M (named for muscle tissue). Different combinations of these subunits create the three CK isoenzymes: BB, MM, and MB. Brain and kidney contain predominantly the BB isoenzyme, skeletal muscle contains MM and some MB, while both MM and MB are found in cardiac muscle (85% CK-MM, 15% CK-MB). Low levels of the MB isoenzyme are also detectable in the intestine, tongue, diaphragm, uterus, and prostate. Because CK-MB can be detected in the blood of healthy subjects, especially in the setting of vigorous physical activity, the cutoff value for elevation is usually set a few units above the normal range for a given laboratory.

Current CK-MB assay methods include highly sensitive and specific mass immunoassays (as opposed to older activity assays) that use monoclonal antibodies directed against CK-MB (8). Following injury, CK-MB is detectable in the serum within 4–6 hours, peaks at 12 to 24 hours, and normalizes within 2–3 days (9). Conservatively, a ratio (relative index) of CK-MB to CK activity of 2.5 is indicative of a myocardial source of CK-MB elevation, although some laboratories use a ratio of 5. As an independent biomarker, an elevated absolute level of CK-MB has been shown to portend adverse outcomes among patients with sus-

Table 1   Non-ACS Causes of Serum CK and CK-MB Elevation

Non-ACS cardiac process
Pericarditis
Myocarditis
Myocardial trauma
Cardiac catheterization or cardiac surgery
Systemic process
Muscular dystrophy
Polymyositis
Collagen vascular disease
Reye's syndrome
Peripheral source
Rhabdomyolysis
Athletic activity
Prostate surgery
Gastrointestinal surgery
Cesarian section
Seizure activity
Intramuscular injection
Miscellaneous
Renal failure
Subarachnoid hemorrhage
Hypothyroidism
Hyperthyroidism
Hypothermia
Hyperthermia
Pulmonary embolism

Source: Adapted from Refs. 4, 5.

pected or confirmed ACS (10), even in the presence of normal CK levels (11–13). However, CK-MB levels may be inaccurate in the setting of acute or chronic skeletal muscle injury, myocarditis, trauma, cardiac surgery or catheterization, gastrointestinal surgery, cesarean section, and shock (Table 1). Regardless, these conditions are usually clinically apparent, and in their absence an elevated absolute level of CK-MB is pathopneumonic for AMI (7).

III. CK ISOFORMS

Isoforms of the MM and MB isoenzymes (CK-MM1, CK-MM2, CK-MM3, CK-MB1, and CK-MB2) have been identified. MM and MB isoforms are formed in the peripheral circulation by the action of carboxypeptidase, which cleaves lysine residues from CK-MM3 and CK-MB2 to form CK-MM2, CK-MM1, and CK-MB1 (7). CK-MB isoenzymes are more sensitive indicators of myocardial damage than are CK isoenzymes. Puelo et al. showed that CK-MB isoforms were accurate markers (95.7% sensitivity) of myocardial infarction in the first 6 hours after the onset of symptoms, compared to the conventional CK-MB assay, which was only 48% sensitive (14). Similarly, Zimmerman et al. reported that CK-MB2 levels greater than 1.0 U/Lr or a ratio of CK-MB2 to CK-MB1 of >2.5 is 46.4% sensitive for diagnosing AMI at 4 hours and 91.5% sensitive at 6 hours (15). Additionally, assays for CK isoforms may permit early detection of successful reperfusion (CK-MB2/CK-MB1 > 3.8 at 2 hours) (16). Overall, although earlier identification of patients with AMI using CK-MB isoenzymes is possible, they are currently utilized only by dedicated research centers. Broader acceptance is limited due to economic and technical constraints.

IV. MYOGLOBIN

Myoglobin is a small, low molecular weight (17,800 D) heme protein found in both cardiac and skeletal muscle. It is released rapidly from injured myocardial cells directly into the coronary circulation (peak serum levels are detectible within 1–4 hours of AMI) and is cleared within 24 hours (16). Serum assays to detect myoglobin are readily available, unlike those for CK-MB isoforms. Among patients with STEMI, elevated myoglobin levels are associated with increased mortality, most likely due to extensive myocardial damage (18). The utility of myoglobin may be limited by lack of cardiac specificity, a brief duration of elevation, and dependence on renal clearance, but a high level of sensitivity, enhanced specificity when combined with CK-MB and cardiac troponins, and early peak after myocardial injury (within 1–4 hours) are helpful features, especially for the very early diagnosis of AMI (19,20). Also, rapid rises in serum myoglobin have been observed after thrombolysis or successful PCI; thus, serial measurements may point to successful reperfusion or correlate with infarct size (17). Finally, elevated levels of serum myoglobin in the setting of ACS may aid in risk stratification by portending increased mortality regardless of baseline clinical characteristics, ECG changes or elevation of other cardiac biomarkers (21), although other studies have not conclusively established an independent correlation (19,22–24).

V. CARDIAC-SPECIFIC TROPONINS

The troponin complex, which regulates the calcium-dependent contractile cycle in striated muscle, consists of three subunits: troponin T (TnT), troponin C (TnC), and troponin I (TnI). Cardiac and skeletal muscles both contain TnT and TnI, but they are encoded by different gene sequences. Thus, monoclonal antibody–based assays can distinguish cardiac-specific TnT (cTnT) and TnI (cTnI). Because TnC has the same isoform in cardiac and smooth muscle, no immunoassays of this subunit have been developed for evaluating ACS. Therefore, reference to "cardiac troponins" implies either cTnI or cTnT. Abnormal levels of cardiac troponins in the setting of ACS provide important prognostic information independent of clinical characteristics, baseline ECG changes, or predischarge exercise stress testing (25–27). Even with normal CK-MB levels, patients who present with NSTEMI as evidenced by elevated cTnT and cTnI levels are at increased risk for death, a risk that is incrementally tied to the measured quantity of cTnT or cTnI (28,29).

Cardiac troponin release in the setting of myocardial ischemia is location dependent. The majority of cTnI and cTnT is structurally bound in the muscle fiber, while only small quantities are found free in the cytoplasm (30,31). Cytoplasmic cardiac troponins are released early and are detectible within 4 hours from the onset of symptoms. Subsequent tissue degeneration leads to a prolonged rise and release over the following days, which can lead to difficulty in determining the exact timing of myocardial damage. The cutoff level for elevated values of cardiac troponins (defined as exceeding that of 99% of a reference control group) (32) is set to slightly above the upper limit of normal for a particular assay, since cardiac troponins are theoretically undetectable in the blood of healthy persons. As a rule, the assays for cTnT are uniform, as they are produced by a single manufacturer, but the assays for cTnI are produced by multiple manufacturers. The sensitivity and threshold values can vary between laboratories, because the majority of cTnI in the bloodstream is complexed with cTnC, which necessitates different antibodies to detect free and complexed cTnI and can alter the cutoff concentration for abnormal levels (33).

Because of their high sensitivity, cardiac troponins can be abnormally elevated without concurrent CK-MB elevation, a finding associated with histological evidence of focal myocyte necrosis in case reports, (34–36), and termed "minor myocardial damage" or "microinfarction" by some investigators (37). Among patients who present with rest pain, normal levels of CK-MB, and no ST segment elevation, approximately 30% would be diagnosed with ACS when assessed with cardiac troponins. This high sensitivity and near absolute myocardial specificity has made cardiac troponins integral to most recent definition of AMI, in particular their serial rise and gradual fall along with either symptoms or ECG changes (38). However, although cardiac troponins are highly sensitive markers of myocardial damage, not all elevations of cTnT or cTnI are due to atherosclerotic coronary artery disease (CAD). Additional precipitants of ACS may be present, including dynamic obstruction (such as coronary spasm or vasoconstriction), inflammation and/or infection, and conditions that alter myocardial metabolic requirements, such as fever, tachycardia, thyrotoxicosis, hypotension, anemia, or hypoxia (39). Therefore, the diagnosis of ACS must be based on ECG changes and clinical findings in addition to elevated cardiac troponins (40). Currently available assays for cTnT and cTnI are equally sensitive and specific for detecting myocardial damage; the choice of which biomarker to measure should be based on cost and institutional preference.

VI. RENAL INSUFFICIENCY

Measurement of cardiac biomarkers in patients with chronic renal insufficiency (CRI) and end-stage renal disease (ESRD) deserves special mention. Although renal dysfunction is an established marker of adverse baseline clinical characteristics and is independently associated with increased risk of death or MI among patients presenting with ACS (41,42), false elevations in CK-MB can be seen in chronic dialysis patients without acute ischemic heart disease (43–47), possibly due to abnormal protein metabolism and muscle wasting. cTnT and cTnI are highly specific for myocardial damage, and elevated cTnT appears to predict adverse outcomes among high-risk patients regardless of creatinine clearance (48), but both markers can also be elevated among dialysis patients without evidence of ongoing myocardial ischemia, especially cTnT (49–52). The etiology for these nonspecific elevations in cardiac troponins is uncertain, although they are likely related to variable expression in extracardiac tissue in combination with impaired renal clearance and excretion. Early cTnT assays demonstrated significant cross-reactivity with skeletal troponin T (52), leading to elevated values in a large percentage of patients (>40%) (49), and improved cTnT assays still yield suboptimal results. With cutoffs ranging from 0.1 to 0.4 ug/L, second-generation assays can show elevated cTnT values in 12–18% of chronic dialysis patients without ACS (41,43,53). Thus, among patients with CRI or ESRD, where incidental elevation of cardiac biomarkers is possible, serial measurements to assess their rise and/or fall may be useful in the appropriate clinical context. In this particular cohort, as with all patients, ACS should not be diagnosed on the basis of an isolated laboratory abnormality.

VII. NEWER CARDIAC BIOMARKERS

Although there are other biochemical markers used to detect myocardial ischemia that are less well studied than those described above, they may provide supplementary diagnostic information that can be incorporated into an overall risk assessment. Elevated markers of coagulation activity are detectible as a result of chronic vascular inflammation secondary to progressive atherosclerosis. They include fibrinopeptide, fibrinogen, serum amyloid A, and interleuken-6 z9il-6), all of which may indicate ACS patients at high risk (54–58). Other investigational markers that may predict increased risk in patients with ACS include circulating soluble adhesion molecules such as intracellular adhesion molecule-1, vascular-cell adhesion molecule-1, and E-selectin (59,60). Multiple recent studies have shown that patients with significantly elevated levels of C-reactive protein (CRP) in the setting of ACS are at increased risk for adverse outcome, with or without concurrent serological evidence of myocardial necrosis (57,61–67). In the TIMI 11A study, early mortality for patients with elevated CRP levels was 5.6%, compared with 0.3% if CRP levels were normal, regardless of cTnT measurements (68). Even among patients with ACS undergoing an early invasive strategy, Mueller et al. (69) showed that elevated levels of CRP were a strong predictor of early and late mortality. Undoubtedly, these newer markers will eventually be integrated into a point-of-care cardiac biomarker panel, but at present they are investigational, and there is no consensus recommendation to support their routine measurement in the setting of ACS.

VIII. CLINICAL USE OF CARDIAC BIOMARKERS: RECOMMENDATIONS

Of all the serum biomarkers, cardiac troponins have gained acceptance as the primary marker in ACS. They provide the greatest diagnostic sensitivity and can identify even small amounts of myocardial necrosis. Also, as noted, even mildly elevated levels of cTnI or cTnT are markers of high risk in patients with ACS. Thus, cardiac troponins provide diagnostic and prognostic information above and beyond clinical presentation, ECG findings, and serum CK-MB measurements. However, for early detection (within 6 hours) of AMI, CK-MB isoforms and myoglobin may be more useful, as cardiac troponins will not become elevated until at least 4 hours after an ischemic insult, and as such may not exclude

Table 2   Cardiac Biomarkers in ACS/NSTEMI: Timing

Marker	Time to initial elevation (h)	Time to peak elevation (h)	Time to return to normal range
Myoglobin	1–4 h	6–7 h	24 h
Cardiac troponins	3–12 h	12–48 h	5–14 days
CK-MB	3–12 h	24 h	48–72 h
CK-MB Isoforms	1–6 h	18 h	Unknown

Source: Adapted from Ref. 7.

a diagnosis of ACS for 8–12 hours after the onset of injury. Myoglobin should not be used in isolation given its poor cardiac specificity and rapid clearance from the bloodstream, but if negative it is helpful for excluding ACS. Although not recommended routinely, serum markers of inflammation such as CRP may provide additional diagnostic and prognostic information.

Obviously, there is significant overlap in the release pattern of the various biochemical cardiac markers, which must be taken into account when evaluating patients for ACS (Tables 2,3). In order to make best use of their respective diagnostic strengths, changes in concentration of cardiac biomarkers should be measured over time. Such a strategy allows for risk stratification; for instance, patients with increasing values and no ST-segment elevation should likely receive GP IIb/IIIa inhibitors, while those with no change over time could undergo early stress testing (70–72). At present, point-of-care testing is available that allows for simultaneous rapid measurement of myoglobin, CK-MB, and cTnI at presentation (70,73,74). With the use of a central laboratory, results should be available within 60 minutes. Point-of-care systems require rigorous quality control and appropriate personnel training, but if properly utilized can reduce transportation and processing delays while expediting appropriate triage and definitive therapy. As they become more widely

Table 3   Cardiac Biomarkers in ACS/NSTEMI: Advantages and Disadvantages

Marker	Advantages	Disadvantages
Myoglobin	Useful for early detection May aid in risk stratification	Low specificity
CK-MB	Rapid Cost-efficient Can detect early reinfarction	Low early and late sensitivity Low specificity in the presence of confounding clinical conditions
CK-MB isoforms	More sensitive than CK-MB Useful for early detection	Expensive Limited availabilty
Cardiac troponins	Powerful risk stratifiers High sensitivity and specificity Can detect late reinfarction Useful for therapy selection	Low early sensitivity May be incidentally elevated in the setting off chronic renal failure If negative, requires repeat measurement

Source: Adapted from Ref. 36.

available, point-of-care systems will continue to evolve and ultimately, along with other diagnostic modalities and newer cardiac biomarkers, will facilitate the diagnosis and treatment of ACS.

REFERENCES

1. Adams J III, Abendschein D, Jaffe A. Biochemical markers of myocardial injury: is CK-MB the choice for the 1990's? Circulation 1993; 88:750–763.
2. Ellis AK. Serum protein measurements and the diagnosis of acute myocardial infarction. Circulation 1991; 83:1107–1109.
3. Gibler WB, Young GP, Hedges JR, Lewis LM, Smith MS, Carleton SC, Aghababian RV, Jorden RO, Allison EJ Jr, Otten EJ. Acute myocardial infarction in chest pain patients with nondiagnostic ECG's: serial CK-MB sampling in the emergency department. The Emergency Medicine Cardiac Research Group. Ann Emerg Med 1992; 21:504–512.
4. Karras DJ, Kane DL. Serum markers in the emergency department diagnosis of acute myocardial infarction. Emerg Med Clin North Am 2000; 19:321-337.
5. Lee TH, Goldman L. Serum enzyme assays in the diagnosis of acute myocardial infarction. Recommendations based on a quantitative analysis. Ann Intern Med 1986; 105:221-233.
6. Roberts R. Enzymatic estimation of infarct size: Thrombolysis induced its demise: Will it now rekindle its renaissance? Circulation 1990; 81:707–710.
7. Antman EM, Braunwald E. Acute myocardial infarction. In: Braunwald E, Zipes DP, Libby P, eds. Heart Disease: A Textbook of Cardiovascular Medicine. Philadelphia: W. B. Saunders Company, 2001:1132.
8. Christenson RH, Vaidya H, Landt Y, Bauer RS, Green SF, Apple FA, Jacob A, Magneson GR, Nag S, Wu AH, Azzazy HM. Standardization of creatine kinase-MB (CK-MB) mass assays: the use of recombinant CK-MB as a reference material. Clin Chem 1999; 45:1414–1423.
9. Lee TH, Goldman L. Serum enzyme assays in the diagnosis of acute myocardial infarction. Ann Intern Med 1986; 105:221.
10. Alexander JH, Sparapani RA, Mahaffey KW, Deckers JW, Newby KL, Ohman ME, Corbalan R, Chierchia SL, Boland JB, Simoons ML, Califf RM, Topol EJ, Harrington RA, for the PURSUIT steering committee. Associations between minor elevations of creatine kinase-MB level and mortality in patients with acute coronary syndromes without ST-segment elevation. JAMA 2000; 283:347–353.
11. Peacock FW, Emerman CL, Mcerlean ES, DeLuca SA, VanLente F, Lowrie M, Rao JS, Nissen SE. Normal CK, elevated MB predicts complications in acute coronary syndromes. J Emerg Med 2001; 20:385–390.
12. Clyne CA, Mederios LJ, Marton KI. The prognostic significance of immunoradiometric CK-MB assay (IRMA) diagnosis of myocardial infarction in patients with low total CK and elevated MB isozymes. Am Heart J 1989; 118:901-906.
13. Hong RA, Licht JD, Wei JY, Heller GV, Blaustein AS, Pasternak RC. Elevated CK-MB with normal creatinine kinase in suspected myocardial infarction: associated clinical findings and early prognosis. Am Heart J 1986; 11:1401-1406.
14. Puelo PR, Meyer D, Wathen C, Tawa CB, Wheeler S, Hamburg RJ, Ali N, Obermueller SD, Triana FJ, Zimmerman JL, Perryman B, Roberts R. Use of rapid assay of subforms of creatine kinase MB to diagnose or rule out acute myocardial infarction. N Engl J Med 1994; 331:561-566.
15. Zimmerman J, Fromm R, Meyer D, Boudreaux A, Wun CC, Smalling R, Davis B, Habib G, Roberts R. Diagnostic marker cooperative study for the diagnosis of myocardial infarction. Circulation 1999; 99:1671-1677.
16. Apple FS. Creatine kinase isoforms and myoglobin: early detection of myocardial infarction and reperfusion. Coron Artery Dis 1999; 10:75–79.
17. Tanasijevic MJ, Cannon CP, Antman EM, Wybenga DR, Fischer GA, Grudzien C, Gibson CM, Winkleman JW, Braunwald E. Myoglobin, creatinine kinase-MB, and cardiac troponin I 60

minute ratios predict infarct-related artery patency after thrombolysis for acute myocardial infarction: results from thrombolysis in myocardial ischemia (TIMI) 10B. J Am Coll Cardiol 1999; 34:739–747.

18. de Lemos JA, Antman, EM, Giugliano RP, Morrow DA, McCabe CH, Charlesworth A, Schroder R, Braun E. Very early risk stratification after thrombolytic therapy using a bedside myoglobin assay and the 12 lead ECG. Am Heart J 2000; 140:373–378.

19. Störk TV, Wu AHB, Müller-Bardorff M, Gareis R, Müller R, Hombach V, Katus H, Möckel M, for the North Württemberg infarction study (NOWSIS) group. Diagnostic and prognostic role of myoglobin in patients with suspected acute coronary syndrome. Am J Cardiol 2000; 86:1371-1374.

20. Newby LK, Storrow AB, Gibler WB, Garvey TL, Tucker JF, Kaplan AL, Schreiber DH, Tuttle RH, McNulty SE, Ohman EM. Bedside multimarker testing for risk stratification in chest pain units: the Chest Pain Evaluation by Creatinine-Kinase-MB, Myoglobin, and Troponin I (CHECKMATE) study. Circulation 2001; 103:1832–1837.

21. de Lemos JA, Morrow DA, Gibson CM, Murphy SA, Sabatine MS, Rifai N, McCabe CH, Antman EM, Cannon CP, Braunwald E. The prognostic value of serum myoglobin in patients with non-ST-segment elevation acute coronary syndromes: results from the TIMI 11B and TACTICS-TIMI 18 studies. J Am Coll Cardiol 2002; 40:238–244.

22. Jurlander B, Clemmensen P, Wagner GS, Grande P. Very early diagnosis and risk stratification of patients admitted with suspected acute myocardial infarction by the combined evaluation of a single serum value of cardiac troponin-T, myoglobin, and creatinine kinase MB (mass). Eur Heart J 2000; 21:382–389.

23. Holmvang L, Luscher MS, Clemmensen P, Thygesen K, Grande P. Very early risk stratification using combined ECG and biochemical assessment in patients with unstable coronary disease (a thrombin inhibition in myocardial ischemia [TRIM] substudy): the TRIM study group. Circulation 1998; 98:2004–2009.

24. Sonel A, Sasseen BM, Fineberg N, Bang N, Wilensky RL. Prospective study correlating fibrinopeptide A, troponin I, myoglobin, and myosin light chain levels with early and late ischemic events in consecutive patients presenting to the emergency department with chest pain. Circulation 2000; 102:1107–1113.

25. Pettijohn TL, Doyle T, Spiekerman AM, Watson LE, Riggs MW, Lawrence ME. Usefulness of positive troponin-T and negative creatine kinase levels in identifying high-risk patients with unstable angina pectoris. Am J Cardiol 1997; 80:510–511.

26. Galvani M, Ottani F, Ferrini D, Ladenson JH, Destro A, Baccos D, Rusticali F, Jaffea S. Prognostic influence of elevated values of cardiac troponin I in patients with unstable angina. Circulation 1997; 95:2053–2059.

27. Lindhal B, Andren B, Ohlsson J, Venge P, Wallentin L. Risk stratification in unstable coronary artery disease: additive value of troponin T determinations and pre-discharge exercise tests. FRISK study group. Eur Heart J 1997; 18:762–770.

28. Ohman EM, Armstrong PW, Christenson RH, Granger CB, Katus HA, Hamm CW, O'Hanesian MA, Wagner GS, Kleinman NS, Harrell FE, Califf RM, Topol EJ for the GUSTO IIA investigators. Cardiac troponin T levels for risk stratification in acute myocardial ischemia. N Engl J Med 1996; 335:1333–1341.

29. Antman EM, Tanasijevic MJ, Thompson B, Schactman M, McCabe CH, Cannon CP, Fischer GA, Fung AY, Thompson C, Wybenga D, Braunwald E. Cardiac-specific troponin I levels to predict the risk of mortality in patients with acute coronary syndromes. N Engl J Med 1996; 335:1342–1349.

30. Cummins B, Auckland ML, Cummins P. Cardiac-specific troponin-I radioimmunoassay in the diagnosis of acute myocardial infarction. Am Heart J 1987; 113:1333–1334.

31. Mair J, Dienstl F, Puschendorf B. Cardiac troponin T in the diagnosis of acute myocardial injury. Crit Rev Clin Lab Sci 1992; 29:31-57.

32. Zhao X-Q, Theroux P, Snapinn SM, Sax FL for the PRISM-PLUS Investigators. Intracoronary thrombus and platelet glycoprotein IIb/IIIa receptor blockade with tirofiban in unstable angina or non-Q-wave myocardial infarction: Angiographic results from the PRISM-PLUS trial

(Platelet Receptor Inhibition for Ischemic Syndrome Management in Patients Limited by Unstable Signs and Symptoms). Circulation 1999; 100:1609–1615.

33. Katrukha AG, Bereznikova AV, Esakova TV, Petterson K, Lovgren T, Severina ME, Pulkki K, Vuopio-Pulkki LM, Gusev NB. Troponin I is released in bloodstream of patients with acute myocardial infarction not in free form but as complex. Clin Chem 1997; 43:1379–1385.

34. Wu AH, Apple FS, Gibler WB, Jesse RL, Warshaw MM, Valdes RJ. National Academy of Clinical Biochemistry Standards of Laboratory Practice recommendations for the use of cardiac markers in coronary artery diseases. Clin Chem 1999; 45:1104–1121.

35. Antman EM, Grudzien C, Mitchell RN, Sacks DB. Detection of unsuspected myocardial necrosis by rapid bedside assay for cardiac troponin T. Am Heart J 1997; 133:596–598.

36. Apple FS, Falahati A, Paulen PR, Miller EA, Sharkey SW. Improved detection of minor ischemic myocardial injury with measurement of serum cardiac troponin I. Clin Chem 1997; 43:2047–2051.

37. Théroux P, Fuster V. Acute coronary syndromes: unstable angina and non-Q-wave myocardial infarction. Circulation 1998; 97:1195–1206.

38. The Joint European Society of Cardiology/American College of Cardiology Committee. Myocardial infarction redefined—a consensus document of the Joint European Society of Cardiology/American College of Cardiology Committee for the Redefinition of Myocardial Infarction. J Am Coll Cardiol 2000; 36:959–969.

39. Braunwald E. Unstable angina: an etiologic approach to management. Circulation 1998; 98:2219–2222.

40. Braunwald E, Antman EM, Beasley JW, Califf RM, Cheitlin MD, Hochman JS, Jones RH, Kereiakes D, Kupersmith J, Levin TN, Pepine CJ, Schaeffer JW, Smith EE III, Steward DE, Théroux P. ACC/AHA 2002 guideline update for the management of patients with unstable angina/non-ST segment elevation myocardial infarction: a report of the American College of Cardiology/American Heart Association Task Force on Practice Guidelines (Committee on the Management of Patients with Unstable Angina). 2002.

41. Apple FS, Sharkey SW, Hoeft P, Skeate R, Voss E, Dahlmeire BA, Preese LM. Prognostic value of serum cardiac troponin I and T in chronic dialysis patients. Am J Kidney Dis 1997; 29:399–403.

42. Al Suwaidi J, Reddan DN, Williams K, Pieper KS, Harrington RA, Califf RM, Granger CB, Ohman EM, Holmes DR for the GUSTO-IIb, GUSTO-III, PURSUIT, and PARAGON-A Investigators. Prognostic implications of abnormalities in renal function in patients with acute coronary syndromes. Circulation 2002; 106:974–980.

43. McLaurin MD, Apple FS, Voss ME, Herzog CA, Sharkey SW. Cardiac troponin I, cardiac troponin T, and creatine kinase MB in dialysis patients without ischemic heart disease: evidence of cardiac troponin T in skeletal muscle. Clin Chem 1997; 43:976–982.

44. Jaffe AS, Ritter C, Meltzer V, Harter H, Roberts R. Unmasking artifactual increases in creatinine kinase isoenzyme in patients with renal failure. J Lab Clin Med 1984; 104:193–202.

45. Chan KM, Landenson JH, Pierce GF, Jaffe AS. Increaed creatinine kinase MB in the absence of acute myocardial infarction. Clin Chem 1986; 32:2044–2051.

46. Lal SM, Nolph KD, Hain H, Moore HL, Khanna R, Van Stone JC, Twardowski ZJ. Total creatinine kinase and isoenzyme fractions in chronic dialysis patients. Int J Artif Organs 1987; 10:72–76.

47. Robbins MJ, Epstein EM, Shah S. Creatine kinase subform analysis in hemodialysis patients without acute coronary syndromes. Nephron 1997; 76:296–299.

48. Aviles RJ, Aksari AT, Lindahl B, Wallentin L, Jia G, Ohman EM, Mahaffey KW, Newby KL, Califf RM, Simoons ML, Topol EJ, Lauer MS. Troponin T levels in patients with acute coronary syndromes, with or without renal dysfunction. N Engl J Med 2002; 346:2047–2052.

49. Hafner G, Thome-Kroner B, Schaube J, Kupferwasser I, Ehrenthal W, Cummins P, Prellwitz W, Michel G. Cardiac troponins in serum in chronic renal failure (lett). Clin Chem 1994; 40:1790–1791.

50. Li D, Keffer J, Corry K, Vazquez M, Jialal I. Nonspecific elevations of troponin T levels in patients with chronic renal failure. Clin Biochem 1995; 28:474–477.

51. Lang K, Schindler S, Forberger C, Stein G, Figulla HR. Cardiac troponins have no prognostic value for acute and chronic cardiac events in asymptomatic patients with end-stage renal failure. Clin Nephrol 2001; 56:44–51.

52. Katus HA, Remppis A, Looser S, Hallermeier K, Scheffold T, Kübler W. Enzyme linked immunoassay of cardiac troponin T for the detection of acute myocardial infarction in patients. J Mol Cell Cardiol 1989; 21:1349–1353.

53. Wayand D, Baum H, Schätzle G, Schärf J, Neumier D. Cardiac troponin T and I in end-stage renal failure. Clin Chem 2000; 46:1345–1350.

54. Ardissino D, Merlini PA, Gamba G, Barberis P, Demicheli G, Testa S, GColombi E, Poli A, Fetiveau R, Montemartini C. Thrombin activity and early outcome in unstable angina pectoris. Circulation 1996; 93:1634–1639.

55. Becker RC, Cannon CP, Bovill EG, Tracy RP, Thompson B, Knatterud GL, Randall A, Braunwald B. Prognostic value of plasma fibrinogen concentration in patients with unstable angina and non-Q-wave myocardial infarction (TIMI IIIB trial). Am J Cardiol 1996; 78:142–147.

56. Biasucci LM, Vitelli A, Liuzzo G, Altamura S, Caligiuri G, Monaco C, Rebuzzi AG, Cilberto G, Maseri A. Elevated levels of interleukin-6 in unstable angina. Circulation 1996; 94:874–877.

57. Sabatine MS, Morrow DA, de Lemos JA, Gibson CM, Murphy SA, Rifai N, McCabe C, Antman EM, Cannon CP, Braunwald E. Multimarker approach to risk stratification in non-ST elevation acute coronary syndromes: simultaneous assessment of troponin I, C-reactive protein, and B-type natriuretic peptide. Circulation 2002; 105:1760–1763.

58. Ikeda U, Ito T, Shimada K. Interleuken-6 and acute coronary syndrome. Clin Cardiol 2001; 24:701-704.

59. Ghaisas NK, Shahi CN, Foley B, Goggins M, Crean P, Kelly A, Kelleher D, Walsh M. Elevated levels of circulating soluble adhesion molecules in peripheral blood of patients with unstable angina. Am J Cardiol 1997; 80:617–619.

60. O'Malley T, Ludlam CA, Riemermsa RA, Fox KA. Early increase in levels of soluble intracellular adhesion molecule 1 (sICAM-1); potential risk factor for the acute coronary syndromes. Eur Heart J 2001; 22:1226–1234.

61. Oltrona L, Ardissino D, Merlini PA, Spinola A, Chiodo F, Pezzano A. C reactive protein elevation and early outcome in patients with unstable angina pectoris. Am J Cardiol 1997; 80:1002–1006.

62. Haverkate F, Thompson SG, Pyke SD, Gallimore JR, Pepys MB, for the European Concerted Action on Thrombosis and Disabilities Angina Pectoris Study Group. Production of C-reactive protein and risk of coronary events in stable and unstable angina. Lancet 1997; 349:462–466.

63. Morrow DA, Rifai N, Antman EM, Weiner DL, McCabe CH, Cannon CP, Braunwald E. C-reactive protein is a potent predictor of mortality independently of an in combination with troponin T in acute coronary syndromes: a TIMI 11A substudy. Thrombolysis in Myocardial Infarction. J Am Coll Cardiol 1998; 31:1460–1465.

64. de Winter RJ, Fischer J, Bholasingh R, van Straalen JP, de Jong T, Tijssen JGP, Sanders GT. C-reactive protein and cardiac troponin T in risk stratification: differences in optimal timing of tests early after the onset of chest pain. Clin Chem 2000; 46:1597–1603

65. Toss H, Lindahl B, Siegbahn A, Wallentin L, for the FRISC Study Group. Prognostic influence of increased fibrinogen and C-reactive protein levels in unstable coronary disease. Circulation 1997; 96:4204–4210.

66. Rebuzzi AG, Quaranta G, Liuzzo G, Caligiuri G, Lanza GA, Gallimore JR, Grillo RL, Cianflone D, Biasucci LM, Maseri A. Incremental prognostic value of serum levels of troponin T and C-reactive protein on admission in patients with unstable angina pectoris. Am J Cardiol 1998; 82:715–719.

67. de Winter RJ, Bholasingh R, Lijmer JG, Koster RW, Gorgels JP, Schouten Y, Hoek FJ, Sanders GT. Independent prognostic value of C-reactive protein and troponin I in patients with unstable angina or non-Q-wave myocardial infarction. Cardiovasc Res 1999; 42:240–245.

68. Morrow DA, Rifai N, Antman EM, Weiner DL, McCabe CH, Cannon CP, Braunwald E. C-reactive protein is a potent predictor of mortality independently and in combination with troponin T in acute coronary syndromes: a TIMI 11A substudy. J Am Coll Cardiol 1998; 31:1460–1465.

69. Mueller C, Buettner HJ, Hodgson JM, Marsch S, Perruchod AP, Roskamm H, Neumann FJ. Inflammation and long term mortality after acute coronary syndrome treated with a very early invasive strategy in 1042 consecutive patients. Circulation 2002; 105:1412–1415.

70. Apple, FS, Christianson RH, Valdes R Jr, Andriak AJ, Berg A, Duh SH, Feng YJ, Jortani SA, Johnson SA, Koplen B, Mascotti K, Wu AH. Simultaneous rapid measurement of whole blood myoglobin, creatine kinase MB, and cardiac troponin I by the triage cardiac panel for detection of myocardial infarction. Clin Chem 1999; 45:199–205.

71. Fesmire FM, Percy RF, Bardoner JB, Wharton DR, Calhoun FB. Serial creatinine kinase (CK) MB testing during the emergency department evaluation of chest pain: utility of a 2–hour delta CK-MB of +1.6 ng/ml. Am Heart J 1998; 136:237–244.

72. Feshire FM. Delta CK-MB outperforms delta troponin I at 2 hours during the initial ER evaluation of chest pain. Am J Emerg Med 2000; 18:1-8.

73. Hamm CW, Goldmann BU, Heeschen C, Kreymann G, Berger J, Meinertz T. Emergency room triage of patients with acute chest pain by means of rapid testing for cardiac troponin T or troponin I. N Engl J Med 1997; 337:1648–1653.

74. Caragher TE, Fernandez BB, Jacobs FL, Barr LA. Evaluation of quantitative cardiac biomarker point-of-care testing in the emergency department. J Emerg Med 2002; 1:1-7.

10-3

Acute Coronary Syndromes: Diagnostic Imaging

Todd C. Kerwin and Robert C. Hendel
Rush Presbyterian–St. Luke's Medical Center, Chicago, Illinois, U.S.A.

Cardiac imaging, in the form of echocardiography and radionuclide myocardial perfusion imaging, has several roles for the evaluation and management of acute coronary syndromes (ACS). Noninvasive imaging can be used to aid in differentiating cardiac from noncardiac pain in patients presenting with chest pain syndromes for which the etiology is not immediately clear following initial routine evaluation. Early risk stratification following presentation with suspected acute coronary syndrome can also be accomplished with noninvasive testing, aiding in decision making regarding treatment strategies. Echocardiography may also assist in the diagnosis of complications following myocardial infarction (MI).

I. IMAGING FOR ACUTE CHEST PAIN SYNDROMES

There are 3 to 5 million Emergency Department visits annually for the complaint of chest pain (1,2). As there is often a low threshold for admission, more than 70% of patients admitted to coronary care units will be found not to have an acute coronary syndrome (3,4). Many of these patients do not have significant obstructive coronary disease and will have a favorable prognosis. However, 2–10% of patients discharged from the emergency department will experience a myocardial infarction soon after discharge (4,5). Additionally, death or other serious complications occurred at a rate nearly twice that of those who were correctly diagnosed initially (4,6).

Although the initial evaluation, consisting of careful history, physical examination, electrocardiogram, and cardiac enzyme markers, will help to risk stratify patients upon presentation, the electrocardiogram is diagnostic in only 40% of cases, and serum biomarkers may require up to 12 hours to be detected (7). Therefore, alternative methods are desirable to improve resource utilization and assist in early identification of high-risk patients.

A. Radionuclide Myocardial Perfusion Imaging

Myocardial perfusion imaging (MPI) is a widely accepted noninvasive modality for the assessment of myocardial blood flow and detection of flow limiting stenoses resulting in myocardial ischemia. MPI was first employed in the setting of acute chest pain syndromes more than 20 years ago using thallium-201 (TI-201) as the imaging agent (8). Thallium initially distributes proportionally to myocardial blood flow, but then demonstrates redistribution of activity with time. Although thallium scintigraphy is a reliable and validated method of detecting myocardial perfusion, the rapid redistribution is a major limitation for imaging transient episodes of acute chest pain. For stable coronary artery disease, technetium 99m (Tc-99m)–labeled perfusion agents have demonstrated similar levels of diagnostic accuracy as thallium but with superior image quality. As with thallium, Tc-99m agents initially distribute proportionally to myocardial blood flow, but there is minimal redistribution of both sestamibi and tetrofosmin, thereby providing a "snapshot" of myocardial blood flow at the time of injection. Imaging may be delayed for up to 3 hours after injection without loss of diagnostic accuracy, providing time for medical stabilization and transport of the patient (9) (Fig. 1).

Rest technetium-99m MPI has been shown to accurately identify patients at high risk for an adverse cardiac event. Multiple studies have revealed a sensitivity in the range of 90–100%, with a specificity of 60–93% (7,10–18) (Table 1). The negative predictive value has been found to be in the range of 90–100%. An abnormal resting perfusion study confers a relative risk of an adverse cardiac event in excess of 10–fold as compared to a normal study (11,18). Additionally a normal resting perfusion study is associated with a very good prognosis. Hilton et. al demonstrated that none of the 82 patients with a normal study suffered a cardiac event within 90 days (13). A low event rate (0–3%) in patients with a normal resting scan has been confirmed in numerous other studies (11,19,20). Hendel and colleagues found that although there were some gender-specific differences, there was a high (97%) negative predictive value of acute rest MPI in both men and women (21). Overall, multiple studies suggest that patients who present with chest pain and have a normal resting myocardial perfusion study are at low risk for

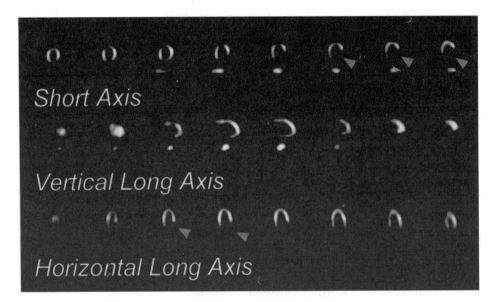

Figure 1 Technetium-99m sestamibi SPECT MPI of a patient presenting to the emergency department with chest pain and a nondiagnostic electrocardiogram. Images demonstrate a moderate-sized perfusion abnormality (arrows) involving the mid to distal inferior and lateral walls. The patient was subsequently diagnosed with an acute myocardial infarction and was found to have a total occlusion of the left circumflex artery at angiography. (Images courtesy of F. Wackers, M.D.)

Table 1 Sensitivity, Specificity, and Negative Predictive Value of Myocardial Perfusion Imaging in Patients with Acute Chest Pain

Author (Ref.)	Year	n	Sensitivity (%)	Specificity (%)	NPV (%)
Wackers, et al. (72)	1979	203	100	63	100
Bilodeau, et al. (7)	1991	45	96	79	94
Varetto, et al. (10)	1993	64	100	92	100
Hilton, et al. (13)	1994	102	94	83	99
Varetto, et al. (15)	1994	27	100	93	—
Stowers, et al. (14)	1995	187	97	78	—
Tatum, et al. (11)	1997	438	100	78	100
Kontos, et al. (18)	1997	532	93	71	99
Heller, et al. (16)	1998	357	90	60	99
Duca, et al. (17)	1999	73	100	73	100
Kontos, et al. (73)	1999	620	92	67	99

Source: Adapted from Ref. 9.

adverse cardiac events, while an abnormal study is associated with an increased risk of subsequent events.

Acute rest MPI has been shown to reduce unnecessary hospitalizations and thereby decrease costs, without compromising appropriate care. In the study by Mather and Shah, perfusion imaging allowed 68% of patients to have their management decisions altered, with 58% of patients being discharged home (1). In a recently published prospective multicenter study, Udelson and colleagues demonstrated that the incorporation of rest Tc-99m sestamibi MPI into the initial work-up of patients presenting to the emergency department with chest pain and a normal or non-diagnostic ECG decreased unnecessary hospitalizations by 20% without reducing appropriate admissions for ACS (22). Heller et al. showed that an abnormal MPI study was the best predictor of ACS among clinical variables studied in emergency department patients with chest pain (16). Acute rest MPI resulted in a 57% reduction in hospitalizations, with a mean cost savings of more than $4,000 per patient. Similarly, a randomized controlled study by Stowers et al. demonstrated that patients initially evaluated with SPECT MPI experienced an average cost savings of $1,843 and a mean decrease in hospital stay of 2 days (23). The cost-effectiveness of acute rest MPI has been shown in several other studies (1,22,24,25), revealing an average cost savings of between $700–$900 per patient.

Although rest MPI is diagnostically accurate and aids in risk assessment, several limitations are present. The timing of injection in relation to chest pain, as well as the duration of chest pain, influence the diagnostic accuracy. Several studies have demonstrated reduced sensitivity if the injection is not administered during the episode of chest pain (7,14). However, it has also been shown that injection of Tc-99m–labeled sestamibi in patients who had an episode of chest pain lasting greater than 30 minutes within the prior 12 hours has a sensitivity of 100% (10). Generally the diagnostic accuracy of acute rest imaging is preserved if the radiopharmaceutical is administered while symptoms persist or within 3 hours of symptom resolution (26). Patients with prior myocardial infarction will not have a normal perfusion scan, even in the absence of an acute process. Therefore, unless a prior imaging study is available, these patients cannot be further risk stratified using this technique. Other limitations of this technique involve logistical aspects, such as administration of the radiopharmaceutical and interpretation of the study, and the availability of such services during nonbusiness hours.

B. Echocardiography

Echocardiography also has potential applications for use in acute chest pain syndromes. Myocardial infarction and ischemia result in decreased systolic wall thickening and endocardial motion when imaged by two-dimensional echocardiography. In the setting of an acute myocardial infarction the wall thickness will be normal, whereas an old infarct scar is characterized by wall thinning and increased echogenicity (Fig. 2). Echocardiography also provides the ability to make alternative diagnoses as the etiology of the chest pain, such as cardiomyopathy, valvular heart disease, pericardial processes, and aortic disease (Fig. 3).

The use of echocardiography to aid in the diagnosis of acute coronary syndrome has been studied by several investigators (15,27–32), who generally demonstrated a high negative predictive value (> 94%), but a low positive predictive value (31–50%) (Table 2). Kontos et al. demonstrated that 2–D echo, when used for patients with suspected acute coronary syndrome but without previous myocardial infarction, had a sensitivity of 97% and a specificity of 84% (30). An abnormal echocardiogram also has important prognostic significance in patients presenting with chest pain. Fleischmann et al. found that left and right ventricular dysfunction, increased end-diastolic dimension, and regional wall motion abnormalities were associated with a significant increase in cardiovascular events (33).

As with the use of radionuclide MPI in the diagnosis of acute chest pain, echocardiography has several limitations. Imaging after symptom resolution will reduce sensitivity; the echocardiographic machine must be in close proximity, and a qualified technician must be immediately available. Additionally, acute treatment should not be delayed in order for the study to be performed. Prior myocardial infarction may not always be accurately differentiated from acute ischemia, although preservation of wall thickness

Figure 2 Apical four-chamber view of a contrast-enhanced 2D echocardiographic image of a patient in the emergency department with chest pain, demonstrating a dyskinetic apex (arrow). The thinning of this region may suggest this is a chronic rather than acute process, but the adjacent segments do appear hyperkinetic.

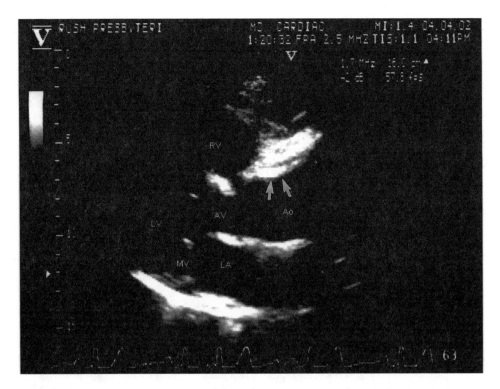

Figure 3 Parasternal long-axis view of a 2D echo image of a patient presenting with severe chest pain of unclear etiology. The image demonstrates a markedly dilated ascending aorta with the suggestion of a dissection flap (arrows).

and normal reflectivity of the myocardium suggest an acute event (5), and hyperkinesis of the uninvolved segments is also indicative of an acute event (34). Another limitation is that smaller areas of ischemia or infarct may not be appreciated by echocardiography.

II. EVALUATION OF COMPLICATIONS FOLLOWING MYOCARDIAL INFARCTION

Complications known to occur following acute myocardial infarction include mitral regurgitation, ventricular septal rupture, and free wall rupture. Echocardiography is the diag-

Table 2 Sensitivity and Specificity of Acute Echocardiography

Author (Ref.)	Year	Sensitivity (%)	Specificity (%)
Loh, et al. (32)	1982	94	100
Horowitz, et al. (31)	1982	94	84
Peels, et al. (27)	1990	88	78
Sabia, et al. (28)	1991	94	46
Varetto, et al. (15)	1994	42	80
Gibler, et al. (29)	1995	47	99
Kontos, et al. (30)	1998	97	84

Source: Adapted from Ref.9.

nostic procedure of choice in the early evaluation of these events and permits the bedside assessment of critically ill patients.

Mitral regurgitation can result from either papillary muscle dysfunction, ischemic dysfunction of the myocardial segment underlying the papillary muscle, or rupture of the papillary muscle or chordal structures. The severity of regurgitation can be assessed by Doppler imaging techniques, and the etiology can usually be determined by two-dimensional imaging. Occasionally transesophageal imaging is helpful, as the mitral valve is a posterior structure.

Ventricular septal rupture occurs as a consequence of myocardial necrosis in a focal area of the interventricular septum. Doppler imaging will demonstrate a high-velocity left-to-right systolic jet. Color flow imaging may also be helpful. Ventricular rupture involving the left ventricular free wall is associated with a high mortality. Echocardiographically, a pericardial effusion, either diffuse or localized, may be seen. Doppler imaging may demonstrate flow at the site of rupture.

III. RISK STRATIFICATION

After the diagnosis of acute coronary syndrome has been made and the patient has been stabilized, management is directed toward risk stratification. One approach for low- or intermediate-risk patients who have not demonstrated evidence of recurrent ischemia is a "conservative" strategy of medical therapy along with noninvasive testing for risk stratification and coronary angiography as dictated by noninvasive test results (35). This may be accomplished by electrocardiographic stress testing if the resting ECG is normal and the patient is capable of exercise. If the ECG is uninterpretable, an imaging modality should be added. If the patient is unable to exercise, pharmacological stress testing with imaging should be utilized. There is evidence to suggest that imaging studies may be superior to exercise ECG in women (36,37). There are no conclusive data regarding the superiority of one imaging modality over the other. Generally test selection should be based on patient characteristics and local availability and expertise (36).

A. Radionuclide Myocardial Perfusion Imaging

The clinical utility of stress MPI has been well established (38–49). In addition to the ability to detect coronary artery disease, stress myocardial perfusion imaging is a powerful tool used to predict disease prognosis. In the Multicenter Study on Silent Myocardial Ischemia, cardiac death rate correlated with defect reversibility and size of defect (47). Vanzetto et al. also found a significant difference in survival based on the number of abnormally perfused segments (44).

The use of stress MPI to assess risk of future cardiac events in post-ACS patients has been well studied. Gibson et al. demonstrated a low 6% event rate in postinfarct patients without ischemia on predischarge Tl-201 stress imaging, whereas patients who had high-risk findings had a 51% event rate (50). Stratmann et al. demonstrated that the presence of a fixed perfusion defect on Tc-99m SPECT imaging following acute MI was an independent predictor of future adverse cardiac events (51). Vasodilator MPI has also been shown to accurately predict future cardiac events in post-ACS patients (52,53–55). Brown et al. compared predischarge dipyridamole MPI to submaximal treadmill exercise in post-MI patients (55). They found that the prognostic value of a dipyridamole study was superior to that of submaximal exercise. Additionally, risk stratification could be performed at day 2 rather than waiting 5–7 days to safely perform exercise in the postinfarction patient. In a study that compared the prognostic ability of predischarge stress echocardiography to Tc-99m tetrofosmin gated SPECT, Candell-Riera et al. found that >15% extent of ischemia by quantitative analysis was predictive of adverse future cardiac events, while no echocardiographic variable had such ability (56).

Stress MPI also has prognostic value in low-risk patients after myocardial infarction. Chiamvimonvat et al. showed that in low-risk post-MI patients who did not require revascularization based on angiographic results, the presence of scintigraphic ischemia on stress MPI had the strongest correlation with future clinical events among the variables studied (57). The presence of scintigraphic ischemia was associated with a 42% 1–year event rate, whereas a scan without reversibility conferred a low 11% event rate with no incidence of death. This study suggested that the physiological data provided by stress MPI may have a more powerful predictive value than the anatomical assessment made by coronary angiography. Currently, the Adenosine Sestamibi Post-Infarction Evaluation (INSPIRE) trial is a multicenter randomized trial examining the potential value of MPI for assessing risk and guiding subsequent therapeutics in stable patients following ACS and should further delineate the role of noninvasive testing after acute myocardial infarction.

B. Echocardiography

Resting echocardiography is a useful tool in assessing prognosis following acute coronary syndrome. Assessment of left ventricular systolic performance is accurately assessed by two-dimensional echocardiography and is an important factor in risk stratification post-ACS (35). Several studies have shown that left ventricular systolic function after an acute myocardial infarction is one of the most important predictors of adverse cardiac events (58–60). Romano and colleagues studied echocardiographic predictors of in-hospital events in patients with non–ST segment elevation myocardial infarction, noting that a lower ejection fraction, a greater number of abnormal segments and a higher end diastolic volume were associated with a higher incidence of in-hospital events (61). In a substudy of the Trandolapril Cardiac Evaluation (TRACE) study, post-ACS patients with an ejection fraction of $g35\%$ who did not experience a recurrent myocardial infarction were followed with serial echocardiograms over 12 months. They found that a decline in left ventricular performance over the follow-up period had significant predictive value in adverse cardiovascular events following AMI (62).

The diagnostic accuracy of stress echocardiography has also been well studied. In numerous studies, the sensitivity ranges from 71 to 97%, with a specificity of 64–100%, with an average of 84% and 86%, respectively (63). Sensitivity is improved in the setting of multivessel disease, where it is > 90% sensitive (64,65). The use of intravenous echocardiographic contrast agents for endocardial border enhancement can facilitate image acquisition and enhance delineation of regional wall motion abnormalities (66).

Stress echocardiography also plays an important role in prognosis. Following acute coronary syndrome, stress echocardiography predicts prognosis with a positive predictive value of 63–80% and a negative predictive value of 78–95% for future cardiac events in the subsequent 12 months (64). A positive dobutamine stress echocardiogram in combination with a resting wall motion abnormality resulted in a 34% incidence of a future cardiac event, where the incidence was 18% if the dobutamine study was negative for inducible ischemia (62). In patients with suspected coronary disease, a normal stress echocardiogram has a high negative predictive value (64).

C. Selection of Management Strategy

Noninvasive imaging is a powerful tool that can be used to help guide in the selection of management strategy following uncomplicated myocardial infarction. With a foundation of multiple clinical trials, the ACC/AHA guidelines do not exclusively recommend an early invasive strategy and routine coronary angiography for patients with non–ST elevation acute coronary syndrome (35). The conservative, or ischemia-guided approach allows patients with recurrent or inducible ischemia on noninvasive testing to proceed to coronary angiography and intervention.

In the TIMI IIIB trial, patients with non–ST elevation acute coronary syndrome treated with either early invasive or conservative strategies had equivalent rates of death, recurrent myocardial infarction, or unsatisfactory results on symptom-limited exercise test at 6 weeks (67). The Medicine versus Angiography in Thrombolytic Exclusion (MATE) trial examined patients with acute coronary syndromes who were ineligible for thrombolytic therapy. They found no difference between patients assigned to an early invasive versus a conservative treatment strategy with regards to death, recurrent myocardial infarction, rehospitalization, or revascularization at 23 months follow-up (68). The Veterans Affairs Non–Q Wave Infarction Strategies in Hospital (VANQWISH) trial randomized patients with non–ST elevation myocardial infarction to early invasive versus conservative treatment strategies (69). They found no difference between the two groups in death or nonfatal infarction with an average follow-up of 23 months. Patients in the early invasive arm had a significantly higher rate of revascularization procedures. Additionally they had a worse clinical outcome in the first year of follow-up, with a higher rate of death and recurrent myocardial infarction. This trial demonstrated that noninvasive stress testing can be used successfully to identify high-risk patients who should undergo coronary angiography.

The Fragmin and Fast Revascularization during Instability in Coronary Artery Disease (FRISC II) trial and the Treat Angina with Aggrastat and Determine Cost of Therapy with Invasive or Conservative Strategy (TACTICS-TIMI 18) trial are two large randomized trials comparing an early invasive to a conservative approach (70,71). Both trials demonstrated that high-risk post-ACS patients with either significant ST segment deviation or elevated cardiac enzyme markers benefit from an early invasive as opposed to a conservative treatment strategy. However, in the TACTICS-TIMI 18 study, patents without high-risk features had similar outcomes regardless of treatment strategy.

IV. CONCLUSION

Both stress echocardiography and radionuclide MPI have been proven accurate and reliable methods of diagnosing coronary artery disease. The use of noninvasive imaging is complementary to the initial evaluation of ACS and enhances diagnostic determinations and triage. Noninvasive imaging is also a powerful tool for the prediction of subsequent cardiac events and can aid in decisions regarding clinical management. High-risk post-ACS patients benefit from early coronary angiography and directed revascularization. The equivalence of a conservative treatment strategy in low-risk patients following acute coronary syndrome utilizing cardiac imaging for determination of ischemia has been verified in multiple large randomized, controlled clinical trials.

REFERENCES

1. Mather PJ, Shah R. Echocardiography, nuclear scintigraphy, and stress testing in the emergency department evaluation of acute coronary syndrome. Emerg Med Clin North Am 2001; 19:339–349.

2. Selker HP. Coronary care unit triage decision aids: how do we know when they work? Am J Med 1989; 87:491–493

3. Schroeder JS, Lamb IK, Harrison DC. Patients admitted to the coronary care unit for chest pain: high risk subgroup for subsequent cardiovascular death. Am J Cardiol 1977; 39:829–832.

4. Lee TH, Juarez G, Cook EF, et al. Ruling out myocardial infarction: a prospective multicenter validation of a 12–hour strategy for patients at low risk. N Engl J Med 1991; 324:1239–1246.

5. Lee TH, Rouan GW, Weisberg MC, et al. Clinical characteristics and natural history of patients with acute myocardial infarction sent home from the emergency room. Am J Cardiol 1987; 60:291–294.

6. McCarthy BD, Beshansky JR, D'Agostino RB, Selker HP. Missed diagnoses of acute myocardial infarction in the emergency department: results from a multicenter study. Ann Emerg Med1993; 22:579–582.

7. Bilodeau L, Theroux P, Gregoire J, et al. Tecnetium-99m sestamibi tomography in patients with spontaneous chest pain: correlations with clinical, electrocardiographic and angiographic findings. J Am Coll Cardiol 1991; 18:1684–1691.

8. Wackers F, Sokole EB, Samson G, et al. Value and limitations of thallium-201 scintigraphy in the acute phase of myocardial infarction. N Engl J Med 1976; 295:1–5.

9. Kim SC, Adams SL, Hendel RC. Role of nuclear cardiology in the evaluation of acute coronary syndromes. Ann Emerg Med 1997; 30:210–218.

10. Varetto T, Cantalupi D, Altieri A, et al. Emergency room technetium-99m sestamibi imaging to rule out acute myocardial ischemic events in patients with nondiagnostic electrocardiograms. J Am Coll Cardiol 1993; 22:1804–1808

11. Tatum JL, Jesse RL, Kontos MC, et al. Comprehensive strategy for the evaluation and triage of the chest pain patient. Ann Emerg Med 1997; 29:116–125.

12. Heller GV, Stowers SA, Hendel RC, et al. Acute emergency department technetium-99m tetrofosmin SPECT imaging in patients with chest pain and nondiagnostic ECG: results of a multicenter trial. Circulation 1996; 94:I-59.

13. Hilton TC, Thompson RC, Williams H, et al. Tecnetium-99m sestamibi myocardial perfusion imaging in the emergency room evaluation of chest pain. J Am Coll Cardiol 1994; 23:1016–1022.

14. Stowers SA, Abuan TH, Szymanski TJ, et al. Technetium-99m sestamibi SPECT and technetium-99m tetrofosmin SPECT in prediction of cardiac events in patients injected during chest pain and following resolution of pain. J Nucl Med 1995; 36:88P-89P.

15. Varetto T, Cantalupi D, Cerruti A. Tc-99m sestamibi and 2D-echo imaging for rule-out of acute ischemia in patients with chest pain and non-diagnostic ECG. Circulation 1994; 90:I-367.

16. Heller GV, Stowers SA, Hendel RC, Herman SD, Daher E, Ahlberg AW, Baron JM, Mendes de Leon CF, Rizzo JA, Wackers FJ. Clinical value of acute rest technetium-99m tetrofosmin tomographic myocardial perfusion imaging in patients with acute chest pain and nondiagnostic electrocardiograms. J Am Coll Cardiol 1998; 31:1011–1017.

17. Duca MD, Giri S, Wu AH, Morris RS, Cyr GM, Ahlberg A, White M, Waters DD, Heller GV. Comparison of acute rest myocardial perfusion imaging and serum markers of myocardial injury in patients with chest pain syndromes. J Nucl Cardiol 1999; 6:570–576.

18. Kontos MC, Jesse RL, Schmidt KL, et al. Value of acute rest sestamibi perfusion imaging for evaluation of patients admitted to the emergency department with chest pain. J Am Coll Cardiol 1997; 30:976–982.

19. Anderson HV, Cannon CP, Stone PH, et al. One-year results of the TIMI-IIIB clinical trial. J Am Coll Cardiol 1995; 26:1643–1650.

20. Boucher CA, Wackers FJ, Zaret BL, et al. Tecnetium-99m sestamibi myocardial imaging at rest for assessment of myocardial infarction and first-pass ejection fraction. Am J Cardiol 1992; 69:22–27.

21. Hendel RC, Gupta A, Ruthazer R, Selker HP, Heller GV, Pope H, Woolard RH, Beshansky JR, Udelson JE. The impact of gender on the diagnostic and prognostic value of myocardial perfusion imaging in patients with acute chest pain. Circulation 2001; 104:II-455.

22. Udelson JE, Beshansky JR, Ballin DS, Feldman JA, Griffith JL, Heller GV, Hendel RC, Pope JH, Ruthazer R, Spiegler EJ, Woolard RH, Handler J, Selker HP. Myocardial perfusion imaging for evaluation and triage of patients with suspected acute cardiac ischemia; a randomized controlled trial. JAMA 2002; 288:2693–2700.

23. Stowers SA, Eisenstein EL, Wackers FJ, Berman DS, Blackshear JL, Jones AD, Szymanski TJ, Lam LC, Simons TA, Natale D, Paige KA, Wagner GS. An economic analysis of an aggressive diagnostic strategy with single photon emission computed tomography myocardial perfusion imaging and early exercise stress testing in emergency department patients who present with chest pain but nondiagnostic electrocardiograms: results from a randomized trial. Ann Emerg Med 2000; 35:17–25.

24. Radensky PW, Stowers SA, Hilton TC, et al. Cost-effectiveness of acute myocardial perfusion imaging with technetium-99m sestamibi for risk stratification of emergency strategies in unstable angina and non-Q wave myocardial infarction. Circulation 1994; 90:I-528.

25. Weissman IA, Dickinson CZ, Dworkin HJ, et al. Cost-effectiveness of myocardial perfusion imaging with SPECT in the emergency department evaluation of patients with unexplained chest pain. Radiology 1996; 199:353–357.

26. Wackers FJ, Brown KA, Heller GV, Kontos MC, Tatum JL, Udelson JE, Ziffer JA. American Society of Nuclear Cardiology position statement on radionuclide imaging in patients with suspected acute ischemic syndromes in the emergency department. J Nucl Cardiol 2002; 9:246–250.

27. Peels CH, Visser CA, Kupper AJ, et al. Usefulness of two-dimensional echocardiography for immediate detection of myocardial ischemia in the emergency room. Am J Cardiol 1990; 65:687–691.

28. Sabia P, Afrookteh A, Touchstone DA, et al. Value of regional wall motion abnormality in the emergency room diagnosis of acute myocardial infarction: a prospective study using two-dimensional echocardiography. Circulation 1991; 84:I85–92.

29. Gibler WB, Runyon JP, Levy RC, et al. A rapid diagnostic and treatment center for patients with chest pain in the emergency department. Ann Emerg Med 1995; 25:1–8.

30. Kontos MC, Arrowood JA, Paulsen WH, et al. Early echocardiography can predict cardiac events in emergency department patients with chest pain. Ann Emerg Med 1998; 31:550–557.

31. Horowitz RS, Morganroth J, Parrotto C. Immediate diagnosis of acute myocardial infarction by two-dimensional echocardiography. Circulation 1982; 65:323–329.

32. Loh IK, Charuzi Y, Beeder C. Early diagnosis of nontransmural myocardial infarction by two-dimensional echocardiography. Am Heart J 1982; 104:963–968.

33. Fleischmann KE, Lee TH, Come PC, et al. Echocardiographic prediction of complications in patients with chest pain. Am J Cardiol 1997; 79:292–298.

34. Otto, CM. The use of echocardiography in patients with ischemic cardiac disease. In: Textbook of Clinical Echocardiography. Philadelphia, PA: W.B. Saunders, 1995:172.

35. Braunwald E, Antman EM, Beasley JW, et al. ACC/AHA 2002 guideline update for the management for the management of patients with unstable angina and non-ST-segment elevation myocardial infarction: a report of the American College of Cardiology/American Heart Association task force on practice guidelines (committee on the management of patients with unstable angina). 2002.

36. Starling MR, Crawford MH, Kennedy GT, et al. Treadmill exercise tests predischarge and six weeks post-myocardial infarction to detect abnormalities of known prognostic value. Ann Intern Med 1981; 94:721–727.

37. Marwick TH, Anderson T, Williams MJ, et al. Exercise echocardiography is an accurate and cost-efficient technique for detection of coronary artery disease in women. J Am Coll Cardiol 1995; 26:335–341.

38. Kiat H, Maddahi J, Roy L, et al. Comparison of technetium-99m methoxy isobutyl isonitrile and thallium-201 for evaluation of coronary artery disease by planar and tomographic methods. Am Heart J 1989; 117:111.

39. Iskandrian AS, Heo J, Long B, et al. Use of technetium-99m isonitrile (RP-30A) in assessing left ventricular perfusion and function at rest and during exercise in coronary artery disease, and comparison with coronary arteriography and exercise thallium-201 SPECT imaging. Am J Cardiol 1989; 64:270.

40. Kahn JK, McGhie I, Akers MS, et al. Quantitative rotational tomography with 201Tl and 99mTc 2–methoxy-isobutyl-isonitrile. Circulation 1989; 79:1282.

41. Solot G, Hermans J, Merlo P, et al. Correlation of 99mTc-sestamibi SPECT with coronary angiography in general hospital practice. Nucl Med Commun 1993; 14:23.

42. Azzarelli S, Galassi AR, Foti R, et al. Accuracy of 99m-Tc-tetrofosmin myocardial tomography in the evaluation of coronary artery disease. J Nucl Cardiol 1999; 6:183.

43. Pierre-Yves M, Danchin N, Durand JF, et al. Long-term prediction of major ischemic events by exercise thallium-201 single-photon emission computed tomography. J Am Coll Cardiol 1995; 26:879.

44. Vanzetto G, Ormezzano O, Fagret D, et al. Long term additive prognostic value of thallium-201 myocardial perfusion imaging over clinical and exercise stress test in low-to-intermediate risk patients. Study in 1,137 patients with 6–year follow-up. Circulation 1999; 100:1521.

45. Mazzanti M, Germano G, Kiat H, et al. Identification of severe and extensive coronary artery disease by automatic measurement of transient ischemic dilation of the left ventricle in dual-isotope myocardial perfusion SPECT. J Coll Cardiol 1996; 27:1612.

46. Sharir T, Germano G, Kavanagh PB, et al. Incremental prognostic value of post-stress left ventricular ejection fraction and volume by gated myocardial perfusion single photon emission computed tomography. Circulation 1999; 100:1035.

47. Bodenheimer MW, Wackers FJTh, Schwartz RG, et al. Prognostic significance of a fixed thallium defect one to six months after onset of acute myocardial infarction or unstable angina. Am J Cardiol 1994; 74:1196.

48. Gill JB, Ruddy TD, Newell JB, et al. Prognostic importance of thallium uptake by the lungs during exercise in coronary artery disease. N Engl J Med 1987; 317:1485.

49. Williams KA, Schneider CM. Increased stress right ventricular activity on dual isotope perfusion SPECT. J Am Coll Cardiol 1999; 34:420.

50. Gibson RS, Watson DD, Craddock GB, et al. Prediction of cardiac events after uncomplicated myocardial infarction: a prospective study comparing predischarge exercise thallium-201 scintigraphy and coronary angiography. Circulation 1983; 68:321–326.

51. Stratmann HG, Mark AL, Amato M, Wittry MD, Younis LT. Risk stratification with pre-hospital discharge exercise technetium-99m sestamibi myocardial tomography in men after acute myocardial infarction. Am Heart J 1998; 136:87–93.

52. Mahmarian JJ, Mahmarian AC, Marks GF, et al. Role of adenosine thallium-201 tomography for defining long-term risk in patients after acute myocardial infarction. J Am Coll Cardiol 1995; 25:1333.

53. Leppo JA, O'Brien J, Rothender JA, Getchell JD, Lee VW. Dipyridamole-thallium-201 scintigraphy in the prediction of future cardiac events after acute myocardial infarction. N Engl J Med 1984; 310:1014–1018.

54. Brown KA, O'Meara J, Chambers CE, Plante DA. Ability of dipyridamole-thallium-201 imaging 1 to 4 hours after acute myocardial infarction to predict in-hospital and later recurrent myocardial ischemic events. Am J Cardiol 1990; 65:160–167.

55. Brown KA, Heller GV, Landin RS, Shaw LJ, Beller GA, Pasquale MJ. Early dipyridamole Tc-99m sestamibi single photon emission computed tomographic imaging 2 to 4 days after acute myocardial infarction predicts in-hospital and postdischarge cardiac events: comparison with submaximal exercise imaging. Circulation 1999; 100:2060–2066.

56. Candell-Riera J, Llevadot J, Santana C, Castrell J, Aguade S, Armadans L. Prognostic assessment of uncomplicated first myocardial infarction by exercise echocardiography and tc-99m tetrofosmin gated SPECT. J Nucl Cardiol 2001; 8:122–128.

57. Chiamvimonvat V, Goodman SG, Langer A, Barr A, Freeman MR. Prognostic value of dipyridamole SPECT imaging in low-risk patients after myocardial infarction. J Nucl Cardiol 2001; 8:136–143.

58. Hammermeister KE, DeRouen TA, Dodge HT. Variables predictive of survival in patients with coronary disease: selection by univariate and multivariate analyses from the clinical, electrocardiographic, exercise, arteriographic, and quantitative angiographic evaluations. Circulation 1979; 59:421–430.

59. Cohn JN, Rector TS. Prognosis of congestive heart failure and predictors of mortality. Am J Cardiol 1988; 62:25A-30A.

60. The Multicenter Post-Infarction Research Group. Risk stratification and survival after myocardial infarction. N Engl J Med 1983; 309:331–336.

61. Romano S, Alessandra D, Penco M, et al. Usefulness of echocardiography in the prognostic evaluation of non-Q-wave myocardial infarction. Am J Cardiol 2000; 86:43G-45G.

62. Korup E, Kober L, Torp-Pedersen C, Toft E. Prognostic usefulness of repeated echocardiographic evaluation after acute myocardial infarction. Am J Cardiol 1999; 83:1559–1562.

63. Cheitlin MD, Alpert JS, Armstrong WF, et al. ACC/AHA Guidelines for the Clinical Application of Echocardiography. A report of the American College of Cardiology/American Heart Association Task Force on Practice Guidelines (Committee on Clinical Application of Echocardiography). Developed in collaboration with the American Society of Echocardiography. Circulation 1997; 95:1686.

64. Otto, CM. The use of echocardiography in patients with ischemic cardiac disease. In: Textbook of Clinical Echocardiography. Philadelphia: W.B. Saunders, 1995:169.

65. Geleijnse ML, Fioretti PM, Roelandt JR. Methodology, feasibility, safety and diagnostic accuracy of dobutamine stress echocardiography. J Am Coll Cardiol 1997; 30:595.

66. Mulvagh SL, DeMaria AN, Feinstein SB, et al. Contrast echocardiography: current and future applications. J Am Soc Echocardiogr 2000; 13:331–342.

67. The TIMI IIB Investigators. Effects of tissue plasminogen activator and a comparison of early invasive and conservative strategies in unstable angina and non Q wave myocardial infarction. Results of the TIMI IIIB trial. Circulation 1994; 89:1545–1556.

68. McCullough PA, O'Neill WW, Graham M, et al. A prospective randomized trial of triage angiography in acute coronary syndromes ineligible for thrombolytic therapy: Results of the MATE trial. J Am Coll Cardiol 1998; 32:596–605.

69. The VANQWISH trial investigators. Outcomes in patients with acute non-Q-wave myocardial infarction randomly assigned to an invasive as compared with a conservative management strategy. N Engl J Med 1998; 338:1785–1792.

70. Cannon CP, Weintraub WS, Demopoulos LA, et al. Comparison of early invasive and conservative strategies in patients with unstable coronary syndromes treated with glycoprotein IIb/IIIa inhibitor tirofiban. N Engl J Med 2001; 344:1879–1887.

71. Fragmin and Fast Revascularization during InStability in Coronary artery disease Investigators. Invasive compared with noninvasive treatment in unstable coronary artery disease: FRISC II prospective randomised multicentre study. Lancet 1999; 354:708–715.

72. Wackers FJ, Lie KI, Liem KL, Sokole EB, Samsom G, van der Schoot J, Durrer D. Potential value of thallium-201 scintigraphy as a means of selecting patients for the coronary care unit. Br Heart J 1979; 41:111–117.

73. Kontos MC, Jesse RL, Anderson FP. Comparison of myocardial perfusion imaging and cardiac troponin I in patients admitted to the emergency department with chest pain. Circulation 1999; 99:2073–2078.

11-1

Thrombogenicity of Prosthetic Heart Valves: History, Design, Characteristics, and Conditions

Jorge M. Balaguer and Richard C. Becker
University of Massachusetts Medical School, Worchester, Massachusetts, and Duke Clinical Research Institute, Durham, North Carolina, U.S.A.

I. INTRODUCTION

Heart valve replacement represents one of the most significant advances in medicine in the modern era—saving lives and improving the quality of life among patients with congenital or acquired valvular heart disease. Its wide acceptance is evidenced by the 2.5 million procedures performed worldwide since 1960 and upward of 90,000 surgeries performed yearly (1). Despite the important contribution that surgical heart valve replacement has made over the past half-century, an existing propensity for localized thrombus formation and systemic thromboembolic events, including fatal and disabling ischemic stroke, remains both an inherent limiting feature and major concern for surgeons, clinicians, and patients alike. The following overview highlights surgical prosthetic heart valve replacement and the complex subject of thrombogenicity, with emphasis on development, device technology, design, and contributing thrombophilic conditions.

II. HISTORICAL BACKGROUND

Early in their development, surgeons recognized the potential devastating consequences of prosthetic heart valve–related thrombosis. The pioneering work of Frater and Ellis quickly brought the problem into full light. Observing valve thrombosis in 19 of 23 dogs receiving a flexible monocusp mitral valve prosthesis, they concluded that "clotting is the major problem" with this procedure (2). Similar findings by several respected investigators reported initially by Frater and Ellis prompted research efforts to better understand the surface properties of prosthetic valve materials and their intrinsic thrombogenicity (3,4). Coupled with an appreciation of blood flow characteristics and its influence on coagulation-related events, the stage was set in the early 1960s for developing the first mechanical valve substitutes for clinical application—the Harken (5) and Starr-Edwards caged-ball valves (6).

In the face of clear technical advances, yet lingering concerns, the problem of mechanical valve thrombosis prompted a relatively rapid turn in the surgical communities' attention toward the use of alternative (biological) materials for constructing replacement devices. Nearly simultaneous with the development of prosthetic caged-ball valves, two celebrated surgeons considered the feasibility of using aortic homografts for human valve replacement. In 1962 Donald Ross performed the first aortic valve replacement using an aortic homograft (7). In 1967 the same surgeon proceeded with the first pulmonary auto-graft (Ross rocedure), a technique wherein the patient's own pulmonic valve is used as an autograft to replace a stenotic or insufficient aortic valve. A pulmonary homograft is then employed to reconstruct the patient's right ventricular outflow tract defect left by procure-ment of the autograft. In the late 1960s, Hancock Laboratories developed porcine valves for routine implantation. The standard Hancock I porcine valve become the first commer-cially successful bioprosthesis.

Over the past 25 years more than 50 heart valve prostheses have been developed for clinical use, but only a handful have been approved by the U.S. Food and Drug Administration (FDA). Of these, approximately 6 are implanted routinely by surgeons practicing in the United States. Although some prostheses are inherently more thrombo-genic than others, the occurrence of thromboembolism has decreased steadily over time. An advancing understanding of valve-related thrombogenicity, associated conditions pre-disposing to thromboembolism and the important role of systemic anticoagulation are responsible for this favorable trend.

III. CARDIAC VALVE SUBSTITUTES

The FDA-approved mechanical and bioprosthetic valves as well as those currently avail-able in other countries are summarized in Tables 1 and 2. Although annuloplasty rings are not considered true valve substitutes, they are made of prosthetic materials and, through exposure to circulating blood, represent a potential site for thrombosis. The FDA-approved annuloplasty rings are listed in Table 3.

A.   Mechanical Valves

1. Caged-Ball Valves

Starr-Edwards Valve.   Initially introduced in 1960, the original design of the Starr-Edwards valve has remained unchanged since its introduction in 1965 (Fig. 1). The

Table 1   Mechanical Prosthetic Heart Valves

Caged-Ball
  Starr-Edwards
Monoleaflet (Tilting—Disk)
  Medtronic Hall[a]
  Omniscience[a]
  Bjork-Shiley Monostrut[a]
  Sorin Monoleaflet Allcarbon
Bileaflet
  St. Jude Medical[a]
  CarboMedics[a]
  Edwards Techna
  ATS
  Sorin Bicarbon
  On-X Mechanical Prosthesis
  Carbomedics KineticUltracor Mechanical

---

[a]FDA-approved and currently in use in the United States.

Table 2 Bioprosthetic Heart Valves

Stented Porcine Valves
 Hankock Porcine Valvea
 Carpentier-Edwards Porcine Valvea
 Medtronic Intact Porcine Valve
 Biocor Porcine Valve
 St. Jude Bioimplant Porcine Valve
 Medtronic Mosaic Porcine Valve
 Labcor Porcine Valve
 Tissue Med Porcine Valve
Stented Pericardial Valves
 Carpentier-Edwards Pericardial Valvea
 Mitroflow Pericardial Valve
 CarboMedics Photofix Pericardial Valve
 Biocor Pericardial Valve
 Sorin Pericarbon Valve
Stentless Porcine and Pericardial Valves
 St. Jude Medical; Toronto SPV Stentless Porcine Valvea
 Medtronic Freestyle Stentless Porcine Valvea
 Cryolife O'Brien Stentless Porcine Valve
 Cryolife O'Brien Stentless (Root) PorcineValve
 Baxter Prima Stentless Porcine Valve
 SorinPericarbon Pericardial Valve
 LabcorStentless Porcine Valve
 Tissue Med Heterograft Roots and Stentless Valve
Homografts
 Cryolife Allograft Root and Valvea
 LifeNET (St. Jude Medical) a
 American Red Cross (Baxter) a

[a]FDA-approved and currently in use.

poppet is molded from silicone rubber and impregnated with barium sulfate to achieve radio-opacity. The pathway of the poppet is protected by a stellite alloy cage, which reduces the possibility of interference with ball motion (6).

2. *Monoleaflet Valves (Tilting-Disk Valves)*

Medtronic-Hall Valve. The Medtronic-Hall tilting-disk valve (Fig. 2) has a central S-shaped guide for leaflet excursion and three struts that protrude through the central orifice. The housing and central guide are made of titanium and the disk of pyrolitic carbon. The prosthesis can be rotated within the sewing ring. The leaflet opens by rotation

Table 3 Annuloplasty Rings

Carpentier-Edwards[a]
Duran[a]
Cosgrove-Edwards[a]
St. Jude Medical (tailor)[a]

[a]FDA-approved annuloplasty rings.

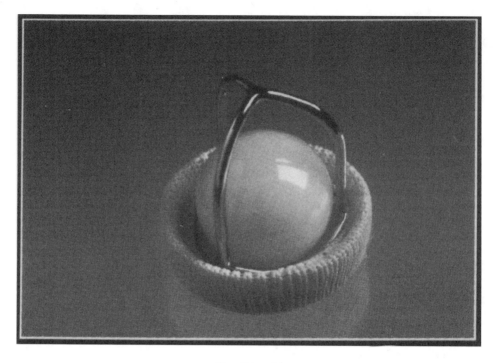

Starr-Edwards
(1964)

Figure 1　The Starr-Edwards "caged-ball" valve was introduced in the early-to-mid 1960s.

and translation, with an opening angle of 70–75 degrees. The disk has a tungsten-loaded substrate for radio-opacity (8,9).

　　　Omnicarbon Valve.　The Omnicarbon valve contains a pyrolite coating over a graphite substrate. The disk, made of pyrolitic carbon, is controlled by short struts with an opening angle of 80 degrees. The housing ring is rotatable within the structure ring; both the housing ring and disk are radio-opaque (8,9).

　　　Bjork-Shiley Monostrut.　In this mechanical monoleaflet prosthesis, the orifice ring and the struts are constructed from a single piece of cobalt-chromium alloy. The tilting disk is made from pyrolytic carbon. The leaflet motion is by rotation and translation. This particular valve has a low-velocity reversed flow for washing of the mechanical components (9).

3.　Bileaflet Valves

　　　St. Jude Valve.　The St. Jude valve, approved by the FDA in 1977, is currently the most widely used valve in the world, accounting for 60% of all prosthetic valve implantations (Fig. 3). The housing and the leaflets are graphite substrate covered by pyrolitic carbon. The leaflets are impregnated with tungsten for radio-opacity. The two leaflets open at 85 degrees by rotation over guarded pivots, resulting in central, near-laminar flow. The

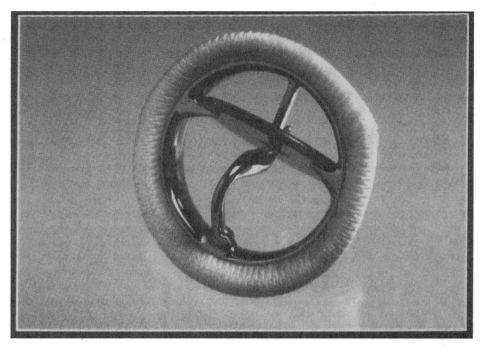

Medtronic-Hall
(1977)

Figure 2 Monoleaflet or tilting disk valves, first introduced in the 1970s, included the Medtronic-Hall (shown), Omnicarbon, and Bjork-Shiley valves.

design allows for some degree of reverse flow that is responsible for washout of the hinge mechanism (8,9).

CarboMedics Valve   The CarboMedics valve is a bileaflet prosthesis with solid pyrolite housing and flat leaflets. It is made of pyrolite carbon over a tungsten-loaded graphite substrate. The opening angle of the leaflets is 78 degrees. The leaflet's hinge mechanism is unique and is located inside the housing without pivot guards or struts. The valve's radio-opacity is based on a titanium stiffening ring and increased tungsten content within the leaflet substrate. The CarboMedics valve received approval by the FDA in 1993 (8,9).

B. Biological Valves

1. Stented Biophrosthesis

Hancock Porcine Valve.   The standard Hancock I porcine valve, a glutaraldehyde-fixed prosthesis available for aortic and mitral valve replacement, was the first commercially successful biological valve. It was recognized early on that, in the aortic position, smaller- sized valves became obstructive (high profile) due to nonmobility of the right coronary cusp. The muscle shell attached to the base of this leaflet made it less flexible, restricting its opening. The MO model (modified orifice) was first implanted in 1976 (8).

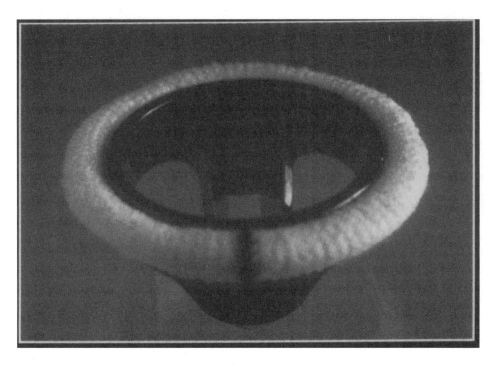

St. Jude Medical
(1977)

Figure 3   The St. Jude valve, one of several bileaflet prosthetic implants, is the most widely used valve worldwide.

This model included the noncoronary leaflet from another porcine root used to replace the right coronary leaflet that contained the muscle shelf. The Hancock II model contains a scalloped sewing ring and, by design, is a reduced profile stent constructed specifically for aortic valve replacement in the supra-annular position (Fig. 4) (8,9).

Carpentier-Edwards Porcine Valve.   The Carpentier-Edwards porcine valve was first introduced in the late 1970s by Carpentier. It is made from porcine aortic roots using high-pressure glutaraldehyde fixation. Models are available for aortic and mitral valve replacement (Fig. 5). The supra-annular model, developed for aortic valve replacement, has a reduced stent profile, and the glutaraldehyde fixation process is performed at low pressure (2–4 mmHg). The tissue is also treated with polysorbate 80, a calcium mitigation agent (8).

Carpentier-Edwards Pericardial Valve.   The Carpentier-Edwards pericardial valve is fabricated with bovine pericardium subjected to low-pressure glutaraldehyde fixation. Optimal leaflet design is achieved with the assistance of computer models to ensure leaflet-to-stent matching and symmetrical leaflet opening. This prosthesis is now available for aortic and mitral valve replacement in the United States (Fig. 6) (8,9).

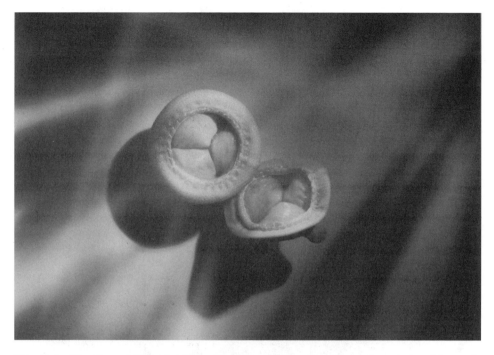

Figure 4 The Hancock II stented bioprosthesis is a porcine valve that has been designed for aortic (scalloped sewing ring) (right upper) or mitral (left lower) surgical implantation.

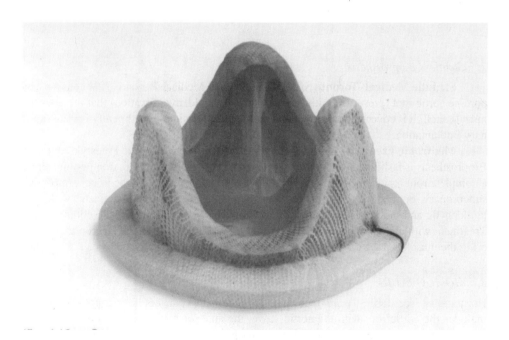

Figure 5 The Carpentier-Edwards Mitral Duraflex Porcine valve is constructed from porcine aortic roots under high-pressure glutaraldehyde fixation.

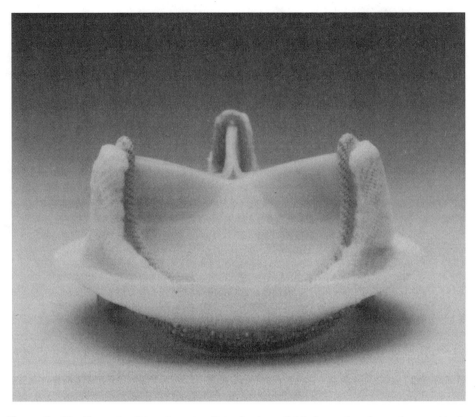

Figure 6 The Carpentier-Edwards pericardial valve is available for aortic valve replacement in the United States.

2. Stentless Bioprosthesis

St. Jude Medical–Toronto SPV. The St. Jude Medical–Toronto SPV consists of a porcine aortic root (preserved with low-pressure glutaraldehyde fixation) that includes the muscle shell. It is covered with a fine Dacron mesh and designed specifically for sub-coronary implantation.

Medtronic Freestyle Stentless Bioprosthesis. The Medtronic Freestyle Stentless Bioprosthesis is fashioned as a porcine aortic root (Fig. 7). Its configuration permits either a complete root replacement or a "tailored" valve replacement as a subcoronary, modified subcoronary, or root inclusion procedure. The tissue is "pressure-free fixed" with glutaraldehyde and the aortic wall is predilated to reduce deformation of the commissures. Treatment with alpha amino oleic acid retards tissue calcification. The Dacron mesh covering the muscle shell forms a fine proximal sewing cuff.

3. HOMOGRAFTS

Homografts (see Table 2) are recovered from human cadavers. The aortic homograft includes the aortic root with the aortic valve, the anterior leaflet of the mitral valve, the stump of the coronary arteries, and the ascending aorta up to the level of the arch (great) vessels. The pulmonary homograft includes the pulmonary root with the pulmonic valve,

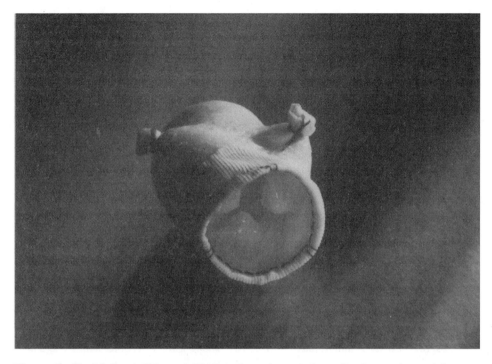

Figure 7 The Medtronic "Freestyle" bioprostheses is a stentless valve that can be used for complete root replacement or tailored valve replacement.

myocardium from the right ventricular outflow tract, and the main pulmonary artery up to and sometimes including the bifurcation.

Homografts were first procured as fresh, antibiotic-treated valves; however, in recent years cryopreservation has traditionally been performed following the current standards of cryobiology. The valve tissue is frozen to –196°C, with the intended goal of preserving viability and collagen strength. Cryopreservation have permitted longer storage times, better distribution, and, in all likelihood, better utilization of aortic and pulmonary homografts.

Aortic homografts can be used as root replacements or they can be implanted in the subcoronary position. Young patients with active lifestyles, patients in whom anticoagulation is contraindicated, and patients affected by aortic valve infective endocarditis (10) are considered the most favored recipients of aortic homografts. In adult patient populations, pulmonary homografts are frequently used for right ventricular outflow tract reconstruction after pulmonary autografting (Ross procedure) or after other pulmonic valve procedures (11).

C. Annuloplasty Rings

1. Carpentier-Edwards

The Carpentier-Edwards annuloplasty ring (Classic model) was the first to be commercially available. Its development followed the pioneering work of the French surgeon Alain Carpentier, who introduced this rigid ring and popularized conservative procedures for patients with mitral valve abnormalities. The incidence of systolic anterior motion of the anterior leaflet and loss of "sphincter-like" function of the mitral annulus lead to the development of a more flexible ring (Physio model) (Fig. 8). These devices are available for mitral and tricuspid annuloplasty procedures.

2. Duran

The Duran ring consists of a flexible circular ring of Dacron fabric. A radio0paque band enables radiological visibility. The flexibility of this device is advantageous in preserving the "sphincter-like" function of the mitral valve. The area and shape of the native mitral annulus decreases 20–50% during systole (12), and the flexible design "adapts" to functional changes that occur during the cardiac (13) cycle. Furthermore, flexible rings place less stress on sutures during systole, minimizing the likelihood of dehiscence.

3. St. Jude Medical "Tailor"

This device is made of double velour polyester. It is flexible and by design can be used as a full ring (similar to the Duran or Carptentier rings) or as a "cut" or "C" ring like the Cosgrove-Edwards (to be described). Barium-impregnated silicone strips allow visualization by chest radiography and fluoroscopy. A holder maintains the ring shape during implantation in either the mitral or tricuspid position (14).

4. Cosgrove-Edwards

The Cosgrove-Edwards annuloplasty device is C-shaped, fully flexible, and, in actuality, an incomplete ring or "band" (Fig. 9). The rationale for its shape is based on current knowledge that plication of the mitral annulus is only necessary in its posterior aspect. The band, covered with polyester velour cloth, is composed of silicone rubber impregnated

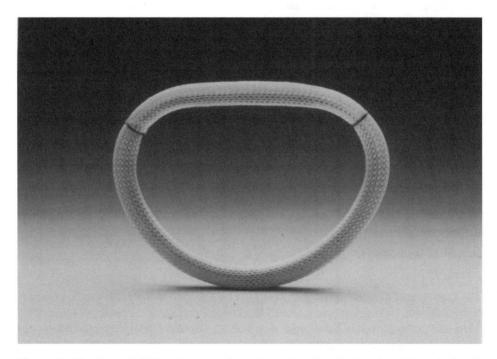

Figure 8   The Carpentier-Edwards annuloplasty ring can be placed in the tricuspid or mitral position. Flexibility has helped maintain normal physiological function of the valve annulus.

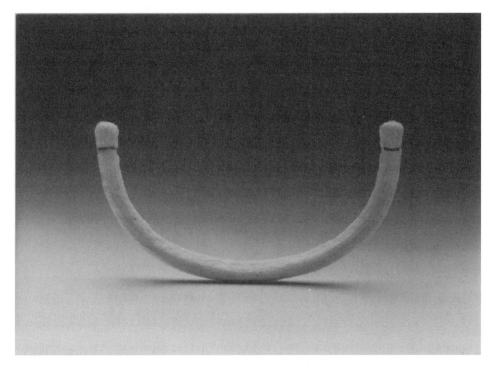

Figure 9 The "incomplete" or Cosgrove-Edwards annuloplasty device is used for plication of the mitral annulus in its posterior anatomical aspect.

with barium sulfate, permitting radiographic visualization. Recently, the manufacturers of the Cosgrove-Edwards and Carpentier-Edwards annuloplasty rings have added a Duraflo treatment to the processing steps, with a goal of reducing platelet aggregation and complement activation. A rigid template is part of the system that serves as a stent for a "measured" annuloplasty. It can be used for mitral or tricuspid valve support.

IV. THROMBOGENICITY INHERENT TO CARDIAC PROSTHESES

Although several patient-related factors, including atrial fibrillation, thrombophilic states, low cardiac output ventricular chamber dilation, and left atrial enlargement, contribute to the risk of thrombosis and thromboembolic events in patients with prosthetic heart valves, the most obvious risk factor is the prosthetic valve itself. This inherent thrombogenicity is collectively determined by the materials used for construction of the prosthesis and the flow conditions through and adjacent to the valve, which are a function of size and prosthetic design.

A. Thrombogenicity of Prosthetic Materials

Conventional heart valve prostheses have three major components: mechanical components, biologic components, and the Sewing ring. Because the interaction between each component and the blood differs, they will be discussed separately (15).

Stentless porcine valves have a polyester cloth partially covering the outer surface of the aortic root, but they do not have either a true sewing ring or stent. Therefore, the host response is directed to the foreign biological tissue (Fig. 10).

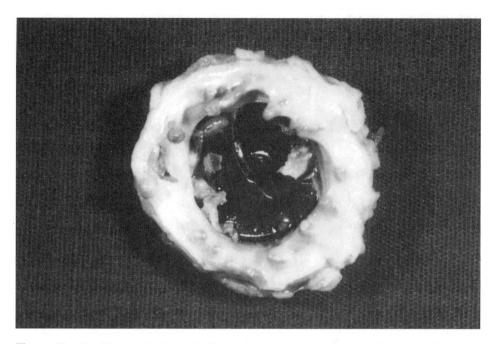

Figure 10 The disk of a Medtronic-Hall valve implanted in the mitral position is partially immobilized by a growing pannus that extends beyond the sewing ring and thrombus within the major and minor orifices.

Annuloplasty rings are used as a stand-alone or complementary intervention for mitral and tricuspid valve repairs. Although they are not replacement devices, when implanted, foreign material is introduced into the circulation, prompting a host response. In reality, the amount of prosthetic material introduced by an annuloplasty ring is substantially lower than a sewing ring alone of any biological or mechanical prosthesis.

Aortic and pulmonary homografts are entirely free of nonbiological prosthetic material.

B. Mechanical Components

1. Materials

The two most common types of material currently used for construction of mechanical valves are metals and carbons. Metals and metallic alloys such as titanium and stellite alloy are used for constructing the cage of caged-ball valves and the housing of several other prostheses. These materials are favored because of their strength, low corrosion rate, and the absence of cytotoxic effects. Carbons, particularly pyrolitic carbon, have become popular for the fabrication of disck, leaflets, and housings and for the coating of other materials such as graphite. Excellent biocompatibility and biostability, high resistance to degradation, very high resistance to wear and a lower degree of thrombogenicity are the outstanding characteristics of these materials (16).

Silastic (silicone rubber) belongs to a group of nondegradable synthetic materials used for the construction of Starr-Edwards ball poppets. Low cost and structural stability represent attractive features of this material. The materials used for the fabrication of widely implanted mechanical prosthetic heart valves are listed in Table 4.

2. Interaction of Circulating Blood with Prosthetic Mechanical Components

Foreign materials provoke an immediate reaction when exposed to circulating blood. Protein adsorption to the housing and moving parts of the mechanical prosthesis represents the initial event, beginning immediately after implantation. Fibrinogen is the first and most prevalent protein involved in this process. Other plasma proteins such as fibronectin, von Willebrand factor, thrombospondin, factor XII, and kininogen quickly join fibrinogen as part of the "protein film." This initial process, known as conditioning of the surface, is characterized by a high degree of thrombogenicity.

After a brief period of dynamic flux, conditioning of the surface reaches a level of equilibrium where the protein coat has a fairly well-defined composition. The composition, in turn, is determined by the binding constants and plasma concentrations of several plasma proteins. The adsorbed proteins subsequently undergo changes in their molecular configuration, promoting variable degrees of platelet adhesion to the protein-coated surface.

The contribution of platelet adhesion to the thrombotic process is variable and influenced strongly by shearing force and flow conditions; however, most prosthetic materials are coated with a monolayer of platelets shortly after exposure to the circulating blood (17).

That initial stage of maximal thrombogenicity is followed by a surface-related event known as passivation. Although the exact mechanism of this phenomenon is not completely understood, accumulating evidence suggests that the protein composition of the adsorbed film changes to a configuration that is less reactive to blood. In general, the greater the concentration of albumin on a protein-coated surface, the more passive the surface becomes. Once the surface has become passivated, it is less prone to thrombosis.

Experimental studies have demonstrated that precoating a given material with albumin accelerates the passivation process. Pyrolytic carbon induces surface passivation more rapidly than other materials, but the exact mechanism remains unclear (15). Minimal molecular alteration of the adsorbed protein coat and a critical surface tension within the biocompatible range are some of the postulated mechanism for its relative thromboresistance (15).

C. Biological Components

1. Tissue Characteristics

The use of biological tissue for valve replacement was undertaken to reduce thrombogenicity. It is known that native tissue thromboresistance is largely determined by normal

Table 4 Individual Components of Mechanical Heart Valves

	Moving parts	Housing	Sewing ring
Starr-Edwards Caged-ball valve	Ball poppet: "cured" Silastic	Cage: stellite alloy and Teflon	Porous knitted propylene
St. Jude Bileaflet	Leaflets: Pyrolytic carbon	Pyrolytic carbon	Dacron
CarboMedics Bileaflet	Leaflets: Pyrolytic carbon	Pyrolytic carbon	Dacron
Omniscience Tilting disk	Disk: Pyrolytic carbon	Titanium	Seamless polyester knit
Medtronic-Hall Tilting disk	Disk: Thin carbon coated	Titanium	Teflon

endothelial cell function. Unfortunately, during the processing of homografts and the preimplantation stages for bioprosthetic valve replacement, the endothelial layer is denuded, with one possible exception—pulmonary autografts.

2. Homograft

Homografts, whether fresh-antibiotic treated or cryopreserved, are considered viable tissue valves. A viable tissue is regarded as one that retains physiological function equal to that of tissues in their normal state. This characteristic may not depend upon cellular viability; in fact, a substantial proportion of the initially "live" cells on a homograft are lost prior to implantation.

The loss of endothelial cells occurs at several specific steps from the time of procurement to the time of implantation. Upon procurement, the standard washing with Ringer's lactate may cause endothelial cell swelling, facilitating their subsequent loss from the surface tissue matrix (18,19). Cold temperatures (4°C) produce a higher degree of endothelial cell loss when compared to preservation at 20°C (20). The antibiotic treatment of homografts, designed to destroy contaminating organisms, results in a variable degree of cell destruction that is directly related to the concentration of antibiotics in the incubation solution (21), duration of the process, and accompanying temperature.

Preservation and storage of homografts contribute to a further decrease in the endothelial cell population. Yankah and colleagues (15) reported that 75% of the endothelial cells were viable after 9 months of cryopreservation if the procurement was performed at 4°C and the tissue was frozen within 2 hours. On the other hand, if the homograft was preserved at 4°C for 7 days, the rate of viable endothelial cells decreased to 10%. Shortening the warm ischemic time during procurement, the use of nontoxic concentrations of antibiotics for graft incubation, slow cooling during the freezing process, and the use of cryoprotective agents such as glycerol and DMSO (dimethyl sulfoxide) are techniques and procedures currently used to promote cellular viability.

Despite intensive efforts to preserve the homograft's endothelial cell layer, once a graft is exposed to circulating blood the endothelium is denuded within 3 months (22). Immunological reactions in all likelihood contribute to this important pathological finding (23).

3. Pulmonary Autograft

Although there are similarities between homografts and autografts, there are also marked differences from a biological perspective. The full complement of histocompatible living cells, the absence of cell and tissue injury related to sterilization or storage, and the short exposure to ischemia upon preparation, have established the pulmonary autograft as a biological gold standard for aortic valve replacement (25).

The cellular (endothelial cells and fibrocytes) and structural components of the autograft, both completely preserved before and after the implantation (23,25), provide an explanation for its attractive track record that includes long-term structural stability, absence of thromboembolic events, and potential for growth.

4. Porcine Bioprosthesis

The preimplantation processing of bioprosthetic materials are necessary to reduce the antigenicity of xenograft tissues, increase their durability, ensure sterility, and reduce the rate of calcification. Chemical treatment involves fixation using low concentrations of glutaraldehyde. This process, accomplished under high (70–80 mmHg) or low (<2 mmHg) pressure, induces collagen-protein cross-linking, which subsequently reduces tissue compliance and increases thermal stability and intrinsic resistance to proteolytic enzyme digestion (26,27). The available evidence supports low-pressure conditions as the best available means to enhance tissue durability.

The procurement and fixation processes largely eliminate the endothelial cell layer from bioprosthetic porcine valves, thereby exposing collagen and the sub-endothelium's basement membrane. These injurious events increase platelet adherence, activation, and aggregation.

5. Pericardial Bioprosthesis

Most pericardial bioprostheses are fabricated from bovine pericardium, with the exception of the Polystan valve, in which porcine pericardium is used. The bovine parietal pericardium is composed of three layers: a serosal layer, consisting of mesothelial cells; the fibrosa, containing collagen bundles and elastic fibers; and the epicardial connective tissue. The fixation process for bovine pericardial tissue is comparable to the technique used for porcine bioprostheses. Unfortunately, the preimplantation process that includes fixation with glutaraldehyde also damages the mesothelial cell layer, exposing collagen within the fibrosa to circulating blood. The components of the currently available stented and stentless bioprostheses and homografts are summarized in Table 5.

6. Interaction of Blood with Biologic Components

With the exception of autografts, the surface of biological valves are largely denuded of endothelial cells, exposing collagen and the basement membrane. This irregular sur-

Table 5 Individual Components of Biological Replacement Heart Valves

	Tissue and preservation	Stent cover	Sewing ring cover
A. Stented bioprosthesis			
Hancock[a] (Medtronic) aortic valve	Glutaraldehyde fixed porcine	Polyester	Dacron
Carpentier-Edwards[a] Porcine (Baxter)	Glutaraldehyde fixed porcine aortic valve	Porous knitted PTFE cloth	Porous seamless PTFE cloth
Carpentier-Edwards[c] Pericardial (Baxter)	Glutaraldehyde fixed bovine pericardium	Woven polyester fabric	Porous seamless PTFE cloth

	Tissue and preservation	Cloth covering	
B. Stentless bioprosthesis (Only available for aortic valve replacement)			
Toronto SPV (St. Jude Medical)	Glutaraldehyde-fixed porcine valve	Polyester[c]	
Freestyle Bioprosthesis (Medtronic)	Porcine aortic root cross-linked in dilute glutaraldehyde	Polyester[c]	

PTFE, polytetrafluoroethylene.
[a]Aortic and mitral valve replacement prosthesis available in the United States.
[b]Only aortic valve replacement prosthesis available in the United States.
[c]Most of the cloth is not exposed to the circulating blood. It is on the outside of the aorta with the root replacement technique or compressed between the porcine valve and the aortic wall if implanted in the subcoronary position. Stentless bioprosthesis do not have stents or sewing rings. The lower edge of the covering cloth becomes a sewing ring.

face is exposed to circulating blood and promptly becomes covered by a thin layer of platelets and fibrin. The concave surface of the valve cusps is most prone to these events because of low shear stress at this particular site. Although under ordinary circumstances platelet adhesion and aggregation would be heightened, manufactured bioprostheses do not initiate a strong platelet-collagen reaction compared with fresh tissue. Pre-treatment with glutaraldehyde may, at least in part, be responsible for this weak response (28).

The endothelial cell layer is reconstituted to variable degrees over time. Although endothelial cells are typically absent during the first year, 70% of bioprostheses implanted for more than 5 years demonstrate an endothelial cell monolayer. The cells are typically grouped in islands and attached to host tissue (fibrin, thrombi, fibrous material). Platelet adhesion is not observed on surfaces containing endothelial cells.

Endothelial cell reconstitution is influenced by valve position and occurs most often on prostheses implanted in the mitral and tricuspid positions. The difference in shear stress to which prostheses are exposed may account for this observation. The reconstitution of a partial endothelial cell layer has not been associated with patient age, presence of infection, thrombus deposition, calcification, stenosis, or regurgitation of the prosthesis.

Several authors have suggested that the endothelial cell layer offers a protective effect in the long-term structural stability of the graft or prosthesis by serving as a biological barrier (15). A barrier for hydrating solvents and ions would allow an increase of phosphate ions in the valve matrix and, therefore, prevent the influx of calcium. Late thrombosis of porcine valves is associated with structural valve degeneration and calcification of the leaflet, leading to increased shearing forces and resulting platelet adherence, activation, and aggregation.

D. Sewing Ring

1. Materials

A variety of materials including silastic and silicone rubber have been used for the fabrication of prosthetic valve sewing rings; however, only the material covering the sewing ring influences host reactions. The most common constituents of covering materials are synthetic: polyethylene terephthalate (Dacron), polypropylene, polyester, and polytetrafluoroethylene (PTFE). Adequate tissue integration, structural stability, and low cost are the most attractive characteristics of these materials (Tables 4, 5).

2. Interaction with Plasma Proteins and Cellular Elements

Plasma protein adsorption represents the host's initial response to implantation, followed soon after by platelet deposition and initiation of the coagulation cascade. The resulting thrombus "organizes," ultimately forming a thin fibrous layer.

There appears to be a relationship between fibrous layer thickness and thromboembolic events. If the thickness is less than 0.5 mm, it is usually well nourished, carrying out physiological metabolic exchange directly with the bloodstream. In contrast, if the fibrous tissue layer exceeds 0.5 mm, the deeper portion is prone to ischemic necrosis and tissue sloughing. This explains why despite the complete incorporation of the sewing ring, it remains a potential source for thromboembolism (25,29). The thickness of the initial covering thrombus correlates directly with the thickness of the fibrous layer (30).

3. Neoendothelium

A monolayer of endothelial cells covers the fibrous layer; however, it rarely evolves to confluence and may not possess normal thromboresistant capabilities. The excessive growth of fibrous tissue can complicate normal incorporation of the sewing ring. This pathological process is known as "tissue ingrowth" or "pannus formation." Excessive fibrous tissue growth advancing beyond the sewing ring surface to invade the prosthesis itself decreases its effective orifice. In the case of mechanical valves, obstruction can impede valve closure and, as a result, cause severe prosthetic valve insufficiency. Prosthetic valves placed in the tricuspid position are particularly prone to tissue ingrowth (15).

E. Annuloplasty Rings

1. Materials

Annuloplasty rings have been used in surgical practice for nearly three decades. Initially made with autologus pericardium or Dacron, they are currently industry-manufactured and sized for more predictable and measured plication of the mitral and tricuspid annulus. The currently FDA-approved annuloplasty rings are summarized in Table 6. In addition to rings, PTFE artificial chords are frequently used when performing "plasty" procedures for mitral valve disease.

2. Interaction of Blood with Annuloplasty Ring and Artificial Chordi

Unlike sewing rings, the bulk of foreign material introduced by annuloplasty rings is relatively small. Nevertheless, the prosthetic material can trigger a similar host response. Incorporation of the annuloplasty ring begins with protein adsorption. Molecular alterations of the protein-coated surface activates several plasma enzymatic systems including the complement pathway, intrinsic coagulation pathway, and the fibrinolytic system. Adsorbed proteins also stimulate platelet adhesion, platelet activation, platelet aggregation, and an acute inflammatory response.

Carpentier-Edwards and Cosgrove-Edwards annuloplasty rings, as previously described, are currently subjected to Duraflo treatment, providing additional bio-compatibility by reducing platelet and complement activation compared to untreated polyester. The overall incorporation process is not adversely influenced by Duraflo treatment (31).

Table 6 Individual Components of Annuloplasty Rings

	Ring material	Ring cover
Carpentier-Edwards[a] (Baxter) "Classic"	Titanium alloy covered by silicone rubber	Polyester knit fabric
Duran[a] (Medtronic)	Circular of Dacron	Ring fabric
Cosgrove-Edwardsa (Baxter) (Duraflo-treated)	Silicone rubber	Polyester velour
St. Jude Medical TailorTM	Silicone rubber (barium impregnated)	Double velour polyester fabric

[a]FDA-approved and currently in the United States.

F. Thrombogenicity Related to Flow Conditions

A comprehensive evaluation of prosthetic valve thrombogenicity must consider existing both hemodynamic and hydrodynamic properties. Ideally, flow should be neither too fast (shear stress) nor too slow (stasis). Unfortunately, and despite substantial improvement in prosthetic heart valve designs introduced during the last three decades, abnormal flow patterns remain a concern. Some general abnormal flow conditions are common to all prostheses; however, specific abnormal flow conditions are typical of some mechanical prosthetic designs.

High-velocity flow and stagnation (stasis) are considered thrombogenic by differing mechanisms (15). High-velocity flow conditions are commonly induced by mechanical prosthetic valves and develop when blood is forced forward through a relatively narrow orifice. The protective regurgitant mechanism (washout between the moving parts) in some mechanical valves and impact of the occluder to the housing are also responsible for erythrocyte damage (hemolysis) and platelet activation.

The release of adenosine diphosphate (ADP) from damaged erythrocytes contributes to the developing "prothrombotic" environment. ADP is a platelet agonist, leading to platelet-fibrin thrombus formation and endothelial cell injury. This firm, relatively insoluble thrombus is highly resistant to fibrinolysis (15).

Stagnation (stasis) occurs in areas of low shear stress and promotes thrombus formation through contact activation of coagulation proteins. In addition, slow flow is associated with erythrocyte-fibrinogen interactions. The combined events yield an erythrocyte-rich thrombus that is loosely connected by a fibrin meshwork. Embolization is more likely to occur under these conditions.

G. Specific Flow Patterns of Mechanical Valves

1. Caged-Ball Valves (Starr-Edwards)

Starr-Edwards prostheses have a large sewing ring and a relatively small effective orifice. These features make it obstructive in small sizes, particularly in the aortic position, causing higher transvalvular pressure gradients when compared to the more modern lower profile prostheses. Leakage volumes are not related to design and, when present, indicate a pathological process. High-velocity forward flow occurs peripherally, causing turbulence in the region of the apex. An area of low-velocity reverse flow occurs at the point of full ball travel (15), creating a zone of relative stagnation that predisposes the cage's apex to thrombus formation (15).

2. Tilting-Disk Valves (Medtronic-Hall, Omniscience)

Tilting-disk valves are less obstructive than caged-ball valves. Early designs were characterized by a low velocity of flow through the minor orifice. Modified versions of the Medtronic-Hall valve have moved the axis of the tilting disk more centrally, facilitating forward flow through the minor orifice and, as a result, decreasing stagnation. Despite this change, the minor orifice remains vulnerable to thrombosis (15). In the Omniscience valve, turbulence is reduced by the disk's curvature, and areas of stasis and shear stress are decreased by the eccentric location of the pivot axis (22).

3. Bileaflet Valves (St. Jude, CarboMedics)

The bileaflet design produces three distinct areas of flow through the prosthetic orifice. Although flow is increased through the two lateral valve orifices, the overall flow is uniform, more laminar, with less turbulence and less impedance than other valve designs. Design modifications have been introduced to further improve hemodynamic performance in small aortic roots. The St. Jude HP (high performance) design has a smaller sewing ring, increasing the effective orifice/annulus ratio. In the Top Hat design of the CarboMedics valve, the housing of the prosthesis sits above the level of the annulus to accommodate a valve two sizes larger than the corresponding annular size. This aortic valve prosthesis is designed for supra-annular implantation.

Bileaflet valve design allows a regurgitant volume for "washing out" the mechanical components. The low-velocity reverse flow that occurs adjacent to each hinge point makes this site prone to thrombus formation. Flow characteristics associated with differing mechanical valve designs are illustrated in Fig. 1.

H. Specific Flow Patterns of Biological Valves

1. Stented Bioprosthesis

Although flow patterns through the valve orifice of stented bioprostheses demonstrate minimal or absent turbulence and vorticeal current formation, the rigidity of the stent and their relative obstructive nature (particularly small sizes in aortic position) lead to abnormal flow characteristics. Rapid flow takes place centrally, but areas of relative stasis exist in the region of concavity (outflow surface) of each cusp. Thrombus formation, when it occurs, is most frequently observed in this specific area (15).

Design modifications have been introduced to improve flow characteristics. The Hancock first-generation porcine valve was found to be obstructive in small sizes due to the nonmobility of the right coronary cusp. The presence of a muscle band at the base of this leaflet limited its opening, causing hemodynamic obstruction. The Hancock MO (modified orifice) was developed in response to this problem (9). Recent modifications of the Carpentier-Edwards porcine and pericardial valve prostheses have included reduced sewing ring models to increase effective orifice to annulus ratio.

2. Stentless Bioprostheses and Homografts

Near ideal hemodynamic results after valve replacement are anticipated with stentless bioprostheses and homografts. Their non-obstructive nature and flexibility cause insignificant gradients across the prosthesis leading to minimal turbulence and maximal laminar flow. These attractive features are achieved with root replacement for implantation versus a sub-coronary technique. The thrombogenicity of stentless bioprostheses and homografts is very low.

V. CLINICAL APPROACH TO PATIENTS WITH PROSTHETIC HEART VALVES

Patients with prosthetic heart valves are at risk for thromboembolism, and many require long-term (lifelong) anticoagulation therapy. It is recognized that the risk of thromboembolism is particularly high with mechanical prosthetic heart valves in descending order of risk: caged-ball, tilting disk, and bileaflet valves. Prosthetic valves in the mitral position also pose greater risk than those in the aortic or other positions. Although biological (tissue) valves and native valves that have undergone repair inherently carry less risk, it is important to consider all associated risk factors for thromboembolism when decisions regarding anticoagulation are being made [e.g., atrial fibrillation, prior thromboembolic events, dilated (>55 mm) left atrium, poor left ventricular performance, and age > 65 years].

VI. CLINICAL EXPERIENCE

A wealth of information is available from clinical trials and clinical experience gained during the past several decades. The incidence of thromboembolism ranges from <1 to 4% per year, with higher rates occurring with mechanical mitral valves and multiple site mechanical valves. The rate of major hemorrhage varies from 0.7 to 5% per year and is highest among older individuals, those with an INR > 4.0, and in the presence of concomitant aspirin use (75). The rates of thromboembolism following valve repair have been difficult to discern in the absence of randomized clinical trials but appear similar to those anticipated with bioprosthetic valves.

VII. MANAGEMENT GUIDELINES

All patients with mechanical prosthetic heart valves should receive oral anticoagulation therapy indefinitely to a target INR of 3.0 (range 2.5–3.5). A higher intensity of antico-

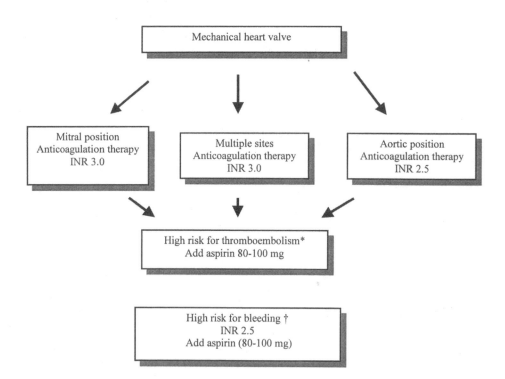

*Patients at high risk for thromboembolism (atrial fibrillation, left atrial enlargement (>55 mm), prior or recurrent thromboemboembolism, reduced left ventricular function (ejection fraction < 35%).
Hemorrhagic events requiring hospitalization, surgical intervention, transfusion, or transient discontinuation of anticoagulation therapy.

Figure 11   Management algorithm for patients with mechanical prosthetic heart valves.

agulation (INR 4.0) might be beneficial among patients at high risk for thromboembolism (caged-ball valve, caged-disk valve, multiple site mechanical valves, recurrent thromboembolism, mitral position, left atrium >55 mm, atrial fibrillation); however, it is preferable to maintain a target INR of 3.0 and add low-dose (80–100 mg) aspirin daily. Low-risk patients (bileaflet prosthetic valve in the aortic position without additional thromboembolic risk factors) can be maintained at an INR of 2.5 (range 2.0–3.0). the combination of oral anticoagulants and aspirin (80–100 mg/d) might reduce thromboembolism but is unlikely to offer added benefit among low-risk patients. Patients with bioprosthetic valves in the mitral position and those with valve repair should receive oral anticoagulants (target INR 2.5) for at least 3 months after insertion. A more prolonged duration of therapy should be considered strongly for those at risk [atrial fibrillation, prior thromboembolism, documented atrial thrombus at the time of surgery, dilated (>55 mm) left atrium, poor ventricular performance]. Patients with biprosthetic valves in the aortic position should receive anticoagulation therapy (target INR 2.5) for the initial 3 months after insertion. Therapy beyond 3 months should be considered for atients with atrial fibrillation, concomitant mitral valve disease, or poor ventricular performance. Long-term therapy with aspirin (80 mg) is recommended for low-risk patients (Figs. 11, 12) (32).

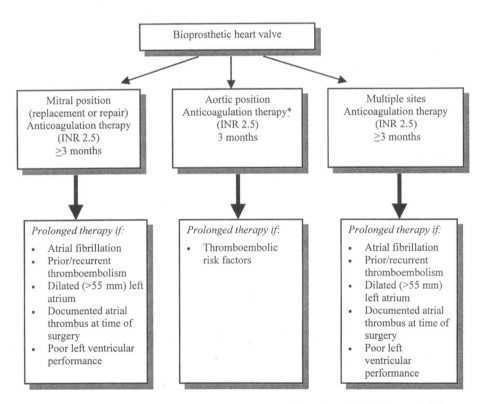

Anticoagulation therapy is strongly recommended in the presence of thromboembolic risk factors including concomitant mitral valve disease, atrial fibrillation, prior thromboembolism, or poor left ventricular performance.

Figure 12 Management algorithm for patients with bioprosthetic heart valves and valve repair.

VIII. SUMMARY

Prosthetic heart valves have contributed substantially to the surgical armemantarium available for patients with congenital or acquired valvular heart disease. An increasing experience, coupled with the development of less thrombogenic materials and, in some
conditions, early intervention that leads to a preservation in left ventricular performance
and maintenance of normal chamber dimensions has reduced the incidence of life-threatening thromboembolic events. However, antithrombotic therapy remains a mainstay in the
prophylaxis of high-risk patients.

REFERENCES

1. Ajit P. Yoganathan. Overview: an engineer's perspective. J Heart Valve Dis 1996;
    5(suppl.I):S3–S6.
2. Frater R, Ellis, Jr, H. Problems in the development of a mitral valve prosthesis. In: Merendino
    KA, ed. Prosthetic Valves for Cardiac Surgery.Springfield, IL: Charles C Thomas, 1961.
3. Kolff W, Seidel W, Akutsu T, Mirkovitch V. Hindberg J. Studies of thrombosis of artificial
    valves In: Merendino KA, ed. Prosthetic Valves for Cardiac Surgery. Springfield, IL: Charles
    C Thomas, 1961.
4. Ross J, Greenfield L, Bowman R, Morrow A. The chemical structure and surface properties of
    certain synthetic polymers and their relationship with valve thrombosis. In: Merendino KA,
    ed.: Prosthetic Valves for Cardiac Surgery. Springfield, IL: Charles C Thomas, 1961.
5. Harken DE, Soroff HS, Taylor WJ, et al. Partial and complete prosthesis in aortic insufficiency.
    J Thorac Cardiovasc Surg 1960; 40:744.
6. Starr A, Edwards M. Mitral replacement: clinical experience with a ball-valve prosthesis. Ann
    Surg 1961; 154:726–40.
7. Ross DN. Homograft replacement of the aortic valve. Lancet 1962; 2:487.
8. Cohn L. Aortic valve prosthesis. Cardiol Rev 1994; 2:5, 219–229.
9. Jamieson E. Cardiac valvular replacement devices: residual problems and innovative inves-
    tigative technologies. Surgical Technology International VII, 1998.
10. Balaguer J, Davaro R. Management of Infective Endocarditis next to the End of the Twentieth
    Century. Rev Argent Cardiol 1999; 67:675–685
11. Balaguer J, Byrne J, Cohn L. Orthotopic pulmonic valve replacement with a pulmonary homo-
    graft as an interposition graft. J Card Surg 1996; 6: 417–420.
12. Orminston J, Shah P, Tei C, et al. Size and motion of the mitral valve annulus in man.
    Circulation 1981; 64:113.
13. Duran CM, Ubago J. Clinical and hemodynamic performance of a totally flexible prosthetic
    ring for atrioventricular valve reconstruction. Ann Thorac Surg 1976; 22:458–463.
14. Sequin J, Demaria R, Rocgier R, Chaptal A. Advance in mitral valve repair using a device flex-
    ible in three dimensions. St. Jude Medical-Sequin Annuloplasty Ring. ASAIO 1996;
    42:M368–M371.
15. Butchart E. Thrombogenesis and anticoagulation in heart valve disease: toward a rational
    approach. J Heart Valve Disease 1993; 1:1–6.
16. Helmus M, Hubbell J. Material selection. Cardiovasc Pathol 1993; 2(2): 1–19.
17. Ruggeri Z. Mechanisms of shear-induced platelet adhesion and aggregation. Thromb
    Haemostasis 1993; 70(1):119–123.
18. Collins G, Bravo-Shugarman M, Teresaki P, et al. Kidney preservation for transplantation.
    Lancet 1969; 2:1219.
19. Acquatella H, Perez Gonzalez M, Morales J, et al. Ionic and histologic changes in the kidney
    after perfusion and storage for transplantation. Transplantation 1972; 14:480.
20. Soldberg S, Larsen T, Jorgensen L, et al. Cold induced endothelial cells detachement in human
    saphenous vein grafts. J Cardiovasc Surg 1987; 28: 571–575.

21. Strickett M, Barrat-Boyes B, MacCullogh D, et al. Disinfection of human heart valve allografts with antibiotics at low concentrations. Pathology 1983; 15:457–462.
22. O'Brien MF, Johnston N, Stafford EG, et al. A study of the cells in the explanted viable cryopreserved allograft valve. J Cardiac Surg 1988,3:279–827.
23. Yankah AC, Hetzer R. Procurement and viability of cardiac valve allografts. In: Cardiac Valve Allografts 1962–1987. Darmstadt: Steinkopff Verlag; New York: Springer-Verlag, 1988
24. Ross D. Evolution of the biological concept in cardiac surgery. A pilgrim's progress. In: Cardiac Valve Allografts 1962–1987. Darmstadt: Steinkopff Verlag; New York: Springer-Verlag, 1988.
25. Buch W, Kosek J, Angell W. The role of rejection and mechanical trauma on valve graft viability. J Thorac Cardiovasc Surg 62; 696–706,1971.
26. Woodroof E. The chemistry and biology of aldehide treated tissue heart valves xenografts. In: Ionescu MI, ed. Tissue Heart Valves. London: Butterworth, 1979:347–362.
27. Cheung D, Perelman N, Ko E, et al. Mechanism of crosslinking of proteins by glutaraldehyde.III. Reactions with collagen in tissues. Connect Tissue Res 1985; 13:109–115.
28. Magilligan D, Oyama C, Flein S, et al. Platelet adherence to bioprosthetic cardiac valves. Am J Cardiol 1984; 53:945–49.
29. Dewanjee M, TrastekV, Tago M, Torianni M, Kaye M. Non-invasive isotopic technique for detection of platelet deposition on bovine pericardial mitral valve prosthesis and in-vivo quantification of visceral microembolism in dogs. Trans Am Soc Artif Intern Organs 1983; 29: 188–193.
30. Berger K, Sauvage L, Wood S, Wesolowski S. Sewing ring healing of cardiac valve prosthesis. Surgery 1967; 61(1):102–117.
31. Hsu L. Biocompatibility in cardiopulmonary bypass. J Cardiothorac Vasc Anesth 1997; 11: 376–382.
32. Sixth ACCP Consensus Conference on Antihrombotic Therapy. Chest/(suppl); 119:1S–370S.

11-2

The Hypercoagulable Evaluation of Patients with Thromboembolic Disease

Michael J. Rohrer and James B. Froehlich
University of Massachusetts Medical School, Worcester, Massachusetts, U.S.A.

I. INTRODUCTION

The clinical identification of the patient with a hypercoagulable state responsible for arterial thromboembolic disease can be a difficult clinical problem since the manifestations of the occlusive disease, be it myocardial infarction, stroke, or limb-threatening ischemia, are frequently the same regardless of the underlying vascular pathology. Furthermore, the therapy treating the clinical emergency may distract the clinician from seeking a diagnosis of a thrombotic tendency, since it is often assumed that atherosclerosis is the underlying pathological problem. It is important to consider the possible presence of a hypercoagulable state in order to appropriately treat the patient's acute event, to help prevent recurrent events, and in some cases to appropriately counsel family members regarding thrombotic risk.

II. IDENTIFICATION OF PATIENTS WITH HYPERCOAGULABLE STATES

Arterial occlusive disease is very common in western societies and is most commonly due to atherosclerosis. The risk factors for atherosclerotic occlusive disease have been well characterized, and clinical studies have demonstrated the benefits of modifying these risk factors. Less well developed is the clinical profile of the patient who presents with arterial thrombotic events due to the presence of a hypercoagulable state.

The initial evaluation of all patients begins with a thorough history and physical examination, which often provides most of the information necessary to consider the diagnosis of a hypercoagulable state. The diagnosis of a hypercoagulable state should be sought in a patient who presents with an arterial thromboembolic event and a family history of thrombotic complications (1), or who presents with a thrombotic event at an especially early age (1,2). In spite of the fact that many hypercoagulable states are genetically based and therefore present at birth, it is unusual for patients to present before young adulthood with a thrombotic problem (3–5).

Like many medical diagnoses, the presence of a clinical entity may remain occult unless specifically sought. Illustrating this point is a study evaluating 20 patients who required lower extremity revascularization for limb-threatening ischemia who were 50 years old or younger. An inherited hypercoagulable state was defined in 30%, and 47% were noted to have abnormally high platelet aggregation profiles (6).

The diagnosis of a hypercoagulable state should also be sought in patients with (a) unusual patterns of vascular disease, (b) arterial thrombosis without an underlying anatomical lesion (2,7), or (c) recurrent or migratory clotting (7). Some historical features suggest specific coagulation abnormalities. A history of warfarin-induced skin necrosis is suggestive of a protein C or protein S deficiency (8,9). Multiple miscarriages may be the clinical manifestation of an antiphospholipid antibody (10–12). Patient characteristics that should prompt a hypercoagulable evaluation are summarized in Table 1.

III. HYPERCOAGULABLE STATES RESPONSIBLE FOR ARTERIAL THROMBOEMBOLIC DISEASE

A. Inherited Hypercoagulable States

Although most biochemically defined hypercoagulable states are predominantly associated with venous thrombosis, arterial thromboses have been reported in patients with antithrombin III (ATIII) deficiency, protein C deficiency, protein S deficiency, activated protein C insensitivity and the factor V Leiden mutation, the prothrombin gene mutation, hyperhomocysteinemia, and other less prominent hypercoagulable states including dysfibrinogenemia, plasminogen deficiency, elevated factor VIII levels, and the presence of plasminogen activator inhibitor (13). Elevated lipoprotein(a) [Lp(a)] levels are primarily associated with the development of arterial occlusive disease and arterial thromboembolic events (14–17).

1. Antithrombin III Deficiency

Antithrombin III (ATIII) has been called the most important inhibitor of activated coagulation enzymes, and heterozygotes for ATIII deficiency have a well-defined hypercoagulable state (18). Plasma concentrations of the activation peptide prothrombin fragment 1+2 are chronically elevated in patients with ATIII deficiency, indicating persistent subclinical activation of the coagulation cascade as a result of deficient neutralization of factor Xa in these patients, even in the absence of clinically apparent thrombotic events (19).

Deficiency of ATIII was described by Egeberg in 1965 (20) and is inherited as an autosomal dominant disorder (21,22). As many as one in 600 people has ATIII deficiency (23), which may be due to either a quantitative deficiency in production of ATIII or be a qualitative abnormality as the result of production of a dysfunctional ATIII molecule. Both of these abnormalities result in diminished ATIII activity on functional assays, although patients with dysfunctional ATIII molecules will have normal measured ATIII protein

Table 1   Characteristics of Patients with Arterial Thromboembolic Disease for Whom a Hypercoagulable Evaluation Should Be Performed

Strong family history of thrombotic events
Thrombotic complications at an unusually young age
Unusual patterns of vascular occlusive disease
No underlying anatomical lesion noted after thrombodissolution
History of recurrent pregnancy loss
Development of skin necrosis after taking warfarin

levels (24,25). Both types of ATIII-deficient patients have an approximate 30–80% lifetime risk of sustaining a thrombotic event (26).

ATIII deficiency is typically manifested by recurrent venous thromboembolism (21,22), which may occur in the absence of precipitating factors or may be associated with pregnancy, estrogen use, trauma, or a surgical procedure. Functional assays of ATIII levels are routinely used to establish the diagnosis of ATIII deficiency because they detect those individuals with both dysfunctional ATIII molecules as well as those with diminished ATIII production. Most ATIII-deficient patients are heterozygotes with approximately 50% of normal activity, although the presence of homozygotes has been reported (27).

Some ATIII-deficient patients require large amounts of heparin to establish a therapeutically prolonged aPTT (26). This is not surprising in light of the fact that heparin's ability to inhibit thrombin is primarily achieved though its binding to ATIII, which changes the latter molecule's configuration and increases its ability to inactivate thrombin and other activated coagulation factors (28). Supplemental ATIII provided as exogenous ATIII concentrate or as fresh frozen plasma may make it easier to achieve therapeutic anticoagulation with heparin in these patients. Patients with recurrent thrombotic events should receive indefinite warfarin therapy at a dosage to maintain a low-intensity International Normalized Ratio (INR) value of 2.0–3.0 (29).

Acquired ATIII deficiency is also associated with numerous disorders, including disseminated intravascular coaglation (DIC) (30), liver disease (30), nephrotic syndrome (31), preeclampsia (32), and in patients taking oral contraceptive agents (33).

2. Protein C Deficiency

Protein C is a vitamin K–dependent plasma protein that inactivates factors Va and VIIIa to inhibit coagulation after being activated by the thrombin-thrombomodulin complex (34). Activated protein C also possesses profibrinolytic activity (35). Protein C deficiency is inherited as an autosomal dominant disorder; hence most patients are heterozygotes with approximately 50% of normal protein C activity. Evidence of subclinical thrombotic activity has been demonstrated in nonanticoagulated asymptomatic protein C–deficient patients using activation peptide assays (36).

The predominant clinical manifestation of protein C–deficient patients is recurrent venous thromboembolism (37), although arterial thrombotic events, including stroke (38), have been reported. Neonatal purpura fulminans is seen in homozygous newborns of heterozygous parents. These children, who have protein C levels <5% of normal, develop DIC at birth, associated with extensive venous and arterial thrombosis (39).

Despite the clear association of protein C deficiency with thrombosis in large epidemiological studies (40), there are also data suggesting that many protein C–deficient patients remain asymptomatic. Several reports have identified an incidence of protein C deficiency of one in 250–500 individuals (41,42). Interestingly, no patient in either of these studies had a history of symptomatic venous thrombosis. These data suggest that additional risk factors may need to be present to provoke thrombosis in heterozygous protein C–deficient patients. In one study, up to 20% of symptomatic protein C–deficient patients had the additional risk factor of activated protein C resistance (43), supporting the concept that many patients with recurrent thrombosis will have more than one risk factor for the development of thrombosis (44).

Warfarin-induced skin necrosis is an unusual syndrome seen in some heterozygotes with protein C deficiency (45). Most patients who develop this syndrome have received relatively large doses of warfarin in the absence of therapeutic heparin anticoagulation. The origin of this clinical problem arises from the fact that protein C and protein S are both vitamin K-dependent factors, as are factors II, VII, IX, and X. It is relevant that the serum half-lives of protein C and protein S are both substantially shorter than those of the coagulation factors. Hence, when warfarin is initially administered (especially in the absence of other anticoagulants such as heparin) and synthesis of all of the vitamin K–dependent molecules is depressed, the circulating levels of protein C and protein S decrease faster than the levels of the coagulation factors, leading to an increase in the coagulation potential. Clinically, this is classically manifested by the presence of skin necrosis due to thrombosis of dermal vessels (46).

A common problem faced by clinicians is the measurement of protein C levels in patients taking oral anticoagulants. Many clinicians forget that protein C is a vitamin K–dependent molecule, and therefore even non–protein C–deficient individuals taking warfarin will have low protein C levels, making the laboratory definition of the diagnosis difficult.

Many patients with protein C deficiency will be asymptomatic, especially those identified in screening studies. Asymptomatic patients need not be treated, but should be considered for prophylaxis when they experience high-risk situations, such as undergoing a surgical procedure operation. Symptomatic protein C–deficient patients should be initially anticoagulated with heparin while long-term anticoagulation with warfarin at an INR of 2.0–3.0 is instituted. Patients with more than one thrombotic event or patients with a single life-threatening thromboembolic event should be considered for indefinite anticoagulation (29).

3. Protein S Deficiency

Protein S is also a vitamin K–dependent plasma protein that mediates the anticoagulant activity of activated protein C and can also inhibit factor Xa activity (47). Like ATIII and protein C deficiencies, protein S deficiency is inherited as an autosomal dominant trait. Most carriers are therefore heterozygotes with approximately 50% of normal protein S activity. Like ATIII and protein C–deficient patients, most patients with symptomatic protein S deficiency will experience venous thromboembolism (48,49). However, unlike other inherited thrombotic disorders, up to 25% of patients with protein S deficiency may experience arterial thrombosis (50). As mentioned previously, many patients with protein S deficiency and thrombosis will have other risk factors for the development of a thrombotic event, including activated protein C resistance, estrogen use, or pregnancy (51). Neonatal purpura fulminans has also been associated with homozygous protein S deficiency (52).

The laboratory diagnosis of protein S deficiency can be complicated (50). C4b-binding protein is an acute-phase reactant and binds to protein S, and only free, unbound protein S has physiological activity. This binding protein is often elevated in patients who have experienced thromboembolic events, resulting in reduced free protein S levels from the patient's true baseline. Consequently, measurement of protein S levels in patients with acute thrombosis may yield misleading results. Because of protein C and protein S interactions, false-positive results may also be seen when functional protein S assays are performed on patients who have activated protein C resistance. Finally, because protein S is a vitamin K–dependent protein, concurrent warfarin therapy poses the same difficulty as described for patients being evaluated for protein C deficiency (53).

Asymptomatic protein S deficient patients are generally not treated, but should be considered for prophylaxis when they are placed in high-risk situations such as undergoing surgical procedures. Protein S–deficient patients who have experienced thrombotic events should be anticoagulated as described for protein C–deficient patients. Patients with recurrent thrombosis or patients with a single life-threatening thromboembolic event should undergo lifelong anticoagulation (29).

4. Resistance to Activated Protein C and Factor V Leiden

Resistance to activated protein C was initially defined in 1993 (54) and has subsequently been defined as the most common underlying hypercoagulable state responsible for venous thrombosis (55). Although unusual in Black and Asian populations, it is present in about 5% of the general population with European ancestry (56) and 18% of patients with venous thromboembolic disease (57,58). Approximately 90% of cases of activated protein C insensitivity were related to the factor V Leiden mutation (59), which renders the activated factor V molecule insensitive to the action of activated protein C, which would ordinarily degrade the molecule.

The presence of factor V Leiden, inherited as an autosomal dominant condition, leads to the clinical syndrome of activated protein C insensitivity. Although classically associated with the presence of venous thrombosis, resistance to activated protein C has been associated with arterial thrombotic events as well (60,61).

Heterozygotes have a two- to sevenfold higher risk of developing DVT than the unaffected population (62–67). Since the incidence of heterozygosity for factor V Leiden is so high, it is not surprising to find that individuals who are homozygous are also present in the population. They have a risk of developing deep venous thrombosis 40–80 times that of unaffected individuals (62–68).

5. Prothrombin 20210

A mutation in the prothrombin gene resulting in a substitution of a single amino acid at position 20210 is present in 2% of asymptomatic individuals and approximately 7% of patients with venous thromboembolic events (69–72). As a result of the mutation, there are increased circulating levels of prothrombin (69). The risk of arterial thrombotic events is poorly defined, but the risk of venous thromboembolic disease is 2-3 fold higher than in unaffected individuals (66,69,72), and increases dramatically with advancing age (72).

6. Hyperhomocysteinemia

Elevated levels of homocysteine, an intermediary in methionine metabolism, have been associated with the development of premature atherosclerotic lesions (73) as well as arterial (74) and venous thromboses (74,75). Hyperhomocysetinemia, defined as fasting plasma levels >15 μM/L, is relatively common in the general population and can result from inherited enzyme deficiencies (76) or acquired disorders such as dietary deficiencies of folate and vitamins B_6 and B_{12}, chronic renal failure, pernicious anemia, and hypothyroidism (76). It has become clear that hyperhomocysteinemia is an independent risk factor for the development of atherosclerosis and atherothrombosis (73).

The presence of hyperhomocysteinemia is evaluated by measuring fasting homocysteine levels. Evaluation of homocysteine levels following a standard methionine loading dose may increase the sensitivity of testing (73). The enzymatic defect can be characterized by testing for the known enzyme deficiencies (73).

Treatment consists of nutritional replacement of folate and vitamins B_6 and B_{12}. Although nutritional supplementation can decrease homocysteine levels, it is still unclear whether the lowering of homocysteine levels will actually decrease the incidence of thrombosis or the other conditions associated with hyperhomocysteinemia such as early atherosclerosis and cerebrovascular disease (75).

7. Lipoprotein(a)

Lipoprotein(a) is a heterogeneous lipoprotein that was first described in 1963 (77). High concentrations of Lp(a) have been identified as a major and independent risk factor for the presence of coronary artery disease and myocardial infarction (78,79) as well as stroke (78,79). Epidemiologically it has been found to play a significant role in the development of premature atherosclerotic occlusive disease (14–17) and is one of the top five or six risk factors for the development of cardiovascular disease (79). Elevated Lp(a) levels have also been demonstrated to be a predictor for restenosis after iliac angioplasty (80). Some authors have found no association between Lp(a) levels and with venous thrombosis (81), although serum Lp(a) levels of >30 mg% were associated with the development of venous thromboembolic disease in one study (82).

The biochemical and physical structure of Lp(a) may help to explain its association with atherogenesis and thrombosis. The apo(a) component of the Lp(a) molecule is composed of multiple loop-shaped units called kringles, the sequence of which is highly similar to the kringle organization in plasminogen (78,83). This structural homology of the Lp(a) molecule with plasminogen endows it with the ability to bind to fibrin and membrane proteins of endothelial cells and monocytes and inhibit the binding of plasminogen and therefore inhibit plasmin generation (84,85). This potential inhibition of fibrinolysis may explain its potential prothrombotic and atherogenic role (86).

Serum Lp(a) can be quantitated quite readily. Levels are largely genetically determined (17,87), and do not appear to be substantially alterable by changes in lifestyle which are known to influence the concentration of other lipoproteins. Numerous studies have demonstrated the lack of impact of exercise (77,88–93) and diet (77,94) on Lp(a) levels. Diets high in *n*-3–polyunsaturated fatty acids may decrease Lp(a) by only 20% (95).

8.   Other Inherited Hypercoagulable States

Other causes of inherited thrombophilia include abnormalities in the proteins of the fibrinolytic system, dysfibrinogenemias, deficiency of heparin cofactor II, abnormal thrombomodulin, and elevated levels of histidine-rich glycoprotein (96).

B.   Acquired Hypercoagulable States

1.   Antiphospholipid Antibody Syndromes

The presence of antiphospholipid antibodies is associated strongly with both arterial and venous thrombosis, the most common of the acquired hypercoagulable states (97). Although often associated with the development of deep venous thrombosis, these antibodies have also been associated with the development of coronary, cerebrovascular, and peripheral vascular thrombotic events (97). One report suggests that up to 18% of patients with premature coronary thrombosis may harbor antiphospholipid antibodies (11). Clinical manifestations of the presence of antiphospholipid antibodies, in addition to the presence of arterial and venous thrombosis, include recurrent fetal loss, thrombocytopenia, livedo reticularis, and neurological symptoms (97).

Although it is known that the antiphospholipid syndrome is caused by a heterogeneous group of antibodies to various proteins complexed with negatively charged phospholipids, the precise mechanism through which these antibodies alter hemostasis remains unclear (97). The presence of antiphospholipid antibodies may be (a) seen as a primary condition, (b) seen in patients with the autoimmune diseases systemic lupus erythematosus and rheumatic arthritis, (c) associated with the use of certain drugs such as procainamide or hydralazine, or (d) seen in the presence of chronic viral infections such as HIV, syphilis, or hepatitis C.

The presence of antiphospholipid antibodies is confirmed by the occurrence of one or more thrombotic events in the presence of positive antibody studies on two occasions more than 3 months apart (98). Studies should be performed to detect the presence of IgG, IgA, and IgM antibodies (11,99).

It is often suggested that patients with a history of thrombosis and the presence of antiphospholipid antibodies are best treated with warfarin with target INR of 3.0–3.5 (vs. the usual target of 2.0–3.0), because of the substantial risk for recurrent thrombosis with less intense anticoagulant regimens (75,100). Some patients will suffer recurrent thromboses while being treated with warfarin and must then be treated with either unfractionated or low molecular weight heparin (99).

2. Heparin-Induced Thrombocytopenia

The frequent exposure to heparin in patients with coronary and peripheral vascular disease means that many patients are potentially subject to the formation of heparin-associated antiplatelet antibodies (HAAPAs). These antibodies, which are formed to the heparin-platelet factor 4 complex (101), bind to the Fc receptor on platelets, causing their activation, aggregation, and subsequent release of procoagulant microparticles (102) leading to thrombin generation and clinical thrombosis (101,103). This platelet aggregation is the reason for the fall in platelet count, which is the hallmark of the disease, and can result in heparin-induced thrombosis (HIT).

The prevalence of clinically important unfractionated heparin-platelet interaction is estimated to be approximately 2%, although the incidence of HAAPA formation with low molecular weight heparin is lower (103). However, in one study of 106 patients undergoing elective arterial reconstruction for peripheral vascular occlusive disease, 21% had development of HAAPAs documented, and those patients with antibody detected had a 2.6-fold increase in the risk of developing a postoperative thrombotic event such as acute graft thrombosis, deep venous thrombosis, or myocardial infarction (104). Another study of vascular surgery patients identified up to a 34% incidence of heparin-platelet factor 4 antibodies, although none of the patients suffered any of the sequelae of HIT (105). Poor outcomes including death, stroke, myocardial infarction, and limb loss are correlated with the lowest platelet counts and the highest heparin-platelet factor 4 antibody titers (106). HIT has been documented to occur 5 or more days after cessation of heparin administration due to the persistence of the IgG antibodies induced by heparin administration (107).

Establishing the presence of HAAPAs is based upon the evaluation of platelet count determinations, which should be performed on a regular basis in individuals receiving any type of heparin preparation, since the development of thrombocytopenia precedes the development of the thrombotic sequelae. Since the development of HAAPAs is an immunological phenomenon, the likelihood of developing antibodies is not necessarily related to the volume of heparin being administered. A precipitous fall in the platelet count, a platelet count of $<100,000/mm^3$, or the development of a thrombotic event should prompt consideration of the presence of heparin-induced thrombosis. Unfortunately, laboratory-based confirmation of a diagnosis is difficult since the diagnostic specificity of both the antigen and activation assays to detect heparin-induced thrombocytopenia is relatively low (105,108,109). Therefore, the clinical evaluation of the patient and an assessment of the clinical context of any thrombocytopenia is important in the determination of the diagnosis of HAAPA and HIT. The availability of effective alternative anticoagulants such as recombinant hirudin (Lepirudin) means that a low threshold to stop heparin in the setting of thrombocytopenia seems prudent to prevent HIT.

Treatment of the hypercoagulable state associated with the presence of HAAPAs requires cessation of heparin and continued anticoagulation in spite of what might be considered (incorrectly) to be a clinical situation with a high risk of bleeding complications because of the depressed platelet count. Although low molecular weight heparins are less likely to induce the formation of heparin induced antiplatelet antibodies (103), the use of low molecular weight heparin molecules is contraindicated as a substitute for unfractionated heparin when HAAPAs are present because of a 60–100% in vitro cross reactivity with unfractionated heparin, and hence a possible progression of the syndrome (110–112). Simple discontinuation of the heparin may fail to prevent subsequent HIT since the antibodies associated with the administration of the heparin persist even after the heparin has been stopped (113).

Treatment with warfarin as an alternate anticoagulant during the period of thrombocytopenia can paradoxically lead to venous limb gangrene (113), presumably because of the relative decrease in the levels of protein C and protein S that occurs acutely after warfarin administration. Heparinoids such as danaproid or direct thrombin inhibitors such as recombinant hirudin (Lepirudin) or argatroban are alternatives to heparin that effectively prevent ongoing thrombosis (113–115). Lepirudin has the advantage of being administered via a constant infusion similar to the manner in which heparin is infused, with the therapeutic goal being elevation of the aPTT to approximately 70 seconds (115). This has been shown to be a safe and effective anticoagulant in clinical experience in patients with HIT (116). Since Lepirudin is eliminated by renal mechanisms, its half-life is markedly prolonged in patients with renal failure (115), and therefore the use of argatroban in patients with renal failure is recommended given the hepatic metabolism of the latter drug (115). Since danaproid is a heparinoid molecule, it is logical to be concerned about the possibility of cross reactivity in the setting of HIT. Danaproid has a 10–15% incidence of cross reactivity with the HIT antibodies in vitro, but in vivo cross reactivity is rare (117). Warfarin may be given as overlapping therapy in the setting of HIT as long as initiation of the warfarin therapy is delayed until platelet counts of 100,000/mm^3 have been documented, low initial doses of Coumadin are used, at least 5 days of overlapping therapy are provided, and the alternative anticoagulant is maintained until the platelet count has normalized (113).

Platelet count monitoring to identify patients who develop the characteristic fall in platelet count prior to developing heparin-induced thrombosis should begin 5–10 days after initiating heparin (108), or sooner if the patient has received heparin within the previous 100 days since preformed circulating HAAPAs from prior heparin exposure may cause rapid-onset HIT with heparin reexposure (108).

It has recently been recognized that the presence of HAAPAs is transient and often does not recur upon subsequent reexposure to heparin. This suggests the possibility that patients with a history of HIT can be considered for a brief reexposure to heparin under exceptional circumstances if HIT antibodies are no longer detectable using sensitive assays (113).

3. Cancer

Although the presence of malignancy-related hypercoagulability is more commonly associated with the presence of venous thromboembolic disease, the presence or arterial thrombosis has also been associated with advanced malignancy (118). Many procoagulant factors such as tissue factor and cancer procoagulant are secreted by or are expressed at the cell surface of many tumors (119). Platelet turnover and activity are also increased (119). Inflammatory cytokines can be released by tumor cells (55). If a hypercoagulable state is suspected as the cause of acute arterial thrombosis, an evaluation for occult malignancy is indicated (118).

4. Other Acquired Hypercoagulable States

The presence of slow blood flow associated with the increased viscosity of unusually high hematocrit values seen in polycythemia vera can result in thrombotic events (120).

IV. LABORATORY TESTING FOR HYPERCOAGULABLE STATES

The presence of ongoing thrombotic processes can be evaluated by measuring activation peptides, enzyme inhibitor complexes, and fibrin/fibrinogen degradation produces, which are markers of hemostatic activation (121). The presence of these prothrombotic markers has been evaluated in patients who are clinically recognized to be at risk for developing thrombotic events, e.g., individuals with a history of myocardial infarction and individuals with advanced malignancies and elevated levels of F1+2, thrombin-antithrombin complexes, and fibrinopeptide A (121). There are, however, specific laboratory tests to define each of the discrete hypercoagulable states that have been recognized.

In theory, the laboratory evaluation of patients with a hypercoagulable state might be tailored to the clinical situation being treated. For example, the laboratory evaluation of an individual with an arterial thromboembolic event with a family history of such events might be limited to congenitally acquired disorders. In practice, the laboratory panel includes some tests to identify acquired pathological states. This practice is justified by the frequent finding of multiple hypercoagulable diagnoses in the same individual, the combination of which have presumably exceeded the threshold of subclinical thrombotic tendency to clinically important thrombotic event. The diagnostic panel submitted to evaluate for the presence of a possible hypercoagulable state is outlined in Table 2.

Combinations of hypercoagulable risk factors can lead to very potent hypercoagulable states manifested by recurrent thrombotic problems (122) and demonstrate the impact of combinations of gene mutations, plasma protein deficiencies, and hyperhomo-

Table 2 Laboratory and Clinical Evaluation of Patients with Arterial Thromboembolic Disease Suspected of Having a Hypercoagulable State

---

Antithrombin III activity
Protein C activity
Protein S total and free levels
Factor V Leiden genetic assay
Activated protein C insensitivity assay
Prothrombin 20210 mutation genetic assay
Homocysteine level
Antiphospholipid antibodies
Plasminogen level
Lipoprotein(a) level

When clinically appropriate:
  Evaluation for occult malignancy
  Heparin-induced antiplatelet antibody assay

---

cysteinemia on thrombotic complications leading to recurrent pregnancy loss (123) and fatal thrombotic consequences (124).

V. CONCLUSIONS

In spite of considerable knowledge regarding hypercoagulable states, only 40–60% of patients with a clinically suggestive thrombotic event will have a diagnosis of a hypercoagulable state made by currently available laboratory testing (44,125). Further work is needed to examine the mechanisms leading to hypercoagulable states, the potential prognostic and treatment implications, and the possible value of quantifying indices of hypercoagulability in clinical practice.

Because an increased number of hypercoagulable states have a relatively high incidence, such as factor V Leiden and prothrombin 20210, it becomes more likely that patients may experience more than one risk factor for the development of pathological thrombotic events. The interaction of these states is a subject for ongoing research.

REFERENCES

1. Perler BA. Review of hypercoagulability syndromes: what the interventionalist needs to know. J Vasc Interv Radiol 1991; 183–193.
2. Levy PJ, Gonzalez FM, Rush DS, Haynes JL. Hypercoagulable states as an evolving risk for spontaneous venous and arterial thrombosis. J Am Coll Surg 1994; 266–270.
3. Jones MP, Alving B. Laboratory testing for hypercoagulable disorders. Curr Opin Hematol 1996; 365–371.
4. Crombleholme TM, Harris BH, Rosenfield CG. Intestinal necrosis from congenital hypercoagulopathy. J Pediatr Surg 1994; 235–236.
5. Chalmers EA. Heritable thrombophilia and childhood thrombosis. Blood Rev 2001; 181–189.
6. Eldrup-Jorgensen J, Flanigan DP, Brace L, Sawchuk AP, Mulder SG, Anderson CP, Schuler JJ, Meyer JR, Durham JR, Schwarcz TH. Hypercoagulable states and lower limb ischemia in young adults. J Vasc Surg 1989; 334–341.
7. Gable DR, Bergamini TM, Livingston CK, Richardson JD. Surgical implications of hypercoagulable syndromes. Am Surg 1997; 163–169.
8. Brigden ML. The hypercoagulable state. Who, how, and when to test and treat. Postgrad Med 1997; 249–6, 259.
9. Chan YC, Valenti D, Mansfield AO, Stansby G. Warfarin induced skin necrosis. Br J Surg 2000; 266–272.
10. Kutteh WH, Park VM, Deitcher SR. Hypercoagulable state mutation analysis in white patients with early first-trimester recurrent pregnancy loss. Fertil Steril 1999; 1048–1053.
11. Bick RL, Arun B, Frenkel EP. Antiphospholipid-thrombosis syndromes. Haemostasis 1999; 100–110.
12. Yamada H, Kato EH, Kobashi G, Ebina Y, Shimada S, Morikawa M, Yamada T, Sakuragi N, Fujimoto S. Recurrent pregnancy loss: etiology of thrombophilia. Semin Thromb Hemost 2001; 121–129.
13. El Hazmi MA. Hematological risk factors for coronary heart disease. Med Princ Pract 2002; 56–62.
14. Scanu AM. The role of lipoprotein(a) in the pathogenesis of atherosclerotic cardiovascular disease and its utility as predictor of coronary heart disease events. Curr Cardiol Rep 2001; 385–390.
15. Stein JH, Rosenson RS. Lipoprotein Lp(a) excess and coronary heart disease. Arch Intern Med 1997; 1170–1176.

16. Scanu AM. Lipoprotein(a). Link between structure and pathology. Ann Epidemiol 1992; 407–412.

17. Sandholzer C, Boerwinkle E, Saha N, Tong MC, Utermann G. Apolipoprotein(a) phenotypes, Lp(a) concentration and plasma lipid levels in relation to coronary heart disease in a Chinese population: evidence for the role of the apo(a) gene in coronary heart disease. J Clin Invest 1992; 1040–1046.

18. Vinazzer H. Hereditary and acquired antithrombin deficiency. Semin Thromb Hemost 1999; 257–263.

19. Bauer KA, Rosenberg RD. The pathophysiology of the prethrombotic state in humans: insights gained from studies using markers of hemostatic system activation. Blood 1987; 343–350.

20. Egeberg O. Inherited antithrombin deficiency causing thrombophilia. Thromb Diath Haemorrh 1965; 516–530.

21. Cosgriff TM, Bishop DT, Hershgold EJ, Skolnick MH, Martin BA, Baty BJ, Carlson KS. Familial antithrombin III deficiency: its natural history, genetics, diagnosis and treatment. Medicine (Baltimore) 1983; 209–220.

22. Marciniak E, Farley CH, DeSimone PA. Familial thrombosis due to antithrombin 3 deficiency. Blood 1974; 219–231.

23. Tait RC, Walker ID, Perry DJ, Islam SI, Daly ME, McCall F, Conkie JA, Carrell RW. Prevalence of antithrombin deficiency in the healthy population. Br J Haematol 1994; 106–112.

24. Lane DA, Mannucci PM, Bauer KA, Bertina RM, Bochkov NP, Boulyjenkov V, Chandy M, Dahlback B, Ginter EK, Miletich JP, Rosendaal FR, Seligsohn U. Inherited thrombophilia: Part 1. Thromb Haemost 1996; 651–662.

25. Rodgers GM, Chandler WL. Laboratory and clinical aspects of inherited thrombotic disorders. Am J Hematol 1992; 113–122.

26. Hirsh J, Piovella F, Pini M. Congenital antithrombin III deficiency. Incidence and clinical features. Am J Med 1989; 34S-38S.

27. Boyer C, Wolf M, Vedrenne J, Meyer D, Larrieu MJ. Homozygous variant of antithrombin III: AT III Fontainebleau. Thromb Haemost 1986; 18–22.

28. Hirsh J, Anand SS, Halperin JL, Fuster V. AHA Scientific Statement: Guide to anticoagulant therapy: heparin: a statement for healthcare professionals from the American Heart Association. Arterioscler Thromb Vasc Biol 2001; E9.

29. Kearon C, Crowther M, Hirsh J. Management of patients with hereditary hypercoagulable disorders. Annu Rev Med 2000; 169–185.

30. Damus PS, Wallace GA. Immunologic measurement of antithrombin III-heparin cofactor and alpha2 macroglobulin in disseminated intravascular coagulation and hepatic failure coagulopathy. Thromb Res 1975; 27–38.

31. Kauffmann RH, Veltkamp JJ, Van Tilburg NH, Van Es LA. Acquired antithrombin III deficiency and thrombosis in the nephrotic syndrome. Am J Med 1978; 607–613.

32. Friedman KD, Borok Z, Owen J. Heparin cofactor activity and antithrombin III antigen levels in preeclampsia. Thromb Res 1986; 409–416.

33. Ball AP, McKee PA. Fibrin formation and dissolution in women receiving oral contraceptive drugs. J Lab Clin Med 1977; 751–762.

34. Esmon CT. The roles of protein C and thrombomodulin in the regulation of blood coagulation. J Biol Chem 1989; 4743–4746.

35. Esmon CT. The regulation of natural anticoagulant pathways. Science 1987; 1348–1352.

36. Bauer KA, Broekmans AW, Bertina RM, Conard J, Horellou MH, Samama MM, Rosenberg RD. Hemostatic enzyme generation in the blood of patients with hereditary protein C deficiency. Blood 1988; 1418–1426.

37. Bovill EG, Bauer KA, Dickerman JD, Callas P, West B. The clinical spectrum of heterozygous protein C deficiency in a large New England kindred. Blood 1989; 712–717.

38. Camerlingo M, Finazzi G, Casto L, Laffranchi C, Barbui T, Mamoli A. Inherited protein C deficiency and nonhemorrhagic arterial stroke in young adults. Neurology 1991; 1371–1373.

39. Marlar RA, Montgomery RR, Broekmans AW. Report on the diagnosis and treatment of homozygous protein C deficiency. Report of the Working Party on Homozygous Protein C Deficiency of the ICTH Subcommittee on Protein C and Protein S. Thromb Haemost 1989; 529–531.

40. Koster T, Rosendaal FR, Briet E, van der Meer FJ, Colly LP, Trienekens PH, Poort SR, Reitsma PH, Vandenbroucke JP. Protein C deficiency in a controlled series of unselected outpatients: an infrequent but clear risk factor for venous thrombosis (Leiden Thrombophilia Study). Blood 1995; 2756–2761.

41. Miletich J, Sherman L, Broze G, Jr. Absence of thrombosis in subjects with heterozygous protein C deficiency. N Engl J Med 1987; 991–996.

42. Tait RC, Walker ID, Reitsma PH, Islam SI, McCall F, Poort SR, Conkie JA, Bertina RM. Prevalence of protein C deficiency in the healthy population. Thromb Haemost 1995; 87–93.

43. Koeleman BP, Reitsma PH, Allaart CF, Bertina RM. Activated protein C resistance as an additional risk factor for thrombosis in protein C deficient families. Blood 1994; 1031–1035.

44. Florell SR, Rodgers GM. Inherited thrombotic disorders: an update. Am J Hematol 1997; 53–60.

45. McGehee WG, Klotz TA, Epstein DJ, Rapaport SI. Coumarin necrosis associated with hereditary protein C deficiency. Ann Intern Med 1984; 59–60.

46. Gailani D, Reese EP, Jr. Anticoagulant-induced skin necrosis in a patient with hereditary deficiency of protein S. Am J Hematol 1999; 231–236.

47. Heeb MJ, Rosing J, Bakker HM, Fernandez JA, Tans G, Griffin JH. Protein S binds to and inhibits factor Xa. Proc Natl Acad Sci U S A 1994; 2728–2732.

48. Comp PC, Esmon CT. Recurrent venous thromboembolism in patients with a partial deficiency of protein S. N Engl J Med 1984; 1525–1528.

49. Schwarz HP, Fischer M, Hopmeier P, Batard MA, Griffin JH. Plasma protein S deficiency in familial thrombotic disease. Blood 1984; 1297–1300.

50. Sie P, Boneu B, Bierme R, Wiesel ML, Grunebaum L, Cazenave JP. Arterial thrombosis and protein S deficiency. Thromb Haemost 1989; 1040.

51. Zoller B, Berntsdotter A, Garcia dF, Dahlback B. Resistance to activated protein C as an additional genetic risk factor in hereditary deficiency of protein S. Blood 1995; 3518–3523.

52. Mahasandana C, Suvatte V, Chuansumrit A, Marlar RA, Manco Johnson MJ, Jacobson LJ, Hathaway WE. Homozygous protein S deficiency in an infant with purpura fulminans. J Pediatr 1990; 750–753.

53. Edson JR, Vogt JM, Huesman DA. Laboratory diagnosis of inherited protein S deficiency. Am J Clin Pathol 1990; 176–186.

54. Dahlback B, Carlsson M, Svensson PJ. Familial thrombophilia due to a previously unrecognized mechanism characterized by poor anticoagulant response to activated protein C: prediction of a cofactor to activated protein C. Proc Natl Acad Sci U S A 1993; 1004–1008.

55. DeLoughery TC. Evaluation of hypercoagulable states. J Thromb Thrombolysis 1998; 43–47.

56. Price DT, Ridker PM. Factor V Leiden mutation and the risks for thromboembolic disease: a clinical perspective. Ann Intern Med 1997; 895–903.

57. Rees DC. The population genetics of factor V Leiden (Arg506Gln). Br J Haematol 1996; 579–586.

58. De S, V, Chiusolo P, Paciaroni K, Leone G. Epidemiology of factor V Leiden: clinical implications. Semin Thromb Hemost 1998; 367–379.

59. Bertina RM, Koeleman BP, Koster T, Rosendaal FR, Dirven RJ, de Ronde H, van der Velden PA, Reitsma PH. Mutation in blood coagulation factor V associated with resistance to activated protein C. Nature 1994; 64–67.

60. Yossepowitch O, Chajek-Shaul T, Rubinow A, Haviv YS, Safadi R. Resistance to activated protein C: arterial thrombosis associated with autoimmune features. Eur J Med Res 1997; 355–357.

61. Rosendaal FR, Siscovick DS, Schwartz SM, Beverly RK, Psaty BM, Longstreth WT, Jr., Raghunathan TE, Koepsell TD, Reitsma PH. Factor V Leiden (resistance to activated protein C) increases the risk of myocardial infarction in young women. Blood 1997; 2817–2821.

62. Martinelli I, Mannucci PM, De S, V, Taioli E, Rossi V, Crosti F, Paciaroni K, Leone G, Faioni EM. Different risks of thrombosis in four coagulation defects associated with inherited thrombophilia: a study of 150 families. Blood 1998; 2353–2358.

63. Simioni P, Sanson BJ, Prandoni P, Tormene D, Friederich PW, Girolami B, Gavasso S, Huisman MV, Buller HR, Wouter tC, Girolami A, Prins MH. Incidence of venous thromboembolism in families with inherited thrombophilia. Thromb Haemost 1999; 198–202.

64. Middeldorp S, Henkens CM, Koopman MM, van Pampus EC, Hamulyak K, van der MJ, Prins MH, Buller HR. The incidence of venous thromboembolism in family members of patients with factor V Leiden mutation and venous thrombosis. Ann Intern Med 1998; 15–20.

65. Lensen RP, Bertina RM, de Ronde H, Vandenbroucke JP, Rosendaal FR. Venous thrombotic risk in family members of unselected individuals with factor V Leiden. Thromb Haemost 2000; 817–821.

66. Martinelli I, Bucciarelli P, Margaglione M, De S, V, Castaman G, Mannucci PM. The risk of venous thromboembolism in family members with mutations in the genes of factor V or prothrombin or both. Br J Haematol 2000; 1223–1229.

67. Simioni P, Tormene D, Prandoni P, Zerbinati P, Gavasso S, Cefalo P, Girolami A. Incidence of venous thromboembolism in asymptomatic family members who are carriers of factor V Leiden: a prospective cohort study. Blood 2002; 1938–1942.

68. Rosendaal FR, Koster T, Vandenbroucke JP, Reitsma PH. High risk of thrombosis in patients homozygous for factor V Leiden (activated protein C resistance). Blood 1995; 1504–1508.

69. Poort SR, Rosendaal FR, Reitsma PH, Bertina RM. A common genetic variation in the 3'-untranslated region of the prothrombin gene is associated with elevated plasma prothrombin levels and an increase in venous thrombosis. Blood 1996; 3698–3703.

70. Zivelin A, Rosenberg N, Faier S, Kornbrot N, Peretz H, Mannhalter C, Horellou MH, Seligsohn U. A single genetic origin for the common prothrombotic G20210A polymorphism in the prothrombin gene. Blood 1998; 1119–1124.

71. Rosendaal FR, Doggen CJ, Zivelin A, Arruda VR, Aiach M, Siscovick DS, Hillarp A, Watzke HH, Bernardi F, Cumming AM, Preston FE, Reitsma PH. Geographic distribution of the 20210 G to A prothrombin variant. Thromb Haemost 1998; 706–708.

72. De S, V, Rossi E, Paciaroni K, Leone G. Screening for inherited thrombophilia: indications and therapeutic implications. Haematologica 2002; 1095–1108.

73. Welch GN, Loscalzo J. Homocysteine and atherothrombosis. N Engl J Med 1998; 1042–1050.

74. Stern JM, Saver JL, Boldy RM, DeGregorio F. Homocysteine associated hypercoagulability and disseminated thrombosis—a case report. Angiology 1998; 765–769.

75. Barger AP, Hurley R. Evaluation of the hypercoagulable state. Whom to screen, how to test and treat. Postgrad Med 2000; 59–66.

76. Gaussem P, Siguret V, Aiach M. [Evaluation of hemostasis in venous thromboembolism pathology]. Ann Biol Clin (Paris) 1998; 49–56.

77. Mackinnon LT, Hubinger L, Lepre F. Effects of physical activity and diet on lipoprotein(a). Med Sci Sports Exerc 1997; 1429–1436.

78. Angles-Cano E, de la Pena DA, Loyau S. Inhibition of fibrinolysis by lipoprotein(a). Ann NY Acad Sci 2001; 261–275.

79. Morrisett JD. The role of lipoprotein[a] in atherosclerosis. Curr Atheroscler Rep 2000; 243–250.

80. Lippi G, Veraldi GF, Dorucci V, Dusi R, Ruzzenente O, Brentegani C, Guidi G, Cordiano C. Usefulness of lipids, lipoprotein(a) and fibrinogen measurements in identifying subjects at risk of occlusive complications following vascular and endovascular surgery. Scand J Clin Lab Invest 1998; 497–504.

81. Lippi G, Bassi A, Brocco G, Manzato F, Marini M, Guidi G. Lipoprotein(a) concentration is not associated with venous thromboembolism in a case control study. Haematologica 1999; 726–729.

82. von Depka M, Nowak-Gottl U, Eisert R, Dieterich C, Barthels M, Scharrer I, Ganser A, Ehrenforth S. Increased lipoprotein (a) levels as an independent risk factor for venous thromboembolism. Blood 2000; 3364–3368.

83. Marcovina SM, Koschinsky ML. Lipoprotein(a) as a risk factor for coronary artery disease. Am J Cardiol 1998; 57U-66U.

84. Pena-Diaz A, Izaguirre-Avila R, Angles-Cano E. Lipoprotein Lp(a) and atherothrombotic disease. Arch Med Res 2000; 353–359.

85. Edelberg JM, Pizzo SV. Lipoprotein (a) in the regulation of fibrinolysis. J Atheroscler Thromb 1995; S5–S7.

86. Marcovina SM, Hegele RA, Koschinsky ML. Lipoprotein(a) and coronary heart disease risk. Curr Cardiol Rep 1999; 105–111.

87. Nakajima K, Hata Y. Intraindividual variations in lipoprotein (a) levels and factors related to these changes. J Atheroscler Thromb 1996; 96–106.

88. Mackinnon LT, Hubinger LM. Effects of exercise on lipoprotein(a). Sports Med 1999; 11–24.

89. Byrne DJ, Jagroop IA, Montgomery HE, Thomas M, Mikhailidis DP, Milton NG, Winder AF. Lipoprotein (a) does not participate in the early acute phase response to training or extreme physical activity and is unlikely to enhance any associated immediate cardiovascular risk. J Clin Pathol 2002; 280–285.

90. Durstine JL, Davis PG, Ferguson MA, Alderson NL, Trost SG. Effects of short-duration and long-duration exercise on lipoprotein(a). Med Sci Sports Exerc 2001; 1511–1516.

91. Imamura H, Katagiri S, Uchid K, Miyamoto N, Nakano H, Shirota T. Acute effects of moderate exercise on serum lipids, lipoproteins and apolipoproteins in sedentary young women. Clin Exp Pharmacol Physiol 2000; 975–979.

92. Hubinger L, Mackinnon LT, Barber L, McCosker J, Howard A, Lepre F. Acute effects of treadmill running on lipoprotein(a) levels in males and females. Med Sci Sports Exerc 1997; 436–442.

93. Gruden G, Olivetti C, Taliano C, Furlani D, Gambino R, Pagano G, Cavallo-Perin P. Lipoprotein(a) after acute exercise in healthy subjects. Int J Clin Lab Res 1996; 140–141.

94. Milionis HJ, Winder AF, Mikhailidis DP. Lipoprotein (a) and stroke. J Clin Pathol 2000; 487–496.

95. Schmidt EB, Klausen IC, Kristensen SD, Lervang HH, Faergeman O, Dyerberg J. The effect of n-3 polyunsaturated fatty acids on Lp(a). Clin Chim Acta 1991; 271–277.

96. Rao AK, Sheth S, Kaplan R. Inherited hypercoagulable states. Vasc Med 1997; 313–320.

97. Bick RL. Antiphospholipid thrombosis syndromes. Hematol Oncol Clin North Am 2003; 115–147.

98. Van Cott EM, Laposata M. Laboratory evaluation of hypercoagulable states. Hematol Oncol Clin North Am 1998; 1141–66, v.

99. Bick RL, Baker WF. Antiphospholipid syndrome and thrombosis. Semin Thromb Hemost 1999; 333–350.

100. Khamashta MA, Cuadrado MJ, Mujic F, Taub NA, Hunt BJ, Hughes GR. The management of thrombosis in the antiphospholipid-antibody syndrome. N Engl J Med 1995; 993–997.

101. Deitcher SR, Carman TL. Heparin-induced thrombocytopenia: natural history, diagnosis, and management. Vasc Med 2001; 113–119.

102. Kelton JG. Heparin-induced thrombocytopenia: an overview. Blood Rev 2002; 77–80.

103. Fabris F, Luzzatto G, Stefani PM, Girolami B, Cella G, Girolami A. Heparin-induced thrombocytopenia. Haematologica 2000; 72–81.

104. Calaitges JG, Liem TK, Spadone D, Nichols WK, Silver D. The role of heparin-associated antiplatelet antibodies in the outcome of arterial reconstruction. J Vasc Surg 1999; 779–785.

105. Lindhoff-Last E, Eichler P, Stein M, Plagemann J, Gerdsen F, Wagner R, Ehrly AM, Bauersachs R. A prospective study on the incidence and clinical relevance of heparin-induced antibodies in patients after vascular surgery. Thromb Res 2000; 387–393.

106. Fabris F, Luzzatto G, Soini B, Ramon R, Scandellari R, Randi ML, Girolami A. Risk factors for thrombosis in patients with immune mediated heparin induced thrombocytopenia. J Intern Med 2002; 149–154.

107. Warkentin TE, Kelton JG. Delayed-onset heparin-induced thrombocytopenia and thrombosis. Ann Intern Med 2001; 502–506.

108. Warkentin TE. Platelet count monitoring and laboratory testing for heparin-induced thrombocytopenia. Arch Pathol Lab Med 2002; 1415–1423.
109. Walenga JM, Jeske WP, Fasanella AR, Wood JJ, Bakhos M. Laboratory tests for the diagnosis of heparin-induced thrombocytopenia. Semin Thromb Hemost 1999; 43–49.
110. Greinacher A, Michels I, Kiefel V, Mueller-Eckhardt C. A rapid and sensitive test for diagnosing heparin-associated thrombocytopenia. Thromb Haemost 1991; 734–736.
111. Keeling DM, Richards EM, Baglin TP. Platelet aggregation in response to four low molecular weight heparins and the heparinoid ORG 10172 in patients with heparin-induced thrombocytopenia. Br J Haematol 1994; 425–426.
112. Kikta MJ, Keller MP, Humphrey PW, Silver D. Can low molecular weight heparins and heparinoids be safely given to patients with heparin-induced thrombocytopenia syndrome? Surgery 1993; 705–710.
113. Warkentin TE. Current agents for the treatment of patients with heparin-induced thrombocytopenia. Curr Opin Pulm Med 2002; 405–412.
114. Farner B, Eichler P, Kroll H, Greinacher A. A comparison of danaparoid and lepirudin in heparin-induced thrombocytopenia. Thromb Haemost 2001; 950–957.
115. Lubenow N, Greinacher A. Hirudin in heparin-induced thrombocytopenia. Semin Thromb Hemost 2002; 431–438.
116. Mudaliar JH, Liem TK, Nichols WK, Spadone DP, Silver D. Lepirudin is a safe and effective anticoagulant for patients with heparin-associated antiplatelet antibodies. J Vasc Surg 2001; 17–20.
117. Keng TB, Chong BH. Heparin-induced thrombocytopenia and thrombosis syndrome: in vivo cross-reactivity with danaparoid and successful treatment with r-Hirudin. Br J Haematol 2001; 394–396.
118. Rigdon EE. Trousseau's syndrome and acute arterial thrombosis. Cardiovasc Surg 2000; 214–218.
119. Lip GY, Chin BS, Blann AD. Cancer and the prothrombotic state. Lancet Oncol 2002; 27–34.
120. Girolami A, Simioni P, Scarano L, Girolami B. Venous and arterial thrombophilia. Haematologica 1997; 96–100.
121. Lopez Y, Paloma MJ, Rifon J, Cuesta B, Paramo JA. Measurement of prethrombotic markers in the assessment of acquired hypercoagulable states. Thromb Res 1999; 71–78.
122. Higginbotham EA, Zimmerman SA, Howard TA, Schanberg L, Kredich D, Ware RE. Effects of inherited thrombophilic mutations in an adolescent with antiphospholipid syndrome and systemic lupus erythematosus. J Rheumatol 2001; 370–372.
123. Raziel A, Kornberg Y, Friedler S, Schachter M, Sela BA, Ron-El R. Hypercoagulable thrombophilic defects and hyperhomocysteinemia in patients with recurrent pregnancy loss. Am J Reprod Immunol 2001; 65–71.
124. Misgav M, Goldberg Y, Zeltser D, Eldor A, Berliner AS. Fatal pulmonary artery thrombosis in a patient with Behcet's disease, activated protein C resistance and hyperhomocysetinemia. Blood Coagul Fibrinolysis 2000; 421–423.
125. Francis JL. Laboratory investigation of hypercoagulability. Semin Thromb Hemost 1998; 111–126.

12-1

Incidence and Management of Complications of Fibrinolytic, Antiplatelet, and Anticoagulant Therapy

Abdallah G. Rebeiz and Christopher B. Granger
Duke Clinical Research Institute, Durham, North Carolina, U.S.A.

Maarten L. Simoons
University Hospital Rotterdam, Rotterdam, The Netherlands

I. INTRODUCTION

The treatment of acute coronary syndromes (ACS) and percutaneous coronary intervention (PCI) encompasses a wide spectrum of pharmacological strategies ranging from clot lysis in ST segment elevation myocardial infarctions to inhibitors of the coagulation cascade and of platelet aggregation in non–ST segment elevation ACS and PCI. Several combinations of these therapies have been studied in large-scale clinical trials with variable degrees of success in improving clinical outcomes, but occasionally showing unacceptably increased rates of hemorrhage, particularly intracranial hemorrhage (1–3). The risk of major hemorrhage may influence the choice of specific fibrinolytic, antithrombotic, and antiplatelet regimens in specific patient subgroups. For each individual patient, the likelihood of intracranial hemorrhage (4,5) and overall mortality (6) can now be predicted, helping in clinical decision making (7). With the ever-growing armamentarium of potent therapies targeted against thrombosis and platelet activation, risk-benefit assessment becomes pivotal in clinical thrombocardiology.

II. HEMORRHAGE

The major complication of fibrinolytic, antithrombotic, and antiplatelet therapies is, not surprisingly, hemorrhage. Many patients with ST segment elevation ACS are treated with fibrinolytic therapy, aspirin, heparin, and early cardiac catheterization with the use of platelet glycoprotein (GP) IIb/IIIa inhibitors and a thienopyridine in the event of percutaneous intervention with stent placement, leading to a substantial risk of hemorrhagic complications. In recent years, emerging data have supported the use of an early invasive strategy in managing patients with non–ST segment elevation acute coronary syndromes (8,9), setting a trend for earlier coronary catheterization, and hence revascularization when indicated, in this patient population, but also increasing the risk of peri-procedural bleeding. The underlying mechanism for fibrinolytic-related hemorrhage is multifactorial, involving mostly fibrin dissolution, but also a systemic hypocoagulable state induced by degradation of factors V, VIII, and circulating fibrinogen, especially with streptokinase use (10). In addition, fibrin degradation products interfere with fibrin polymerization and platelet function.

It was hoped that the rates of hemorrhagic complications would be reduced with the use of fibrin-specific agents such as alteplase, which have greater activity in plasminogen conversion to plasmin at the fibrin clot surface and cause a greater decrease in circulating fibrinogen. Although there is a relationship between lower risk of systemic bleeding with greater degree of fibrin specificity, intracranial hemorrhage is not lower with fibrin-specific agents. Regimens combining thrombolysis and platelet GP IIb/IIIa inhibition in acute myocardial infarction have also shown some alarming trends in the risk of major bleeding, especially in the elderly. The main mechanism for hemorrhage, especially intracranial hemorrhage, appears to involve the local lysis of fibrin in the hemostatic plug rather than a systemic hypocoagulable state induced by fibrinolytic therapy. This is supported by the fact that alteplase confers a higher risk of intracranial hemorrhage and only a slightly lower risk of noncerebral hemorrhage than does streptokinase (5,11).

A. Intracranial Hemorrhage

The most catastrophic complication of fibrinolytic therapy is intracranial hemorrhage, occurring in 0.3–1.0% of patients (5,12–15). In the Fibrinolytic Therapy Trialists (FTT) Collaboration overview (12), probable cerebral hemorrhage occurred in 0.4% of patients treated with fibrinolytic therapy vs. 0.01% in placebo-treated patients. There is considerable variability in the rate of intracranial hemorrhage from each of the major placebo-controlled fibrinolytic trials (Table 1), due in part to inconsistencies in reporting and in documentation of the type of stroke (16–22). In trials where computed tomography (CT) and magnetic resonance imaging (MRI) were systematically obtained for suspected strokes, intracranial hemorrhage rates ranged from 0.4 to 0.9% (Table 2) (5,11,15,23,24). In a registry conducted in the Netherlands in 1988–1989, the rate was even higher at 1% (25). It should be noted that the risk of embolic stroke is reduced with fibrinolytic therapy, therefore balancing the increased rate of intracerebral bleeding and leading to only a slight increase in the overall stroke rate (3.9 per 1000 patients) (12).

Table 1 Intracranial Hemorrhage in Randomized, Controlled Thrombolytic Trials of Over 1000 Patients

Trial (Ref.)	Agent	Intracranial hemorrhage rate % (n/n)	
		Thrombolytic	Control
GISSI-1 (16)	Streptokinase	0.14% (8/5860)	0% (0/5852)
ISIS-2 (17)	Streptokinase	0.08% (7/8592)	0% (0/8595)
ISAM (18)	Streptokinase	0.47% (4/859)	0% (0/882)
EMERAS (19)	Streptokinase	0.81% (18/2234)	0.18% (4/2259)
ASSET (20)	Alteplase	0.28% (7/2512)	0.08% (2/2493)
LATE (21)	Alteplase	0.85% (24/2836)	0.21% (6/2875)
AIMS (22)	Anistreplase	0.32% (2/624)	0.12% (1/634)
Pooled		0.30% (70/23,517)	0.06% (13/23,590)
95% Confidence Interval		0.23–0.37%	0.03–0.09%

[a] Probable intracranial hemorrhage.

Table 2 Intracranial Hemorrhage Rates in Comparative Thrombolytic Trials

Trial (Ref.)	n	Rate (n)	n	Rate (n)	Difference
		Streptokinase		*Alteplase*[a]	*Alteplase vs. Streptokinase*
GISSI-2/International Study (14)	10,396	0.29% (30)	10,372	0.42% (44)	+0.23%
ISIS-3 (23)	12,848	0.30% (39)	12,841	0.72% (92)	+0.42%
GUSTO-I (5)	20,213	0.51% (104)	10,376	0.70% (73)	+0.19%
		Streptokinase		*Reteplase*	*Reteplase vs. Streptokinase*
INJECT (24)	3006	0.37% (11)	3004	0.77% (23)	+0.40%
		Alteplase		*Reteplase*	*Reteplase vs. Alteplase*
GUSTO-III (25)	4921	0.87%	10,138	0.91%	+0.04%

[a] Alteplase 100 mg over 3 h in GISSI-2; duteplase 0.6 MU/kg over 4 h in ISIS-3; alteplase 100 mg over 90 minutes in GUSTO-I.

The underlying mechanism of intracranial hemorrhage after fibrinolytic therapy is not fully understood. Fibrin-specific fibrinolytic agents are associated with a higher rate of intracranial hemorrhage, suggesting that the main mechanism is the dissolution of hemostatic plugs in the cerebral circulation. Underlying abnormalities of the cerebral vasculature seem to be associated with a higher risk for intracranial hemorrhage, such as amyloid angiopathy (26), which places the patient at risk for cerebral bleeding both with (27,28) and without (29,30) thrombolysis. Lacunar infarcts are common findings in areas distinct from the hemorrhage among patients with intracranial hemorrhage (31). Minor head trauma with little disruption of the cerebral vasculature also appears to increase the risk of hemorrhage (32).

The majority (75%) of intracranial hemorrhagic events occur within 24 hours of thrombolysis, with the median time of onset at 10–15 hours following administration (5,13). The most common initial symptom is impaired level of consciousness (26), which is particularly problematic given that many patients with acute myocardial infarction are treated with concomitant narcotics and sedatives, leading to potentially fatal delays in diagnosis and management. The most common anatomical sites of hemorrhage are the major cerebral lobes in 70–80% of cases (26,31), the cerebellum being the second most common. Half the patients with intracranial hemorrhage have intraventricular blood, while 15–20% have subdural blood (isolated or in addition to intracerebral blood) (31). Roughly a third of patients have multifocal hemorrhagic sites, suggesting a diffuse underlying process predisposing to bleeding.

Intracranial hemorrhage is associated with a 30-day mortality of 50–70% (5,15,25,33). Among the survivors, 63% are left with moderate to severe disability, and 33% have mild or no disability. Of all the patients with intracranial hemorrhage, only 13% survive with no significant disability.

B. Nonintracranial Hemorrhage

Due to varying definitions, data collection methods, use of invasive strategies, and threshold for transfusions, it is difficult to interpret and compare overall rates of hemorrhage across trials of fibrinolytic, antithrombotic, and antiplatelet therapies. Major hemorrhage is generally defined as bleeding that is life threatening or requires transfusion (12). In randomized controlled trials, fibrinolytic therapy was associated with a two- to threefold increase in the rate of major hemorrhage, from 0.4% to 1.1%. However, the use of heparin and aspirin was not routine in most of the early placebo-controlled trials of thrombolysis. In the early TIMI (34) and TAMI (35) trials, however, protocols dictated full-dose intravenous heparin and early cardiac catheterization, leading to blood transfusions in 20–30% of enrolled patients. Most bleeding events in these trials were related to percutaneous or surgical revascularization procedures, and bleeding was associated with higher fibrin-degradation products (34) and lower fibrinogen levels (35). In the TIMI II trial, early angiography in the first 24 hours led to an incidence of major bleeding (hemoglobin drop of 5 g/dL or more) of 18.5%, compared to 12.8% in patients treated with a conservative approach ($p < 0.001$) (36). Bleeding was associated with the degree of fibrinogen degradation, prolonged activated partial thromboplastin time (aPTT), and peak alteplase level. Among the non–bypass-related bleeding causes, the most common was a decrease in hemoglobin with no obvious source (1.5%), followed by catheterization access site (1.2%), gastrointestinal (0.7%), needle puncture sites (0.5%), and genitourinary (0.2%).

In GUSTO I, severe bleeding (resulting in hemodynamic instability) occurred in 1.1% of patients, and moderate bleeding (requiring transfusion) in 11.4% (37). Most common bleeding sources were bypass surgery related (3.6%), catheterization access sites (2.0%), and gastrointestinal (1.0%).

C. Hemorrhage Rates with Specific Fibrinolytic Agents

1. Intracranial Hemorrhage

Despite its fibrin specificity, alteplase was not shown to have an improved safety profile as was initially hoped, with a consistently greater (0.2–0.4% higher) risk of intracranial hemorrhage than streptokinase, probably related to a greater potency (Table 2) (38). Anistreplase (11) and reteplase (23) appear to be associated with intracranial hemorrhage rates close to the alteplase range (Table 2).

The risk of intracranial bleeding is influenced by the dose and speed of fibrinolytic administration. In the TIMI II trial, a 150 mg dose of alteplase was associated with an alarmingly high rate of intracranial hemorrhage in the 1.5% range, leading to premature discontinuation of the dose (1,39). Dose reduction to 100 mg led to a decrease in the hemorrhage rate to 0.4% (13). Among patients randomized to a lower dose of alteplase (0.8 mg/kg, not to exceed 80 mg), the intracranial bleeding rate was 0.55% (40), slightly lower than the average rate seen with the 100 mg dose across multiple trials. In the COBALT trial, there was a nonsignificantly higher risk of intracranial hemorrhage with two 50 mg boluses of alteplase than with an accelerated alteplase regimen (41). Tenecteplase, a genetically engineered variant of alteplase, was associated with intracranial hemorrhages in 3 of 78 patients enrolled in TIMI-10B when given as a 50 mg bolus (the highest dose), a dose that was discontinued early (42). In more recent trials, tenecteplase given in a weight-adjusted fashion was associated with an overall intracranial hemorrhage rate in the 0.9% range (43,45).

2. Noncerebral Hemorrhage

Fibrin-specific fibrinolytic agents such as alteplase, reteplase, and tenecteplase confer a consistently reduced risk of nonintracranial bleeding when compared to streptokinase, in contrast to the higher rates of cerebral hemorrhage seen with these drugs versus streptokinase (Table 3) (11,23,24,37,44). There was a 15–20% relative reduction in major hemorrhage with both alteplase and reteplase compared with streptokinase and a 25% relative reduction with tenecteplase (the most fibrin-specific) compared with alteplase (45).

Table 3 Hemorrhage Rates (Other than Intracranial) in Comparative Thrombolytic Trials

Trial (Ref.)	n	Major[a] hemorrhage (n)	n	Major[a] hemorrhage (n)	Difference
		Streptokinase		*Alteplase*[b]	*Alteplase vs. Streptokinase*
GISSI-2 (43)	10,386	0.9% (96)	10,372	0.6% (64)	–0.3%
ISIS-3 (23)	13,607	0.9% (118)	13,569	0.8% (109)	–0.1%
GUSTO-I (37)	20,196	12.9% (2611)	10,366	11.1% (1155)	–1.8%
		Streptokinase		*Reteplase*	*Reteplase vs. Streptokinase*
INJECT (24)	3006	1.0%	3004	0.7%	–0.3%
		Alteplase		*Reteplase*	*Reteplase vs. Alteplase*
GUSTO-III (25)	4921	6.8%	10,138	6.9%	+0.2%

[a] Major hemorrhage is defined as receiving or requiring transfusion.
[b] Alteplase 100 mg over 3 h in GISSI-2; duteplase 0.6 MU/kg over 4 h in ISIS-3; alteplase 100 mg over 90 minutes in GUSTO-I.

D. Hemorrhage with Antithrombotic Therapy

1. Intracranial Hemorrhage

Acute coronary syndrome patients treated with heparin and aspirin without fibrinolytic therapy have a small risk of intracranial hemorrhage. In the FTT overview there was a 0.05% rate of probable or definite intracranial hemorrhage (12). In the GUSTO IIb trial there were no reported intracranial bleeding events (95% CI < 0.07%) among 4343 patients with non–ST segment elevation ACS treated with aspirin and full-dose heparin (without thrombolysis) (46). In the ESSENCE trial of enoxaparin vs. unfractionated heparin in unstable angina, none of the patients in the enoxaparin arm ($n = 1607$) and one patient in the unfractionated heparin arm ($n = 1564$) experienced intracranial hemorrhage (47). In the TIMI-11B trial, 2 of 1936 patients treated with unfractionated heparin and 1 of 1938 patients randomized to enoxaparin experienced intracranial bleeding (48). The risk of intracranial hemorrhage in patients treated with full-dose aspirin and heparin appears to be on the order of one in 2000.

Hirudin, a more potent antithrombotic agent, was associated with a 0.1% (95% CI 0.01–0.2%) rate of intracranial hemorrhage even without concomitant fibrinolytic therapy (46).

The addition of antithrombotic therapy to fibrinolytic agents confers an added risk of intracranial hemorrhage (49), in contrast to conventional dose aspirin, which does not affect the cerebral bleeding rate when given in addition to fibrinolytic therapy (17). In ISIS-3, heparin given subcutaneously at 12,500 U twice a day was associated with a 0.15% absolute increase in definite intracranial hemorrhage ($p < 0.05$) (11). In the GUSTO I trial, full-dose intravenous heparin was associated with a 0.11% absolute increase in intracranial hemorrhage ($p =$ NS) compared to subcutaneous heparin (5). The ASSENT-3 trial randomized patients presenting with ST segment elevation myocardial infarction to either full-dose tenecteplase and intravenous unfractionated heparin administered as a 60 U/kg bolus then a 12 U/kg/h infusion, or tenecteplase and enoxaparin given as a 30 mg/kg intravenous bolus followed by 1 mg/kg given subcutaneously every 12 hours (the third treatment arm in the trial was a combination of abciximab with half-dose tenecteplase). There were no significant differences in the rates of intracranial hemorrhage among treatment arms, with a 0.93% incidence in the unfractionated heparin arm, compared to 0.88% in the enoxaparin arm (43).

The risk of intracranial hemorrhage after fibrinolytic therapy is greatly affected by the dose of concomitant heparin therapy as well as the APTT achieved (Fig. 1) (50). In the GUSTO IIa and TIMI-9a trials, higher doses of heparin (initial infusion rates of 1000–1300 U/h) were administered following thrombolysis with a target APTT of 60–90 seconds, resulting in a 10-second increase in the median APTT in the hours following fibrinolytic therapy and a doubling in the rate of intracranial hemorrhage to 1.5% (2,3). In GUSTO IIb and TIMI-9b, the initial heparin infusion rate was reduced to 1000 U/h, resulting in a 15- to 20-second reduction in the median APTT and a decrease in the rate of intracranial hemorrhage to 0.7% (51).

The elderly, who are at especially high risk of intracranial hemorrhage, had a lower than expected rate of intracranial hemorrhage with the fully weight-adjusted dosing of unfractionated heparin with tenecteplase in the ASSENT-3 trial. With a bolus of 60 units/kg (maximum 4000) and initial infusion of 12 units/kg/h (maximum 1000 units/h), the rate of intracranial hemorrhage was only 0.74% among patients over the age of 75 (45). Using the same dosing regimen of tenecteplase and unfractionated heparin, the rate of intracranial hemorrhage among patients over age 75 was 0.75% in the ASSENT-3 Plus trial (52). Compared to the higher doses of unfractionated heparin used in ASSENT-2, the rate of noncerebral hemorrhage in ASSENT-3 with tenecteplase was 50% lower (43,56).

The use of hirudin and other direct thrombin inhibitors with thrombolysis has been shown to carry a substantially higher risk of intracranial hemorrhage in several trials (9,10,49,50). However, a 50% reduction in the hirudin dose was associated with a significant reduction in reinfarction compared with heparin, with no increase in the risk of intracranial hemorrhage (51).

2. Nonintracranial Hemorrhage

The reported rates of nonintracranial hemorrhage with heparin therapy when given without fibrinolytics vary widely, due in part to differences in definitions, dosing regimens, and use of invasive strategies. In a meta-analysis of the TIMI-11B and ESSENCE trials, major hemorrhage while on therapy (defined as bleeding resulting in death, transfusion of ≥2 units blood, a decrease in hemoglobin of ≥3 mg/L, intracranial, intraocular, or retroperitoneal) occurred in 1.1% of patients treated with unfractionated heparin and 1.3% of those treated with enoxaparin (p = NS). During the same treatment period, the pooled rate of minor hemorrhage was 10% in the enoxaparin arm and 4.3% in the unfractionated heparin arm (p < 0.0001), a difference accounted for by injection site ecchymoses (53). In the ESSENCE cohort, the overall rate of major hemorrhage at 30 days was comparable between the two groups (6.5% for enoxaparin, 7.0% for unfracionated heparin; p = NS). Most bleeding episodes were associated with bypass surgery, with a substantially higher risk of major hemorrhage among patients who underwent coronary bypass within 12 hours of cessation of treatment (56% for enoxaparin, 46% for unfractionated heparin) (54).

The addition of heparin to fibrinolytic therapy increases the overall hemorrhage risk. In ISIS-3 (11) and GISSI-2 (44), subcutaneous heparin given twice daily at 12,500 U increased the incidence of major hemorrhage from 0.7 to 1.0% (p < 0.001). The addition of intravenous heparin therapy to thrombolysis increased the overall bleeding rate from 16 to 23% (OR = 1.55, 95% CI = 1.2–2.0) (49) and in another overview was associated with an excess of 3–13 major hemorrhages per 1000 patients treated (55). Recent trials comparing unfractionated heparin to enoxaparin with fibrinolytic therapy have shown no significant difference in the rate of major bleeding complications between the two groups. In ASSENT-3, enoxaparin was associated with a 3.0% rate of major noncerebral hemorrhage vs. 2.2% in the heparin group (p = NS). Blood transfusion rates were 3.4% for enoxaparin and 2.3% for unfractionated heparin (p = NS) (43).

A

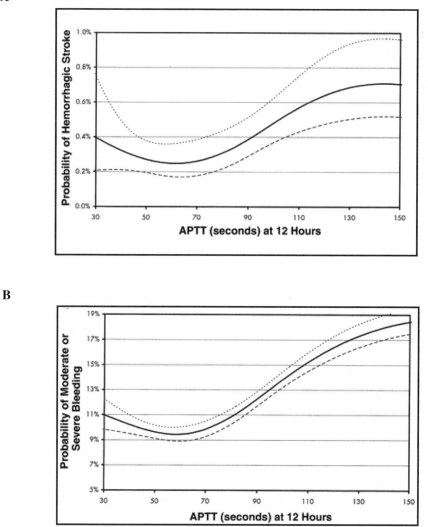

B

Figure 1   Predicted probability and 95% confidence intervals (CI) of intracranial hemorrhage (**A**) and of moderate and severe bleeding (**B**) according to activated partial thromboplastin time (aPTT) at 12 hours among patients treated with thrombolytic therapy and intravenous heparin in the GUSTO-I trial. (From Ref. 50.)

Not surprisingly, the bleeding risk conferred by heparin therapy is affected by the dose and route of administration of the drug. When given in addition to fibrinolytic therapy, higher-dose intravenous heparin increases the risk of hemorrhage over lower-dose subcutaneous heparin from 11.8% to 14.0% ($p = 0.0001$) (37). Among patients treated with intravenous heparin, there is an almost direct correlation between the aPTT and the rate of bleeding, with a 1% increase in the risk or moderate to severe hemorrhage with every 7-second increase in aPTT above 75 seconds (Fig. 1) (50). In the ASSENT-2 trial of tenecteplase vs. alteplase in patients with ST segment elevation myocardial infarction, a higher and not fully weight-adjusted dose of heparin was associated with a higher rate of major hemorrhage than the fully weight-adjusted dose used in ASSENT-3 (4.7% vs. 2.2%) (43,56). These findings support the use of a fully weight-adjusted dose of heparin as recommended in the ACC/AHA guidelines (57), with earlier monitoring of the aPTT at 3 hours following the bolus dose. As with unfractionated heparin, the dose of enoxaparin is also related to the bleeding risk. In the TIMI-11a trial of enoxaparin in non–ST segment elevation ACS, the major hemorrhage rate was 6.5% among patients receiving 1.2 mg/kg twice daily compared with 1.9% for the 1.0 mg/kg dose (58). Patients who bled had higher anti-Xa levels than those without bleeding events. The risk of bleeding with hirudin is also dose-dependent. There was a doubling of the rate of major noncerebral hemorrhage with high-dose hirudin compared to heparin (7.0% vs. 3.0%; $p = 0.02$) (3). With a reduction of the hirudin dose, however, rates of serious hemorrhage were comparable to heparin (1.2% vs. 1.1%) (46,59).

E.   Hemorrhage with Antiplatelet Therapy

1.   Intracranial Hemorrhage

The early trials of platelet GP IIb/IIIa receptor inhibitors in angioplasty showed an excess of bleeding complications secondary to the high doses of concomitant heparin therapy (60), a trend that was corrected with a more judicious use of heparin (61–63). The use of GP IIb/IIIa inhibitors in managing patients with acute coronary syndromes has been extensively investigated (64–66). In the PRISM trial, there was no difference in the rate of intracranial hemorrhage between the tirofiban and heparin arms (0.12% in both arms) (64). There were no reported intracranial bleeding events in the PRISM PLUS trial (65). In the PURSUIT trial, patients treated with heparin and eptifibatide had a comparable incidence of intracranial hemorrhage to those treated with heparin only (0.06% in both arms) (66). In GUSTO IV ACS, abciximab administered for 24 hours was associated with a nonsignificantly higher rate of intracranial hemorrhage than placebo (0.15% vs. 0.04%) (67). In a meta-analysis of all trials of GP IIb/IIIa inhibition in coronary syndromes (without thrombolysis), treatment with a GP IIb/IIIa inhibitor in addition to heparin and aspirin was associated with a 0.09% incidence of intracranial bleeding (pooled data) (68).

The use of GP IIb/IIIa inhibitors as "adjuncts" to fibrinolytic therapy in ST elevation coronary syndromes has recently been studied in large clinical trials. In GUSTO V, there were similar rates of intracranial hemorrhage with abciximab and half-dose reteplase compared with full-dose reteplase (0.6% in both arms). Treatment with abciximab plus reteplase was associated with a 2.1% incidence of intracranial bleeding among elderly patients (>75 years), however, compared to 1.1% with reteplase alone ($p = 0.69$) (69). In ASSENT-3, patients treated with tenecteplase and abciximab had a 0.94% rate of intracranial hemorrhage vs. 0.93% with heparin and 0.88% with enoxaparin ($p = 0.98$) (43).

The thienopyridine derivatives ticlopidine and clopidogrel are antiplatelet agents that are almost universally used following percutaneous interventions with stent placement. Clopidogrel use is becoming more widespread, with large trials showing improved outcome in patients with vascular disease (70). In the CURE trial of clopidogrel, given in addition to conventional therapy, in patients with unstable angina, there was a 0.1% incidence of hemorrhagic stroke in both the clopidogrel and placebo arms (71).

2.   Non-Intracranial hemorrhage

When used in the setting of percutaneous coronary intervention, GP IIb/IIIa inhibitors are associated with a higher rate of procedural bleeding than placebo. In the EPIC trial there was a 14% rate of major hemorrhage with 12 hours of abciximab vs. 7% with placebo, mostly driven by groin and retroperitoneal bleeding (60). The use of lower heparin doses and target activated clotting times has reduced the rates of severe hemorrhagic complications. The rate of major hemorrhage was 1.5% in patients treated with abciximab in the EPISTENT trial vs. 2.2% with placebo (72). In trials of GP IIb/IIIa inhibitors in unstable coronary syndromes, rates of major hemorrhage are generally increased with GP IIb/IIIa inhibition. Pooled data from the major tirofiban and eptifibatide trials shows a significantly higher incidence of major noncerebral hemorrhage with the use of GP IIb/IIIa inhibitors compared to placebo (1.6% vs. 1.0%, OR = 1.64, 95% CI = 1.30–2.07) (68). In GUSTO IV ACS, patients treated with abciximab for 24 hours had a 4.7% incidence of intracranial hemorrhage vs. 2.8% for placebo (OR = 1.72, 95% CI = 1.28–2.32) (67).

The use of the GP IIb/IIIa inhibitor abciximab in combination with fibrinolytic therapy is associated with a doubling in the incidence of noncerebral major hemorrhage. In the GUSTO V trial, patients treated with abciximab and reteplase had a 4.6% rate of moderate or severe nonintracranial bleeding, compared to 2.3% with reteplase alone ($p <$ 0.0001), and a significantly higher rate of transfusions (5.7% vs. 4.0%; $p < 0.0001$) (69). In ASSENT-3 abciximab was associated with a 4.4% incidence of major non-cerebral hemorrhage, compared with 2.2% and 3.0% for heparin and enoxaparin, respectively ($p =$ 0.0005) (43).

In the CURE trial, major bleeding was significantly more common in the clopidogrel group (3.7% compared with 2.7%; $p = 0.001$) (71). Overall, there was no significant increase in the rate of hemorrhage following coronary bypass surgery (1.3% vs. 1.1%; $p =$ NS). However, in a subgroup of patients whose medications were discontinued within 5 days before surgery, the rate of major bleeding was 9.6% in the clopidogrel group and 6.3% in the placebo group ($p = 0.006$) (71). In the CURE cohort of patients who underwent PCI, there was no significant difference in major hemorrhage between the clopidogrel and placebo groups (1.6% vs. 1.4% at 30 days; $p =$ NS) (73).

F. Prediction of Hemorrhage

1. Intracranial Hemorrhage

Three predictive models of fibrinolytic-associated intracranial bleeding have been developed from large databases (4,5,45). Age (>65 years), low body weight (<70 kg), hypertension on admission, and type of fibrinolytic agent (use of alteplase vs. streptokinase) have all been shown to be independently associated with the risk of intracranial hemorrhage (4).

The most important predictor of intracranial hemorrhage is older age (4,5,45,74,75), with a steeper slope above the age of 65, reaching about 2% in risk at age 80 (Fig. 2) (5). Lower body weight is the second most important predictor of intracranial hemorrhage, even when alteplase or tenecteplase are given in a weight-adjusted dose (Fig. 2) (5,45). The higher bleeding rate seen with lower body weights reinforces the need for weight-adjusted dosing of potent antithrombotic agents. Hypertension at presentation is consistently shown to be an important predictor of intracranial hemorrhage following thrombolysis (45,74–76). There appears to be a continuous relationship between blood pressure and risk of hemorrhage, without a clear-cut value above which risk abruptly increases (77). Whether treating the hypertension prior to initiating thrombolysis reduces the risk of intracranial hemorrhage is not known, but doing so would be prudent. Finally, the use of more potent fibrinolytic regimens (alteplase vs. streptokinase, combined alteplase streptokinase vs. either alone) is, not surprisingly, associated with a higher risk of intracranial hemorrhage.

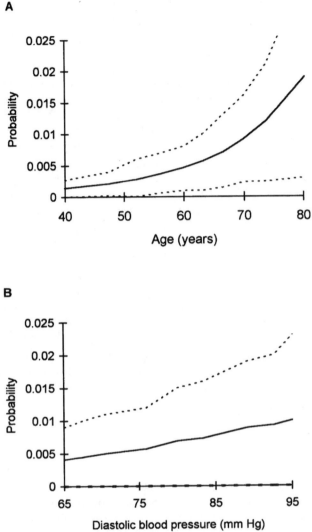

Figure 2 Predicted probability (solid line) and 95% confidence intervals (dashed lines) of intracranial hemorrhage according to patient age (**A**) and weight (**B**) in the GUSTO-I trial. (From Ref. 5.)

Two trials have shown an association between risk of intracranial hemorrhage and history of cerebrovascular disease (stroke or transient ischemic attacks) (5,13). Recent stroke is listed among exclusion criteria for thrombolysis in the ACC/AHA guidelines (57), but there are no data regarding the bleeding risk conferred by a more remote stroke. Female sex was shown to be an independent predictor in GISSI 2/International Study (78), but not in other studies after adjustment for age, weight, and blood pressure (4,5). Warfarin use at presentation was an independent predictor in the Netherlands registry report (25), but not in a larger analysis (4). A history of head trauma within 2 weeks carries a 7.6-fold increase in the risk of intracranial hemorrhage (95% CI = 2.9–20), and dementia is associated with a 3.4-fold increase in risk (95% CI = 1.2–10) (32).

2. Nonintracranial Hemorrhage

Predictive models of noncerebral hemorrhage after fibrinolytic therapy have been developed from four large databases (Table 4) (35–37,45). The most important predictors of nonintracranial bleeding are invasive procedures, older age, low body weight, and female sex. In GUSTO I age was the most important predictor of hemorrhage after accounting for whether invasive procedures were performed. The risk of bleeding among GUSTO I patients not undergoing invasive procedures increased by 40% with every 10 additional years of age (37). That risk increased by 30% with every 10 kg decrease in weight (37). The bleeding risk among women was twice that seen among men after adjusting for other variables (36,37). African American patients had a 30% higher risk of hemorrhage than other races in GUSTO I, mostly in the alteplase arm (37).

Most trials have identified hypertension as a risk factor, albeit a less important one, for hemorrhage (25,35,37). However, hypertension was not a significant risk factor in the TAMI trial (79). Other factors associated with an increased hemorrhage risk include fibrinogen depletion (35,36), thrombocytopenia (36,39), and higher serum levels of alteplase (36).

3. Special Patient Groups

The use of fibrinolytic or potent antithrombotic therapy for myocardial infarction has been met with concerns about a potentially increased risk of hemorrhage in certain subgroups of patients. Among 135 patients who received fibrinolytics following cardiopulmonary resuscitation (including patients having received prolonged resuscitation), none experienced hemorrhage attributable to the resuscitative efforts (80–82). Accordingly, cardiopulmonary resuscitation should not be a contraindication to thrombolysis.

Menstruating women are another subgroup of patients in which the perceived bleeding risk has deterred treatment. In a series of 12 menstruating women presenting with acute myocardial infarction, no serious or life-threatening bleeding events were reported, and three patients required transfusions (83). Thus, the risk of serious hemorrhage from menstruation seems low and should not deter thrombolysis.

The risk of ocular bleeding resulting in vision loss or disability is extremely low, with no reported hemorrhagic events among >6000 diabetic patients in the GUSTO-I cohort, 300 of which had proliferative retinopathy (84). Thus, diabetic retinopathy should not preclude thrombolysis in patients with myocardial infarction.

G. Management of Hemorrhage

With the advent of more potent antithrombotic and antiplatelet agents, in addition to fibrinolytic therapy, and the trend for a more invasive strategy in managing patients with acute coronary syndromes, the management of serious bleeding complications is of critical importance. Optimal management of hemorrhage is based on early identification and control of bleeding, reversing the underlying causes, and prompt resuscitation when indicated (10). Immediate measures should be undertaken in reversing any antithrombotic effect in patients with an abrupt-onset neurological deficit within 24 hours of thrombolysis, pending CT imaging of the head.

When managing severe hemorrhage with hemodynamic instability, venous access with two large-bore lines should be secured, and fluid and packed red cell transfusions should be initiated. When an obvious bleeding source is identified, local compression should be used to control the hemorrhage. Antithrombotic and antiplatelet agents should be discontinued, and protamine should be used to reverse

Table 4 Baseline Patient Predictors of Bleeding Complications from Multivariable Logistic Regression Models

	TAMI (35)	TIMI (36)	GUSTO-I (37)	ASSENT-2 (45)
Patients in the model	386	1424	40,903	16,949
Patients (n) with hemorrhage[a]	14% (55)	7% (58)	12.6% (5154)	5.3% (898)
Angiography	100% (acute)	50% within 42 days	55% in-hospital	24% angioplasty in-hospital
Predictors of bleeding:				
Bypass surgery	Bleeding (#1 predictor)	Not reported	Bleeding (#1 predictor); $\chi^2 = 775$;[b] OR = 3.8–7.2	Higher bleeding in U.S. vs. non-U.S.
Angiography or angioplasty	All patients underwent angiography	Bleeding (angiography) ($p < 0.001$)	Bleeding $\chi^2 = 48$; OR = 1.2–1.6	Higher bleeding in U.S. vs. non-U.S.
Advanced age	Blood loss ($p = 0.095$)	Bleeding (invasive strategy arm)[c] ($p < 0.001$)	Bleeding (#1 nonprocedure predictor) $\chi^2 = 267$; OR = 1.4/10 y	OR 1.4 per 10 years
Lower body weight	Bleeding ($p = 0.02$)	Combined major and minor bleeding ($p < 0.001$)	Bleeding (#2 nonprocedure predictor); $\chi^2 = 218$; OR = 1.3/10 kg	OR 1.38 for <67 kg vs. ≥67 kg
Female sex	Increased blood loss ($p = 0.01$)	Combined major and minor bleeding ($p < 0.001$)	Bleeding (#3 nonprocedure predictor) $\chi^2 = 136$; OR = 1.7	OR 1.48
African ancestry	Not evaluated	Not evaluated	Bleeding; $\chi^2 = 42$; OR = 1.9	Not significant
History of hypertension	Blood loss ($p = 0.091$)	Bleeding ($p < 0.001$), OR = 3.2	Bleeding; $\chi^2 = 11$; OR = 1.1	Not significant
Cardiac decompensation	Not evaluated	Bleeding ($p < 0.04$), OR = 2.0	Bleeding, patients without invasive procedures; $\chi^2 = 30$	Not significant
Low fibrinogen	Increased blood loss ($p = 0.005$)	Combined major and minor bleeding ($p = 0.001$)	Not evaluated	Not evaluated
Platelet ≤ 100,00/mL	Not evaluated	Bleeding ($p < 0.001$), OR = 7.5	Not evaluated	Not evaluated
Alteplase level ≥ 1500 ng/mL	Not evaluated	Bleeding ($p < 0.001$), OR = 3.3	Not evaluated	Not evaluated

OR = odds ratio.

[a] Major bleeding in TIMI and TAMI; moderate or severe bleeding in GUSTO-I.

[b] $\chi^2 > 6$ corresponds to $p < 0.05$; the greater the χ^2, the more statistically significant the predictive power.

[c] "Conservative strategy" patients received 100 mg alteplase.

the heparin effect. Each milligram of protamine sulfate neutralizes about 90 U of heparin, and thus an initial dose of 20–30 mg is needed for patients on intravenous heparin infusions. If bleeding persists after thrombolysis, 10 U of cryoprecipitate should be given to replete fibrinogen and factor VIII, both degraded by activated plasmin. Once fibrinogen levels normalize, fresh frozen plasma transfusions can be used as a source of factors V and VIII.

Potent inhibitors of platelet aggregation have become pivotal in the management of acute coronary syndromes. Platelet dysfunction is even more pronounced in patients receiving fibrinolytic agents because of the inhibitory effects of fibrin degradation products (10). When managing life-threatening hemorrhage following thrombolysis, platelet transfusions should be considered even in the absence of thrombocytopenia. The therapeutic value of platelet transfusions in patients treated with GP IIb/IIIa inhibitors and suspected of having serious bleeding depends on the specific agent used. Abciximab has a short plasma half-life, on the order of 20–30 minutes (85), but results in sustained inhibition of platelet aggregation given its high affinity to GP IIb/IIIa (86). Accordingly, in the event of severe hemorrhage on abciximab, the infusion should be discontinued, and platelet transfusions intiated. On the other hand, eptifibatide has a longer plasma half-life, on the order of 2-1/2 hours, with much lower affinity for the GP IIb/IIIa receptor (86). Thus, platelet transfusions following eptifibatide discontinuation are of little benefit.

Antifibrinolytic lysine-analogue agents such as e-aminocaproic acid are only used for severe hemorrhage early after thrombolysis that is not controlled with other measures. These agents inhibit the binding of plamsin to fibrin (via lysine-binding sites) but carry a high risk of severe refractory thrombosis, especially among patients with disseminated intravascular coagulation (DIC) (87), diabetes, or with prior protamine exposure.

The role of neurosurgical evacuation of intracranial hemorrhage following thrombolysis is unclear. In one observational study, neurosurgical evacuation conferred a better survival, especially in managing cerebellar hemorrhages (88).

III. HEMATOLOGICAL COMPLICATIONS

Hematological complications, such as thrombocytopenia or neutropenia, occur at a relatively low incidence with various antithrombotic and antiplatelet agents, yet a prompt recognition is critical given serious and potentially life-threatening sequelae.

Thrombocytopenia is a known complication of specific antiplatelet and antithrombotic therapies, and can be an isolated finding or part of systemic syndromes such as heparin-induced thrombocytopenia of thrombotic thrombocytopenic purpura (TTP). In the GUSTO IV ACS trial, abciximab was associated with a 2% incidence of serious thrombocytopenia (platelet count < 50,000 per mL), compared to virtually none in the placebo arm (67). In the PURSUIT trial, profound thrombocytopenia (platelet count < 20,000 per mL) was more common in the eptifibatide arm as compared to placebo (0.2% vs. <0.1%, RR = 5, 95% CI = 1.3–32.4) (66). The incidence of thrombocytopenia appears to be similar between aspirin- and thienopyridine-treated patients. In the CAPRIE cohort, thrombocytopenia was identical in the clopidogrel and aspirin groups (0.26%), with the rates of severe thrombocytopenia being 0.19% and 0.10%, respectively (p = NS) (89). In a randomized comparison of clopidogrel and ticlopidine, there were similar rates of thrombocytopenia in both groups (0.57% for ticlopidine vs. 1.01% for clopidogrel; p = 0.43) (90). In the CLASSICS trial, clopidogrel had a more favorable safety profile with a lower combined incidence of major bleeding, neutropenia, thrombocytopenia, or early discontinuation (4.6% vs. 9.1%; p = 0.005) (91). Neutropenia is the most common side effect of ticlopidine therapy, with an incidence of 1.0–2.4% in most clinical trials (92,93), compared to virtually no cases with clopidogrel therapy. Physicians are encouraged to closely monitor complete blood cell counts at 2-week intervals with ticlopidine use.

TTP is a life-threatening, multisystem disease characterized by thrombocytopenia, microangiopathic hemolytic anemia, fever, neurological changes, and renal failure (94). TTP is a rare but serious complication of thienopyridine therapy. The estimated rate of ticlopidine-associated TTP is one in 1600, while its mortality rate is 33% (95,96). The incidence of TTP with clopidogrel is much lower, on the order of one in 250,000 (97). TTP tends to occur earlier with clopidogrel therapy (within 2 weeks of initiation of the drug) than with ticlopidine (usually at weeks 2–12 following initiation of therapy) (95–97). The management of TTP includes prompt discontinuation of the offending drug and initiation of plasma exchange therapy.

The most feared and serious complication of heparin therapy is heparin-induced thrombocytopenia and thrombosis (HITT). Heparin-associated thrombocytopenia, or type I heparin-induced thrombocytopenia (HIT I), occurs in around 10–20% of patients (98), usually 1–4 days after initiation of therapy, and is a benign form of mild thrombocytopenia (100,000–130,000 per mL) that resolves spontaneously (99–102). It is caused by direct interaction between heparin and platelets rather than an immune-mediated effect (103). Heparin-induced thrombocytopenia and thrombosis (HITT), or type II HIT, is the more serious form of the condition, occurring in 2–3% of patients, usually 5–8 days after initiation of heparin therapy, or earlier in patients with prior exposure to heparin. It carries a 50% risk of thrombotic complications and a mortality rate as high as 30% (104,105). Type II HIT is often associated with more severe thrombocytopenia (platelet count < 100,000 per mL) and is caused by an antibody (usually immunoglobulin G)–mediated platelet aggregation (106,107). In a series of orthopedic patients, unfractionated heparin was associated with a sevenfold greater risk of HIT than enoxaparin (108). It is recommended that the platelet count be measured twice weekly in the first week or two of heparin therapy to detect HIT early with the intent of then being able to prevent thrombosis (109). The diagnosis of immune HIT should be considered in any patient with a 50% reduction of platelet count while on heparin after 4 days, or upon readministration if exposed to heparin in the prior 3 months. There are multiple available diagnostic modalities to confirm the suspicion of HITT, such as the platelet aggregation test (PAT), the serotonin release assay (SRA), or enzyme-linked immunosorbent assay (ELISA). The initial management of patients with HITT is based on withdrawal of heparin, treatment with an alternative anticoagulant, and treatment of thrombotic complications. All forms of heparin should be discontinued, including coated catheters and flushes. Although no randomized trials of alternative antithrombotic agents have been conducted for treatment of HITT patients with acute coronary syndromes or needing PCI, direct thrombin inhibitors, such as argatroban, lepirudin, or bivalirudin, currently offer the most promising option (110).

IV. IMMUNOLOGICAL COMPLICATIONS

Streptokinase and anistreplase are both derived from group C streptococci and thus have the potential to cause immunological reactions. On the other hand, alteplase and reteplase are derived from the human plasminogen activator protein and are not antigenic. Circulating *Streptococcus* antibody is present in nearly all patients given the ubiquity of the *Streptococcus* bacterium (111,112). Mild allergic reactions are estimated to occur in 4% of patients treated with streptokinase (17,113). The incidence of true anaphylactic shock ranges from 0.1 to 0.7% (16,113). Other immune-mediated reactions such as renal injury (114), serum sickness (115), and lung injury (116) have been reported but are rare. Since about half of patients treated with streptokinase will have significant levels of neutralizing antibodies for at least 4 years (117), it is recommended that such patients be treated with alteplase or reteplase if they suffer a new myocardial infarction during this time. Hypotension occurs in around 6% of patient after streptokinase administration (118), probably secondary to kallikrein activation and bradykinin release.

V. CONCLUSION

The overall benefits of fibrinolytic, antithrombotic, and antiplatelet therapies for management of acute coronary syndromes have been well established, but they come with a cost of risk of serious complications, especially intracranial hemorrhage, in a subgroup of patients. Individualized risk assessment should be undertaken for specific patients prior to decision on the optimal management strategy to adopt in managing coronary syndromes. With the advent of more specific and potent antithrombotic and antiplatelet agents, research is ongoing to develop combination therapies aiming at optimizing clinical outcomes while minimizing the risk of serious complications.

REFERENCES

1. Braunwald E, Knatterud GL, Passamani E, Robertson TL, Solomon R. Update from the thrombolysis in myocardial infarction trial (abstr). J Am Coll Cardiol 1987; 10:970.
2. The Global Use of Strategies to Open Occluded Coronary Arteries (GUSTO) IIa Investigators. Randomized trial of intravenous heparin versus recombinant hirudin for acute coronary syndromes. Circulation 1994; 90:1631–1637.
3. Antman EM, for the TIMI 9A Investigators. Hirudin in acute myocardial infarction: safety report from the Thrombolysis and thrombin inhibition In Myocardial Infarction (TIMI) 9A trial. Circulation 1994; 90:1624–1630.
4. Simoons ML, Maggioni AP, Knatterud G, et al. Individual risk assessment for intracranial haemorrhage during thrombolytic therapy. Lancet 1993; 342:1523–1528.
5. Gore JM, Granger CB, Sloan MA, et al. Stroke after thrombolysis: mortality and functional outcomes in the GUSTO-I trial. Circulation 1995; 92:2811–2818.
6. Lee KL, Woodlief LH, Topol EJ, et al. Predictors of 30-day mortality in the era of reperfusion for acute myocardial infarction: results from an international trial of 41,021 patients. Circulation 1995; 91:1659–1668.
7. Boersma H, van der Vlugt JJ, Arnold AER, Deckers JW, Simoons ML. Estimated gain in life expectancy: a simple tool to select optimal reperfusion treatment in individual patients with evolving myocardial infarction. Eur Heart J 1996; 17:64–75.
8. Wallentin L, Lagerqvist B, Husted S, Kontny F, Stahle E, Swahn E. Outcome at 1 year after an invasive compared with a non-invasive strategy in unstable coronary-artery disease: the FRISC II invasive randomised trial. Lancet 2000; 356:9–16.
9. The TACTICS-TIMI 18 investigators. Comparison of early invasive and conservative strategies in patients with unstable coronary syndromes treated with the glycoprotein IIb/IIIa inhibitor tirofiban. N Engl J Med 2001; 344:1879–1887
10. Sane DC, Califf RM, Topol EJ, Stump DC, Mark DB, Greenberg CS. Bleeding during thrombolytic therapy for acute myocardial infarction: mechanisms and management. Ann Intern Med 1989; 111:1010–1022.
11. ISIS-3 (Third International Study of Infarct Survival Collaborative Group). ISIS-3: a randomised comparison of streptokinase vs tissue plasminogen activator vs anistreplase and of

aspirin plus heparin vs aspirin alone among 41,299 cases of suspected acute myocardial infarction. Lancet 1992; 339:753–770.

12. Fibrinolytic Therapy Trialists' (FTT) Collaborative Group. Indications for fibrinolytic therapy in suspected acute myocardial infarction: collaborative overview of early mortality and major morbidity results from all randomised trials of more than 1000 patients. Lancet 1994; 343:311–322.

13. Gore JM, Sloan M, Price TR, et al. Intracerebral hemorrhage, cerebral infarction, and subdural hematoma after acute myocardial infarction and thrombolytic therapy in the Thrombolysis in Myocardial Infarction study: Thrombolysis In Myocardial Infarction, Phase II, pilot and clinical trial. Circulation 1991; 83:448–459.

14. Maggioni AP, Franzosi MG, Farina ML, et al. Cerebrovascular events after myocardial infarction: analysis of the GISSI trial. Br Med J 1991; 302:1428–1431.

15. Maggioni AP, Franzosi MG, Santoro E, et al. The risk of stroke in patients with acute myocardial infarction after thrombolytic and antithrombotic treatment. N Engl J Med 1992; 327:1–6.

16. Gruppo Italiano per lo Studio della Streptochinasi nell'Infarto Miocardico (GISSI). Effectiveness of intravenous thrombolytic treatment in acute myocardial infarction. Lancet 1986; 1:397–402.

17. ISIS-2 (Second International Study of Infarct Survival) Collaborative Group. Randomised trial of intravenous streptokinase, oral aspirin, both, or neither among 17,187 cases of suspected acute myocardial infarction: ISIS-2. Lancet 1988; 2:349–360.

18. The ISAM Study Group. A prospective trial of intravenous streptokinase in acute myocardial infarction (ISAM). Mortality, morbidity, and infarct size at 21 days. N Engl J Med 1986; 314:1465–1471.

19. EMERAS (Estudio Multicentrico Estreptoquinasa Republicas de America del Sur) Collaborative Group. Randomised trial of late thrombolysis in patients with suspected acute myocardial infarction. Lancet 1993; 342:767–772.

20. Wilcox RG, von der Lippe G, Olsson CG, Jensen G, Skene AM, Hampton JR. Trial of tissue plasminogen activator for mortality reduction in acute myocardial infarction. Anglo-Scandinavian Study of Early Thrombolysis (ASSET). Lancet 1988; 2:525–530.

21. LATE Study Group. Late assessment of thrombolytic efficacy (LATE) study with alteplase 6–24 hours after onset of acute myocardial infarction. Lancet 1993; 342:759–766.

22. AIMS Trial Study Group. Effect of intravenous APSAC on mortality after acute myocardial infarction: preliminary report of a placebo-controlled clinical trial. Lancet 1988; 1:545–549.

23. International Joint Efficacy Comparison of Thrombolytics. Randomised, double-blind comparison of reteplase double-bolus administration with streptokinase in acute myocardial infarction (INJECT): trial to investigate equivalence. Lancet 1995; 346:329–336.

24. The Global Use of Strategies to Open Occluded Infarct Arteries (GUSTO-III) Investigators. An international, multicenter, randomized comparison of reteplase and tissue plasminogen activator for acute myocardial infarction. N Engl J Med 1997; 337:1118–1123.

25. de Jaegere PP, Arnold AA, Balk AH, Simoons ML. Intracranial hemorrhage in association with thrombolytic therapy: incidence and clinical predictive factors. J Am Coll Cardiol 1992; 19:289–294.

26. Sloan MA, Price TR, Petito CK, et al. Clinical features and pathogenesis of intracerebral hemorrhage after rt-PA and heparin therapy for acute myocardial infarction: the thrombolysis in myocardial infarction (TIMI) II pilot and randomized clinical trial combined experience. Neurology 1995; 45:649–658.

27. Ramsey DA, Penswick JL, Robertson DM. Fatal streptokinase-induced intracerebral hemorrhage in amyloid angiopathy. Can J Neurol Sci 1990; 17:336–341.

28. LeBlanc R, Haddad G, Robitaille Y. Cerebral hemorrhage from amyloid angiopathy and coronary thrombolysis. Neurosurgery 1992; 31:586–590.

29. Itoh Y, Yamada M, Hayakawa M, Otomo E, Miyatake T. Cerebral amyloid angiopathy: a significant cause of cerebellar as well as lobar cerebral hemorrhage in the elderly. J Neurol Sci 1993; 116:135–141.

30. Kalyan-Raman UP, Kalyan-Raman K. Cerebral amyloid angiopathy causing intracranial hemorrhage. Ann Neurol 1984; 16:321–329.

31. Gebel JM, Sila CA, Sloan MA, Granger CB, Mahaffey KW, Weisenberger J, Green CL, White HD, Gore JM, Weaver WD, Califf RM, Topol EJ. Thrombolysis-related intracranial hemorrhage: a radiographic analysis of 244 cases from the GUSTO-1 trial with clinical correlation. Global Utilization of Streptokinase and Tissue Plasminogen Activator for Occluded Coronary Arteries. Stroke 1998; 29:563–569.

32. Granger C, White H, Simoons M, et al. Risk factors for stroke following thrombolytic therapy: case-control study from the GUSTO trial (abstr). J Am Coll Cardiol 1995; 25:232A.

33. Kase CS, Pessin MS, Zivin JA, et al. Intracranial hemorrhage after coronary thrombolysis with tissue plasminogen activator. Am J Med 1992; 92:384–390.

34. Rao AK, Pratt C, Berke A, et al. Thrombolysis in Myocardial Infarction (TIMI) trial—phase 1; hemorrhagic manifestations and changes in plasma fibrinogen and the fibrinolytic system in patients treated with recombinant tissue plasminogen activator and streptokinase. J Am Coll Cardiol 1988; 11:1–11.

35. Califf RM, Topol EJ, George BS, et al. Hemorrhagic complications associated with the use of intravenous tissue plasminogen activator in treatment of acute myocardial infarction. Am J Med 1988; 85:353–359.

36. Bovill EG, Terrin ML, Stump DC, et al. Hemorrhagic events during therapy with recombinant tissue-type plasminogen activator, heparin, and aspirin for acute myocardial infarction. Ann Intern Med 1991; 115:256–265.

37. Berkowitz SD, Granger CB, Pieper KS, et al. Incidence and predictors of bleeding after contemporary thrombolytic therapy for myocardial infarction. Circulation 1997; 95:2508–2516.

38. Granger CB, Becker R, Tracy RP, et al. Thrombin generation, inhibition and clinical outcomes in patients with acute myocardial infarction treated with thrombolytic therapy and heparin: results from the GUSTO trial. J Am Coll Cardiol 1998; 31:497–505.

39. TIMI Study Group. Comparison of invasive and conservative strategies after treatment with intravenous tissue plasminogen activator in acute myocardial infarction. Results of the Thrombolysis In Myocardial Infarction (TIMI) phase II trial. N Engl J Med 1989; 320:618–627.

40. The TIMI IIIB Investigators. Effects of tissue plasminogen activator and a comparison of early invasive and conservative strategies in unstable angina and non-Q-wave myocardial infarction: results of the TIMI IIIB trial. Circulation 1994; 89:1545–1556.

41. The COBALT investigators. A comparison of continuous infusion alteplase with double-bolus administration for acute myocardial infarction. N Engl J Med 1997; 337:1124–1130.

42. Braunwald E. TIMI-10B preliminary results. TIMI 10-B Investigators Meeting, Boston, Massachusetts, June 1997.

43. The ASSENT-3 investigators. Efficacy and safety of tenecteplase in combination with enoxaparin, abciximab, or unfractionated heparin: the ASSENT-3 randomised trial in acute myocardial infarction. Lancet 2001; 358:605–613.

44. Gruppo Italiano per lo Studio della Sopravvivenza nell'Infarto Miocardico. GISSI-2: A factorial randomised trial of alteplase versus streptokinase and heparin versus no heparin among 12 490 patients with acute myocardial infarction. Lancet 1990; 336:65–71.

45. Van de Werf F, Barron HV, Armstrong PW, Granger CB, Berioli S, Barbash G, Pehrsson K, Verheugt FWA, Myer J, Betriu A, Califf RM, Li X, Fox NL. Incidence and predictors of bleeding events after fibrinolytic therapy with fibrin-specific agents: a comparison of TNK-tPA and rt-PA. *European Heart J* 2001; 22(24):2253–2261.

46. The Global Use of Strategies to Open Occluded Coronary Arteries (GUSTO) IIb Investigators. A comparison of recombinant hirudin with heparin for the treatment of acute coronary syndromes. N Engl J Med 1996; 335:775–782.

47. Cohen M, Demers C, Gurfinkel EP, et al. A comparison of low molecular weight heparin with unfractionated heparin for unstable coronary artery disease (the ESSENCE trial). N Engl J Med 1997; 337:447–452.

48. The TIMI-11B investigators. Enoxaparin prevents death and cardiac ischemic events in unstable angina/non-Q-wave myocardial infarction: results of the TIMI-11B trial. Circulation 1999; 100:1593–1601.

49. Mahaffey KW, Granger CB, Collins R, et al. Overview of randomized trials of intravenous heparin in patients with acute myocardial infarction treated with thrombolytic therapy. Am J Cardiol 1996; 77:551–556.

50. Granger CB, Hirsh J, Califf RM, et al. Activated partial thromboplastin time and outcome after thrombolytic therapy for acute myocardial infarction: results from the GUSTO-I trial. Circulation 1996; 93:870–878.

51. Simes RJ, Granger CB, Antman EM, Califf RM, Braunwald E, Topol EJ. Impact of hirudin versus heparin on mortality and (re)infarction in patients with acute coronary syndromes: a prospective meta-analysis of the GUSTO-IIb and TIMI 9b trials. Circulation 1996; 94:I-430. Abstract.

52. Wallentin L. Preliminary Results of the ASSENT-3 Plus Trial. Scientific Sessions 2002 of the American Heart Association, Chicago, IL, November 2002.

53. Antman E, Cohen M, Radley D, et al. Assessment of the treatment effect of enoxaparin for unstable angina/non-Q-wave myocardial infarction: TIMI-11B-ESSENCE meta-analysis. Circulation 1999; 100:1602–1608.

54. Berkowitz S, Stinnett S, Cohen M, et al. Prospective comparison of hemorrhagic complications after treatment with enoxaparin versus unfractionated heparin for unstable angina pectoris or non-ST-segment elevation acute myocardial infarction. Am J Cardiol 2001; 88:1230–1234.

55. Collins R, MacMahon S, Flather M, et al. Clinical effects of anticoagulant therapy in suspected acute myocardial infarction: systematic overview of randomised trials. Br Med J 1996; 313:652–659.

56. The ASSENT-2 investigators. Single-bolus tenecteplase compared with front-loaded alteplase in acute myocardial infarction: the ASSENT-2 double-blind randomised trial. Lancet 1999; 354:716–722.

57. Ryan TJ, Antman EM, Brooks NH, et al. 1999 update: ACC/AHA guidelines for the management of patents with acute myocardial infarction: executive summary and recommendations. A report of the American College of Cardiology/American Heart Association Task Force on Practice Guidelines. Circulation 1999; 100:1016–1030.

58. Antman EM, McCabe CH, Marble SJ, et al. Dose ranging trial of enoxaparin for unstable angina: results of TIMI 11A. Circulation 1996; 94:I–554. Abstract.

59. Antman EM. Hirudin in acute myocardial infarction–thrombolysis and thrombin in myocardial infarction (TIMI) 9B trial. Circulation 1996; 94:911–921.

60. EPIC Investigators. Use of a monoclonal antibody directed against the platelet glycoprotein IIb/IIIa receptor in high-risk coronary angioplasty. N Engl J Med 1996; 330:956–961.

61. The CAPTURE Investigators. Randomised placebo-controlled trial of abciximab before and during coronary intervention in refractory unstable angina: the CAPTURE study. Lancet 1997; 349:1429–1435.

62. Tcheng JE. Glycoprotein IIb/IIIa receptor inhibitors: putting the EPIC, IMPACT II, RESTORE, and EPILOG trials into perspective. Am J Cardiol 1996; 78:35–40.

63. The IMPACT-II Investigators. Randomised placebo-controlled trial of effect of eptifibatide on complications of percutaneous coronary intervention—IMPACT-II. Lancet 1997; 349:1422–1428.

64. The PRISM Study Investigators. A comparison of aspirin plus tirofiban with aspirin plus heparin for unstable angina. N Engl J Med 1998; 338:1498–1505.

65. The PRISM-PLUS Study Investigators. Inhibition of the platelet glycoprotein IIb/IIIa receptor with tirofiban in unstable angina and non-Q-wave myocardial infarction. Platelet Receptor Inhibition in Ischemic Syndrome Management in Patients Limited by Unstable Signs and Symptoms. N Engl J Med 1998; 338:1488–1497.

66. The PURSUIT Trial Investigators. Inhibition of platelet glycoprotein IIb/IIIa with eptifibatide in patientd with acute coronary syndromes. N Engl J Med 1998; 339:436–443.

67. The GUSTO IV-ACS investigators. Effect of glycoprotein IIb/IIIa receptor blocker abciximab on outcome in patients with acute coronary syndromes without early coronary revascularization: the GUSTO IV-ACS randomised trial. Lancet 2001; 357:1915–1924.

68. Boersma E, Harrington RA, Moliterno DJ, et al. Platelet glycoprotein IIb/IIIa inhibitors in acute coronary syndromes: a meta-analysis of all major randomised clinical trials. Lancet 2002; 359:189–198.

69. The GUSTO-V Investigators. Reperfusion therapy for acute myocardial infarction with fibrinolytic therapy or combination reduced fibrinolytic therapy and platelet glycoprotein IIb/IIIa inhibition: the GUSTO V randomised trial. Lancet 2001; 357:1905–1914.

70. The CAPRIE Steering Committee. A randomised, blinded, trial of clopidogrel versus aspirin in patients at risk of ischaemic events (CAPRIE). Lancet 1996; 348:1329–1339.

71. The CURE Trial Investigators. Effects of clopidogrel in addition to aspirin in patients with acute coronary syndromes without ST-segment elevation. N Engl J Med 2001; 345:494–502.

72. The EPISTENT Investigators. Randomised placebo-controlled and balloon-angioplasty-controlled trial to assess safety of coronary stenting with use of platelet glycoprotein-IIb/IIIa blockade. Lancet 1998; 352:87–92.

73. Mehta SR, Yusuf S, Peters RJ, et al. Effects of pretreatment with clopidogrel and aspirin followed by long-term therapy in patients undergoing percutaneous coronary intervention: the PCI-CURE study. Lancet 2001; 358:527–533.

74. Anderson JL, Karagounis L, Allen A, Bradford MJ, Menlove RL, Pryor TA. Older age and elevated blood pressure are risk factors for intracerebral hemorrhage after thrombolysis. Am J Cardiol 1991; 68:166–170.

75. O'Connor CM, Califf RM, Massey EW, et al. Stroke and acute myocardial infarction in the thrombolytic era: clinical correlates and long-term prognosis. J Am Coll Cardiol 1990; 16:533–540.

76. White HD, Barbash GI, Califf RM, et al. Age and outcome with contemporary thrombolytic therapy: results from the GUSTO-I trial. Circulation 1996; 94:1826–1833.

77. Aylward PE, Wilcox RG, Horgan JH, et al. Relation of increased arterial blood pressure to mortality and stroke in the context of contemporary thrombolytic therapy for acute myocardial infarction. Ann Intern Med 1996; 125:891–900.

78. White HD, Barbash GI, Modan M, et al. After correcting for worse baseline characteristics, women treated with thrombolytic therapy for acute myocardial infarction have the same mortality and morbidity as men except for a higher incidence of hemorrhagic stroke. Circulation 1993; 88:2097–2103.

79. Wall TC, Califf RM, Ellis SG, et al. Lack of impact of early catheterization and fibrin specificity on bleeding complications after thrombolytic therapy. The TAMI Study Group. J Am Coll Cardiol 1993; 21:597–603.

80. Tenaglia AN, Califf RM, Candela RJ, et al. Thrombolytic therapy in patients requiring cardiopulmonary resuscitation. Am J Cardiol 1991; 68:1015–1019.

81. Scholz KH, Tebbe U, Herrmann C, et al. Frequency of complications of cardiopulmonary resuscitation after thrombolysis during acute myocardial infarction. Am J Cardiol 1992; 69:724–728.

82. van Campen LC, van Leeuwen GR, Verheugt FW. Safety and efficacy of thrombolysis for acute myocardial infarction in patients with prolonged out-of-hospital cardiopulmonary resuscitation. Am J Cardiol 1994; 73:953–955.

83. Karnash SL, Granger CB, White HD, et al. Treating menstruating women with thrombolytic therapy: insights from the Global Utilization of Streptokinase and Tissue Plasminogen Activator for Occluded Coronary Arteries (GUSTO-I) trial. J Am Coll Cardiol 1995; 26:1651–1656.

84. Mahaffey KW, Granger CB, Stebbins AL, Califf RM, GUSTO-I Investigators. Diabetic retinopathy should not be a contraindication to thrombolytic therapy: Quantification of risk of 6011 patients (abstr). Circulation 1995; 92 (suppl):I-417.

85. Kleiman NS, Raizner AE, Jordan R, et al. Differential inhibition of platelet aggregation induced by adenosine diphosphate or a thrombin receptor-activating peptide in patients treated

with bolus chimeric 7E3 Fab: implication for inhibition of the internal pool of GPIIb/IIIa receptors. J Am Coll Cardiol 1995; 26:1665–1671.

86. Jordan RE, Wagner CL, Mascelli MA, et al. Preclinical development of c7E3 Fab: a mouse/human chimeric monoclonal antibody fragment that inhibits platelet function by blockade of GP IIb/IIIa receptors with observations on the immunogenicity of c7E3 Fab in humans. In: Horton MA, ed. Adhesion Receptors as Therapeutic Targets. Boca Raton, FL: CRC Press, 1996:281–305.

87. Naeye RL. Thrombotic state after a hemorrhagic diathesis, a possible complication of therapy with epsilon-amino caproic acid. Blood 1962; 19:694–701.

88. Mahaffey KW, White HD, Granger CB, et al. Neurosurgical evacuation for intracranial hemorrhage associated with improved outcome in GUSTO (abstr). J Am Coll Cardiol 1995; 25:232A–233A.

89. Harker LA, Boissel JP, Pilgrim AJ, Gent M. Comparative safety and tolerability of clopidogrel and aspirin: results from CAPRIE. Drug Safety 1999; 21(4):325–335.

90. Taniushi M, Kurz HI, Lasala JM. Randomized comparison of ticlopidine and clopidogrel after intracoronary stent implantation in a broad patient population. Circulation 2001; 104(5):539–543.

91. Bertrand ME, Rupprecht HJ, Urban P, et al. Double-blind study of the safety of clopidogrel with and without a loading dose in combination with aspirin compared with ticlopidine in combination with aspirin after coronary stenting: the clopidogrel aspirin stent international cooperative study (CLASSICS). Circulation 2000; 102:624–629.

92. Gent M, Easton JD, Hachinski VC, et al. The Canadian American ticlopidine study (CATS) in thromboembolic stroke. Lancet 1989; 1:1215–1220.

93. Hass WK, Easton JD, Adams HP, ct al. A randomized trial comparing tclopidine hydrochloride with aspirin for the prevention of stroke in high-risk patients (TASS). N Engl J Med 1989; 321:501–507.

94. Amorosi E, Ultmann J. Thrombotic thrombocytopenic purpura: report of 16 cases and review of the literature. Medicine 1996; 45:139–159.

95. Bennet CL, Kiss JE, Weinberg PD, et al. Thrombotic thrombocytopenic purpura after stenting and ticlopidine. Lancet 1998; 352:1036–1037.

96. Bennet CL, Weinberg PD, Rozenberg-Ben-Dror K, et al. Thrombotic thrombocytopenic purpura associated with ticlopidine: a review of 60 cases. Ann Intern Med 1998; 128:541–544.

97. Bennet CL, Connors JM, Carwile JM, et al. Thrombotic thrombocytopenic purpura associated with clopidogrel. N Engl J Med 2000; 342:1773–1777.

98. Brieger DB, Mak KH, Kottke-Marchant K, et al. Heparin-induced thrombocytopenia. J Am Coll Cardiol 1998; 31:1449–1459.

99. Bell WR, Tomasulo PA, Alving BM, Duffy TP. Thrombocytopenia occurring during administration of heparin: a prospective study of 52 patients. Ann Intern Med 1975; 85:155–160.

100. King DJ, Kelton JG. Heparin associated thrombocytopenia. Ann Intern Med 1984; 100:535–540.

101. Powers PJ, Kelton JG, Carter CJ. Studies on the frequency of heparin associated thrombocytopenia. Thromb Res 1984; 33:439–443.

102. Cines DB, Kaywin P, Bina M, et al. Heparin associated thrombocytopenia. N Engl J Med 1980; 303:788–795.

103. Chong BH. Heparin-induced thrombocytopenia. Austr NZ Med 1992; 22:145–152.

104. Aster RH. Heparin-induced thrombocytopenia and thrombosis. N Engl J Med 1995; 332:1374–1376.

105. Greinacher A. Antigen generation in heparin-associated thrombocytopenia; the nonimmunologic type and the immunologic type are closely linked in their pathogenesis. Thromb Haemost 1995; 21:106–116.

106. Kelton JG, Smith JW, Warkentin TE, et al. Immunoglobulin G from patients with heparin-induced thrombocytopenia binds to a complex of heparin and platelet factor 4. Blood 1994; 83:3232–3229.

107. Visentin GP, Ford SE, Scott JP, et al. Antibodies from patients with heparin-induced throm-bocytopenia/thrombosis are specific for platelet factor 4 complexed with heparin or bound to endothelial cells. J Clin Invest 1994; 93:81–88.
108. Warkentin TE, Levine MN, Hirsh J, et al. Heparin-induced thrombocytopenia in patients treated with low-molecular-weight heparin or unfractionated heparin. N Engl J Med 1995; 332:1330–1335.
109. Chong B. Heparin-induced thrombocytopenia. Br J Haematol 1995; 89:431–439.
110. Mahaffey KW. Anticoagulation for acute coronary syndromes and percutaneous coronary intervention in patients with heparin-induced thrombocytopenia. Curr Cardiol Rep 2001; 3:362–370.
111. Vaughan DE, Van Houtte E, Declerck PJ, Collen D. Streptokinase-induced platelet aggrega-tion. Circulation 1991; 84:84–91.
112. Lynch M, Pentecost BL, Littler WA, Stockley RA. Overt and subclinical reactions to strep-tokinase in acute myocardial infarction. Am J Cardiol 1994; 74:849–852.
113. The GUSTO Investigators. An international randomized trial comparing four thrombolytic strategies for acute myocardial infarction. N Engl J Med 1993; 329:673–682.
114. Murray N, Lyons J, Chappell M. Crescentic glomerulonephritis: a possible complication of streptokinase treatment for myocardial infarction. Br Heart J 1986; 56:483–485.
115. Toty WG, Romano T, Bemian GM, Gilula LA, Sherman LA. Serum sickness following strep-tokinase therapy. Am J Radiol 1982; 138:143–144.
116. Le SP, Chatterjee K, Wolfe CL. Adult respiratory distress syndrome following thrombolytic therapy with APSAC for acute myocardial infarction. Am Heart J 1992; 123:1368–1369.
117. Elliott JM, Cross DB, Cederholm-Williams SA, et al. Neutralizing antibodies to streptokinase four years after intravenous thrombolytic therapy. Am J Cardiol 1993; 71:640–645.
118. Lew AS, Laramee P, Cercek B, Shah PK, Ganz W. The hypotensive effect of intravenous streptokinase in patients with acute myocardial infarction. Circulation 1985; 72:1321–1326.

13-1

Percutaneous Coronary Intervention in Acute Myocardial Infarction

Paul Edwards and Youssef G. Chami
Harper University Hospital, Wayne State University, Detroit, Michigan, U.S.A.

David M. Larson
Ridgeview Medical Center, Waconia, Minnesota; and Minneapolis Heart Institute Foundation, Minneapolis, Minnesota, U.S.A.

Over the past two decades, percutaneous coronary intervention (PCI) has emerged as an effective method of treating ST elevation myocardial infarctions (MI). ST elevation MI most commonly results from the rupture of vulnerable plaque with subsequent thrombotic occlusion of an epicardial vessel (1). The rapid and complete restoration of forward flow within the coronary artery has been shown to decrease morbidity and mortality (2,3). Initial approaches to restoring coronary patency relied on the administration of thrombolytic therapy, but much data has accumulated over the past 10 years to document the superiority of emergency angioplasty in the setting of acute ST elevation MI.

PCI in the setting of ST elevation can be divided into three categories:

1. Establishing initial reperfusion as an alternative to thrombolytic therapy (primary PCI)
2. Achieving reperfusion after the failure of initial thrombolytic therapy (rescue angioplasty)
3. Immediate or delayed PCI of significant stenosis after successful thrombolysis

I. PRIMARY ANGIOPLASTY

Several trials have been published comparing the strategies of primary angioplasty (PTCA) and thrombolytic therapy. One of the earlier studies, the Mayo Clinic trial (4), established that myocardial salvage as determined by Sestamibi imaging was similar, when primary PTCA was compared to a reteplase (t-PA) infusion over 3 hours. In this relatively small study (108 patients), the two treatments were similar. Another early trial from Zwolle, the Netherlands (5), compared primary PTCA with streptokinase. In this study of 142 patients, primary PTCA was found to result in higher patency rates of the infarct-related artery, better left ventricular function, and less recurrent ischemia and infarction. The Zwolle authors in 1999 reported on 395 patients with a mean follow-up of 5 years (6). Again, the reduction in mortality and ischemic events was noted and a durable benefit was maintained. The major limitation of these studies is that streptokinase is a less effective thrombolytic agent than the front-loaded t-PA regimen.

The first multicenter trial (PAMI) was published in 1993 (7). This study enrolled 395 patients at 12 centers. Primary PTCA was compared to a t-PA infusion over 3 hours. Primary PTCA was noted to be effective, with procedural success in 97% (TIMI 2 or 3 flow). The in-hospital mortality was not statistically different in the two groups (2.6% PTCA vs. 6.5% t-PA PTCA; $p = 0.06$). However, the combined endpoint of death and nonfatal reinfarction at discharge was reduced in the PTCA group, 5.1%, versus 12% in the t-PA group ($p = 0.02$). PTCA remained superior at 6-month follow-up (8).

The GUSTO investigators published the largest study comparing PTCA and thrombolytic therapy (9). This study used the most effective thrombolytic regimen (front-loaded t-PA) (10) and included 57 centers. One thousand one hundred and thirty-eight patients were randomized to t-PA or PTCA. PTCA was again noted to be effective therapy with a procedural success rate of 93% and with TIMI-3 flows in 73% of patients. The primary endpoint was the combined incidence of death, nonfatal reinfarction, and nonfatal disabling stroke at 30 days. The primary endpoint was met in 9.6% of PTCA patients and 13.6% of thrombolytic patients ($p = 0.03$), but at 6 months there was no significant difference between the two groups. There were no differences between the two groups with respect to the secondary endpoints, which included death, reinfarction, or disabling stroke. Overall bleeding complications were more frequent in the PTCA group, with the exception of intracranial bleeding, which was higher in the t-PA group. This study was felt to reflect community practice in terms of the skills of the PTCA operators.

The findings of the GUSTO investigators suggested that the benefit observed with PTCA was short-lived. Weaver et al. (11) published a meta-analysis of the randomized trials

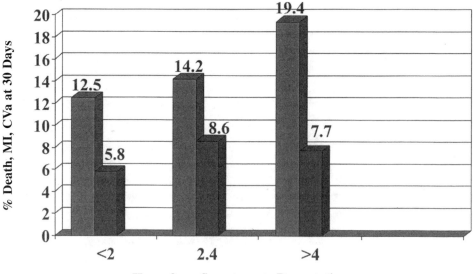

Figure 1 Primary PTCA (dark bars) vs. intravenous thrombolysis (lighter bars).

comparing thrombolytic therapy with PTCA. Ten trials involving 2606 patients were analyzed. There were differences in the type of thrombolytic regimen used (streptokinase, t-PA, and front-loaded t-PA), the patient population, the skill and experience of the operator, and the length of follow-up. The use of primary PTCA was associated with a 34% reduction in mortality at 30 days or less (4.4% vs. 6.5% thrombolytic therapy; $p = 0.02$) The rates of death and nonfatal reinfarction were also significantly reduced by PTCA (7.2% vs. 11.9%; $p < 0.001$), as were the risks of hemorrhagic and nonhemorraghic stroke.

A review of 10 randomized trials by Zijlstra et al. (2635 patients) comparing primary PTCA to intravenous thrombolysis examined clinical characteristics and outcomes based on time from symptom onset to presentation (12). Major adverse cardiac events (death, reinfarction, or stroke) were lower in the primary PTCA groups compared to thrombolysis without regard to time from symptom onset to treatment. With increasing time from onset of symptoms to presentation, there was a significant increase in major adverse cardiac events in the thrombolysis groups. However, this was not found in the primary PTCA treated groups (Fig. 1).

II. ADVANTAGES OF PCI OVER THROMBOLYTIC THERAPY

A. Availability

One of the major advantages of thrombolytic therapy as compared to primary PCI is the widespread availability of thrombolytic therapy and its ease of use. Less than 20% of hospitals in the United States have the facilities to perform primary PCI, and even fewer have the ability to deliver this on a 24-hour basis (13). Effective primary PTCA requires not only the physical infrastructure but also experienced angiographers and technical staff (14). An important criticism of primary PTCA is that large trials for the most part were performed in large centers with high volumes and experienced operators. It remains to be seen whether these results can be widely duplicated in the community setting, although some reports have been promising (15).

The Atlantic Cardiovascular Patient Outcomes Research Team (C-PORT) trial is a randomized, prospective trial that compared primary PCI with thrombolysis in 11 community hospitals from Massachusetts and Maryland without on-site cardiac surgery. The incidence of the composite endpoint of death, recurrent MI, or stroke was less in the primary PTCA group at 6 weeks (10.7% vs. 17.7%; $p = 0.03$) and at 6 months (12.4% vs. 19.9%; $p = 0.03$) (16).

Despite the ease of use and availability of thrombolytic therapy, there remain significant barriers to patients getting timely reperfusion therapy when PTCA is not an option. The presence of contraindications to thrombolytic therapy has been estimated to be as high as 40% in some subgroups. In some instances contraindications to thrombolytic therapy, i.e., recent surgery, active bleeding, or elderly patients, indicate a higher risk of myocardial infarction. The contraindications to primary PTCA are less frequent and often relative but include the inability to use heparin, acute renal failure, unsuitable coronary anatomy (unprotected left main), and contrast allergy. O'Keefe et al. in a report of primary PTCA in 1000 patients found that only 4% had contraindications to PTCA (17). Even in patients without contraindications, thrombolytic therapy may be underutilized. In the NRMI database, 24% of thrombolysis eligible patients were not offered therapy (18). In contrast, most patients with contraindications to thrombolytic therapy can safely be offered PCI.

Approximately two thirds of patients with an acute myocardial infarction present to hospitals without a cardiac catheter laboratory (19). Transferring these patients acutely for primary or rescue PTCA has been shown to be feasible and safe (20–22). Three other recent randomized controlled trials further support the concept of transferring MI patients for primary PCI from community hospitals that do not have PCI capabilities.

The first of these was the PRAGUE study, a multicenter, randomized controlled trial from the Czech Republic designed to find the best reperfusion strategy for patients with acute MI presenting to community hospitals without catheterization labs (23). Three hundred patients were randomized into three groups: (a) on-site thrombolysis (streptokinase) at the community hospital, (b) thrombolysis during transfer for immediate facilitated PCI, and (c) immediate transfer for primary PCI without pretreatment with a thrombolytic drug. The lowest rate of death, MI, or stroke at 30 days occurred in the group transferred for primary PCI without thrombolysis (8% vs. 23% for thrombolysis without transfer, and 15% for the thrombolysis and transfer for facilitated PCI; $p < 0.02$). There were no deaths during transfers. The mean door-to-balloon (from the community hospital) time was 95 minutes in the primary PCI group vs. 108 minutes in the thrombolysis and transfer group. In the group randomized to thrombolysis without transfer, the mean door-to-drug time was 82 minutes.

The more recent DANAMI-2 study is a Danish national, multicenter, randomized controlled trial comparing primary PCI to thrombolysis for the treatment of acute ST elevation MI (24). Participating in this trial were 24 referral hospitals (without PTCA capability) and 5 invasive centers. The distance from the referral hospitals to the invasive centers ranged from 35 to 95 miles. The preliminary results show an overall statistically significant reduction of the primary endpoint of death, reinfarction, or stroke at 30 days for patients treated with primary PTCA (8.0% for primary PTCA vs. 13.7% for thrombolysis; $p < 0.001$). Of the 1572 patients enrolled, 1129 (72%) presented initially to the referral hospitals and were randomized to thrombolysis with front-loaded t-PA vs. transfer for primary PTCA without the thrombolytic. The results favoring primary PTCA also held true for those who presented initially to the referral hospitals (8.5% for transfer for primary PTCA vs. 14.2% for thrombolysis; ($p = 0.002$). There were no deaths during transfer from the referral hospitals to the invasive centers.

A recent U.S. multicenter randomized study, the Air-PAMI study, also compared thrombolysis to transfer for primary PTCA (25). Patients with high-risk acute myocardial infarctions who presented to hospitals without PTCA capabilities were randomized to on-site thrombolysis versus transfer for primary PTCA. The study was prematurely terminated after 39 months and 132 patients due to the inability to recruit the necessary sample size. The mean distance from the referral hospitals to the PTCA center was 32 ± 36 miles. Compared to the PRAGUE and DANAMI-2 studies, a much longer time was needed to transfer the patients. The mean door-to-balloon time in the group transferred for primary PTCA was 174 ± 80 minutes. This delay was largely due to the time taken from randomization and initiation of transfer (mean door to randomization, 52 ± 57 minutes; door to transfer, 104 ± 114 minutes). Despite these delays, there was still a non-statistically significant 38% reduction in major adverse cardiac events (death, reinfarction, or stroke) in the primary PTCA group at 30 days (8.4% vs. 13.6%; $p = 0.331$). The data from these three randomized trials favor transferring patients acutely from hospitals without cardiac catheterization capabilities to regional hospitals that perform primary PTCA. Transferring such patients is safe and feasible. In order to optimize treatment and keep the recommended door-to-balloon times of 90 minutes or less, there needs to be an efficient, coordinated system of regionalized cardiac care, perhaps similar to the trauma system model.

B. Efficacy

Several trials have established that the rapidity and completeness with which reperfusion can be achieved are intimately related to the subsequent mortality and morbidity. This is true whether the method of reperfusion is thrombolytic therapy or PTCA (3,26). Timely restoration of normal antegrade flow in the infarct-related artery (TIMI-3 flow) is associated with better outcomes than either an absence of patency in the infarct related artery (TIMI-0 or TIMI-1 flow) or a patent artery with poor (TIMI-2) flow. The GUSTO angiographic investigators found that TIMI-0 or TIMI-1 flow at 90 minutes was associated with a 30-day mortality of 8.9%. TIMI-2 and TIMI-3 flow were associated with 30-day mortalities of 7.4% and 4.4%, respectively (3). The most effective thrombolytic regimen accelerated or front-loaded t-PA with intravenous heparin has a patency rate at 90 minutes of 81%, whereas the rate of TIMI-3 flow is only 54% (3). The PTCA trials have consistently achieved patency rates of over 90%. The PAMI trial achieved patency rates of 97% (7). The patency rate in GUSTO-2b was 93%, with a TIMI-3 flow rate of 73% (8).

Although PCI is more effective at achieving arterial patency than thrombolytic therapy, the latter therapy is usually quicker to administer, particularly during off-hours. In GUSTO-2b the time from randomization to the administration of the t-PA bolus was a mean of 20 minutes as compared to a median of 76 minutes from randomization to balloon inflation in the angioplasty arm. Shorter randomization to inflation times were noted in the PAMI trial (7) (mean 60 min), but in the NMRI database, which is probably more reflective of real-world practice, the median time from hospital arrival to balloon inflation was 111 minutes (27). It is unclear whether this time advantage of thrombolytic therapy can be translated into better clinical outcomes. If GUSTO efficacy for t-PA is assumed at 110 minutes (20 min for bolus + 90 min), 54% of patients will have TIMI-3 flow. At the same point in time, 73% of the PCI group will have TIMI-3 flow.

Other important considerations include the rates of recurrent ischemia and late reocclusions. Several trials, including the Mayo Clinic, Zwolle, and PAMI, have shown a decrease in the incidence of recurrent ischemia (4, 6, 7). In the case of the PAMI study, this benefit was still present at 6 months. The Zwolle, Netherlands, study reported that the persistent benefit of PTCA in survival free of reinfarction remained at a mean of 5 years of follow-up (6).

With regards to late reocclusion, STENT-PAMI (28) found that at 6-month angiographic follow-up, 9.3% of the PTCA group had occluded the infarct-related artery. This rate was even lower in the stent arm—5.1%. This compares to rates of late reocclusion of 25% at 3 months in the Apricot study (29) and 46% at 6 months in TAMI-6 (30). Although the thrombolytic agents used—streptokinase, anistreplase (APRICOT), and a 3-hour t-PA infusion (TAMI-6)—are less effective than front-loaded t-PA, these results included only patients with patent arteries following thrombolysis.

C. Complications

Both PTCA and thrombolytic therapy are associated with complications. The major concern with thrombolytic therapy is the risk of bleeding (particularly intracranial) with subsequent cerebrovascular accidents (CVA). Accelerated t-PA in the GUSTO trial had a CVA risk of 1.6% with a 0.72% risk of hemorrhagic CVA (10). In the PAMI trial the total CVA rate was 2% in the thrombolytic arm versus 0% in the PTCA arm (7). The risk for hemorrhagic CVA in the thrombolytic arm was 1.5%.

With respect to bleeding in other locations, PCI has generally higher rates. In the GUSTO 2 trial the incidence of all bleeding, severe or life-threatening bleeding, and transfusion was higher in the PTCA arm (40.3, 2.7, and 11.3%, respectively) compared to 34.2, 1.9, and 8.9% in the thrombolytic arms (8). In the PAMI study the risk of bleeding was higher in the PTCA arm, but if the patients who underwent CABG were excluded, the bleeding in the invasive arm was mostly secondary to access site and retroperitoneal hematoma. In this study, GI bleeding was higher in the thrombolytic group.

Weaver et al. in a meta-analysis noted higher incidences of CVA (2.0% vs. 0.7) and hemorraghic CVA (1.1% vs. 0.1) in the thrombolytic arm (11). In this analysis there was no significant difference between overall bleeding complications in both arms.

Angiography also carries small risks of neurovascular injury, contrast allergy, and renal failure, but these have not been significantly different compared to thrombolytic therapy in the randomized trials. This lack of difference may be related to the low absolute risk and the relatively small sample size.

D. Cost

A few studies have examined the relative costs of primary PCI vs. thrombolytic therapy. Stone et al. (31) reviewed the economic data from the PAMI trial. In this study, despite the cost of cardiac catheterization the total hospital charges were similar in the two study arms ($27,653 ± 13,709 vs. $30,227 ± 18,903; $p = 0.21$). The initial cost of the procedure and the associated professional fees in the PTCA arm were counterbalanced by the reduction in morbid events and in duration of hospital stay while in the hospital. In follow-up study up to 2.1 years, posttrial events were the same in the two groups leading to the assumption that posthospital charges were similar. Zijlstra et al. (6) looked at the medical charges for a 2-year period in their comparison of streptokinase with PTCA. They included charges for the initial hospital stay, readmissions, procedures, professional fees, and medications. At the end of the 2-year period, again the costs were similar, with $16,090 for the PTCA arm compared with $16,813 for the thrombolytic arm ($p = 0.05$). Additional considerations in U.S. patients include the fact that hospital DRGs are higher when PCI is performed and the reduced need for noninvasive evaluation.

A substudy of PAMI-2 (32) assessed early discharge in low-risk patients who underwent primary PCI for ST elevation MI. The low-risk patient was defined by the following criteria (age < 70 years, ejection fraction > 45%, one- or two-vessel disease, successful PTCA, and no ventricular arrythmias). The patients were randomized to accelerated or traditional care. The accelerated-care patients were managed in a non–intensive care setting and were discharged at day 3. There were no differences in either in-hospital morbidity or mortality or at 6-month follow-up. The accelerated care patients were discharged 3 days earlier with mean hospital costs of $9,658 ± $5,287 versus $11,604 ± $6,125 ($p = 0.002$).

E. Patients in Shock

Patients with shock in the setting of acute MI have a high mortality (33). In this population the efficacy of thrombolytic therapy is known to be diminished (34). Several non-randomized trials have examined the question of the optimal therapy of MI complicated by shock. These studies have suggested that primary PCI is more effective therapy in this setting when compared to thrombolytics (35). However, these trials are prone to selection bias, with healthier patients more likely to undergo PTCA.

In the SHOCK trial, which randomized patients to an early invasive strategy versus medical therapy (thrombolytic therapy + intra-aortic balloon pump) (36), the success rate of PCI was 77% (TIMI-2 and -3) flow in the invasive arm and 80% in patients in the medical arm who received PCI. Successful PCI was associated with a 30-day mortality of 38% as compared to the mortality of 79% in those in whom PCI was unsuccessful. Of interest is the association of TIMI-3 flow achieved after PTCA with subsequent mortality. In those patients in whom TIMI-3 flow was achieved the in hospital mortality was 33%. This compared to mortality rates of 50 and 86% in those with TIMI-2 and TIMI-1/TIMI-0, respectively (37). The procedural success rate in this group of patients (77%)

is lower when compared to other primary PTCA trials, most likely indicating the high-risk nature of these patients.

III. STENTS

The early trials of primary PCI compared balloon PTCA to thrombolytic therapy. One of the major limitations of balloon PTCA is the potential for restenosis. Nakagawa et al. performed serial angiographic follow-up on patients who received primary PTCA (38). The restenosis rate was 20% at 3 weeks and 47% at one year. The reocclusion rate was 14% at one year. Recent years have seen an increase in the use of routine stenting. The benefits of routine stenting include larger luminal diameters, less acute closure, and less restenosis (39). Trials have been performed to determine if these benefits translate into better clinical outcome in the setting of acute myocardial infarction.

One of the larger studies Stent-Pami (28) randomized 900 patients to PTCA alone or with the routine use of a heparin-coated Palmaz-Schatz stent. Procedural success was obtained in 99.3% of the stent group and 98.4% of the PTCA group. The stent group had larger minimal luminal diameters of 2.56 ± 0.44 mm versus 2.12 ± 0.45 mm ($p \leq 0.001$), less residual stenosis of $11.1 \pm 11.6\%$ versus $25.1 \pm 11.9\%$, and less dissection of 11.9 versus 30.8. The rates of TIMI-2 or TIMI-3 flow were similar in the two groups—99.3% stent versus 98.3 PTCA alone ($p = 0.22$). If TIMI-3 flow rates alone were considered, there was a trend towards lower TIMI-3 flow rates in the stent arm compared to the PTCA arm—89.4% versus 92.7% ($p = 0.1$). During hospitalization, bleeding complications, rates of recurrent ischemia, and lengths of stay were similar in both groups.

The primary endpoint of death, reinfarction, disabling stroke, or target vessel revascularization for ischemia at 6 months was significantly reduced in the stent group—12.6% versus 20.1% ($p < 0.01$). This difference was driven primarily by the differences in the rates of target vessel revascularization—7.7% in the stent arm versus 17% in the PTCA arm ($p \leq 0.0010$). All individual components of the primary endpoint were not significantly different at 6 months. Angiographic follow-up performed at 6 months revealed a restenosis rate of 20.3% in the stent arm versus 33.5% in the PTCA arm ($p \leq 0.001$).

The superiority of stenting compared to balloon PTCA was confirmed in the FRESCO study, which randomized 150 patients to stenting or no further therapy after optimal PTCA (40). Optimal acute results (<30% residual and TIMI-3 flow) were obtained in 100% of the stent arm and 98.5% of the PTCA arm. The primary endpoint was a composite of death, reinfarction, or target vessel revascularization secondary to ischemia. At 6 months, freedom from the composite endpoint was 87% in the stent arm versus 68% in the PTCA arm ($p = 0.002$). Again, this difference was principally attributable to a significant reduction in TVR for ischemia.

The largest trial of stenting in acute myocardial infarction is the CADILLAC trial (41). This multicenter trial studied 2665 patients randomized to four groups: primary stenting, primary PTCA with bailout stenting, stenting + abciximab, and PTCA + abciximab. The primary endpoint was a composite of death, reinfarction, disabling CVA, or the need for a repeat procedure for ischemia at 6 months. The primary endpoint was achieved in 20% of the PTCA-only group versus 10.9% of the stent group. The rates of death, reinfarction, or disabling CVA were the same in all group, but target vessel revascularization for ischemia was much less in the stent group—7.4% versus 14.2% in the PTCA group.

The STAT trial compared primary PTCA with stenting to front-loaded t-PA (42). The clinical endpoint in this trial was a composite of death, reinfarction, CVA, or repeat TVR for ischemia. The composite endpoint at 6 months was 24.2% in the stent arm versus 55.7% in the thrombolytic arm ($p < 0.001$).

IV. OTHER DEVICES

For the most part balloon PTCA in combination with routine stenting is the mainstay of interventional therapy of ST elevation myocardial infarction. The use of atherectomy devices has been disappointing. In a small study of directional atherectomy by Saito et al., DCA was associated with a higher incidence of restenosis when compared to balloon PTCA despite a larger minimal luminal diameter at the end of the procedure (43). Rotational atherectomy is contraindicated as it is associated with a higher incidence of distal embolization and microvascular obstruction, resulting in the no-reflow phenomenon (44). This syndrome of poor epicardial flow despite a patent artery is also seen with balloon PTCA and stenting in the setting of acute MI and has been associated with poor outcome (45,46).

Two newer devices may reduce the incidence of no reflow. These are the Angiojet thrombectomy device and distal protection devices. The Angiojet Catheter (Possis Medical Inc., Minneapolis, MN) is a rheolytic thrombolytic device. Saline jets are used to create a Venturi effect at the catheter tip. This vortex of negative pressure causes fragmentation of the thrombus, which can then be aspirated, lowering thrombus burden prior to treatment of the lesion. One of the earlier reports from Nakagawa et al. reviewed 31 selected patients (47). The use of the Angiojet device resulted in the increase in mean TIMI grade flow from 0.7 to 2.61. This was followed by balloon PTCA or stenting (40%) with no adverse events.

Silva et al. presented the results of Angiojet use in 89 patients, noting a 7% incidence of death, reinfarction, or revasularization at 30 days (48). Percentage diameter stenosis was reduced from 82 to 50%. Procedural complications included distal embolization (2%), no reflow (2%), and abrupt closure (2%). Other small nonrandomized studies have concluded that the device may be used safely with abciximab. However, larger randomized studies are needed to confirm the safety and efficacy of this device in this setting.

Another device with promise in decreasing the incidence of the no reflow phenomenon is the Percusurge Gaurdwire Plus (AVE/Medtronic) (49). This is a distal protection device consisting of a guidewire with an occluding balloon at the distal end. The balloon is positioned beyond the stenosis and inflated before PTCA is performed. Debris is aspirated prior to deflation of the balloon. The device is currently approved only for saphenous vein grafts. Small studies have suggested that use of this device may result in improved blush scores and TIMI frame counts post-PCI. However, more data are needed, and several other distal protection devices are under investigation. Therefore, both the distal protection device and Angiojet may have a role in reducing distal embolization, the no-reflow phenomenon, and ultimately in improving patient outcome.

It is clear that if primary PCI can be performed in a timely fashion by experienced operators, it is superior to thrombolytic therapy for reperfusion. It has been suggested that the method of initial reperfusion in ST elevation myocardial infarction should be tailored to the risk of subsequent morbidity and mortality. Patients at low risk will do well with either thrombolytic therapy or primary PCI. The GUSTO investigators identified anterior myocardial infarction, age > 70 years, systolic blood pressure < 100 mmHg, heart rate greater than 100, and cardiogenic shock as risk factors for poor outcome after thrombolysis (50). In our opinion, primary PCI, when available in qualified centers, should be the method of choice for initial reperfusion, particularly in the high-risk patient.

V. RESCUE PCI

The use of thrombolytic therapy for reperfusion of ST elevation MI is associated with failure in a significant number of patients, often resulting in continued clinical signs or electrocardiographic evidence of ischemia. However, predicting failure of thrombolysis remains a difficult task. The GUSTO angiographic investigators recorded an overall incidence of 30% of failure in the thrombolytic therapy group (defined as TIMI grade 0 or 1 flow at 90 min) (50). This failure rate is even higher if TIMI-3 flow is considered as the marker for successful thromblysis. This group of patients is at higher risk of mortality compared to those in whom thrombolytic therapy is successful (3). Rescue PCI is performed in the setting of failed thrombolysis in an attempt to achieve coronary patency with the hope of decreasing subsequent morbidity and mortality. Randomized trials of rescue PCI are difficult to perform as many physicians are reluctant to randomize patients who have failed thrombolysis in the conservative arm.

The initial use of PTCA in this group was somewhat controversial as intervention in the postthrombolytic millieu was thought to be less effective and prone to higher complications rates. One of the earlier reports to review the use of PTCA in this setting was the CORAMI trial (51). The authors described their experience in rescue PTCA in a group of patients who had failed thrombolytic therapy. The failure rate (TIMI grade 0 or 1 flow) of thrombolysis was 29% (72 patients). PTCA was attempted in 90% of those in whom lysis failed with a procedural success rate of 90%. There was no mortality difference between failed and successful PTCA in this small nonrandomized study. Patients received aspirin and IV heparin during the PTCA procedure, but there is no information regarding the level of anticoagulation achieved during the procedure. The survival rate of the patients who failed thrombolysis as a whole was 92% at 18 months, which is higher than reported in other trials (50).

The RESCUE investigators in a nonrandomized subset analysis (52) randomized 151 patients with anterior MI who had failed thrombolytic therapy to rescue PTCA or medical therapy. The procedural success rate was 92%. The primary combined endpoint of death and congestive heart failure was reduced in the PTCA group (6% in the PTCA group and 17% in the medical arm).

The GUSTO angiographic investigators in a nonrandomized subset analysis (50) compared the use of rescue PTCA in 198 patients who had failed thrombolytic therapy with patients who were managed conservatively (266 patients) (42). Failure of thrombolysis was diagnosed by angiography 90 minutes after lysis, and the decision to perform PTCA was at the discretion of the angiographer. This study confirmed the efficacy of PTCA in this setting with procedural success in 88.4% of cases with TIMI-3 flow rates in 68%. Significantly, the rates of major bleeding, surgical repair, stroke, and emergency CABG were the same as the group managed conservatively. The left ventricular function was superior in the group undergoing successful rescue PTCA as compared to the arm managed conservatively, but the 30-day mortality was similar in the two arms. Both left ventricular function and mortality were lower than in those with initially successful thrombolytic therapy. Of note, the mortality in the patients with unsuccessful PTCA was 30.4% (7 of 23), including 5 of the 7 patients in cardiogenic shock prior to PTCA.

An interesting hybrid approach was studied by the PACT investigators (53). Six hundred and six patients with ST elevation were randomized to half-dose rt-PA or placebo. All patients were then taken to immediate angiography. Patients with TIMI flows 0–2 underwent rescue PCI (thrombolysis patients) or primary PCI in those given placebo. The patients given thrombolytics were twice as likely to have patent IRAs (TIMI-2 or TIMI-3 flow) as compared to those given placebo (61% vs. 34%; $p < 0.001$) with TIMI-3 flow rates of 33% (thrombolytic group) versus 15% (placebo group). The success of PCI was similar in the thrombolytic and placebo groups. The primary endpoint of the study, left ventricular function, was highest in the group that had TIMI-3 flow at the time of angiography. The lowest ejection fractions were noted in those patients who never regained TIMI-3 flows. Of note, successful PCI with TIMI-3 flow within one hour of study drug administration had the same outcome as in patients who were initially found to have TIMI-3 flow. The rates of major bleeding were the same in the placebo and thrombolytic arms (13.5% vs. 12.9%; $p = 0.84$)

The above studies suggest that PTCA can be performed safely and effectively in the postthrombolytic period with acceptable risk. Based on available data, there appears to be improved outcome in patients in whom rescue PCI is successful. Thus, we would recommend cardiac catheterization for patients with ongoing chest pain, persistent ST elevation, or hemodynamic instability after thrombolysis. However, unsuccessful attempts at PCI portend a poor outcome for this high-risk patient subgroup.

VI. ROUTINE PTCA AFTER THROMBOLYSIS

In contrast to the proven efficacy of PTCA in the setting of primary PCI or failed thrombolysis, available studies do not support the routine use of PCI after successful thrombolysis in the absence of either spontaneous or inducible recurrent ischemia. The use of routine PTCA has been looked at as early (within 18–24 hours postthrombolysis) or delayed up to 7 days.

The European Cooperative Study Group (54) assessed the use of immediate PCI versus conservative management following rt-PA infusion. PTCA was attempted in the invasive arm if a coronary stenosis of >60% was present irrespective of TIMI flow rates. The trial was stopped early because of a trend towards higher mortality in the invasive arm. The primary endpoint of enzymatically determined infarct size and left ventricular function was similar in both arms.

The TIMI-2A substudy compared three strategies in 586 patients who had received a 6-hour infusion of t-PA (55). One arm underwent immediate angiography and PTCA if the infarct-related vessel was not patent, the second arm underwent deferred angiography at 18–24 hours after lysis, and the third arm was managed conservatively with angiography undertaken for spontaneous ischemia or predischarge. The primary endpoint of left ventricular ejection fraction at discharge was the same in all arms. The success rate of PTCA in the immediate angiography arm was low by current standards (76.6%). In the deferred angiography arm the success rate was somewhat higher (89.7%). The important limitations of this study were: (a) aspirin started as late as day 2 and many patients not on aspirin at time of PTCA procedure, (b) unknown level of anticoagulation, and (c) exclusion of patients with occluded arteries.

In the conservative arm 12.2% of patients had ischemia that was refractory to medical therapy by day 5 and thus underwent angiography. At discharge angiography the invasive arms had less stenosis of the infarct related artery but similar ejection fractions as compared to the conservative arm. At 6 weeks there was a trend towards more inducible ischemia on exercise testing in the conservative arm. At one year the rates of death, fatal or nonfatal myocardial infarction, CABG, and inducible ischemia on stress testing were similar in all groups. However, it should be noted that half of the deaths in the invasive arm occurred prior to PTCA. The invasive groups at one year still had a higher rate of PTCA than the conservative arm. The immediate invasive arm also had a higher requirement for transfusion as compared to the delayed invasive and conservative arms.

The TIMI-2 trial compared the strategies of routine coronary angiography with PTCA within 18–24 hours after thrombolytic therapy versus a conservative therapy in which angiography was reserved for those patients with evidence of spontaneous ischemia (56). A total of 3262 patients were randomized. The success rate of PTCA was 93%. Of the patients randomized to the conservative arm, 32.7% underwent angiography within 14 days and 13.3% had PTCA. The primary endpoint of death and reinfarction at 42 days was not statistically different in the two arms (10.9% invasive vs. 9.7% conservative; $p = 0.25$). The conservative arm had a higher incidence of inducible ischemia at hospital discharge resulting in angiography and PTCA (12.8% invasive vs. 17.7% conservative; $p < 0.001$) At 6 weeks the left ventricular ejection fraction and inducible ischemia on exercise testing was the same.

Two studies that have looked at a routine delayed invasive strategy after successful thrombolysis are the SWIFT and TAMI studies. The SWIFT study (57) looked at 800 patients after thrombolysis with anistreplase and IV heparin. The patients were random- ized to a conservative or invasive strategy within 12 hours of thrombolysis. The invasive arm required coronary angiography within 48 hours with PTCA attempted for lesions of >50% at the discretion of the operator. Angiography in the conservative arm was permitted for recurrent ischemia or a positive stress test. One hundred and sixty-nine patients in the invasive arm (43%) underwent PTCA as compared to 3% of the conservative group. At 12 months mortality, anginal symptoms and left ventricular function were the same in both groups.

The TAMI trial (58) studied patients postthrombolysis who had immediate angiog- raphy. Patients who had a patent artery with >50% stenosis were randomized to immediate PTCA versus delayed PTCA at 7 days. The PTCA success rates were similar in the two groups, as was the follow-up left ventricular ejection fraction. Only 51% of patients ini- tially randomized to deferred PTCA underwent PTCA. In 15% of these patients there was no longer a significant lesion noted, and 13% underwent CABG.

In contrast to the routine use of PCI in angiographically significant stenosis post- thrombolysis, selective revascularization in patients who have either spontaneous or inducible ischemia has been shown to be of benefit. A large multicenter trial, the DANAMI trial, was performed at 43 centers in Denmark (59). This study randomized 1008 patients who had received thrombolytics for acute myocardial infarction and who had either spon- taneous or inducible ischemia (on predischarge exercise stress testing) to a conservative versus invasive strategy. Revascularization in the invasive arm (PTCA in 52.9% and CABG in 29%) was performed within 2 weeks of randomization.

The primary endpoints of the study were death, reinfarction, and admission for unstable angina. After 2.4 years of follow-up, there was no significant difference in mor- tality, but reinfarction was lower in the invasive arm (5.6% vs. 10.5%; $p = 0.0038$), as was admission for unstable angina (17.9% vs. 29.5%; $p < 0.00001$). The patients in the inva- sive arm also had less ischemia as measured by anginal class and use of anti-ischemia medications. The authors concluded that in selected patients a strategy of delayed revacu- larization may be beneficial in patients with inducible ischemia.

Despite the absence of improved clinical outcome in the strategy of routine PCI fol- lowing successful thrombolysis, several studies have suggested that there are important ben- efits to be derived from opening the infarct-related artery. Reductions in ventricular excitability (60) infarct expansion (61), and ventricular remodeling (62) have been described, especially with regard to the left anterior descending artery. It should also be noted that most of the clinical outcome data come from a time when stenting was used infrequently and adju- vant therapy such as GP IIb/IIIa inhibitors were unavailable. However, based on available data, the use of angiography after successful reperfusion with thrombolytics should be reserved for patients with recurrent ischemia, inducible ischemia, impaired left ventricular function, or patients at high risk for subsequent morbidity or mortality.

VII. SUMMARY

Primary PCI is effective therapy for the treatment of ST elevation MI, offering significant benefits compared to thrombolytic therapy if it can be performed in a timely fashion by experienced operators. Rescue PCI is safe and may offer some benefit to patients who have ongoing ischemia or are unstable after thrombolysis. Current data do not support routine PCI after successful thrombolysis in patients without recurrent ischemia or high-risk clinical features.

REFERENCES

1. Davies MJ, Thomas AC. Plaque fissuring—the cause of acute MI, sudden ischemic death and crescendo angina. Br Heart J 1985; 53:363.
2. The GISSI Authors. Effectiveness of intravenous thrombolytic treatment in acute myocardial infarction. Lancet 1986; 1:397-401.
3. The GUSTO Angiographic Investigators. The effects of tissue plasminogen activator, streptokinase or both on coronary artery patency, ventricular function, and survival after acute myocardial infarction. N Engl J Med 1993; 329:1615–1622.
4. Gibbons RJ, Holmes DR, Reeder GS, Bailey KR, Hopfenspirger MR, Gersh BJ. Immediate angioplasty compared with the administration of a thrombolytic agent followed by conservative treatment for myocardial infarction. N Engl J Med 1993; 328:685–691.
5. Zijlstra F, Jan De Boer M, Hoorntje JCA, Reiffers S, Reiber JHC, Suryapranata H. A comparison of immediate coronary angioplasty with intravenous streptokinase in acute myocardial infarction. N Engl J Med 1993; 328:680–684.
6. Zijlstra F, Hoorntje JCA, Jan de Boer M, Reiffers S, Miedema K, Ottervanger JP, et al. Long term benefit of primary angioplasty as compared with thrombolytic therapy for acute myocardial infarction. N Engl J Med 1999; 341:1413–1419.
7. Grines CL, Browne KF, Marco j, Rothbaum D, Stone GW, O'Keefe J, Overlie P, et al. A comparison of immediate angioplasty with thrombolytic therapy for acute myocardial infarction. N Engl J Med 1993; 328:673–679.
8. Stone GW, Grines CL Browne KF, Marco J, Rothbaum D and O'Keefe J, et al. Predictors of in-hospital and 6 month outcome after acute myocardial infarction in the reperfusion era: the Primary Angioplasty in Myocardial Infarction (PAMI) trial. J Am Coll Cardiol 1995; 25:370–377.
9. The Global Use of Strategies To Open Occluded Coronary Arteries in Acute Coronary Syndromes (GUSTO IIB) Angioplasty Substudy Investigators. N Engl J Med 1997; 336:1621–1628.
10. The GUSTO Investigators. An international randomized trial comparing 4 thrombolytic strategies for myocardial infarction. N Engl J Med 1993; 329:673–682.
11. Weaver WD, Simes J, Betriu A, Grines CL, Zijlstra F, Garcia E, et al. Comparison of primary coronary angioplasty and intravenous thrombolytic therapy for acute myocardial infarction. A quantitative review. JAMA. 1997; 278:2093–2098.
12. Zijlstra F, Patel A, Jones M, Grines C, et al. Clinical characteristics and outcome of patients with early (>2h), intermediate (2–4h) and late (>4h) presentation treated by primary coronary angioplasty or thrombolytic therapy for acute myocardial infarction. Eur Heart J 2002; 23:550–557.
13. Ryan TJ, Antman E M, Brooks N H, Califf R M, Hillis L D, Hrratzka L F, et al. ACC/AHA guidelines for the management of patients with acute myocardial infarction. J Am Coll Cardiol 1996; 28:1328–1428.

14. Bashore TM, Bates ER, Kern MJ, Berger PB, Laskey WK, Clark DA. American College of Cardiology/Society for Cardiac Angiography and Interventions Clinical Expert Consensus. Doucment on Cardiac Catheterization Laboratory Standards. J Am Coll Cardiol 2001; 37:2170–214.

15. Ashmore RC, Luckasen GJ, Larson DG, Miller WE, Whitsitt TB, Downes TR, et al. Immediate angioplasty for acute myocardial infarction. A community hospitals experience. J Invasive Cardiol 1999; 11:61–65.

16. Aversano T, et al. Thrombolytic therapy vs primary percutaneous coronary intervention for myocardial infarction in patients presenting to hospitals without on-site cardiac surgery. A randomized controlled trial. JAMA 2002; 287(15):1943–1951.

17. O'Keefe Jr, JH, Bailey WL, Rutherford BD, Hartzier GO. Primary angioplasty for acute myocardial infarction in 1000 consecutive patients. Results in an unselected population and high risk subgroups. Am J Cardiol 1993; 72:107G–115G.

18. Barron HV, Bowlby LJ, Breen T, Rogers WJ, Canto JG, Zhang Y, et al. Use of reperfusion therapy for acute myocardial infarction in the United States. Data from the National Registry of Myocardial Infarction. Circulation 1998; 97:1150–1156.

19. Thiemann DR, Coresh J, Oetgen W, Powe N. The association between hospital volume and survival after acute myocardial infarction in elderly patients. NEJM 1999; 340:1640–1648.

20. Zijlstra F, van't Hof W, Liem A, et al. Transferring patients for primary angioplasty: a retrospective analysis of 104 selected high risk patients with acute myocardial infarction. Heart 1997; 78:333–336.

21. Straumann E, Yoon S, Naegeli J. Hospital transfer for primary coronary angioplasty in high risk patients with acute myocardial infarction. Heart 1999; 82:415–419.

22. Vermeer F, Oude Ophius A, vd Berg E, et al. Prospective randomized comparison between thrombolysis, rescue PTCA, and primary PTCA in patients with extensive myocardial infarction admitted to a hospital without PTCA facilities: a safety and feasibility study. Heart 1999; 82:426–431.

23. Widimsky P, Groch L, Zelizko M. Multicentre randomized trial comparing transport to primary angioplasty vs. immediate thrombolysis vs. combined strategy for patients with acute myocardial infarction presenting to a community hospital without a catheterization laboratory. The PRAGUE Study. Eur Heart J 2000; 21:823–831.

24. Anderson HR. The Danish multicenter randomized study on thrombolytic therapy versus acute coronary angioplasty in acute myocardial infarction (DANAMI-2). American College of Cardiology Scientific Sessions, Atlanta, GA, March 20, 2002.

25. Grines C, Westerhausen D, Grines L, et al. A randomized trial of transfer for primary angioplasty versus on-site thrombolysis in patients with high-risk myocardial infarction. The Air Primary Angioplasty in Myocardial Infarction Study. J Am Coll Cardiol 2002; 39:1713–1719.

26. Cannon CP, Gibson CM, Lambrew CT, Shoultz DA, Levy D, French WJ, et al. Relationship of symptom onset to balloon time and door to balloon time with mortality in patients undergoing angioplasty for acute myocardial infarction. JAMA 2000; 283(22):2941–2947.

27. Tiefenbrunn AJ, Chandra NC, French WJ, Gore JM and Rogers WJ. Clinical experience with primary percutaneous transluminal coronary angioplasty compared with alteplase (recombinant tissue type plasminogen activator) in patients with acute myocardial infarction. A report from the second national registry of myocardial infarction (NRMI-2). J Am Coll Cardiol 31(6):1240–1245.

28. Grines CL, Cox DA, Stone GW, Garcia E, Mattos LA, Giambartolomei A et al. Coronary angioplasty with or without stent implantation for acute myocardial infarction. N Engl J Med; 341:1949–1956.

29. Meijer A, Verheugt FW, Werter CJ, Kie KI, Van der Pol JM, Van Eenige MJ. Aspirin versus coumadin in the prevention of reocclusion and recurrent ischemia after successful thrombolysis; a prospective placebo controlled angiographic study. Results of the APRICOT Study. Circulation 1993; 87(5):1524–1530.

30. Topol EJ, Ellis SG, Wall TC, et al. Does late reperfusion therapy for myocardial infarction improve left ventricular function? Preliminary results of the TAMI-6 randomised controlled trial. J Am Coll Cardiol 1991; 17:45A.

31. Stone GW, Grines CL, Rothbaum D, Browne KF, O'Keefe J, Overlie PA, et al. Analysis of the relative costs and effectiveness of primary angioplasty versus tissue-type plasminogen activator: the primary angioplasty in myocardial infarction (PAMI) trial. J Am Coll Cardiol 1997; 29:901–907.

32. Grines CL, Marsalese DL, Brodie B, Griffin J, Donohue B, Costantini CR, et al. Safety and cost effectiveness of early discharge after primary angioplasty in low risk patients with acute myocardial infarction. PAMI-II investigators. Primary angioplasty in myocardial infarction. J Am Coll Cardiol 1998; 31:967–972.

33. Goldberg R, Gore J, Alpert J, Osganian V, de Groot J, Bade J, et al. Cardiogenic Shock after acute myocardial infarction. Incidence and mortality from a community wide perspective, 1975 to 1988. N Engl J Med 1991; 325:1117–1122.

34. Brewitt RM, Gu S, Gareber PJ, Ducas J. Marked systemic hypotension depresses coronary thrombolysis induced by intracoronary administration of recombinant tissue type plasminogen activator. J Am Coll Cardiol 1992; 20:1626–1633.

35. Hesdai D, Topol E J, Califf RM, Berger PB, Holmes DR. Cardiogenic shock complicating acute coronary syndromes. Lancet 2000; 356:749–756.

36. Hochman JS, Sleeper LA, Webb JG, Sanborn TA, White HD, Talley JD, et al. Early revascularization in acute myocardial infarction complicated by cardiogenic shock. Shock Investigators. Should we emergently revascularize occluded coronaries for cardiogenic shock. N Engl J Med 1999; 341(9):625–634.

37. Webb JG, Sanborn TA, Sleeper LA, Carere RG, Buller CE, Slater JN, et al. Percutaneous coronary intervention for cardiogenic shock in the Shock trial registry. Am Heart J 2001; 141:964–970.

38. Nakagawa Y, Iwasaki Y, Kimura T, Tamura T, Yokoi H, Yokoi H, et al. Serial angiographic follow-up after successful direct angioplasty for acute myocardial infarction. Am J Cardiol 1996; 78:980–984.

39. Weaver WD, Reisman MA, Griffin JJ, Buller CE, Leimgruber PP, Henry T, et al. Optimum percutaneous transluminal coronary angioplasty compared with routine stent strategy trial (OPUS-1): a randomised trial. Lancet 2000 24; 355:2199–2203.

40. Antoniucci D, Santoro GM, Bolognese L, Valenti R, Trapani M, Fazzini F. A clinical trial comparing primary stenting of the infarct related artery with optimal primary angioplasty for acute myocardial infarction. J Am Coll Cardiol 1998; 31:1234–1239.

41. Stone GW, Grines CL, Cox DA, et al. for the CADILLAC Investigators. Comparison of angioplasty with stenting, with or without abciximab, in acute myocardial infarction. N Engl J Med 2002; 346:957–966.

42. Le May MR, Labinaz M, Davies RF, Marquis JF, Laramee LA, O'Brien ER, et al. Stenting versus thrombolysis in acute myocardial infarction trial (STAT). J Am Coll Cardiol 2001; 37:985–991.

43. Saito S, Kim K Hosokawa G, Tanaka S, Miyake S, Harada K, et al. Short and long term clinical effects of primary directional coronary atherectomy for acute myocardial infarction. Cathet Cardiovasc Diagn 1996; 39:166–167.

44. Abbo KM, Dooris M, Glazier S, O'Neil WW, Byrd D, Grines CL, et al. Features and outcome of no reflow after percutaneous coronary intervention. Am J Cardiol 75(12):778–782.

45. Mercho N, Eldin AM, Shareef B, Glazier JJ, Abbas S A, et al. Angiographic complications of primary angioplasty (abstr). J Am Coll Cardiol 1996; 61A.

46. Ito H, Maruyama A, Iwakura K, Takiuchi S, Masuyama T, Hori M, et al. Clinical implications of the "no reflow" phenomenon. A predictor of complications and left ventricular remodelling in reperfused anterior wall myocardial infarction. Circulation 1996; 93(2):223–228.

47. Nakagawa Y, Matsuo S, Kimura T, Yokoi H, Tamura T, Hamasaki N, et al. Thrombectomy with Angiojet catheter in native coronary arteries for patients with acute or recent myocardial infarction. Am J Cardiol 1999; 83:1–6.

48. Silva JA, Ramee SR, Kuntz R, Dandreo K, Popma J. Mechanical thrombectomy using the Angiojet catheter in the treatment of acute myocardial infarction. J Am Coll Cardiol 1998; 31:410A–411A.

49. Baim D, Wahr D, George B, Leon MB, Greenberg J, Cutlip DE, et al. Randomized trial of a distal embolic protection device during percutaneous intervention of saphenous vein aorto-coronary bypass grafts. Circulation 2002; 105:r13–r18.

50. Ross A M, Lundergan C F, Rohrbeck S C, Boyle D H, Van Den Brand M, Buller C H. Rescue angioplasty after failed thrombolysis: technical and clinical outcomes in a large thrombolysis trial. J Am Coll Cardiol 1998; 31:1511–1517.

51. The CORAMI Study Group. Outcome of attempted rescue coronary angioplasty after failed thrombolysis for acute myocardial infarction. Am J Cardiol 1994; 74(2):172–174.

52. Ellis SG, Da Silva ER, Heyndrickx G, Talley JD, Cernigliaro C, Sleg G, et al. Randomised comparison of rescue angioplasty with conservative management of patients with early failure of thrombolysis for acute anterior myocardial infarction. Circulation 1994; 90:2280–2284.

53. Ross AM, Coyne KS, Reiner JS, Greenhouse SW, Fink C, Frey A, et al. A randomized trial comparing primary angioplasty with a strategy of short acting thrombolysis and immediate planned rescue angioplasty in acute myocardial infarction: the PACT trial. J Am Coll Cardiol 1999; 34:1954–1962.

54. De Bono DP. The European Cooperative Study Group trial of intravenous recombinant tissue type plasminogen activator (rt-PA) and conservative therapy versus rt-PA and immediate coronary angioplasty. J Am Coll Cardiol 1988; 12(suppl A):20A–23A.

55. Rogers WJ, Baim DS, Gore JM, Brown G, Roberts R, Williams DO, et al. Comparison of immediate invasive, delayed invasive and conservative strategies after tissue-type plasminogen activator. Circulation 1990; 81:1457–1476.

56. The TIMI Study Group. Comparison of invasive and conservative strategies after treatment with intravenous tissue plasminogen in acute myocardial infarction. N Engl J Med 1989; 320:618–627.

57. The SWIFT (Should We Intervene Following Thrombolysis) Trial Study Group. SWIFT trial of delayed elective intervention versus conservative treatment after thrombolysis with anistreplase in acute myocardial infarction. Br Med J 1991; 302:555–558.

58. Topol EJ, Califf RM, Kereiakes DJ, George LS. Thmbolysis and Angioplasty in Myocardial Infarction (TAMI) trial. J Am Coll Cardiol 1987; 10:65B–74B.

59. Madsen J K, Grande P, Saunamaki K, Thayssen P, Kassis E, Erikssen U, et al. Danish multicenter study of invasive versus conservative treatment in patients with inducible ischemia after thrombolysis in acute myocardial infarction. Circulation 1997; 96:748–755.

60. Boehrer JD, Glamann DB, Lange RA, Willard JE, Brogan WC 3rd, Eichorn EJ, et al. Effect of coronary angioplasty on late potentials one to two weeks after acute myocardial infarction. Am J Cardiol 1992; 70:1515–1519.

61. Jeremy RW, Hackworthy RA, Bautovich G, Hutton BF, Harris PJ. Infarct artery perfusion and changes in left ventricular volume in the month after acute myocardial infarction. J Am Coll Cardiol 1987; 9:989–995.

62. Pizzetti G, Belotti G, Margonato A, Cappelletti A, Chierchia SL. Coronary recanalization by elective angioplasty prevents ventricular dilation after anterior myocardial infarction. J Am Coll Cardiol 1996; 28:846–848

14-1

Adjunctive Anticoagulant Therapy During Percutaneous Coronary Intervention

John J. Young, Wojciech Mazur, and Dean J. Kereiakes
The Lindner Center for Research & Education and The Ohio Heart Health Center, Cincinnati, Ohio, U.S.A.

I. INTRODUCTION

Thrombosis plays a central role in the pathogenesis of the acute ischemic syndromes and the complications of percutaneous coronary revascularization. Rupture of atherosclerotic plaque initiates thrombosis and occurs spontaneously in the acute ischemic syndromes or is induced by percutaneous revascularization devices. Plaque rupture exposes thrombogenic subendothelial components, which leads to platelet aggregation and initiation of the coagulation cascade. Propagation of thrombus may lead to partial or complete arterial occlusion and end-organ ischemia or infarction. Moreover, platelet-thrombus formation may be important in the progression of stable atherosclerotic plaque. In addition to cellular migration and proliferation, episodic plaque rupture, thrombus formation, and incorporation of thrombus into the plaque may contribute to gradual, step-wise progression of arterial lumen compromise. Antithrombotic agents are therefore integral to management strategies for acute and chronic coronary artery disease.

II. PERCUTANEOUS CORONARY INTERVENTION

The acute success rate of percutaneous coronary intervention (PCI) has continued to increase since its introduction, despite a widening scope of indications (1–3). The processes of balloon dilatation and ablative new technologies denude the arterial endothelial barrier, exposing atherosclerotic material and connective tissue elements to circulating blood (4–6). Tissue factor from the disrupted plaque combines with factor VII in the presence of platelet phospholipid membrane to produce activated factor X (Xa), which in turn converts prothrombin to thrombin (classic extrinsic coagulation pathway) (7–9). Thrombin converts fibrinogen to fibrin, directly activates platelets, and binds antithrombin. The formation of thrombin-antithrombin III complexes depletes endogenous antithrombin capacity and may contribute to a prothrombotic milieu.

   Following deep arterial wall injury, platelets adhere to exposed collagen, von Willebrand factor, and fibrinogen via specific cell receptors [glycoprotein (GP) Ia/IIa, GP Ib-IX, GP IIb/IIIa, respectively] and become activated by independent mediators including collagen, thromboxane, serotonin, epinephrine, adenosine diphosphate (ADP), and thrombin (9–11) (Fig. 1). Activated platelets degranulate and secrete chemotaxins, clotting factors, and vasoconstrictors that promote further thrombin generation, vasospasm, and platelet aggregation (12–14). Clinical and laboratory investigations have demonstrated that the coagulation cascade is activated during balloon angioplasty with thrombin production and thrombus deposition at the site of arterial wall injury (15–21). Hence, myocardial ischemic complications related to thrombus are observed to complicate 4–12% of PCI procedures (22–26).

Abrupt vessel closure during or shortly after balloon angioplasty was still observed in 2–5% of patients undergoing catheter-based revascularization procedures (23–29). Abrupt vessel closure may result in myocardial infarction (10–35%) or death (2–5%) despite attempts at urgent reintervention. (23–29). Coronary artery stents are currently placed in more than 70% of elective interventions, in part because they are very effective in preventing abrupt vessel closure (30). Stenting, however, is associated with a unique and potentially devastating complication, subacute thrombosis, which follows 1–4% of procedures (31,32). Unfortunately, the majority of patients who experience this complication suffer myocardial infarction (MI) and/or die. Thrombosis plays a major role in acute/subacute vessel closure following both balloon angioplasty and stenting. This chapter will review the current status of anticoagulant therapy to prevent thrombotic complications associated with PCI.

III. UNFRACTIONATED HEPARIN

Unfractionated heparin (UFH) is a glycosaminoglycan composed of a heterogeneous mixture of molecules of different molecular weights. The anticoagulant action of UFH is

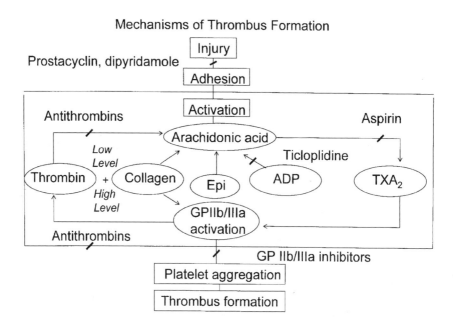

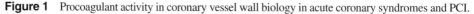

Figure 1   Procoagulant activity in coronary vessel wall biology in acute coronary syndromes and PCI.

derived from the binding of approximately one third of UFH molecules to antithrombin III (AT-III), leading to a conformational change that markedly enhances the affinity of the UFH AT-III complex to inactivate thrombin (33). UFH avidly binds to endothelial cells, macrophages, and plasma proteins, which results in two distinct clearance phases from the body. An initial rapid equilibration phase is followed by a slower, saturable elimination phase (34). The binding capacity for UFH varies by individual as heparin-binding proteins are largely acute phase reactants. Thus, the half-life of UFH is both variable and dose dependent (33). Natural inhibitors of UFH (platelet factor 4) may be released from thrombus and further alter UFH dose-response relationship, especially when large amounts of thrombus are present (33).

Controversy exists with regard to appropriate periprocedural dosing and strategies to monitor procedural UFH therapy in clinical practice. The three main tests used to monitor UFH anticoagulation have been the whole blood clotting time, the activated clotting time (ACT), and the activated partial thromboplastin time (aPTT) (35–37). The term activated refers to the use of agents which activate factor XII during performance of the assay. The whole blood clotting time may be less reproducible and is more dependent on the degree of contact activation (35–38). The aPTT has been traditionally used to monitor UFH therapy but has limited responsiveness to changes in UFH concentration, especially at higher levels of anticoagulation (39–42). In addition, the use of a platelet-poor preparation during measurement of the aPTT ignores the potential UFH-neutralizing effects of platelet factor 4 (PF4) (33). These concerns are less applicable to measurement of the ACT. The added appeal of a rapidly available "point-of-care" assay has contributed to making the ACT the standard for assessing UFH anticoagulation in catheterization laboratories (43,44).

Guidelines for UFH use during PCI have been the subject of discussion and controversy (45–48). Initially, empirically derived intravenous bolus doses of 5000–10,000 units of UFH prior to PCI were widely utilized. The variable adequacy of anticoagulation with this regimen led to the subsequent formation of weight-adjusted bolus dose regimens and to dose adjustment based on close monitoring of in-laboratory ACT values (43,49). Early recommendations for UFH dosing during PCI came from studies demonstrating that an ACT of more than 300–400 seconds is required to prevent fibrin deposition within the extracorporeal circuit in patients undergoing cardiopulmonary bypass (50). Retrospective analyses of clinical series demonstrated an inverse relationship between the intensity of UFH anticoagulation during PCI as reflected by the ACT and the occurrence of ischemic complications including abrupt vessel closure, emergency bypass surgery, and death (51–58). However, the risk of serious bleeding complications also increased at progressively higher ACT levels (52,56,59,60). Although an optimal "target" or threshold for ACT could not be identified from these data, the consensus recommendation was made for achieving an ACT level of ≥300 seconds during PCI.

Nevertheless, subsequent studies have suggested equivalence in clinical outcomes for patients undergoing PCI who receive lower doses of UFH (5000 unit bolus or 100 U/kg) compared with patients receiving higher doses (15,000 unit bolus) of UFH (61–63). These studies have enrolled patients undergoing elective PCI and often excluded patients with acute coronary syndromes. Furthermore, the use of coronary stents, which scaffold dissections and provide more laminar flow within the arterial lumen, thus potentially decreasing the degree of platelet thrombus formation, may have contributed to the relative safety of PCI in the context of lower levels of UFH anticoagulation.

Recently, a meta-analysis that combined data from six randomized controlled trials was performed to determine the relationship of periprocedural ACT with clinical outcomes (64. This analysis included 6146 patients derived from studies of novel adjunctive

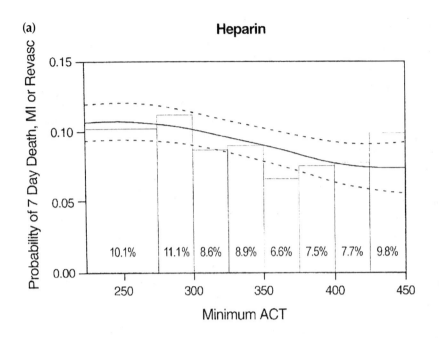

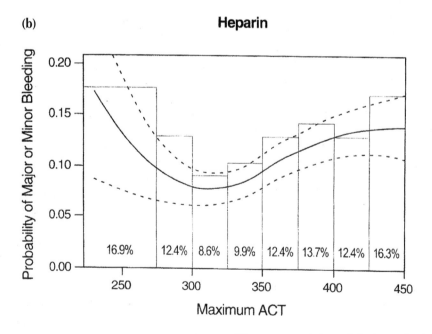

Figure 2 (a) Relationship between minimum ACT at or around time of device activation and death, MI, or urgent revascularization (Revasc.) at 7 days. (b) Relationship between maximum ACT and major or minor bleeding events at 7 days. Lowest smoothing estimate and 95% confidence intervals are indicated by solid and dotted lines, respectively. Percentages represent actual event rates observed. (From Ref. 64.)

antithrombotic regimens in which UFH constituted the control arm and ACT data were available on 5216 patients. An ACT of 350–375 seconds during PCI was associated with the lowest composite event rate (death, MI, revascularization) to 7 days follow-up (6.6%) (64) (Fig. 2a). The lowest incidence of major or minor bleeding events was observed for ACTs in the range of 300–325 seconds (8.6%) and progressively increased at 350–375 seconds (12.4%) (Fig. 2b). This analysis concluded that, contrary to prior reports, the optimal suppression of ischemic events with UFH therapy in patients undergoing PCI requires ACT levels substantially higher than previously appreciated. These data suggest that the optimal level of periprocedural ACT is in the range of 350–375 seconds for preventing ischemic complications while minimizing bleeding complications during PCI.

The dose of UFH should be reduced using a weight-adjusted algorithm if concomitant platelet glycoprotein (GP) IIb/IIIa receptor inhibitor therapy is administered. Through an interaction at the level of the GP IIb/IIIa receptor, GP IIb/IIIa blocking agents further prolong the ACT in the presence of UFH (65,66). In the Evaluation of c7E3 for the Prevention of Ischemic Complications (EPIC) trial, markedly elevated ACT levels were observed following the administration of non–weight-adjusted UFH in combination with abciximab and were associated with frequent major bleeding complications and transfusion requirements (26). Subsequent utilization of a reduced dose weight-adjusted UFH regimen in conjunction with early vascular access sheath removal resulted in a marked reduction in both bleeding and transfusion events for abciximab-treated patients (67). The safety and efficacy of this reduced-dose UFH regimen (70 U/kg bolus) in combination with abciximab was subsequently confirmed in a large, multicenter randomized trial [Evaluation of PTCA to Improve Long-term Outcome by c7E3 GP IIb/IIIa receptor blockade (EPILOG)] (68). Mean and median maximum in-laboratory ACT values observed with this regimen were 270 and 299 seconds, respectively. Although subsequent clinical trials and empirical clinical experience have suggested enhanced safety (fewer bleeding complications) with maintenance of efficacy at an even lower doses of weight-adjusted UFH without concomitant GP IIb/IIIa blockade [65 U/kg (69) or 60 U/kg (70) UFH] or with concomitant GP IIb/IIIa blockade [50 U/kg (71) or [≤1000 units] (72) UFH] to target ACT values of 200 seconds during PCI, these regimens have not been compared in large-scale randomized trials.

Intravenous UFH treatment for 1–4 days preceding PCI may improve procedural outcomes in patients with unstable coronary syndromes (73–76). However, postprocedural administration of UFH is not supported by data from clinical trials, and prolonged UFH infusions following PCI are associated with increased cost and bleeding complications without reduction in subsequent ischemic events (77–80). Prolonged intravenous UFH infusions can be even more problematic when employed in conjunction with platelet GP IIb/IIIa blockade therapy (26). The subcutaneous administration of a low molecular weight heparin may provide a more safe means of extending antithrombin therapy if clinically indicated when compared with prolonged infusion of UFH (81).

IV. LOW MOLECULAR WEIGHT HEPARIN

Low molecular weight heparins (LMWHs)are produced by enzymatic or chemical depolymerization of UFH and have saccharide chains with molecular weights of 4000–6500 daltons (average 5000 D or 15 saccharide units) (82–85). Due to their relatively small molecular size, LMWHs have a greater capacity for inactivating factor Xa relative to thrombin (factor IIa). Thus, compared with UFH, which has a ratio for factor Xa to IIa inactivation of 1:1, LMWHs exhibit antifactor Xa to IIa ratios of between 2 and 4:1

(84,85). As early ("upstream") events are greatly magnified during the coagulation cascade, factor Xa likely contributes more to the procoagulant activity of thrombus in situ than does thrombin (IIa). Furthermore, inhibition of factor Xa may be of greater importance in acute coronary syndromes (ACS) and during PCI.

Unlike UFH, LMWHs have little nonspecific plasma protein and cellular binding, which contributes to a more predictable dose response and a longer pharmacologic half-life (84,85). Furthermore, the bioavailability of LMWH following subcutaneous (SQ) injection approximates 90% (vs. 30% for UFH) (84). This combination of more predictable anticoagulant response, high bioavailability, and long half-life suggests that a reliable anticoagulant response can be achieved following twice-daily SQ injection using a weight-adjusted dose regimen in the absence of routine laboratory monitoring. In addition, animal models of thrombosis have shown LMWH to be associated with less bleeding (enhanced safety), which may in part be explained by a lower affinity for platelets and less consequent inhibition of platelet function (85,86). Heparin-induced thrombocytopenia also occurs less commonly with LMWH than UFH (Table 1).

Several studies have evaluated the efficacy of LMWH in the setting of unstable angina and coronary intervention (83,87,88). In the Efficacy and Safety of Subcutaneous Enoxaparin in Non-Q-wave Coronary Events (ESSENCE) trial, 3171 patients with unstable angina or non–Q-wave MI were randomly assigned to receive either aspirin and SQ enoxaparin (1 mg/kg every 12h) therapy or aspirin and intravenous UFH (adjusted by aPTT) (83). The composite primary endpoint of death, MI, or recurrent angina was significantly reduced ($p = 0.016$) to 30 days after treatment with enoxaparin and relative benefit extended to 1 year. Similar results were found in the Thrombolysis in Myocardial Infarction (TIMI) 11B trial (87). In TIMI 11B, enoxaparin was administered as a 30 mg intravenous bolus followed by 1 mg/kg SQ every 12 hours, and UFH was administered as a 70 U/kg intravenous bolus followed by a 15 U/kg per hour infusion with dose titration based on aPTT measurements. In the prospectively planned meta-analysis of the ESSENCE and TIMI 11B trials, the composite endpoint of death, myocardial infarction, or urgent revascularization was reduced from 25.8% (UFH) to 23.3% (enoxaparin; $p = 0.008$) at one-year follow-up. Each individual component of the composite endpoint was directionally consistent in favoring enoxaparin (versus UFH) therapy (89).

In the Fragmin during Instability in Coronary Artery Disease (FRISC) trial, 1506 patients with unstable angina randomly received treatment with either SQ dalteparin (120 U/kg, maximum 10,000 U) twice daily for 6 days followed by 7500 U daily for 35–45 days or placebo injections (88). The composite endpoint of death, MI, and revascularization was reduced at 40 days by dalteparin. Although no differences in outcomes were evident in the overall study between treatment groups at 5-month follow-up, patients with a troponin T level $10.1 mg/L on enrollment demonstrated a reduction in the composite endpoint of death or MI that was sustained to 5 months following treatment with dalteparin (90). A

Table 1 Advantages of Low Molecular Weight Heparins over Conventional Unfractionated Heparin

Pharmacological effects	Clinical benefit
Quick and predictable subcutaneous absorption	More reliable level of anticoagulation
More stable dose response	Eliminates need for monitoring
Resistant to inhibition by platelet factor 4	Decreased incidence of thrombocytopenia
Depressed antiheparin antibody production by 70%	Greater antithrombotic effects
Greater anti-Xa activity	Potential to reduce bleeding
Less anti-IIa activity	Absence of rebound

subsequent evaluation of SQ dalteparin versus standard UFH in a randomized trial of 1482 patients with unstable angina of non–Q-wave MI [Fragmin in unstable coronary artery disease (FRIC) study] demonstrated equivalent efficacy and concluded that dalteparin was a safe and effective alternative to UFH in the treatment of unstable coronary heart disease (91). In the FRISC II trial, 2267 patients with unstable angina or non–Q-wave MI were administered dalteparin 120 U/kg SQ twice daily for 5–7 days and were randomly assigned to either an invasive or a noninvasive treatment strategy at 2–7 days following enrollment (92). Following randomization to revascularization strategy, a second random allocation to either dalteparin 7500 U or placebo SQ twice-daily therapy for 90 days was employed. A reduction in the composite endpoint of death or MI was observed in patients who received dalteparin (vs. placebo), particularly in association with the invasive revascularization strategy (93).

LMWH has not been shown to reduce angiographic restenosis following PCI. Enoxaparin 40 mg administered SQ daily for 1 month following successful PCI resulted in no difference in the incidence of angiographic restenosis or in the occurrence of clinical events compared with placebo injections [Enoxaparin Restenosis after Angioplasty (ERA) trial) (94). A randomized comparison of reviparin with standard UFH administered during and following PCI [Restenosis prevention after PTCA Early administration of LMWH LU47311 in a Double-blind Unfractionated heparin and placebo Controlled Evaluation (REDUCE) trial] demonstrated no difference in major clinical events or angiographic restenosis over 30 weeks of follow-up (95). Although clinical trials have demonstrated the superiority of LMWH over UFH for the treatment of patients with non–ST segment elevation ACS, no effect on restenosis or reocclusion after PCI has been observed.

Enoxaparin has been administered both with and without adjunctive abciximab to patients undergoing PCI in the National Investigator Collaborating on Enoxaparin (NICE) trials. In the NICE 1 pilot trial, 60 patients were randomly assigned to receive either UFH (10,000 U intravenous bolus followed by supplemental UFH to target an ACT of 300 seconds) or enoxaparin (1 mg/kg intravenously) prior to PCI (96). No differences in procedural success or bleeding events were observed between treatment groups. Enoxaparin had minimal effect on the ACT and the anti-factor Xa activity was similar between these two regimens. The NICE 1 study evaluated 828 patients undergoing PCI while receiving enoxaparin (1 mg/kg intravenously) without concomitant GP IIb/IIIa blockade and demonstrated a low incidence of major bleeding (0.5%), transfusion (1.3%), or ischemic events (death, MI, urgent revascularization) to 30 days following enrollment (97).

In the NICE 4 study, enoxaparin 0.75 mg/kg was administered intravenously in combination with standard dose abciximab to 818 patients undergoing PCI with an FDA approved device (excluding rotational atherectomy). Multivessel PCI was performed in 52% and stent deployment in 88% of the PCI procedures (98). Major (0.4%) and minor (7.0%) bleeding (TIMI study group definition) or transfusion (1.8%) to 30 days following enrollment was uncommon. A comparison of bleeding events not related to coronary bypass surgery with historical benchmarks [the EPILOG trial, abciximab plus low-dose weight-adjusted UFH cohort; or the Evaluation of Platelet IIb/IIIa Inhibitor for Stenting (EPISTENT) trial, stent plus abciximab cohort] demonstrated fewer bleeding events with bolus and 12-hour infusion of abciximab administered in combination with 0.75 mg/kg enoxaparin compared with UFH (98,99) (Fig. 3).

Further experience with combination enoxaparin and platelet GP IIb/IIIa inhibitor therapy initiated "upstream" before cardiac catheterization for patients presenting with ACS has been obtained in the NICE 3 study. In NICE 3, 661 patients with non–ST-segment elevation ACS were administered aspirin and enoxaparin (1.0 mg/kg SQ every 12h) plus a GP IIb/IIIa inhibitor (abciximab, $n = 147$; eptifibatide, $n = 252$; tirofiban, $n = 217$)

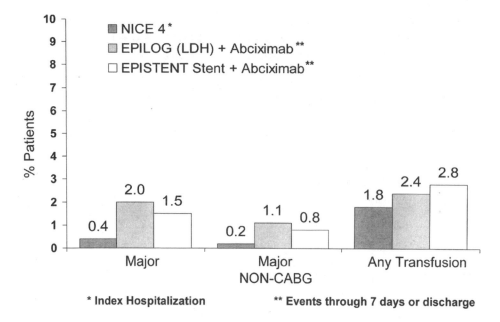

Figure 3 Major bleeding events with and without events related to coronary artery bypass surgery (CABG) and the requirement for blood product transfusion in the NICE 4 study, EPILOG low-dose weight-adjusted heparin (LDH) + abciximab, and EPISTENT stent + abciximab cohorts, respectively. (From Ref. 98.)

(100). The allocation of platelet GP IIb/IIIa inhibitor was not randomized, and 45 patients received aspirin and enoxaparin alone. The major objectives of NICE 3 were to assess the safety profile of enoxaparin and a platelet GP IIb/IIIa antagonist in combination as well as the feasibility and safety of taking patients to the cardiac catheterization laboratory with combination therapy. The primary endpoint [occurrence of major in-hospital non-surgery related bleeding (TIMI definition)] was observed in 1.9% of all patients receiving combination enoxaparin plus platelet GP IIb/IIIa inhibitor therapy (0.7% abciximab, 3.2% eptifibatide, 1.4% tirofiban) (100).

The relative safety of enoxaparin versus UFH in patients undergoing PCI treated with eptifibatide was assessed in the Coronary Revascularization Using Integrilin and Single bolus Enoxaparin (CRUISE) study (101). In the CRUISE study, 261 patients undergoing elective or urgent PCI treated with eptifibatide (180 μg bolus x 2, 10 minutes apart, 2.0 μg/kg infusion for 18–20 hours) were randomly assigned to treatment with either UFH (60 U/kg intravenous bolus; n = 132) or enoxaparin (0.75 mg/kg intravenous bolus; n = 129). No significant differences with respect to either TIMI or GUSTO bleeding indices were observed between randomly assigned treatment regimens, although a trend (p = 0.08) toward total reduction in TIMI major plus minor bleeding was observed in enoxaparin treated patients. (101). At both 48 hours and 30 days postenrollment, no differences in adverse ischemic endpoints were observed between randomly assigned treatment groups. Of note, vascular closure devices were utilized in 42% of enoxaparin-treated and 34% of UFH-treated patients. TIMI major bleeding events were observed in 2.6% of patients treated with UFH in whom a vascular closure device was used and in none of the enoxaparin-treated patients following closure device use.

The cumulative experience from the NICE and CRUISE trials suggests that adjunctive enoxaparin therapy for PCI (with or without concomitant platelet GP IIb/IIIa therapy) is safe and effective. Safety (as reflected by the occurrence of major bleeding events) of combination therapy is enhanced following reduced dose enoxaparin plus abciximab for PCI compared with historical cohorts administered reduced dose UFH in combination with abciximab (85). Data in support of dalteparin administration during PCI are more limited and will require confirmation in a larger population of PCI patients.

Despite the theoretical pharmacodynamic advantages of LMWH versus UFH, which include a more predictable and reliable level of anticoagulation, the adoption of LMWH for use during PCI has been slow primarily due to uncertainty about the level of anticoagulation and a lack of comfort in the transition from medical therapy (medical service) to procedural anticoagulation (cath lab) (85). Larger-scale, more definitive pharmacokinetic, safety, and efficacy studies are needed for individual LMWH agents. In the recently presented Aggrastat to Zocor (A to Z) study, 3987 patients with non–ST segment elevation acute coronary syndrome were treated with intravenous tirofiban plus aspirin (102). Patients were then randomly assigned to receive enoxaparin (1 mg/kg SQ every 12h; $n = 2026$) or weight-adjusted UFH intravenously with dose titration based on aPTT measurement ($n = 1961$). Aggressive versus conservative care was instituted per local practice. The primary endpoint of the A to Z study was the composite occurrence of death, myocardial infarction, and refractory ischemia to 7 days following enrollment. The primary hypothesis (that enoxaparin is not "inferior" to UFH in the treatment of non–ST segment elevation ACS) was satisfied and the primary endpoint was observed in 8.4% of enoxaparin-treated ($n = 169$ events) versus 9.4% of UFH-treated patients ($n = 184$ events) at 7 days following enrollment (102). Subgroup analysis of the A to Z study revealed that those patients with the greatest risk profile (ST segment change ≥ 1 mm, elevated serum troponin, TIMI risk score ≥ 3) manifest the greatest relative benefit in favor of enoxaparin versus UFH. Another study with enoxaparin, the SYNERGY (A Prospective, Randomized, Open-Label, Multicenter Study in Patients Presenting with Acute Coronary Syndromes) trial, plans to randomize 8000 high-risk ACS patients to therapy with either enoxaparin or UFH, both with or without platelet GP IIb/IIIa inhibition, in a 2 X 2 factorial design (103). The primary endpoint is the composite occurrence of death or nonfatal MI to 30 days. This trial will provide important data in validating an algorithm for the transition or "bridge" between medical therapy and invasive interventional care.

Recent meta-analyses of trials that have randomly compared enoxaparin versus UFH therapy following fibrinolytic treatment for acute ST segment elevation myocardial infarction have demonstrated enhanced efficacy (reduction in death, recurrent myocardial infarction, or recurrent ischemia) as well as similar rates of major bleeding in patients who were randomly assigned to treatment with enoxaparin (104). The odds ratio for occurrence of death, recurrent myocardial infarction and recurrent ischemia was 0.80 (CI 0.68–0.95) in favor of enoxaparin (vs. UFH) in a meta-analysis of the ASSENT-3 (Assessment of the Safety and Efficacy of a New Thrombolytic Regimen), HART-II (Heparin and Aspirin Reperfusion Therapy), and ENTIRE (Enoxaparin as Adjunctive Antithrombin Therapy for ST-Elevation Myocardial Infarction)-TIMI 23 trials (105) (Table 2).

V. DIRECT THROMBIN INHIBITORS

Newer, direct-acting thrombin inhibitors (DITs) have been evaluated in patients with ACS and during PCI. These agents (hirudin, bivalirudin, argatroban, efegatran) do not require antithrombin as a cofactor, bind directly to both free and clot-bound thrombin, are not neutralized by PF4, and thus provide a more predictable dose response (106–110). In animal models of deep arterial injury simulating PCI, direct antithrombins were superior to UFH

Table 2 Meta-analysis of ASSENT-3, HART-II, and ENTIRE-TIMI 23 Trials

Enoxaparin vs. UFH	Death/ReMI/RI OR (95% CI)	Death/ReMI OR (95% CI)	Major bleeding OR (95% CI)
ASSENT-3 n = 4078	0.81 (0.68–0.95)	0.86 (0.70–1.05)	1.42 (0.96–2.01)
ENTIRE n = 242	0.38 (0.19 – 0.79)	0.24 (0.09 – 0.62)	0.76 (0.16 –4.58)
HART-II n = 400	1.21 (0.70–2.10)	1.00 (0.49–2.06)	1.18 (0.39–3.57)
TOTAL n = 4717	0.80 (0.68–0.95)	0.74 (0.51–1.09)	1.34 (0.93–1.95)

UFH = unfractionated heparin; ReMI = recurrent myocardial infarction; RI = refractory ischemia; OR = odds ratio; CI = confidential interval.
Source: Ref. 105

in inhibiting thrombus formation (111). Randomized comparative trials with intravenous UFH in patients undergoing PCI have demonstrated that direct antithrombin agents were associated with similar or fewer ischemic complications and a lower incidence of bleeding complications (112–116).

Hirudin has been evaluated in large-scale clinical trials in the clinical settings of ACS and PCI. Despite the theoretical advantages of direct thrombin inhibition in these settings, many of these studies failed to show benefit for hirudin relative to UFH. In three trials— GUSTO (Global Use of Strategies to Open Occluded Coronary Arteries)-IIb, TIMI 9, and HIT (randomized r-Hirudin for Improvement of Thrombolysis)—which cumulatively enrolled over 15,000 patients with acute MI or unstable angina, hirudin therapy conferred no substantive advantage and provided a nonsignificant reduction ($g 10%) in the risk of death or reinfaction compared with UFH (117–119). Moreover, the therapeutic window for safety with hirudin appeared narrow, with an excess risk of intracranial hemorrhage evident when higher doses of hirudin were administered in combination with fibrinolytic therapy (120,121).

In the Hirudin in a European restenosis prevention trial VErsus heparin Treatment In PTCA patients (HELVETICA) trial, which was a randomized comparison of hirudin versus UFH for patients undergoing PTCA, a reduction in early (96 h) ischemic events in favor of hirudin was observed (116). However, late (6 months) follow-up showed no difference in clinical outcomes. In the bivalirudin (hirulog) angioplasty study, similar clinical outcomes and lower rates of serious bleeding events accompanied bivalirudin therapy compared with standard UFH (114,115). In a prespecified cohort of patients with postinfarction angina, bivalirudin reduced the incidence of procedural failure (5.1% vs. 10.8% for UFH; $p = 0.004$) as well as the composite endpoints of death or MI, and death, MI, or revascularization compared with UFH (115). In addition, bivalirudin was associated with significantly fewer major ($p $g 0.001) and minor ($p $g 0.001) bleeding events compared with UFH (122). Hirudin, bivalirudin and a synthetic, direct-acting antithrombin agent, argatroban, have also been used for antithrombin therapy in patients with heparin-induced thrombocytopenia and thrombosis syndrome who require PCI (123–125).

The Randomized Evaluation in PCI Linking Angiomax to Reduced Clinical Events (REPLACE)-2 trial randomly assigned 6010 patients to receive either intravenous bivalirudin (0.75 mg/kg bolus plus 1.75 mg/kg/h infusion for duration of PCI), with provisional GP IIb/IIIa inhibition ($p = 2999$) or UFH (65 U/kg bolus) with planned GP IIb/IIIa inhibition ($n = 3011$) (69). The primary quadruple composite endpoint was the incidence of death, MI, urgent revascularization to 30 days, or in-hospital major bleeding, with the key secondary triple composite endpoint of death, MI, or urgent revascularization to 30 days. Provisional GP IIb/IIIa blockade was administered to 7.2% of patients in the bivalirudin group (3.7% eptifibatide, 3.5% abciximab), and planned GP IIb/IIIa blockade was administered to 96.5% of patients in the UFH group (eptifibatide 53.4%, abciximab 42.9%). By 30 days, the primary composite endpoint had occurred in 9.2% of patients in the bivalirudin group versus 10.0% in the UFH-plus-GP IIb/IIIa group ($p = 0.32$) (69). The secondary composite endpoint occurred in 7.6% of patients in the bivalirudin versus 7.1% in the UFH-plus-GP IIb/IIIa groups ($p = 0.40$) (69). Prespecified statistical criteria for noninferiority of bivalirudin versus UFH-plus-GP IIb/IIIa were satisfied for bivalirudin by both composite endpoints. In-hospital major bleeding rates were significantly reduced in bivalirudin-treated patients (2.4% vs. 4.1% UFH + GP IIb/IIIa; $p \$g 0.001$) (69). The REPLACE-2 study concluded that bivalirudin with provisional GP IIb/IIIa blockade was not inferior to UFH plus planned GP IIb/IIIa blockade during contemporary PCI with regard to ischemic endpoints and was associated with fewer bleeding complications (Fig. 4). The results of the REPLACE-2 trial are supported by recent pooled analyses involving multiple ($n = 10$) prospective PCI trials. In 6134 patients ($n = 3277$ bivalirudin vs. $n = 2857$ UFH), adverse ischemic events (death, myocardial infarction, target vessel revascularization) were reduced in patients who received bivalirudin (7.4%) versus UFH (13%; $p \$g 0.0001$) (126). In addition, hemorrhagic events were less frequent in bivalirudin (2.8%)– versus UFH (7.6%; $p \$g 0.0001$)–treated patients (126).

The Direct Thrombin Inhibitor Trialists Collaborative Group plans on combining the data from more than 30 randomized trials involving more than 40,000 patients with ACS and undergoing PCI treated with DTIs in an effort to obtain reliable estimates of the treatment effects of DTIs on death, MI, major bleeding, refractory or recurrent ischemia, and need for

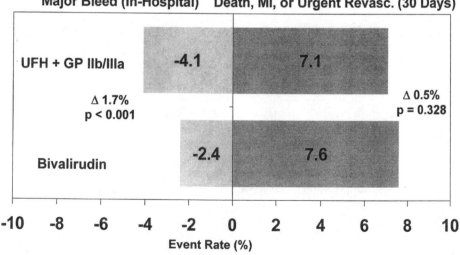

Figure 4 Event rates of major bleeding (in-hospital) and death, MI, or urgent revascularization to 30 days in the REPLACE-2 trial. (Adapted from Ref. 69.)

revascularization (127). These data are now merged into a master database for analysis and provide important information about the appropriate use of these therapeutic agents.

VI. OTHER ANTICOAGULANT AGENTS

Restenosis after successful PCI leads to repeat intervention in at least one fifth of patients. The pathogenesis of restenosis is complex and incompletely understood. Debate persists as to whether mural thrombosis plays an important role in the restenotic process. The Balloon Angioplasty and Anticoagulation Study (BAAS) assigned 261 patients to receive aspirin alone and 270 patients to receive aspirin plus coumarins beginning 1 week prior to undergoing PCI (128). At 6 months the minimal luminal diameter by quantitative angiography was similar in both treatment groups and there was no significant difference in restenosis rates. Interestingly, event-free survival (freedom from death, MI, revascularization, or stroke) was improved and recurrent angina was less common in the aspirin plus coumarin group compared with aspirin alone (128) (Fig. 5).

These data are consistent with recent evidence that demonstrates a beneficial effect of warfarin therapy both following MI and in postcoronary artery bypass grafting patients (129,130). Following a MI, therapy with warfarin in combination with aspirin (vs. aspirin alone) was associated with an approximate 30% risk reduction in the composite endpoint of death, nonfatal MI, and thromboembolic stroke in medically treated patients (129). The main benefit of warfarin plus aspirin in this patient population was the prevention of nonfatal reinfarction and thromboembolic stroke. To date, no beneficial effect on mortality has been demonstrated. The clinical benefit of coumadin is derived at the cost of increased bleeding. A fourfold increase in major bleeding episodes was observed in patients receiving aspirin and warfarin compared to aspirin therapy alone (129,130). Furthermore, the combination of aspirin and warfarin was associated with more frequent bleeding episodes than treatment with warfarin alone.

Animal models have demonstrated that warfarin may exhibit antiproliferative effects as well as enhancing apoptosis of smooth muscle and endothelial cells (130). Oral thrombin inhibitors in clinical evaluation such as ximelagatran, as well as dual antiplatelet therapy (aspirin plus clopidogrel), may provide clinical benefit in addition to less bleeding risk for patients with cardiovascular disease. The durable benefits of warfarin should become better characterized by future studies of oral direct thrombin inhibitors compared with warfarin.

The need for antithrombotic agents with more specific activity and a broader therapeutic range has motivated active investigation. These efforts have led to the design of recombinant molecules and monoclonal antibodies that interrupt activation of the coagulation cascade at several strategically important points. Synthetic inhibitors of factor Xa inhibit coagulation induced by tissue factor and lipopolysaccharide and are effective in the prophylaxis of venous thromboembolic complications following orthopedic surgery (131,132). Transmembrane signaling through G protein–coupled receptors modulates a diverse array of cellular processes including blood coagulation. Novel cell-penetrating peptides, termed pepducins, act as intracellular inhibitors of signal transference from surface receptors to G proteins (133). Attachment of these agents to protease-activated receptor 1 (PAR1) or PAR 4 provides potent inhibition of thrombin-mediated platelet aggregation 134). Infusion of the anti-PAR4 pepducin into mice prolonged bleeding time and blocked systemic platelet activation (134). A potential benefit of this new class of antithrombins (anti-PAR agents) is inhibition of thrombin-mediated platelet activation with enhanced safety compared to DTIs since they allow fibrin formation to occur unperturbed. The relationship between clinical benefit and cost increment related to these new molecules remains to be seen.

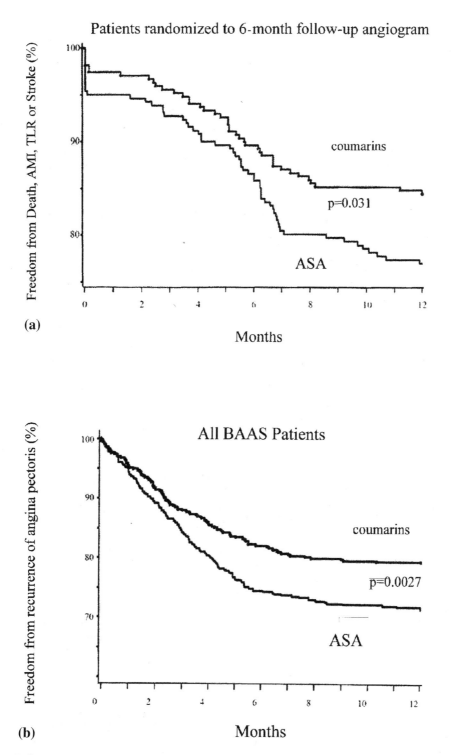

Figure 5   (a) Event-free survival of the patients treated with aspirin alone (ASA) or with the combination of ASA and coumarins (coumarius). AMI, acute myocardial infarction; TLR, target lesion revascularization. (b) Time to recurrence of angina pectoris in the patients treated with ASA alone (ASA) or with combination of ASA and coumarins (coumarins). (From Ref. 128.)

REFERENCES

1. Bittl JA. Advances in coronary angioplasty. N Engl J Med. 1996; 335:1290–1302.
2. Serruys PW, van Hout B, Bonnier H, et al. Randomised comparison of implantation of heparin-coated stents with balloon angioplasty in selected patients with coronary artery disease. Lancet 1998; 352:673–681.
3. Lincoff AM, Califf RM, Moliterno DJ, et al. Complementary clinical benefits of coronary-artery stenting and blockade of platelet glycoprotein IIb/IIIa receptors. N Engl J Med. 1999; 341:319–327.
4. Uchida Y, Hasegawa K, Kawamura K, et al. Angioscopic observation of the coronary luminal changes induced by percutaneous transluminal coronary angioplasty. Am Heart J. 1989; 177:769–776.
5. Waller BF, Gorfinkel HJ, Rogers FJ, et al. Early and late morphologic changes in major epicardial coronary arteries after percutaneous transluminal coronary angioplasty. Am J Cardiol. 1984: 33:42C-47C.
6. Waller BF, Pinkerton CA, Orr CM, et al. Morphologic observations late ($130 days) after clinically successful coronary angioplasty: an analysis of 20 necropsy patients and review of 41 necropsy patients with coronary angioplasty restenosis. Circulation. 1991: 83:I-28 – I-41.
7. Ferguson JJ. Conventional antithrombotic approaches. Am Heart J. 1995; 130:651–657.
8. Barasch E, Wilson JM, Ferguson JJ. Anticoagulation and PTCA. Dev Cardiol. 1994; 4:91–103.
9. Wilcox JM, Smith KM, Schwartz SM, Gordon D. Localization of tissue factor in the normal vessel wall and in the atherosclerotic plaque. Proc Natl Acad Sci USA. 1989; 86:2839–2843.
10. Wilentz JR, Sanborn TA, Haudenschild C, et al. Platelet accumulation experimental angioplasty: time course in relation to vascular injury. Circulation. 1987; 75:636–642.
11. Nelken NA, Soifer SJ, Okeff J, et al. Thrombin receptor expression in normal and atherosclerotic human arteries. J Clin Invest. 1992; 90:1614–1621.
12. Barry WL, Sarembock IJ. Antiplatelet and anticoagulant therapy in patients undergoing percutaneous transluminal coronary angioplasty. Cardiol Clin. 1994; 12:517–535.
13. Smyth SS, Joneckis CC, Parise LV. Regulation of vascular integrins. Blood. 1993; 81: 2827–2843.
14. Bar-Shavit R, Eldor A, Vlodavsky I. Binding of thrombin to subendothelial extracellular matrix: protection and expression of functional properties. J Clin Invest. 1989; 84:1096–1104.
15. Lam JYT, Chesebro JH, Steele PM, et al. Antithrombotic therapy for deep arterial injury by angioplasty. Efficacy of common platelet inhibition compared with thrombin inhibition in pigs. Circulation. 1991; 84:814–820.
16. Jackson CL, Raines EW, Ross R, et al. Role of endogenous platelet-derived growth factor in arterial smooth muscle cell migration after balloon catheter injury. Arterioscler Thromb Vasc Biol. 1993; 13:1218–1226.
17. Marmur JD, Rossikhina M, Guha A, et al. Tissue factor is rapidly induced in arterial smooth muscle after balloon injury. J Clin Invest. 1993; 91:2253–2259.
18. Peltonen S, Lassila R, Heikkila J. Activation of coagulation and fibrinolysis despite heparinization during successful elective coronary angioplasty. Thromb Res. 1996; 82:459–468.
19. Heras M, Chesebro JH, Penny WJ, et al. Importance of adequate heparin dosage in arterial angioplasty in a porcine model. Circulation. 1988; 78:654–660.
20. Owen J, Hunter-Laszlo M, Williams JK, et al. Thrombin activity induced by balloon angioplasty of the coronary artery in *Macaca fascicularis* (cynomolgus monkey). Blood Coagul Fibrinolysis. 1990; 1(4–5):505–507.
21. Hafner G, Rupprucht HJ, Luz M, et al. Recombinant hirudin as a periprocedural antithrombotic in coronary angioplasty for unstable angina pectoris. Eur Heart J. 1996; 8:1207–1215.
22. deFeyter PJ, vandenBrand M, Jaarman G, et al. Acute coronary occlusion during and after percutaneous transluminal coronary angioplasty. Circulation. 1991; 83:927–936.
23. Lincoff AM, Popma JJ, Ellis SG, et al. Abrupt vessel closure complicating coronary angioplasty: clinical, angiographic and therapeutic profile. J Am Coll Cardiol. 1992; 19:926–935.

24. Detre KM, Holmes DRG, Holubkov R, et al. Incidence and consequences of periprocedural occlusion: the 1985–1986 National Heart, Lung and Blood Institute percutaneous coronary angioplasty registry. Circulation. 1990; 82:739–750.

25. Ellis SG, Roubin GS, King SB, et al. Angiographic and clinical predictors of acute closure after native vessel angioplasty. Circulation. 1988; 77:372–379.

26. The EPIC investigators: Use of a monoclonal antibody directed against the platelet glycoprotein IIb/IIIa receptor in high risk coronary angioplasty. N Engl J Med. 1994; 330: 956–961.

27. Narins CR, Hillegass WB, Nelson CL, et al. Relation between activated clotting time during angioplasty and abrupt closure. Circulation. 1996; 93:667–671.

28. Haude M, Hopp HW, Rupprecht HJ, et al. Immediate stent implantation versus conventional techniques for the treatment of abrupt vessel closure or symptomatic dissections after coronary balloon angioplasty. Am Heart J. 2000; 140:e26.

29. Piana RN, Ahmed WH, Chaitman B, et al. Effect of transient abrupt vessel closure during otherwise successful angioplasty for unstable angina on clinical outcome at six months. J Am Coll Cardiol. 1999; 33:73–78.

30. Topol EJ. Coronary-artery stents—gauging, gorging, and gouging. N Engl J Med. 1998; 339:1702–1704.

31. Mak KH, Belli G, Ellis SG, et al. Subacute stent thrombosis: evolving issues and current concepts. J Am Coll Cardiol. 1996; 27:494–503.

32. Cutlip DE, Baim DS, Ho KKL, et al. Stent thrombosis in the modern era. A pooled analysis of multicenter coronary stent clinical trials. Circulation 2001; 103:1967–1971.

33. Hirsch J: Heparin. N Engl J Med. 1991; 324:1565–1574.

34. deSwart CAM, Nijmeyer B, Roelogs JMM, et al. Kinetics of intravenously administered heparin in normal humans. Blood. 1982; 60:1251–1258.

35. Bowers J, Ferguson JJ. The use of activated clotting times to monitor heparin therapy during and after interventional procedures. Clin Cardiol. 1994; 17:357–361.

36. Ferguson JJ, Wilson JM. Early and late ischemic complications of PTCA. J Invasive Cardiol. 1994; 6:3A-12A.

37. Schriever HG, Epstein SE, Mintz MD. Statistical correlation and heparin sensitivity of activated partial thromboplastin time, whole blood coagulation time, and an automated coagulation time. Am J Clin Pathol. 1973; 60:323–329.

38. Noureddine SM. Research review: use of activated clotting time to monitor heparin therapy in coronary patients. Am J Crit Care. 1995; 4:272–279.

39. Blumenthal RS, Carter AJ, Resar JR, et al. A comparison of bedside and hospital laboratory coagulation studies during and after coronary intervention. Cathet Cardiovasc Diagn. 1995; 35:9–17.

40. Dougherty KG, Gaos CM, Bush HS, et al. Activated clotting times and activated partial thromboplastin times in patients undergoing coronary angioplasty who received bolus doses of heparin. Cathet Cardiovasc Diagn. 1992; 26:260–263.

41. Vacek JL, Hibiya K, Rosamond TL, et al. Validation of a bedside method of activated partial thromboplastin time measurement with clinical range guidelines. Am J Cardiol. 1991; 68:557–559.

42. Grill HP, Spero JE, Granato JE. Comparison of activated partial thromboplastin time to activated clotting time for adequacy of heparin anticoagulation just before percutaneous transluminal coronary angioplasty. Am J Cardiol. 1993; 71:1219–1220.

43. Ogilby JD, Kopelman HA, Klein LW, et al. Adequate heparinization during PTCA: assessment using activated clotting times. Cathet Cardiovasc Diagn. 1989; 18:206–209.

44. Rath B, Bennett DH. Monitoring the effect of heparin by measurement of activated clotting time during and after percutaneous transluminal coronary angioplasty. Br Heart J. 1990; 63:18–21.

45. Rund MM, Smith DD, DeLuca SA, et al. For the IMPACT II study coordinators/investigators: heparin during coronary angioplasty: are there any rules? Circulation. 1994; 90:I487.

46. Ferguson JJ, Dohman P, Wilson JM, et al. Results of a national survey on anticoagulation for PTCA. J Invas Cardiol. 1995; 7:136–141.

47. Smith SC, Dove JT, Jacobs AK, et al. ACC/AHA guidelines for percutaneous coronary intervention: a report of the American College of Cardiology/American Heart Association Task Force on Practice Guidelines (committee to revise the 1993 guidelines for percutaneous transluminal coronary angioplasty). J Am Coll Cardiol. 2001; 37:2215–2239.

48. Popma JJ, Ohman EM, Weitz J, et al. Antithrombotic therapy in patients undergoing percutaneous coronary intervention. Chest. 2001; 119:321S-336S.

49. Blumenthal RS, Wolff MR, Resar JR, et al. Pre-procedural anticoagulation does not reduce angioplasty heparin requirements. Am Heart J. 1993; 125:1221–1225.

50. Bull MH, Huse WM, Bull BS. Evaluation of tests used to monitor heparin therapy during extra-corporeal circulation. Anesthesiology. 1975; 43:346–353.

51. Vaitkus PT, Herrmann HC, Laskey WK. Management and immediate outcome of patients with intracoronary thrombus during percutaneous transluminal coronary angioplasty. Am Heart J. 1992; 124:1–8.

52. McGarry TF, Gottlieb RS, Morganroth J, et al. The relationship of anticoagulation level and complications after successful percutaneous transluminal coronary angioplasty. Am Heart J. 1992; 123:1445–1451.

53. Frierson JH, Dimas AP, Simpendoerfer CC, et al. Is aggressive heparin necessary for elective PTCA ? Cathet Cardiovasc Diagn. 1993; 28:279–282.

54. Ferguson JJ, Dougherty KG, Gaos CM, et al. Relationship between procedural activated coagulation time and outcome after percutaneous transluminal coronary angioplasty. J Am Coll Cardiol. 1994; 23:1061–1065.

55. Laskey MAL, Deutsch E, Barnathan E, et al. Influence of heparin therapy on percutaneous transluminal coronary angioplasty outcome in unstable angina pectoris. Am J Cardiol. 1990; 65:1425–1429.

56. Laskey MAL, Deutsch E, Hirshfeld JW, et al. Influence of heparin therapy on percutaneous transluminal coronary angioplasty outcome in patients with coronary arterial thrombus. Am J Cardiol. 1990; 65:179–182.

57. Mooney MR, Mooney JF, Goldenberg If, et al. Percutaneous transluminal coronary angioplasty in the setting of large intracoronary thrombi. Am J Cardiol. 1990; 65:427–431.

58. Satler LF, Leon MB, Kent KM, et al. Strategies for acute occlusion after coronary angioplasty. J Am Coll Cardiol. 1992; 19:936–938.

59. Avendano A, Ferguson JJ. Comparison of Hemochron and Hemotech activated coagulation time target values during percutaneous transluminal coronary angioplasty. J Am Coll Cardiol. 1994; 23:907–910.

60. Hillegass WB, Narins CR, Brott BC, et al. Activated clotting time predicts bleeding complications from angioplasty. J Am Coll Cardiol. 1994; 23:184A.

61. Boccara A, Beenamer H, Juliard JM, et al. A randomized trial of a fixed high dose vs. a weight adjusted low dose of intravenous heparin during coronary angioplasty. Eur Heart J. 1997; 18:631–635.

62. Koch KT, Piek JJ, deWinter RJ, et al. Safety of low dose heparin in elective coronary angioplasty. Heart. 1997; 77:517–522.

63. Vianer J, Fleisch M, Gunnes P, et al. Low dose heparin for routine coronary angioplasty and stenting. Am J Cardiol. 1996; 78:964–966.

64. Chew DP, Bhatt DL, Lincoff AM, et al. Defining the optimal activated clotting time during percutaneous coronary intervention. Circulation. 2001; 103:961–966.

65. Ammar T, Scudder LE, Coller BS. In vitro effects of the platelet glycoprotein receptor antagonist c7E3 on the activated clotting time. Circulation. 1997; 95:614–617.

66. Moliterno DJ, Califf RM, Aguirre FE, et al. Effects of glycoprotein IIb/IIIa endocrine blockade on activated clotting time during percutaneous transluminal coronary angioplasty or directional atherectomy. Am J Cardiol. 1995; 75:559–562.

67. Lincoff AM, Tcheng JE, Califf RM, et al. Standard vs. low dose weight adjusted heparin in patients treated with the platelet glycoprotein IIb/IIIa receptor antibody fragment abciximab during percutaneous coronary revascularization. Am J Cardiol. 1997; 79:286–291.

68. Platelet glycoprotein IIb/IIIa receptor blockade and low-dose heparin during percutaneous coronary revascularization. The EPILOG investigators. N Engl J Med. 1997; 336:1689–1696.

69. Lincoff AM, Bittl JA, Harrington RA, et al. Bivalirudin and provisional glycoprotein IIb/IIIa blockade compared with heparin and planned glycoprotein IIb/IIIa blockade during percutaneous coronary intervention. REPLACE-2 randomized trial. JAMA. 2003; 289:853–863.

70. Tolleson TR, O'Shea JC, Bittl JA, et al. Relationship between heparin anticoagulation and clinical outcomes in coronary stent intervention: observations from the ESPRIT trial. J Am Coll Cardiol. 2003; 41:386–393.

71. Kereiakes DJ, Broderick TM, Abbottsmith C, et al. Bleeding risks and vascular complications following abciximab therapy for percutaneous coronary intervention: a new look at an old problem. J Invas Cardiol. 2000; 12:95–98.

72. Denardo SJ, Davis KE, Reid PR, et al. Efficacy and safety of minimal dose (> or = 1,000 units) unfractionated heparin with abciximab in percutaneous coronary intervention. Am J Cardiol. 2003; 91:1–5.

73. Hettleman BDL, Aplin RL, Sullivan PR, et al. Three days of heparin pretreatment reduces major complications of coronary angioplasty in patients with unstable angina. J Am Coll Cardiol. 1990; 15:154A.

74. Pow TK, Varrichione TR, Jacobs AK, et al. Does pretreatment with heparin prevent abrupt closure following PTCA? J Am Coll Cardiol. 1988; 11:238A.

75. Sugrue DD, Holmes DR, Smith HC, et al. Coronary artery thrombus as a risk factor for acute vessel occlusion during percutaneous transluminal coronary angioplasty: improving results. Br Heart J. 1986; 53:363–373.

76. Klein LW, Wahid F, VadenBurg BJ, et al. Comparison of heparin therapy for ≤ 48 hours to > 48 hours in unstable pectoris. Am J Cardiol. 1997; 79:259–263.

77. Ellis SG, Rubin GS, Willentz J, et al. Effective 18–24 hour heparin administration for prevention of restenosis after uncomplicated coronary angioplasty. Am Heart J. 1989; 117:777–782.

78. Saenz CB, Baxley WA, Bulle TM, et al. Early and late effect of heparin infusion following elective angioplasty. Circulation. 1988; 78:II-98.

79. Walford GD, Midei MM, Aversano TR, et al. Heparin after PTCA: increased early complications and no clinical benefit. Circulation. 1991; 84:II-592

80. Friedman HZ, Cragg DR, Glazier SM, et al. Randomized prospective evaluation of prolonged vs. abbreviated intravenous heparin therapy after coronary angioplasty. J Am Coll Cardiol. 1994; 24:1214–1219.

81. Chow WH, Fan K, Chow TC. Use of low molecular weight heparin in postangioplasty management. Int J Cardiol. 1997; 58:83–85.

82. Turpie AGG. Successors to heparin: new antithrombotic agents. Am Heart J. 1997; 134:S71–S77.

83. Cohen M, Demers C, Gurfinkel EP, et al. A comparison of low molecular weight heparin with unfractionated heparin for unstable coronary artery disease. N Engl J Med. 1997; 337:447–452.

84. Weitz JI. Low-molecular-weight heparins. N Engl J Med. 1997; 337:688–698.

85. Young JJ, Kereiakes DJ. Low-molecular-weight heparin in percutaneous coronary intervention: ready for prime time? ACC Current Journal Review. Mar/Apr. 2002.

86. Choo JK, Kereiakes DJ. Low molecular weight heparin therapy for percutaneous coronary intervention: a practice in evolution. J Thromb Thrombolysis. 2001; 11:235–246.

87. Antman EM, McCabe CH, Gurfinkel P, et al. For the TIMI 11B investigators: Enoxaparin prevents death and cardiac ischemic events in unstable angina/non-Q-wave myocardial infarction—results of the Thrombolysis in Myocardial Infarction (TIMI) 11B trial. Circulation. 1999; 100:1593–1601.

88. Low-molecular weight heparin during instability in coronary artery disease. Fragmin during Instability in Coronary Artery Disease (FRISC) study group. Lancet. 1996; 347:561–568.

89. Antman EM, Cohen M, McCabe C, et al. Enoxaparin is superior to unfractionated heparin for preventing clinical events at 1–year follow-up of TIMI 11B and ESSENCE. Eur Heart J. 2002; 23:308–314.

90. Lindahl B, Venge P, Wallentin L. The FRISC experience with troponin T. Use as decision tool and comparison with other prognostic markers. Eur Heart J. 1998; 19(Suppl N):N41–N58.

91. Klein W, Buchwald A, Hillis SE, et al. Comparison of low molecular weight heparin with unfractionated heparin acutely and with placebo for 6 weeks and the management of unstable coronary artery disease. Fragmin in unstable coronary artery disease study (FRIC). Circulation. 1997; 96:61–68.

92. FRISC II Investigators: Long-term low-molecular-mass heparin in unstable coronary artery disease: FRISC II prospective randomized multicentre study. Lancet. 1999; 354:701–707.

93. FRISC II Investigators: Invasive compared with non-invasive treatment in unstable coronary artery disease: FRISC II prospective randomized multicentre study. Lancet. 1999; 354:708–715.

94. Faxon DP, Spiro TE, Minor S, et al. Low molecular weight heparin in prevention of restenosis after angioplasty: results of enoxaparin restenosis (ERA) trial. Circulation. 1994; 90:908–914.

95. Karsch KR, Preisack MB, Baildon R, et al. Low molecular weight heparin (reviparin) in percutaneous transluminal coronary angioplasty: results of a randomized, double blind, unfractionated heparin in placebo controlled, multi-center trial (REDUCE). J Am Coll Cardiol. 1996; 28:1437–1443.

96. Rabah MM, Premmereur J, Graham M, et al. Usefulness of intravenous enoxaparin for percutaneous coronary intervention in stable angina pectoris. Am J Cardiol. 1999; 84:1391–1395.

97. Kereiakes DJ, Grines C, Fry E, et al. Abciximab-enoxaparin interaction during percutaneous coronary intervention: results of the NICE 1 and 4 trials. J Am Coll Cardiol. 2000; 35:92A.

98. Kereiakes DJ, Grines C, Fry E, et al. For the NICE 1 and NICE 4 investigators: Enoxaparin and abciximab adjunctive pharmacotherapy during percutaneous coronary intervention. J Invas Cardiol. 2001; 13:272–278.

99. Young JJ, Kereiakes DJ, Grines CL. Low-molecular-weight heparin therapy in percutaneous coronary intervention: The NICE 1 and NICE 4 trials. J Invas Cardiol. 2000; 12(suppl E):E14–E18.

100. Ferguson J, Antman E, Bates E, et al. and the NICE 3 Investigators. The use of enoxaparin and IIb/IIIa antagonists in acute coronary syndromes, including PCI: The NICE 3 study. Am J Cardiol. 2000; 86:16i.

101. Bhatt DL, Lee BI, Casterella PJ, et al. Safety of concomitant therapy with eptifibatide and enoxaparin in patients undergoing percutaneous coronary intervention: results of the Coronary Revascularization Using Integrilin and Single bolus Enoxaparin Study. J Am Coll Cardiol. 2003; 41:20–25.

102. Blazing MA, deLemos JA, White HA, et al. A-phase of the Aggrastat to Zocor (A to Z) study: comparison of the safety and efficacy of unfractionated heparin versus enoxaparin in combination with tirofiban and aspirin in individuals who present with non-ST elevation acute coronary syndromes. Late Breaking Trials presentation at the ACC 52nd Annual Scientific Session, Chicago, IL, March 30–April 2, 2004.

103. SYNERGY Executive Committee. Superior yield of the new strategy of enoxaparin, revascularization and glycoprotein IIb/IIIa inhibitors. The SYNERGY trial: study design and rationale. Am Heart J. 2004; 143:952–960.

104. Theroux P, Welsh R. Meta-analysis of randomized trials comparing enoxaparin versus unfractionated heparin as adjunctive therapy to fibrinolysis in ST-elevation acute myocardial infarction. Am J Cardiol. 2003; 91:860–864.

105. Sinnaeve PR, Antman EM, Ross AM, Hasselbladv, Vande WerfFJ,Granger CB, Enoxaparin is superior to unfractionated heparin after fibrinolysis in acute myocardial infarction: meta-analysis of ASSENT-3, HART-II, and ENTIRE-TIMI-23 Trials. J Am Coll Cardiol. 2003;14:334A.

106. Phillippides GJ, Loscalzo J. Potential advantages of direct acting thrombin inhibitors. Coron Artery Dis. 1996; 7:497–507.

107. Ali MN, Villarreal-Levy G, Schaefer AI. The role of thrombin and thrombin inhibitors in coronary angioplasty. Chest. 1995; 108:1409–1419.

108. Cannon CP, Braunwald E. Hirudin: initial results in acute myocardial infarction, unstable angina and angioplasty. J Am Coll Cardiol. 1995; 25:30S-37S.

109. Bittl JA. Clinical trials of hirulog in patients undergoing high risk percutaneous transluminal coronary angioplasty. Coron Artery Dis. 1996; 7:449–454.

110. Agnelli G. Thrombin plays a pivotal role in vascular reocclusion after PTCA and coronary thrombolysis. Cardiovasc Res. 1996; 31:232–234.

111. Kaiser B, Simon A, Markwardt F. Antithrombotic effects of recombinant hirudin in experimental angioplasty needed for vascular thrombolysis. Thromb Haemost. 1990; 63:44–47.

112. Topol EJ, Bonan R, Jewitt D, et al. Use of a direct antithrombin hirulog in place of heparin during coronary angioplasty. Circulation. 1993; 87:1622–1629.

113. Rupprecht HJ, Terres WI, Ozbek C, et al. Recombinant hirudin prevents troponin T release after coronary angioplasty in patients with unstable angina. J Am Coll Cardiol. 1995; 26:1637–1642.

114. Bittl JA, Strony J, Brinker JA, et al. for the Hirulog Angioplasty Study Investigators. Treatment with bivalirudin (hirulog) as compared with heparin during coronary angioplasty for unstable or post infarction angina. N Engl J Med. 1995; 333:764–769.

115. Bittl JA. Comparative safety profiles of hirulog and heparin in patients undergoing angioplasty. Am Heart J. 1995; 130:658–665.

116. Serruys PW, Herrman JP, Simon R, et al. For the Helvetica investigators: A comparison of hirudin with heparin in the prevention of restenosis after coronary angioplasty. N Engl J Med. 1995; 333:757–763.

117. Global Use of Strategies to Open Occluded Coronary Arteries (GUSTO) IIb Investigators. A comparison of recombinant hirudin with heparin for the treatment of acute coronary syndromes. N Engl J Med. 1996; 335:775–782.

118. Antman E, for the TIMI 9B Investigators. Hirudin in acute myocardial infarction. Thrombolysis and Thrombin Inhibition in Myocardial Infarction (TIMI) 9B Trial. Circulation. 1996; 94:911–921.

119. Neuhaus KL, Essen RV, TebbeU, et al. Safety observations from the pilot phase of the randomized r-hirudin for improvement of thrombolysis (HIT-III) study: a study of the Arbeitsgemeinschaft Leitender Kardiologischer Krankenhausarzte (ALKK). Circulation. 1994; 90:1638–1642.

120. GUSTO II Investigators. Randomized trial of intravenous heparin versus recombinant hirudin for acute coronary syndromes: the Global Use of Strategies to Open Occluded Coronary Arteries (GUSTO) IIa Investigators. Circulation. 1994; 90:1631–1637.

121. Antman EM, for the TIMI 9A Investigators. Hirudin in acute myocardial infarction: safety report from the thrombolysis and thrombin inhibition in myocardial infarction (TIMI) 9A trial. Circulation. 1994; 90:1642–1630.

122. Bittl JA, Feit F, for the Hirulog Angioplasty Study Investigators. A randomized comparison of bivalirudin and heparin in patients undergoing coronary angioplasty for postinfarction angina. Am J Cardiol. 1998; 82:43P-49P.

123. Schiele F, Villemenot A, Kramerz P, et al. Use of recombinant hirudin as antithrombotic treatment in patients with heparin induced thrombocytopenia. Am J Hematol. 1995; 50:20–25.

124. Chamberlin JR, Lewis V, Leya F, et al. Successful treatment of heparin associated thrombocytopenia and thrombosis using Hirulog. Can J Cardiol. 1995; 11:511–514.

125. Lewis BE, Ferguson JJ, Grassman ED, et al. Successful coronary interventions performed with argatroban anticoagulation in patients with heparin induced thrombocytopenia and thrombosis syndrome. J Invas Cardiol. 1996; 8:410–417.

126. Feit F, Bittl JA, Lincoff AM, et al. Bivalirudin reduces ischemic and hemorrhagic complications of percutaneous coronary intervention: pooled data from 10 prospective studies in 6,134 patients. J Am Coll Cardiol. 2003; 41:25A

127. Direct Thrombin Inhibitor Trialists' Collaborative Group. Direct thrombin inhibitors in acute coronary syndromes and during percutaneous coronary intervention: design of a meta-analysis based on individual patient data. Am Heart J. 2001; 141:2.

128. tenBerg JM, Kelder JC, Suttorp MJ, et al. A randomized trial assessing the effect of coumarins started before coronary angioplasty on restenosis: results of the 6–month angiographic substudy of the Balloon Angioplasty and Anticoagulation Study (BAAS). Am Heart J. 2003; 145:58–65.

129. Hurlen M, Abdelnoor M, Smith P, et al. Warfarin, aspirin, or both after myocardial infarction. N Engl J Med. 2002; 347:969–974.

130. Askew K, Wallin R, Sane D. Warfarin: mechanisms for durable effects in coronary artery disease. HeartDrug. 2002; 2:184–191.

131. Asakura H, Ichino T, Yoshida T, et al. Beneficial effect of JTV-803, a new synthetic inhibitor of activated factor X, against both lipopolysaccharide-induced and tissue factor-induced disseminated intravascular coagulation in rat models. Blood Coagul Fibrinolysis. 2002; 13:233–239.

132. Bauer KA, Eriksson BI, Lassen MR, et al. Fondaparinux compared with enoxaparin for the prevention of venous thromboembolism after elective major knee surgery. N Engl J Med. 2001; 345:1305–1310.

133. Covic L, Gresser AL, Talavera J, et al. Activation and inhibition of G protein-coupled receptors by cell-penetrating membrane-tethered peptides. Proc Natl Acad Sci USA. 2002; 99:643–648.

134. Covic L, Misra M, Badar J, et al. Pepducin-based intervention of thrombin-receptor signaling and systemic platelet activation. Nat Med. 2002; 8:1161–1165.

14-2

Adjunctive Use of Antiplatelet Therapy During Percutaneous Coronary Intervention

John J. Young and Dean J. Kereiakes
The Lindner Center for Research & Education and The Ohio Heart Health Center, Cincinnati, Ohio, U.S.A.

I. INTRODUCTION

The past decade has seen major advances in adjunctive pharmacotherapy for percutaneous coronary intervention (PCI). Pharmacotherapeutic advances have resulted from a greater understanding of the pathophysiological mechanisms underlying platelet activation and aggregation, thrombin generation, and thrombus formation. Specifically, refinements in the use of unfractionated heparin (UFH), developments in the use of low molecular weight heparin (LMWH) and direct thrombin inhibitors (DTIs), as well as improvement in both oral and parenteral adjunctive antiplatelet therapies have occurred.

Periprocedural myocardial ischemic events primarily related to thrombus formation complicate up to 4–12% of PCIs (1–3). The thrombotic cascade responsible for these events involves a complex interaction between platelets and other coagulation factors. All current PCI techniques denude the arterial endothelium, thereby exposing atherosclerotic material and connective tissue elements to circulating blood (4–6). This deep arterial wall injury initiates the coagulation cascade, which includes platelet adherence to exposed collagen, von Willebrand factor, or fibrinogen via specific cell membrane receptors [glycoprotein (GP) Ia/IIa, GP Ib/IX, and GP IIb/IIIa, respectively] with subsequent platelet activation and aggregation (7,8). The end product for both the intrinsic and extrinsic coagulation pathways is the generation of thrombin that initiates conversion of fibrinogen to fibrin (formation of "red" thrombus) and is a potent stimulus for platelet aggregation (formation of "white" thrombus). Optimal pharmacological strategies to minimize periprocedural ischemic complications during PCI have become increasingly focused on neutralizing both platelet and pro-coagulant pathways. This chapter will review the value of antiplatelet therapy in preventing thrombotic complications associated with PCI.

II. ASPIRIN

Aspirin exerts its effect primarily by interfering with the biosynthesis of cyclic prostanoids [e.g., thromboxane A_2 (TXA$_2$), prostacyclin], often referred to as prostaglandins. Prostaglandins are generated by the enzymatically catalyzed oxidation of arachidonic acid, which itself is derived from membrane phospholipids (9). Arachidonic acid is further metabolized by the enzyme prostaglandin H synthase (PGH synthase), commonly referred to as cyclooxygenase (COX). COX exists as two isomers: COX-1 and COX-2. COX-1 results in the synthesis of prostaglandins responsible for normal homeostatic functions, such as gastric mucosal protection, maintenance of blood flow, and the regulation of platelet activation and aggregation (9). COX-2 is an inducible enzyme and produces prostaglandins, which contribute to the inflammatory response (10,11). Interestingly, researchers have recently identified a third distinct COX isoenzyme (COX-3) (12). Unlike COX-1 and COX-2, COX-3 is selectively inhibited by analgesic/antipyretic agents such as acetaminophen.

Aspirin exerts its primary antithrombotic effects through the inhibition of PGH synthase enzyme by the irreversible acetylation of a serine residue at position 529 (13,14). In addition, aspirin is approximately 170-fold more potent in inhibiting COX-1 than COX-2 (15). In the presence of aspirin, COX-1 is completely inactivated, whereas COX-2 cannot convert arachidonic acid to subsequent metabolites. The net result is that neither COX isoform is capable of converting arachidonic acid to metabolites necessary for the production of prostaglandins. By inhibiting prostaglandin synthesis, aspirin's therapeutic effects (e.g., inhibition of platelet aggregation, vasodilation, anti-inflammatory) are manifest. These actions also account for aspirin's adverse gastrointestinal profile secondary to the inhibition of prostaglandin synthesis related to gastric mucosal protection.

Across the spectrum of atherosclerotic vascular disease (coronary, cerebral, and peripheral vascular), aspirin has been demonstrated to reduce the risk of adverse ischemic events by 15–25% (16). In the setting of acute myocardial infarction (MI), the benefit of coadministration of aspirin with fibrinolytic therapy was unequivocally demonstrated in the ISIS-2 (Second International Study of Infarct Survival) study (17). Aspirin was associated with a 23% reduction in mortality to 5 weeks following enrollment, which was equivalent to the mortality reduction attributable to streptokinase alone (25%) and additive when streptokinase and aspirin were combined (42% mortality reduction) (17). Among patients with unstable angina in four placebo-controlled trials, aspirin (in doses ranging from 75 to 1320 mg/day) was associated with a consistent reduction in the risk of death or MI by 30–50% (18–21).

The efficacy of aspirin in reducing the ischemic complications of coronary angioplasty has also been established. In a retrospective analysis (22), occlusive intracoronary thrombi following balloon dilation were less frequent among patients pretreated with aspirin (1.8% vs. 10.7%). In a prospective randomized trial (23), periprocedural Q-wave MI was significantly lower (1.6% vs. 6.9%) among patients who had received antiplatelet therapy. In addition, daily doses of aspirin ranging from 80 to 1500 mg appeared equally efficacious in reducing the incidence of abrupt coronary closure following PCI by 50–75% (22,24,25). In the stable phase of coronary artery disease, aspirin therapy reduces the risk of vascular death, reinfarction, and stroke by up to 25% (16). Recent data have prompted important changes in the American Heart Association (AHA) guidelines for primary prevention of cardiovascular disease and stroke, and have confirmed that the recommended daily dose of aspirin (75–160 mg) is as effective as higher doses of aspirin and is associated with less bleeding risk (26–28).

III. THIENOPYRIDINES: TICLOPIDINE AND CLOPIDOGREL

Thienopyridine derivatives (ticlopidine and clopidogrel) irreversibly bind to adenosine diphosphate (ADP) receptors on the platelet and, thus, inhibit ADP-mediated GP IIb/IIIa receptor activation and platelet aggregation (29–32) (Fig. 1). A systematic overview of 39

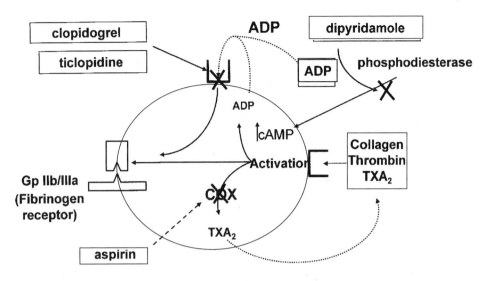

Figure 1   Mechanism of action of oral antiplatelet agents. ADP = adenosine diphosphate; TXA_2 = thromboxane A_2; COX = cyclooxygenase. Adapted from: Schafer AI. Antiplatelet therapy. (Adapted from Ref. 31.)

placebo-controlled trials of ticlopidine in patients with vascular disease demonstrated a significant 33% reduction in the risk of ischemic events, similar to the beneficial treatment effect that was provided by aspirin therapy (25–30%) (16). In three small trials that compared aspirin directly to ticlopidine among a cumulative total of 3500 high-risk patients with coronary or cerebral vascular disease, a nonsignificant advantage for ticlopidine (10% approximate reduction in adverse events) was observed (16).

The addition of ticlopidine to aspirin and UFH has been demonstrated to reduce both the indices of procedural platelet activation (serotonin release, P-selectin expression) as well as the correlates of thrombin generation (fibrinopeptide A, prothrombin fragment 1.2, thrombin-antithrombin complexes) following PCI (33–36). The combination of aspirin and ticlopidine has proven superior to aspirin alone or the combination of aspirin and warfarin for reducing ischemic events and hemorrhagic complications after elective coronary stenting (37–39). Combination antiplatelet therapy appears to provide optimal adjunctive pharmacology after "bailout" or unplanned stent deployment as well (37–42). These observations led to the previously established recommendation that ticlopidine be administered in a dose of 250 mg orally twice daily for at least 2 weeks (up to 4 weeks) in combination with aspirin 325 mg orally once daily following intracoronary stent deployment (43). Important disadvantages of therapy with ticlopidine include skin rash, gastrointestinal intolerance, bone marrow suppression, thrombocytopenia (including potentially fatal thrombotic thrombocytopenia purpura) as well as a delay in peak pharmacodynamic action of 3–5 days or more after initiation of treatment (44,45).

Clopidogrel is a thienopyridine derivative that is closely related structurally to ticlopidine. In a study of over 19,000 patients with coronary, peripheral, or cerebral vascular disease, clopidogrel was found to be modestly superior to aspirin with regard to the long-term risk of ischemic events (vascular death, MI, or ischemic stroke) (5.32 vs. 5.83%, respectively) over a mean 1.9-year follow-up ($p = 0.043$) (46). Clopidogrel was not associated with bone marrow suppression or gastrointestinal intolerance in this trial. The CLASSICS (Clopidogrel Aspirin Stent International Cooperative Study) trial, which compared ticlopidine 250 mg orally twice daily (plus aspirin) versus clopidogrel 75 mg orally daily (with or without a 300 mg oral loading dose) plus aspirin following coronary stent deployment, demonstrated no differences in clinical outcomes but better tolerability with clopidogrel (47).

The efficacy of the combination of clopidogrel and aspirin in reducing long-term ischemic complications among patients with non–ST segment elevation acute coronary syndromes was described in the CURE (Clopidogrel in Unstable angina to prevent Recurrent ischemic Events) trial (48). Among 12,562 patients randomized to receive aspirin alone versus aspirin plus clopidogrel who were followed for 6–12 months, the composite endpoint of cardiovascular death, MI, or stroke was reduced from 11.4 to 9.3% (p < 0.001) (48). The prospectively planned substudy, PCI-CURE (Percutaneous Coronary Intervention-CURE), analyzed 2658 of the patients with non-ST elevation ACS who had PCI (nonrandomized) by their randomly assigned pharmacological treatment strategy (clopidogrel, n = 1313; placebo, n = 1345) (49). Patients were pretreated with aspirin and study drug for a median of 6 days before PCI, and the primary substudy endpoint was the composite occurrence of cardiovascular death, MI, or urgent revascularization to 30 days post-PCI. Pretreatment with clopidogrel was associated with a reduction in the primary endpoint in the clopidogrel patients compared with aspirin alone (4.5% vs. 6.4% respectively; p = 0.03) (49). In addition, longer-term administration of clopidogrel (≥8 months) following PCI was associated with durable enhanced benefit and a lower incidence of cardiovascular death or myocardial infarction (p = 0.047).

Oral loading doses of 300–450 mg clopidogrel result in early (2–6 h) marked platelet inhibition and appear to be well tolerated (50–52). Oral thienopyridine loading (clopidogrel 300 mg) administered to patients who present with non-ST elevation ACS has been demonstrated to reduce major adverse cardiovascular events (MACE) in patients undergoing PCI (49). The clinical benefit of clopidogrel appears additive for further reducing periprocedural ischemic events even when periprocedural platelet GP IIb/IIIa inhibition is administered (53–55). The benefit of clopidogrel pretreatment appears greatest in those patients with plaque inflammation as reflected by elevation in serum C-reactive protein (53). Based on randomized comparative trials and meta-analyses demonstrating enhanced safety, efficacy, and tolerability for clopidogrel (vs. ticlopidine) when administered in combination with aspirin following coronary stent deployment, clopidogrel has become the thienopyridine treatment of choice (56).

The American College of Cardiology/American Heart Association (ACC/AHA) guidelines for PCI currently recommend continuation of oral aspirin and thienopyridine therapy for 30 days following stent deployment (57). The recent updated guidelines for unstable angina and non-ST elevation MI patients, however, recommend continued thienopyridine therapy in combination with aspirin for at least 1 month (Class 1, Level of evidence A) following presentation with an ACS, and for up to 9 months (Class 1, Level of Evidence B) whether PCI has been performed or not (58). Recently, The Clopidogrel for the Reduction of Events During Observation (CREDO) trial added important insight into the optimal duration of combination oral antiplatelet therapy following PCI (59). CREDO randomized 2116 patients undergoing elective PCI to receive either a 300mg clopidogrel oral loading dose (n = 1053) or placebo (n = 1063) 3–24 hours before PCI. All patients then received clopidogrel (75 mg/d) through day 28. After 28 days, patients in the clopidogrel loading-dose group continued to receive clopidogrel (75 mg/d) through 12 months, while those in the control group received placebo. Both treatment groups received aspirin throughout the study. Although the loading dose of clopidogrel before PCI did not reduce ischemic events (death, MI, urgent revascularization) to 28 days, subgroup analysis suggested that those patients with a longer interval (≥ 6 h) between the loading dose and PCI did have a reduction in adverse events (59). At 1-year follow-up, long-term clopidogrel therapy was associated with a 26.9% relative reduction in the combined endpoint of death, MI, or stroke ($p = 0.02$) (59) (Fig. 2). The results of the CREDO trial are consistent with current ACC/AHA guidelines and suggest that in patients undergoing PCI, clopidogrel (in combination with aspirin) therapy should be continued for at least 1 year and leads to a significant reduction in atherothrombotic events.

IV. PLATELET GP IIB/IIIA BLOCKADE

A variety of antibody, peptide, peptidomimetic, and nonpeptide compounds have been shown to interfere with platelet aggregation by blocking the glycoprotein (GP) IIb/IIIa receptor (60–62). Following platelet activation, this transmembrane heterodimer receptor undergoes a conformational change with consequent high-affinity binding to adhesive proteins (fibrinogen, von Willebrand factor, fibronectin, vitronectin), which bridge platelet GP IIb/IIIa receptors and result in platelet aggregation. Adjunctive therapy with GP IIb/IIIa blockade, in addition to aspirin and heparin during PCI, significantly reduces the composite occurrence of death, MI, or additional coronary revascularization in hospital and to 30 days and 6 months following PCI (63) (Fig. 3). GP IIb/IIIa receptor blocking drugs differ in their duration of action at the platelet target receptor and in receptor affinity [GP IIb/IIIa vs. $\alpha_v\beta_3$ (vitronectin) vs. CD11b/18 (MAC 1)] (64,65).

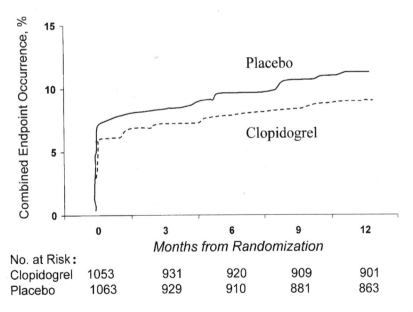

No. at Risk:					
Clopidogrel	1053	931	920	909	901
Placebo	1063	929	910	881	863

Figure 2 Combined endpoint (death, MI, stroke) results at 1 year for clopidogrel versus placebo in the CREDO trial. The relative risk reduction for clopidogrel compared with placebo is 26.9% (95% CI 3.9–44.4%; $p = 0.02$). (From Ref. 59.)

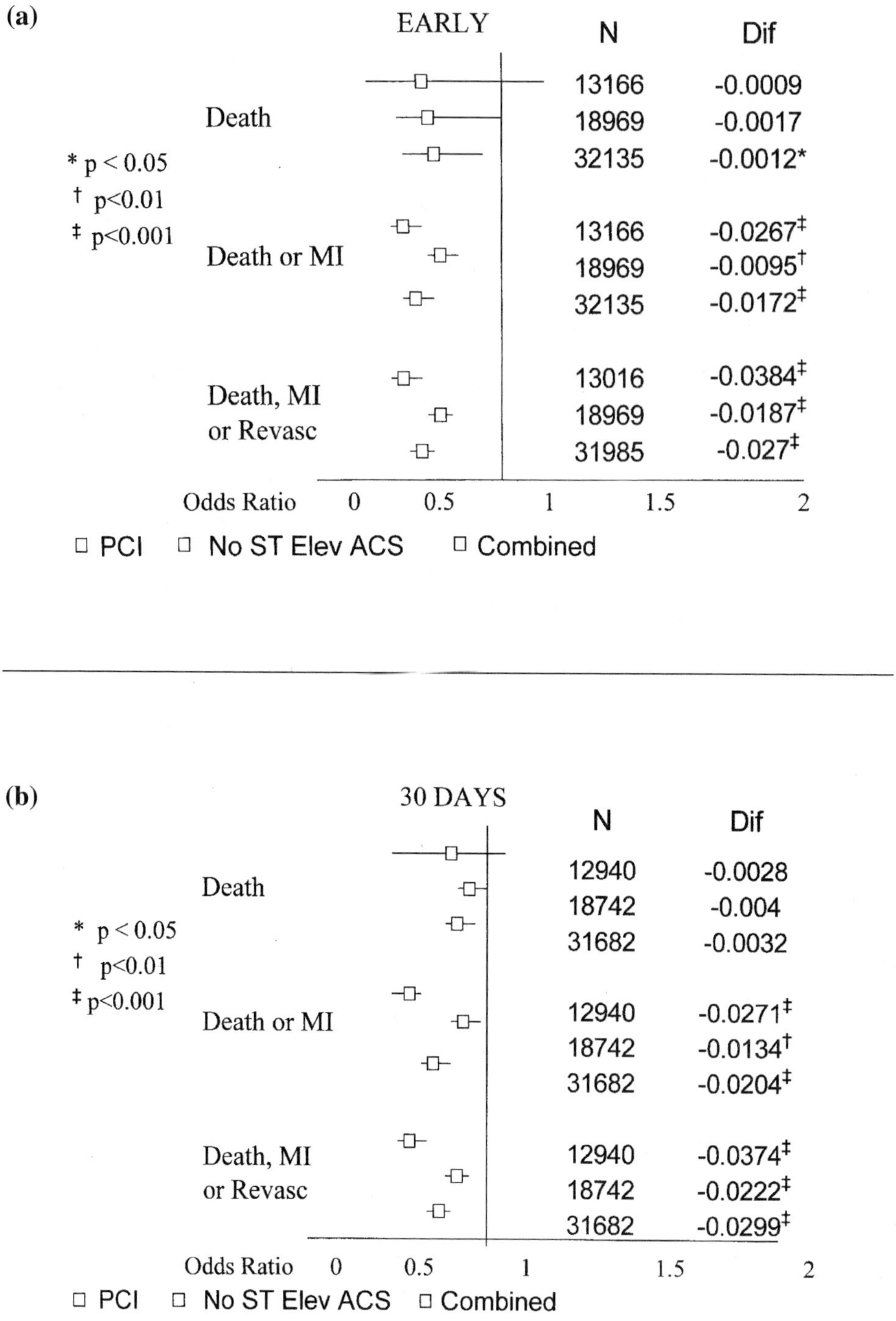

(a)

EARLY   N   Dif

Death	13166	-0.0009
	18969	-0.0017
	32135	-0.0012*
Death or MI	13166	-0.0267‡
	18969	-0.0095†
	32135	-0.0172‡
Death, MI or Revasc	13016	-0.0384‡
	18969	-0.0187‡
	31985	-0.027‡

* $p < 0.05$
† $p < 0.01$
‡ $p < 0.001$

Odds Ratio   0   0.5   1   1.5   2

□ PCI   □ No ST Elev ACS   □ Combined

(b)

30 DAYS   N   Dif

Death	12940	-0.0028
	18742	-0.004
	31682	-0.0032
Death or MI	12940	-0.0271‡
	18742	-0.0134†
	31682	-0.0204‡
Death, MI or Revasc	12940	-0.0374‡
	18742	-0.0222‡
	31682	-0.0299‡

* $p < 0.05$
† $p < 0.01$
‡ $p < 0.001$

Odds Ratio   0   0.5   1   1.5   2

□ PCI   □ No ST Elev ACS   □ Combined

Figure 3 Odds ratios and 95% confidence intervals for the occurrence of death; death or myocardial infarction (MI); or death, MI, or coronary revascularization (Revasc) for all randomized trials of platelet GP IIb/IIIa blockade versus placebo in hospital **(a)** and at 30 days **(b)** and 6 months **(c;** facing page) after enrollment. Odds ratios are for trials of PCI, non-ST elevation ACS, or combination of all. PCI = percutaneous coronary intervention; No ST Elev ACS = non–ST segment elevation acute coronary syndrome. (From Ref. 63.)

(c)

6 MONTHS

		N	Dif
Death		12790	-0.0021
		15145	-0.0002
		27935	-0.0015

* p < 0.05
† p<0.01
‡ p<0.001

Death or MI		12790	-0.023†
		15145	-0.0155†
		27935	-0.0196‡

Death, MI or Revasc		12790	-0.0281†
		15145	-0.0198†
		27935	-0.0232‡

Odds Ratio 0   0.5   1   1.5   2

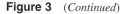

□ PCI   □ No ST Elev ACS   □ Combined

Figure 3 (*Continued*)

A. Abciximab

The Evaluation of 7E3 for the Prevention of Ischemic Complications (EPIC) trial was the first study to test the efficacy of adjunctive GP IIb/IIIa receptor blockade for PCI (60). Eligible patients were randomly assigned to receive abciximab intravenous bolus only, abciximab bolus plus 12-hour infusion, or placebo (no abciximab). Treatment with abciximab bolus plus infusion was associated with a 35% reduction in the primary endpoint of death, nonfatal MI, or need for urgent revascularization (vs. placebo) through 30 days. Three-year follow-up demonstrated sustained clinical benefit (66). A more recent analysis by intention to treat at 7-year follow-up demonstrated a significant and similar reduction in mortality for all abciximab-treated patients (mortality 17.3% bolus plus 12-h infusion, 16.1% bolus only, and 20.1% placebo) (67) (Fig. 4). This observation suggests a beneficial effect of abciximab to reduce mortality in excess of that explained solely by suppression of early periprocedural ischemic events. Indeed, abciximab bolus only was associated with only 10% reduction (p = NS) in the primary study endpoint to 30 days and yet appeared to provide a similar survival advantage to 7 years as observed with bolus plus 12-hour infusion therapy.

The Evaluation in PTCA to Improve Long-term Outcome with Abciximab Glycoprotein IIb/IIIa blockade (EPILOG) study investigated whether the benefits of abciximab could be extended to a broader spectrum of patients undergoing angioplasty and whether a low-dose, weight-adjusted regimen for concomitant UFH administration would reduce the excessive bleeding rates observed in the EPIC trial without a loss of clinical efficacy (68). Eligible patients were randomly assigned to receive one of three regimens: abciximab plus standard-dose (100 U/kg) UFH, abciximab plus reduced-dose (70 U/kg)

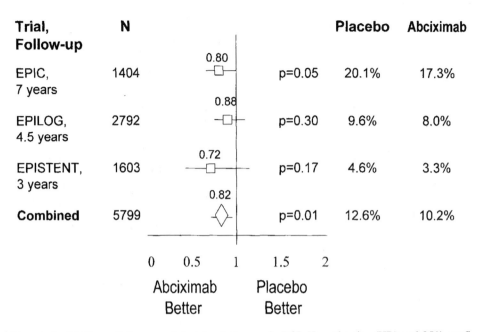

Figure 4   Multiyear follow-up of abciximab therapy in PCI. Hazard ratios (HR) and 95% confidence intervals (CI) for each of the three trials at maximum follow-up. (From Ref. 67.)

UFH, or standard-dose heparin alone (no abciximab). Treatment with abciximab plus reduced-dose UFH was associated with a 55% reduction in death, nonfatal MI, or urgent revascularization through 30 days. The primary endpoint event rates observed with abciximab and standard-dose UFH were nearly identical to those observed in the group receiving abciximab and low-dose UFH. As with EPIC, long-term follow-up data confirmed a durable benefit on primary endpoint events to 1-year follow-up (69). Furthermore, the rate of major bleeding was similar between all three treatment groups. A recent analysis of all EPILOG trial patients by intention to treat with follow-up through 4.5 years demonstrated a trend toward reduction in late mortality associated with abciximab bolus plus infusion (8%) versus placebo (9.6%) (67) (Fig. 4).

In the Evaluation of Platelet GP IIb/IIIa Inhibitor for Stenting (EPISTENT) trial, patients with ischemic heart disease and suitable coronary lesions were randomly assigned to stenting plus placebo, stenting plus abciximab, or balloon angioplasty plus abciximab (70). Abciximab was administered as a standard bolus plus 12-hour infusion, and all patients who received abciximab were also treated with reduced-dose weight-adjusted (70 U/kg) UFH. The primary clinical endpoint was the composite occurrence of death, MI, or urgent revascularization through 30 days. The primary endpoint was observed in 10.8% of patients in the stent-placebo group, 5.3% in the stent-abciximab group, and 6.9% in the balloon-abciximab group (70). The outcomes most dramatically reduced by abciximab included the composite occurrence of death and large MI (>5-fold upper limit of normal creatine kinase – MB fraction elevation), which was observed in 7.8% of the stent-placebo group, 3.0% of the stent-abciximab group, and 4.7% of the balloon-abciximab group. At 1-year follow-up, 1% of patients in the stent-abciximab group had died, compared with 2.4% of patients in the stent-placebo group. The combined endpoint of death or MI was observed in 5.3% and 11% of stented patients who received abciximab or placebo, respectively. A prospectively defined substudy was performed in diabetics, with the endpoint being the composite occurrence of death, MI, or target-vessel revascularization (TVR) through 6 months (71). Abciximab therapy, irrespective of revascularization strategy (PTCA or stent), significantly reduced the rate of death or MI to 6 months in the diabetic cohort. The 1-year mortality rate for diabetic patients was 4.1% in the stent-placebo and 1.2% in stent-abciximab treatment groups (72). A recent analysis of all patients by intention to treat with follow-up through 3 years demonstrated a trend toward reduction in mortality associated with abciximab, especially in combination with stenting (stent + placebo, 4.8%; balloon + abciximab, 4.6%; stent + abciximab, 3.3%) (67) (Fig. 4).

Clinical studies of the benefits of abciximab as an adjunct to primary angioplasty in patients with ST-segment elevation MI (STEMI) include ReoPro in Acute Myocardial Infarction and Primary PTCA Organization and Randomization Trial (RAPPORT) (73), Intracoronary Stenting and Antithrombotic Regimen 2 (ISAR-2) (74), Abciximab before Direct Angioplasty and Stenting in Myocardial Infarction Regarding Acute and Long-term Follow-up (ADMIRAL) (75), and Controlled Abciximab and Device Investigation to Lower Late Angioplasty Complications (CADILLAC) (76). In all four trials abciximab significantly decreased the incidence of death, reinfarction, and the need for urgent target vessel revascularization (TVR) at the cost of increased bleeding mainly at sites of vascular access (Fig. 5). In the CADILLAC trial, the combination of stent plus abciximab provided optimal outcomes, with 96.7% of patients achieving thrombolysis in MI (TIMI) grade 3 flow following PCI and very low mortality rates (76). The Abciximab and Carbostent Evaluation in Acute Myocardial Infarction (ACE) trial enrolled 400 patients with STEMI to treatment with stenting (Carbostent) with or without abciximab therapy (77). Preliminary results demonstrate an improvement in the primary composite endpoint of death, reinfarction, TVR, or stroke to 30 days in abciximab treated patients.

Abciximab in combination with reduced-dose fibrinolysis for acute STEMI was initially studied in the Thrombolysis In Myocardial Infarction (TIMI)-14 and Strategies for

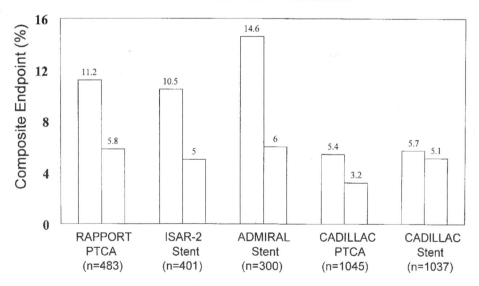

Figure 5 Composite endpoint (death, MI, urgent revascularization) reduction by 30-days in trials of abciximab during primary PCI for acute MI. (From Ref. 67.)

Patency Enhancement in the Emergency Department (SPEED) trials (78,79). The recently completed GUSTO-V trial examined the clinical efficacy and safety of half-dose reteplase and full-dose abciximab compared to full-dose reteplase in an open label design (80). At 30 days mortality (all cause) was similar between the two groups (reteplase plus abciximab, 5.6%; reteplase alone, 5.9%) (80). However, at 7 days recurrent ischemia, reinfarction, and the need for urgent coronary intervention were all significantly less frequent in the reduced-dose reteplase plus abciximab group. The frequency of major cardiac complications following MI was significantly reduced in the reteplase plus abciximab group. No significant difference in the incidence of intracranial hemorrhage (ICH) was seen in the overall population, although a trend toward more frequent ICH was present in elderly patients (age > 75 years; 2.1% combination vs. 1.1% monotherapy) (80). The occurrence of nonintracranial bleeding and thrombocytopenia was higher with combination therapy. Combination therapy with abciximab and half-dose reteplase did not reduce mortality over 1 year compared with fibrinolytic therapy with reteplase alone (81).

Thus, the GUSTO V trial demonstrated "noninferiority" of an alternative reperfusion strategy (vs. fibrinolytic monotherapy) and substantiates the concept of combined fibrinolysis and platelet GP IIb/IIIa inhibition in the management of STEMI. The attractiveness of the combination therapy approach is that for patients who fail to achieve prompt pharmacological reperfusion, this strategy facilitates a smooth transition from medical to catheter-based (PCI) revascularization. The Facilitated Intervention with Enhanced Reperfusion Speed to Stop Events (FINESSE) trial, which compares reduced-dose reteplase plus abciximab with abciximab alone before primary stenting, will provide another step toward evaluating a facilitated PCI strategy for acute MI.

B. Eptifibatide

The clinical benefit of adjunctive eptifibatide for PCI was demonstrated by the IMPACT-II (Integrilin to Minimize Platelet Aggregation and Prevent Coronary Thrombosis II) (61) and ESPRIT (Enhanced Suppression of the Platelet IIb/IIIa Receptor with Integrilin Therapy) (82) trials. In the IMPACT-II trial the primary study endpoint was the composite occurrence of death, MI, unplanned coronary revascularization, or coronary stent implantation for abrupt or threatened coronary closure to 30 days. By 24 hours post-enrollment treatment with eptifibatide was associated with a statistically significant 25% reduction in the primary endpoint, but by 30 days no difference between treatment groups was observed (61). Eptifibatide treatment did not increase rates of major bleeding or transfusion.

The ESPRIT trial was a randomized, placebo-controlled trial to assess whether a novel, double-bolus dosing strategy for eptifibatide (180 mg/kg bolus x 2, 10 min apart followed by 2.0 mg/kg infusion for 18–24 h) could improve the clinical outcomes of patients undergoing coronary stenting compared with placebo (no eptifibatide) (82). The primary endpoint was the composite occurrence of death, MI, urgent TVR, or the requirement for bailout GP IIb/IIIa inhibitor therapy to treat thrombotic complications through 48 hours after randomization. The secondary endpoint was the composite occurrence of death, MI, or urgent TVR to 30 days. The primary endpoint was reduced by 37% (10.5% placebo vs. 6.6% eptifibatide) (82). The secondary endpoint was reduced by 35% (10.5% placebo vs. 6.8% eptifibatide) (82). At 6-month follow-up the beneficial effect of eptifibatide was persistent primarily due to the early (<48 h after initiation of therapy) suppression of adverse events (83). At 12-month follow-up the composite endpoint of death or MI was observed in 8.0% of eptifibatide-treated patients and 12.4% of placebo-treated patients ($p = 0.001$) (84). Similarly, the composite occurrence of death, MI, or TVR was 17.5% in eptifibatide-treated patients versus 22.1% in placebo-treated patients ($p = 0.007$). Comparisons of 6-

month and 1-year outcomes following coronary artery stenting in diabetic versus nondiabetic patients from the ESPRIT trial have demonstrated somewhat discrepant and confusing results. For example, sequential publications have cited variable numbers of patients in the diabetic cohort and variable endpoint event rates. The composite occurrence of death or MI to 6 months follow-up has been reported as 10.2% placebo vs. 6.3% eptifibatide (p = NS) in 419 diabetic patients 83 as well as 12.5% (placebo) vs. 6.9% eptifibatide in 466 diabetic patients (85). Similarly, the prevalence of target vessel revascularization at 6 months (14.9% eptifibatide vs. 10.2% placebo) was considerably different (16.1% eptifibatide vs. 18.1% placebo) by 1-year follow-up coincident with the increased number of patients included in the diabetic cohort. This variability makes comparison of outcomes achieved with other GP IIb/IIIa inhibitors in diabetic patients problematic (83,85).

Eptifibatide therapy has also been evaluated for treatment of patients with STEMI. The Integrilin to Manage Platelet Aggregation and Combat Thrombolysis in Acute Myocardial Infarction (IMPACT-AMI) trial was a dual phase, dose-ranging, randomized, placebo-controlled trial that examined various dose regimens of eptifibatide in patients receiving full-dose alteplase, aspirin, and intravenous UFH for acute MI (86). Therapy with the highest doses of eptifibatide in combination with full-dose alteplase resulted in superior TIMI grade 2 and 3 coronary patency rates at 90 minutes following initiation of therapy compared with alteplase alone. The subsequent Integrilin and Low-dose Thrombolysis in Acute Myocardial Infarction (INTRO-AMI) trial evaluated even higher doses of eptifibatide than those employed in IMPACT-AMI in conjunction with a reduced dose of alteplase (87). Angiography demonstrated TIMI grade 3 flow rates of up to 65% at 60 minutes and 78% at 90 minutes for patients who received eptifibatide plus reduced-dose alteplase. The INTRO-AMI trial concluded that compared to standard dose alteplase alone, double-bolus eptifibatide followed by a 48-hour infusion in combination with reduced-dose alteplase is associated with improved velocity and extent of coronary reperfusion.

Recently, combination reperfusion therapy with eptifibatide and reduced dose tenecteplase (TNK) for STEMI was reported from a phase II angiographic trial. The Integrilin and Tenecteplase in Acute Myocardial Infarction (INTEGRITI) trial enrolled 438 patients with STEMI of <6 hours duration into either a dose-finding (n = 189) arm, which evaluated different dosing combinations of double-bolus eptifibatide and reduced-dose TNK, or a dose-confirmation (n = 249) arm, where patients were randomized 1:1 to either double-bolus eptifibatide in combination with reduced-dose TNK or to standard-dose TNK monotherapy (88). All patients received aspirin and weight-adjusted UFH, and the primary study endpoint was TIMI grade 3 epicardial flow rates at 60 minutes following enrollment. In the dose-finding arm, TIMI grade 3 flow rates were similar across dose groups with a trend toward improved arterial patency at the highest dose of eptifibatide evaluated in combination with reduced-dose TNK. In the dose-confirmation arm, combination eptifibatide plus reduced dose TNK therapy demonstrated a trend toward enhanced TIMI 3 flow rates (59% vs. 49%; p = 0.15), arterial patency (85% vs. 77%; p = 0.17), and ST segment resolution (71% vs. 61%; p = 0.08) compared with TNK monotherapy but was associated with more major hemorrhage (7.6% vs. 2.5%; p = 0.14) and transfusions (13.4% vs. 4.2%; p = 0.02) (88). The authors concluded that further study is needed before this combination can be recommended for general use. The ADVANCE MI (Addressing the Value of Primary Angioplasty after Combination Therapy or Eptifibatide Monotherapy in Acute Myocardial Infarction) study is intended to investigate the safety and efficacy of eptifibatide administered with reduced-dose TNK in patients with STEMI who will proceed to direct PCI in a "facilitated PCI" model.

Of note, a recent study of adjunctive eptifibatide therapy for PCI in acute MI demonstrated a relatively high rate of subacute thrombosis (SAT) within 3–5 days of the procedure. The Integrilin in Acute Myocardial Infarction (INAMI) Stenting study was a prospective, multicenter feasibility and efficacy study that assigned 55 consecutive patients with STEMI to primary PCI with eptifibatide therapy (double bolus 180 µg/kg 10 min. apart; 24-h infusion 2.0 µ/kg/min) (89). Angiographic patency of the infarct vessel with TIMI flow rates, TIMI myocardial perfusion grade (TMPG), and corrected TIMI frame counts were assessed at the end of the procedure and before hospital discharge. At 30-days follow-up, the primary endpoint of the trial (composite of death, MI, and urgent TVR) was observed in 12.7% of patients, which compares unfavorably with similar 30-day composite endpoint rates of 6.0% in the ADMIRAL trial and 4.4% in the CADILLAC trial. TIMI grade 3 (normal) flow and TMPG grade 3 (normal) perfusion was observed in 93% and 86% of patients, respectively, immediately following PCI and declined to 86% and 78%, respectively ($p < 0.05$), before hospital discharge (89). There were five (9.1%) instances of SAT, which presented as acute MI and required urgent TVR within 3–5 days of the primary PCI procedure. The authors concluded that although administration of eptifibatide during primary PCI for STEMI is associated with high TIMI grade 3 flow and TMPG grade 3 rates acutely, these salutory effects are not maintained even in short-term follow-up. The dosage and duration of infusion of eptifibatide in patients with STEMI undergoing PCI needs further evaluation. Ongoing studies, such as Time to Integrilin Therapy in Acute Myocardial Infarction (TITAN)-TIMI 34, will provide more data on appropriate use and duration of therapy with eptifibatide in acute MI patients.

C. Tirofiban

The Randomized Efficacy Study of Tirofiban for Outcomes and Restenosis (RESTORE) trial was a randomized, double-blind, placebo-controlled trial of tirofiban (10 µg/kg bolus; 0.15 µg/kg/min infusion for 36 h) in patients undergoing PCI (balloon angioplasty or directional atherectomy) within 72 hours of presentation with an ACS (62). The primary endpoint of the study was the composite occurrence of death, MI, coronary bypass surgery due to angioplasty failure or recurrent ischemia, repeat target-vessel angioplasty for recurrent ischemia, and insertion of a stent due to actual or threatened abrupt closure of the dilated artery. The primary composite endpoint at 30 days was reduced from 12.2% in placebo-treated patients to 10.3% in tirofiban-treated patients (relative reduction of 16%) (62). However, when repeat angioplasty or coronary artery bypass surgery procedures were included only if performed on an urgent or emergency basis, the composite 30-day event rates were 10.5% in placebo-treated patients and 8.0% in tirofiban-treated patients for a relative reduction of 24%. At 6 months the composite endpoint was not significantly different between the two groups (90).

To date, only one large-scale, randomized clinical comparison of platelet GP IIb/IIIa inhibitors during PCI has been performed. The TARGET (Do Tirofiban and ReoPro Give Similar Efficacy Outcomes Trial) study compared tirofiban (in the RESTORE trial dose regimen) to standard-dose abciximab in patients undergoing planned stent deployment and tested a "not inferior" hypothesis for tirofiban (vs. abciximab) (55). All patients received a loading dose of clopidogrel (300 mg) orally 2–6 hours before PCI. By 30 days there was a significant excess of composite primary endpoint events (death, MI, or urgent revascularization) in the tirofiban group (7.6% vs. 6.0% in the abciximab group) (55) (Fig. 6). The individual endpoints that comprised this composite endpoint were also reduced by abciximab compared with tirofiban. The benefit of abciximab was evident in the first 48–72

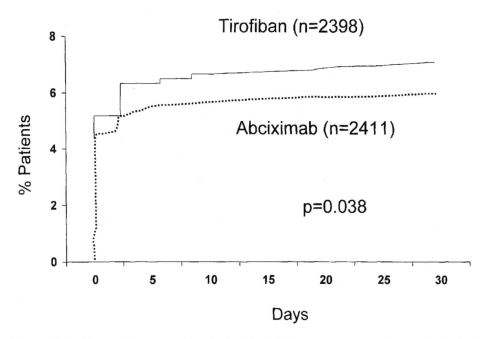

Figure 6 Incidence of the composite endpoint (death, MI, urgent target vessel revascularization) in the first 30 days after enrollment in the TARGET trial. 7.6% in the tirofiban group vs. 6.0% in the abciximab group (CI 1.01–1.57%; $p = 0.03$). (From Ref. 55.)

hours of treatment. Adequate platelet inhibition (>80% inhibition by Accumetrics Rapid Platelet Function Analyzer) was confirmed at both 5 minutes and 4–12 hours following initiation of tirofiban in a small substudy cohort of patients. This trial concluded that tirofiban was inferior to abciximab, which remained the reference standard for PCI.

Recently, the TIGER-PA (Tirofiban Given in the Emergency Room before Primary Angioplasty) pilot trial demonstrated improvement in angiographic outcomes with early administration of tirofiban (RESTORE trial dose regimen) initiated in the emergency department (91). The TIGER-PA pilot trial was a single-center randomized study to evaluate the safety, feasibility, and utility of early tirofiban administration before planned primary PCI in patients presenting with STEMI. One hundred patients with STEMI were randomized to either early administration of tirofiban in the emergency room or later administration in the catheterization laboratory. The primary outcome measures were TIMI grade flow, corrected TIMI frame count, and TMPG on the initial angiogram. MACE to 30 days was also assessed. Significant improvement in initial TIMI flow, corrected TIMI frame counts, and TMPG was observed when tirofiban was administered early (in the emergency room) versus late (in the cath lab) before PCI (91). The occurrence of MACE to 30 days also trended in favor of the earlier administration of tirofiban in the emergency room. Larger studies will be required to confirm the findings of this pilot trial.

V. FUTURE ANTIPLATELET THERAPY

Over the past decade the platelet has emerged as being pivotally important in the pathophysiology of cardiovascular diseases. Indeed, the "preeminence of the platelet" has prompted development of a variety of drugs that have been demonstrated in large-scale randomized trials to improve outcomes for both ACS and PCI. Although the platelet was initially perceived as a "bystander" in hemostasis, it is now well appreciated that it is a key mediator of thrombosis as well as inflammation. A greater understanding of platelet biology has contributed to novel and more precise targets for therapeutic modulation of platelet function.

The concept of a purinergic signaling system that utilizes purine nucleotides and nucleosides as extracellular messengers was first proposed over 30 years ago (92). These molecules mediate both short-term (acute) signaling functions in neurotransmission, secretion, and vasodilation as well as long-term (chronic) signaling functions in development, regeneration, proliferation, and cell death. The thienopyridines (ticlopidine and clopidogrel), which act via metabolites on the platelet ADP receptor subtype now designated P2Y(12), are part of this purinergic signaling system (93,94). Both the P2Y(12) and P2Y(1) ADP receptors are important in modulating shear-induced platelet aggregation as well as platelet aggregation subsequent to initial adhesion via von Willebrand factor. Experimental models have demonstrated that more profound platelet inhibition accompanies blockade of both receptors, and, thus, a combination of antagonists may provide potentially more effective antiplatelet/antithrombotic therapy (95). Orally active agents that target these receptors and that may be more effective than clopidogrel are being developed.

The transmembrane signaling process through G protein–coupled receptors has also generated great interest. Novel cell-penetrating peptides, termed pepducins, may act as intracellular inhibitors of signal transference from surface receptors to G proteins (96). The attachment of pepducins to protease-activated receptors (PARs) provides potent inhibition of thrombin-mediated platelet aggregation (97). A potential advantage of this new class of antithrombin/antiplatelet agent (anti-PAR agents) is inhibition of thrombin-mediated platelet activation that may be achieved with enhanced safety in comparison to other anticoagulants since fibrin formation is unaltered. Other potential future platelet-related targets include the CD40-CD40 ligand system, P-selectin, RANTES, and the GP Ib/IX–von Willebrand factor complex (98). Newer insights at both the cellular and genomic level will hopefully generate novel therapeutic agents to inhibit platelet function more effectively and safely than previously thought possible.

REFERENCES

1. deFeyter PJ, van den Brand M, Laarman GJ, et al. Acute coronary artery occlusion during and after percutaneous transluminal coronary angioplasty. Frequency, prediction, clinical course, management, and follow-up. Circulation. 1991; 83:927–936.
2. Lincoff AM, Popma JJ, Ellis SG, et al. Abrupt vessel closure complicating coronary angioplasty: clinical, angiographic and therapeutic profile. J Am Coll Cardiol. 1992; 19:926–935.
3. Detre KM, Holmes DR, Holubkov R, et al. Incidence and consequences of periprocedural occlusion. The 1985–1986 National Heart, Lung, and Blood Institute Percutaneous Transluminal Coronary Angioplasty Registry. Circulation. 1990; 82:739–750.
4. Uchida Y, Hasegawa K, Kawamura K, et al. Angioscopic observation of the coronary luminal changes induced by percutaneous transluminal coronary angioplasty. Am Heart J. 1989; 117:769–776.
5. Waller BF, Gorfinkel HJ, Rogers FJ, et al. Early and late morphologic changes in major epicardial coronary arteries after percutaneous transluminal coronary angioplasty. Am J Cardiol. 1984; 53:C42–C47.
6. Waller BF, Pinkerton CA, Orr CM, et al. Morphological observations late (greater than 30 days) after clinically successful coronary balloon angioplasty. Circulation. 1991; 83:128–141.
7. Ferguson JJ. Conventional antithrombotic approaches. Am Heart J. 1995; 130:651–657.

8. Wilcox JN, Smith KM, Schwartz SM, et al. Localization of tissue factor in the normal vessel wall and in the atherosclerotic plaque. Proc Natl Acad Sci USA. 1989; 86:2839–2843.

9. Smith WL. Prostanoid biosynthesis and the mechanism of action. Am J Physiol. 1992; 263:F118–F191.

10. Xie WL, Chipman JG, Robertson DL, et al. Expression of a mitogen-responsive gene encoding prostaglandin synthase is regulated by mRNA splicing. Proc Natl Acad Sci USA. 1991; 88:2692–2696.

11. Kujubu DA, Fletcher BS, Varnum BC, et al. TIS10, a phorbol ester tumor promoter-inducible mRNA from Swiss 3T3 cells, encodes a novel prostaglandin synthase/cyclooxygenase homologue. J Biol Chem. 1991; 266:12866–12872.

12. Chandrasekharan NV, Dai H, Roos KL, et al. COX-3, a cyclooxygenase-1 variant inhibited by acetaminophen and other analgesic/antipyretic drugs: cloning, structure and expression. Proc Natl Acad Sci USA. 2002; 99:13926–13931.

13. Roth GJ, Majerus PW. The mechanism of the effect of aspirin on human platelets: acetylation of a particulate fraction protein. J Clin Invest. 1975; 56:624–632.

14. Loll PJ, Picot D, Garavito RM. The structural basis of aspirin activity inferred fromm the crystal structure of inactivated prostaglandin H2 synthase. Nat Struct Biol. 1995; 2:637–643.

15. Vane JR, Bakhle YS, Botting RM. Cyclooxygenases 1 and 2. Ann Rev Pharmacol Toxicol. 1998; 38:97–120.

16. Antiplatelet Trialists' Collaboration. Collaborative overview of randomized trials of antiplatelet therapy: prevention of death, myocardial infarction, and stroke by prolonged antiplatelet therapy in various categories of patients. BMJ. 1994; 308:81–106.

17. ISIS-2 (Second International Study of Infarct Survival) Collaborative Group. Randomized trial of intravenous streptokinase, oral aspirin, both, or neither among 17,187 cases of suspected acute myocardial infarction: ISIS-2. Lancet. 1988; 2:349–360.

18. Lewis HDJ, Davis JW, Archibald DG, et al. Protective effects of aspirin against acute myocardial infarction and death in men with unstable angina: results of the Veterans Administration Cooperative Study. N Engl J Med. 1983; 309:396–403.

19. Cairns JA, Gent M, Singer J, et al. Aspirin, sulfinpyrazone, or both in unstable angina. N Engl J Med. 1985; 313:1369–1375.

20. Theroux P, Ouimet H, McCans J, et al. Aspirin, heparin, or both to treat acute unstable angina. N Engl J Med. 1988; 319:1105–1111.

21. RISC Group. Risk of myocardial infarction and death during treatment with low dose aspirin and intravenous heparin in men with unstable coronary artery disease. Lancet. 1990; 336:827–830.

22. Barnathan ES, Schwartz JS, Taylor L, et al. Aspirin and dipyridamole in the prevention of acute coronary thrombosis complicating coronary angioplasty. Circulation. 1987; 76:125–134.

23. Schwartz L, Bourassa MG, Lesperance J, et al. Aspirin and dipyridamole in the prevention of restenosis after percutaneous transluminal coronary angioplasty. N Engl J Med. 1988; 318:1714–1719.

24. Kent KM, Ewels CJ, Kehoe MK, et al. Effect of aspirin on complications during transluminal coronary angioplasty. J Am Coll Cardiol. 1988; 11:132A.

25. Mufson L, Black A, Roubin GS, et al. A randomized trial of aspirin in PTCA: effect of high vs. low dose aspirin on major complications of restenosis. J Am Coll Cardiol. 1988; 11:236A.

26. Antithrombotic Trialists' Collaboration. Collaborative meta-analysis of randomized trials of antiplatelet therapy for prevention of death, myocardial infarction, and stroke in high-risk patients. BMJ. 2002; 324:71–86.

27. Peters RJG, Zao F, Lewis BS, et al. For the CURE Investigators. Aspirin dose and bleeding events in the CURE study (abstract suppl.). Eur Heart J. 2002; 4:510.

28. Mangano DT. For the Multicenter Study of Perioperative Ischemia Research Group. Aspirin and mortality from coronary bypass surgery. N Engl J Med. 2002; 347:1309–1317.

29. Cattaneo M, Akkawat B, Lecchi A, et al. Ticlopidine selectively inhibits human platelet response to adenosine diphosphate. Thromb Haemost. 1991; 66:694–699.

30. McTavish D, Faulds D, Goa KL. Ticlopidine: an updated review of its pharmacology and therapeutic use in platelet dependent disorders. Drugs. 1990; 40:238–259.

31. Harker LA, Bruno JJ. Ticlopidine mechanism of action on human platelets. In Hass WK, Easton JD, eds. Ticlopidine. Platelets and Vascular Disease. New York: Springer Verlag, 1991:41–51.

32. Quinn MJ, Fitzgerald DJ. Ticlopidine and clopidogrel. Circulation. 1999; 100:1667–1672.

33. Gregorini L, Marko J, Fajadet J, et al. Ticlopidine and aspirin pretreatment reduces coagulation of platelet activation during coronary dilatation procedures. J Am Coll Cardiol. 1997; 29:13–20.

34. Gawaz M, Neumann FJ, Ott I, et al. Changes in membrane glycoprotein as circulating platelets after coronary stent implantation. Heart 1996; 76:166–172.

35. Kruse KR, Greenburg CS, Tanguay JF, et al. Thrombin and fibrin activity in patients treated with enoxaparin, ticlopidine and aspirin vs. the conventional coumadin regimen after elective stenting: the ENTICES trial. J Am Coll Cardiol. 1996; 27:334A.

36. Gregorini L, Marko J, Fajadet J, et al. Ticlopidine attenuates post stent implantation thrombin generation. J Am Coll Cardiol. 1996; 27:334A.

37. Leon MB, Baim DS, Popma JJ, et al. A clinical trial comparing three antithrombotic-drug regimens after coronary-artery stenting. Stent Anticoagulation Restenosis Study Investigators. N Engl J Med. 1998; 339:1665–1671.

38. Schomig A, Neumann FJ, Kastrati A, et al. A randomized comparison of antiplatelet and anticoagulant therapy after the placement of coronary artery stents. N Engl J Med. 1996; 334:1084–1089.

39. Bertrand M, Legrand V, Boland J, et al. Full anticoagulation versus ticlopidine plus aspirin after stent implantation: a randomized multi-center European study; the FANTASTIC trial. Circulation. 1996; 94:I-685.

40. Schuhlen H, Hadimitzky M, Walter H, et al. Major benefit of antiplatelet therapy for patients at high risk for adverse cardiac events after coronary Palmaz-Schatz stent placement: analysis of a prospective risk stratification protocol in the intracoronary stenting and antithrombotic regimen (ISAR) trial. Circulation. 1997; 95:2015–2021.

41. van Belle E, McFadden EP, LaBlanche JM, et al. Two-pronged antiplatelet therapy with aspirin and ticlopidine without systemic anticoagulation: an alternative therapeutic strategy after bailout stent implantation. Coron Artery Dis. 1995; 6:341–345.

42. Urban P, Macaya C, Rupprecht HJ, et al. Randomized evaluation of anticoagulation versus antiplatelet therapy after coronary stent implantation in high-risk patients. Circulation. 1998; 98:2126–2132.

43. Berger PB, Bell MR, Hasdai D, et al. Safety and efficacy of ticlopidine for only 2 weeks after successful intracoronary stent placement. Circulation. 1999; 99:248–253.

44. Quinn MJ, Fitzgerald DJ. Ticlopidine and clopidogrel. Circulation. 1999; 100:1667–1672.

45. Lincoff AM. Anticoagulant and antiplatlet drugs. Cathet Cardiovasc Interv. 2001; 54:514–520.

46. CAPRIE Steering Committee. A randomized, blinded trial of clopidogrel versus aspirin in patients at risk of ischaemic events (CAPRIE). Lancet. 1996; 348:1329–1339.

47. Bertrand ME, Rupprecht HJ, Gershlick AH, for the CLASSICS Investigators. Double-blind study of the safety of clopidogrel with and without a loading dose in combination with aspirin compared with ticlopidine in combination with aspirin after coronary stenting: the clopidogrel aspirin stent international cooperative study (CLASSICS). Circulation. 2000; 102:624–629.

48. Clopidogrel in Unstable Angina to Prevent Recurrent Events Trial Investigators. Effects of clopidogrel in addition to aspirin in patients with acute coronary syndromes without ST-segment elevation. N Engl J Med. 2001; 345:494–502.

49. Mehta SR, Yusuf S, Peters RJG, et al. for the CURE Investigators. Effects of pretreatment with clopidogrel and aspirin followed by long-term therapy in patients undergoing percutaneous coronary intervention: the PCI-CURE study. Lancet. 2001; 358:527–533.

50. Helft G, Osende JI, Worthley SG, et al. Acute antithrombotic effect of a front-loaded regimen of clopidogrel in patients with atherosclerosis on aspirin. Arterioscler Thromb Vasc Biol. 2000; 20:2316–2321.

51. Seyfarth HJ, Koksch M, Roething G, et al. Effect of 300– and 450–mg clopidogrel loading doses on membrane and soluble P-selectin in patients undergoing coronary stent implantation. Am Heart J. 2002; 143:118–123.

52. Gurbel PA, Malinin AI, Callahan KP, et al. Effect of loading with clopidogrel at the time of coronary stenting on platelet aggregation and glycoprotein IIb/IIIa expression and platelet-leukocyte aggregate formation. Am J Cardiol. 2002; 90:312–315.

53. Chew DP, Bhatt DL, Robbins MA, et al. Effect of clopidogrel added to aspirin before percutaneous coronary intervention on the risk associated with C-reactive protein. Am J Cardiol. 2001; 88:672–674.

54. Assali AR, Salloum J, Sdringola S, et al. Effects of clopidogrel pretreatment before percutaneous coronary intervention in patients treated with glycoprotein IIb/IIIa inhibitors (abciximab or tirofiban). Am J Cardiol. 2001; 88:884–886.

55. Topol EJ, Moliterno DJ, Herrmann HC, et al. Comparison of two platelet glycoprotein IIb/IIIa inhibitors, tirofiban and abciximab, for the prevention of ischemic events with percutaneous coronary revascularization. N Engl J Med. 2001; 344:1888–1894.

56. Bhatt DL, Bertrand ME, Berger PB, et al. Meta-analysis of randomized and registry comparisons of ticlopidine with clopidogrel after stenting. J Am Coll Cardiol. 2002; 39:9–14.

57. Smith SC, Dove JT, Jacobs AK, et al. ACC/AHA Guidelines for Percutaneous Coronary Intervention [revision of the 1993 PTCA guidelines—executive summary]. Circulation. 2001; 103:3019–3041.

58. Braunwald E, Antman EM, Beasley JW, et al. ACC/AHA 2002 Guideline update for the management of patients with unstable angina and non-ST-segment elevation myocardial infarction—summary article: a report of the American College of Cardiology/American Heart Association task force on practice guidelines. J Am Coll Cardiol. 2002; 40:1366–1374.

59. Steinhubl SR, Berger PB, Mann JT, et al. Early and sustained dual oral antiplatelet therapy following percutaneous coronary intervention. JAMA. 2002; 288:2411–2420.

60. EPIC Investigators. Use of a monoclonal antibody directed against the platelet glycoprotein IIb/IIIa receptor in high-risk coronary angioplasty. N Engl J Med. 1994; 330:956–961.

61. The IMPACT-II Investigators. Randomised placebo-controlled trial of effect of eptifibatide on complications of percutaneous coronary intervention: IMPACT-II. Lancet. 1997; 349:1422–1428.

62. RESTORE Investigators. Effects of platelet glycoprotein IIb/IIIa blockade with tirofiban on adverse cardiac events in patients with unstable angina or acute myocardial infarction undergoing coronary angioplasty. Circulation. 1997; 96:1445–1453.

63. Kong DF, Califf RM, Miller DP, et al. Clinical outcomes of therapeutic agents that block the platelet glycoprotein IIb/IIIa integrin in ischemic heart disease. Circulation. 1998; 98:2829–2835.

64. Coller BS. Blockade of platelet GP IIb/IIIa receptors as an antithrombotic strategy. Circulation. 1995; 92:2373–2380.

65. Ezratty AM, Loscalzo J. New approaches to antiplatelet therapy. Blood Coagul. Fibrinolysis. 1991; 2:317–327.

66. Topol EJ, Ferguson JJ, Weisman HF, et al. Long-term protection from myocardial ischemic events in a randomized trial of brief integrin beta-3 blockade with percutaneous coronary intervention. EPIC Investigator Group. Evaluation of Platelet IIb/IIIa Inhibition for Prevention of Ischemic Complication. JAMA. 1997; 278:479–484.

67. Topol EJ, Lincoff AM, Kereiakes DJ, et al. Multi-year follow-up of abciximab therapy in three randomized placebo-controlled trials of percutaneous coronary revascularization. Am J Med. 2002; 113:1–6.

68. EPILOG Investigators. Platelet glycoprotein IIb/IIIa blockade with abciximab with low-dose heparin during percutaneous coronary revascularization. N Engl J Med. 1997; 336:1689–1696.

69. Lincoff AM, Tcheng JE, Califf RM, et al. Sustained suppression of ischemic complications of coronary intervention by platelet GP IIb/IIIa blockade with abciximab: one-year outcome in the EPILOG trial. Evaluation in PTCA to Improve Long-term Outcome with Abciximab GP IIb/IIIa Blockade. Circulation. 1999; 99:1951–1958.

70. EPISTENT Investigators. Randomised placebo-controlled and balloon-angioplasty-controlled trial to assess safety of coronary stenting with use of platelet glycoprotein IIb/IIIa blockade. Lancet. 1998; 352:87–92.

71. Lincoff AM, Califf RM, Moliterno DJ, et al. Complementary clinical benefits of coronary artery stenting and blockade of platelet glycoprotein IIb/IIIa receptors. Evaluation of Platelet IIb/IIIa Inhibition in Stenting Investigators. N Engl J Med. 1999; 341:319–327.

72. Bhatt DL, Marso SP, Lincoff AM, et al. Abciximab reduces mortality in diabetics following percutaneous coronary intervention. J Am Coll Cardiol. 2000; 35:922–928.

73. Brener SJ, Barr LA, Burchenal JE, et al. Randomized, placebo-controlled trial of platelet glycoprotein IIb/IIIa blockade with primary angioplasty for acute myocardial infarction. ReoPro and Primary PTCA Organization and Randomized Trial (RAPPORT) Investigators. Circulation. 1998; 98:734–741.

74. Neumann FJ, Kastrati A, Schmitt C, et al. Effect of glycoprotein IIb/IIIa receptor blockade with abciximab on clinical and angiographic restenosis rate after the placement of coronary stents following acute myocardial infarction. J Am Coll Cardiol. 2000; 35:915–921.

75. Montalescot G, Barragan P, Wittenberg O, et al. Platelet glycoprotein IIb/IIIa inhibition with coronary stenting for acute myocardial infarction. The Abciximab Before Direct Angioplasty and Stenting in Myocardial Infarction Regarding Acute and Long-term Follow-up (ADMIRAL) trial. N Engl J Med. 2001; 344:1895–1903.

76. Stone GW, Grines CL, Cox DA, et al. Comparison of angioplasty with stenting, with or without abciximab, in acute myocardial infarction. Controlled Abciximab and Device Investigation to Lower Late Angioplasty Complications (CADILLAC) Investigators. N Engl J Med. 2002; 346:957–966.

77. Antoniucci D. Abciximab and Carbostent Evaluation in Acute Myocardial Infarction (ACE) trial. Presented at Transcatheter Therapeutics (TCT) 2002.

78. Antman EM, Giugliano RP, Gibson CM, et al. Abciximab facilitates the rate and extent of thrombolysis: results of the thrombolysis in myocardial infarction (TIMI) 14 trial. The TIMI 14 Investigators. Circulation. 1999; 99:2720–2732.

79. Strategies for Patency Enhancement in the Emergency Department (SPEED) Group. Trial of abciximab with and without low-dose reteplase for acute myocardial infarction. Circulation. 2000; 101:2788–2794.

80. GUSTO V Investigators. Reperfusion therapy for acute myocardial infarction with fibrinolytic therapy or combination reduced fibrinolytic therapy and platelet glycoprotein IIb/IIIa inhibition: the GUSTO V randomized trial. Lancet. 2001; 357:1905–1914.

81. GUSTO V Randomized Trial. Mortality at 1 year with combination platelet glycoprotein IIb/IIIa inhibition and reduced-dose fibrinolytic therapy vs. conventional fibrinolytic therapy for acute myocardial infarction. JAMA. 2002; 288:2130–2135.

82. The ESPRIT Investigators. Novel dosing regimen of eptifibatide in planned coronary stent implantation (ESPRIT): a randomized, placebo-controlled trial. Enhanced Suppression of the Platelet IIb/IIIa Receptor with Integrilin Therapy. Lancet. 2000; 356:2037–2044.

83. O'Shea JC, Hafley GE, Greenberg S, et al. Platelet glycoprotein IIb/IIIa integrin blockade with eptifibatide in coronary stent intervention: the ESPRIT trial: a randomized controlled trial. JAMA. 2001; 285:2468–2473.

84. O'Shea JC, Buller CE, Cantor WJ, et al. for the ESPRIT Investigators. Long-term efficacy of platelet glycoprotein IIb/IIIa integrin blockade with eptifibatide in coronary stent intervention. JAMA. 2002; 287:618–621.

85. Labinaz M, Madan M, O'Shea JO, et al. for the ESPRIT Investigators. Comparison of one-year outcomes following coronary artery stenting in diabetic versus nondiabetic patients (from the Enhanced Suppression of the Platelet IIb/IIIa Receptor with Integrilin Therapy [ESPRIT] Trial). Am J Cardiol. 2003; 90:585–590.

86. Ohman EM, Kleiman NS, Gacioch G, et al. Combined accelerated tissue-plasminogen activator and platelet glycoprotein IIb/IIIa integrin receptor blockade with Integrilin in acute myocardial infarction. Results of a randomized, placebo-controlled, dose-ranging trial. IMPACT-AMI Investigators. Circulation. 1997; 95:846–854.

87. Brener SJ, Zeymer U, Adgey AAJ, et al. Eptifibatide and low-dose tissue plasminogen activator in acute myocardial infarction. The Integrilin and Low-dose Thrombolysis in Acute Myocardial Infarction (INTRO-AMI) trial. J Am Coll Cardiol. 2002; 39:377–386.

88. Giugliano RP, Roe MT, Harrington RA, et al. Combination reperfusion therapy with eptifibatide and reduced dose tenecteplase for ST-elevation myocardial infarction: results of the Integrilin and Tenecteplase in Acute Myocardial Infarction (INTEGRITI) Phase II Angiographic Trial. J Am Coll Cardiol. 2003; 41:1251–1260.

89. Kaul U, Gupta RK, Haridas KK, et al. Platelet glycoprotein IIb/IIIa inhibition using eptifibatide with primary coronary stenting for acute myocardial infarction: a 30 day follow-up study. Integrilin in Acute Myocardial Infarction (INAMI) Stenting Study Investigators. Cathet Cardiovasc Intervent. 2002; 57:497–503.

90. Gibson CM, Goel M, Cohen DJ, et al. Six-month angiographic and clinical follow-up of patients prospectively randomized to receive either tirofiban or placebo during angioplasty in the RESTORE trial. Randomized Efficacy Study of Tirofiban for Outcomes and Restenosis. J Am Coll Cardiol. 1998; 32:28–34.

91. Lee DP, Herity NA, Hiatt BL, et al. Adjunctive platelet glycoprotein IIb/IIIa receptor inhibition with tirofiban before primary angioplasty improves angiogrpahic outcomes. Results of the Tirofiban Given in the Emergency Room before Primary Angioplasty (TIGER-PA) Pilot Trial. Circulation. 2003; 107:1497–1501.

92. Burnstock G. Potential therapeutic targets in the rapidly expanding field of purinergic signaling. Clin Med. 2002; 2:45–53.

93. Storey F. The P2Y12 receptor as a therapeutic target in cardiovascular disease. Platelets. 2001; 12:197–209.

94. Storey RF, Newby LJ, Heptinstall S. Effects of P2Y(1) and P2Y(12) receptor antagonists on platelet aggregation induced by different agonists in human whole blood. Platelets 2001; 12:443–447.

95. Remijn JA, Wu YP, Jeninga EH, et al. Role of ADP receptor P2Y(12) in platelet adhesion and thrombus formation in flowing blood. Arterioscler Thromb Vasc Biol. 2002; 22:686–691.

96. Covic L, Gresser AL, Talavera J, et al. Activation and inhibition of G protein-coupled receptors by cell-penetrating membrane-tethered peptides. Proc Natl Acad Sci USA. 2002; 99:643–648.

97. Covic L, Misra M, Badar J, et al. Pepducin-based intervention of thrombin-receptor signaling and systemic platelet activation. Nat Med. 2002; 8:1161–1165.

98. Bhatt DL, Topol EJ. Scientific and therapeutic advances in antiplatelet therapy. Nat Rev Drug Discov. 2003; 2:15–28.

15-1

Coronary Stents

Briain D. MacNeill, Ik-Kyung Jang, and Philip Wong
Massachusetts General Hospital, Harvard Medical School, Boston, Massachusetts, U.S.A.

I. INTRODUCTION

The concept of a splint to stabilize tissue was developed by a nineteenth-century dentist, Charles R. Stent (1845–1901), to support skin grafting. Although the first percutaneous application of this concept was proposed by Dotter in 1969 for peripheral arterial intervention (1), it was not until 1986 that the first coronary stent was placed. The following year, 1987, a landmark report by Sigwart et al. was published on the early and late reduction in restenosis of the first 29 patients treated with self-expanding coronary Wallstents (2). Subsequently, coronary stents have been established as the single most important development in percutaneous coronary intervention (PCI), and consequently their use has grown explosively.

Sigwart et al.'s initial experience with stenting was complicated by the development of thrombosis, demonstrating the potential of stent insertion within a thrombogenic mileau to create a nidus for thrombus formation. Changes in stent design, a greater understanding of arterial responses to stenting, and improved antithrombotic therapy have been central to the evolution of stent practice, resulting in stent placement in over 80% of PCI. This chapter will provide an overview of the various trials that led to this evolution and that support current indications for stenting in PCI.

II. FOCAL LESIONS

Several randomized controlled trials have compared coronary stenting with angioplasty (Table 1) (3–8). The two most significant studies in the early development of stenting were the STRESS and the BENESTENT trials (3,4). In the STRESS (STent REStenosis Study) trial, 410 patients with symptomatic coronary artery disease were randomly assigned to angioplasty alone or angioplasty and stenting with a Palmaz-Schatz™ stent (3). Inclusion criteria encompassed stable or unstable presentations of focal stenosis (≤15 mm) in moderate-sized coronary arteries (≥3.0 mm diameter). Recent acute myocardial infarction (AMI), reduced left ventricular function (EF < 40%), and several angiographic variables, including the suspicion of thrombus, formed the most significant exclusion criteria. Restenosis at 6 months, defined angiographically as a ≥ 50% diameter narrowing, was significantly reduced in the stent group compared to angioplasty group (31.6% vs. 42.1%; *p*

Table 1 Studies Comparing Coronary Stenting with Balloon Angioplasty in Native Arteries (>3.0 mm)

Study (Ref.)	Follow-up	Numbers		Angiographic restenosis (%)			Target vessel revascularization (%)			Death, MI, or TVR (%)	
		Stent	PTCA	Stent	PTCA	p-value	Stent	PTCA	p-value	Stent	PTCA
STRESS (3)	6	205	202	31.6	42.1	0.046	10.2	15.4	0.06	19.5	23.8
BENESTENT (4)	7/60	259	257	22	32	0.02	13.5	23.3	<0.05	20.1	29.6
START (5)	48	229	223	22	37	<0.002	12	24.6	<0.002	16.9	29.9
OCBAS (6)	7	57	59	18.8	16.6	—	17.5	9.2	—	19.2	16.9
Versaci (7)	12	60	60	19	40	0.02	6.6	22	—	—	—

= 0.046). Moreover, a reduction in major adverse clinical events (MACE) and in the rate of subsequent target vessel revascularization (TVR) was found in the stent group (3). Significant, however, was the high rate of bleeding and vascular complications resulting from aggressive antithrombotic therapy comprising a combination of aspirin, dipyridamole, dextran, and warfarin for 1 month (3).

The BElgian NEtherlands STENT (BENESTENT) trial randomized 520 patients with stable symptomatic single vessel coronary artery disease to stenting, with a Palmaz-Schatz stent, or balloon angioplasty alone for focal de novo lesions in moderate sized coronary arteries (≥3.0 mm diameter) (4). The composite clinical endpoint of death, myocardial infarction, cerbrovascular accident, or TVR was significantly reduced in the stent arm compared to the angioplasty arm (20% vs. 30%; $p = 0.02$) (Fig. 1). The primary angiographic endpoint of restenosis occurred in 22% of the stent group, as compared to 32% of the angioplasty group ($p = 0.02$) (4). As with the STRESS trial, complications of antithrombotic therapy were more common in the stent group (3.1% vs. 1.5%; $p = 0.001$) (3,4).

Although the STRESS and BENESTENT trials demonstrated a benefit, both trials were limited by short follow-up (3,4). The long-term clinical effect of stenting was studied in the START trial, which performed 4-year follow-up on 452 patients with

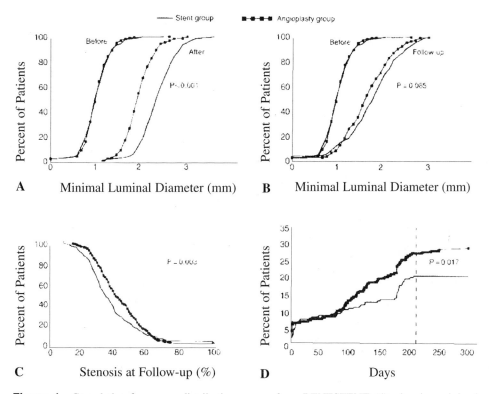

Figure 1 Cumulative frequency distribution curves from BENESTENT (4), showing minimal luminal diameters measured before and after intervention and at follow-up, the percentage of stenosis at follow-up, and the percentage of patients with clinical end points. Signifcant differences were apparent that consistently favored the stent group over the angioplasty group with respect to the increased minimal luminal diameter at intervention (Panel A) and follow-up (Panel B), the percentage of stenosis at follow-up (Panel C), and the incidence of major clinical events (Panel D). The vertical dashed line in Panel D indicates the end of the study.

stable or unstable angina, treated by stent or balloon angioplasty (5). At 6-month angiography, restenosis rates comparable to both the STRESS and BENESTENT trials were found: 22% for the stent arm, 37% for the PTCA arm ($p < 0.002$). At 4-year follow up, mortality (2.7% vs. 2.4%) and nonfatal MI (2.2% vs. 2.8%) were similar in both groups, but the requirement for TVR was significantly reduced in the stent group (12% vs. 25%; $p = 0.0006$). This study demonstrated the persistence of a benefit of stenting in reducing restenosis and TVR compared to angioplasty alone for 4 years after PCI (5). Subsequent studies have demonstrated a small but significant increase in minimal lumen diameter (MLD) after the initial 6-month period after stent insertion (9), and it was determined that concerns of stent migration, metal fatigue, or aneurysm formation were unfounded (9,10). Ironically, stenting resulted in significantly more neointimal hyperplasia than angioplasty alone, effecting most of the benefit by preventing elastic recoil and late negative remodeling (11).

Subsequent improvements in stent deployment and antithrombotic therapy permitted less severe antithrombotic regimes, resulting in a reduction in hemorrhagic complications and a relative increase in the benefit of stenting (12–15). The results of the STRESS, BENESTENT and START trials, were echoed in the other randomized trials of coronary stenting, demonstrating that stenting *de novo* lesions in vessels > 3.0 mm results in less restenosis, fewer procedural complications and less subsequent target lesion revascularization than angioplasty alone (figure 2 & 3) (3-8). These results were consistent even when optimal balloon angiographic result (*stent-like result*) was obtained (16).

Recommendations: The data strongly support the use of coronary stents, if the coronary anatomy is favorable, for de novo lesions in vessels >3.0 mm in caliber, regardless of the balloon angioplasty results.

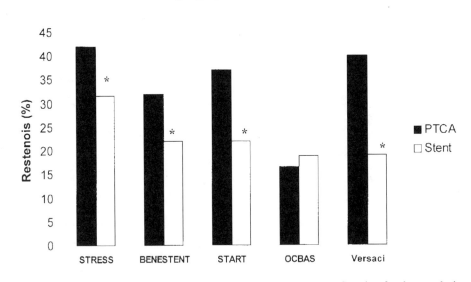

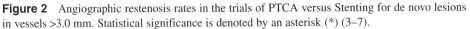

Figure 2 Angiographic restenosis rates in the trials of PTCA versus Stenting for de novo lesions in vessels >3.0 mm. Statistical significance is denoted by an asterisk (*) (3–7).

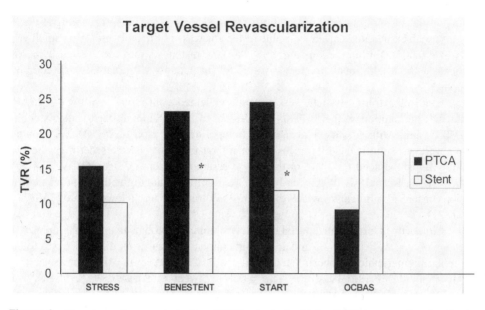

Figure 3 Target vessel revascularization (TVR) rates in the trials of PTCA versus Stenting for de novo lesions in vessels >3.0 mm. Statistical significance is denoted by an asterisk (*) (3–6).

III. NON-STRESS/BENESTENT LESIONS

A. Restenotic Lesions Following Prior Angioplasty

Soon after the emergence of coronary angioplasty, two significant complications developed that limited the clinical application of percutaneous coronary therapy. The first, abrupt vessel closure, formed the initial indication for stent insertion, termed bail-out stenting (17–20). The second complication of early angioplasty was restenosis, arising from the combination of elastic recoil of the vessel wall and late negative remodeling (21–23). Balloon angioplasty of restenotic lesions traditionally resulted in angiographic restenosis rates of 50–70%, preventing effective percutaneous therapy. The growing evidence of a reduction in restenosis for de novo lesions logically led to studies of stenting for the treatment of restenotic lesions following prior balloon angioplasty.

The Restenosis Sten. Study was a randomized study of 383 patients treated for clinical and angiographic evidence of restenosis with balloon angioplasty or stenting with a Palmaz-Schatz stent. Restenosis rates were significantly lower in the stent group than in the angioplasty group (18% vs. 32%; $p = 0.03$). Similarly, the need for TVR at 6 months was significantly lower in the stent group (10% vs. 27%; $p = 0.001$) (24).

Recommendations: Evidence supports the use of stents over angioplasty for restenotic lesions following prior balloon angioplasty.

B. Small Vessels

Although effective for treatment of vessels with a caliber of ≥3 mm, several trials identified reference vessel size as an independent predictor of adverse events following stenting and demonstrated an inverse relationship between vessel size and angiographic restenosis rate, raising the question of the role of stenting in smaller arteries (25,26). A study of 2602 patients with successful stent implantation examined rates of restenosis according to vessel size. As with earlier studies, angiographic restenosis was significantly greater in small vessels ($p < 0.001$). Within the small artery group, the restenosis rate varied from 29.6% in patients without additional risk factors to 53.5% in patients with diabetes and complex lesions (27).

Controlled trials of small vessel stenting yielded conflicting results. The ISAR-SMART trial randomized 404 patients with lesions of 2.0–2.8 mm in size to either stenting or PTCA, both with adjunctive abciximab, ticlopidine, and aspirin (28). After 7 months, there were no significant differences in the infarct-free survival rates between the two study groups, the need for TVR, or the rate of restenosis (stent, 35.7%; PTCA, 37.4%; $p = 0.74$) (28). Reanalysis of this study found a significant angiographic improvement in lesions of >15 mm in length, which did not did not translate into a lower rate of TVR at 1 year (29).

Similarly, in a randomized trial of 351 symptomatic patients to either angioplasty or stenting of vessels between 2.3 and 2.9 mm in caliber, no significant difference was found in either angiographic restenosis (stent, 28% vs. PTCA, 32.9%; $p = 0.36$) or in need for TVR (stent, 17.8% vs. PTCA, 20.3%; $p = 0.54$) between either arm, suggesting equivalence of angioplasty and stenting in coronary arteries <3.0 mm (30). Challenging this result was a similar randomized study of stenting versus angioplasty in 381 patients with symptomatic de novo focal lesions in small coronary arteries (<3 mm). Despite similar peri-procedural success and adverse event rates, angiographic restenosis at 6 months was significantly lower in the stent group compared to the angioplasty group ($p = 0.0001$). Similarly, the requirement for TVR was significantly lower in the stent group (13% vs. 25%; $p = 0.0006$) (31). The Stenting in Small Coronary Arteries (SISCA) trial randomized patients to elective stenting with a heparin-coated BeStent™ or optimum angioplasty for the treatment of focal de novo lesions (diameter = 2.1–3.0 mm). A reduction in restenosis was found in the stent arm at 6-month angiography (22.7% vs. 48.5%; $p < 0.001$) along with a lower rate of TVR (13% vs. 25%; $p = 0.02$) (32). One-year follow-up of the SISCA trial demonstrated a sustained benefit in event-free survival in the stent arm (90.5% vs. 76.1%; $p = 0.016$) (33).

With conflicting results from the current literature, practice guidelines remain unclear. It is likely that stent design plays a more significant role in smaller vessels, providing potential for the varied results obtained and necessitating further controlled trials for clarification.

Recommendations: There is no unifying consensus on recommendations for stenting in vessels of <3.0 mm. Although angiographic benefit is seen, particularly in lesions longer than 15 mm, this does not translate into clinical benefit at follow-up. It is likely that newer stent design, specifically aimed at smaller vessel caliber, will improve the outcome of small vessel stenting, but there is currently no evidence for benefit above optimal angioplasty.

C. Chronic Occlusions

Recanalizing occluded vessels has been proven to reduce angina, improve left ventricular function, and lower subsequent referral for coronary artery bypass grafting (CABG) (34,35), but successfully recanalized occluded coronary arteries were complicated by reocclusion in up to 45% (36). To explore the role of stenting in this setting, the Stenting in Chronic Coronary Occlusion (SICCO) trial was commenced. Following a satisfactory recanalization of a chronic occlusion, 119 patients were randomized to stenting (Palmaz-Schatz) or optimum angioplasty. At 6-month follow-up, the stent group were more likely to be symptom-free (57% vs. 24%; $p < 0.001$) and free of restenosis (32% vs. 74%; $p <$

0.001) compared to the angioplasty group (37). Clinical follow-up of these groups at 33 months demonstrated that the early benefit of stenting for chronic total occlusions persisted, with a reduction in MACE ($p = 0.0002$) and TVR ($p = 0.002$) (38).

Similarly, the Total Occlusion Study of Canada (TOSCA) randomized 410 patients with nonacute native coronary occlusions to PTCA or primary stenting with the heparin-coated Palmaz-Schatz stent. As with the earlier two trials, vessel occlusion at 6-month angiography was lower in the stent group (10.9% vs. 19.5%; $p = 0.024$), as was target-vessel revascularization (8.4% vs. 15.4%; $p = 0.03$) (39). These studies and others support the recommendation of stenting following successful recanalization of chronic total occlusions (40–43).

Recommendations: We recommend the use of coronary stents following the recanalization of chronically occluded arteries to reduce reocclusion, restenosis, and need for TVR.

D. Acute Myocardial Infarction

The evidence supporting the "open artery hypothesis" as a means of reducing the complications of acute myocardial infarction (AMI), combined with the acceptance of the limitations of thrombolytic regimes to achieve and maintain patency of infarct-related vessels without excessive thrombotic risk, led to interest in trials of primary angioplasty (44).

The Primary Angioplasty in Myocardial Infarction (PAMI) study compared primary angioplasty with thrombolytic therapy in the form of tissue plasminogen activator (t-PA) within 12 hours of AMI. Primary angioplasty was successful in 97% and resulted in a significantly lower rate of major adverse events (MACE) than the t-PA group (5.1% vs. 12.0%; $p = 0.02$) (45). This initial benefit was sustained at 6-month ($p = 0.02$) and at 24-month follow-up ($p = 0.034$) (46). Furthermore, multivariate analysis isolated angioplasty as an independent predictor of a reduction in death, reinfarction, or TVR ($p = 0.0001$) (46). Although these findings were mirrored by two further prospective randomized trials of primary angioplasty (47,48), it contradicted registry-based comparisons of the two treatment strategies (49,50), suggesting a discrepancy between trial conditions and clinical practice. Ultimately, a meta-analysis of 10 trials comparing primary angioplasty to thrombolysis demonstrated that a strategy of primary angioplasty was associated with a lower mortality (4.4% vs. 6.5%; $p = 0.02$), fewer composite endpoints of death or reinfarction (7.2% vs. 11.9%; $p < 0.001$), and a reduction in stroke (0.7% vs. 2.0%; $p = 0.07$) (51).

The success of the primary angioplasty trials combined with the growing acceptance of stenting as a method to improve PCI led to trials of stenting for AMI (47,48). The Stent PAMI Study was a multicenter randomized trial comparing stenting with optimal angioplasty for AMI. Patients ($n = 900$) presenting with AMI were randomly assigned to receive either angioplasty alone or angioplasty and stenting with a heparin-coated Palmaz-Schatz stent (52). Stenting resulted in a greater acute mean luminal diameter than angioplasty ($p < 0.001$), less angina at 6-month follow-up (11.3% vs. 16.9%; $p = 0.02$), and lower rates of TVR (7.7% vs. 17.0%; $p < 0.001$). Restenosis was significantly lower in the stent group than in the angioplasty group (20.3% vs. 33.5%; $p < 0.001$) (52). Furthermore, a strategy of primary stenting was shown to expedite discharge, resulting in substantial cost savings (53). An interesting observation in this trial was the lower rate of thrombolysis in myocardial infarction (TIMI) grade 3 flow that was achieved by stenting compared to angioplasty, thought to relate to distal embolization of thrombus. The adjunctive use of glycoprotein (GP) IIb/IIIa inhibition (54) and novel techniques of rheolytic thrombectomy (55) have subsequently been shown to protect the micro-circulation during primary angioplasty, thus improving TIMI 3 flow following stenting.

The success of the PAMI stent trial was seen in other randomized trials confirming the benefits of stenting in AMI (Table 2; Fig. 4) (56–63).

Recommendations: On the basis of these data the use of stents following primary angioplasty is strongly advised. To further improve TIMI grade 3 flow rates, adjunctive GP IIb/IIIa inhibition and mechanical devices to reduce thrombus load or embolism should be considered.

E.   Saphenous Vein Grafts

In the last two decades coronary artery bypass graft procedures have increased such that vein graft degeneration has become a new disease entity, for which treatment options are limited. Repeat CABG carries double the mortality rate of initial surgery and results in less complete relief of symptoms and a higher rate of saphenous vein graft (SVG) attrition (64). Percutaneous treatments are complicated by distal embolization and restenosis, resulting in a higher morbidity than standard PCI (65). Balloon angioplasty of SVG lesions is associated with a high rate of restenosis and major adverse events (66), while adjunctive atherectomy results in distal embolization (65,67). As a result, the role of stenting for SVG treatment was explored. The Palmaz-Schatz Stent Study examined the safety and efficacy of SVG stenting of focal lesions in 589 symptomatic patients. Angiography restenosis at 6 months was 29.7%, and the 12-month actuarial event-free survival was 76.3% (68). Comparing these results with the angioplasty arm of the Coronary Angioplasty Versus Excisional Atherectomy Trial II (CAVEAT II), the stent group had a lower in-hospital MACE (10% vs. 17%; $p = 0.059$) and a lower TVR at 1-year follow-up (23% vs. 45%; $p < 0.001$) (69).

These favorable results led to the SAVED study, in which 220 patients with de novo SVG lesions were randomly assigned to stenting with a Palmaz-Schatz stent or optimum balloon angioplasty. As compared with the angioplasty arm, the stent group had a lower

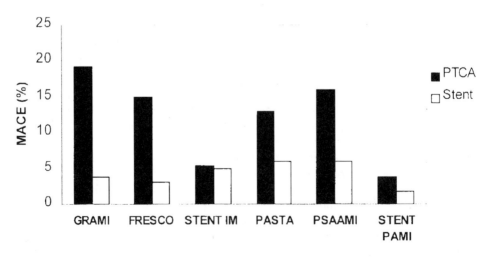

Figure 4   Major adverse clinical event rates (MACE) in the trials of PTCA versus stenting for acute myocardial infarction (AMI) (52,56–58,60, 61).

Table 2 Trials of PTCA Versus Stenting for AMI

Study	Year	Follow-up (Months)	Stent/ PTCA(%)	Success	Early events (<30 days)				Death	Late events, cumulative (%)		
					Death	Reinfarction	TVR	MACE		Reinfarction	TVR	MACE
GRAMI (56)	1998	12	52/52	98/94.2	3.8/7.6	0/7.6	0/5.7	3.8/19.2	—	—	14/21	17/35
FRESCO (57)	1998	6	75/75	99	0/0	1.3/2.6	1.3/12	3/15	1/0	1/3	7/25	13/32
STENTIM 2(58)	2000	12	101/101	95/94.5	1/0	4/3.6	5/5.4	5/5.4	3/1.9	4/5.5	17.8/28.2	12.9/20
Suryapranata (59)	1998	6	112/115	98/96	2/3	1/4	—	—	2/3	1/7	4/17	5/20
PASTA (60)	1999	12	67/69	99/97	3/7	3/4	6/13	6/19	5/9	—	—	22/49
PSAAMI (61)	2001	23	44/44	—	2/5	0/2	0/9	5/11	9/18	2/9	16/34	23/43
STENT PAMI (52)	1999	3	452/448	89.4/92.7	3.5/1.8	0.4/1.1	1.8/3.8	4.6/5.8	4.2/2.7	2.4/2.2	7.7/17	12.6/20.1

Source: Modified from Ref. 117.

rate of major adverse events (58% vs. 73%; $p = 0.03$) and a reduction, albeit nonsignificant, in restenosis (37% vs. 46%; $p = 0.24$) when analyzed on the basis of intention to treat. Hemorrhagic complications were higher in the stent arm (17% vs. 5%; $p < 0.01$), reflecting an aggressive anticoagulation regime that included aspirin, dipyridamole, dextran, and heparin acutely, followed by warfarin, aspirin, and dipyridamole for 1 month (70). In a similar design, the VENESTENT study randomized 150 patients to stenting or optimum SVG angioplasty with similar initial success rates in each arm (71). At 6-month follow-up, however, TVR was lower in the stent arm (11.5% vs. 25%; $p = 0.03$). Angiographic follow-up in 82% of the population demonstrated a nonsignificant reduction in angiographic restenosis (21.9% vs. 36.6%; $p = 0.09$) (71). Despite failing to demonstrate a significant reduction in restenosis, these trials suggest that stenting effectively reduces the high MACE and TVR associated with SVG angioplasty.

Recommendations: Stenting is recommended for SVG intervention, as it has been shown to be reduce adverse events and the need for future TVR. Furthermore, the use of distal protection devices should be considered to minimize distal embolization during intervention.

F.   Left Main Coronary Disease

Protected left main stem disease, where a patent graft supplies one or both of the LAD or Circumflex arteries, is amenable to balloon angioplasty, albeit with high peri-procedural mortality rates (72). In this group, adjunctive stenting appears to reduce long-term mortality (73). Stenting "unprotected" left main disease, although technically feasible, is associated with a high late mortality presumed to arise from global ischemia after high-grade restenosis (74). A recent report of unprotected left main coronary artery stenosis, including a large cohort of patients unsuitable for CABG, confirmed the high mortality complicating unselected left main stem PCI (75). Patients under 65 years of age with left ventricular ejection fraction of >30% were defined as having low procedural risk and tended to do substantially better, with a 1-year mortality of only 3.4% (75). Similar results have been shown in other reports (76).

Various patterns of left main disease exist, each with unique challenges for intervention and stenting (77). Although some patterns are unlikely to ever be amenable to percutaneous therapy, certain patterns of low-risk patients may benefit from stenting. Controlled trials are needed to further evaluate the potential of stenting for this indication.

Recommendations: Protected left main stenosis, that is, where a patent graft supplies the LAD or Circumflex, can be treated with stenting, albeit at a higher peri-procedural complication rate than standard stenting. There is currently insufficient evidence to support the use of stenting for unprotected left main stem disease.

IV.   NEW DEVELOPMENTS IN STENTING

A.   Stent Design and Deployment

Stent design has progressed dramatically since the first generation of stents (Palmaz-Schatz, Wallstents, Gianturco-Roubin). The ideal stent should be flexible, trackable, poorly thrombogenic, visible by x-ray, and of course affordable. Currently more than 50 stent configurations are available worldwide, with varying characteristics of flexibility, surface area coverage, composition, and strut configuration. Previously, trials of stent design have generally shown equivalence between the different designs available (78), such that the decision to use one stent design over another has often been a matter of operator preference. Recently, however, the importance of stent design and its relationship to tissue reaction has been realized such that stent design has become an important research focus.

Although it is accepted that stent caliber (25,26) and length (79) are important determinants of restenosis, there is little research on the effect of stent geometry on outcome. The interaction between stent design, postdilatation geometry, and restenosis rates of different stent configurations were recently studied (38). Significantly less mural thrombus and neointima was found with increasing number of stent struts per cross-sectional area, suggesting that vessel geometry, dictated by stent design, determines neointimal thickness (80). Similarly, the effect of stent strut thickness was studied in the recently presented ISAR-STEREO-2 trial (81). Stents designed with a strut thickness of 50 μm resulted in a lower restenosis rate at 6 months than stents designed with thicker (140 μm) struts (17.9% vs. 31.4%; $p < 0.001$) (81). These studies provide some insight into the mechanisms of stent-induced vascular injury, which are of increasing importance in the era of small-vessel stenting and drug-coated stents.

The role of adjunctive intravascular ultrasound (IVUS) remains controversial. Previous trials have demonstrated that despite excellent angiographic appearances, suboptimal stent expansion at traditionally accepted inflation pressures is common (82,83), leading to inadequate stent apposition and higher rates of stent thrombosis. IVUS-guided optimum stent deployment allowed for less aggressive antithrombotic therapy at a time when hemorrhagic complications threatened to limit coronary stenting (84,85). Subsequent high deployment pressures without IVUS guidance proved sufficient to accomplish low stent thrombosis rates, moving clinicians away from routine IVUS (86), although later studies infer that this benefit arose from novel antithrombotic regimes rather than deployment techniques (87). Novel imaging modalities, including optical coherence tomography, have expanded our understanding of the interaction between the arterial wall and stent geometry (Fig. 5) (88).

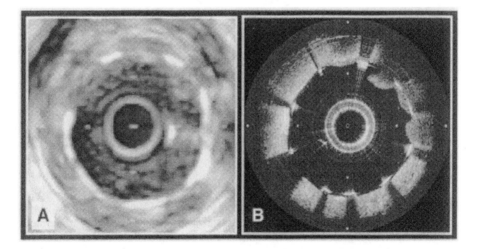

Figure 5 Intravascular ultrasound (A) and optical coherence tomography (B) images of an invivo stent in a right coronary artery. Although IVUS showed a well-deployed stent, the detailed structure around the stent struts is not well visualized. In addition, OCT clearly visualized tissue prolapse between the stent struts (12 to 3 o'clock). The tissue prolapse occurred mainly in an area with lower OCT signal intensity, which is suggestive of a plaque with a large lipid content. (From Ref. 118.)

B. Coated Stents

The potential to coat coronary stents with pharmacologically active materials to exert a localized action at the site of stent deployment has obvious appeal (89,90). The success of brachytherapy in preventing restenosis (91) led to interest in anti-proliferative drugs as potential antirestenotic stent coatings (92). Two agents in particular have shown promising results in the reduction of restenosis. The first, sirolimus, found on streptomyces fungi, causes smooth muscle cell cycle arrest. Following successful preliminary results in which negligible restenotic responses were observed angiographically and using IVUS, a randomized trial was undertaken. The resultant RAVEL trial randomized 238 patients undergoing PCI for de novo lesions to receive a sirolimus-covered Velocity™ stent or a conventional stent. Remarkably, at 6 months there was no restenosis detected in the sirolimus group (0% vs. 26%; $p < 0.0001$) (93,94). A further randomized trial of sirolimus-coated stents, the SIRIUS trial, is underway.

The second antiproliferative agent tested was paclitaxel, which is derived from the yew tree and causes microtubular disruption within proliferating cells. A blinded controlled trial, the Taxus trial, compared paclitaxel coated stents with noncoated stents for de novo lesions in 3.0–3.5 mm arteries (95). At 18-month follow-up there was no binary restenosis in the paclitaxel group compared to 10% in the noncoated stent group. Similarly, major adverse cardiac events were lower in the paclitaxel-coated group as compared to the noncoated group (3% vs. 14%). IVUS imaging at follow-up demonstrated neointima covering stent struts but at a significantly reduced volume compared to the noncoated group. Furthermore, systemic paclitaxel levels were undetectable. Taxus III studied paclitaxel-coated stents for the treatment of instent restenosis in 29 patients (96). Restenosis was found in 4 of 25 patients (16%), the majority occurring in lesions that were not adequately covered by the paclitaxel-coated stent (96).

These remarkable results raise important issues, such as (a) the optimum agent, (b) toxicity, (c) the potential for delayed restenosis or thrombosis, (d) the effect of stent design on drug delivery, (e) the cost of PCI, and (f) which patient cohort will benefit most.

C. Covered Stents

In an effort to address distal embolization and restenosis, covered stents have been proposed, with the rationale that a lining material or polymer would reduce embolization of friable atheroma or thrombus and possibly reduce neointimal formation. Materials tested as stent coats include autologous tissue and synthetic materials (97,98). Autologous stent covering using venous and arterial tissue lining a conventional stent demonstrated favorable results, indicating a potential clinical application (99), but the need for a harvest procedure and the unpredictable profile of a tissue-covered stent confines its use to emergent or specialized indications (97, 100, 101).

Initial synthetic materials tested as potential stent coats included silicone, Dacron, and polyurethane layers covering coil tantalum stents (98). Despite reasonable acute angiographic results, each stent design was hampered by late occlusion. Histology of the stented vessel demonstrated intense inflammation characterized by the presence of multinucleated giant cells and macrophages surrounding proteinaceous debris and thrombus (98).

Polytetrafluoroethylene (PTFE) has been successfully used in surgical practice with good long-term results and a predictable tissue response. Initial coronary experience with first-generation PTFE-covered stents for vein graft disease demonstrated a reduction in major adverse events and in the need for target vessel revascularization as compared to standard angioplasty (102,103). Neointimal proliferation was predominantly found at the stent edges, which in the first-generation design was not covered by PTFE, as compared to uniform longitudinal neointimal formed on bare stents (102,103).

A multicenter study reporting on a large series of patients observed a low rate of periprocedural complications and instent restenosis. Target lesion revascularization and vein graft occlusion were also considerably lower than in historical reports (104). A multicenter randomized controlled trial of PTFE-covered stents for saphenous vein grafts is currently underway.

V. Stenting vs. Surgery

The optimum choice of revascularization for multivessel coronary artery disease is a complex issue, with treatment options influenced greatly by patient preference and co-morbidities. Several randomized trials compared multivessel balloon angioplasty with CABG, showing that, at least for the early follow-up period, there was no difference in mortality (105–108). An increased need for subsequent TVR in patients treated with angioplasty was found. Moreover, diabetic patients benefited significantly from an initial surgical approach for multivessel disease (109–111).

Using the National Heart, Lung, and Blood Institute (NHLBI) Dynamic Registry, a comparison was made between the angioplasty practice in 1997 and that of 1987 (12). The analysis demonstrated that despite both higher-risk patients and procedures, the success rate had increased and complication rates were reduced (12), suggesting that the advent of newer technologies, particularly stenting, had a role for multivessel therapy.

Coronary Angioplasty with Stenting versus Coronary Bypass Surgery in patients with Multiple-Vessel Disease (ERACI II) randomized 450 patients to PCI with stenting or CABG. Only patients with multivessel disease and indications for revascularization were enrolled. During the first month the PCI arm had lower major adverse events compared with CABG arm (3.6% vs. 12.3%; $p = 0.002$). At 18-month follow-up, survival was 96.9% in the PCI arm compared with 92.5% in CABG ($p < 0.017$), although a higher requirement for TVR was seen in the PCI arm (16.8% vs. 4.8%; $p < 0.002$) (112).

The Arterial Revascularization Therapies Study (ARTS) found that patients randomized to either stenting or CABG had similar rates of mortality after 1 year (113). Despite a similar rate of TVR compared to other stent trials, the CABG arm, particularly the diabetic cohort, performed significantly better in terms of TVR. The Stent or Surgery (SoS) study found a lower mortality at 1 year in those undergoing CABG instead of PCI (0.8% vs. 2.5%) (114). Interestingly, the low surgical mortality and higher incidence of cancer deaths in the PCI arm have been used by some to explain the benefits of CABG in the SoS trial. The SoS study has yet to report the quality of life and neuropsychiatric outcomes.

From these three trials the role of stenting for multivessel disease remains unclear. Both procedures have similar outcomes, with little difference in mortality. CABG is more invasive, complicated by higher MACE and decline in cognitive function associated with cardiopulmonary bypass (115). Stenting is associated with a greater need for a repeat procedure and a higher rate of recurrent angina. The need for subsequent TVR appears to be decreasing and is likely to reduce further with novel stent therapy (94), while adjunctive GPIIb/IIIa inhibition to reduce complications following stenting may also alter the outcome of multivessel stenting in the near future (116).

VI. CONCLUSIONS

The addition of coronary stenting to interventional cardiology has reduced the complications and increased the clinical application of PCI. Convincing evidence supports the use of stents for the treatment of de novo and restenotic lesions, acute myocardial infarction, saphenous vein grafts, and following recanalization of chronic total occlusions. Currently there is no strong evidence to support the use of stenting above optimum angioplasty in small-vessel intervention and limited evidence supporting left main coronary artery stenting. Progress in stent design and adjunctive mechanical and pharmacological therapies provides a constantly changing field, necessitating ongoing basic and clinical research that will likely increase the indications for stenting in the future.

REFERENCES

1. Dotter C, Transluminally placed coilspring endarterial tube grafts. Long term patency in canine popliteal artery. Invest. Radiol. 1969. 4(3):29–32.
2. Sigwart U, Puel J, Mirkovitch V, et al., Intravascular stents to prevent occlusion and restenosis after transluminal angioplasty. N Engl. J Med., 1987; 316(12):701–706.
3. Fischman D, Leon M, Baim D, et al., A randomized comparison of coronary-stent placement and balloon angioplasty in the treatment of coronary artery disease. Stent Restenosis Study Investigators. N Engl. J Med., 1994; 331(8):496–501.
4. Serruys P, de Jaegere P, Kiemeneij F, et al., A comparison of balloon-expandable-stent implantation with balloon angioplasty in patients with coronary artery disease. Benestent Study Group. N Engl. J Med., 1994; 331(8):489–495.
5. Betriu A, Masotti M, Serra A, et al., Randomized comparison of coronary stent implantation and balloon angioplasty in the treatment of de novo coronary artery lesions (START): a four-year follow-up. J Am Coll Cardiol, 1999; 34(5):1498–1506.
6. Rodriguez A, Ayala F, Bernardi V, et al., Optimal coronary balloon angioplasty with provisional stenting versus primary stent (OCBAS): immediate and long-term follow-up results. J Am Coll Cardiol, 1998; 32(5):1351–1357.
7. Versaci F, Gaspardone A, Tomai F, et al., A comparison of coronary-artery stenting with angioplasty for isolated stenosis of the proximal left anterior descending coronary artery. N Engl. J Med., 1997; 336(12):817–822.
8. George CJ, Baim DS, Brinker JA, et al., One-year follow-up of the Stent Restenosis (STRESS I) Study. Am J Cardiol, 1998; 81(7):860–865.
9. Kimura T, Yokoi H, Nakagawa Y, et al., Three-year follow-up after implantation of metallic coronary-artery stents. N Engl. J Med., 1996; 334(9):561–566.
10. Slota PA, Fischman DL, Savage MP, et al., Frequency and outcome of development of coronary artery aneurysm after intracoronary stent placement and angioplasty. STRESS Trial Investigators. Am J Cardiol, 1997; 79(8):1104–1106.
11. Al Suwaidi J, Berger PB, Holmes DR, Jr., Coronary artery stents. JAMA, 2000; 284(14):1828–1836.
12. Laskey WK, Williams DO, Vlachos HA, et al., Changes in the practice of percutaneous coronary intervention: a comparison of enrollment waves in the National Heart, Lung, and Blood Institute (NHLBI) Dynamic Registry. Am J Cardiol, 2001; 87(8):964–969.
13. Leon M, Baim D, Popma J, et al., A clinical trial comparing three antithrombotic-drug regimens after coronary-artery stenting. Stent Anticoagulation Restenosis Study Investigators. N Engl. J Med., 1998; 339(23):1665–1671.
14. Bertrand M, Legrand V, Boland J, et al., Randomized multicenter comparison of conventional anticoagulation versus antiplatelet therapy in unplanned and elective coronary stenting. The full anticoagulation versus aspirin and ticlopidine (fantastic) study. Circulation, 1998; 98(16):1597–1603.
15. Urban P, Macaya C, Rupprecht H, et al., Randomized evaluation of anticoagulation versus antiplatelet therapy after coronary stent implantation in high-risk patients: the multicenter aspirin and ticlopidine trial after intracoronary stenting (MATTIS). Circulation, 1998; 98(20):2126–2132.

16. Holmes DR, Jr., Kip KE, Yeh W, et al., Long-term analysis of conventional coronary balloon angioplasty and an initial "stent-like" result. The NHLBI PTCA Registry. J Am Coll Cardiol, 1998; 32(3):590–595.

17. Sigwart U, Urban P, Golf S, et al., Emergency stenting for acute occlusion after coronary balloon angioplasty. Circulation, 1988; 78(5 pt 1):1121–1127.

18. Carrozza JP, Jr., Schatz RA, George CJ, et al., Acute and long-term outcome after Palmaz-Schatz stenting: analysis from the New Approaches to Coronary Intervention (NACI) registry. Am J Cardiol, 1997; 80(10A):78–88.

19. Colombo A, Goldberg SL, Almagor Y, et al., A novel strategy for stent deployment in the treatment of acute or threatened closure complicating balloon coronary angioplasty. Use of short or standard (or both) single or multiple Palmaz-Schatz stents. J Am Coll Cardiol, 1993; 22(7):1887–1891.

20. Maiello L, Colombo A, Gianrossi R, et al., Coronary stenting for treatment of acute or threatened closure following dissection after coronary balloon angioplasty. Am Heart J, 1993; 125(6):1570–1575.

21. Gruntzig A, Schneider HJ, The percutaneous dilatation of chronic coronary stenoses—experiments and morphology. Schweiz Med Wochenschr, 1977; 107(44):1588.

22. Gruntzig AR, Senning A, Siegenthaler WE, Nonoperative dilatation of coronary-artery stenosis: percutaneous transluminal coronary angioplasty. N Engl. J Med., 1979; 301(2):61–68.

23. Gruntzig AR, Percutaneous transluminal angioplasty in coronary occlusion. Hosp Pract, 1981; 16(11):129–136.

24. Erbel R, Haude M, Hopp HW, et al., Coronary-artery stenting compared with balloon angioplasty for restenosis after initial balloon angioplasty. Restenosis Stent Study Group. N Engl. J Med., 1998; 339(23):1672–1678.

25. Keane D, Azar AJ, de Jaegere P, et al., Clinical and angiographic outcome of elective stent implantation in small coronary vessels: an analysis of the BENESTENT trial. Semin Interv Cardiol, 1996; 1(4):255–262.

26. Akiyama T, Moussa I, Reimers B, et al., Angiographic and clinical outcome following coronary stenting of small vessels: a comparison with coronary stenting of large vessels. J Am Coll Cardiol, 1998; 32(6):1610–1618.

27. Elezi S, Kastrati A, Neumann FJ, et al., Vessel size and long-term outcome after coronary stent placement. Circulation, 1998; 98(18):1875–1880.

28. Kastrati A, Schomig A, Dirschinger J, et al., A randomized trial comparing stenting with balloon angioplasty in small vessels in patients with symptomatic coronary artery disease. ISAR-SMART Study Investigators. Intracoronary Stenting or Angioplasty for Restenosis Reduction in Small Arteries. Circulation, 2000; 102(21):2593–2598.

29. Hausleiter J, Kastrati A, Mehilli J, et al., Comparative analysis of stent placement versus balloon angioplasty in small coronary arteries with long narrowings (the Intracoronary Stenting or Angioplasty for Restenosis Reduction in Small Arteries [ISAR-SMART] Trial). Am J Cardiol, 2002; 89(1):58–60.

30. Doucet S, Schalij MJ, Vrolix MC, et al., Stent placement to prevent restenosis after angioplasty in small coronary arteries. Circulation, 2001; 104(17):2029–2033.

31. Koning R, Eltchaninoff H, Commeau P, et al., Stent placement compared with balloon angioplasty for small coronary arteries: in-hospital and 6-month clinical and angiographic results. Circulation, 2001; 104(14):1604–1608.

32. Moer R, Myreng Y, Molstad P, et al., Stenting in small coronary arteries (SISCA) trial. A randomized comparison between balloon angioplasty and the heparin-coated beStent. J Am Coll Cardiol, 2001; 38(6):1598–1603.

33. Moer R, Myreng Y, Molstad P, et al., Clinical benefit of small vessel stenting: one-year follow-up of the SISCA trial. Scand Cardiovasc J, 2002; 36(2):86–90.

34. Puma JA, Sketch MH, Jr., Tcheng JE, et al., Percutaneous revascularization of chronic coronary occlusions: an overview. J Am Coll Cardiol, 1995. 26(1):1–11.

35. Sirnes PA, Myreng Y, Molstad P, et al., Improvement in left ventricular ejection fraction and wall motion after successful recanalization of chronic coronary occlusions. Eur Heart J, 1998; 19(2):273–281.

36. Smyth DW, Jewitt DE, Angioplasty of occluded coronary arteries: is it worth the effort? Br Heart J, 1994; 72(1):1–2.

37. Sirnes PA, Golf S, Myreng Y, et al., Stenting in Chronic Coronary Occlusion (SICCO): a randomized, controlled trial of adding stent implantation after successful angioplasty. J Am Coll Cardiol, 1996; 28(6):1444–1451.

38. Sirnes PA, Golf S, Myreng Y, et al., Sustained benefit of stenting chronic coronary occlusion: long-term clinical follow-up of the Stenting in Chronic Coronary Occlusion (SICCO) study. J Am Coll Cardiol, 1998; 32(2):305–310.

39. Buller CE, Dzavik V, Carere RG, et al., Primary stenting versus balloon angioplasty in occluded coronary arteries: the Total Occlusion Study of Canada (TOSCA). Circulation, 1999; 100(3):236–242.

40. Suttorp MJ, Mast EG, Plokker HW, et al., Primary coronary stenting after successful balloon angioplasty of chronic total occlusions: a single-center experience. Am Heart J, 1998; 135(2 Pt 1):318–322.

41. Rubartelli P, Niccoli L, Verna E, et al., Stent implantation versus balloon angioplasty in chronic coronary occlusions: results from the GISSOC trial. Gruppo Italiano di Studio sullo Stent nelle Occlusioni Coronariche. J Am Coll Cardial, 1998; 32(1):90–96.

42. Lotan C, Rozenman Y, Hendler A, et al., Stents in total occlusion for restenosis prevention. The multicentre randomized STOP study. The Israeli Working Group for Interventional Cardiology. Eur Heart J, 2000; 21(23):1960–1966.

43. Sievert H, Rohde S, Utech A, et al., Stent or angioplasty after recanalization of chronic coronary occlusions? (The SARECCO Trial). Am J Cardiol, 1999; 84(4):386–390.

44. Kim CB, Braunwald E, Potential benefits of late reperfusion of infarcted myocardium. The open artery hypothesis. Circulation, 1993; 88(5 Pt 1):2426–2436.

45. Grines CL, Browne KF, Marco J, et al., A comparison of immediate angioplasty with thrombolytic therapy for acute myocardial infarction. The Primary Angioplasty in Myocardial Infarction Study Group. N Engl. J Med., 1993; 328(10):673–679.

46. Nunn CM, O'Neill WW, Rothbaum D, et al., Long-term outcome after primary angioplasty: report from the primary angioplasty in myocardial infarction (PAMI-I) trial. J Am Coll Cardiol, 1999; 33(3):640–646.

47. Zijlstra F, de Boer MJ, Hoorntje JC, et al., A comparison of immediate coronary angioplasty with intravenous streptokinase in acute myocardial infarction. N Engl. J Med., 1993; 328(10):680–684.

48. Zijlstra F, Beukema WP, van't Hof AW, et al., Randomized comparison of primary coronary angioplasty with thrombolytic therapy in low risk patients with acute myocardial infarction. J Am Coll Cardiol, 1997; 29(5):908–912.

49. Every NR, Parsons LS, Hlatky M, et al., A comparison of thrombolytic therapy with primary coronary angioplasty for acute myocardial infarction. Myocardial Infarction Triage and Intervention Investigators. N Engl. J Med., 1996; 335(17):1253–1260.

50. Tiefenbrunn AJ, Chandra NC, French WJ, et al., Clinical experience with primary percutaneous transluminal coronary angioplasty compared with alteplase (recombinant tissue-type plasminogen activator) in patients with acute myocardial infarction: a report from the Second National Registry of Myocardial Infarction (NRMI-2). J Am Coll Cardiol, 1998; 31(6):1240–1245.

51. Weaver WD, Simes RJ, Betriu A, et al., Comparison of primary coronary angioplasty and intravenous thrombolytic therapy for acute myocardial infarction: a quantitative review. JAMA, 1997; 278(23):2093–2098.

52. Grines CL, Cox DA, Stone GW, et al., Coronary angioplasty with or without stent implantation for acute myocardial infarction. Stent Primary Angioplasty in Myocardial Infarction Study Group. N Engl. J Med., 1999; 341(26):1949–1956.

53. Grines CL, Marsalese DL, Brodie B, et al., Safety and cost-effectiveness of early discharge after primary angioplasty in low risk patients with acute myocardial infarction. PAMI-II

Investigators. Primary Angioplasty in Myocardial Infarction. J Am Coll Cardiol, 1998; 31(5):967–972.

54. Stone GW, Grines CL, Cox DA, et al., Comparison of angioplasty with stenting, with or without abciximab, in acute myocardial infarction. N Engl. J Med., 2002; 346(13):957–966.

55. Silva JA, Ramee SR, Cohen DJ, et al., Rheolytic thrombectomy during percutaneous revascularization for acute myocardial infarction: experience with the AngioJet catheter. Am Heart J, 2001; 141(3):353–389.

56. Rodriguez A, Bernardi V, Fernandez M, et al., In-hospital and late results of coronary stents versus conventional balloon angioplasty in acute myocardial infarction (GRAMI trial). Gianturco-Roubin in Acute Myocardial Infarction. Am J Cardiol, 1998; 81(11):1286–1291.

57. Antoniucci D, Santoro GM, Bolognese L, et al., A clinical trial comparing primary stenting of the infarct-related artery with optimal primary angioplasty for acute myocardial infarction: results from the Florence Randomized Elective Stenting in Acute Coronary Occlusions (FRESCO) trial. J Am Coll Cardiol, 1998; 31(6):1234–1239.

58. Maillard L, Hamon M, Khalife K, et al., A comparison of systematic stenting and conventional balloon angioplasty during primary percutaneous transluminal coronary angioplasty for acute myocardial infarction. STENTIM-2 Investigators. J Am Coll Cardiol, 2000; 35(7):1729–1736.

59. Suryapranata H, van't Hof AW, Hoorntje JC, et al., Randomized comparison of coronary stenting with balloon angioplasty in selected patients with acute myocardial infarction. Circulation, 1998; 97(25):2502–2505.

60. Saito S, Hosokawa G, Tanaka S, et al., Primary stent implantation is superior to balloon angioplasty in acute myocardial infarction: final results of the primary angioplasty versus stent implantation in acute myocardial infarction (PASTA) trial. PASTA Trial Investigators. Catheter Cardiovasc Interv, 1999; 48(3):262–268.

61. Scheller B, Hennen B, Severin-Kneib S, et al., Long-term follow-up of a randomized study of primary stenting versus angioplasty in acute myocardial infarction. Am J Med, 2001; 110(1):1–6.

62. van't Hof AW, Liem A, Suryapranata H, et al., Angiographic assessment of myocardial reperfusion in patients treated with primary angioplasty for acute myocardial infarction: myocardial blush grade. Zwolle Myocardial Infarction Study Group. Circulation, 1998; 97(23):2302–2306.

63. SoRelle R, Stents are the CADILLAC of care. Controlled Abciximab and Device Investigation to Lower Late Angioplasty Complications. Circulation, 2002; 105(14):9094–9095.

64. Cameron A, Kemp HJ, Green G, Cameron A, Kemp HG Jr, Green GE. Reoperation for coronary artery disease: 10 years of clinical follow-up. Circulation, 1988; 78(suppl 1):158–162.

65. Lefkovits J, Holmes D, Califf R, et al., Predictors and sequelae of distal embolization during saphenous vein graft intervention from the CAVEAT-II trial. Coronary Angioplasty Versus Excisional Atherectomy Trial. Circulation, 1995; 92(4):734–740.

66. de Feyter PJ, van Suylen RJ, de Jaegere PP, et al., Balloon angioplasty for the treatment of lesions in saphenous vein bypass grafts. J Am Coll Cardiol, 1993; 21(7):1539–1549.

67. Hong MK, Popma JJ, Pichard AD, et al., Clinical significance of distal embolization after transluminal extraction atherectomy in diffusely diseased saphenous vein grafts. Am Heart J, 1994; 127(6):1496–1503.

68. Wong SC, Baim DS, Schatz RA, et al., Immediate results and late outcomes after stent implantation in saphenous vein graft lesions: the multicenter U.S. Palmaz-Schatz stent experience. The Palmaz-Schatz Stent Study Group. J Am Coll Cardiol, 1995; 26(3):704–712.

69. Brener SJ, Ellis SG, Apperson-Hansen C, et al., Comparison of stenting and balloon angioplasty for narrowings in aortocoronary saphenous vein conduits in place for more than five years. Am J Cardiol, 1997; 79(1):13–18.

70. Savage MP, Douglas JS, Jr., Fischman DL, et al., Stent placement compared with balloon angioplasty for obstructed coronary bypass grafts. Saphenous Vein De Novo Trial Investigators. N Engl. J Med., 1997; 337(11):740–747.

71. Hanekamp C, Koolen J, Heyer P, et al., A Randomized Comparison Between Balloon Angioplasty and Elective Stent Implantation in Venous Bypass Grafts; the Venestent Study. Suppl J Am Coll Cardiol 2000; 35(2, suppl A):9.

72. O'Keefe JH, Jr., Hartzler GO, Rutherford BD, et al., Left main coronary angioplasty: early and late results of 127 acute and elective procedures. Am J Cardiol, 1989; 64(3):144–147.

73. Lopez JJ, Ho KK, Stoler RC, et al., Percutaneous treatment of protected and unprotected left main coronary stenoses with new devices: immediate angiographic results and intermediate-term follow-up. J Am Coll Cardiol, 1997; 29(2):345–352.

74. Ellis SG, Tamai H, Nobuyoshi M, et al., Contemporary percutaneous treatment of unprotected left main coronary stenoses: initial results from a multicenter registry analysis 1994–1996; Circulation, 1997; 96(11):3867–3872.

75. Tan WA, Tamai H, Park SJ, et al., Long-term clinical outcomes after unprotected left main trunk percutaneous revascularization in 279 patients. Circulation, 2001; 104(14):1609–1614.

76. Nageh T, Thomas MR, Wainwright RJ, Safety and efficacy of unprotected left main coronary artery stenting. Circulation, 2002; 105(14):85.

77. Oesterle SN, Whitbourn R, Fitzgerald PJ, et al., The stent decade: 1987 to 1997. Stanford Stent Summit faculty. Am Heart J, 1998; 136(4 pt 1):578–599.

78. Holmes DR, Jr., Hirshfeld J, Jr., Faxon D, et al., ACC Expert Consensus document on coronary artery stents. Document of the American College of Cardiology. J Am Coll Cardiol, 1998; 32(5):1471–1482.

79. Kobayashi Y, De Gregorio J, Kobayashi N, et al., Stented segment length as an independent predictor of restenosis. J Am Coll Cardiol, 1999; 34(3):651–659.

80. Garasic JM, Edelman ER, Squire JC, et al., Stent and artery geometry determine intimal thickening independent of arterial injury. Circulation, 2000; 101(7):812–818.

81. Schulen H, Intracoronary Stenting and Angiographic Results; Strut Thickness Effect on Restenosis Outcome 2 (ISAR-STEREO-2) trial. Suppl J Am Coll Cardiool 2002; 39(5, suppl A).

82. Albiero R, Rau T, Schluter M, et al., Comparison of immediate and intermediate-term results of intravascular ultrasound versus angiography-guided Palmaz-Schatz stent implantation in matched lesions. Circulation, 1997; 96(9):2997–3005.

83. Mudra H, Klauss V, Blasini R, et al., Ultrasound guidance of Palmaz-Schatz intracoronary stenting with a combined intravascular ultrasound balloon catheter. Circulation, 1994; 90(3):1252–1261.

84. de Lemos J, Antman E, Giugliano R, et al., Comparison of a 60- versus 90-minute determination of ST-segment resolution after thrombolytic therapy for acute myocardial infarction. In TIME-II Investigators. Intravenous nPA for Treatment of Infarcting Myocardium Early-II. Am J Cardiol, 2000; 86(11):1235–1237.

85. Serruys P, Deshpande N, Is there MUSIC in IVUS guided stenting? Is this MUSIC going to be a MUST? Multicenter Ultrasound Stenting in Coronaries Study. Eur Heart J, 1998; 19(8):1122–1124.

86. Nakamura S, Hall P, Gaglione A, et al., High pressure assisted coronary stent implantation accomplished without intravascular ultrasound guidance and subsequent anticoagulation. J Am Coll Cardiol, 1997; 29(1):21–27.

87. Dirschinger J, Kastrati A, Neumann FJ, et al., Influence of balloon pressure during stent placement in native coronary arteries on early and late angiographic and clinical outcome: A randomized evaluation of high-pressure inflation. Circulation, 1999; 100(9):918–923.

88. Jang IK, Tearney G, Bouma B, Visualization of tissue prolapse between coronary stent struts by optical coherence tomography: comparison with intravascular ultrasound. Circulation, 2001; 104(22):2754.

89. Serruys PW, Emanuelsson H, van der Giessen W, et al., Heparin-coated Palmaz-Schatz stents in human coronary arteries. Early outcome of the Benestent-II Pilot Study. Circulation, 1996; 93(3):412–422.

90. Serruys PW, van Hout B, Bonnier H, et al., Randomised comparison of implantation of heparin-coated stents with balloon angioplasty in selected patients with coronary artery disease (Benestent II). Lancet, 1998; 352(9129):673–681.

91. Waksman R, Bhargava B, White L, et al., Intracoronary beta-radiation therapy inhibits recurrence of in-stent restenosis. Circulation, 2000. 101(6):1895–1898.

92. Serruys PW, Regar E, Carter AJ, Rapamycin eluting stent: the onset of a new era in interventional cardiology. Heart, 2002; 87(4):305–307.

93. Fajadet J, Perin M, Ban Hayashi E, et al., 210-day follow-up of the RAVEL study: a randomized study with the sirolimus-eluting Bx VELOCITY™ balloon-expandable stent in the treatment of patients with de novo native coronary artery lesions. Suppl J Am Coll Cardiol 2002; 39(5, suppl. A).

94. Morice MC, Serruys PW, Sousa JE, et al., A randomized comparison of a sirolimus-eluting stent with a standard stent for coronary revascularization. N Engl. J Med., 2002; 346(23):1773–80.

95. Grube E. Taxus: paclitaxel eluting stent program. Clinical update. In: The Paris Course in Revascularization. 2002; Paris.

96. Grube E, Serruys P, Safety and performance of a paclitaxel-eluting stent for the treatment of in-stent restenosis: preliminary results of the Taxus III trial. Suppl J Am Coll Cardiol 2002; 39(5, suppl. A).

97. Stefanadis C, Toutouzas K, Tsiamis E, et al., Total reconstruction of a diseased saphenous vein graft by means of conventional and autologous tissue-coated stents. Cathet Cardiovasc Diagn, 1998; 43(3):318–321.

98. van der Giessen WJ, Lincoff AM, Schwartz RS, et al., Marked inflammatory sequelae to implantation of biodegradable and nonbiodegradable polymers in porcine coronary arteries. Circulation, 1996; 94(7):1690–1697.

99. Stefanadis C, Toutouzas K, Vlachopoulos C, et al., Stents wrapped in autologous vein: an experimental study. J Am Coll Cardiol, 1996; 28(4):1039–1046.

100. Stefanadis C, Toutouzas K, Vlachopoulos C, et al., Autologous vein graft-coated stent for treatment of coronary artery disease. Cathet Cardiovasc Diagn, 1996; 38(2):159–170.

101. Colon P, Ramee S, Mulingtapang R, et al., Percutaneous bailout therapy of a perforated vein graft using a stent-autologous vein patch. Cathet Cardiovasc Diagn, 1996; 38(2):175–178.

102. Baldus S, Koster R, Reimers J, et al., Membrane-covered stents: a new treatment strategy for saphenous vein graft lesions. Catheter Cardiovasc Interv, 2001; 53(1):1–4.

103. Briguori C, De GJ, Nishida T, et al., Polytetrafluoroethylene-covered stent for the treatment of narrowings in aorticocoronary saphenous vein grafts. Am J Cardiol, 2000; 86(3):343–6.

104. Baldus S, Koster R, Elsner M, et al., Treatment of aortocoronary vein graft lesions with membrane-covered stents: A multicenter surveillance trial. Circulation, 2000; 102(17):2024–2027.

105. Comparison of coronary bypass surgery with angioplasty in patients with multivessel disease. The Bypass Angioplasty Revascularization Investigation (BARI) Investigators. N Engl. J Med., 1996; 335(4):217–225.

106. Hamm CW, Reimers J, Ischinger T, et al., A randomized study of coronary angioplasty compared with bypass surgery in patients with symptomatic multivessel coronary disease. German Angioplasty Bypass Surgery Investigation (GABI). N Engl. J Med., 1994; 331(16):1037–1043.

107. King SB, 3rd, Lembo NJ, Weintraub WS, et al., A randomized trial comparing coronary angioplasty with coronary bypass surgery. Emory Angioplasty versus Surgery Trial (EAST). N Engl. J Med., 1994; 331(16):1044–1050.

108. Rodriguez A, Boullon F, Perez-Balino N, et al., Argentine randomized trial of percutaneous transluminal coronary angioplasty versus coronary artery bypass surgery in multivessel disease (ERACI): in-hospital results and 1-year follow-up. ERACI Group. J Am Coll Cardiol, 1993; 22(4):1060–1067.

109. Writing Group for the Bypass Angioplasty Revascularization Investigation (BARI) Investigators. Five-year clinical and functional outcome comparing bypass surgery and angioplasty in patients with multivessel coronary disease. A multicenter randomized trial. JAMA, 1997; 277(9):715–721.

110. Henderson RA, Pocock SJ, Sharp SJ, et al., Long-term results of RITA-1 trial: clinical and cost comparisons of coronary angioplasty and coronary-artery bypass grafting. Randomised Intervention Treatment of Angina. Lancet, 1998; 352(9138):1419–1425.

111. Rodriguez A, Mele E, Peyregne E, et al., Three-year follow-up of the Argentine Randomized Trial of Percutaneous Transluminal Coronary Angioplasty Versus Coronary Artery Bypass Surgery in Multivessel Disease (ERACI). J Am Coll Cardiol, 1996; 27(5):1178–1184.

112. Rodriguez A, Bernardi V, Navia J, et al., Argentine Randomized Study: Coronary Angioplasty with Stenting versus Coronary Bypass Surgery in patients with Multiple-Vessel Disease (ERACI II): 30-day and one-year follow-up results. ERACI II Investigators. J Am Coll Cardiol, 2001; 37(1):51–58.

113. de Feyter PJ, Serruys PW, Unger F, et al., Bypass surgery versus stenting for the treatment of multivessel disease in patients with unstable angina compared with stable angina. Circulation, 2002; 105(20):2367–2372.

114. Stables R, SoS Results. Presented at the Annual Meeting of the American College of Cardiology, 2001. Orlando, Florida. Circulation, 2001; 27(2-suppl A.):1A–648A.

115. Van Dijk D, Jansen EW, Hijman R, et al., Cognitive outcome after off-pump and on-pump coronary artery bypass graft surgery: a randomized trial. JAMA, 2002; 287(11):1405–1412.

116. Topol E, Mark D, Lincoff A, et al., Outcomes at 1 year and economic implications of platelet glycoprotein IIb/IIIa blockade in patients undergoing coronary stenting: results from a multicentre randomised trial. EPISTENT Investigators. Evaluation of Platelet IIb/IIIa Inhibitor for Stenting. Lancet, 1999; 354(9195):2019–2024.

117. Smith SC, Jr., Dove JT, Jacobs AK, et al., ACC/AHA guidelines of percutaneous coronary interventions (revision of the 1993 PTCA guidelines)—executive summary. A report of the American College of Cardiology/American Heart Association Task Force on Practice Guidelines (committee to revise the 1993 guidelines for percutaneous transluminal coronary angioplasty). J Am Coll Cardiol, 2001; 37(8):2215–2239.

15-2

Antithrombotic Therapy for Coronary Stenting

Briain D. MacNeill and Ik-Kyung Jang

Massachusetts General Hospital, Harvard Medical School, Boston, Massachusetts, U.S.A.

Patients received 250 to 500 mg of aspirin daily and 75 mg of dipyridamole three times a day; this treatment was started the day before the procedure and was continued for six months. During the procedure, patients receiving a stent were treated with a continuous infusion of dextran (1000 ml) and a bolus dose of 10,000 U of heparin, repeated if necessary, followed by a combination of heparin and oral anticoagulation therapy (with warfarin) after the removal of the sheath and titrated by measuring the prothrombin time and either the activated partial-thromboplastin time or the activated clotting time. The dose of heparin was decreased progressively after the prothrombin time had been in the therapeutic range (international normalized ratio, 2.5 to 3.5) for at least 36 hours. Warfarin therapy was continued for three months (1).

I. INTRODUCTION

Over the last decade numerous anatomical and technical limitations have been resolved, resulting in an explosive increase in percutaneous coronary interventions (PCIs). With the advent of intracoronary stenting, acute vessel closure, a potentially fatal complication, and restenosis, the Achilles' heel of coronary angioplasty, became manageable (1,2). Initial reports confirmed procedural success of stenting for both failed angioplasty and peri-procedural abrupt vessel closure, but a prohibitively high rate of thrombosis in the early post-procedural period demonstrated that metal stents and balloon-disrupted endothelium present a perfect nidus for platelet accumulation and subsequent thrombosis (3,4).

During this time the pathophysiology of acute stent thrombosis was unclear, resulting in a paucity of clinical guidelines for poststenting antithrombotics. Initial experience with either antithrombotics or antiplatelet agents used in isolation displayed persistent acute and subacute thrombosis, prompting all-encompassing treatment strategies, often incorporating heparin, dextran, aspirin, dipyridamole, and warfarin. Predictably, this aggressive regime caused high rates of hemorrhagic complication, increased mortality, and prolonged hospitalization, all for the sake of a device designed to improve patient outcome (1,2). The reluctance that ensued saw intracoronary stents reserved predominantly for bailout procedures or failed angioplasty (5).

Two landmark trials of intracoronary stenting, the Belgium-Netherlands Stent Study (BENESTENT) and the Stent Restenosis Study (STRESS), displayed significant improvement in angiographic and clinical endpoints corresponding to a dramatic reduction in the need for repeat target vessel revascularization. Low rates of stent thrombosis were achieved in both trials, but at the expense of hemorrhagic complications, reflecting aggressive anticoagulation (1,2). Nevertheless, the reduction of restenosis was of such significance as to warrant FDA approval of Palmaz-Schatz stents for de novo lesions.

Adjunctive use of intravascular ultrasound (IVUS) taught us that despite excellent angiographic appearances, suboptimal stent expansion at traditionally accepted inflation pressures was common (6,7). Inadequate stent apposition to the coronary wall leads to plaque protrusion, strut irregularity, and turbulent coronary flow, all promoting thrombosis. This concept led investigators to examine less aggressive anticoagulation following IVUS-guided stent deployment with successful results using a combination of heparin, aspirin, dextran, and dipyridamole (8). The Multicenter Ultrasound Stenting In Coronaries Study (MUSIC) trial further reduced the level of poststent treatment to aspirin alone following IVUS-guided stent deployment with low rates of both stent thrombosis and hemorrhagic complications (9,10).

Enhanced understanding of the pathophysiology of stenting coupled with pharmacological advances have expanded the armamentarium available to prevent and treat stent thrombosis including low molecular weight heparin (LMWH), thienopyridines, direct thrombin inhibitors, and glycoprotein IIb/IIIa inhibitors.

II. PATHOPHYSIOLOGY OF STENT THROMBOSIS

Endothelial disruption, atherosclerotic plaque rupture, foreign metal material, and activated platelets provide the perfect environment for thrombus formation following intracoronary stent insertion (11). Platelet activation and aggregation are key steps in the dynamic thrombotic process that occurs (12). Exposure of procoagulant matrix following plaque rupture or balloon injury causes initial binding of platelets to von Willebrand factor, collagen, and soluble adhesion molecules. Once bound, platelets can be activated by agonists including adenosine diphosphate, collagen, thrombin, and thromboxane A_2, all acting through one of three pathways: phospholipase C causing a calcium influx, phospholipase A_2 causing an increase in arachadonic acid, and finally inhibition of adenylate cyclase. Regardless of the mechanism of activation, the end result is a change in platelet morphology, degranulation, and activation of the GP IIb/IIIa receptors. Binding of fibrinogen to GP IIb/IIIa receptors causes cross-linking of neighboring platelets, creating a platelet-rich clot. Inhibition of this process of activation can be achieved at any stage of the process with varying degrees of efficacy.

III. HEPARINOIDS

Although heparin has been used routinely as an adjunct to PCI, data from controlled trials are lacking. Extensive evidence from animal studies, observation studies, and randomized trials of heparin's effect in acute coronary syndromes provide surrogate data to support its continued use and define heparin as the standard against which other agents are compared (13,14). As with all anticoagulants, the efficacy of heparin in reducing ischemic events is counterbalanced by hemorrhagic complications. The recommended dose of heparin used during PCI varies from center to center, but an activated clotting time (ACT) of 300 seconds is commonly used as a guide for heparin monotherapy (15). Combining heparin with other antiplatelet agents requires further adjustment. In the Evaluation of 7E3 for the Prevention of Ischemic Complications (EPIC) trials the combination of heparin (100 units/kg) and abciximab caused an excess of hemorrhagic complications that was significantly reduced in the Evaluation in PTCA to Improve Long-Term Outcome with Abciximab GP IIb/IIIa Blockade (EPILOG) trial using lower doses of intravenous heparin (70 units/kg), aiming for an ACT of 200 seconds (16,17).

Low molecular weight heparin is derived by enzymatic or chemical depolymerization of unfractionated heparin (UFH), producing a compound one-third the size. Smaller molecules have less plasma protein binding, ultimately producing a longer half-life and improved bioavailability. Unlike UFH, LMWH is resistant to platelet factor 4 and has minimal binding to acute phase reactants and vascular endothelial cells (18,19). LMWH bonds in a similar manner as UFH with antithrombin III (AT III), although its smaller size does not allow for simultaneous AT III and thrombin binding, making it less effective as a catalyst for AT III. Instead, the majority of its antithrombin effect is achieved primarily through inactivating factor Xa (20).

LMWH has proven efficacious for management of unstable coronary syndromes in a safer and more clinically applicable manner than UFH and has been adopted into practice guidelines (21–24). A longer half-life and the lack of readily available monitoring for LMWH lead interventional cardiologists to be weary of its use before and during PCI (25). Preliminary recommendations for the use of LMWH suggest that LMWH can be continued during diagnostic studies but should be changed to UFH during PCI. A lower ACT should be targeted if the last dose of LMWH was within 6 hours of the intervention (26). A recently presented preliminary study on the use of LMWH during PCI suggested that ACT could be used for rapid monitoring with a lower target ACT of 180 seconds during PCI (27). Data from the National Investigators Collaborating on Enoxaparin (NICE) trials have demonstrated the safety of combining enoxaparin with GP IIb/IIIa inhibitors in patients undergoing PCI (28). Trials are underway to add further information to combination therapy (29,30).

Continued treatment with LMWH following PCI was also studied. Prolonged treatment with Dalteparin for 45 days following an episode of unstable angina led to a reduction of 43% in the incidence of death or myocardial infarction compared to control groups in the Fast Revascularization during Instability in Coronary artery disease II (FRISC II) trial (31). Continuing the treatment to 90 days, however, showed no further benefit.

In vitro evidence of reduced smooth muscle proliferation with LMWH raised the hypothesis that LMWH, in addition to acting as an anticoagulant, could act as an antiproliferative, thereby decreasing restenosis following stenting. However, LMWH in isolation and in combination with fish oils following stent insertion failed to show any benefit in the prevention of restenosis (32–34).

IV. DIRECT THROMBIN INHIBITORS

Thrombin is the most potent platelet activator known, stimulating the production of platelet-derived growth factor (PDGF) and the secretion of platelet activating factor, prostacycline, and plasminogen-activator inhibitor. Thrombin induces lymphocytes and vascular smooth muscle mitosis, raising suspicion of a role in the development of restenosis. Advantages of direct thrombin inhibitors over heparin include (a) a more constant anticoagulant effect necessitating less monitoring, (b) a mode of action independent of the cofactor AT III, (c) the ability to bind clot-bound as well as free thrombin, and (d) resistance to platelet factor 4 (35).

The two subtypes are distinguishable. The first, specific thrombin inhibitors such as hirudin and bivalirudin, bind to active sites and substrate sites on thrombin, allowing for a high specificity. The second, active site inhibitors including argatroban, inogatran, and efegatran, bind only to the thrombin active site (36,37).

In combination with thrombolysis for acute myocardial infarction (AMI), high doses of hirudin resulted in significant hemorrhagic complications, particularly intracranial hemorrhage; although subsequently reduced dose regimes yielded a safer side effect profile, no statistically significant benefit over heparin was achieved (38–41). The Global Use of Strategies to Open Occluded Coronary Arteries in Acute Coronary Syndromes (GUSTO-IIb) trial focused on acute coronary syndromes, randomizing patients to 72 hours of either heparin or intravenous hirudin. Despite a 39% reduction in the 24-hour combined endpoint of death or MI and an 18% reduction in MI at 30 days, the results did not reach statistical significance. Moreover, a 14% higher rate of bleeding complications was seen in the hirudin-treated group (42).

Initially, hirudin treatment during PCI compared favorably to heparin in terms of antithrombin activity and safety profile (43). Moreover, hirudin appeared to be superior to heparin in reducing troponin T elevation following PCI (44). Both of these trials paved the way for the Hirudin in a European Restenosis Prevention Trial, Versus Heparin Treatment in the Prevention of Coronary Angioplasty (HELVETICA) study, comparing hirudin with heparin in the prevention of restenosis following coronary angioplasty. A total of 1141 patients scheduled for angioplasty for unstable angina were randomized to receive either heparin or hirudin prior to angioplasty. Although a significantly lower rate of early cardiac events occurred in the first 96 hours of hirudin treatment, there was no reduction in the development of restenosis and no apparent benefit at 7 months. The authors concluded that the antithrombin effect as assayed following the angioplasty was suboptimal compared to the heparin group, inferring an overcautious dosing regime (45,46).

There are possible explanations for the lack of an observed benefit of hirudin over heparin. Although hirudin has a greater ability to inhibit thrombin activity, this capacity can be exceeded, thus allowing thrombosis, while heparin, the effect of which occurs upstream in the coagulation cascade, results in lower concentrations of thrombin generation (Fig. 1). Also, hirudin binds thrombin with a tight 1:1 stoichiometric mechanism, while heparin acts as a catalytic inhibitor with weaker bonds, allowing one molecule of heparin to catalyze the effect of multiple molecules of AT III. Furthermore, the inability of hirudin to adequately passivate the site of endothelial injury could explain the beneficial effects seen in the first 24 hours of the GUSTO-IIb, which did not persist beyond the hirudin infusion, as well as the transient benefit found in the above trials (42).

Hirulog as an adjunct to PCI was first studied by Topol et al., who demonstrated its potential and safety as a substitute for heparin (47). In the subsequent study by Bittl et al., 4098 patients undergoing PCI for unstable or postinfarct angina were randomized to receive either hirulog or heparin. Although no significant reduction in the endpoints of death, MI, or abrupt vessel closure occurred, a significant reduction in bleeding complications (9.8% to 3.8%) was found in the hirulog group. The subgroup of patients with postinfarct angina received a significant acute benefit from bivalirudin, but once again this was no longer significant at 6-month follow-up (48,49). Reanalysis of this study based on the intention-to-treat principles and modified endpoints of death, revascularization, or myocardial infarction was recently published, demonstrating a more significant reduction both in ischemic events (6.2% vs. 7.9%; $p = 0.039$) and hemorrhagic complications (3.5% vs. 9.3%) (50).

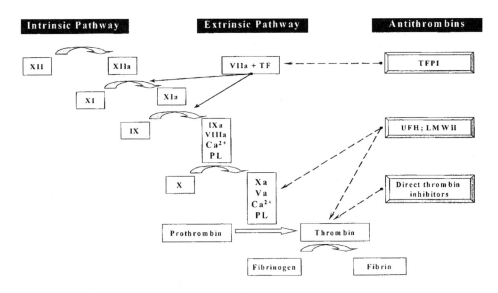

Figure 1 Schema of intrinsic and extrinsic activation pathways of the coagulation cascade. TF = tissue factor; TFPI = tissue factor pathway inhibitor; UFH = unfractionated heparin; LWMH = low molecular weight heparin; PL = platelets.

Preliminary results from the Comparison of Abciximab Complications with Hirulog Events Trial (CACHET) lend further support to the use of hirulog as an adjunct to PCI by demonstrating a stable and predictable anticoagulant effect, a reduction in adverse clinical events, and a reduction in bleeding complications (51–53). Further trials, including REPLACE, are awaited for further clarification of the role of hirulog in PCI.

Argatroban, a synthetic competitive thrombin inhibitor, derived from L-arginine is equally effective against fluid phase and clot bound thrombin (54). Animal studies of thrombosis demonstrated argatroban's efficacy in attenuating arterial thrombus (55,56). Argatroban treatment as an adjunct to thrombolysis has shown enhanced reperfusion of infarct related vessels and was shown to be as safe as heparin (57,58). Limited trials on the effect of argatroban during PCI have shown success in reducing thrombotic complications (59–61), supporting its indication for use as an alternative to heparin in patients undergoing PCI (62). Further trials are underway to assess argatroban's efficacy, as an alternative to heparin, in combination with Abciximab during PCI.

V. THIENOPYRIDINES

Thienopyridines inhibit adenosine diphosphate (ADP) induced platelet aggregation by noncompetitive antagonism of platelet ADP receptors (Fig. 2). ADP, released from activated platelets, red blood cells, and injured endothelium, induces platelet adhesion and aggregation through membrane-bound receptors (63). Although the exact mechanism of action remains unclear, it is thought that thienopyridines inhibit expression, occupation, or function of the platelet membrane ADP receptor (64). Inhibiting ADP release from platelet granules confers the additional effect of reducing platelet aggregation by other agonists, including platelet activation factor, collagen, and thrombin, at low concentrations. At

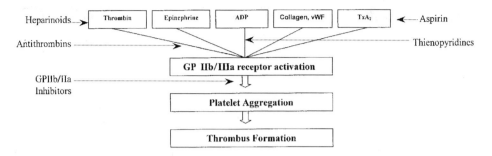

Figure 2   Mechanism of platelet activation and sites of platelet inhibition. ADP = adenosine diphosphate; vWF = von Willebrand factor; TxA_2 = thromboxane A_2.

higher agonist concentrations, platelet aggregation occurs independent of ADP, reducing the effect of ADP antagonism (65).

Ticlopidine and clopidogerol are thienopyridines with similar structural design and pharmacokinetics. Ticlopidine, the first marketed of the two, has been compared to various anticoagulant regimes. The Stent Anticoagulation Restenosis Study (STARS) group randomized low-risk patients after successful stent implantation to receive ticlopidine and aspirin for 28 days followed by aspirin alone (n = 546), warfarin combined with aspirin (n = 550), or aspirin alone (n = 546). Death, revascularization, angiographically detected thrombus, and nonfatal MI were significantly reduced by 85% compared to the aspirin monotherapy group and 80% compared to the combined warfarin aspirin group (66) (Table 1).

The Full Anticoagulation Versus Aspirin and Ticlopidine (FANTASTIC) trial, designed primarily to demonstrate the relative safety of the combination of ticlopidine and aspirin, found a significant reduction in cardiac events for patients undergoing elective stenting treated with ticlopidine compared to a strategy of aspirin and initial heparinization followed by warfarin for 6 weeks. Results from the subgroup of patients in whom coronary stenting was performed as a bailout for failed or suboptimal PTCA showed no significant benefit (67).

The Multicenter Aspirin and Ticlopidine Trial After Intracoronary Stenting (MATTIS) study similarly examined ticlopidine compared to oral anticoagulants, with a target international normalized ratio (INR) of 2.5–3 following coronary stenting in a study

Table 1   Prevention of Major Cardiac Events Following Coronary Stent Insertion: Ticlopidine Versus Anticoagulation Therapy

Study (Ref.)	Patient no.	Population	Risk reduction, %(p)
STARS (66)	1652	Low	1.9 (<0.05)
FANTASTIC (67)	485	Mixed	2.56 (0.37)
MATTIS (68)	350	High	5.4 (0.07)
ISAR (69)	517	Mixed	4.6 (0.01)

Cardiac events included death due to cardiac causes, myocardial infarction, repeat PTCA of the stented vessel, or bypass surgery at 30 days in the ISAR, MATTIS, and STARS studies. In the FANTASTIC study, cardiac events (death, myocardial infarction, and stent occlusion) were secondary endpoints and did not include repeat PTCA or bypass surgery.

population defined as high risk on the basis of abrupt vessel closure, suboptimal angiographic result, long stents, or deployment with a balloon diameter of ≤ 2.5 mm. A reduction of 49% in the endpoints of death, revascularization, and MI was demonstrated in the ticlopidine/aspirin group, a result that did not achieve statistical significance ($p = 0.07$), possibly due to the small numbers ($n = 517$) (68).

Again, a ticlopidine/aspirin combination was compared with an anticoagulant/aspirin combination in the Intracoronary Stenting and Antithrombotic Regimen (ISAR) study (69). Risk stratification using 18 clinical, procedural, and angiographic variables was used to define groups as low ($n = 165$), intermediate ($n = 148$), or high risk ($n = 204$). Within a 30-day follow-up, cardiac event rate (death, myocardial infarction, repeat intervention) was 6.4% for high-risk, 3.4% for intermediate-risk, and 0% for low-risk patients ($p < 0.01$). Stent vessel occlusion occurred in 5.9, 2.7, and 0%, respectively ($p < 0.01$). Low- and intermediate-risk patients did equally well on either anticoagulation or antiplatelet therapy. In high-risk patients, however, the cardiac event rate was 12.6% with anticoagulant therapy and 2.0% with antiplatelet therapy ($p = 0.007$), and the rate of stent vessel occlusion was 11.5 and 0%, respectively ($p < 0.001$) (69).

An important issue in these trials was the timing and length of treatment. In both the FANTASTIC and ISAR studies, ticlopidine treatment was withheld until after stent insertion, accounting for a delay in the relative benefit of the ticlopidine/aspirin combination, leading to a higher rate of acute stent occlusion (67,69). These findings are consistent with the pharmacodynamics of platelet activation, which peaks at 48–72 hours post-PCI, and the antiplatelet effects of ticlopidine, which is maximal after 3–5 days treatment (64). This was further supported by the demonstration of a lower incidence of procedure-related non–Q-wave MI following pretreatment with ticlopidine (70).

Clopidogrel is closely related to ticlopidine in structure, differing only by the addition of a carboxymethyl side group. In the Clopidogrel versus Aspirin in Patients at Risk of Ischemic Events (CAPRIE) trial, clopidogrel demonstrated superiority over aspirin in reduction of vascular death, MI, and fatal and nonfatal stroke in high-risk atherosclerotic patients (recent ischemic stroke, recent myocardial infarction, or symptomatic peripheral arterial disease) without risk of neutropenia compared to aspirin treatment.

Evidence of efficacy of clopidogrel and ticlopidine in animal models and the prominent side effect profile of ticlopidine led to comparative trials between the thienopyridines following stenting (71–76). The use of clopidogrel, with and without a loading dose, was compared to ticlopidine in the CLopidogrel ASpirin Stent International Cooperative Study (CLASSICS) study (77). The primary endpoint, which consisted of major peripheral bleeding, neutropenia, thrombocytopenia, and noncardiac adverse event necessitating discontinuation of treatment, occurred in 9.1% of patients ticlopidine group and 4.6% of the clopidogrel group. Major adverse cardiac events were low and comparable between treatment groups, suggesting that the safety of clopidogrel is superior to that of ticlopidine with comparable efficacy with regard to cardiac events after successful stenting. The safety and efficacy of clopidogrel was further proven in three trials, which together displayed that compared to ticlopidine, clopidogrel had a lower rate of adverse events and was more likely to be tolerated by the patient (77).

The platelet suppression of clopidogrel preceded by a loading dose is significantly higher compared to standard clopidogrel or ticlopidine, without an increase in complications. Bolus dose clopidogrel displayed a 75% greater inhibition of ADP-induced platelet aggregation, an effect that was evident within 2 hours of the loading dose, compared to standard clopidogrel or ticlopidine (78).

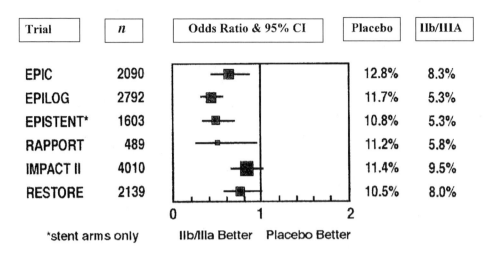

Trial	*n*	Odds Ratio & 95% CI	Placebo	IIb/IIIA
EPIC	2090		12.8%	8.3%
EPILOG	2792		11.7%	5.3%
EPISTENT*	1603		10.8%	5.3%
RAPPORT	489		11.2%	5.8%
IMPACT II	4010		11.4%	9.5%
RESTORE	2139		10.5%	8.0%

*stent arms only   IIb/IIIa Better   Placebo Better

Figure 3   Odds ratio analysis of placebo controlled GPIIb IIIa inhibition trials.

VI. GLYCOPROTEIN IIB/IIIA INHIBITORS

The benefit of GP IIb/IIIa receptor antagonism was first demonstrated in the EPIC trial (Fig. 3) in which patients undergoing relatively high-risk coronary angioplasty were randomized to receive abciximab or placebo (Table 2). A 35% reduction in mortality, myocardial infarction, or recurrent ischemic events occurred in the abciximab-treated group. The benefit persisted at 3-year follow-up and was most significant in patients treated for an unstable coronary syndrome (16). Analysis of the 64 cases randomized in the EPIC trial that underwent primary angioplasty in the EPIC-AMI study showed a significant 83% reduction in major adverse coronary events at 1 month, a benefit that became even more pronounced at 6-month follow-up and was predominantly due to a decreased need for repeat revascularization (79).

The EPIC trial was noteworthy for high rates of hemorrhagic complications that occurred in the abciximab-treated group (16). This feature was addressed in the follow-up study of the EPILOG trial by using a lower dose and a shorter infusion of weight-adjusted

Table 2   Placebo-Controlled Trials Comparing GPIIb/IIIa Inhibitors

Trial	Drug	*n*	Indication	Placebo (%)	GPIIb IIIa (%)	Reduction (%)	*p*-value	Ref.
EPIC	Abciximab	2099	PTCA	12.8	8.3	35	0.008	16
EPILOG	Abciximab	2792	PTCA	11.7	5.2	56.	0.001	17
CAPTURE	Abciximab	1252	PTCA	15.9	11.3	29	0.012	84
EPISTENT	Abciximab	1603	Stent	10.8	5.3	51.	0.007	80
ADMIRAL	Abciximab	300	Stent, Acute MI	14.6	6.0	59	0.01	99
IMPACT II	Eptifibatide	4010	PTCA	11.4	9.2	19	0.06	88
ESPRIT	Eptifibatide	1206	STENT	11.5	7.5	35	0.02	90
RESTORE	Tirofiban	2139	PTCA	12.2	10.3	16	0.16	91

heparin (17). This study was designed to include less unstable patients than had been studied in the original EPIC trial. Again, a significant reduction was seen in all major end-points, which persisted to follow-up at 1 year, with a reduced rate of bleeding complications compared to the EPIC trial.

These trials demonstrated that abciximab improved outcome in PCI. The trials were not designed, however, to study the effect on coronary stenting. The EPIC trial had a stent placement rate of only 0.6 % in both the abciximab and the control group, while the more recent EPILOG trial included stenting in 11% of the 935 patients randomized to receive abciximab (16,17). Of this group, 19 (2%) of the cases were planned stenting, and the remaining 81(9%) were unplanned. The Evaluation of Platelet IIb/IIIa Inhibitor for Stenting (EPISTENT) trial was designed, therefore, to study the effect of the combination of GP IIb/IIIa inhibition and stenting, randomizing patients undergoing coronary stenting to receive either abciximab or placebo (80). A synergistic effect was found between abciximab, which reduced mortality and infarction rates, and stenting, which reduced the requirement for target vessel revascularization (81). Follow up at 1 year demonstrated a continued benefit with a reduction in mortality from 2.4 to 1% in the abciximab group. A greater benefit was perceived in patients presenting with unstable symptoms compared to patients undergoing elective PCI and diabetics (82). Subsequently, the synergism between abciximab and stenting has been demonstrated in other studies (83).

The c7E3 Fab Antiplatelet Therapy in Unstable Refractory Angina (CAPTURE) trial studied abciximab in a placebo-controlled trial as an adjunct to PCI, in which coronary stenting was not encouraged (84). Patients with unstable angina refractory to conventional medical therapy were randomized following angiography to receive an 18- to 24-hour infusion of abciximab or placebo prior to the PCI. Although coronary stenting was performed in only 27.4%, the trial design allowed the effect of abciximab and PCI to be analyzed separately. Abciximab demonstrated a significant resolution of coronary thrombus prior to the procedure with a corresponding reduction of MI leading up to PCI. Moreover, it afforded a reduction in periprocedural infarction and a reduction of post-PCI MACE. As in GP IIb/IIIa trials, in other settings the maximum benefit was found in higher-risk patients, as stratified by raised serum troponin levels (84–86).

The effect of abciximab on the prevention of in-stent restenosis in humans was studied in the Evaluation of ReoPro" And Stenting to Eliminate Restenosis (ERASER) trial, in which patients ($n = 245$) were randomized to receive a placebo or 12-hour or 24-hour infusion of abciximab (87). Follow-up evaluation by quantitative coronary angiography (QCA) and intravascular ultrasound at 6 months, however, revealed no difference in restenosis, definitively quashing the theory that abciximab reduces in-stent restenosis. The results of this well-designed trial again raise the question of origin of the late benefit seen in the EPIC and EPISTENT trials, if not from prevention of restenosis.

Eptifibatide as an adjunct to balloon angioplasty was examined in the Integrilin to Minimize Platelet Aggregation and Coronary Thrombosis II (IMPACT II) trial, which demonstrated a significant reduction in major adverse cardiac events without incidence of hemorrhagic complications experienced in trials of abciximab (88). This led to the Enhanced Suppression of the Platelet IIb/IIIa Receptor with Integrilin Therapy (ESPRIT) trial, which showed the efficacy of adjunctive, double-bolus eptifibatide therapy (bolus of 180 mg/kg × 2 given 10 min apart) in reducing ischemic complications of nonurgent coronary stent implantation (89,90). Patients ($n = 2064$) were randomly assigned to receive placebo or double-bolus eptifibatide commenced immediately before stent implantation and continued for 18–24 hours. Follow-up at 6 months revealed a reduction in death or MI in the eptifibatide group compared to the placebo group (7.5% vs. 11.5%). Similarly, the composite endpoint of death, MI, or target vessel revascularization was 14.2% in eptifi-batide-treated patients versus 18.3% in placebo-treated patients. Most of this benefit occurred within the first 48 hours, but it was maintained to 6 month follow-up (89,90).

Tirofiban, although not studied with coronary stenting, was the focus of the Randomized Efficacy Study of Tirofiban for Outcomes and Restenosis (RESTORE) trial, in which stenting was permitted as a bailout in high-risk patients randomized to receive tirofiban or placebo as adjunctive treatment for PCI (91). Coronary stents were required in only 4% of the study population. Composite endpoints at 30 days occurred in 10.5% of the placebo group and 8.0% of the tirofiban group, a relative reduction of 24% ($p = 0.052$), a value that did not achieve statistical significance. No significant increase was found in adverse events or bleeding complications in the tirofiban-treated group. Angiographic follow-up at 6 months demonstrated no reduction in restenosis in the tirofiban-treated group (92).

Several oral GP IIb/IIIa inhibitors were examined in various phase I and II trials (93–95). The rationale proposed was that a drug such as aspirin, despite weak antiplatelet effect, could have a dramatic impact on reducing ischemic deaths, and by maximizing platelet inhibition using a receptor with proven effects, over a long period could reduce mortality. In practice, oral GP IIb/IIIa inhibitors led to significant adverse effects and excess mortality. Fluctuations in drug concentration causing variable levels of GP IIb/IIIa inhibition combined with partial agonist action at low concentration were thought to explain some aspects of the failure of these agents (96–98).

Primary or direct infarct angioplasty and rescue angioplasty have resulted in a dra-matic change in our treatment of myocardial infarction and raised questions about the effect of coronary stenting in combination with a GP IIb/IIIa inhibitor. These questions were further addressed in the Abciximab before Direct Angioplasty and Stenting for Myocardial Infarction Regarding Acute and Long-Term Follow-up (ADMIRAL) trial (99). In a randomized placebo-controlled design, 300 patients received either abciximab or placebo prior to coronary intervention. The results demonstrated a significant reduction in the composite endpoint of death, reinfarction, or target vessel revascularization as well as improved left ventricular function and a higher procedural success rate. Further trials con-firmed the positive results in combining GP IIb/IIIa inhibition with primary angioplasty (100–102).

With the weight of evidence supporting the role of GP IIb/IIIa inhibitors in inter-ventional cardiology (56), the issues of which drug to prescribe and at what cost are impor-tant. The optimum agent in this new class of drugs is a source of much debate, leading to laboratory and clinical trials to clarify the issue.

Measurement of platelet activity at the time of PCI was used as a benchmark by which the three agents could be compared (103,104). Results from two trials in which this design was used contradicted each other. The first trial used flow cytometry, ADP-induced aggregometry, and rapid platelet function assays as markers of platelet aggregation in patients treated by standard recommended doses of the three GP IIb/IIIa antagonists (103). No difference in the effects of the three drugs was found. The second study employed dif-ferent techniques to record platelet activity by increasing the concentration of ADP used as an agonist and changing the anticoagulant to achieve a more physiological concentra-tion of calcium (104). Under these conditions eptifibatide achieved >80% platelet inhibi-tion more consistently than did abciximab, while tirofiban failed to achieve this level of platelet inhibition through most of the infusion, suggesting that the dose of the tirofiban was too low or, alternatively, that tirofiban is less efficacious.

Thus far the only head-to-head trial involving GP IIb/IIIa inhibitors is the TARGET trial comparing tirofiban with abciximab in the setting of PCI, using death, MI, and need for revascularization as an endpoint (105). In a trial design powered to show the noninferiority of tirofiban compared to abciximab, 4809 patients undergoing PCI with the intention of stent insertion were randomized to receive one of the two agents. Despite the design of the trial, the results favored abciximab and demonstrated that tirofiban offered less protection from ischemic events following PCI (105).

VII. RISKS OF STENT THROMBOSIS

In an era of aggressive antiplatelet therapy, new-generation stents and high-pressure deployment of stents, thrombosis have become less common. Analysis of stent thrombosis has identified features that confer a higher risk of thrombosis and can be broadly divided into patient and procedural factors.

Stent thrombosis is increased during intracurrent illness especially in patients with thrombocytemia or receiving chemotherapy (106,107). Several genetic markers have been tested both retrospectively and prospectively. Higher rates of coronary stent thrombosis were found in patients with polymorphisms of the platelet glycoprotein IIIa gene (P1A) (108,109) but not in the glycoprotein IIb (110). Polymorphism in the G protein beta3 subunit gene have been associated with arterial hypertension, coronary artery disease, and MI but have been shown to have no predictive value in the development of stent thrombosis (111).

Procedural features can significantly increase the risk of stent thrombosis. In a meta-analysis of six stent trials, Cutlip et al. studied the rate of and risks for stent thrombosis. Factors conferring increased risk for thrombosis were persistent dissection following stent insertion, longer stented regions, and smaller instent lumen diameters. Also apparent from this study is the high mortality and morbidity that ensues following stent thrombosis, with death or myocardial infarction occurring in 64.4% and a 6-month mortality rate of 8.9% (112).

Ultrasound evaluation of stent thrombosis found that the most significant predictor of stent thrombosis is the plaque burden prior to stenting, suggesting that the stimulus of thrombosis is the residual plaque surrounding or protruding through the stent struts (113). In the STARS registry higher rates of 30-day mortality and peri-procedural non–Q-wave MI occurred following stent insertion that was described as "suboptimal," as defined by a residual diameter stenosis of >10%, evidence of poststent thrombus or severe dissection, abrupt closure, or slow flow (114).

The incidence of acute and subacute stent thrombosis was also studied retrospectively in groups undergoing PCI using nonionic versus ionic contrast medium. The combined endpoint of coronary artery bypass grafting, target lesion revascularization, and overall mortality was significantly reduced by the use of ionic contrast at 1-year follow-up, suggesting that stent thrombosis occurs more frequently with the use of nonionic contrast (115). This has not been confirmed by other authors in prospective studies (116–118).

VIII. COMPLICATIONS OF ANTITHROMBOTICS

Complications of antithrombotic therapy can be defined as general or specific. Effective and safe treatment requires a fine balance between prevention of clotting and the development of bleeding. Hemorrhagic complications are common to all antithrombotic agents and occur more frequently when used in combination, requiring dose reduction (16). In general, to reduce arterial access complications, prompt sheath removal is advised once ACT falls to 150–180 seconds.

Specific complications, although infrequent, can be significant. An uncommon but significant complication of UFH is the development of heparin-induced thrombocytopenia (HIT), occurring in 1–3% of cases (119,120). HIT is mediated through IgG antibodies targeting heparin–platelet factor 4 (PF4) complexes, causing platelet activation and degranulation, which releases further PF4. Newly released PF4 binds to heparin, stimulating an escalating immune response, and to heparin-like molecules on the endothelial surface causing immune-mediated endothelial damage (121). Presentation typically occurs 5–7 days after commencement of heparin with arterial or venous thrombosis (122). Clinical suspicion is raised in patients who develop unexplained thrombocytopenia or thrombosis following heparin therapy. Confirmatory tests detecting heparin-dependent antiplatelet antibodies have a false-negative rate of 15%.

Rebound thrombogenicity has been found following cessation of heparin infusion in patients treated for unstable angina and following PCI. This procoagulant phase creates reactivation of coronary ischemia, resulting in an increased need for urgent intervention (123–125). This rebound phenomenon has been biochemically correlated with increased fibrinopeptide A and prothrombin fragment 1.2, indicative of augmented thrombin production and activity. The mechanism, although unclear, may relate to an accumulation of procoagulant factors and a relative inactivity of AT III following heparin withdrawal.

Along with high rates of gastrointestinal side effects, ticlopidine causes an increase in cholesterol of approximately 9%, cholestatic jaundice, and abnormal liver function tests. More life-threatening is the association with neutropenia and thrombotic thrombocytopenic purpura (TTP). Neutropenia occurs in 1–2% of patients, more commonly following longer periods of treatment. Berger et al. demonstrated the safety of a 3-week course of ticlopidine following stenting in a report of 827 cases with a 0.7% stent thrombosis rate, none of which occurred after 14 days (126). Postmarket surveillance of ticlopidine has reported TTP in 40 patients (127); 15% occurred within 2 weeks and 80% within 4 weeks of commencing treatment, with a high mortality rate of 33%. Subsequent analysis of the EPISTENT group reported 9 cases of TTP from the 43,322 cases treated with ticlopidine (0.02%) (128). One in five of these cases developed TTP during a 2-week course, and the overall mortality was 21%, with survivors more commonly requiring plasmapheresis. This study demonstrated that TTP associated with ticlopidine therapy occurred more frequently than in the general population (0.02% vs. 0.0004%), carries a high rate of mortality, and is not prevented by limiting treatment to 2 weeks (128).

Clopidogrel is better tolerated than ticlopidine, although significant side effects have been reported, including aplastic anemia, profound thrombocytopenia, and the hemolytic uremic syndrome (129–131). Clopidogrel-associated thrombotic thrombocytopenic purpura, although rare, is a recognized, potentially fatal complication (132).

Abciximab is antigenic, with human antichimeric antibodies (HACA) detected in approximately 6% of patients after primary administration and 20% after repeat administration. The clinical significance of HACA is uncertain, though reports from the ReoPro Readministration Registry suggest that despite the higher risk of thrombocytopenia, repeat use of abciximab is safe (133).

Thrombocytopenia, including profound thrombocytopenia with platelet counts of <50,000 cells/mL, can complicate abciximab administration. This typically develops within several hours of administration and is self-limiting, with spontaneous increases in platelet count averaging 20,000–25,000 cells/mL per day following the nadir count. For this reason platelet counts should be measured at baseline and 2–4 hours following the bolus dose, and again at 24 hours or prior to discharge. Drug cessation and occasionally platelet transfusion are required in cases of severe thrombocytopenia associated with abciximab therapy.

IX. RECOMMENDATIONS FOR ANTITHROMBOTIC THERAPY DURING STENT INSERTION

Aspirin: Aspirin (80–325 mg) commenced prior to and continuing post-PCI. In aspirin-sensitive patients, treatment with clopidogrel alone may be considered.

Thienopyridines: Clogidogerol (loading dose 300 mg; daily dose 75 mg) commenced prior to PCI and continued for 14–30 days. Chronic treatment as a replacement in aspirin sensitive patients is justified.

Heparinoids: Unfractionated heparin (60–100 IU/kg) given intravenously at the commencement of the PCI to achieve an ACT of 250–350 seconds for the duration of the procedure. Repeat ACT measurements are required to ensure continued adequate anticoagulation. If used in combination with a GP IIb/IIIa inhibitor, a lower ACT (250 seconds) should be targeted. LMWH is currently not recommended as a replacement for UFH during PCI. When possible, LMWH should be with held for 12 hours prior to PCI.

GP IIb/IIIa Inhibitors: Medical decisions to withhold or prescribe treatments are by necessity founded on the dynamics of efficacy, safety, and cost-effectiveness. Efficacy and safety data are convincing, while economic analysis after 1-year follow-up of the EPISTENT trial estimated that the combination of stenting and abciximab yielded significant reductions in major adverse events to such a degree as to make it an attractive strategy by conventional health economics (82). Other trials have also found this, with a more favorable cost analysis in high-risk or diabetic patients (134,135). Abciximab should be considered in all patients undergoing primary PCI for acute MI. Abciximab or eptifibitide should be considered in patients with unstable coronary syndromes or in high-risk patients undergoing PCI.

Direct Thrombin Inhibitors: Argatroban may be used as an alternative to heparin in heparin-sensitive or HIT patients. Bivalirudin can also be considered as an alternative to heparin. Argatroban in combination with abciximab is currently being tested.

X. CONCLUSION

Since the introduction of intracoronary stenting, acute and subacute stent thrombosis has become a rare event despite the escalating numbers of stents used. This is due to a combination of mechanical and pharmacological discoveries, which in isolation afford small advantage, but when taken together have shown synergistic benefit. Further work is required on the use of existing drugs in combination, such as LMWH or direct thrombin inhibitors in combination with GP IIb/IIIa inhibitors during PCI, as well as developing newer agents such as tissue pathway factor inhibitors.

REFERENCES

1. Serruys P, de Jaegere P, Kiemeneij F, et al. A comparison of balloon-expandable-stent implantation with balloon angioplasty in patients with coronary artery disease. Benestent Study Group. N Engl J Med. 1994. 331(8):489–495.
2. Fischman D, Leon M, Baim D, et al. A randomized comparison of coronary-stent placement and balloon angioplasty in the treatment of coronary artery disease. Stent Restenosis Study Investigators. N Engl J Med. 1994. 331(8):496–501.
3. Serruys P, Strauss B, Beatt K, et al. Angiographic follow-up after placement of a self-expanding coronary-artery stent. N Engl J Med. 1991. 324(1):13–17.
4. Sigwart U, Puel J, Mirkovitch V, Joffre F, and Kappenberger L., Intravascular stents to prevent occlusion and restenosis after transluminal angioplasty. N Engl J Med 1987 Mar 19;316(12):701-6, 1987. 316(12):701–706.
5. Roubin G, Cannon A, Agrawal S, et al. Intracoronary stenting for acute and threatened closure complicating percutaneous transluminal coronary angioplasty. Circulation, 1992. 85(3):916–927.
6. Albiero R, Rau T, Schluter M, et al. Comparison of immediate and intermediate-term results of intravascular ultrasound versus angiography-guided Palmaz-Schatz stent implantation in matched lesions. Circulation, 1997. 96(9):2997–3005.
7. Mudra H, Klauss V, Blasini R, et al. Ultrasound guidance of Palmaz-Schatz intracoronary stenting with a combined intravascular ultrasound balloon catheter. Circulation, 1994. 90(3):1252–1261.
8. Colombo A, Hall P, Nakamura S, et al. Intracoronary stenting without anticoagulation accomplished with intravascular ultrasound guidance. Circulation, 1995. 91(6):1676–1688.
9. deLemos J, Antman EM, Giuliano DA et al. Comparison of a 6- vs. 90-minute determination of SI-segment resolution after thrombolytic therapy for acute myocardial infarction. In TIME-II Investigators. Intravenous nPA for Treatment of Infarcting Myocardium Early-II. Am J Cardiol, 2000. 86(11):1235–1237, A5.
10. Serruys P and Deshpande N, Is there MUSIC in IVUS guided stenting? Is this MUSIC going to be a MUST? Multicenter Ultrasound Stenting in Coronaries Study. Eur Heart J, 1998. 19(8):1122–1124.
11. Marmur J, Merlini P, Sharma S, et al. Thrombin generation in human coronary arteries after percutaneous transluminal balloon angioplasty. J Am Coll Cardiol, 1994. 24(6):1484–1491.
12. Gawaz M, Neumann F, Ott I, May A, and Schomig A., Platelet activation and coronary stent implantation. Effect of antithrombotic therapy. Circulation, 1996. 94(3):279–285.
13. Heras M, Chesebro J, Penny W, et al. Importance of adequate heparin dosage in arterial angioplasty in a porcine model. Circulation, 1988. 78(3):654–660.
14. Laskey M, Deutsch, E, Hirshfeld, J, Kussmaul, W, Barnathan, E, and Laskey, W, Influence of heparin therapy on percutaneous transluminal coronary angioplasty outcome in patients with coronary arterial thrombus. Am J Cardiol, 1990. 65(3):179–182.
15. Garachemani, A. and Meier, B, Heparin for coronary angioplasty: high dose, low dose, or no dose? Heart, 1998. 80:3–4.
16. Use of a monoclonal antibody directed against the platelet glycoprotein IIb/IIIa receptor in high-risk coronary angioplasty. The EPIC Investigation. N Engl J Med. 1994. 330(14):956–961.
17. Platelet glycoprotein IIb/IIIa receptor blockade and low-dose heparin during percutaneous coronary revascularization. The EPILOG Investigators. N Engl J Med. 1997. 336(24):1689–1696.
18. Hirsh, J. and Levine, M, Low molecular weight heparin: laboratory properties and clinical evaluation. A review. Eur J Surg Suppl, 1994(571):9–22.
19. Young, E, Venner, T, Ribau, J, Shaughnessy, S, Hirsh, J, and Podor, T, The binding of unfractionated heparin and low molecular weight heparin to thrombin-activated human endothelial cells. Thromb Res, 1999. 96(5):373–381.

20. Hirsh, J, Warkentin, T, Raschke, R, Granger, C, Ohman, E, and Dalen, J, Heparin and low-molecular-weight heparin: mechanisms of action, pharmacokinetics, dosing considerations, monitoring, efficacy, and safety. Chest, 1998. 114(5 Suppl):489S–510S.

21. Satre, H, Holmvang, L, Wagner, G, Lindahl, B, and Wallentin, L, Reduction of myocardial damage by prolonged treatment with subcutaneous low molecular weight heparin in unstable coronary artery disease. FRISC study group. Fragmin during Instability in Coronary Artery Disease. Eur Heart J, 1999. 20(9):645–652.

22. Cohen, M, Demers, C, Gurfinkel, E, et al. Low-molecular-weight heparins in non-ST-segment elevation ischemia: the ESSENCE trial. Efficacy and Safety of Subcutaneous Enoxaparin versus intravenous unfractionated heparin, in non-Q-wave Coronary Events. Am J Cardiol, 1998. 82(5B):19L–24L.

23. Mark, D, Cowper, P, Berkowitz, S, et al. Economic assessment of low-molecular-weight heparin (enoxaparin) versus unfractionated heparin in acute coronary syndrome patients: results from the ESSENCE randomized trial. Efficacy and Safety of Subcutaneous Enoxaparin in Non-Q wave Coronary Events [unstable angina or non-Q-wave myocardial infarction]. Circulation, 1998. 97(17):1702–1707.

24. Braunwald, E, Antman, E, Beasley, J, et al. ACC/AHA guidelines for the management of patients with unstable angina and non-ST-segment elevation myocardial infarction: executive summary and recommendations. A report of the American College of Cardiology/American Heart Association task force on practice guidelines (committee on the management of patients with unstable angina). Circulation, 2000. 102(10):1193–1209.

25. Kessler, C, Esparraguera, I, Jacobs, H, et al. Monitoring the anticoagulant effects of a low molecular weight heparin preparation. Correlation of assays in orthopedic surgery patients receiving ardeparin sodium for prophylaxis of deep venous thrombosis. Am J Clin Pathol, 1995. 103(5):642–648.

26. Cohen, M, Goodman, S, and Samuels, L.E.: Scribner Education, 1998, Management of Unstable Angina or non Q-wave Myocardial Infarction: A Practical Guide for Intergrating enoxaparin into the AHCPR Guidelines. 1998, Cincinnati, OH: Scribner Education.

27. Marmur, J, Anand, S, Bagga, R, Fareed, J, Sharma, S, and Richard, M, Intravenous dalteparin during percutaneous coronary intervention can be monitored using the activated clooting time. Am J Cardiol, 2001:98G.

28. Young, J, Kereiakes, D, and Grines, C, Low-molecular-weight heparin therapy in percutaneous coronary intervention: the NICE 1 and NICE 4 trials. National Investigators Collaborating on Enoxaparin Investigators. J Invasive Cardiol, 2000. 12(suppl E):E14–18.

29. Blazing, M, De, L.J, Dyke, C, Califf, R, Bilheimer, D, and Braunwald, E, The A-to-Z Trial: Methods and rationale for a single trial investigating combined use of low-molecular-weight heparin with the glycoprotein IIb/IIIa inhibitor tirofiban and defining the efficacy of early aggressive simvastatin therapy. Am Heart J, 2001. 142(2):211–217.

30. Ferguson, J, Combining low-molecular-weight heparin and glycoprotein IIb/IIIa antagonists for the treatment of acute coronary syndromes: the NICE 3 story. National Investigators Collaborating on Enoxaparin. J Invasive Cardiol, 2000. 12 Suppl E:E10–13.

31. Wallentin, L, Lagerqvist, B, Husted, S, Kontny, F, Stahle, E, and Swahn, E, Outcome at 1 year after an invasive compared with a non-invasive strategy in unstable coronary-artery disease: the FRISC II invasive randomised trial. FRISC II Investigators. Fast Revascularisation during Instability in Coronary artery disease. Lancet, 2000. 356(9223):9–16.

32. Karsch, K, Preisack, M, Baildon, R, et al. Low molecular weight heparin (reviparin) in percutaneous transluminal coronary angioplasty. Results of a randomized, double-blind, unfractionated heparin and placebo-controlled, multicenter trial (REDUCE trial). Reduction of Restenosis After PTCA, Early Administration of Reviparin in a Double-Blind Unfractionated Heparin and Placebo-Controlled Evaluation. J Am Coll Cardiol, 1996. 28(6):1437–1443.

33. Gimple, L, Herrmann, H, Winniford, M, and Mammen, E, Usefulness of subcutaneous low molecular weight heparin (ardeparin) for reduction of restenosis after percutaneous transluminal coronary angioplasty. Am J Cardiol, 1999. 83(11):1524–1529.

34. Cairns, J, Gill, J, Morton, B, et al. Fish oils and low-molecular-weight heparin for the reduction of restenosis after percutaneous transluminal coronary angioplasty. The EMPAR Study. Circulation, 1996. 94(7):1553–1560.

35. Antman, E, The search for replacements for unfractionated heparin. Circulation, 2001. 103(18):2310–2314.

36. Hirsh, J. and Weitz, J, New antithrombotic agents. Lancet, 1999. 353(9162):1431–1436.

37. Weitz, J, Califf, R, Ginsberg, J, Hirsh, J, and Theroux, P, New antithrombotics. Chest, 1995. 108(4 suppl):471S–485S.

38. Antman, E, Hirudin in acute myocardial infarction. Safety report from the Thrombolysis and Thrombin Inhibition in Myocardial Infarction (TIMI) 9A Trial. Circulation, 1994. 90(4):1624–1630.

39. Neuhaus, K, von, E.R, Tebbe, U, et al. Safety observations from the pilot phase of the randomized r-Hirudin for Improvement of Thrombolysis (HIT-III) study. A study of the Arbeitsgemeinschaft Leitender Kardiologischer Krankenhausarzte (ALKK). Circulation, 1994. 90(4):1638–1642.

40. Antman, E, Hirudin in acute myocardial infarction. Thrombolysis and Thrombin Inhibition in Myocardial Infarction (TIMI) 9B trial. Circulation, 1996. 94(5):911–921.

41. Neuhaus, K, Molhoek, G, Zeymer, U, et al. Recombinant hirudin (lepirudin) for the improvement of thrombolysis with streptokinase in patients with acute myocardial infarction: results of the HIT-4 trial. J Am Coll Cardiol, 1999. 34(4):966–973.

42. Metz, B, White, H, Granger, C, et al. Randomized comparison of direct thrombin inhibition versus heparin in conjunction with fibrinolytic therapy for acute myocardial infarction: results from the GUSTO-IIb Trial. Global Use of Strategies to Open Occluded Coronary Arteries in Acute Coronary Syndromes (GUSTO-IIb) Investigators. J Am Coll Cardiol, 1998. 31(7):1493–1498.

43. van den Bos, A.A, Deckers, J.W, Heyndrickx, G.R, et al. Safety and efficacy of recombinant hirudin (CGP 39 393) versus heparin in patients with stable angina undergoing coronary angioplasty. Circulation, 1993. 88(5 Pt 1):2058–2066.

44. Rupprecht, H, Terres, W, Ozbek, C, et al. Recombinant hirudin (HBW 023) prevents troponin T release after coronary angioplasty in patients with unstable angina. J Am Coll Cardiol, 1995. 26(7):1637–1642.

45. Herrman, J, Simon, R, Umans, V, et al. Evaluation of recombinant hirudin (CGP 39,393/TMREVASC) in the prevention of restenosis after percutaneous transluminal coronary angioplasty. Rationale and design of the HELVETICA trial, a multicentre randomized double blind heparin controlled study. Eur Heart J, 1995. 16 Suppl L:56–62.

46. Serruys, P, Herrman, J, Simon, R, et al. A comparison of hirudin with heparin in the prevention of restenosis after coronary angioplasty. HELVETICA Investigators. N Engl J Med. 1995. 333(12):757–763.

47. Topol, E, Bonan, R, Jewitt, D, et al. Use of a direct antithrombin, hirulog, in place of heparin during coronary angioplasty. Circulation, 1993. 87(5):1622–1629.

48. Bittl, J, Strony, J, Brinker, J, et al. Treatment with bivalirudin (Hirulog) as compared with heparin during coronary angioplasty for unstable or postinfarction angina. Hirulog Angioplasty Study Investigators. N Engl J Med. 1995. 333(12):764–769.

49. Bittl, J, Comparative safety profiles of hirulog and heparin in patients undergoing coronary angioplasty. The Hirulog Angioplasty Study Investigators. Am Heart J, 1995. 130(3 pt 2):658–665.

50. Bittl, J.A, Chaitman, B.R, Feit, F, Kimball, W, and Topol, E.J, Bivalirudin versus heparin during coronary angioplasty for unstable or postinfarction angina: Final report reanalysis of the Bivalirudin Angioplasty Study. Am Heart J, 2001. 142(6):952–959.

51. Topol, E, Evolution of improved antithrombotic and antiplatelet agents: genesis of the Comparison of Abciximab Complications with Hirulog [and back-Up Abciximab] Events Trial (CACHET). Am J Cardiol, 1998. 82(8B):63P–68P.

52. Kleiman, N, Lincoff, A, Sapp, S, Maresh, K, and Topol, E. Pharmacodynamics of a direct thrombin inhibitor combined with a GPIIb-IIIA antagonist: first experience in humans. AHA. 1999: Circulation.

53. Kleiman, N, Lincoff, A, Harrington, R, Sapp, S, Wolski, C, and Topol, E. Antithrombin, antiplatelet therapy or both during PCI: A preliminary randomized trail. J Am Coll Cardiol, 2001.

54. Fitzgerald, D. and Murphy, N, Argatroban: a synthetic thrombin inhibitor of low relative molecular mass. Coron Artery Dis, 1996. 7(6):455–458.

55. Jang, I, Gold, H, Ziskind, A, Leinbach, R, Fallon, J, and Collen, D, Prevention of platelet-rich arterial thrombosis by selective thrombin inhibition. Circulation, 1990. 81(1):219–225.

56. Sabatine, M, Tu, T, and Jang, I, Combination of a direct thrombin inhibitor and a platelet gly-coprotein IIb/IIIa blocking peptide facilitates and maintains reperfusion of platelet-rich thrombus with alteplase. J Thromb Thrombolysis, 2000. 10(2):189–196.

57. Jang, I, Brown, D, Giugliano, R, et al. A multicenter, randomized study of argatroban versus heparin as adjunct to tissue plasminogen activator (TPA) in acute myocardial infarction: myocardial infarction with novastan and TPA (MINT) study. J Am Coll Cardiol, 1999. 33(7):1879–1885.

58. Vermeer, F, Vahanian, A, Fels, P, et al. Argatroban and alteplase in patients with acute myocardial infarction: the ARGAMI Study. J Thromb Thrombolysis, 2000. 10(3):233–240.

59. Suzuki, S, Matsuo, T, Kobayashi, H, et al. Antithrombotic treatment (argatroban vs. heparin) in coronary angioplasty in angina pectoris: effects on inflammatory, hemostatic, and endothelium-derived parameters. Thromb Res, 2000. 98(4):269–279.

60. Suzuki, S, Sakamoto, S, Adachi, K, et al. Effect of argatroban on thrombus formation during acute coronary occlusion after balloon angioplasty. Thromb Res, 1995. 77(4):369–373.

61. Sakamoto, S, Hirase, T, Suzuki, S, et al. Inhibitory effect of argatroban on thrombin-antithrombin III complex after percutaneous transluminal coronary angioplasty. Thromb Haemost, 1995. 74(2):801–802.

62. Matthai, W, Use of argatroban during percutaneous coronary interventions in patients with heparin-induced thrombocytopenia. Semin Thromb Hemost, 1999. 25 Suppl 1:57–60.

63. Foster, C, Prosser, D, Agans, J, et al. Molecular identification and characterization of the platelet ADP receptor targeted by thienopyridine antithrombotic drugs. J Clin Invest, 2001. 107(12):1591–1598.

64. Quinn, M. and Fitzgerald, D, Ticlopidine and clopidogrel. Circulation, 1999. 100(15):1667–1672.

65. Solet, D, Zacharski, L, and Plehn, J, The role of adenosine 5¢-diphosphate receptor blockade in patients with cardiovascular disease. Am J Med. 2001. 111(1):45–53.

66. Leon, M, Baim, D, Popma, J, et al. A clinical trial comparing three antithrombotic-drug regimens after coronary-artery stenting. Stent Anticoagulation Restenosis Study Investigators. N Engl J Med. 1998. 339(23):1665–1671.

67. Bertrand, M, Legrand, V, Boland, J, et al. Randomized multicenter comparison of conventional anticoagulation versus antiplatelet therapy in unplanned and elective coronary stenting. The full anticoagulation versus aspirin and ticlopidine (fantastic) study. Circulation, 1998. 98(16):1597–1603.

68. Urban, P, Macaya, C, Rupprecht, H, et al. Randomized evaluation of anticoagulation versus antiplatelet therapy after coronary stent implantation in high-risk patients: the multicenter aspirin and ticlopidine trial after intracoronary stenting (MATTIS). Circulation, 1998. 98(20):2126–2132.

69. Schuhlen, H, Hadamitzky, M, Walter, H, Ulm, K, and Schomig, A, Major benefit from antiplatelet therapy for patients at high risk for adverse cardiac events after coronary Palmaz-Schatz stent placement: analysis of a prospective risk stratification protocol in the Intracoronary Stenting and Antithrombotic Regimen (ISAR) trial. Circulation, 1997. 95(8):2015–2021.

70. Steinhubl, S, Ellis, S, Wolski, K, Lincoff, A, and Topol, E, Ticlopidine pretreatment before coronary stenting is associated with sustained decrease in adverse cardiac events: data from the Evaluation of Platelet IIb/IIIa Inhibitor for Stenting (EPISTENT) Trial. Circulation, 2001. 103(10):1403–1409.

71. Harker, L, Marzec, U, Kelly, A, et al. Clopidogrel inhibition of stent, graft, and vascular thrombogenesis with antithrombotic enhancement by aspirin in nonhuman primates. Circulation, 1998. 98(22):2461–2469.

72. Herbert, J, Dol, F, Bernat, A, Falotico, R, Lale, A, and Savi, P, The antiaggregating and antithrombotic activity of clopidogrel is potentiated by aspirin in several experimental models in the rabbit. Thromb Haemost, 1998. 80(3):512–518.

73. Makkar, R, Eigler, N, Kaul, S, et al. Effects of clopidogrel, aspirin and combined therapy in a porcine ex vivo model of high-shear induced stent thrombosis. Eur Heart J, 1998. 19(10):1538–1546.

74. Moussa, I, Oetgen, M, Roubin, G, et al. Effectiveness of clopidogrel and aspirin versus ticlopidine and aspirin in preventing stent thrombosis after coronary stent implantation. Circulation, 1999. 99(18):2364–2366.

75. Muller, C, Buttner, H, Petersen, J, and Roskamm, H, A randomized comparison of clopidogrel and aspirin versus ticlopidine and aspirin after the placement of coronary-artery stents. Circulation, 2000. 101(6):590–593.

76. Rupprecht, H, Darius, H, Borkowski, U, et al. Comparison of antiplatelet effects of aspirin, ticlopidine, or their combination after stent implantation. Circulation, 1998. 97(11):1046–1052.

77. Bertrand, M, Rupprecht, H, Urban, P, Gershlick, A, and Investigators, f, Double-blind study of the safety of clopidogrel with and without a loading dose in combination with aspirin compared with ticlopidine in combination with aspirin after coronary stenting: the clopidogrel aspirin stent international cooperative study (CLASSICS). Circulation, 2000. 102(6):624–629.

78. Savcic, M, Hauert, J, Bachmann, F, Wyld, P, Geudelin, B, and Cariou, R, Clopidogrel loading dose regimens: kinetic profile of pharmacodynamic response in healthy subjects. Semin Thromb Hemost, 1999. 25(suppl 2):15–19.

79. Lefkovits, J, Ivanhoe, R, Califf, R, et al. Effects of platelet glycoprotein IIb/IIIa receptor blockade by a chimeric monoclonal antibody (abciximab) on acute and six-month outcomes after percutaneous transluminal coronary angioplasty for acute myocardial infarction. EPIC investigators. Am J Cardiol, 1996. 77(12):1045–1051.

80. Randomised placebo-controlled and balloon-angioplasty-controlled trial to assess safety of coronary stenting with use of platelet glycoprotein-IIb/IIIa blockade. The EPISTENT Investigators. Evaluation of Platelet IIb/IIIa Inhibitor for Stenting. Lancet, 1998. 352(9122):87–92.

81. Lincoff, A, Califf, R, Moliterno, D, et al. Complementary clinical benefits of coronary-artery stenting and blockade of platelet glycoprotein IIb/IIIa receptors. Evaluation of Platelet IIb/IIIa Inhibition in Stenting Investigators. N Engl J Med. 1999. 341(5):319–327.

82. Topol, E, Mark, D, Lincoff, A, et al. Outcomes at 1 year and economic implications of platelet glycoprotein IIb/IIIa blockade in patients undergoing coronary stenting: results from a multicentre randomised trial. EPISTENT Investigators. Evaluation of Platelet IIb/IIIa Inhibitor for Stenting. Lancet, 1999. 354(9195):2019–2024.

83. Cura, F, Bhatt, D, Lincoff, A, et al. Pronounced benefit of coronary stenting and adjunctive platelet glycoprotein IIb/IIIa inhibition in complex atherosclerotic lesions. Circulation, 2000. 102(1):28–34.

84. Randomised placebo-controlled trial of abciximab before and during coronary intervention in refractory unstable angina: the CAPTURE Study. Lancet, 1997. 349(9063):1429–1435.

85. Januzzi, J, Chae, C, Sabatine, M, and Jang, I, Elevation in serum troponin predicts the benefit of tirofiban J Thromb Thrombolysis 2001. 11(3):211–215.

86. Sabatine, M, Januzzi, J, Snapinn, S, Theroux, P, and Jang, I, A risk score system for predicting adverse outcomes and magnitude of benefit with glycoprotein IIb/IIIa inhibitor therapy in patients with unstable angina pectoris. Am J Cardiol, 2001. 88(5):488–492.

87. The ERASER Investigators. Acute platelet inhibition with abciximab does not reduce in-stent restenosis (ERASER study). Circulation, 1999. 100(8):799–806.

88. Randomised placebo-controlled trial of effect of eptifibatide on complications of percutaneous coronary intervention: IMPACT-II. Integrilin to Minimise Platelet Aggregation and Coronary Thrombosis-II. Lancet, 1997. 349(9063):1422–1428.

89. Blankenship, J, Tasissa, G, O'Shea, J, et al. Effect of glycoprotein IIb/IIIa receptor inhibition on angiographic complications during percutaneous coronary intervention in the ESPRIT trial. J Am Coll Cardiol, 2001. 38(3):653–658.

90. O'Shea, J, Hafley, G, Greenberg, S, et al. Platelet glycoprotein IIb/IIIa integrin blockade with eptifibatide in coronary stent intervention: the ESPRIT trial: a randomized controlled trial. JAMA, 2001. 285(19):2468–2473.

91. The RESTORE Investigators. Effects of platelet glycoprotein IIb/IIIa blockade with tirofiban on adverse cardiac events in patients with unstable angina or acute myocardial infarction undergoing coronary angioplasty. Randomized Efficacy Study of Tirofiban for Outcomes and Restenosis. Circulation, 1997. 96(5):1445–1453.

92. Gibson, C, Goel, M, Cohen, D, et al. Six-month angiographic and clinical follow-up of patients prospectively randomized to receive either tirofiban or placebo during angioplasty in the RESTORE trial. Randomized Efficacy Study of Tirofiban for Outcomes and Restenosis. J Am Coll Cardiol, 1998. 32(1):28–34.

93. Cannon, C, McCabe, C, Borzak, S, et al. Randomized trial of an oral platelet glycoprotein IIb/IIIa antagonist, sibrafiban, in patients after an acute coronary syndrome: results of the TIMI 12 trial. Thrombolysis in Myocardial Infarction. Circulation, 1998. 97(4):340–349.

94. Kereiakes, D, Kleiman, N, Ferguson, J, et al. Sustained platelet glycoprotein IIb/IIIa blockade with oral xemilofiban in 170 patients after coronary stent deployment. Circulation, 1997. 96(4):1117–1121.

95. Catella-Lawson, F, Kapoor, S, Moretti, D, et al. Oral glycoprotein IIb/IIIa antagonism in patients with coronary artery disease. Am J Cardiol, 2001. 88(3):236–242.

96. Peter, K, Schwarz, M, Nordt, T, and Bode, C, Intrinsic activating properties of gp iib/iiia blockers Thromb Res, 2001. 103(suppl 1):S21–27.

97. Peter, K, Schwarz, M, Ylanne, J, et al. Induction of fibrinogen binding and platelet aggregation as a potential intrinsic property of various glycoprotein IIb/IIIa (alphaIIbbeta3) inhibitors. Blood, 1998. 92(9):3240–3249.

98. Verstraete, M, Exit of platelet glycoprotein-IIb/IIIa-receptor inhibitors? Lancet, 2001. 357(9267):1535.

99. Montalescot, G, Barragan, P, Wittenberg, O, et al. Platelet glycoprotein IIb/IIIa inhibition with coronary stenting for acute myocardial infarction. N Engl J Med. 2001. 344(25):1895–1903.

100. Kastrati, A, Pache, J, Dirschinger, J, et al. Primary intracoronary stenting in acute myocardial infarction: long-term clinical and angiographic follow-up and risk factor analysis. Am Heart J, 2000. 139(2 Pt 1):208–216.

101. Schomig, A, Neumann, F, Walter, H, et al. Coronary stent placement in patients with acute myocardial infarction: comparison of clinical and angiographic outcome after randomization to antiplatelet or anticoagulant therapy. J Am Coll Cardiol, 1997. 29(1):28–34.

102. Giri, S, Mitchel, J, Hirst, J, et al. Synergy between intracoronary stenting and abciximab in improving angiographic and clinical outcomes of primary angioplasty in acute myocardial infarction. Am J Cardiol, 2000. 86(3):269–274.

103. Neumann, F, Hochholzer, W, Pogatsa-Murray, G, Schomig, A, and Gawaz, M, Antiplatelet effects of abciximab, tirofiban and eptifibatide in patients undergoing coronary stenting. J Am Coll Cardiol, 2001. 37(5):1323–1328.

104. Proimos, G, Platelet aggregation inhibition with glycoprotein IIb-IIIa inhibitors. J Thromb Thrombolysis, 2001. 11(2):99–110.

105. Topol, E, Moliterno, D, Herrmann, H, et al. Comparison of two platelet glycoprotein IIb/IIIa inhibitors, tirofiban and abciximab, for the prevention of ischemic events with percutaneous coronary revascularization. N Engl J Med. 2001. 344(25):1888–1894.

106. Smith, S, Winters, K, and Lasala, J, Stent thrombosis in a patient receiving chemotherapy. Cathet Cardiovasc Diagn, 1997. 40(4):383–386.

107. Turgut, T, Harjai, K, Edupuganti, R, et al. Acute coronary occlusion and in-stent thrombosis in a patient with essential thrombocythemia. Cathet Cardiovasc Diagn, 1998. 45(4):428–433.

108. Kastrati, A, Koch, W, Gawaz, M, et al. P1A polymorphism of glycoprotein IIIa and risk of adverse events after coronary stent placement. J Am Coll Cardiol, 2000. 36(1):84–89.

109. Walter, D, Schachinger, V, Elsner, M, Dimmeler, S, and Zeiher, A, Platelet glycoprotein IIIa polymorphisms and risk of coronary stent thrombosis. Lancet, 1997. 350(9086):1217–1219.

110. Bottiger, C, Kastrati, A, Koch, W, et al. Polymorphism of platelet glycoprotein IIb and risk of thrombosis and restenosis after coronary stent placement. Am J Cardiol, 1999. 84(9):987–991.

111. von Beckerath, N, Kastrati, A, Koch, W, et al. G protein beta3 subunit polymorphism and risk of thrombosis and restenosis following coronary stent placement. Atherosclerosis, 2000. 149(1):151–155.

112. Cutlip, D, Baim, D, Ho, K, et al. Stent thrombosis in the modern era: a pooled analysis of multicenter coronary stent clinical trials. Circulation, 2001. 103(15):1967–1971.

113. Werner, G, Gastmann, O, Ferrari, M, et al. Risk factors for acute and subacute stent thrombosis after high-pressure stent implantation: a study by intracoronary ultrasound. Am Heart J, 1998. 135(2 pt 1):300–309.

114. Cutlip, D, Leon, M, Ho, K, et al. Acute and nine-month clinical outcomes after "suboptimal" coronary stenting: results from the STent Anti-thrombotic Regimen Study (STARS) registry. J Am Coll Cardiol, 1999. 34(3):698–706.

115. Scheller, B, Hennen, B, Pohl, A, Schieffer, H, and Markwirth, T, Acute and subacute stent occlusion; risk-reduction by ionic contrast media. Eur Heart J, 2001. 22(5):385–391.

116. Grabowski, E, Head, C, and Michelson, A, Nonionic contrast media. Procoagulants or clotting innocents? Invest Radiol, 1993. 28(suppl 5):S21–24.

117. Grabowski, E, Jang, I, Gold, H, et al. Platelet degranulation induced by some contrast media is independent of their nonionic vs ionic nature. Acta Radiol Suppl, 1995. 399:182–184.

118. Grabowski, E, Jang, I, Gold, H, Head, C, Benoit, S, and Michelson, A, Variability of platelet degranulation by different contrast media. Acad Radiol, 1996. 3(suppl 3):S485–487.

119. Aster, R, Heparin-induced thrombocytopenia and thrombosis. N Engl J Med. 1995. 332(20):1374–1376.

120. Januzzi, J.J. and Jang, I, Fundamental concepts in the pathobiology of heparin-induced thrombocytopenia. J Thromb Thrombolysis, 2000. 10(suppl 1):7–11.

121. Kelton, J, Smith, J, Warkentin, T, Hayward, C, Denomme, G, and Horsewood, P, Immunoglobulin G from patients with heparin-induced thrombocytopenia binds to a complex of heparin and platelet factor 4. Blood, 1994. 83(11):3232–3239.

122. Boon, D, Michiels, J, Stibbe, J, van, V.H, and Kappers-Klunne, M, Heparin-induced thrombocytopenia and antithrombotic therapy. Lancet, 1994. 344(8932):1296.

123. Theroux, P, Waters, D, Lam, J, Juneau, M, and McCans, J, Reactivation of unstable angina after the discontinuation of heparin. N Engl J Med. 1992. 327(3):141–145.

124. Granger, C, Miller, J, Bovill, E, et al. Rebound increase in thrombin generation and activity after cessation of intravenous heparin in patients with acute coronary syndromes. Circulation, 1995. 91(7):1929–1935.

125. Smith, A, Holt, R, Fitzpatrick, J, et al. Transient thrombotic state after abrupt discontinuation of heparin in percutaneous coronary angioplasty. Am Heart J, 1996. 131(3):434–439.

126. Berger, P, Bell, M, Hasdai, D, Grill, D, Melby, S, and Holmes, D, Safety and efficacy of ticlopidine for only 2 weeks after successful intracoronary stent placement. Circulation, 1999. 99(2):248–253.

127. Bennett, C, Davidson, C, Raisch, D, Weinberg, P, Bennett, R, and Feldman, M, Thrombotic thrombocytopenic purpura associated with ticlopidine in the setting of coronary artery stents and stroke prevention. Arch Intern Med. 1999. 159(21):2524–2528.

128. Steinhubl, S, Tan, W, Foody, J, and Topol, E, Incidence and clinical course of thrombotic thrombocytopenic purpura due to ticlopidine following coronary stenting. EPISTENT Investigators. Evaluation of Platelet IIb/IIIa Inhibitor for Stenting. JAMA, 1999. 281(9):806–810.

129. Trivier, J, Caron, J, Mahieu, M, Cambier, N, and Rose, C, Fatal aplastic anaemia associated with clopidogrel. Lancet, 2001. 357(9254):446.

130. Elmi, F, Peacock, T, and Schiavone, J, Isolated profound thrombocytopenia associated with clopidogrel. J Invasive Cardiol, 2000. 12(10):532–535.

131. Moy, B, Wang, J, Raffel, G, and Marcoux, J, Hemolytic uremic syndrome associated with clopidogrel: a case report. Arch Intern Med. 2000. 160(9):1370–1372.
132. Bennett, C, Connors, J, Carwile, J, et al. Thrombotic thrombocytopenic purpura associated with clopidogrel. N Engl J Med. 2000. 342(24):1773–1777.
133. Tcheng, J, Kereiakes, D, Lincoff, A, et al. Abciximab readministration: results of the ReoPro Readministration Registry. Circulation, 2001. 104(8):870–875.
134. Zwart-van, R.J, Klungel, O, Leufkens, H, Broekmans, A, Schrijver-van, V.S, and Umans, V, Costs and effects of combining stenting and abciximab (ReoPro) in daily practice. Int J Cardiol, 2001. 77(2-3):299–303.
135. Zwart-van, R.J. and van, H.B, Cost-efficacy in interventional cardiology; results from the EPISTENT study. Evaluation of Platelet IIb/IIIa Inhibitor For Stenting Trial. Eur Heart J, 2001. 22(16):1476–1484.

15-3

Clinician Update: Direct Thrombin Inhibitors and Low Molecular Weight Heparins in Acute Coronary Syndromes

Joanna J. Wykrzykowska, Sekar Kathiresan, and Ik-Kyung Jang
Massachusetts General Hospital, Harvard Medical School, Boston, Massachusetts, U.S.A.

Thrombin plays a central role in the pathogenesis of acute coronary syndromes (ACS) including both unstable angina (UA) and acute myocardial infarction (AMI) (1). It promotes platelet aggregation, its own autocatalysis, and catalysis of fibrinogen to fibrin (2,3). Antithrombin and antiplatelet therapies have become the cornerstones of the treatment of cardiovascular disease. The usual medical regimen for non–ST segment elevation MI includes intravenous unfractionated heparin (UFH), aspirin, thienopyridine, and glycoprotein IIb/IIIa inhibitors, and for ST-elevation MI, aspirin, UFH, and thrombolytic agents.

UFH has been the thrombin inhibitor of choice in both the catheterization laboratory and medical management of ACS (4). The widespread use of UFH, however, has made its deficiencies very apparent. Some of these deficiencies are intrinsic to UFH's mechanism of action, which is indirect and requires antithrombin III as a cofactor. It is ineffective against clot-bound thrombin (5) and is readily inactivated by platelet factor 4 (PF4) and plasma proteins. In consequence, it has a rather unpredictable dose response (6), necessitating frequent monitoring of the activated partial thromboplastin time (aPTT). In addition, UFH use is associated with a significant risk of major bleeding—7.7% in a study of 12,000 patients with ST segment elevation MI (STEMI) and non–ST elevation MI (NSTEMI) treated with UFH (7). More importantly, up to 14% of patients receiving UFH in the setting of procedures develop antibodies to PF4, and 5% of them manifest thrombocytopenia with thrombotic complications: heparin-induced thrombocytopenia (HIT) and heparin-induced thrombocytopenia with thrombotic syndrome (HITTS) (8).

I. DIRECT THROMBIN INHIBITORS

Development of direct thrombin inhibitors (DTIs), agents that are capable of inactivating thrombin without a need for the cofactor antithrombin III, raised hopes for more potent, more predictable, and safer anticoagulation in patients with ACS. In contrast to UFH, DTIs inhibit both clot-bound and fluid-phase thrombin (9). The prototypical agent hirudin was derived from the medicinal leech (10) and is now made with recombinant technology and marketed as lepirudin or Refludan®. The N-terminal portion of hirudin inhibits thrombin's active site, while the C-terminal portion inhibits thrombin's fibrinogen-binding site. Two other DTIs studied in the United States are bivalirudin (Angiomax®) and argatroban. Bivalirudin is synthesized by joining the N-terminal and C-terminal active peptides of hirudin with a synthetic linker. Meanwhile, argatroban, an arginine derivative, is a small molecule that inhibits the thrombin's active site (11).

The initial studies of hirudin and bivalirudin in the clinical settings of AMI, UA, and percutaneous coronary intervention (PCI) conducted in the early 1990s proved to be disappointing. Hirudin and bivalirudin showed no advantage over UFH in potency, and in the case of hirudin an increase in bleeding complications was noted (7,12). The enthusiasm for DTIs waned for a number of years. However, the need for better anticoagulants persisted. As the knowledge of more appropriate use of these drugs progressed, there was a renewed interest in DTIs, particularly in the face of the increasing number of patients with HIT/HITTS. Herein we will review the clinical studies assessing hirudin, bivalirudin, and argatroban in the settings of AMI, UA, and PCI.

A. HIRUDIN

1. Hirudin in AMI

Thrombolytic regimens of front-loaded tissue plasminogen activator (t-PA) or streptokinase (SK) in combination with UFH and aspirin proved to be unsatisfactory in ensuring vessel patency in acute STEMI (13). Depending on the agent, only 30–55% of patients achieved Thrombolysis in Myocardial Infarction (TIMI) grade 3 flow at 90 minutes. The initial pilot studies TIMI 5 and 6 assessed whether hirudin in combination with t-PA or SK could improve coronary patency rates. The initial results of these small studies were promising. In TIMI 5 (14), when compared with UFH and t-PA, the combination of hirudin with t-PA showed an 8% increase in TIMI grade 3 flow and a decrease in angiographic reocclusion rate. The TIMI 6 (15) trial studied the combination of hirudin with SK and showed a 7% decrease in the incidence of major bleeding when compared with the SK and UFH regimen. Thus, both promises of greater efficacy and improved safety seemed to be fulfilled.

Three larger phase III trials of hirudin in combination with thrombolytics were all stopped prematurely because of unacceptably high increases in major bleeding in the hirudin group when compared to the UFH group. The GUSTO IIa (Global Use of Strategies to Open Occluded Coronary Arteries IIa) (16) enrolled patients within 12 hours of onset of ischemia. It randomized them to 72- to 120-hour infusion of heparin with a goal PTT of 60–90 (5000 U bolus and 1000–1300 U/h infusion) versus high-dose hirudin (0.6 mg/kg bolus and 0.2 mg/kg/h infusion) in combination with t-PA and SK. The recruitment of 12,000 patients stopped at 2500 because of increased bleeding risk in the hirudin group. There was a 1.7% risk of intracranial hemorrhage (ICH) in patients treated with t-PA and hirudin versus 0.9% in the UFH group. Risk of ICH was 3.2% in patients treated with SK and hirudin versus 2.7% in patients treated with SK and UFH. TIMI 9A (17) used the same high-dose regimen of hirudin, and enrollment of patients with AMI was stopped at 757 patients after increased major hemorrhage was noted in both the hirudin and UFH group (7.0 vs. 3.0%; $p = 0.02$). The rates of hemorrhage were higher than those observed in the TIMI 5 and 6 trials. The third of the trials, HIT III (Hirudin for Improvement of Thrombolysis III) (18a), planned to randomize 7000 patients within 6 hours of AMI to UFH (70 U/kg bolus and 15 U/kg/h infusion) versus hirudin (0.4 mg/kg bolus and 0.15 mg/kg/h infusion) in addition to t-PA. The trial was stopped after enrollment of 300 patients secondary to higher number of intracranial bleeds in the hirudin group as well as higher number of in-hospital deaths.

Subsequently, in TIMI 9B (12) and GUSTO IIb (7) the dosages of UFH and hirudin were markedly reduced and titrated to maintain the aPTT between 55 and 85 seconds. TIMI 9B enrolled 3002 patient with STEMI of <12 hours duration. They were randomized to either accelerated t-PA or SK, followed by either UFH for 96 hours (5,000 U/bolus and 1000 U/h infusion) or low-dose hirudin (0.1 mg/kg bolus and 0.1 mg/kg/h infusion). Although aPTT values were more predictably achieved in the hirudin group, this did not translate into a better clinical safety profile. Primary outcome of death or reinfarction was slightly higher in the hirudin group at 12.9% versus 11.9% in the UFH group, but the difference was not statistically significant. Further, there was no advantage of hirudin over UFH at 30 days with respect to mortality or reinfarction in the overall trial and in all subgroups analyzed.

It was hypothesized that the lack of benefit with hirudin may have been related to the timing of administration of hirudin. Since hirudin has a weak ability to bind to clot-bound thrombin, once the coronary artery is occluded with thrombus, hirudin may not be as efficacious. Thus, early infusion, perhaps even prior to thrombolysis, could be particularly important. There was no statistically significant difference in the rate of intracranial hemorrhage or major bleeding with either of the drugs used at low dose. One must note, however, that the trial enrolled predominantly men averaging 60 years of age and thus lacked the group at highest risk for intracranial hemorrhage with thrombolysis, elderly women.

The largest trial to date of hirudin in AMI and UA, GUSTO IIb (7) enrolled 4131 patients with STEMI as well as 8011 patients with UA and NSTEMI. Patients with STEMI received front-loaded t-PA or SK and low-dose UFH or hirudin. This trial demonstrated a small, albeit statistically significant, advantage of hirudin over UFH at 24 hours with respect to mortality and risk of MI (1.3% vs. 2.1%; $p = 0.001$). The difference in primary endpoints persisted at 30 days after treatment (8.9 vs. 9.8%; $p = 0.06$). While a 14% decrease in a composite endpoint of death and MI across both the AMI and UA groups was demonstrated at 30 days with hirudin versus UFH, these differences were no longer statistically significant when AMI and UA patients were analyzed separately. Subgroup reanalysis of the GUSTO IIb trial demonstrated benefit of hirudin over UFH only when used with SK but no added advantage when used with the more potent lytic t-PA.

In the HIT-IV (Hirudin for Improvement of Thrombolysis-IV) study (18b), 1200 patients were treated with SK for AMI within 6 hours of presentation. They were randomized to lower doses of subcutaneous hirudin (0.2 mg/kg IV bolus and 0.5 mg/kg bid for 5–7 days) and UFH (placebo bolus followed by s.c. injections of 12,500 U bid for 5–7 days). The primary endpoint was angiographic TIMI 3 flow at 90 minutes. It was achieved in equivalent numbers of patients treated with hirudin and UFH (40% vs. 33%; $p = 0.16$). The additional endpoint of ST segment resolution at 90 minutes was achieved in 28% of patients treated with hirudin versus 22% of patients treated with UFH ($p = 0.05$). The difference was no longer significant at 180 minutes. There was no significant difference in mortality (6.8 vs. 6.4%) or reinfarction rate (4.6% vs. 5.1%) at 30 days. The rate of hemorrhagic stroke was low in both groups (0.2 vs. 0.3%). The safety profile of hirudin when used in conjunction with SK was improved at the expense of efficacy. The result is rather difficult to interpret because of the placebo bolus in the UFH-treated group as well as the subcutaneous formulation of the drug.

Given the problems with safety shown in the majority of the studies, hirudin is not approved in the United States for use with thrombolytics in acute STEMI. It appears from all three phase III trials that hirudin has a very narrow therapeutic window. At the high doses required to show benefit over UFH, hirudin caused an unacceptably high rate of bleeding complications, and at lower doses the drug was no longer more efficacious.

2. Hirudin in UA

As described above, GUSTO IIb enrolled 8011 patients with NSTEMI and randomized them to UFH (5000 U bolus and 1000 U/h) versus hirudin (0.1 mg/kg bolus and 0.1 mg/kg/h infusion) administered for 3–5 days. There was no difference in the rate of death or reinfarction at 30 days post-MI (9.1% vs. 8.3%; $p = 0.22$). There was, however, an increased rate of severe bleeding in the hirudin group (1.3% vs. 0.9%; $p = 0.06$) as well as increased rate of intracranial hemorrhage (0.2% vs. 0.02%; $p = 0.06$).

In addition to GUSTO IIb (8011 patients), the Organization to Assess Strategies for Ischemic Syndromes (OASIS) (pilot, 1997) (19) and OASIS 2 (10,141 patients, 1999) (20) trials explored the effectiveness of hirudin alone versus UFH in patients with NSTEMI and UA. In OASIS, 900 patients with NSTEMI were given either UFH (5000 U bolus and 15 U/kg/h infusion) or hirudin (two doses: high-dose, 0.4 mg/kg bolus + 0.15 mg/kg/h infusion, or low-dose, 0.2 mg/kg bolus + 0.1 mg/kg/h infusion). Both infusions were continued for 72 hours. At 7 days, combined risk of MI or death was lower in the high-dose hirudin group (2.6% in the hirudin group vs. 4.9% in the UFH group; $p = 0.07$). At 35 days follow-up, the difference in combined outcome was no longer statistically significant (6.1% vs. 8.6%; $p = 0.15$). OASIS 2 enrolled 10,000 patients with UA or suspected NSTEMI and randomized them to high-dose hirudin versus UFH. There was a small, nonsignificant difference in the combined endpoint of death and MI at 7 days (3.6% in the hirudin group vs. 4.3% in the UFH group; $p = 0.077$). The number of patients requiring coronary interventions, intra-aortic balloon pump or thrombolysis was lower in the hirudin group (6.8% vs. 8.1%; $p = 0.016$). At 35 days, the risk reduction for the combined endpoints persisted (6.8% vs. 7.7%; $p = 0.06$).

Similar to GUSTO IIb, the OASIS 2 trial showed only a marginal decrease in the death and MI rate in the hirudin arm of the study. Meta-analysis of the OASIS trials showed that compared with UFH, hirudin use in UA was associated with a 20% reduction in cardiovascular deaths and a 17% reduction in need for interventions within 7 days (20).

Thus, hirudin has not been consistently shown to be more efficacious than UFH. Multiple hypotheses have been proposed to explain the failure to show a benefit of hirudin over UFH. First, since hirudin binds to thrombin in a 1:1 stoichiometric fashion, its supply may be exhausted more easily, necessitating longer infusion times to prevent rebound thrombosis. Second, rebound thrombosis with shorter infusion time could also have been a result of hirudin's inability to inhibit the generation of thrombin. Hirudin can only bind to thrombin directly and inhibit its activity but does not affect the upstream coagulation cascade. Lastly, hirudin can bind only weakly to clot-bound thrombin, which reduces its potential advantage over UFH (21). Thus, rebound hypercoagulability appears to be of major concern with hirudin even after infusions as long as 96 hours.

3. Hirudin in PCI

Only two major trials of hirudin in PCI have been conducted. HELVETICA (22) enrolled 1141 patients with UA scheduled to undergo angioplasty. It compared three regimens: (a) intravenous UFH (10,000 U bolus followed by 15 U/kg/h infusion for 24 hours and subcutaneous placebo for 3 days), (b) intravenous hirudin (40 mg hirudin bolus followed by 0.2 mg/kg/h infusion for the first 24 h), and (c) subcutaneous hirudin (40 mg subcutaneous bid doses up to 72 h). The combination of intravenous and subcutaneous hirudin postprocedure led to a reduction in all cardiac events at 96 hours when compared with UFH (5.6% vs. 11% for any event including MI, need for intervention or death; RR 0.61 in the combined hirudin groups; $p = 0.023$). There was no benefit of hirudin over UFH at 7 months postprocedure with respect to cardiac events (32.0% in combined subcutaneous and intravenous hirudin vs 32.7% in the UFH group; $p = 0.61$) or degree of restenosis. In fact, Kaplan-Meier curves of event-free survival for hirudin and UFH appeared to intersect at 3 months, resulting in slightly worse outcomes at 7 months in the hirudin group. The measurement of prothrombin fragments postprocedure indicated that hirudin, even at high doses, was incapable of adequately inhibiting thrombin generation. Dosage of UFH used, on the other hand, was adequate to inhibit thrombin generation. A small pilot trial of 61 patients undergoing angioplasty for UA (23) suggested that at higher doses, hirudin compared with UFH may reduce serum cardiac troponin T levels. Both of the trials were conducted prior to widespread use of glycoprotein IIb/IIIa inhibitors, and thus the safety profile of hirudin in combination with glycoprotein IIb/IIIa inhibitors is unknown.

B. HIRULOG

1. Hirulog in AMI

Hirulog (bivalirudin or Angiomax[*]) has been proposed as a safer direct antithrombin than hirudin. Thrombin can cleave the Arg-Pro bond of bivalirudin, thereby reactivating its own active site and allowing for subsequent hemostasis. This would prevent major bleeding events observed with hirudin. An early pilot study of hirulog versus UFH with SK in 45 patients with AMI showed higher TIMI grade 3 flow rates at 120 minutes in the hirulog group compared with the UFH group (87% vs. 47%; $p < 0.01$) (24). Another study of 70 patients compared SK combined with two different regimens of hirulog and UFH (25). The two hirulog regimens were the following: a 12-hour infusion of 1 mg/kg/h of hirulog followed by placebo versus 0.5 mg/kg/h infusion for 12 hours followed by long 0.1 mg/kg/h infusion for up to 4–6 days. TIMI grade 3 flow at 120 minutes was achieved in 92% of patients treated with hirulog compared to only 46% of patients in the UFH group ($p = 0.014$). RR for achieving TIMI 3 flow with hirulog was 1.73 at 120 min ($p = 0.02$). At 4–6 days postlysis, TIMI grade 3 flow in the culprit vessel was achieved in 96% of low-dose/long infusion hirulog-treated patients versus 83% of UFH treated patients. Interestingly, the outcomes for the 12-hour high-dose hirulog group were worse than for UFH, again suggesting that direct antithrombins are incapable of inhibiting generation of new thrombin and predispose to "rebound" thrombosis, especially after short duration of therapy. Improved angiographic patency with hirulog also translated into better clinical outcomes with recurrent ischemia occurring in only 7% of patients treated with low-dose hirulog versus 23% of patients treated with UFH ($p = $ NS). Superior efficacy of prolonged low-dose hirulog infusion over UFH was not accompanied by any compromise in safety. In fact, hirulog appeared to have a better safety profile with bleeding complications observed in 22% (5% requiring transfusions) of patients in the hirulog group versus 31% (31% requiring transfusions; $p = 0.02$) of patients on UFH.

The encouraging data from these two small European pilot studies were subsequently confirmed by two larger multicenter trials from the Hirulog Early Reperfusion/Occlusion (HERO) Trial Investigators. HERO enrolled 412 patients presenting with STEMI who were all treated with SK. It compared the following adjunctive regimens: (a) UFH (5000 U bolus followed by 60-h 1000–1200 U/h infusion; (b) low-dose hirulog (0.125 mg/kg bolus followed by 12-h infusion of 0.25 mg/kg/h and 0.125 mg/kg/h infusion); and (c) high-dose hirulog (0.25 mg/kg bolus followed by 12-h infusion of 0.5 mg/kg/h and 0.25 mg/kg/h infusion). The trial showed a 37% improvement in early TIMI grade 3 flow rates in both low-dose and high-dose hirulog compared with the UFH group (26). Notably in this study, overall TIMI grade 3 flow was achieved in a much smaller percentage of patients than in the pilot studies (35% of UFH-treated patients and 46% of hirulog-treated patients). The benefit of hirulog was more appreciable in patients treated within 3 hours of the symptom onset (70% rate of TIMI grade 3 flow). Higher incidence of bleeding and need for rescue angioplasty was noted in the UFH group. The study was not powered to show statistical significance of increased cardiovascular events in the UFH group.

Meanwhile, the HERO-2 trial (27) enrolled 17,000 patients with STEMI and was powered to show a mortality difference between adjunctive hirulog versus UFH. At 30 days, the mortality rates in the hirulog and UFH groups were no different (10.5% vs. 10.9%; $p = 0.46$). There was a nonsignificant decrease in the risk of stroke in the hirulog group. It is unclear why HERO-2 failed to replicate the improved efficacy and safety seen with the previous smaller trials. The shorter time of drug infusion (average of 48 h in HERO-2 vs. 4–6 days in HERO-1) with consequent rebound thrombosis has been posited as a possible explanation. It is also possible that SK does not require an antithrombin for increased efficacy. The safety profile of hirulog remained favorable even at higher doses, especially when compared to the high rates of major bleeding observed in hirudin-treated patients. It must be noted, however, that hirudin trials included patients treated with the more potent thrombolytic alteplase, whereas hirulog in acute MI was tested with less potent SK.

2. Hirulog in Medical Management of UA

Data on hirulog in medical management of UA is rather sparse, with only one study published to date, the TIMI 7 (410 patients) trial. In TIMI 7 (28), patients received a 72-hour infusion of hirulog at four different doses: 0.02, 0.25, 0.5, and 1.0 mg/kg/h. There was no difference in mortality or risk of MI between the four groups through the duration of treatment. Of note, 46% of patients received UFH infusion after hirulog at the discretion of the treating physician. Thirty-two percent of patients treated with high-lose hirulog infusion were subsequently treated with UFH for several days. In-hospital death or MI occurred in 10% of patients treated with the 0.02 mg/kg/h hirulog dose (equivalent to placebo) and in only 3.2% ($p = 0.008$) of patients in all three higher-dose hirulog groups (0.25, 0.5, and 1.0 mg/kg/h). This benefit persisted at 6 weeks (12.5% rate of death or MI in placebo group vs. 5.2% rate in the hirulog group; $p = 0.009$). There were no intracranial hemorrhages in any of the patients, and the rate of major hemorrhage was 0.5%. This study is limited by the lack of a head-to-head comparison with UFH.

3. Hirulog in PCI

The Bivalirudin Angioplasty Study compared hirulog to high-dose UFH during coronary angioplasty for UA (29). Hirulog was given as a 1.0 mg/kg bolus followed by 2.5 mg/kg/h infusion for 4 hours and then 0.2 mg/kg/h infusion for 20 hours. UFH, on the other hand, was given as a high-dose bolus of 175 U/kg followed by 24 hours of a 15 U/kg infusion with a goal activated clotting time (ACT) of 350–400 seconds. The study demonstrated a statistically significant reduction in composite endpoint of death, MI, and need for revascularization in the hirulog group compared with the UFH group (4.9% vs. 9.9%; $p = 0.009$). This benefit was particularly pronounced in patients undergoing angioplasty for post-infarction angina (9.1 vs. 14.2%; $p = 0.04$). The risk of major hemorrhage was also lower in the hirulog group (3.8% vs. 9.8%; $p < 0.001$), as was the need for transfusions (2.0% vs. 5.7%; $p < 0.001$). However, this decreased risk of bleeding must be interpreted with caution since UFH was given as a high-dose bolus with slightly higher ACT values. One should note that current recommendation for ACT goals in the setting of PCI is much lower than those used in the study. Reanalysis of the data at 90 and 180 days postinfusion showed a sustained but waning benefit of hirulog over UFH (17.5% vs. 24.3% for the composite endpoint at 90 days; $p < 0.001$ and 24.5% vs. 30.3% at 180 days; $p < 0.001$).

This study of bivalirudin (29,30) was conducted in patients treated with angioplasty without stenting. It excluded all patients who received stents and did not evaluate this drug in conjunction with glycoprotein IIb/IIIa inhibitors. In patients with UA there was no significant difference in the primary endpoint of death or MI between the UFH and bivalirudin-treated groups (11.4% vs. 12.2%; $p = 0.44$). However, there was a clear benefit of bivalirudin over UFH in patients treated for postinfarction angina (9.1% vs. 14.2% rate of death or MI; $p = 0.04$). However, this difference was no longer statistically significant at 6 months (25.7% vs. 26.6%; $p = 0.54$). There was no effect on the restenosis rate on follow-up coronary angiography at 6 months. In both UA and postinfarction angina patients, the risk of bleeding was lower in the bivalirudin group compared with the UFH group (3.8% vs. 9.8% in the UA patients; $p < 0.001$ and 3.0% vs. 11.1% in the postinfarction angina patients; $p < 0.001$).

The recent Comparison of Abciximab Complications with Hirulog for Ischemic Events Trial (CACHET) assessed the additive value of bivalirudin in the modern era of routine stent and glycoprotein IIb/IIIa inhibitor use (31). CACHET randomized 268 patients to three treatment groups: (a) full-dose bivalirudin with planned abciximab (1.0 mg/kg bolus + 2.5 mg/kg/h 4-hour infusion; (b) half-dose bivalirudin (0.5 mg/kg bolus + 1.75 mg/kg/h 4-hour infusion) with provisional abciximab; and (c) weight-adjusted UFH at 70 U/kg bolus with planned abciximab. Provisional abciximab (given to 24% of patients in provisional group) was used only in "rescue" situations when stenting and antithrombin therapy did not result in patency of the vessel. The ACT goal in this study was 200–250 seconds, and infusions of bivalirudin were stopped at 4 hours. Stents were used in 88% of patients, and all patients receiving stents also received clopidogrel in addition to aspirin. The rate of death and MI in the pooled bivalirudin groups was lower than in the UFH group (3.4% vs. 10.6%; $p = NS$ and $p = 0.018$ for pooled hirulog groups) at 7 days postintervention. The study was too small to show statistical significance for individual hirulog doses. There was no evidence of increased risk of bleeding in bivalirudin group (3.5% vs. 9.3%; $p = NS$). Most importantly, this suggested that bivalirudin could be safely used with potent glycoprotein IIb/IIIa inhibitors.

The larger study of 6000 patients with UA undergoing PCI entitled REPLACE (Randomized Evaluation Linking Angiomax to reduced Clinical Events) was published recently (32). The trial was designed to test noninferiority of bivalirudin alone against heparin with planned IIb/IIIa inhibitor. The primary "quadruple" endpoint combined both safety (major bleeding) and efficacy (death, MI, or ischemia requiring intervention at 30 days from the index procedure) measures. The study randomized 3000 patients into the bivalirudin group (0.75 mg/kg bolus followed by 1.75 mg/kg/h infusion for the duration of the procedure) and an equivalent number of patients received a heparin bolus (65 U/kg) with either abciximab (0.25 mg/kg bolus followed by 0.125 mg/kg/min infusion for 12 h) or eptifibatide (two 180 mg/kg boluses 10 minutes apart followed by 2.0 mg/kg/min infusion for 18 h). Heparin was not continued as an infusion together with IIb/IIIa inhibitor. Seven percent of the patients in the bivalirudin group received "rescue" IIb/IIIa inhibitor for indications such as occlusion of the side branch vessel, thrombus, slow flow, dissection, unplanned stent placement, prolonged ischemia, or other clinical instability. There was no statistically significant difference in the quadruple endpoint of safety and efficacy between bivalirudin and heparin + IIb/IIIa groups at 30 days after PCI (9.2% vs. 10%, respectively; $p = 0.32$). However, in the bivalirudin group, there were more non–Q-wave MIs (195 vs. 172; $p = 0.43$). The secondary "triple" endpoint of efficacy showed statistically nonsignificant superiority of UFH and IIb/IIIa inhibitor (7.1% vs. 7.6%; OR 1.09, p

= 0.40). The noninferiority of lower-dose bivalirudin alone lies mostly in the safety profile and lower rate of the major bleeding (2.4% vs. 4.1%; $p < 0.001$). The indirect comparison of UFH and bivalirudin was imputed using a random effects meta-analysis of the data sets from previous trials of heparin versus heparin and IIb/IIIa inhibitors (33,34). The authors attempted to promote bivalirudin alone as an economically attractive alternative to UFH and IIb/IIIa inhibitor for uncomplicated PCI in patients with UA.

C.   Univalent Direct Thrombin Inhibitors

1.   Argatroban in Acute MI

The Myocardial Infarction with Novastan and t-PA study (MINT) treated 125 patients with STEMI with front-loaded full-dose alteplase and aspirin. For adjunctive antithrombin therapy, patients were randomized into three groups (35): (a) low-dose weight-based UFH, (b) low-dose argatroban (100 mg/kg bolus + 1 mg/kg/min infusion), or (c) high-dose argatroban (100 mg/kg bolus + 3 mg/kg/min infusion). There was a dose-dependent benefit of argatroban over UFH in TIMI grade 3 flow at 90 minutes postlysis (59.5% patency in high-dose agratroban and 55.5% with low-dose argatroban vs. 41.9% TIMI grade 3 flow with UFH). This translated into a decreased rate of death and MI at 30 days in the argatroban group (25.5% in high-dose argatroban, 32% with low-dose argatroban vs. 37.5% in the UFH group). The incidence of major bleeding was much lower in the argatroban group (2.6% with low-dose argatroban, 4.6% with high-dose argatroban, and 10% with UFH).

Meanwhile, the ARGatroban in Acute Myocardial Infarction (ARGAMI) study failed to show any immediate benefit of argatroban over UFH with respect to angiographic patency (36). It randomized 127 patients to low-dose UFH (5000 U bolus + 1000 U/h infusion) versus high-dose argatroban (100 mg/kg bolus + 3.0 mg/kg/min infusion) as an adjunct to alteplase. Ninety-minute angiographic patency was 76% in UFH group and 82% in the argatroban group, and this difference did not reach statistical significance. There was no difference in the rate of bleeding between the two groups. ARGAMI-2 (results published only in abstract form) (37) randomized 1200 patients receiving alteplase and SK to high-dose and low-dose argatroban infusions (2 and 4 mg/kg/min) versus UFH. It assessed the risk for mortality, MI, and angiographic patency at 30 days after the index event. The low-dose argatroban arm was terminated due to lack of efficacy. Comparison of high-dose argatroban infusion versus UFH at 30 days showed no significant difference in mortality or rate of reinfarction (20 vs. 19%). However, there were fewer bleeding complications with argatroban (0.4% vs. 1.2%). The Argatroban in Myocardial Infarction (AMI) study randomized 910 patients with acute MI to placebo versus high-dose (3 mg/kg/min) or low-dose argatroban (1 mg/kg/min) infusions for 72 hours in conjunction with SK. The rate of MI, heart failure, or death was nonsignificantly higher in both argatroban groups compared with the placebo group (19.9% vs. 16%; $p = $ NS).

Thus, the small MINT study appears to be the only study that showed a clear benefit of adjunctive argatroban in the setting of STEMI. The other larger studies examining argatroban in combination with either alteplase or less potent SK failed to show any benefit.

2.   Argatroban in UA

Argatroban has been studied in UA in a single small phase I trial involving 43 patients (38). Nine of 43 patients experienced recurrent unstable angina after cessation of infusion.

Thrombin generation was not decreased with increasing doses of argatroban, raising concerns about the ability of argatroban to passivate the thrombogenic endothelial surface.

3. Argatroban in PCI

The only published study to date enrolled 91 HIT patients who underwent 112 PCIs while on intravenous argatroban (25 mg/kg/min infusion after a 350 mg/kg initial bolus) (39). Outcomes on intravenous argatroban were compared with historical control patients treated with UFH. Satisfactory outcome of the procedure and adequate anticoagulation during PCI were the major endpoints. Among patients undergoing initial PCIs with argatroban (n = 91), 94.5% had a satisfactory outcome of the procedure and 97.8% achieved adequate anticoagulation. Death (zero patients), MI (four patients), or revascularization (four patients) at 24 hours after PCI occurred in seven (7.7%) patients overall. One patient (1.1%) experienced periprocedural major bleeding.

Argatroban has been recently evaluated in conjunction with glycoprotein IIb/IIIa inhibitors in a multicenter prospective study of 101 patients (40). Patients received a 250 mg/kg bolus followed by 15 mg/kg/min infusion during the procedure with a goal ACT of 275–325 seconds. The primary endpoint of death, MI, or need for repeat revascularization at 30 days poststenting occurred in 3% of patients. This low rate of primary adverse events suggests that argatroban may provide adequate anticoagulation levels during PCI. Longer-term follow-up data are currently unavailable.

4. Efegatran in AMI and UA

Efegatran is a tripeptide arginine-derived antithrombin, which binds to the active site of thrombin and is capable of inactivating clot-bound thrombin. It was shown to have good therapeutic index in canine models (41). Efegatran was studied in three European studies, all of which failed to show any benefit over UFH. PRIME (42) randomized 336 patients with AMI at 33 sites to receive one of five doses of efegatran sulfate or UFH for 72–96 hours, both with accelerated alteplase and aspirin. There was no difference in the primary endpoint of thrombolytic failure (death, reinfarction, or TIMI grade 0–2 flow in the infarct artery from 90 minutes to discharge or 30 days) between UFH and efegatran. The lowest-dose efegatran arm was terminated because of an unacceptably increased rate of thrombolytic failure. The primary endpoint occurred in 53.0% of patients treated with UFH, in 53.8% of patients treated with efegatran overall ($p = 0.90$), and in 55.4% of patients given intermediate-dose efegatran ($p = 0.74$). ESCALAT (43) compared the efficacy of efegatran plus SK versus UFH plus accelerated alteplase in the setting of STEMI. It was a randomized, dose-finding study of 245 patients that explored four doses of efegatran sulfate in combination with SK (1.5 million U) given intravenously within 12 hours of symptom onset. The optimal dosage group of 0.5 mg/kg/h was expanded and compared with UFH plus accelerated alteplase. The study showed lower angiographic patency (TIMI 2 or 3 flow) with combination of efegatran and SK versus UFH and alteplase (73% vs. 79%; p = NS). Furthermore, in-hospital mortality rate was 5% for the efegatran/SK group versus 0% for the UFH/alteplase group (p = NS). Major bleeding occurred in 23% of patients in the efegatran/SK group versus 11% in the UFH/alteplase group (p = NS). The results of this study may be difficult to interpret given that the differences between UFH and efegatran may be confounded by the differences between SK and more potent alteplase. Lastly, a study of 430 patients evaluated the ability of efegatran versus UFH to suppress ischemia in patients with UA and failed to show any benefit of efegatran over UFH (44).

II. LOW MOLECULAR WEIGHT HEPARINS

LMWHs are produced by enzymatic depolymerization of UFH chains to chains of 4000–6000 Da. The activity of LMWHs is dependent on the pentasaccharide that binds to antithrombin III (AT III). Only a small percentage of LMWH chains contain the additional 13 residues necessary for the ternary complex formation with thrombin, and therefore the anticoagulant properties rely on the anti-factor Xa activity (45). Like UFH, LMWH cannot inactivate clot-bound thrombin or factor Xa once it is part of the prothrombinase complex. In contrast to UFH, it cannot be inactivated by platelet factor 4, it is less likely to bind to acute phase reactants or endothelial cells, and therefore it has a more predictable anticoagulation effect. It does not cause platelet activation, has longer plasma half-life (3–6 h), and is somewhat less likely to cause HITTS. While its anticoagulation effect cannot be monitored with aPTT, such monitoring is rarely necessary except for patients with reduced renal function and those at extremes of weight. The subcutaneous route additionally offers ease of administration. Given these potential advantages over UFH, there has been an interest in exploring LMWHs as potential agents in the treatment of ACS (46).

A. LMWHs in Unstable Angina

LMWHs were most extensively studied in the medical management of UA/NSTEMI. The first small open-label study enrolled 219 patients with UA within 6 hours of the onset of chest pain and randomized them to aspirin alone, aspirin and UFH (400 U/kg/day), or aspirin and LMWH nadroparin (214 U/kg sc bid) (47). The endpoints of recurrent angina, MI, urgent revascularization, and death as well as major bleeding were evaluated. Recurrent angina (ischemia) was significantly less frequent in the LMWH group (21%) compared to the UFH (44%; OR 3.07; $p = 0.002$) and placebo groups (37%; OR 2.26; $p = 0.03$). Risk of MI and need for urgent revascularization was also lower, and there was no excess bleeding observed in the LMWH group. Following these encouraging results, LMWHs were tested against UFH in large randomized trials and several meta-analyses.

The Fragmin during Instability in Coronary Artery Disease (FRISC) Study enrolled 1506 patients with NSTEMI and randomized them to LMWH (120 U/kg sc bid for 5–7 days followed by 7500 U sc bid for 35–45 days or placebo) (48). LMWH group had lower combined rate of death and MI at 6 days (1.7% vs. 4.7%; $p = $ NS), mostly due lower MI rate. There was also a reduction in the need for revascularization in the LMWH group by 67%. This benefit was attenuated at 40 days due to an increase in the rate of death and MI in the LMWH group after its dose was lowered to 7500 U bid (25% benefit of LMWH, 10.7 to 8%; $p = 0.007$). At 150 days rate of death was reduced only from 15.5 to 14%, and the difference was no longer statistically significant. There was no increased risk of major bleeding in the dalteparin group.

FRISC II randomized 2267 Scandinavian patients with UA to dalteparin sc bid injections for 3 months versus placebo after open-label administration of dalteparin sc for 6 days (49). During the 3 months there was a nonsignificant decrease in composite endpoint of death and MI in the dalteparin group (6.7 vs. 8%; $p = 0.17$) and a significant decrease in combined triple endpoint of death, MI, and revascularization (29 vs. 33.4%; $p = 0.031$). This benefit was not sustained, however, at 6 months, 3 months after dalteparin was stopped. Interestingly, the same study evaluated the benefits of early invasive versus conservative strategy in patients with UA and found that this benefit of early PTCA in reducing recurrent angina was independent and did not interact with administration of dalteparin. The same study also offered insight into risk stratification of patients with UA based on the level of troponin T as a strong predictor of mortality.

Fragmin in Unstable Coronary Artery Disease (FRIC) compared dalteparin to UFH rather than placebo in 1482 patients with UA (50). The LMWH regimen used was identical to that in the FRISC study. UFH was given iv with goal PTT 1.5 times the control value for 48 hours followed by either continued iv infusion or high sc doses for additional 4 days. There was no difference in the rate of death or MI at 6 days (3.9 vs. 3.6%; RR 1.07; p = NS) or up to 45 days (12.3% in both groups; RR 1.01; p = NS). There was also no difference in major bleeding complications. It did not appear that prolonged administration of dalteparin offered any benefit over UFH.

Enoxaparin in Non-Q-Wave Coronary Events (ESSENCE) trial enrolled 3171 patients with UA and either EKG changes or documented history of CAD and randomized them to either enoxaparin 1 mg/kg sc bid or UFH iv infusion titrated to PTT 55–85 for 2–8 days (51). At 14 days the combined risk of death, MI, and recurrent angina was lower in the enoxaparin group (16.6 vs. 19.8%; p = 0.019). The benefit of enoxaparin over UFH persisted at 30 days (19.8 vs. 23.3%; p = 0.016). This benefit was most significant in the reduction of recurrent angina at 14 days and the reduction of the risk of MI as well as recurrent angina at 30 days. Enoxaparin also significantly decreased the need for revascularization with PTCA (27 vs. 32.2%; p = 0.001). There was no significant risk of major bleeding associated with enoxaparin use (6.5 vs. 7%; p = 0.57) but risk of minor bleeding was somewhat increased. The effects on rate of MI and death were much lower than in the FRISC trial, where comparison was made with placebo. The benefit of enoxaparin over UFH was greater than that of dalteparin in the FRIC trial, possibly owing to the greater anti-Xa/anti-IIa activity ratio of enoxaparin.

TIMI 11B enrolled 3910 patients with UA/NQWMI (52). It randomized them to enoxaparin (30 mg IV bolus, followed by 1 mg/kg sc bid dosing for 2–8 days, and followed by 40–60 mg sc bid for 35 days), or UFH (70 U/kg bolus, followed by 15 U/kg/hr iv infusion for 2–8 days, and followed by placebo). The combined mortality and reduction in MI rate benefit of enoxaparin was noted at 8 hours. At 48 hours the event rate was 5.5% in the enoxaparin versus 7.3% in the UFH group (p = 0.048). At 14 days (after both drugs were stopped) there was still a benefit of enoxaparin (14.2 vs. 16.7% event rate; p = 0.029). In the subgroup analysis the greatest benefit was noted in the patients with ST depressions and those who were treated with aspirin in the previous 24 hours. At 43 days the Kaplan-Meier curves for enoxaparin and UFH remained parallel, denoting no additional benefit of continued subcutaneous enoxaparin over placebo, but persistent benefit of initial enoxaparin administration over UFH. The risk of major bleeding in the initial phase of treatment was equal in the UFH and enoxaparin groups (1–1.5%; p = 0.741), but it was increased in the long-term administration of enoxaparin phase.

The meta-analysis of ESSENCE and TIMI 11B showed a reduction of MI and death rate of 20% in the enoxaparin group, which was not quite as impressive as the initial open-label pilot of 219 patients suggested (>50% reduction) (53).

The Fraxiparin in Ischemic Syndromes (FRAXIS) trial enrolled 3468 patients with UA and randomized them to short-term nadroparin (0.1 mL/10 kg sc bid for 6 days), long-term nadroparin (14 days), or UFH iv infusion (6 days) (54). The primary endpoint of death, MI and revascularization at 14 days was similar in all three groups (17.8% vs. 20% vs. 18.1%, respectively; p = 0.85). There was no difference in the risk of major hemorrhage between short-term nadroparin and UFH, but this risk was increased with long-term nadroparin administration.

In summary, it appears from the phase III trials of LMWHs that they are at least equivalent to UFH in prevention of recurrent angina and MI in patients with UA. Enoxaparin may be even superior to UFH, as shown in ESSENCE and TIMI 11B. This is likely due to its higher activity against factor Xa compared to other LMWHs. The magnitude of the benefit, however, is not as great as projected from the initial pilot study. There is furthermore no benefit in treatment beyond the acute phase of 2–8 days. Follow-up studies and reanalysis suggest that high-risk patients with ST changes may benefit most from LMWHs over UFH. These encouraging results with LMWH in UA led to its studies in combination with IIb/IIIa inhibitors.

B.   LMWHs in Conjunction with IIb/IIIa Inhibitors for Medical Management of UA

LMWHs owing to their smaller size are less likely to activate platelets. It was therefore hypothesized that they would afford more potent platelet inhibition when used in combination with IIb/IIIa inhibitors in the medical management of UA and NSTEMI. This hypothesis was proven in the Antithrombotic Combination Using Tirofiban and Enoxaparin (ACUTE I) trial (55) and was subsequently evaluated in five other trials.

The ACUTE II trial enrolled 525 patients with UA/NSTEMI treated with tirofiban and aspirin and randomized them to UFH or enoxaparin bid injections for 24–96 hours (56). Bleeding complications were assessed at 24 hours, with major bleeding being lower in the enoxaparin group (0.3 vs. 1%; p = NS). There was a higher incidence of nuisance bleeding in the patients treated with enoxaparin. There was no difference in death and MI at 30 days in the two groups (9 vs. 9.2%; p = NS). However, there was a significantly lower rate of refractory ischemia requiring urgent intervention (0.6 vs. 4.3%; p = 0.01) and rehospitalization (1.6 vs. 7.1%; p = 0.02) in the enoxaparin arm.

Similar data were obtained in the INTERACT study, which enrolled 746 patients within 24 hours of the onset of rest ischemic chest pain and concomitant CK elevation or ST segment deviation (57). All patients were treated with aspirin and eptifibatide (180 mg/kg bolus and 2 mg/kg/h infusion). They were randomized to enoxaparin 1 mg/kg bid or UFH (70 U/kg bolus followed by 15 U/kg/h infusion) for 48 hours. Major bleeding incidence was assessed at 96 hours and was significantly lower in the LMWH group (1.8 vs. 4.6%; p = 0.003). Conversely, minor bleeding risk was higher in the enoxaparin group (30.3 vs. 20.8%; p = 0.003). The rate of recurrent ischemia was significantly lower in the enoxaparin arm within the first 48 hours (14.3 vs. 25.4%; p = 0.0002) and after 48 hours post–index event (12.7 vs. 25.9%; p < 0.0001). In addition in this study there was also a demonstrable 30-day mortality benefit of LMWH (5 vs. 9%; p = 0.031).

GUSTO IV–ACS enrolled 7800 patients with chest pain and ST depressions or TnT or I elevation and randomized them to placebo, abciximab bolus, and 24- or 48-hour infusion (58). All patients in this study received UFH (70U/kg bolus and 15 U/kg/h infusion) except for a substudy population (646 patients), who were given 120 U/kg sc injections of dalteparin twice daily for 5–7 days. The overall conclusion of this study was that patients with NSTEMI (troponin leaklet MI) do not benefit from abciximab. The substudy of LMWH showed equivalent efficacy (death or MI at 30 days endpoint) to UFH (9.5 vs. 8%; p = NS). There was no difference in the rates of major or minor bleeding with LMWH in either the placebo or abciximab group.

PARAGON B (Platelet IIb/IIIa Antagonist for the Reduction of Acute coronary syndrome events in a Global Organization Network B) enrolled patients with NSTEMI and randomized them to placebo or lamifaban (59). The substudy of PARAGON B randomized 805 of patients receiving lamifaban to LMWH (at unspecified dose) versus UFH. LMWH group tended to have lower rates of death, MI, and recurrent ischemia at 30 days (10.2% vs. 12% in the whole study population). This trend towards a benefit was sustained at 6 months (11.9 vs. 13.8% composite rate of death and MI). There was also a trend to lower need for revascularization at 6 months (42.8 vs. 51.2%) in the group receiving LMWH. There was no significant difference in bleeding risk.

The conclusion of the trials combining IIb/IIIa inhibitors with LMWH versus UFH is that it is certainly safe to do so in terms of the risk of major bleeding. The major and consistent benefit appears to be lower risk of recurrent ischemia and need for reintervention in the LMWH groups, which is a worthwhile trade-off for the slightly higher rate of "nuisance" minor bleeding.

SYNERGY (Superior Yield of the New strategy of Enoxaparin, Revascularization and Glycoprotein IIb/IIIa inhibitors) will enroll 8000 patients with NSTEMI treated with early invasive strategy and randomize them to LMWH and UFH (60). It will be the largest randomized multicenter trial to date to assess the safety and efficacy of LMWH in combination with IIb/IIIa inhibitors and early invasive strategy.

C. LMWHs in AMI/STEMI

Five major trials evaluated the effect of adjunctive LMWH on coronary artery patency after fibrinolysis: AMI-SK, HART II, ENTIRE-TIMI23, ASSENT-3, and ASSENT-3 PLUS.

AMI-SK enrolled 496 patients who received SK for STEMI and randomized them to 30 mg IV bolus followed by 1 mg/kg bid subcutaneous injections of enoxaparin versus placebo for 3–8 days (61). Complete ST segment resolution at 180 minutes was achieved in 36 versus 25% of patients treated with enoxaparin and placebo, respectively. Corresponding to this, TIMI 3 flow was achieved in 70% of patients treated with enoxaparin versus 58% of patients in the placebo arm ($p = 0.01$). This translated into lower rates of death, MI, and recurrent angina at 30 days (13 vs. 21%; $p = 0.03$). There was no significant difference in safety endpoints.

The HART II (Heparin Adjunctive to Recombinant Tissue Plasminogen Activator Thrombolysis and Aspirin) trial enrolled 400 patients treated with accelerated t-PA and randomized them to 3-day treatment with enoxaparin (30 mg IV bolus and 1 mg/kg bid sc injections) or UFH (4000–5000 U bolus and 15 U/kg infusion) (62). TIMI 2 or 3 flow at 90 minutes was achieved in 80% versus 75% of patients treated with enoxaparin versus UFH. The reocclusion rate at 5–7 days (TIMI 3 to TIMI 0 flow) was lower in the enoxaparin arm (3.1 vs. 9.1%; $p = 0.12$). Although this trial was designed to demonstrate noninferiority of LMWH, results approach criteria for superiority. Enoxaparin and UFH were similar with respect to safety endpoints as well as the rate of death at 30 days (4.5 vs. 5%).

ENTIRE 23 (Enoxaparin as Adjunctive Antithrombin Therapy for ST-Elevation Myocardial Infarction) enrolled 483 patients presenting within 6 hours of onset of STEMI who were treated with full-dose tenecteplase (TNK). It randomized them to enoxaparin (30 mg iv bolus and 1 mg/kg bid sc injections) or UFH (60 U/kg bolus and 12 U/kg/h infusion) (63). Another arm of the study randomized patients to half-dose TNK and abciximab with lower-dose UFH (40 U/kg bolus + 7 U/kg/h infusion) or enoxaparin (30 mg IV bolus and 0.3–0.37 mg/kg sc bid injection). The endpoints in this study were TIMI 3 flow at angiography 60 minutes after TNK, ST segment resolution on EKG at 180 minutes, and combined rate of death/MI at 30 days. Across both TNK and the TNK/abciximab combination treatment groups, 50% of patients achieved TIMI 2–3 flow in the UFH group versus 51% patients in the enoxaparin group (p = NS). The ST segments had resolved completely in 45% of patients receiving UFH and 51% of patients treated with enoxaparin at 180 minutes. At 30 days there was a marked difference in the combined endpoint of death and MI between UFH and enoxaparin in the full-dose TNK arm of the study (15.9% in the UFH group vs. 4.4% in the LMWH group; $p = 0.005$). The difference was largely due to rates of MI (12.2 vs. 1.9%; $p = 0.003$). The benefit of enoxaparin over UFH was much smaller in the combination therapy arm (6.5 vs. 5.5%; p = NS). There were no differences in rates of major hemorrhage between the UFH and enoxaparin groups, except for the combination therapy arm, where enoxaparin was associated with slightly higher rates of bleeding (5.2% with UFH and 8.5% with enoxaparin; overall rate 4.8% across the study population). Thus, the benefit of enoxaparin was seen mostly in long-term recurrence of ischemia/MI when used with fibrinolytic therapy alone. This could potentially be due to lower platelet activation rates by enoxaparin, which occurs due to released thrombin products postfibrinolysis. When a potent platelet IIb/IIIa inhibitor was used there was no added benefit of enoxaparin over UFH.

The ASSENT 3 trial studied three different reperfusion regimens in 6095 patients with AMI (64). The three groups were (a) full-dose TNK with enoxaparin (weight-adjusted bolus of 30–50 mg iv followed by 1 mg/kg sc bid dosing), (b) half-dose TNK with abciximab and UFH (lower dose adjusted to PTT 50–70 given co-administration of abciximab), and (c) full-dose TNK with UFH (4000 U bolus and 12 U/h infusion for 48 h). The endpoint was 30-day mortality, reinfarction, or recurrent ischemia. The primary endpoint was reached in 6.1% of patients treated with TNK and enoxaparin, 5.2% of patients treated with half-dose TNK and abciximab, and 8.8% of patients treated with TNK and UFH (p < 0.0001). These results, like the TIMI23 findings, suggested that the benefit of enoxaparin was lower rates of platelet and coagulation cascade activation after fibrinolysis. The rate of major bleeding events in the enoxaparin group was not significantly higher that in the UFH group when combined with TNK alone.

The ASSENT-3 PLUS trial (65) enrolled 1639 patient with STEMI and randomized them to prehospital administration of enoxaparin (30–50 mg iv bolus and 1 mg/kg sc bid dosing) for 7 days versus weight-adjusted UFH (60 U/kg bolus and 12 U/kg/h infusion) for 48 hours in combination with TNK. While the composite endpoint of death/MI/ischemia was lower in the enoxaparin group (14.2 vs. 17.8%; p = 0.08), the rate of major hemorrhage and stroke was higher (2.9 vs. 1.3%; p = 0.026). The increase in stroke rate was mostly observed in patients older than 75 years (9.4%).

The study by Baird et al. enrolled 300 patients with acute MI treated with SK or t-PA (66) Patients were randomized to UFH (5000 U bolus and 30,000 U/h infusion) and enoxaparin (40 mg bolus and 40 mg sc bid) for 4 days. At 90 days the composite endpoint of death, MI, or recurrent ischemia was reached in 36% of patients treated with UFH and in 25% of patients treated with enoxaparin (p = 0.04). There was no significant difference in the rates of major bleeding.

Lastly, BIOMACS II (67) evaluated another LMWH dalteparin versus placebo in conjunction with SK in 101 patients with STEMI. Dalteparin was administered as two injections of 100 and 120 IU/kg, separated by 12 hours. Patients treated with dalteparin had slightly higher TIMI 3 flow rates (68 vs. 51%; p = 0.1) and lower rates of recurrent ischemia in the first 24 hours (16 vs. 38%; p = 0.04). However, 24–72 hours post-MI, after the dalteparin was withdrawn, there were more reinfarctions in the dalteparin-treated patients. These reinfarctions were attributed to too short treatment with antithrombotics and rebound prothrombotic state as well as to a lower anti-Xa:IIa ratio of dalteparin. There was no significant increase in bleeding with dalteparin.

LMWH enoxaparin appears to be safe when used in conjunction with thrombolytics for AMI. It has a potential advantage over UFH in reducing recurrent ischemia by virtue of reducing thrombin generation and platelet activation after fibrinolysis. This advantage is no longer apparent when it is used in combination with IIb/IIIa inhibitors. The ASSENT-3 PLUS trial of prehospital administration of enoxaparin raised concerns of increased bleeding complications (65). The safety of enoxaparin in the elderly at a reduced dose will be investigated further by the EnoXaparin and Thrombolysis Reperfusion for Acute myocardial infarction Trial (EXTRACT) (46).

D. LMWHs in PCI

The initial hesitation in using LMWHs for PCI stemmed from an inability to follow activated clotting time (ACT) and partial thromboplastin time (PTT) in the catheterization lab. In addition, protamine, while able to fully reverse the antithrombin activity of LMWHs, can only counteract 60% of its anti-Xa activity (68). Predictable levels of anticoagulation were achieved, however, in three observational studies (registries), namely, the National Investigators Collaborating on Enoxaparin (NICE) 1, 3, and 4 (69). NICE-1 established that a dose of 1 mg/kg of IV enoxaparin could be used in PCI, whereas NICE-4 showed safety of reduced dose 0.75 mg/kg in combination with abciximab during PCI. Bleeding events and ischemic outcomes in-hospital and at 30 days post-PCI were comparable to historical controls.

The Coronary Revascularization Using Integrilin and Single Bolus Enoxaparin (CRUISE) study was the first randomized trial that looked at bleeding and procedural complications of enoxaparin compared to UFH used in conjunction with eptifibatide in PCI (70). It enrolled 261 patients undergoing both elective and urgent PCI. The primary safety endpoint was the bleeding index defined as a change in hemoglobin corrected for the number of units of blood transfused in the first 24 hours postprocedure. This index was 0.8 in the enoxaparin group and 1.1 in the UFH group (p = NS). There were no statistically significant differences in other groin or closure device complications. Further, there were no differences between groups in the composite efficacy endpoint of death, MI, or need for urgent revascularization at 48 hours and 30 days.

Collet et al.'s study enrolled 451 patients with UA/NSTEMI who had been treated with enoxaparin for 48 hours (1 mg/kg sc bid) (71). It evaluated the safety of intervention in 132 of these patients who underwent PCI within 8 hours of the last dose of LMWH when the anti-Xa level activity is highest. Outcomes were compared between PCI- and non–PCI-treated groups, but there was no comparison to UFH or placebo. The rate of major hemorrhage was very low, 0.8%, in the PCI group and 0.7% in the whole patient population. In addition, this study showed mortality benefit of PCI in patients with positive troponins.

Choussat et al.'s study looked at outcomes and anti-Xa levels in 242 patients undergoing elective PCI who were treated with single iv bolus of enoxaparin (72). Anti-Xa levels of >0.5 IU/mL were achieved in 97.5% of patients. The group included patients over age of 75 (33 patients) and with renal insufficiency (30 patients). Of the group, 169 patients received a stent and 64 patients were treated with eptifibatide. Eptifibatide had no effect on the anti-Xa levels. The rate of composite endpoint of death, MI, and urgent revascularization was 2.5% but did not correlate with anti-Xa levels. Only one major bleeding event occurred in the entire cohort.

The invasive arm of FRISC II randomized 1222 patients who had been receiving open-label dalteparin at 120 IU/kg sc bid for 5 days to further treatment for 90 days with dalteparin or placebo (49). The rate of major bleeding was 1.5% in the LMWH group. The results of several smaller studies corroborate these data.

The lack of large randomized trials and an inability to monitor the level of anticoagulation during the procedure limit the widespread use of LMWH in cardiac catheterization laboratories. Although large randomized trials are lacking, it appears from the above-mentioned preliminary data that it would be a safe alternative to UFH in PCI. Its predictable anticoagulation profile would obviate the need for ACT measurement, and one might see lower rates of rebound thrombosis than with UFH. As hypothesized by the ATLAS trial of LMWH in patients at high risk of stent thrombosis, LMWHs may offer advantages over UFH in terms of lower activation of von Willebrandt factor and lower platelet activation (73).

III. SUMMARY AND FUTURE DIRECTIONS

The first phase II studies of hirudin were not powered to select the appropriate dose. In consequence, large phase III trials of hirudin in combination with powerful thrombolytics for acute STEMI showed unacceptably high bleeding. Subsequent lower-dose trials failed to show any benefit over UFH. Given the significant risk of bleeding documented in thrombolysis trials, no trials of hirudin in combination with glycoprotein IIb/IIIa inhibitors have been conducted. Further studies of hirudin as an alternative to UFH seem unlikely to prove fruitful.

Unlike hirudin, bivalirudin proved to have an excellent safety profile when given with SK for STEMI. In patients with UA given a long infusion of 4–6 days, it showed a 30% mortality benefit at 30 days. With shorter infusions of hirulog as an adjunct to SK in patients with NSTEMI in the HERO-2 trial, the 30-day mortality benefit was no longer present despite initial short-term reduction in the rate of reinfarction.

In contrast to hirudin, data on bivalirudin, especially in combination with glycoprotein IIb/IIIa inhibitors during PCI, look promising. The CACHET trial of low-dose bivalirudin with abciximab showed superior angiographic results and lower reinfarction rates compared to UFH without increased risk of bleeding. The recently published REPLACE-2 trial unfortunately looked only at the combined safety and efficacy of bivalirudin alone compared to heparin with IIb/IIIa inhibitor. For a very select group of patients with UA undergoing uncomplicated PCI, it appears that bivalirudin alone with "rescue" IIb/IIIa inhibitor may be equivalent to heparin with IIb/IIIa inhibitor. Data regarding the safety of bivalirudin when combined with IIb/IIIa inhibitors in higher-risk PCI, such as patients with STEMI, are still unavailable. Hirulog is approved in the United States for use in PCI.

Argatroban, the univalent direct thrombin inhibitor, has not been adequately studied to establish its efficacy. It has a good safety profile compared to UFH, as shown in the MINT study. The data regarding its efficacy in combination with thrombolytics are rather conflicting. The studies of argatroban during PCI demonstrated safety in HIT patients, and our preliminary data on argatroban use with glycoprotein IIb/IIIa inhibitors show an excellent safety profile and a 3% rate of infarction at 30 days. It would appear that univalent DTIs such as argatroban would merit further investigation. It is premature to discount the univalent DTIs given the paucity of data and their potential utility in PCI (74,75).

The initial expectations of using DTIs to replace UFH thus far have not been met. Except for bivalirudin, there are no data to show a better safety profile of DTIs. None of them are markedly more potent and their therapeutic window is still fairly narrow, requiring careful aPTT monitoring. Given their inability to inhibit generation of thrombin, rebound thrombosis appears to be of even greater concern than with UFH.

LMWHs, in contrast to DTIs, have proven to be safe and to prevent rebound ischemia. They offer predicatable anticoagulation levels as well as ease of subcutaneous administration, the only caveat being heterogeneity within the class with respect to anti-Xa:IIa activity. LMWHs such as enoxaparin with higher anti-Xa:IIa appear to be most advantageous compared to UFH. LMWHs are approved as an alternative to UFH in UA and in combination with thrombolytics for AMI. Although larger trials are still needed, preliminary results suggest that LMWHs would be safe in PCI including coadministration with IIb/IIIa inhibitors in the setting of high-risk stenting. More data are required to support the routine use of LMWH in cardiac catheterization laboratories.

Table 1 Summary of Hirudin Trials in AMI, UA, and PCI[a]

Trial	Clinical setting	No. of patients	Regimen	Result (efficacy; safety)
TIMI 5	AMI (with t-PA) 2	46	Hirudin (dose 1: 0.15 mg/kg bolus + 0.05 mg/kg/h infusion; dose 2: 0.1 mg/kg bolus + 0.1 mg/kg/h infusion; dose 3: 0.3 mg/kg bolus + 0.1 mg/kg/h infusion; dose 4: 0.6 mg/kg bolus + 0.1 mg/kg/h infusion) vs. UFH 5000 U bolus + 1000 U/h infusion	Efficacy: 8% increase in TIMI 3 flow; Safety: 3.5% decrease in major hemorrhage rate
TIMI 6	AMI (with SK)	193	Hirudin (dose 1: 0.15 mg/kg bolus + 0.05 mg/kg/h infusion; dose 2: 0.3 mg/kg bolus + 0.1 mg/kg/h infusion; or dose 3: 0.6 mg/kg bolus + 0.2 mg/kg/h infusion) vs. UFH (5000 U bolus, followed by a 1000 U/h infusion)	Efficacy: no effect; Safety: 7% decrease in the incidence of major bleeding in the hirudin group
HIT III	AMI	302	Hirudin (0.4 mg/kg bolus + 0.15 mg/kg infusion) vs. UFH (70 U/kg bolus + 15 U/kg infusion)	Efficacy: no effect; Safety: increased rate of intracranial bleeding in hirudin group
HIT IV	AMI	1200	Hirudin (0.2 mg/kg IV bolus + 0.5 mg/kg sc bid injection for 5–7 days) vs. UFH (placebo bolus + 12,500 U sc bid for 5–7 days)	Efficacy: no mortality effect; better initial ST segment resolution in hirudin group; Safety: equivalent
TIMI 9A	AMI	757	Hirudin (0.6 mg/kg bolus + 0.2 mg/kg infusion) vs. UFH (5000 U bolus + 1300 U/h)	Efficacy: unable to assess, trial terminated early; Safety: 7% rate of major hemorrhage in hirudin group
GUSTO IIA	AMI	2564	Hirudin (0.6 mg/kg bolus and 0.2 mg/kg/h infusion) vs. UFH (5000 U bolus and 1000–1300 U/h infusion)	Efficacy: unable to assess, trial terminated early; Safety: increased risk of major bleeding with hirudin, especially in group that received t-PA
TIMI 9B	AMI	3002	Hirudin (0.1 mg/kg bolus + 0.1 mg/kg/h infusion) vs. UFH (5000 U bolus and 1000 U/h infusion)	Efficacy: greater incidence of reinfarction and death in hirudin group (not statistically significant); Safety: no effect

(*Continued*)

Table 1 Summary of Hirudin Trials in AMI, UA, and PCIa (*Continued*)

Trial	Clinical setting	No. of patients	Regimen	Result (efficacy; safety)
CUSTO IIB	AMI	4131	Hirudin (0.1 mg/kg bolus + 0.1 mg/kg/h infusion) vs. UFH (5000 U bolus and 1000 U/h infusion)	Efficacy: Benefit of hirudin with SK but no added benefit with t-PA; Safety: no effect
	UA	8011		Efficacy: 14% reduction in composite endpoint of death and MI at 30 days; Safety: no effect
OASIS I	UA	909	Hirudin at two doses (high: 0.4 mg/kg bolus + 0.15 mg/kg/h infusion; low: 0.2 mg/kg bolus + 0.1 mg/kg/h infusion) vs. UFH (5000 U bolus + 15 U/kg/h infusion)	Efficacy: No statistically significant difference in combined endpoint of death and MI at 35 days; Safety: no effect
OASIS II	UA	10141	Hirudin (0.4 mg/kg bolus + 0.15 mg/kg/h infusion) vs. UFH (5000 U bolus + U/kg/h infusion)	Efficacy: 12% decrease in MI, death, and need for reintervention at 35 days; Safety: no effect
HELVETICA	PCI	1141	Hirudin sc (40 mg bolus + bid injections for 72 h) vs. UFH (10,000 U bolus + 15 U/h infusion)	Efficacy: decreased need for reintervention at 96 h but no benefit at 7 months; Safety: no effect

[a]Total number of patients studied was 12,400 with AMI, 19,200 with UA, and 1,300 patients undergoing PCI.

Table 2 Summary of Hirulog Trials in AMI, UA, and PCI[a]

Trial	Clinical setting	No. of patients	Regimen	Result (efficacy; safety)
Theroux et al.	AMI	70	Hirulog (1 mg/kg/h for 12 h) vs. hirulog 0.5 mg/kg/h for 12 h followed by 0.1 mg/kg/h infusion for 4–6 days vs. UFH (5000 U bolus + 1000 U/h infusion	Efficacy: increased TIMI 3 flow and lower rate of recurrent ischemia in low dose/long infusion log; worse outcomes in high dose/short infusion hirulog than in UFH group; Safety: advantage of hirulog
HERO	AMI	412	Hirulog (0.125 mg/kg bolus followed by 0.25 mg/kg/h for 12 h and then 0.125 mg/kg/h) vs. hirulog (0.25 mg/kg bolus followed by 0.5 mg/kg/h for 12 h and then 0.25 mg/kg/h) vs. UFH (5000 U bolus + 1000–1200 U/h)	Efficacy: improved TIMI 3 flow in both low- and high-dose hirulog group (not statistically significant); Safety: less major bleeding in hirulog group
HERO-2	AMI	17,000	Hirulog (0.25 mg/kg bolus followed by 0.5 mg/kg/h for 12 h and then, 0.25 mg/kg/h) vs. UFH (5000 U bolus + 1000–1200 U/h)	Efficacy: no difference in mortality at 30 days but slightly lower incidence of reinfarction at 96 h in hirulog group; Safety: good safety profile of hirulog
TIMI 7	UA	410	Hirulog at 4 different doses for 72 h (0.02-placebo equivalent, 0.25, 0.5, 1 mg/kg/h)	Efficacy: lower incidence of in-hospital death and MI at 6 weeks in the combined hirulog groups 0.25, 0.5, and 1 mg/kg/h versus 0.02-placebo equivalent group; Safety: good safety profile of hirulog
BAS	UA/PCI	4312	Hirulog (1 mg/kg bolus followed by 2.5 mg/kg/h infusion for 4 h and then 0.2 mg/kg/h for 20 h) vs. UFH (175 U/kg bolus + 15 U/h infusion for 24 h)	Efficacy: reduced combined endpoint of MI/revascularization/death in the hirulog group; marginal benefit at 90 and 180 days; Safety: decreased risk of major bleeding

(Continued)

Table 2   Summary of Hirulog Trials in AMI, UA, and PCI[a] (*Continued*)

Trial	Clinical setting	No. of patients	Regimen	Result (efficacy; safety)
CACHET	PCI	300	Hirulog (1 mg/kg bolus + 2.5 mg/kg/h infusion for 4 h with provisional abciximab) vs. hirulog (0.5 mg/kg bolus + 1.75 mg/kg/h for 4 h with planned abciximab) vs. UFH (70 U/kg bolus with planned abciximab)	Efficacy: lower rate of MI and death in the pooled hirulog groups at 7 days; Safety: good safety profile with Iib/IIIa inibitor
REPLACE-2	PCI	6000	Hirulog (0.75 mg/kg bolus + 1.75 mg/kg/h infusion) vs. UFH (65 U/kg bolus + abciximab or eptifibatide)	Efficacy and safety combined: noninferiority of hirulog alone compared to UFH + IIb/IIIa inhibitor in the combined safety and efficacy quadruple endpoints of major bleeding, revascularization, MI, death; increased number of NSTEMI in the hirulog group

[a]Total number of patients studied was 17,400 with AMI, 4,700 with UA, and 10,900 patients undergoing PCI.

Table 3 Summary of Argatroban Studies in AMI, UA, and PCI

Trial	Clinical setting	No. of patients	Regimen	Result (efficacy; safety)
MINT	AMI (with t-PA)	125	Argatroban (100 µg/kg bolus + 1 µg/kg/min infusion) vs. agratroban (100 µg bolus + 3 µg/kg/h infusion) vs. UFH (70 U/kg bolus + 15 U/kg/h infusion)	Efficacy: 18% increase in TIMI 3 flow at 90 min and decreased rate of death and MI at 30 days in agratroban group; Safety: lower rate of major bleeding with argatroban
ARGAMI	AMI (with t-PA)	127	Argatroban (100 µg/kg bolus + 3 µg/kg/min infusion) vs. UFH (5000 U bolus + 1000 U/h infusion)	Efficacy: no difference in angiographic patency; Safety: no difference in rate of bleeding
ARGAMI-2	AMI (with t-PA and SK)	1200	Argatroban (2 µg/kg/min and 4 µg/kg/min) vs. UFH (5000 U bolus + 1000 U/h infusion)	Efficacy: no difference in mortality at 30 days; Safety: decreased bleeding with agratroban
AMI	AMI (with SK)	910	Argatroban (1 µg/kg/min and 3 µg/kg/min) vs. placebo	Efficacy: no difference in rate of death or MI between agratroban and placebo group; Safety: no effect
Gold et al.	UA	43	Argatroban (doses ranging from 0.5 to 5 µg/kg/min) for 4 h	Efficacy: 9/43 patients had recurrent ischemia; Safety: satisfactory
Lewis et al.	PCI	91	Argatroban (350 µg/kg bolus + 25 µg/kg/h infusion) vs. historical controls treated with UFH	Efficacy and safety: Satisfactory outcomes postprocedure
Jang et al.	PCI (with IIb/IIIA inhibitor)	101	Argatroban (250 µg/kg bolus + 15 µg/kg/min infusion)	Efficacy: very low rate of MI or death postprocedure and at 30 days (3%); adequate anticoagulation; Safety: no increased incidence of bleeding

[a]Total number of patients studied was 2500.

Table 4   Summary of Low Molecular Weight Heparin Trials in UA, AMI, and PCI

Trial	Clinical setting	No. of patients	Regimen	Result (efficacy; safety)
ACUTE I	UA	219	Nadroparin 214 U/kg sc bid vs. UFH 400 U/kg/day vs. placebo	Efficacy: 50% reduction in recurrent ischemia; Safety: no excess bleeding
FRISC	UA	1506	Fragmin 120 U/kg sc bid for 5–7 days followed by 7500 U sc bid for 35–45 days vs. placebo	Efficacy: lower short-term MI rate but no significant benefit long term; Safety: no excess bleeding
FRISC II	UA/PCI	2267	Dalteparin 120 U/kg sc bid for 6 days (open label) and then for 3 months vs. placebo	Efficacy: reduction in combined endpoint of death/MI/revascularization; no significant benefit of long-term administration; Safety: no increased major bleeding risk short-term; increased risk of minor bleeding
FRIC	UA	1482	Dalteparin 120 U/kg sc bid for 6 days vs. UFH IV (adjusted to PTT 1.5 × control) for 48 h and then IV or high-dose sc for 4 days	Efficacy: no difference; Safety: no excess bleeding
ESSENCE	UA	3171	Enoxaparin 1 mg/kg sc bid vs. UFH IV (PTT goal 55–85) for 2–8 days	Efficacy: lower recurrent ischemia rate and MI rate at 30 days with enoxaparin; Safety: no excess bleeding
TIMI11B	UA	3910	Enoxaparin 30 mg IV bolus, followed by 1 mg/kg sc bid for 2–8 days, followed by 40–60 mg sc bid for 35 days vs. UFH 70U/kg bolus and 15 U/kg/h infusion for 2–8 days followed by placebo	Efficacy: sustained reduction in mortality and MI rate at 14 days and 43 days; no additional advantage of long-term enoxaparin administration; Safety: no excess bleeding in the initial 2–8 days
FRAXIS	UA	3468	Nadroparin 0.1 mL/10 kg sc bid for 6 days vs. 14 days vs. UFH IV for 6 days	Efficacy: no difference between groups; Safety: no difference with short-term administration
ACUTE II	UA	525	Enoxaparin 1 mg/kg sc bid vs. UFH IV for 24–96 h with tirofiban and aspirin	Efficacy: no mortality benefit but decreased rate of ischemia; Safety: increased nuisance bleeding

(*Continued*)

Table 4 Summary of Low Molecular Weight Heparin Trials in UA, AMI, and PCI (*Continued*)

Trial	Clinical setting	No. of patients	Regimen	Result (efficacy; safety)
INTERACT	UA	746	Enoxaparin 1 mg/kg sc bid or UFH (70 U/kg IV bolus + 15 U/kg/h infusion) for 48 h with eptifibatide	Efficacy: lower rate of ischemia at 48 h and lower mortality at 30 days; Safety: lower rate of major bleeding with enoxaparin but increased minor bleeding
GUSTO IV–ACS	UA	646 (substudy of 7800 patients)	Dalteparin 120 U/kg sc bid for 5–7 days vs. UFH 70 U/kg bolus + 15 U/kg/hr infusion with abciximab	Efficacy: equivalent; Safety: no difference in bleeding rates
PARAGON B	UA	805 (substudy)	LMWH (dose and type not specified) vs. UFH with lamifaban	Efficacy: lower rate of death and MI at 30 days and 6 months; Safety: equivalent
AMI-SK	AMI	496	Enoxaparin 30 mg IV bolus followed by 1 mg/kg sc bid for 3–8 days vs. placebo with SK	Efficacy: lower rates of death/MI/angina at 30 days; Safety: equivalent
HART II	AMI	400	Enoxaparin 30 mg IV bolus followed by 1 mg/kg sc bid for 3 days vs. UFH (4000–5000 U bolus + 15 U/kg/h infusion) with t-Pa	Efficacy: noninferiority in reocclusion rate; Safety: equivalent
ENTIRE 23	AMI	483	Enoxaparin 30 mg IV bolus and 1 mg/kg sc bid vs. UFH (60 U/kg bolus + 12 U/kg/h infusion) with TNK; another arm half-dose TNK with abciximab and with reduced-dose enoxaparin and UFH	Efficacy: lower rate of death/MI at 30 days; Safety: lower rates of hemorrhage with full-dose TNK and enoxaparin but higher in the combination with abciximab arm
ASSENT 3	AMI	6095 (2040)	Enoxaparin (30–50 mg iv bolus followed by 1 mg sc bid) with TNK vs. UFH (4000 U bolus + 12 U/kg for 4 days) vs. reduced-dose UFH with half-dose TNK in combination with abciximab	Efficacy: lower rate of infarction and recurrent ischemia at 30 days with enoxaparin; Safety: no difference

(*Continued*)

Table 4 Summary of Low Molecular Weight Heparin Trials in UA, AMI, and PCI (*Continued*)

Trial	Clinical setting	No. of patients	Regimen	Result (efficacy; safety)
ASSENT 3 PLUS	AMI	1639	Enoxaparin 30 mg IV bolus followed by 1 mg/kg sc bid for 7 days vs. weight-adjusted UFH for 48 h with TNK	Efficacy: lower composite rate of death/MI/ischemia in enoxaparin group; Safety: significantly higher rate of major bleeding/stroke in patients >75 year old
Baird et al.	AMI	300	Enoxaparin (40 mg IV bolus and 40 mg sc bid) vs. UFH (5000 U IV bolus and 30,000 U/h infusion for 4 days after SK or t-PA	Efficacy: lower rate of recurrent ischemia at 90 days; Safety: no difference
BIOMACS	AMI	101	Dalteparin 100 and 120 IU separated by 12 h versus placebo with SK	Efficacy: higher TIMI 3 rates but more recurrent ischemia in dalteparin group; Safety: no increased bleeding
CRUISE	PCI	261	Enoxaparin 0.75 mg/kg iv X1 dose with eptifibatide	Efficacy: no difference; Safety: no difference
Collet et al.	PCI	451	Enoxaparin 1 ma/kg sc bid	Efficacy: no assessed; Safety: low rates of bleding
Choussat et al.	PCI	242	Enoxaparin 0.5 mg/kg iv X1 dose	Efficacy: low rate of death/MI/ischemia; Safety: one major bleeding event observed
FRISC II	PCI	1,222	Dalteparin 120 IU/kg sc bid for 5 days and then additional 90 days (vs. placebo)	Safety: low rate of major bleeding

[a]Total number of patients studied: 18,500 patients with UA, 9500 patients with AMI, and 1000 patients treated with PCI.

REFERENCES

1. Gotoh K, Minamino T, Katoh O, et al. The role of intracoronary thrombus in unstable angina: angiographic assessment and thrombolytic therapy during ongoing anginal attacks. Circulation 1988; 77:526–534.
2. Falk E, Shah PK, Fuster V. Coronary plaque disruption. Circulation 1995; 92:657–671.
3. Fuster V. Mechanisms leading to myocardial infarction: insights from studies of vascular biology. Circulation 1994; 90:2126–2146.
4. Theroux P, Ouimet H, McCans J, et al. Aspirin, heparin, or both to treat acute unstable angina. N Engl J Med 1994; 319:1105–1111.
5. Liaw PC, Becker DL, Stafford AR, et al. Molecular basis for the susceptibility of fibrin-bound thrombin inactivation by heparin cofactor II in the presence of dermatan sulfate but not heparin. J Biol Chem. 2001; 276:20959–20965.
6. Hirsh J, Raschke R, Warkentin TE, et al. Heparin: mechanism of action, pharmacokinetics, dosing considerations, monitoring, efficacy, and safety. Chest 1995; 108:258S–275S.
7. GUSTO IIb Investigators. A comparison of recombinant hirudin with heparin for the treatment of acute coronary syndromes. N Engl J Med 1996; 335:775–782.
8. Warkentin TE, Sheppard JI, Horsewood P, et al. Impact of patient population on the risk of heparin-induced thrombocytopenia. Blood 2000; 96:1703–1708.
9. Berry CN, Girardot C, Lecoffre C, et al. Effects of synthetic thrombin inhibitor argatroban on fibrin- or clot-incorporated thrombin: comparison with heparin and recombinant hirudin. Thromb Haemost. 1994; 72:381–386.
10. Wallis RB. Hirudins: from leeches to man. Semin Thromb Hemost 1996; 22:185–196.
11. Kathiresan S, Shiomura J, Jang IK, Argatroban. J. Thrombosis and Thrombolysis 2002; 13(1):41–47.
12. Antman EM, for the TIMI 9B Investigators. Hirudin in acute myocardial infarction. Circulation 1996; 94:911–921.
13. The TIMI IIIB Investigators. Effects of tissue plasminogen activator and a comparison of early invasive and conservative strategies in unstable angina and non-Q wave myocardial infarction. Circulation 1994; 89:1545–1556.
14. Cannon CP, McCabe CH, Henry TD, et al. A pilot trial of recombinant desulfatohirudin compared with heparin in conjunction with tissue type plasminogen activator and aspirin in acute myocardial infarction: results of the Thrombolysis in Myocardial Infarction (TIMI) 5 trial. J Am Coll Cardiol 1994; 23:993–1003.
15. Lee LV. Initial experience with hirudin and streptokinase in acute myocardial infarction: results of TIMI 6 trial. Am J Cardiol 1995; 75:7–13.
16. GUSTO IIa Investigators. Randomized trial of intravenous heparin versus recombinant hirudin for acute coronary syndromes. Circulation 1994; 90: 1631–1637.
17. Antman EM for the TIMI 9A Investigators. Hirudin in acute myocardial infarction: safety report from the TIMI 9A trial. Circulation 1994; 90:1624–1630.
18. (a) Neuhaus KL, von Essen R, Tebbe U, et al. Safety observations from the pilot phase of the randomized r-Hirudin for Improvement of Thrombolysis (HIT-III) study. Circulation 1994; 90:1638–1642; (b) Neuhaus KL, Molhoek GP, Zeymer U, et al. Recombinant hirudin (lepirudin) for the improvement of thrombolysis with streptokinase in patients with acute myocardial infarction: results of the HIT-4 trial. J. Am. Coll. Cardiol. 1999; 34(4):966–973.
19. OASIS-2 Investigators. Effects of recombinant hirudin (lepirudin) compared with heparin on death, myocardial infarction, refractory angina, and revascularization procedures in patients with acute myocardial ischemia without ST elevation: randomized trial. Lancet 1999; 353:429–438.
20. Antman EA. The search for replacement for unfractionated heparin. Circulation 2001; 103:2310–2314.
21. Organization to Assess Strategies for Ischemic Syndromes (OASIS). Comparison of the effects of two doses of recombinant hirudin compared with heparin in patients with acute myocardial ischemia without ST elevation: a pilot study. Circulation 1997; 96:769–777.

22. Serruys PW, Herrman JP, Simon R, et al. A comparison of hirudin with heparin in the prevention of restenosis after coronary angioplasty. HELVETICA Investigators. N Engl J Med 1995; 333:757–763.

23. Rupprecht HJ, Terres W, Ozbek C, et al. Recombinant hirudin (HBW023) prevents troponin T release after coronary angioplasty in patients with unstable angina. J Am Coll Cardiol 1995; 26(7):1637–1642.

24. Lindon RM, Theroux P, Lesperance J, et al. A pilot, early angiographic patency study using a direct thrombin inhibitor as adjunctive therapy to streptokinase in acute myocardial infarction. Circulation 1994; 89:1567–1572.

25. Theroux P, Perez-Villa F, Waters D, et al. Randomized double-blind comparison of two doses of hirulog with heparin as adjunctive therapy to streptokinase to promote early patency of the infarct-related artery in acute myocardial infarction. Circulation 1995; 91:2132–2139.

26. White HD, Aylward PE, Frey MJ, et al. Randomized, double-blind comparison of hirulog versus heparin in patients receiving streptokinase and aspirin for acute myocardial infarction (HERO). Circulation 1997; 96:2155–2161.

27. White HD and the Hirulog and Early Reperfusion or Occlusion (HERO)-2 trial. Thrombin-specific anticoagulation with bivalirudin versus heparin in patients receiving fibrinolytic therapy for acute myocardial infarction: the HERO-2 randomised trial. Lancet 2001; 358(9296):1855–1863.

28. Fuchs J and Cannon CP for TIMI7 Investigators. Hirulog in the treatment of unstable angina. Results of the TIMI 7 trial. Circulation 1995; 92:727–733.

29. Bittl JA, Strony J, Brinker JA, et al. Treatment with bivalirudin (hirulog) as compared with heparin during coronary angioplasty for unstable or postinfarction angina. N Engl J Med 1995; 333:764–769.

30. Bittl JA, Chairman BR, Feit F, et al. Bivalirudin versus heparin during coronary angioplasty for unstable or postinfarction angina: Final report reanalysis of the Bivalirudin Angioplasty Study. Am Heart J 1001; 142(6): 952–990.

31. Lincoff AM, Kleiman NS, Meierson ES, et al. Bivalirudin with planned or provisional abciximab versus low-dose heparin and abciximab during percutaneous coronary revascularization: results of the Comparison of Abciximab Complications with Hirulog for Ischemic Events Trial (CACHET). Am Heart J 2002; 143(5):847–853.

32. Lincoff AM, Bittle JA, Harrington RA, et al., for the REPLACE-2 Investigators. Bivalirudin and provisional glycoprotein IIb/IIIa blockade compared with heparin and planned glycoprotein IIb/IIIa blockade during percutaneous coronary intervention. JAMA 2003; 289(7):853–863.

33. The EPISTENT Inverstigators. Randomised placebo-controlled and balloon-angioplasty-controlled trial to assess safety of coronary stenting with use of platelet glycoprotein-IIb/IIIa blockade. Lancet 1998; 352:87–92.

34. The ESPRIT Investigators. Novel dosing regimen of eptifibatide in planned coronary stent implantation (ESPRIT): a randomised, placebo-controlled trial. Lancet 2000; 356:2037–2044.

35. Jang IK, Brown DF, Giugliano RP, et al. A multicenter randomized study of argatroban versus heparin as adjunct to tissue plasminogen activator (t-PA) in acute myocardial infarction: myocardial infarction with novastan and t-PA (MINT) study. J Am Coll Cardiol 1999; 33:1880–1885.

36. Vermeer F, Vahanian A, Fels PW, et al. Argatroban and anteplase in patients with acute myocardial infarction: the ARGAMI study. J Thromb Thrombolysis 2000; 10:233–240.

37. Behar S, Hod H, Kaplinsky E for the ARGAMI-2 Study Group. Argatroban versus heparin as adjuvant therapy to thrombolysis for acute myocardial infarction: safety considerations—ARGAMI-2 study. Circulation 1998; 98(1, suppl):1453–1454.

38. Gold HK, Torres FW, Garabedian HD, et al. Evidence for a rebound coagulation phenomenon after cessation of a 4-hour infusion of a specific thrombin inhibitor in patients with unstable angina pectoris. J Am Coll Cardiol 1993; 21:1039–1047.

39. Lewis BE, Wallis DE, Berkowitz SD, et al. Argatroban anticoagulant therapy in patients with heparin-induced thrombocytopenia. Circulation 2001; 103: 1838–1843.

40. Jang IK, Lewis BE, Matthai WH, et al. Combination of a direct thrombin inhibitor, argatroban and glycoprotein IIb/IIIa inhibitor is effective and safe in patients undergoing percutaneous coronary intervention. ACC 2002 (submitted abstract).

41. Shetler TJ, Crowe VG, Bailey BD, et al. Antithrombotic assessment of the effects of combination therapy with the anticoagulants efegatran and heparin and the glycoprotein IIb-IIIa platelet receptor antagonist 7E3 in a canine model of coronary artery thrombosis. Circulation 1996; 94:1719–1725.

42. Multicenter, dose-ranging study of efegatran sulfate versus heparin with thrombolysis for acute myocardial infarction: the Promotion of reperfusion in Myocardial Infarction Evolution (PRIME) trial. Am Heart J 2002, 143(1):95–105.

43. Fung AY, Lorch G, Cambier PA, et al. Efegatran sulfate as an adjunct to streptokinase versus heparin as an adjunct to tissue plasminogen activator in patients with acute myocardial infarction. ESCALAT Investigators. Am Heart J 1999; 138(4 pt 1):696–704.

44. Klootwijk P, Lenderink T, Meij S, et al. Anticoagulant properties, clinical efficacy and safety of efegatran, a direct thrombin inhibitor, in patients with unstable angina. Eur Heart J 1999; 20(15):1101–1111.

45. Sabatine MS, Jang IK. Antithrombotic therapy in acute coronary syndromes. Acta Cardiol 1999; 54(1):3–29.

46. Wong GC, Giugliano RP, Antman EM Use of low-molecular-weight heparins in the management of acute coronary artery syndromes and percutaneous coronary intervention. JAMA 2003; 289(3):331–342.

47. Gurfinkel EP, Manos EJ, Mejail RI, et al. Low molecular weight heparin versus regular heparin or aspirin in the treatment of unstable angina and silent ischemia. J Am Coll Cardiol 1995; 26(2):313–318.

48. Swahn E and Wallentin L. Low-molecular-weight heparin (Fragmin) during instability in coronary artery disease (FRISC). FRISC Study Group. Am J Cardiol 1997; 80(5A):25E–29E.

49. Fragmin and Fast Revascularization during InStability in Coronary artery disease (FRISC) Investigators. Long-term low-molecular-mass heparin in unstable coronary-artery disease: FRISC II prospective randomised multicenter study. Lancet 1999; 354:701–707.

50. Klein W, Buchwald A, Hillis SE, et al. Comparison of low-molecular-weight heparin with unfractionated heparin acutely and with placebo for 6 weeks in the management of unstable coronary artery disease. Fragmin in unstable coronary disease study (FRIC). 1997; 96(1):61–68.

51. Cohen M, Demers C, Gurfinkel EP, et al. for the Efficacy and Safety of Subcutaneous Enoxaparin in Non-Q-Wave Coronary Events Study Group. A comparison of low-molecular-weight heparin with unfractionated heparin for unstable coronary artery disease. N Eugl J Med 1997; 337(7):447–452.

52. Antman EM, McCabe CH, Gurfinkel EP, et al., for the TIMI 11B Investigators. Enoxaparin prevents death and cardiac ischemic events in unstable angina/non-Q-wave myocardial infarction. Results of the Thrombolysis in Myocardial Infarction (TIMI) 11B trial. Circulation 1999; 100:1593–1601.

53. Antman EM, Cohen M, Radley D, et al., for the TIMI 11 B and ESSENCE Investigators. Assessment of the treatment effect of enoxaparin for unstable angina/non-Q-wave myocardial infarction. TIMI 11B-ESSENCE Meta-Analysis. Circulation 1999; 100:1602–1608.

54. FRAXIS Investigators. Comparison of two treatments of durations (6 days and 14 days) of low molecular weight heparin with a 6-day treatment of unfractionated heparin in the initial management of unstable angina or non-Q-wave myocardial infarction. Fraxiparine in Ischaemic Syndrome. Eur Heart J 1999; 20(21):1553–1562.

55. Cohen M, Theroux P, Weber S, et al. Combination therapy with tirofiban and enoxaparin in acute coronary syndromes. Int J Cardiol 1999; 71:273–281.

56. Cohen M, Theroux P, Borzak S, et al. Randomized double-blind safety study of enoxaparin versus unfractionated heparin in patients with non-ST elevation acute coronary syndromes treated with tirofiban and aspirin: the ACUTE II study: the Antithrombotic Combination Using Tirofiban and Enoxaparin. Am Heart J 2002; 144:470–477.

57. Goodman S, Fitchett D, Armstrong P, et al. Randomized evaluation of the safety and efficacy of enoxaparin versus unfractionated heparin in high-risk patients with non-ST-segment elevation acute coronary syndromes receiving the glycoprotein IIb/IIIa inhibitor eptifibatide. Circulation 2003; 107:238–244.

58. James S, Armstrong P, Califf R, et al. Safety and efficacy of abciximab combined with dalteparin in treatment of acute coronary syndromes. Eur Heart J 2002; 23:1538–1545.

59. Mukherjee D, Mahaffey KW, Moliterno DJ, et al. Promise of combined low molecular weight heparin and platelet glycoprotein IIb/IIIa inhibition: results from Platelet IIb/IIIa Antagonist for the Reduction of Acute coronary syndrome events in a Global Organization Network B (PARAGON B). Am Heart J. 2002; 144:995–1002.

60. SYNERGY Executive Committee. Superior Yield of the New strategy of Enoxaparin, Revascularization and G1Y coprotein IIb/IIIa inhibitors. The SYNERGY trial: study design and rationale. Am Heart J 2002; 143(6):952–960.

61. Simoons M, Krzeminska-Pakula M, Alonso A, et al. Improved reperfusion and clinical outcome with enoxaparin as an adjunct to streptokinase thrombolysis in acute myocardial infarction: the AMI-SK study. Eur Heart J 2002; 23:1282–1290.

62. Ross AM, Molhoek P, Lundergan, C, et al. Randomized comparison of enoxaparin, a low-molecular-weight heparin, with unfractionated heparin adjunctive to recombinant tissue plasminogen activator thrombolysis and aspirin: second trial of Heparin and Aspirin Reperfusion Therapy (HART II). Circulation 2001; 104:648–652.

63. Antman EM, Louwerenburg HW, Baars HF, et al. Enoxaparin as adjunctive antithrombin therapy for ST-elevation myocardial infarction: results of the ENTIRE-Thrombolysis in Myocardial Infarction (TIMI) 23 Trial. Circulation 2002; 105:1642–1649.

64. Van de Werf H, for The Assessment of the Safety and Efficacy of a New Thrombolytic Regimen (ASSENT)-3 Investigators. Efficacy and safety of tenecteplase in combination with enoxaparin, abciximab, or unfractionated heparin: the ASSENT-3 randomized trial in acute myocardial infarction. Lancet 2001; 358:605–613.

65. Wallentin L, Goldstein P, Armstrong PW, et al. Efficacy and safety of tenecteplase in combination with the low molecular-weight heparin enoxaparin or unfractionated heparin in the prehospital setting: the Assessment of the Safety and Efficacy of a New Thrombolytic Regimen (ASSENT)-3 PLUS randomized trial in acute myocardial infarction. Circulation 2003; 108(2):135–142.

66. Baird SH, Menown BA, McBride SJ, et al. Randomized comparison of enoxaparin with unfractionated heparin following fibrinolytic therapy for acute myocardial infarction. Eur Heart J 2002; 23:627–632.

67. Frostfeld G, Ahlberg G, Gustafsson G, et al. Low molecular weight heparin (Dalteparin) as adjuvant treatment to thrombolysis in acute myocardial infarction—a pilot study: biochemical markers in acute coronary syndromes (BIOMACS II). J Am Coll Cardiol. 1999; 33(3):627–633.

68. Gram J, Mercker S, Bruhn HD. Does protamine chloride neutralize low molecular weight heparin sufficiently? Thromb Res 1988; 52:353–359.

69.   (a) Kereiakes DJ, Grines C, Fry E, et al. Enoxaparin and abciximab adjunctive pharmacotherapy during percutaneous coronary intervention. J Invasive Cardiol. 2001; 13:272–278; (b) Ferguson JJ. The use of enoxaparin and IIb/IIIa antagonists in acute coronary syndromes including PCI: final results of the NICE 3 study. J Am Coll Cardiol. 2001; 37(suppl A):365A.

70. Bhatt DL, Lee DI, Casterella PJ, et al. Safety of concomitant therapy with eptifibatide and enoxaparin in patients undergoing percutaneous coronary intervention—results of the CRUISE study. J Am Coll Cardiol. 2003; 41:20–25.

71. Collet JP, Montalescot G, Lison L, et al. Percutanous coronary intervention after subcutaneous enoxaparin pretreatment in patients with unstable angina pectoris. Circulation 2001; 103:658–663.

72. Choussat R, Montalescot G, Collet JP, et al. A unique, low dose of intravenous enoxapirin in elective percutaneous coronary intervention. J Am Coll Cardiol. 2002; 40:1943–1950.

73. Batchelor WB, Mahaffey KW, Berger PB, et al. A randomized, placebo-controlled trial of enoxaparin after high-risk coronary stenting: the ATLAS trial. J Am Coll Cardiol. 2001; 38:1608–1613.
74. Jang IK. Direct thrombin inhibitors in acute coronary syndromes. Lancet 2002; 360(9331):491–492..
75. Direct Thrombin Inhibitor Trialists' Collaborative Group. Direct thrombin inhibitors in acute coronary syndromes: principal results of a meta-analysis based on individual patients' data. Lancet 2002; 359:294–302.

16-1

Facilitating Perfusion Strategies in Acute Myocardial Infarction

Robert V. Kelly, Mauricio G. Cohen, and E. Magnus Ohman
The University of North Carolina at Chapel Hill, Chapel Hill, North Carolina, U.S.A.

I. BACKGROUND

Every year almost 1 million Americans suffer an acute myocardial infarction (AMI), and 225,000 of these patients have a fatal outcome (1). Thrombolytic therapy (TT) is a very effective treatment for AMI, especially if these patients can be identified early. It reduces mortality and establishes early coronary artery patency, limits myocardial damage, and improves left ventricular (LV) systolic function. However, TT is not without limitations. Only 60–80% of patients achieve patency of the infarct-related artery (IRA) within 90 minutes of the initiation of treatment. TIMI 3 flow is established in only 30–55% of patients, and 13% of patients may experience early reocclusion of the culprit artery (2–4). In addition, there is a significant risk of stroke and bleeding with TT (5,6).

Mechanical reperfusion is an alternative option by means of primary percutaneous coronary intervention (PCI). According to the results of two large meta-analyses, the use of primary PCI was associated with smaller infarct size, a reduced risk of reinfarction and stroke, and lower hospital mortality compared with TT (7,8). However, the negative impact caused by frequent long delays and in performing primary PCI may blunt the potential benefits of such a strategy.

A third treatment alternative is the combination of pharmacological and mechanical reperfusion strategies.

II. FACILITATED ANGIOPLASTY IN AMI

The term "facilitated PCI" was coined by the SPEED (Strategy for Patency Enhancement in the Emergency Department) investigators to designate immediate PCI following pharmacologic perfusion therapies (9). Facilitated angioplasty refers to the use of pharmacological reperfusion strategies to restore infarct-related artery patency before planned angioplasty in acute ST elevation myocardial infarction patients. It differs from rescue PCI in that it is a planned intervention in all AMI patients following pharmacological reperfusion therapy and not just in those patients who clinically fail to achieve reperfusion with thrombolytic therapy. It differs from primary angioplasty as it combines pharmacological and mechanical reperfusion strategies rather than adopting a mechanical strategy alone.

The initial results using this strategy suggest similar outcomes compared with primary angioplasty and far superior outcomes to TT alone (9–12). Furthermore, facilitated PCI provides an opportunity to start treating AMI patients in hospitals that do not have primary intervention facilities and simultaneously transferring these patients to tertiary referral centers for mechanical intervention treatment.

III. PHARMACOLOGICAL REPERFUSION STRATEGIES

TT has been the mainstay of treatment of AMI for over 20 years. In all trials of TT compared to placebo, TT has been associated with a significant reduction in 30-day mortality (9.6% vs. 11.5%; $p < 0.0001$). Patients treated early after symptom onset had the greatest reduction in mortality (5,13). The ISIS-2 (International Study of Infarc Survival) trial showed that streptokinase reduced mortality by 53% when given within 4 hours of symptom onset compared with a 33% reduction in mortality when given between 4 and 24 hours (14). GUSTO (Global Utilization of Streptokinase and t-PA for Occluded Coronary Arteries) I found that t-PA improved outcomes compared with streptokinase and that this was dependent on the degree of myocardial perfusion at 90 minutes (15). TT has the major advantage that it is widely available without the need for complex equipment and specialized staff and it can be given in the field, either in the ambulance or even at home (16–19). However, not every patient is suitable for TT, and in some cases there is an increased risk of stroke and major bleeding (5). This is a concern, particularly with an aging population of AMI patients (Fig. 1). In a study including 7864 Medicare beneficiaries, TT was not associated with improved survival. In fact, patients over the age of 75 years had more strokes and required more blood transfusions compared to patients aged 65–75 years (20).

Furthermore, over 50% of all TT patients who fail to achieve early complete reperfusion are subject to a twofold higher mortality rate. An additional 20% of patients fail to

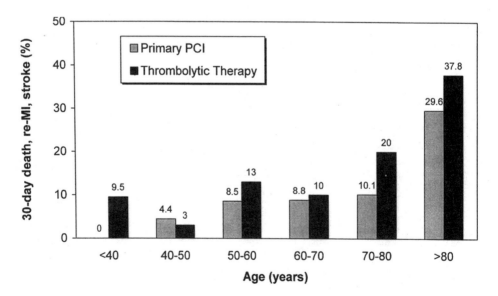

Figure 1   Differential effect in 30-day mortality, reinfarction, and stroke of primary PCI vs. thrombolytic therapy in the GUSTO IIb study.

Trial	n	Agent	Control	Active
FTT *	58,600	Placebo vs. SK	11.28	9.00
GUSTO I	41,021	SK vs. t-PA	7.30	6.30
INJECT	6,010	SK vs. r-PA	9.50	9.00
COBALT	7,169	t-PA Inj vs. t-PA Bolus	7.53	7.98
GUSTO III	15,059	t-PA vs. r-PA	7.24	7.47
ASSENT-2	16,950	t-PA vs. TNK	6.15	6.18
In TIME-II	15,078	t-PA vs. n-PA	6.60	6.80
ASSENT-3	6,095	TNK vs. ½TNK + Abx	6.00	6.60
GUSTO V	16,588	r-PA vs. ½r-PA + Abx	5.90	5.60

RR

0.60   0.80   1.0   1.20

Active Better   Control Better

* < 6 hs

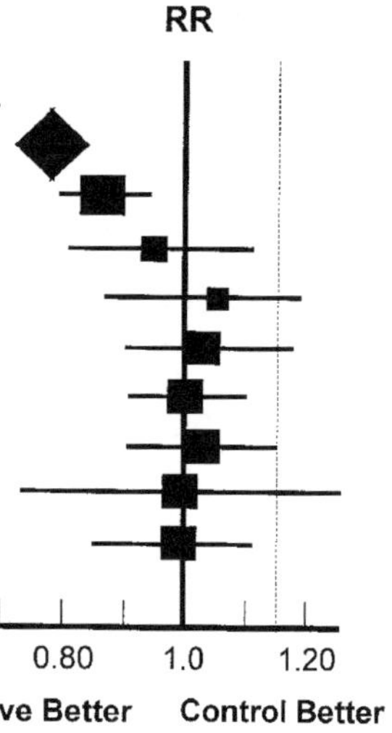

Figure 2   Phase 3 thrombolytic trials and 30-day mortality.

reperfuse at the myocardial tissue level, and 5–10% of TT patients reinfarct despite initially successful reperfusion (4). New investigations over the last 10 years of alternative TT molecules with longer half-lives have failed to show superiority over front loaded t-PA (Fig. 2) (21–23). Combining t-PA with glycoprotein receptor antagonists as in GUSTO V (24), which studied abciximab plus half-dose reteplase versus full-dose reteplase alone, did not show a survival benefit with the combined strategy, despite angiography showing better patency with combination therapy in phase II trials (25,26). Combination therapy leads to higher bleeding rates, including higher intracranial hemorrhage, especially among elderly patients (24,27).

IV. MECHANICAL PERFUSION AS AN ALTERNATIVE TO THROMBOLYSIS

Mechanical means of perfusion, i.e., primary angioplasty, have been in place since 1982 as an alternative to TT for patients with acute myocardial infarction (28). In 1993, the first randomized clinical trials comparing primary PCI versus TT showed lower mortality and reinfarction rates in patients treated with primary PCI (29). Subsequently, a number of small randomized studies have shown a consistent benefit of primary PCI over different thrombolytic agents (30).

In a comprehensive meta-analysis that compared PCI with TT in 2606 patients, 30-day mortality was 4.4% for the PCI group and 6.5% for the TT group ($p = 0.02$). The rate of death or nonfatal reinfarction was lower in PCI-treated patients compared with TT group (7.2% vs. 11.9%; $p < 0.001$). PCI was associated with a significant reduction in total stroke (0.7% vs. 2%; $p = 0.007$) and intracranial hemorrhage (0.1% vs. 1.1%; $p < 0.001$) (7). In a more contemporary meta-analysis of 7739 AMI patients, including trials using coronary stents and intravenous glycoprotein IIb/IIIa receptor blockers, it was found that primary PCI was superior to TT at reducing overall short-term mortality (7% vs. 9%; $p = 0.0002$), nonfatal reinfarction (3% vs. 7%; $p < 0.0001$), stroke (1% vs. 2%; $p = 0.0004$) and the combined endpoint of death, nonfatal MI, and stroke (8% vs. 14%; $p < 0.0001$).

These outcomes with PCI remained superior to those with TT at one-year follow-up, and this was independent of the type of thrombolytic agent used and whether or not the patient was transferred for primary PCI (8). In the Zwolle randomized trial, the benefit of primary PCI was sustained after 5 years with a decreased risk of death (RR 0.54; 95% CI 0.36–0.87), reinfarction (RR 0.27, 95% CI 0.15–0.52), heart failure, and rehospitalization among patients treated with primary PCI (30). Based on these data, the current ACC/AHA guidelines for the management of myocardial infarction consider primary PCI as an alternative to TT (1). Similar benefits of primary PCI over TT have been reported in the MIR (Myocardial Infarction Registry) and MITRA (Myocardial Individual Therapy in Acute Myocardial Infarction) German registries, which were more representative of every day clinical practice, enrolling 9906 patients (31). In fact, these data have shown a significant reduction in hospital mortality from 1994 to 1998 in patients treated with primary PCI across all subgroups, a trend that was not observed with TT. Moreover, there was a continuously increasing benefit with primary angioplasty, reaching statistical significance in 1997 and in 1998, highlighting the positive effect of the progress in interventional techniques, equipment, and adjuvant antithrombotic therapies during the last decade (32).

However, primary angioplasty like TT has several limitations. First, there is an inherent delay in performing primary PCI. Only 50% of patients receive reperfusion therapy within 2 hours of presenting to the emergency department (ED). According to NRMI-2 (Second National Registry of Myocardial Infarction), the median door-to-balloon time is 111 minutes in U.S. hospitals, with only 8% of patients treated within 60 minutes, which is well outside the guideline boundaries recommended for primary PCI treatment. In fact, door-to-balloon time beyond 2 hours was associated with a significantly increased 30-day mortality, compared to < 2 hours (9.2% vs. 4.3%; $p = 0.04$), and with worse left ventricular function despite equivalent degrees of coronary flow after primary PCI (33).

Second, there is a shortage of facilities and personnel to offer primary PCI to all AMI patients. Only 15–20% of U.S. and 10% of European hospitals have the facilities and the staff needed to provide a primary angioplasty service (1). Transferring AMI patients to these centers is fraught with delays. In fact, the strongest independent predictors of delay are hospital transfer, nondaytime presentation, and low-volume centers (34). Delay in initiation of therapy is important, especially for primary PCI-treated patients, probably as this delay reflects quality of care. Organizational skills, logistical expertise, and optimal use of all aspects of care are likely to have a major impact on outcome. Prehospital triage of patients can reduce ischemic times and improve door-to-balloon times (35). More immediate solutions to improving access and availability of PCI include providing community hospital–based primary PCI at sites without surgical backup or direct transfer to PCI centers (10,36–40).

In the situation where on-site PCI is not available, transfer to tertiary care centers for PCI is superior to local TT. The DANAMI-2 (Danish Study in Acute Myocardial Infarction) trial randomized AMI patients to TT at their local hospital versus transfer for PCI. Patients who were transferred for PCI had significantly lower reinfarction rates (1.6% vs. 6.3%; $p < 0.001$) and similar stroke and mortality rates compared with TT patients. The primary endpoint of 30-day death, reinfarction, or disabling stroke was reached in 8.5% of PCI patients compared with 14.2% of TT patients ($p < 0.0001$). Over 95% of transferred PCI patients reached the referral hospital within 2 hours of randomization. Median door-to-balloon time was 112 minutes. There were no deaths during transfer, but there were 14 cases of atrial fibrillation and 8 cases of ventricular arrhythmias (40).

The PRAGUE-2 (Primary Angioplasty in patients transferred from General community hospitals to specialized PTCA Units with or without Emergency thrombolysis) study randomized 850 patients to on-site thrombolysis or transfer for primary PCI. Median door-to-balloon time was 97 minutes. During hospital transfer there was a 1.4% ventricular fibrillation risk and 2.1% mortality rate. The results showed a non-significant 30-day mortality difference (10% in the on-site thrombolysis group vs. 6.8% in the primary PCI group; $p = 0.68$). However, patients arriving after more than 3 hours of symptoms had a significantly lower mortality with primary PCI than with thrombolytic therapy (6% vs. 15.3%, respectively; $p < 0.02$), whereas patients enrolled within 3 hours of symptom onset had equivalent mortality rates (7.4% in the primary PCI vs 7.3% in the on-site thrombolysis group; $p = NS$) (39).

The Air-PAMI trial suggested that high-risk AMI patients (age > 70, anterior MI, Killip class II/III, HR > 100/min or SBP < 100 mmHg) should also be transferred for primary PCI rather than receive TT on site in a predominantly North American setting. The mean door-to-balloon time was 155 minutes, substantially longer than in the European trials. This study was terminated after 39 months for poor enrollment, recruiting only 32% of the estimated sample size. Even though the transfer for primary PCI strategy was associated with a 38% relative reduction in the occurrence of death, reinfarction, and disabling stroke compared with on-site thrombolysis, this difference was not statistically significant due to lack of power (38). A recent meta-analysis based on 3750 patients enrolled in six clinical trials comparing primary angioplasty after interhospital transfer and on-site thrombolysis found that PCI patients had a statistically significant 42% relative risk reduction in the composite of 30-day death, reinfarction, and stroke, compared with TT patients ($p < 0.001$). Transfer time was always less than 3 hours across the analyzed trials (41).

Even though there is little question about the superiority of PCI, TT seems to have similar efficacy if given within the first 2–3 hours of symptom onset (42). In the CAPTIM (Comparison of Angioplasty and Prehospital Thrombolysis in Acute Myocardial Infarction) trial, patients were given prehospital TT within a median time of 130 minutes from the onset of symptoms, while primary PCI was performed at a median time of 190 minutes. While there was no difference in the composite of 30-day death, nonfatal MI, and nonfatal stroke (8.2% vs. 6.2% for PCI; $p = 0.29$) or mortality (3.8% vs. 4.8%, $p = 0.61$) between patients treated within or after 2 hours of the onset of chest pain, there was a strong trend toward lower mortality (2.2% vs. 5.7%; $p = 0.058$) and a reduction of cardiogenic shock (1.3% vs. 5.3%; $p = 0.032$) in patients treated with prehospital TT within 2 hours of symptom onset (43). It appears that low molecular weight heparin (LMWH) may have incremental adjunctive effect on thrombolysis for coronary reperfusion. In the ASSENT-3 (Assessment of the Safety of a New Thrombolytic) study, prehospital administration of TT and enoxaparin within 2 hours of symptom onset was associated with a reduction in 30-day mortality (7.5% vs. 6.0%; $p = 0.8$), recurrent ischemia (4.4% vs. 6.5%; $p = 0.067$), and reinfarction (3.5% vs. 5.8%; $p = 0.028$) compared to a conventional regimen of TT with unfractionated heparin. However, this was at the expense of a higher rate of stroke and intracranial bleeding with LMWH (19). Therefore, in early AMI it is very important to decide promptly on the reperfusion strategy, since if PCI is delayed excessively, its efficacy may well be inferior to very early TT. This issue has been further examined in a recent publication combining data from 22 randomized clinical trials. It appears that the salutatory effect of primary PCI on 4- to 6-week mortality is offset by time delays if the difference between the door-to-needle and door-to-balloon times is expected to be greater than one hour. According to this report, the absolute mortality reduction associated with primary PCI decreases by 0.94% for every 10-minute delay. In fact, TT and primary PCI become equivalent with regard to mortality when PCI-related delays are longer than 62 minutes (44).

V. CORONARY STENTING IN ACUTE MYOCARDIAL INFARCTION

Coronary stenting reduces restenosis and the abrupt closure rates seen with balloon angioplasty alone and is now routinely used in the majority of patients undergoing primary PCI for AMI. Stent implantation is associated with a 50% reduction in target vessel revascularization (TVR) at 6–12 months (OR 0.43, 95% CI 0.36–0.52) (45). However, other clinical outcomes are not affected by stent implantation. As a matter of fact, the STENT-PAMI trial has shown a trend towards increased 6-month mortality in the stent arm (4.2%) in comparison with the balloon arm (2.7%), possibly related to less attainment of final TIMI grade 3 flow in the stent arm (46). In the CADILLAC (Controlled Abciximab and Device Investigation to Lower Late Angioplasty Complications) trial, a 2×2 factorial design was used to assess the effect of more flexible stents and abciximab in primary PCI. Interestingly, the 6-month results in the abciximab arms paralleled the STENT-PAMI results, with a mortality of 4.2% in the stent group and 2.5% in the balloon group (47). Stent implantation may result in microvascular dysfunction, related to the release of vasoactive mediators, such as serotonin and endothelin-1, attenuated NO activity, and platelet microembolization, resulting in a proinflammatory state with free radical production and microvascular plugging (48–51). In addition, coronary stenting carries the risk of mobilizing thrombogenic material, causing distal embolization. This correlates with decreased left ventricular ejection fraction (51% vs. 42%; $p = 0.009$) and less favorable clinical outcomes (52). Stenting plus abciximab however has been showed to improve myocardial perfusion compared to thrombolysis or balloon angioplasty and this correlates to better clinical outcomes as well (Fig. 3) (53–56). Increased attention has been turned into the potential of new drug-eluting stents for reducing long-term revascularization procedures in acute MI patients. The recently reported RESEARCH (Rapamycin Eluting Stent. Evaluated at Rotterdam Cardiology Hospital) registry showed that sirolimus-eluting stents are associated with a similar incidence of subacute stent thrombosis compared with

		Mortality (%)	
	n	Stent	Balloon
Suryapranata et al.	227	2.0	3.0
STENT-PAMI	900	4.2	2.7
STENTIM-2	211	2.0	1.0
CADILLAC	1030	4.5	3.0
Pooled	**2368**	**3.9**	**2.6**
	n	Abciximab	Placebo
RAPPORT	483	4.1	4.2
ISAR-2	401	2.0	4.5
ADMIRAL	300	3.4	7.3
CADILLAC	2082	3.3	3.7
ACE	400	4.5	8.0
Pooled	**3666**	**3.9**	**5.0**

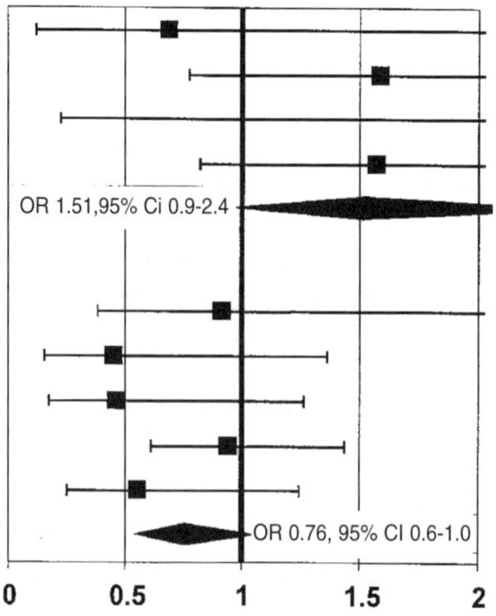

Figure 3 The effect of stents and abciximab on long-term mortality in primary PCI trials.

bare metal stents. In addition, the rates of death and reinfarction at one year were 8.8% and 10.4% for drug-eluting stents and bare metal stents, respectively (p =NS). However, the TVR rates were substantially lower in patients treated with drug-eluting stents (1.1% vs. 8.2%; $p < 0.02$) (57). These results are to be interpreted cautiously because there are no randomized data available assessing the efficacy and safety of drug-eluting stents in the setting of acute MI.

VI. THE ROLE OF GLYCOPROTEIN IIB IIIA INHIBITORS IN ACUTE MYOCARDIAL INFARCTION

A. Glycoprotein IIb IIIa Inhibitors and Thrombolytic Therapy

The use of glycoprotein IIb IIIa inhibitors in the setting of acute myocardial infarction is based on the pivotal role of platelets as a cause of occlusive thrombi (58). Abciximab possesses an intrinsic ability to reperfuse acutely occluded vessels during myocardial infarction in a time-dependent fashion (25,26,59,60). Improvements in culprit artery patency with abciximab may be due to the reduced size of platelet aggregates and increased fibrin exposure in platelet-rich thrombi, thereby improving endogenous fibrinolysis (61). Small molecule glycoprotein IIb IIIa inhibitors have also been tested prior to primary PCI (62). The use of glycoprotein IIb IIIa inhibitors as part of a pharmacological reperfusion strategy is based on the fact that TT exacerbates platelet activation through several mechanisms. These include incomplete lysis, platelet release of PAI-1 and thromboxane A2, exposure of clot-bound thrombin, and direct platelet activation, generating a state of "thrombolysis resistance," which in turn may create favorable conditions for rethrombosis or reocclusion (63). An ex vivo study has demonstrated the synergistic effect of abciximab and t-PA by increasing the binding velocity of the thrombolytic agent and lysis rate in platelet-rich areas of the thrombus (64). Another study evaluated platelet activation and aggregation in 20 controls and 51 patients with acute myocardial infarction before and after reperfusion with either t-PA or reteplase or a combination of a reduced-dose of these agents with abciximab. Here, abciximab did not have a role in preventing platelet activation, whereas patients treated with full-dose thrombolytic therapy had increased platelet aggregability at 90 minutes. However, those treated with combined abciximab and reduced-dose reteplase or t-PA achieved more than 80% inhibition of platelet aggregation at 90 minutes, which was sustained at 24 hours. The major conclusions of this study were that the addition of abciximab does not prevent platelet activation, but it adequately inhibits platelet aggregation during the first 24 hours following myocardial infarction (65). An angiographic study comparing 732 patients treated with half-dose thrombolytic therapy plus abciximab and 1662 patients treated with stand-alone thrombolytic therapy has found that patients treated with combination therapy were significantly less likely to have a visible thrombus at 90-minute angiography (25.5% vs. 35.4%; $p < 0.001$). In addition, the absence of an angiographically evident thrombus was associated with an increased frequency of complete ST-segment resolution at 90 minutes (66).

Unfractionated heparin has long been considered an integral adjunct to TT despite a paucity of randomized clinical data to support its use (67). There is evidence that GP IIb IIIa inhibitors help to prevent fibrinolytic induced thrombin generation, although not completely in vitro (68). In IMPACT-AMI (Integrilin to Minimize Platelet Aggregation and Coronary Thrombosis in Acute Myocardial Infarction), eptifibatide had no effect on thrombin generation when heparin was delayed (69). Immediate heparin administration not only reduced thrombin generation but also improved the rate of TIMI 3 flow. In

SPEED and TIMI-14 (Thrombolysis in Myocardial Infarction) (25,26), lower dose heparin was associated with lower TIMI 3 flow rates. Therefore, heparin therapy seems to be necessary when glycoprotein IIb IIIa inhibitors are combined with TT. Lower-doses of heparin than are conventionally used appear to be effective, although the optimal dose remains to be determined.

The safety and efficacy of the combination of full- or reduced-dose thrombolytic therapy and glycoprotein IIb IIIa inhibitors has been studied in a number of clinical trials (Fig. 4) (25,26,69–74). In TIMI-14, TIMI 3 flow in the infarct-related artery at 90 minutes was achieved in 32% of patients treated with abciximab alone, in 62% of patients treated with full-dose t-PA, and in 77% of patients treated with half-dose t-PA and abciximab. There was no increase in major bleeding. The combination of low-dose streptokinase and abciximab was associated with modest improvement of TIMI grade 3 flow as compared with abciximab alone, but with an unacceptable rate of bleeding complications (26).

In the SPEED trial, the primary endpoint of TIMI grade 3 flow at 60 minutes in the infarct-related artery was achieved in 27% of patients treated with abciximab alone, 47% in patients treated with full-dose reteplase, and 62% in patients treated with abciximab and reteplase administered in 2 boluses of 5 U each. The overall mortality of the trial was low (3.8%), with no substantial differences between groups in the occurrence of death and ischemic complications. The combination of abciximab and reteplase was associated with a nonsignificant trend toward increased major bleeding (3.3% in the abciximab-only group versus 9.2% in all combination therapy groups; $p = 0.11$) (25).

Full-dose TT versus combination therapy has been evaluated in GUSTO V. The primary endpoint of 30-day death occurred in 5.9% in the full-dose TT (reteplase) group and 5.6% in the combination therapy (abciximab + 5 U double-bolus reteplase) group ($p = 0.43$). However, there was a 1% absolute increase in intracranial hemorrhage in patients older than 75 years. Other bleeding complications and transfusions occurred more often in

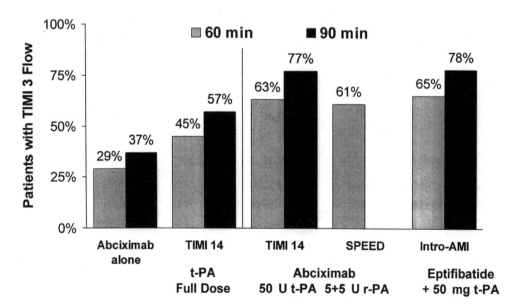

Figure 4 Phase 2 studies with combination of thrombolytic therapy and GP IIb IIIa inhibitors; TIMI 3 grade flow at 60 and 90 minutes.

the combination therapy group (24). The 1-year mortality was identical in both groups (8.4%) (75).

Other trials, including a European study (Integrilin and Low-Dose Thrombolysis in Acute Myocardial Infarction), INTRO-AMI and INTEGRITI, (Results of the Integrilin and Tenecteplase in Acute Myocardial Infarction), with eptifibatide; FASTER-TIMI 24, with tirofiban; and ENTIRE-TIMI 23 and ASSENT-3, with abciximab, have evaluated combination therapy with different TT regimes (streptokinase, alteplase, tenecteplase). Overall, combination therapy causes a modest improvement in TIMI 3 flow compared to TT alone. However, in studies using eptifibatide there were no differences in reinfarction or death rates, but there were increased bleeding complications associated with combination therapy. The use of LMWH has been studied in the ASSENT 3 and the ENTIRE-TIMI 23 studies. In the latter, LMWH actually reduced mortality among patients not undergoing PCI. In ASSENT-3, patients treated with enoxaparin in combination with tenecteplase had similar rates of death, reinfarction, and recurrent ischemia compared with abciximab plus tenecteplase (11.4% vs. 11.1%; p = NS) (72–74,76,77). In summary, these trials suggest that the administration of reduced-dose thrombolytic therapy combined with glycoprotein IIb IIIa inhibitors is associated with higher patency rates compared with stand-alone thrombolysis and is not associated with increased bleeding rates when TT consists of a low-dose fibrin-specific agent. However, the higher patency rates obtained with combination therapy have not translated into improved clinical outcomes in a large phase III trial.

B. Glycoprotein IIb IIIa Inhibitors and Primary PCI

The beneficial effect of abciximab as adjuvant antithrombotic therapy during primary PCI is well established and consistent across randomized clinical trials (53,78–80). A number of studies have reported a stepwise relationship between TIMI 3 flow and time to receiving glycoprotein IIb IIIa receptor inhibitors (Fig. 5). In the GRAPE study, 18% of AMI patients study achieved TIMI 3 flow at a median time of 45 minutes after bolus abciximab in the ED (TIrofibian Given in the Emergency Room before Primary Angioplasty) (60).

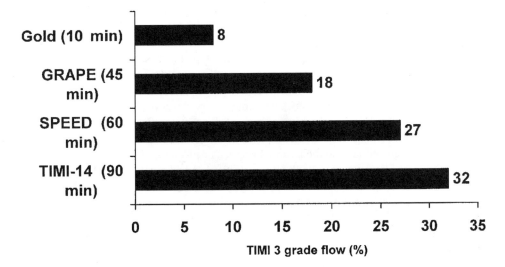

Figure 5 Stepwise relationship between time of abciximab administration and patency of the infarct-related vessel.

The TIGER pilot trial showed that tirofiban administration in the ED 33 minutes prior to coronary angiography in AMI patients was associated with a TIMI 3 grade flow rate of 32%, with significant improvement in myocardial perfusion grade ($p = 0.001$) and corrected TIMI frame count ($p = 0.005$) compared with tirofiban administration in the catheterization laboratory (81). In the RAPPORT study, 483 patients with AMI treated with primary balloon angioplasty were randomized to abciximab or placebo. The use of abciximab was associated with a significant reduction in the incidence of death, reinfarction, or urgent TVR at 30 and 180 days (11.2% vs. 5.8%; $p = 0.03$, and 17.8% vs. 11.6%; $p = 0.05$, respectively) (78). The ISAR-2 (Intracoronary Stenting and Antithrombotic Regimen) study randomized 401 patients with myocardial infarction undergoing PCI within 48 hours of symptom onset to abciximab or placebo before making a decision for stent implantation. At 30 days, the use of abciximab was associated with a 53% relative reduction in the incidence of death or nonfatal reinfarction. This beneficial effect was maintained at 1-year follow-up (79). The ISAR investigators also found that abciximab was associated with a greater increase in coronary Doppler peak flow velocity and improvement in left ventricular wall motion at 2 weeks, compared with placebo. Interestingly, the multivariable analysis showed that the two independent predictors for myocardial wall motion recovery were abciximab administration ($p = 0.017$) and TIMI grade flow prior to intervention ($p = 0.007$) (53).

In the ADMIRAL (Abciximab before Direct angioplasty and stenting in Myocardial Infarction Regarding Abciximab and Long-term follow-up) trial, 300 AMI patients undergoing primary PCI with stent implantation were randomly assigned to abciximab or placebo. At baseline angiography, abciximab-treated patients had higher patency rates compared with placebo (25.8% vs. 10.8%; $p = 0.006$). The procedural success rates were 95.1% and 84.3% in the abciximab and placebo groups, respectively ($p = 0.01$). At 6 months, reocclusion occurred in 2.9% of patients treated with abciximab and in 12.1% treated with placebo ($p = 0.01$). The combined 30-day primary endpoint of death, reinfarction, and urgent TVR occurred in 6% in the abciximab group and in 14.6% in the placebo group ($p = 0.01$). At 6 months, the difference was maintained with 7.4% combined events with abciximab group and 15.9% with placebo ($p = 0.02$) (80).

The CADILLAC trial assessed the efficacy of abciximab and coronary stenting in the setting of myocardial infarction. This was the largest interventional trial in acute myocardial infarction with a total enrollment of 2082 patients allocated in a 2×2 factorial design to stent or balloon angioplasty, and open-label abciximab, or standard anticoagulation with unfractionated heparin. The combination of death, reinfarction, ischemic TVR, or disabling stroke was significantly reduced with abciximab (7.0% vs. 4.6%; $p = 0.01$). Subacute thrombosis was also reduced with abciximab (1.5% vs. 0.4%; $p = 0.01$). The effect of treatment on clinical outcomes was not sustained over time. However, at one year the difference in the combined endpoint was no longer significant (18.4% control vs. 16.9% abciximab; $p = 0.29$). Bleeding rates did not differ between groups (82). The modest effect of abciximab and the lack of sustained benefit in CADILLAC should be cautiously interpreted because abciximab administration was open-labeled and patients were randomized in the catheterization laboratory. Furthermore, patients enrolled in the CADILLAC trial were at lower risk compared with those in the ADMIRAL trial, with higher rates of TIMI grade 3 flow at baseline. A recent meta-analysis of all interventional trials evaluating adjunctive abciximab therapy in acute myocardial infarction has found a 46% significant reduction in the combination of death, reinfarction and ischemic TVR and a nonsignificant trend towards a reduction in the combination of death or reinfarction (OR 0.72, 95% CI 0.49–1.05) (83).

The recently published ACE trial randomized 400 patients to primary stenting with a carbofilm-coated tubular stent alone or stenting plus abciximab. Randomization occurred once the culprit lesion was identified and deemed feasible for stenting. The primary outcome measure was the composite of death, reinfarction, TVR, or stroke at one month. Even though the study design was similar to the CADILLAC trial, with abciximab being administered in the catheterization laboratory, the results were more comparable with the ADMIRAL trial. The primary endpoint occurred in 4.5% in the abciximab group vs. 10.5% in the stenting alone group $(p = 0.023)$. In addition, surrogates for myocardial tissue-level reperfusion showed better ST segment resolution at 30 minutes and smaller scintigraphic infarct size in the abciximab group (Fig. 3) (56).

VII. COMBINING PHARMACOLOGICAL AND MECHANICAL STRATEGIES

More than a decade ago, a number of studies assessed various strategies of PCI following TT (including rescue angioplasty). The TIMI IIA trial randomized 389 patients to immediate balloon angioplasty versus delayed angioplasty 18–48 hours after TT. There were no differences between the groups in ejection fraction at discharge, the primary study endpoint (84). Immediate angioplasty was associated with increased rates of bleeding complications and coronary artery bypass surgery. The TAMI-1 trial was designed to address the same question as TIMI IIA. A total of 386 patients were treated with alteplase achieving a 90-minute patency rate of 75%. Subsequently, 197 patients with an open infarct-related artery were randomized to immediate or delayed angioplasty 7–10 days later. The results showed no differences in left ventricular function recovery and reocclusion rates, but recurrent ischemia occurred more often in the delayed angioplasty group compared with the immediate angioplasty group (16% vs. 5%; $p = 0.01$) (85). In the ECSG study, 367 patients were randomized to immediate balloon angioplasty versus conservative management after thrombolytic therapy administration with alteplase. Patients managed conservatively had lower rates of death, recurrent ischemia, and bleeding complications. The rates of reocclusion (transient or sustained) and recurrent ischemia in the angioplasty group were 23% and 17%, respectively. There were no differences in left ventricular ejection fraction at 10–22 days (86). Finally, a meta-analysis including these and other smaller studies showed no additional benefit with immediate balloon angioplasty following thrombolytic therapy in comparison with a more conservative strategy (87).

The role of intentional TT before PCI has also been assessed. In the SAMI trial, full-dose streptokinase infusion given prior to primary PCI produced identical angioplasty success rate and left ventricular function recovery at 6 months compared to the PCI group alone. However, patients treated with streptokinase needed more emergency bypass surgery (10.3% vs. 1.6%; $p = 0.03$) and more blood transfusions (39% vs. 8%; $p = 0.0001$) when compared with the placebo group (88). The PACT (Plasminogen-activator Angioplasty Compatibility Trial) trial randomized 606 patients with myocardial infarction to a reduced dose of alteplase (50 mg bolus) or placebo, followed by coronary angiography and PCI if TIMI flow grade was 2 or less. If TIMI grade 3 flow was present in the infarct-related artery, another 50 mg bolus of alteplase was administered and the intervention deferred at the discretion of the physician caring for the patient. The results showed that TIMI grade 2 or 3 flow at 49 minutes after thrombolytic therapy administration was present in 61% of patients in the alteplase group and 34% in the placebo group ($p < 0.0001$). Angioplasty procedures were equally successful in the alteplase and placebo groups.

Stents were used in 26% of patients and abciximab in 10%. At 1-week follow-up, there were no differences in left ventricular function between groups, but the timing of complete flow restoration in the infarct-related artery correlated with improvements in left ventricular function. Patients with TIMI 3 flow upon arrival to the catheterization laboratory had a predischarge ejection fraction of 62.4%, patients without TIMI 3 flow upon arrival but with successful mechanical restoration had an ejection fraction of 57.9% *(p < 0.004)*, and patients in whom complete flow restoration was never achieved had an ejection fraction of 54.7%. There were no differences in adverse events between the placebo and alteplase groups. Therefore, PACT was the first randomized clinical trial that demonstrated a favorable effect of adjunctive PCI on left ventricular function preservation (89). There are many reasons to explain the differences in outcomes that were observed in the older trials and PACT. In the first place, a fibrin-specific agent was used in PACT, and this may account for the differences in bleeding rates. Second, streptokinase administration is associated with higher levels of PAI-1 than alteplase, which may correlate with higher reocclusion rates (90). Streptokinase before angioplasty has also been evaluated in the PRAGUE-1 study (transfer for PCI vs. TT vs. combined strategy). Bleeding rates were higher among patients treated with streptokinase than with the other strategies *(p < 0.001)* (91). These event rates were significantly reduced when PCI was performed without prior streptokinase administration, with an incidence of 30-day death and reinfarction rates of 7% and 1%, respectively. Even though stents were implanted in 79% of the cases, PCI performed after streptokinase infusion did not reduce the incidence of reinfarction. Apparently, streptokinase is not appropriate adjuvant thrombolytic therapy. Furthermore, if procedural angiographic complications do occur, then the use of additional intravenous antiplatelet therapies may not be an option because of the unacceptable bleeding rates observed with the administration of glycoprotein IIb IIIa inhibitors after streptokinase infusion (26,72).

In stark contrast, alteplase and immediate stenting have recently been shown to reduce reinfarction compared to TT and delayed PCI. In SIAM III (Southwest German Interventional study in Acute MI), a randomized study of transfer for immediate versus delayed stenting two weeks after TT in AMI patients, immediate stenting was associated with a significant reduction in the combined endpoint of death, MI, and TVR (25.6 vs. 50.6%; *p* = 0.001), which was mainly driven by a reduction in ischemic events (4.9% vs. 28.4%). This was the first study showing superiority of an early invasive strategy after TT (10). More recently, the results of the GRACIA-2 study support this early invasive stenting strategy immediately after TT. A total of 205 patients with ST elevation MI were randomized to TT and primary PCI versus primary PCI alone within 3–12 hours of symptoms. TIMI 3 flow was achieved in 59% of combination therapy patients compared to 14% of primary PCI patients at baseline angiography. The combined endpoints of death, nonfatal infarction, and ischemia-driven TVR were 9% for combination therapy compared to 12% for primary PCI patients. The results of this trial indicate that TT followed by immediate PCI is as effective as primary PCI alone, suggesting that TT may be able to prolong the window to PCI in AMI patients. Further encouragement for this strategy is supported by the lower bleeding rates with facilitated PCI compared to primary PCI (2 vs. 3 %) (11). The SIAM III and GRACIA-2 studies support a combined pharmacological and mechanical reperfusion approach to managing AMI patients.

VIII.   IMPORTANCE OF TIMI 3 FLOW BEFORE PRIMARY PCI

In the SPEED trial, which assessed various doses of reteplase in combination with abciximab, 88% of patients underwent coronary angiography at a median time of 63 minutes. Immediate or facilitated PCI was attempted in 323 (61%) patients, with stents used in 78% of the cases, and an overall success rate of 88%. Compared to conservative management, facilitated PCI was associated with a significant reduction in the combination of death, reinfarction, and recurrent ischemia requiring urgent revascularization (5.6% vs. 16%; $p < 0.001$). Of note, safety endpoints were also reduced with facilitated PCI compared with conservative management. The incidences of major bleeding and transfusion rates were 6.5% versus 8.6% ($p = $ NS) and 9% versus 16% ($p < 0.05$), with facilitated PCI and conservative management, respectively. A major contribution of SPEED was the analysis of PCI procedural outcomes by baseline coronary flow, with higher success rates when PCI was performed on a patent infarct-related artery in comparison to an occluded artery (9). Similar findings were observed in a subanalysis of the PACT trial, with a dramatic reduction of adverse events when TIMI grade 3 flow restoration with thrombolytic therapy was followed by immediate PCI. The composite of death, reinfarction, emergency TVR, and recurrent ischemia occurred in 0% of the 32 patients treated with adjunctive PCI and 43% of the 109 patients managed conservatively ($p < 0.01$) (92).

The importance of an open artery at baseline angiography was further explored in a pooled analysis of the four PAMI trials with a total of 2327 patients with myocardial infarction and fewer than 12 hours of symptoms. This was the first study to demonstrate an association between baseline TIMI 3 flow and 6-month mortality, although these patients were not pretreated with thrombolytic or intravenous antiplatelet agents before arrival at the catheterization laboratory. At baseline, TIMI grade 3 flow was present in 15.7% of infarct-related arteries, TIMI 2 flow in 12.6%, and TIMI 0–1 in 71.2%. Patients with complete spontaneous reperfusion (TIMI grade 3 flow) presented more often in Killip class I and had a more benign hospital course with less heart failure, hypotension, and need for mechanical ventilation compared with patients without complete reperfusion (TIMI grade 2 flow or less). Long-term mortality significantly correlated with lower grades of preprocedural TIMI flow (4.4% in patients with initial TIMI 0/1 flow, 2.8% with TIMI 2 flow, and 0.5% with initial TIMI 3 flow; p for trend = 0.009). Multivariable analysis showed that advanced age, female gender, anterior myocardial infarction location, and preprocedural TIMI grade 2 flow or less were independently associated with a higher long-term mortality. In addition, the presence of a patent infarct-related artery at baseline was associated with better postprocedural outcomes, which in turn was associated with improved 6-month survival. Six-month mortality was 22.2% in patients with postprocedural TIMI 0–1 flow, 6.1% in patients with TIMI 2 flow, and 2.6% in patients with TIMI 3 flow ($p < 0.0001$) (93).

The ON-TIME study recently reported a non statistically significant difference in baseline TIMI 3 flow in patients who received tirofiban before interhospital transfer for primary PCI compared with patients who received tirofiban at the time of PCI (19% vs. 15%; $p = 0.22$). A strategy of early tirofiban was associated with a reduction in TIMI 0 flow rates (44% vs. 59%; $p = 0.0013$) and a reduction in the presence of coronary thrombus (25% vs. 32%; $p = 0.06$) compared with the delayed tirofiban strategy (94).

An observational study carried out in the Netherlands showed similar findings. In the HEAP study, 860 patients with acute myocardial infarction transferred for primary PCI from rural hospitals and pretreated with 500 mg of aspirin and a heparin bolusof ≥5000 U were compared to 842 patients who presented to the emergency room of a tertiary care center. TIMI grade 3 flow was observed in 17% of patients in the transfer group and 10% of patients in the emergency room patients. These results suggest that heparin and aspirin have a modest effect in recanalizing the infarct-related artery. Even though there were no differences in procedural or clinical outcomes between groups, the presence of TIMI grade

3 flow at baseline angiography was significantly correlated with improved procedural results, left ventricular function, and clinical outcomes (95).

IX. MICROVASCULAR FLOW AS A DETERMINANT OF CLINICAL OUTCOMES

Even though successful culprit vessel recanalization is strongly associated with improved clinical outcomes in acute myocardial infarction, it appears that epicardial flow restoration is not enough to achieve sustained clinical benefits. Flow must be restored at the myocardial tissue level. This hypothesis has been tested with various angiographic techniques for myocardial reperfusion assessment beyond epicardial flow (96–99). The corrected TIMI frame count (cTFC) is a reproducible method that allows an objective definition of epicardial flow by quantifying the number of cine frames needed for the contrast to reach standardized distal landmarks (100). A pooled analysis of the TIMI 4, 10A, and 10B trials has shown that a higher cTFC at 90 minutes in the culprit vessel is independently correlated with in-hospital and 30- to 42-day mortality (98). The TIMI myocardial perfusion (TMP) or "myocardial blush" grades consist of a semi-quantitative assessment of the filling and clearance of myocardial contrast after selective coronary injection (TMP 0–3) (99). In a study of patients with myocardial infarction undergoing primary PCI, Stone and colleagues showed that epicardial TIMI grade flow 3 was restored in 94.2% of patients. However, myocardial "blush" grade 3 was present in only 30% of patients. Mortality at 1 year was strongly associated with both epicardial and microvascular flow, with rates of 6.8% with blush grade 3, 13% with blush grade 2, and 22% with blush grade 0 or 1 ($p <$ 0.001) (101). In addition, the angiographic substudy of the TIMI 10B trial has shown a positive relationship between an open microvasculature at 90 minutes and improved post-procedural clinical outcomes. Multivariable analysis adjusting for traditional mortality predictors (age, sex, heart rate, anterior location, and any PCI during the index hospitalization) demonstrated that preprocedural TIMI flow grade 2 or 3 (hazard ratio = 0.32; $p <$ 0.001), cTFC ($p = 0.01$), and pre-TMP grade 2 or 3 (hazard ratio = 0.46; $p = 0.02$) were independent predictors for 2-year mortality (102). Similar findings have been reported from the Zwolle group showing that blush grade post-PCI is the strongest predictor of death at 16 months (RR 2.9, 95% CI 1.4–5.8; $p <$ 0.003) (103).

Data from the STOP-AMI (Stent vs. Thrombolysis for Occluded coronary arteries in Patients with Acute Myocardial Infarction) trials indicate that myocardial salvage/perfusion as assessed by Tc-99m sestamibi scintigraphy depends on the type of reperfusion therapy. Coronary stenting seems to be superior to TT independently of the time to treatment intervals, and this difference in benefit increases with more prolonged time from symptom onset. Furthermore, TT but not PCI was associated with a time-dependent increase in infarct size ($p=0.04$), whereas myocardial salvage decreased in TT but not PCI patients ($p = 0.03$) even as time increased beyond 280 minutes (104). Other studies have shown consistent results, with better ST segment resolution and improved long-term clinical outcomes in patients treated with primary PCI compared with TT (105,106).

An important question to be answered is whether or not primary PCI with stent implantation provides any additional benefit in achieving myocardial tissue–level flow restoration after thrombolytic therapy. As part of the LIMIT-AMI study, 118 patients underwent immediate PCI following thrombolysis. Angiography at 90 minutes showed that TIMI grade 3 flow was present in 54.2% of patients and improved to 87.2% after stent placement ($p < 0.001$). As expected, the median cTFCs decreased from 38 to 21 ($p <$ 0.001). However, microvascular reperfusion was improved in 24%, remained unchanged in 57%, but worsened in 20% of patients. There was a trend towards decreased TMP grade 3 (36.1% to 28.6%) after stent implantation (107). These data suggest that coronary stent implantation after thrombolytic therapy may be associated with a significant increase in epicardial coronary flow, but it is uncertain whether or not this effect is translated into better myocardial tissue–level flow.

There is evidence suggesting that glycoprotein IIb IIIa inhibitors are associated with improved microvascular reperfusion. Data from the TIMI-14 trial has shown that patients treated with combined thrombolytic and abciximab therapies have a more complete ($\geq$70%) ST segment resolution at 90 minutes compared with thrombolytic therapy alone (59% with combination therapy vs. 37% with thrombolysis alone; $p < 0.0001$) (108). The continuous ST segment monitoring substudy of GUSTO V has demonstrated increased speed and stability of ST segment resolution in patients treated with combination therapy versus thrombolytic therapy alone (109). Clinical evidence of the effect of glycoprotein IIb IIIa inhibitors emerge from a subgroup analysis from the ADMIRAL trial suggests that early administration of abciximab is associated with maximal clinical benefit. In 26% of patients who received abciximab in the ambulance or emergency department, the 30-day primary endpoint (death, reinfarction, and urgent TVR) was 2.5% with abciximab versus 21.1% in patients treated with placebo ($p = 0.004$). In contrast, when abciximab was administered in the catheterization laboratory, there were no statistical differences in the occurrence of the primary endpoint between abciximab and placebo (8.3% vs. 12.4%; $p = 0.31$) (80).

Facilitated PCI is currently being assessed in a number of ongoing clinical trials randomizing patients to various pharmacological strategies before PCI versus primary PCI (Table 1).

X. MODULATORS OF RESPONSE TO THERAPY: NECROSIS, INFLAMMATION, PRECONDITIONING

The importance of cardiac and inflammatory biomarkers in risk stratification may help to identify patients who would benefit more from these facilitated reperfusion strategies. There is evidence that the combination of troponin T at baseline and TIMI flow post-PCI predicts mortality and reinfarction risk (110). Elevated CRP at baseline is associated with mortality but not reinfarction. Fibrinogen at admission, PAI, and von Willebrand factor post-MI also predict outcome (111,112). Oxidative stress is present during MI, but its prognostic value is unknown (113). The presence of coronary collateral circulation has no impact on outcome, but a history of preinfarction angina is associated with better ST segment resolution and better TIMI 3 flow (114). It is important, therefore, while we await

Table 1 Ongoing Facilitated PCI Trials in Acute Myocardial Infarction.

	n	Comparison	IIb/IIIa	Enoxaparin
CARESS	2500	PCI vs. tPA 1/2 + IIb/IIIa	Abciximab	
FINESS	4000	PCI vs. rPA 1/2 + IIb/IIIa		
		vs. IIb IIIa alone	Abciximab	
TIGER	6000	PCI vs. TNK 1/2 + IIb/IIIa	Eptifibatide	All
ASSENT-4	4000	PCI vs. TNK + PCI	Avoid with TNK	With TNK
Total	16,500			

ongoing trials that our current strategy takes care of those patients most likely to benefit from it. Elderly, female, renal failure, heart failure, and diabetic patients, patients with previous CABG and prior PCI, as well as AMI patients who present late might be a productive starting point (42,115–117).

XI. NEWER FACILITATING PERFUSION STRATEGIES

A. Beyond Reperfusion: Myocardial Cytoprotectants

Establishing coronary artery flow after recent occlusion is associated with multiple changes in the myocardial tissue bed. Adequate perfusion of the myocardium is essential for a favorable prognosis following revascularization. Several pharmacological agents to prevent myocardial reperfusion injury, including P-selectin inhibitors, magnesium, glucose-insulin-potassium (GIK) infusions, Na+/H+ exchange, inhibitors, adenosine, and complement inhibitors, have been evaluated, with differing outcomes in primary angioplasty AMI patients. Table 2 summarizes the major results of these studies (118–132).

Other pharmacological therapies have specifically been evaluated in stent-related outcomes in AMI patients. Alpha-adrenergic blockade with phentolamine has been associated with improvement in myocardial perfusion and postischemic LV dysfunction (133). Ketanserin, a serotonin antagonist, has been shown to improve microvascular function (48). Targeted deletion of matrix metalloproteinase-9 gene protects the heart from the no-reflow phenomenon post-MI, and nicorandil, a potassium channel blocker, has also been shown to improve microvascular function (134,135). Antiplatelet agents, in particular glycoprotein receptor antagonists, have led to a 50% reduction in primary endpoints when used in association with coronary stents, especially in high-risk patients (80,82). Clopidogrel is currently being evaluated in AMI patients in the CLARITY and COMMIT trials.

Other novel approaches for myocardial function recovery include the injection of intracoronary autologous bone marrow cells. In a small randomized trial, 30 patients underwent autologous bone marrow cell injection into the infarct-related coronary artery using a balloon catheter between 4 and 8 days post-MI. The results were promising, with a significant improvement in left ventricular function at 5–6 months (136).

B. New Approaches and Technologies

Distal embolization occurs in 9–15% of primary PCI, and it is associated with a 44% 5-year mortality rate (52,137). Efforts to prevent distal embolization have included the deployment of distal protection devices, thrombus aspiration, as well as adjunctive pharmacotherapy with glycoprotein IIb IIIa inhibitors, calcium and potassium channel blockers, adenosine, nitroprusside, and intracoronary thrombolytic therapy (138–145).

Studied distal protection devices in the AMI setting include the FilterWire-EX and the Guardwire (Percusurge). A recent study compared 53 AMI patients treated with stenting and distal embolic protection with the use of a FilterWire, with matched controls. The embolic protection device was associated with improved TIMI frame count, blush grade, and ST segment resolution, as well as lower peak CK levels and increased LV wall motion indices and ejection fraction. The FilterWire was successfully deployed in 89% of patients, and inspection of the filter postprocedure revealed macroscopic particles in 34% of the cases. Distal embolization occurred in 2% of patients with the FilterWire and 15% in PCI-alone patients (138). The Guardwire has only been tested in a small number of AMI

Table 2 Studies with Agents to Prevent Myocardial Reperfusion Injury Following Reperfusion Therapy

Trial	Agent	Mechanism of action	n	Endpoint	Results
TAMI 9	Fluosol	↓ neutrophils, ↑ O_2 delivery	430	Infarct size, EF	Negative (22% vs. 17%)
ISIS-4	Magnesium	Membrane stabilization	58,050	35-day mortality	Negative (7.6 vs.7.2%)
MAGIC			6,213	30-day mortality	Negative (16.3% vs. 16.2%)
CORE Pilot	RheothRx	↑ O_2 delivery	114	Infarct size	Positive (16 vs. 26%)
CORE			2,607	Death, shock, re-MI	Negative (14.0 vs. 12.6%)
ECLA-GIK	GIK	Metabolic protection	407	Death, CHF, V.Fib	Positive (11.9% vs. 20.1%)
ECLA-GIK 2			10,000	30-day mortality	Ongoing
DIGAMI			620	3.4 years	Positive (33% vs. 44%)
GIPS			940	30-day mortality	Negative (4.8% vs. 5.8%)
CREATE	2 × 2 Factorial LMWH and GIK		15,000	7-day death, reinfarction, stroke	Ongoing
EMIP-FR	Trimetazidine	↓H^+, free radicals, neutrophils	19,665	35-day mortality	Negative (12.2% vs. 12.3%)
Flaherty	hSOD	↓Free radicals	120	EF	Negative (no effect)
RAPSODY	rPSGL-Ig	P-selectin inhibitor	598	Infarct size	Negative (no effect)
AMISTAD	Adenosine	↓neutrophils, vasodilator, metabolic modulation	236	Infarct size	Positive (20% vs. 13%)
AMISTAD-2			2,118	6-month death/CHF	Negative (16% vs. 18%)
HALT/LIMIT	Anti-CD18	↓neutrophils	400+	Infarct size	Negative (no effect)
Rupprecht	Cariporide	Na^+/H^+ exchange inhibitor	100	EF, infarct size	Positive (50% vs. 40%)
ESCAMI	Eniporide		1,389	Infarct size	Negative (no effect)
COMPLY	Pexelizumab + TT	Complement inhibitor	960	Infarct size	Negative (no effect)
COMMA	Pexelizumab + PCI		943	Infarct size	Negative primary endpoint Mortality benefit (1.8 vs. 5.9%; $p = 0.014$)

patients with 88% procedural success (141). Nonrandomized data have shown that the use of the Guardwire in the setting of primary angioplasty is associated with significant improvement in myocardial perfusion and 30-day outcomes, compared with the combination of angioplasty and tirofiban (146). Further evaluation is still needed before any firm conclusions are drawn with the use of this device.

Adjunctive intracoronary thrombectomy with devices such as X-sizer or Angiojet has been shown to be associated with improved ST segment resolution and myocardial perfusion in AMI patients (143,147). Beran et al. reported 83% ST segment resolution rates and 90% TIMI 3 flow using the X-sizer catheter compared to 52% and 84% in controls, respectively. MACE rates (6.1%) were identical in both groups. The device could not be advanced in 3 of the 30 X-sizer patients (142).

Nakagawa and colleagues (144) have reported 94% TIMI 3 flow at 6-month follow up using the Angiojet thrombectomy catheter in 31 AMI patients. In 94% of patients, adjunctive PCI was performed after Angiojet, with 40% of patients requiring stents. However, restenosis occurred in 21% of patients, possibly due to lower stent use. There was no major in-hospital or follow-up events. Angiojet was successfully deployed in all intended patients, although a change of guide catheter was initially required at first in two patients. One patient had a coronary perforation and three patients had a branch occlusion, but no cases of no-reflow were observed. In a study enrolling 91 acute MI patients assessing the Intracoronary Aspiration Thrombectomy (ICAT) catheter, 43 patients underwent ICAT followed by PCI and 48 underwent PCI alone. Recanalization of the culprit vessel was achieved in 58% of patients with ICAT alone and 91% after adjunctive PCI. Thrombi were aspirated in 70% of patients. However, no differences in procedural success and complication rates were observed with either strategy (145). Another aspiration device is the "rescue" percutaneous thrombectomy system, which is a 4.5 F aspiration catheter with an oblique tip to facilitate passage through the lesion. The proximal end has an extension tube connected to a vacuum pump with a collection bottle. The catheter can be moved to different positions within the vessel to remove embolized material. In a small study with 50 AMI patients, TIMI 3 flow was established after thrombus aspiration in 82% of the cases (148). Kaplan et al. (149) reported the application of the transluminal extraction catheter (TEC), which cuts and aspirates thrombus and atheromatous material, in 100 patients with acute coronary syndromes including primary reperfusion for AMI in 32% of cases, postinfarct angina in 28% of cases, thrombolytic failure in 40% of cases, and cardiogenic shock in 11% of cases. Overall procedural success was achieved in 94% of patients. Distal embolization, no reflow, or both occurred in 6% of patients. The use of adjunctive angioplasty substantially improved the residual stenosis after TEC from 56 to 28% ($p < 0.001$), and the TIMI 2 or 3 flow after TEC from 89 to 96% with an in-hospital mortality of 5% (149).

Ultraviolet excimer light at 308 nm can potentially vaporize thrombus and ablate the underlying plaque, enhancing thrombolytic therapy and glycoprotein IIb IIIa inhibitor efficacy. Small case series have reported the feasibility and safety of laser-guided thrombectomy (150).

Endovascular ultrasound fibrinolysis to dissolve coronary thrombus and reduce distal embolization showed early promise, but its use in saphenous vein grafts has been associated with poor angiographic outcomes and increased incidence of acute ischemic complications. Higher success rates (98%) have been seen in native vessels. In a pilot study, ultrasound lysis achieved TIMI 3 flow in 87% of AMI patients. Adjunct PCI after ultrasound thrombolysis produced a final residual stenosis of 20%. TIMI 3 flow was maintained at 24-hour angiographic follow-up. One patient developed recurrent ischemia at 5 days with reocclusion at the treated site, requiring emergent CABG. The ACUTE trial to assess ultrasound lysis in acute myocardial infarction is ongoing (151).

Transcutaneous low-energy ultrasound has been shown to facilitate systemic thrombolysis inducing a structural alteration of the fibrin network. These changes seem to enhance fluid permeation, increasing the transport of a thrombolytic agent into the thrombus. A pilot study designed to evaluate the feasibility and safety of adjunctive transcutaneous ultrasound therapy with TT in 25 AMI patients showed a 90-minute patency rate of 84% (152).

Catheter-delivered low-dose fibrinolytic therapy as a routine adjunct to PCI is another logical treatment option. Delivering fibrinolytic therapy to the site of a fibrin-rich red thrombus may be another way to facilitate perfusion in AMI patients (140). Other treatment strategies including aqueous oxygen and cooling catheters may also facilitate reperfusion and myocardial preservation in AMI patients (153,154).

XII. CONCLUSION

Randomized data consistently show that primary PCI is the preferred strategy for managing AMI. As more data emerge from randomized clinical trials favoring a transfer for PCI strategy over on-site thrombolytic therapy at remote rural hospitals, it is expected that transfer to tertiary care centers for primary PCI will become the standard of care for patients with acute myocardial infarction in the near future (Fig. 6). Therefore, more patients with ongoing myocardial necrosis will be exposed to significant treatment delays during transport. In fact, the 30-day mortality of the transferred patients in the DANAMI-2 and PRAGUE-2 trials was approximately 6%, substantially higher than the 3% mortality reported for similar patients enrolled in the PAMI, ADMIRAL, and CADILLAC trials (155). Recent studies suggest that early PCI with stenting is safe and effective after administration of low-dose thrombolysis with fibrin-specific agents combined with glycoprotein IIb IIIa inhibitors. Moreover, different studies consistently show that primary PCI on a

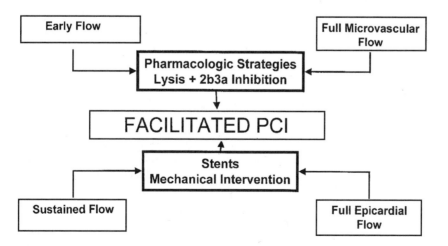

Figure 6 Synergy between pharmacological and mechanical reperfusion strategies in acute myocardial infarction.

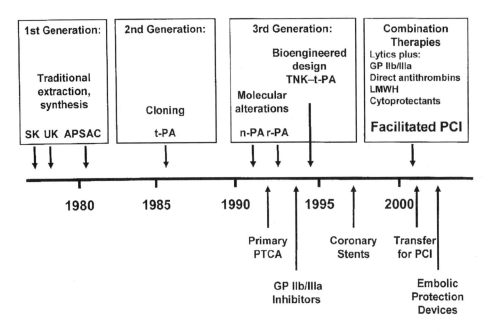

Figure 7 Evolution of reperfusion therapies.

patent infarct-related artery is associated with improved angiographic and clinical outcomes. Direct stenting after full-dose TT is reemerging as a potential perfusion strategy, but issues with bleeding need to be overcome first. It appears also that glycoprotein IIb IIIa inhibition attenuates the microvascular dysfunction associated with reperfusion and stent implantation, achieving higher degrees of myocardial tissue–level reperfusion.

Facilitated angioplasty may soon become the ultimate step in reperfusion strategies for acute myocardial infarction, offering the unique ability to achieve synergism between pharmacological and mechanical strategies (Fig. 7). However, the role of facilitated PCI needs to be established in large multicenter randomized clinical trials. The role of adjunctive mechanical and pharmacological strategies such as distal protection devices, thrombectomy, ultrasound, cooling catheters, cytoprotectant agents, and newer antithrombotic agents in facilitating perfusion in acute myocardial infarction patients requires further evaluation.

REFERENCES

1. Ryan TJ, Antman EM, Brooks NH, Califf RM, Hillis LD, Hiratzka LF, et al. 1999 update: ACC/AHA guidelines for the management of patients with acute myocardial infarction. A report of the American College of Cardiology/American Heart Association Task Force on Practice Guidelines (Committee on Management of Acute Myocardial Infarction). J Am Coll Cardiol 1999; 34(3):890–911.
2. Ross AM, Coyne KS, Moreyra E, Reiner JS, Greenhouse SW, Walker PL, et al. Extended mortality benefit of early postinfarction reperfusion. GUSTO-I Angiographic Investigators. Global Utilization of Streptokinase and Tissue Plasminogen Activator for Occluded Coronary Arteries Trial. Circulation 1998; 97(16):1549–1556.
3. Ohman EM, Califf RM, Topol EJ, Candela R, Abbottsmith C, Ellis S, et al. Consequences of reocclusion after successful reperfusion therapy in acute myocardial infarction. TAMI Study Group. Circulation 1990; 82(3):781–791.

4. Lincoff AM, Topol EJ. Illusion of reperfusion. Does anyone achieve optimal reperfusion during acute myocardial infarction? Circulation 1993; 88(3):1361–1374.

5. Indications for fibrinolytic therapy in suspected acute myocardial infarction: collaborative overview of early mortality and major morbidity results from all randomised trials of more than 1000 patients. Fibrinolytic Therapy Trialists' (FTT) Collaborative Group. Lancet 1994; 343(8893):311–322.

6. Gebel JM, Sila CA, Sloan MA, Granger CB, Mahaffey KW, Weisenberger J, et al. Thrombolysis-related intracranial hemorrhage: a radiographic analysis of 244 cases from the GUSTO-1 trial with clinical correlation. Global Utilization of Streptokinase and Tissue Plasminogen Activator for Occluded Coronary Arteries. Stroke 1998; 29(3):563–569.

7. Weaver WD, Simes RJ, Betriu A, Grines CL, Zijlstra F, Garcia E, et al. Comparison of primary coronary angioplasty and intravenous thrombolytic therapy for acute myocardial infarction: a quantitative review. JAMA 1997; 278(23):2093–2098.

8. Keeley EC, Boura JA, Grines CL. Primary angioplasty versus intravenous thrombolytic therapy for acute myocardial infarction: a quantitative review of 23 randomised trials. Lancet 2003; 361(9351):13–20.

9. Herrmann HC, Moliterno DJ, Ohman EM, Stebbins AL, Bode C, Betriu A, et al. Facilitation of early percutaneous coronary intervention after reteplase with or without abciximab in acute myocardial infarction: results from the SPEED (GUSTO-4 Pilot) trial. J Am Coll Cardiol 2000; 36(5):1489–1496.

10. Scheller B, Hennen B, Hammer B, Walle J, Hofer C, Hilpert V, et al. Beneficial effects of immediate stenting after thrombolysis in acute myocardial infarction. J Am Coll Cardiol 2003; 42(4):634–641.

11. Aviles FF. Randomised trial comparing primary PCI versus facilitated intervention (TNK + stenting) in patients with STEAMI (Gracia 2 trial). In: European Congress of Cardiology; 2003; Vienna.

12. Loubeyre C, Lefevre T, Louvard Y, Dumas P, Piechaud JF, Lanore JJ, et al. Outcome after combined reperfusion therapy for acute myocardial infarction, combining pre-hospital thrombolysis with immediate percutaneous coronary intervention and stent. Eur Heart J 2001; 22(13):1128–1135.

13. Boersma E, Maas AC, Deckers JW, Simoons ML. Early thrombolytic treatment in acute myocardial infarction: reappraisal of the golden hour. Lancet 1996; 348(9030):771–775.

14. Randomised trial of intravenous streptokinase, oral aspirin, both, or neither among 17,187 cases of suspected acute myocardial infarction: ISIS-2. ISIS-2 (Second International Study of Infarct Survival) Collaborative Group. Lancet 1988; 2(8607):349–360.

15. The GUSTO Angiographic Investigators. The effects of tissue plasminogen activator, streptokinase, or both on coronary-artery patency, ventricular function, and survival after acute myocardial infarction. N Engl J Med 1993; 329(22):1615–1622.

16. Morrow DA, Antman EM, Sayah A, Schuhwerk KC, Giugliano RP, deLemos JA, et al. Evaluation of the time saved by prehospital initiation of reteplase for ST-elevation myocardial infarction: results of The Early Retavase-Thrombolysis in Myocardial Infarction (ER-TIMI) 19 trial. J Am Coll Cardiol 2002; 40(1):71–77.

17. Rawles J. GREAT: 10 year survival of patients with suspected acute myocardial infarction in a randomised comparison of prehospital and hospital thrombolysis. Heart 2003; 89(5):563–564.

18. Bonnefoy E, Lapostolle F, Leizorovicz A, Steg G, McFadden EP, Dubien PY, et al. Primary angioplasty versus prehospital fibrinolysis in acute myocardial infarction: a randomised study. Lancet 2002; 360(9336):825–829.

19. Wallentin L, Goldstein P, Armstrong PW, Granger CB, Adgey AA, Arntz HR, et al. Efficacy and safety of tenecteplase in combination with the low-molecular-weight heparin enoxaparin or unfractionated heparin in the prehospital setting: the Assessment of the Safety and Efficacy of a New Thrombolytic Regimen (ASSENT)-3 PLUS randomized trial in acute myocardial infarction. Circulation 2003; 108(2):135–142.

20. Thiemann DR, Coresh J, Schulman SP, Gerstenblith G, Oetgen WJ, Powe NR. Lack of benefit for intravenous thrombolysis in patients with myocardial infarction who are older than 75 years. Circulation 2000; 101(19):2239–2246.

21. Intravenous NPA for the treatment of infarcting myocardium early; InTIME-II, a double-blind comparison of single-bolus lanoteplase vs accelerated alteplase for the treatment of patients with acute myocardial infarction. Eur Heart J 2000; 21(24):2005–2013.

22. Single-bolus tenecteplase compared with front-loaded alteplase in acute myocardial infarction: the ASSENT-2 double-blind randomised trial. Assessment of the Safety and Efficacy of a New Thrombolytic Investigators. Lancet 1999; 354(9180):716–722.

23. A comparison of reteplase with alteplase for acute myocardial infarction. The Global Use of Strategies to Open Occluded Coronary Arteries (GUSTO III) Investigators. N Engl J Med 1997; 337(16):1118–1123.

24. Topol EJ. Reperfusion therapy for acute myocardial infarction with fibrinolytic therapy or combination reduced fibrinolytic therapy and platelet glycoprotein IIb/IIIa inhibition: the GUSTO V randomised trial. Lancet 2001; 357(9272):1905–1914.

25. Trial of abciximab with and without low-dose reteplase for acute myocardial infarction. Strategies for Patency Enhancement in the Emergency Department (SPEED) Group. Circulation 2000; 101(24):2788–2794.

26. Antman EM, Giugliano RP, Gibson CM, McCabe CH, Coussement P, Kleiman NS, et al. Abciximab facilitates the rate and extent of thrombolysis: results of the thrombolysis in myocardial infarction (TIMI) 14 trial. The TIMI 14 Investigators. Circulation 1999; 99(21):2720–2732.

27. Savonitto S, Armstrong PW, Lincoff AM, Jia G, Sila CA, Booth J, et al. Risk of intracranial haemorrhage with combined fibrinolytic and glycoprotein IIb/IIIa inhibitor therapy in acute myocardial infarction. Dichotomous response as a function of age in the GUSTO V trial. Eur Heart J 2003; 24(20):1807–1814.

28. Hartzler GO, Rutherford BD, McConahay DR, Johnson WL, Jr., McCallister BD, Gura GM, Jr., et al. Percutaneous transluminal coronary angioplasty with and without thrombolytic therapy for treatment of acute myocardial infarction. Am Heart J 1983; 106(5 pt 1):965–973.

29. Grines CL, Browne KF, Marco J, Rothbaum D, Stone GW, O'Keefe J, et al. A comparison of immediate angioplasty with thrombolytic therapy for acute myocardial infarction. The Primary Angioplasty in Myocardial Infarction Study Group. N Engl J Med 1993; 328(10):673–1419.

30. Zijlstra F, Hoorntje JC, de Boer MJ, Reiffers S, Miedema K, Ottervanger JP, et al. Long-term benefit of primary angioplasty as compared with thrombolytic therapy for acute myocardial infarction. N Engl J Med 1999; 341(19):1413–1419.

31. Zahn R, Schiele R, Schneider S, Gitt AK, Wienbergen H, Seidl K, et al. Primary angioplasty versus intravenous thrombolysis in acute myocardial infarction: can we define subgroups of patients benefiting most from primary angioplasty? Results from the pooled data of the Maximal Individual Therapy in Acute Myocardial Infarction Registry and the Myocardial Infarction Registry. J Am Coll Cardiol 2001; 37(7):1827–1835.

32. Zahn R, Schiele R, Schneider S, Gitt AK, Wienbergen H, Seidl K, et al. Decreasing hospital mortality between 1994 and 1998 in patients with acute myocardial infarction treated with primary angioplasty but not in patients treated with intravenous thrombolysis. Results from the pooled data of the Maximal Individual Therapy in Acute Myocardial Infarction (MITRA) Registry and the Myocardial Infarction Registry (MIR). J Am Coll Cardiol 2000; 36(7):2064–2071.

33. Cannon CP, Gibson CM, Lambrew CT, Shoultz DA, Levy D, French WJ, et al. Relationship of symptom-onset-to-balloon time and door-to-balloon time with mortality in patients undergoing angioplasty for acute myocardial infarction. JAMA 2000; 283(22):2941–2947.

34. Angeja BG, Gibson CM, Chin R, Frederick PD, Every NR, Ross AM, et al. Predictors of door-to-balloon delay in primary angioplasty. Am J Cardiol 2002; 89(10):1156–1161.

35. Van de Werf F, Ardissino D, Betriu A, Cokkinos DV, Falk E, Fox KA, et al. Management of acute myocardial infarction in patients presenting with ST-segment elevation. The Task Force on the Management of Acute Myocardial Infarction of the European Society of Cardiology. Eur Heart J 2003; 24(1):28–66.

36. Aversano T, Aversano LT, Passamani E, Knatterud GL, Terrin ML, Williams DO, et al. Thrombolytic therapy vs primary percutaneous coronary intervention for myocardial infarc-

tion in patients presenting to hospitals without on-site cardiac surgery: a randomized controlled trial. JAMA 2002; 287(15):1943–1951.

37. Vermeer F, Oude Ophuis AJ, vd Berg EJ, Brunninkhuis LG, Werter CJ, Boehmer AG, et al. Prospective randomised comparison between thrombolysis, rescue PTCA, and primary PTCA in patients with extensive myocardial infarction admitted to a hospital without PTCA facilities: a safety and feasibility study. Heart 1999; 82(4):426–431.

38. Grines CL, Westerhausen DR, Jr., Grines LL, Hanlon JT, Logemann TL, Niemela M, et al. A randomized trial of transfer for primary angioplasty versus on-site thrombolysis in patients with high-risk myocardial infarction: the Air Primary Angioplasty in Myocardial Infarction study. J Am Coll Cardiol 2002; 39(11):1713–1719.

39. Widimsky P, Budebreve, sbreve, nsky T, Voracbreve, Groch L, et al. Long distance transport for primary angioplasty vs immediate thrombolysis in acute myocardial infarction. Final results of the randomized national multicentre trial-PRAGUE-2. Eur Heart J 2003; 24(1):94–104.

40. Andersen HR, Nielsen TT, Rasmussen K, Thuesen L, Kelbaek H, Thayssen P, et al. A comparison of coronary angioplasty with fibrinolytic therapy in acute myocardial infarction. N Engl J Med 2003; 349(8):733–742.

41. Dalby M, Bouzamondo A, Lechat P, Montalescot G. Transfer for primary angioplasty versus immediate thrombolysis in acute myocardial infarction: a meta-analysis. Circulation 2003; 108(15):1809–1814.

42. Zijlstra F, Patel A, Jones M, Grines CL, Ellis S, Garcia E, et al. Clinical characteristics and outcome of patients with early (<2 h), intermediate (2–4 h) and late (>4 h) presentation treated by primary coronary angioplasty or thrombolytic therapy for acute myocardial infarction. Eur Heart J 2002; 23(7):550–557.

43. Steg PG, Bonnefoy E, Chabaud S, Lapostolle F, Dubien PY, Cristofini P, et al. Impact of time to treatment on mortality after prehospital fibrinolysis or primary angioplasty: data from the CAPTIM randomized clinical trial. Circulation 2003; 108(23):2851–2856.

44. Nallamothu BK, Bates ER. Percutaneous coronary intervention versus fibrinolytic therapy in acute myocardial infarction: is timing (almost) everything? Am J Cardiol 2003; 92(7):824–826.

45. Zhu MM, Feit A, Chadow H, Alam M, Kwan T, Clark LT. Primary stent implantation compared with primary balloon angioplasty for acute myocardial infarction: a meta-analysis of randomized clinical trials. Am J Cardiol 2001; 88(3):297–301.

46. Grines CL, Cox DA, Stone GW, Garcia E, Mattos LA, Giambartolomei A, et al. Coronary angioplasty with or without stent implantation for acute myocardial infarction. Stent Primary Angioplasty in Myocardial Infarction Study Group. N Engl J Med 1999; 341(26):1949–1956.

47. Stone GW, Grines CL, Cox DA, Garcia E, Tcheng JE, Griffin JJ, et al. Comparison of angioplasty with stenting, with or without abciximab, in acute myocardial infarction. N Engl J Med 2002; 346(13):957–966.

48. Leosco D, Fineschi M, Pierli C, Fiaschi A, Ferrara N, Bianco S, et al. Intracoronary serotonin release after high-pressure coronary stenting. Am J Cardiol 1999; 84(11):1317–1322.

49. Aymong ED, Curtis MJ, Youssef M, Graham MM, Shewchuk L, Leschuk W, et al. Abciximab attenuates coronary microvascular endothelial dysfunction after coronary stenting. Circulation 2002; 105(25):2981–2985.

50. Serrano CV, Jr., Ramires JA, Venturinelli M, Arie S, D'Amico E, Zweier JL, et al. Coronary angioplasty results in leukocyte and platelet activation with adhesion molecule expression. Evidence of inflammatory responses in coronary angioplasty. J Am Coll Cardiol 1997; 29(6):1276–1283.

51. Mukherjee D, Moliterno DJ. Achieving tissue-level perfusion in the setting of acute myocardial infarction. Am J Cardiol 2000; 85(8A):39C-46C.

52. Henriques JP, Zijlstra F, Ottervanger JP, de Boer MJ, van 't Hof AW, Hoorntje JC, et al. Incidence and clinical significance of distal embolization during primary angioplasty for acute myocardial infarction. Eur Heart J 2002; 23(14):1112–1117.

53. Neumann FJ, Blasini R, Schmitt C, Alt E, Dirschinger J, Gawaz M, et al. Effect of glycoprotein IIb/IIIa receptor blockade on recovery of coronary flow and left ventricular function after

the placement of coronary-artery stents in acute myocardial infarction. Circulation 1998; 98(24):2695–2701.

54. Schomig A, Kastrati A, Dirschinger J, Mehilli J, Schricke U, Pache J, et al. Coronary stenting plus platelet glycoprotein IIb/IIIa blockade compared with tissue plasminogen activator in acute myocardial infarction. Stent versus Thrombolysis for Occluded Coronary Arteries in Patients with Acute Myocardial Infarction Study Investigators. N Engl J Med 2000; 343(6):385–391.

55. Kastrati A, Mehilli J, Dirschinger J, Schricke U, Neverve J, Pache J, et al. Myocardial salvage after coronary stenting plus abciximab versus fibrinolysis plus abciximab in patients with acute myocardial infarction: a randomised trial. Lancet 2002; 359(9310):920–925.

56. Antoniucci D, Rodriguez A, Hempel A, Valenti R, Migliorini A, Vigo F, et al. A randomized trial comparing primary infarct artery stenting with or without abciximab in acute myocardial infarction. J Am Coll Cardiol 2003; 42(11):1879–1885.

57. Saia F, Lemos PA, Lee CH, Arampatzis CA, Hoye A, Degertekin M, et al. Sirolimus-eluting stent implantation in ST-elevation acute myocardial infarction: a clinical and angiographic study. Circulation 2003; 108(16):1927–1929.

58. Collet JP, Montalescot G, Lesty C, Soria J, Mishal Z, Thomas D, et al. Disaggregation of in vitro preformed platelet-rich clots by abciximab increases fibrin exposure and promotes fibrinolysis. Arterioscler Thromb Vasc Biol 2001; 21(1):142–148.

59. Gold HK, Garabedian HD, Dinsmore RE, Guerrero LJ, Cigarroa JE, Palacios IF, et al. Restoration of coronary flow in myocardial infarction by intravenous chimeric 7E3 antibody without exogenous plasminogen activators. Observations in animals and humans. Circulation 1997; 95(7):1755–1759.

60. van den Merkhof LF, Zijlstra F, Olsson H, Grip L, Veen G, Bar FW, et al. Abciximab in the treatment of acute myocardial infarction eligible for primary percutaneous transluminal coronary angioplasty. Results of the Glycoprotein Receptor Antagonist Patency Evaluation (GRAPE) pilot study. J Am Coll Cardiol 1999; 33(6):1528–1532.

61. Collet JP, Montalescot G, Lesty C, Mishal Z, Soria J, Choussat R, et al. Effects of Abciximab on the architecture of platelet-rich clots in patients with acute myocardial infarction undergoing primary coronary intervention. Circulation 2001; 103(19):2328–2331.

62. Cutlip DE, Cove CJ, Irons D, Kalaria V, Le M, Cronmiller H, et al. Emergency room administration of eptifibatide before primary angioplasty for ST elevation acute myocardial infarction and its effect on baseline coronary flow and procedure outcomes. Am J Cardiol 2001; 88(1):A6, 62–64.

63. Cannon CP. Overcoming thrombolytic resistance: rationale and initial clinical experience combining thrombolytic therapy and glycoprotein IIb/IIIa receptor inhibition for acute myocardial infarction. J Am Coll Cardiol 1999; 34(5):1395–1402.

64. Collet JP, Montalescot G, Lesty C, Weisel JW. A structural and dynamic investigation of the facilitating effect of glycoprotein IIb/IIIa inhibitors in dissolving platelet-rich clots. Circ Res 2002; 90(4):428–434.

65. Coulter SA, Cannon CP, Ault KA, Antman EM, Van de Werf F, Adgey AA, et al. High levels of platelet inhibition with abciximab despite heightened platelet activation and aggregation during thrombolysis for acute myocardial infarction: results from TIMI (Thrombolysis in Myocardial Infarction) 14. Circulation 2000; 101(23):2690–2695.

66. Gibson CM, de Lemos JA, Murphy SA, Marble SJ, McCabe CH, Cannon CP, et al. Combination therapy with abciximab reduces angiographically evident thrombus in acute myocardial infarction: a TIMI 14 substudy. Circulation 2001; 103(21):2550–2554.

67. Collins R, Peto R, Baigent C, Sleight P. Aspirin, heparin, and fibrinolytic therapy in suspected acute myocardial infarction. N Engl J Med 1997; 336(12):847–860.

68. Campbell KR, Ohman EM, Cantor W, Lincoff AM. The use of glycoprotein IIb/IIIa inhibitor therapy in acute ST-segment elevation myocardial infarction: current practice and future trends. Am J Cardiol 2000; 85(8A):32C-38C.

69. Ohman EM, Kleiman NS, Gacioch G, Worley SJ, Navetta FI, Talley JD, et al. Combined accelerated tissue-plasminogen activator and platelet glycoprotein IIb/IIIa integrin receptor

blockade with Integrilin in acute myocardial infarction. Results of a randomized, placebo-controlled, dose-ranging trial. IMPACT-AMI Investigators. Circulation 1997; 95(4):846–854.

70. Kleiman NS, Ohman EM, Califf RM, George BS, Kereiakes D, Aguirre FV, et al. Profound inhibition of platelet aggregation with monoclonal antibody 7E3 Fab after thrombolytic therapy. Results of the Thrombolysis and Angioplasty in Myocardial Infarction (TAMI) 8 Pilot Study. J Am Coll Cardiol 1993; 22(2):381–389.

71. Combining thrombolysis with the platelet glycoprotein IIb/IIIa inhibitor lamifiban: results of the Platelet Aggregation Receptor Antagonist Dose Investigation and Reperfusion Gain in Myocardial Infarction (PARADIGM) trial. J Am Coll Cardiol 1998; 32(7):2003–2010.

72. Ronner E, van Kesteren HA, Zijnen P, Altmann E, Molhoek PG, van der Wieken LR, et al. Safety and efficacy of eptifibatide vs placebo in patients receiving thrombolytic therapy with streptokinase for acute myocardial infarction. A phase II dose escalation, randomized, double-blind study. Eur Heart J 2000; 21(18):1530–156.

73. Brener SJ, Zeymer U, Adgey AA, Vrobel TR, Ellis SG, Neuhaus KL, et al. Eptifibatide and low-dose tissue plasminogen activator in acute myocardial infarction: the integrilin and low-dose thrombolysis in acute myocardial infarction (INTRO AMI) trial. J Am Coll Cardiol 2002; 39(3):377–386.

74. Giugliano RP, Roe MT, Harrington RA, Gibson CM, Zeymer U, Van de Werf F, et al. Combination reperfusion therapy with eptifibatide and reduced-dose tenecteplase for ST-elevation myocardial infarction: results of the integrilin and tenecteplase in acute myocardial infarction (INTEGRITI) Phase II Angiographic Trial. J Am Coll Cardiol 2003; 41(8):1251–1260.

75. Lincoff AM, Califf RM, Van de Werf F, Willerson JT, White HD, Armstrong PW, et al. Mortality at 1 year with combination platelet glycoprotein IIb/IIIa inhibition and reduced-dose fibrinolytic therapy vs conventional fibrinolytic therapy for acute myocardial infarction: GUSTO V randomized trial. Jama 2002; 288(17):2130–2135.

76. Efficacy and safety of tenecteplase in combination with enoxaparin, abciximab, or unfractionated heparin: the ASSENT-3 randomised trial in acute myocardial infarction. Lancet 2001; 358(9282):605–613.

77. Antman EM, Louwerenburg HW, Baars HF, Wesdorp JC, Hamer B, Bassand JP, et al. Enoxaparin as adjunctive antithrombin therapy for ST-elevation myocardial infarction: results of the ENTIRE-Thrombolysis in Myocardial Infarction (TIMI) 23 Trial. Circulation 2002; 105(14):1642–1649.

78. Brener SJ, Barr LA, Burchenal JE, Katz S, George BS, Jones AA, et al. Randomized, placebo-controlled trial of platelet glycoprotein IIb/IIIa blockade with primary angioplasty for acute myocardial infarction. ReoPro and Primary PTCA Organization and Randomized Trial (RAPPORT) Investigators. Circulation 1998; 98(8):734–741.

79. Neumann FJ, Kastrati A, Schmitt C, Blasini R, Hadamitzky M, Mehilli J, et al. Effect of glycoprotein IIb/IIIa receptor blockade with abciximab on clinical and angiographic restenosis rate after the placement of coronary stents following acute myocardial infarction. J Am Coll Cardiol 2000; 35(4):915–921.

80. Montalescot G, Barragan P, Wittenberg O, Ecollan P, Elhadad S, Villain P, et al. Platelet glycoprotein IIb/IIIa inhibition with coronary stenting for acute myocardial infarction. N Engl J Med 2001; 344(25):1895–1903.

81. Lee DP, Herity NA, Hiatt BL, Fearon WF, Rezaee M, Carter AJ, et al. Adjunctive platelet glycoprotein IIb/IIIa receptor inhibition with tirofiban before primary angioplasty improves angiographic outcomes: results of the TIrofiban Given in the Emergency Room before Primary Angioplasty (TIGER-PA) pilot trial. Circulation 2003; 107(11):1497–1501.

82. Tcheng JE, Kandzari DE, Grines CL, Cox DA, Effron MB, Garcia E, et al. Benefits and risks of abciximab use in primary angioplasty for acute myocardial infarction: the Controlled Abciximab and Device Investigation to Lower Late Angioplasty Complications (CADILLAC) trial. Circulation 2003; 108(11):1316–1323.

83. Kandzari DE, Hasselblad V, Tcheng JE, Stone GW, Califf RM, Brener SJ, et al. Improved clinical outcomes with abciximab therapy in acute myocardial infarction: a systematic overview of randomized clinical trials. J Am Coll Cardiol 2003; 41(6):333A.

84. Immediate vs delayed catheterization and angioplasty following thrombolytic therapy for acute myocardial infarction. TIMI II A results. The TIMI Research Group. JAMA 1988; 260(19):2849–2858.

85. Topol EJ, Califf RM, George BS, Kereiakes DJ, Abbottsmith CW, Candela RJ, et al. A randomized trial of immediate versus delayed elective angioplasty after intravenous tissue plasminogen activator in acute myocardial infarction. N Engl J Med 1987; 317(10):581–588.

86. Simoons ML, Arnold AE, Betriu A, de Bono DP, Col J, Dougherty FC, et al. Thrombolysis with tissue plasminogen activator in acute myocardial infarction: no additional benefit from immediate percutaneous coronary angioplasty. Lancet 1988; 1(8579):197–203.

87. Michels KB, Yusuf S. Does PTCA in acute myocardial infarction affect mortality and reinfarction rates? A quantitative overview (meta-analysis) of the randomized clinical trials. Circulation 1995; 91(2):476–485.

88. O'Neill WW, Weintraub R, Grines CL, Meany TB, Brodie BR, Friedman HZ, et al. A prospective, placebo-controlled, randomized trial of intravenous streptokinase and angioplasty versus lone angioplasty therapy of acute myocardial infarction. Circulation 1992; 86(6):1710–1717.

89. Ross AM, Coyne KS, Reiner JS, Greenhouse SW, Fink C, Frey A, et al. A randomized trial comparing primary angioplasty with a strategy of short-acting thrombolysis and immediate planned rescue angioplasty in acute myocardial infarction: the PACT trial. PACT investigators. Plasminogen-activator Angioplasty Compatibility Trial. J Am Coll Cardiol 1999; 34(7):1954–1962.

90. Paganelli F, Alessi MC, Morange P, Maixent JM, Levy S, Vague IJ. Relationship of plasminogen activator inhibitor-1 levels following thrombolytic therapy with rt-PA as compared to streptokinase and patency of infarct related coronary artery. Thromb Haemost 1999; 82(1):104–108.

91. Widimsky P, Groch L, Zelizko M, Aschermann M, Bednar F, Suryapranata H. Multicentre randomized trial comparing transport to primary angioplasty vs immediate thrombolysis vs combined strategy for patients with acute myocardial infarction presenting to a community hospital without a catheterization laboratory. The PRAGUE study. Eur Heart J 2000; 21(10):823–831.

92. Ross AM, Coyne KS, Reiner JS, Traboulsi M, Fung AY, Thompson C, et al. Very early PTCA of infarct arteries with TIMI 3 flow is associated With improved clinical outcomes. J Am Coll Cardiol 2000; 35(2, suppl. A):403.

93. Stone GW, Cox D, Garcia E, Brodie BR, Morice MC, Griffin J, et al. Normal flow (TIMI-3) before mechanical reperfusion therapy is an independent determinant of survival in acute myocardial infarction: analysis from the primary angioplasty in myocardial infarction trials. Circulation 2001; 104(6):636–641.

94. van't Hof AW. Does pre-transportation treatment with tirofiban improve patency in acute myocardial infarction patients who are referred for percutaneous coronary intervention (ON-TIME)? In: European Congress of Cardiology; 2003; Vienna; 2003.

95. Zijlstra F, Ernst N, de Boer MJ, Nibbering E, Suryapranata H, Hoorntje JC, et al. Influence of prehospital administration of aspirin and heparin on initial patency of the infarct-related artery in patients with acute ST elevation myocardial infarction. J Am Coll Cardiol 2002; 39(11):1733–1737.

96. Ito H, Maruyama A, Iwakura K, Takiuchi S, Masuyama T, Hori M, et al. Clinical implications of the 'no reflow' phenomenon. A predictor of complications and left ventricular remodeling in reperfused anterior wall myocardial infarction. Circulation 1996; 93(2):223–228.

97. Wu KC, Zerhouni EA, Judd RM, Lugo-Olivieri CH, Barouch LA, Schulman SP, et al. Prognostic significance of microvascular obstruction by magnetic resonance imaging in patients with acute myocardial infarction. Circulation 1998; 97(8):765–772.

98. Gibson CM, Murphy SA, Rizzo MJ, Ryan KA, Marble SJ, McCabe CH, et al. Relationship between TIMI frame count and clinical outcomes after thrombolytic administration. Thrombolysis In Myocardial Infarction (TIMI) Study Group. Circulation 1999; 99(15):1945–1950.

99. Gibson CM, Cannon CP, Murphy SA, Ryan KA, Mesley R, Marble SJ, et al. Relationship of TIMI myocardial perfusion grade to mortality after administration of thrombolytic drugs. Circulation 2000; 101(2):125–130.

100. Gibson CM, Cannon CP, Daley WL, Dodge JT, Jr., Alexander B, Jr., Marble SJ, et al. TIMI frame count: a quantitative method of assessing coronary artery flow. Circulation 1996; 93(5):879–888.

101. Stone GW, Peterson MA, Lansky AJ, Dangas G, Mehran R, Leon MB. Impact of normalized myocardial perfusion after successful angioplasty in acute myocardial infarction. J Am Coll Cardiol 2002; 39(4):591–597.

102. Gibson CM, Cannon CP, Murphy SA, Marble SJ, Barron HV, Braunwald E. Relationship of the TIMI myocardial perfusion grades, flow grades, frame count, and percutaneous coronary intervention to long-term outcomes after thrombolytic administration in acute myocardial infarction. Circulation 2002; 105(16):1909–1913.

103. Henriques JP, Zijlstra F, Van 't Hof AW, De Boer MJ, Dambrink JH, Gosselink M, et al. Angiographic assessment of reperfusion in acute myocardial infarction by myocardial blush grade. Circulation 2003; 107(16):2115–2119.

104. Schomig A, Ndrepepa G, Mehilli J, Schwaiger M, Schuhlen H, Nekolla S, et al. Therapy-dependent influence of time-to-treatment interval on myocardial salvage in patients with acute myocardial infarction treated with coronary artery stenting or thrombolysis. Circulation 2003; 108(9):1084–1088.

105. Zeymer U, Schroder R, Machnig T, Neuhaus KL. Primary percutaneous transluminal coronary angioplasty accelerates early myocardial reperfusion compared to thrombolytic therapy in patients with acute myocardial infarction. Am Heart J 2003; 146(4):686–691.

106. Berrocal DH, Cohen MG, Spinetta AD, Ben MG, Rojas Matas CA, Gabay JM, et al. Early reperfusion and late clinical outcomes in patients presenting with acute myocardial infarction randomly assigned to primary percutaneous coronary intervention or streptokinase. Am Heart J 2003; 146(6):E22.

107. Gibson CM, Frisch D, Murphy SA, Gourlay SG, Gibbons R, Baran KW, et al. The relationship of intracoronary stent placement following thrombolytic therapy to tissue level perfusion. J Thromb Thrombolysis 2002; 13(2):63–68.

108. de Lemos JA, Antman EM, Gibson CM, McCabe CH, Giugliano RP, Murphy SA, et al. Abciximab improves both epicardial flow and myocardial reperfusion in ST-elevation myocardial infarction. Observations from the TIMI 14 trial. Circulation 2000; 101(3):239–243.

109. Krucoff MW, Green CL, Langer A, Gibler WB, Armstrong PW, Trollinger KM, et al. The Abciximab ST-Recovery ON AMI (ASTRONAMI) GUSTO V substudy: enhanced early speed, stability, and quality of reperfusion with anti-platelet augmented thrombolytic therapy for ST-Elevation AMI. J Am Coll Cardiol 2002; 39, (suppl A (5):

110. Giannitsis E, Muller-Bardorff M, Lehrke S, Wiegand U, Tolg R, Weidtmann B, et al. Admission troponin T level predicts clinical outcomes, TIMI flow, and myocardial tissue perfusion after primary percutaneous intervention for acute ST-segment elevation myocardial infarction. Circulation 2001; 104(6):630–635.

111. De Sutter J, De Buyzere M, Gheeraert P, Van de Wiele C, Voet J, De Pauw M, et al. Fibrinogen and C-reactive protein on admission as markers of final infarct size after primary angioplasty for acute myocardial infarction. Atherosclerosis 2001; 157(1):189–196.

112. Collet JP, Montalescot G, Vicaut E, Ankri A, Walylo F, Lesty C, et al. Acute release of plasminogen activator inhibitor-1 in ST-segment elevation myocardial infarction predicts mortality. Circulation 2003; 108(4):391–394.

113. Diaz-Araya G, Nettle D, Castro P, Miranda F, Greig D, Campos X, et al. Oxidative stress after reperfusion with primary coronary angioplasty: lack of effect of glucose-insulin-potassium infusion. Crit Care Med 2002; 30(2):417–421.

114. Takahashi T, Anzai T, Yoshikawa T, Maekawa Y, Asakura Y, Satoh T, et al. Effect of preinfarction angina pectoris on ST-segment resolution after primary coronary angioplasty for acute myocardial infarction. Am J Cardiol 2002; 90(5):465–469.

115. Lee KL, Woodlief LH, Topol EJ, Weaver WD, Betriu A, Col J, et al. Predictors of 30-day mortality in the era of reperfusion for acute myocardial infarction. Results from an international trial of 41,021 patients. GUSTO-I Investigators. Circulation 1995; 91(6):1659–1668.

116. Morrow DA, Antman EM, Giugliano RP, Cairns R, Charlesworth A, Murphy SA, et al. A simple risk index for rapid initial triage of patients with ST-elevation myocardial infarction: an InTIME II substudy. Lancet 2001; 358(9293):1571–1575.

117. Thiemann DR. Primary angioplasty for elderly patients with myocardial infarction: theory, practice and possibilities. J Am Coll Cardiol 2002; 39(11):1729–1732.

118. Early administration of intravenous magnesium to high-risk patients with acute myocardial infarction in the Magnesium in Coronaries (MAGIC) Trial: a randomised controlled trial. Lancet 2002; 360(9341):1189–1196.

119. Kopecky SL, Aviles RJ, Bell MR, Lobl JK, Tipping D, Frommell G, et al. A randomized, double-blinded, placebo-controlled, dose-ranging study measuring the effect of an adenosine agonist on infarct size reduction in patients undergoing primary percutaneous transluminal coronary angioplasty: the ADMIRE (AmP579 Delivery for Myocardial Infarction REduction) study. Am Heart J 2003; 146(1):146–152.

120. Rupprecht HJ, vom Dahl J, Terres W, Seyfarth KM, Richardt G, Schultheibeta HP, et al. Cardioprotective effects of the Na(+)/H(+) exchange inhibitor cariporide in patients with acute anterior myocardial infarction undergoing direct PTCA. Circulation 2000; 101(25):2902–2908.

121. Zeymer U, Suryapranata H, Monassier JP, Opolski G, Davies J, Rasmanis G, et al. The Na(+)/H(+) exchange inhibitor eniporide as an adjunct to early reperfusion therapy for acute myocardial infarction. Results of the evaluation of the safety and cardioprotective effects of eniporide in acute myocardial infarction (ESCAMI) trial. J Am Coll Cardiol 2001; 38(6):1644–1650.

122. Mahaffey KW, Puma JA, Barbagelata NA, DiCarli MF, Leesar MA, Browne KF, et al. Adenosine as an adjunct to thrombolytic therapy for acute myocardial infarction: results of a multicenter, randomized, placebo-controlled trial: the Acute Myocardial Infarction STudy of ADenosine (AMISTAD) trial. J Am Coll Cardiol 1999; 34(6):1711–1720.

123. Ross AM. Acute Myocardial Infarction Study of Adenosine II (Amistad II). In: American College of Cardiology, 51st Annual Scientific Session; 2002; Atlanta.

124. Sodi-Pallares D, Testelli M, Fishleder F. Effects of an intravenous infusion of a potassium-insulin-glucose solution on the electrocardiographic signs of myocardial infarction. Am J Cardiol 1962; 9:166–181.

125. Malmberg K. Prospective randomised study of intensive insulin treatment on long term survival after acute myocardial infarction in patients with diabetes mellitus. DIGAMI (Diabetes Mellitus, Insulin Glucose Infusion in Acute Myocardial Infarction) Study Group. BMJ 1997; 314(7093):1512–1515.

126. Diaz R, Paolasso EA, Piegas LS, Tajer CD, Moreno MG, Corvalan R, et al. Metabolic modulation of acute myocardial infarction. The ECLA (Estudios Cardiologicos Latinoamerica) Collaborative Group. Circulation 1998; 98(21):2227–2234.

127. van der Horst IC, Zijlstra F, van't Hof AW, Doggen CJ, de Boer MJ, Suryapranata H, et al. Glucose-insulin-potassium infusion inpatients treated with primary angioplasty for acute myocardial infarction: the glucose-insulin-potassium study: a randomized trial. J Am Coll Cardiol 2003; 42(5):784–791.

128. Granger CB, Mahaffey KW, Weaver WD, Theroux P, Hochman JS, Filloon TG, et al. Pexelizumab, an anti-C5 complement antibody, as adjunctive therapy to primary percutaneous coronary intervention in acute myocardial infarction: the COMplement inhibition in Myocardial infarction treated with Angioplasty (COMMA) trial. Circulation 2003; 108(10):1184–1190.

129. Mahaffey KW, Granger CB, Nicolau JC, Ruzyllo W, Weaver WD, Theroux P, et al. Effect of pexelizumab, an anti-C5 complement antibody, as adjunctive therapy to fibrinolysis in acute myocardial infarction: the COMPlement inhibition in myocardial infarction treated with thromboLYtics (COMPLY) trial. Circulation 2003; 108(10):1176–1183.

130. Wall TC, Califf RM, Blankenship J, Talley JD, Tannenbaum M, Schwaiger M, et al. Intravenous Fluosol in the treatment of acute myocardial infarction. Results of the Thrombolysis and Angioplasty in Myocardial Infarction 9 Trial. TAMI 9 Research Group. Circulation 1994; 90(1):114–120.

131. Effects of RheothRx on mortality, morbidity, left ventricular function, and infarct size in patients with acute myocardial infarction. Collaborative Organization for RheothRx Evaluation (CORE). Circulation 1997; 96(1):192–201.

132. Tanguay JF, Krucoff MW, Gibbons RJ, Chavez E, Sosa-Liprandi A, Molina-Viamonte V, et al. Efficacy of a novel P-selectin antagonist, rPSGL-Ig for reperfusion therapy in acute myocardial infarction: the RAPSODY trial. J Am Coll Cardiol 2003; 41(6):404A.

133. Gregorini L, Marco J, Kozakova M, Palombo C, Anguissola GB, Marco I, et al. Alpha-adrenergic blockade improves recovery of myocardial perfusion and function after coronary stenting in patients with acute myocardial infarction. Circulation 1999; 99(4):482–490.

134. Romanic AM, Harrison SM, Bao W, Burns-Kurtis CL, Pickering S, Gu J, et al. Myocardial protection from ischemia/reperfusion injury by targeted deletion of matrix metalloproteinase-9. Cardiovasc Res 2002; 54(3):549–558.

135. Ito H, Taniyama Y, Iwakura K, Nishikawa N, Masuyama T, Kuzuya T, et al. Intravenous nicorandil can preserve microvascular integrity and myocardial viability in patients with reperfused anterior wall myocardial infarction. J Am Coll Cardiol 1999; 33(3):654–660.

136. Wollert KC. Randomized-controlled clinical trial of intracoronary autologous bone marrow cell transplantation post myocardial infarction. In: American Heart Association Scientific Sessions 2003; November 9–12, 2003; Orlando, FL.

137. Topol EJ, Yadav JS. Recognition of the importance of embolization in atherosclerotic vascular disease. Circulation 2000; 101(5):570–580.

138. Limbruno U, Micheli A, De Carlo M, Amoroso G, Rossini R, Palagi C, et al. Mechanical prevention of distal embolization during primary angioplasty: safety, feasibility, and impact on myocardial reperfusion. Circulation 2003; 108(2):171–176.

139. Michaels AD, Appleby M, Otten MH, Dauterman K, Ports TA, Chou TM, et al. Pretreatment with intragraft verapamil prior to percutaneous coronary intervention of saphenous vein graft lesions: results of the randomized, controlled vasodilator prevention on no-reflow (VAPOR) trial. J Invasive Cardiol 2002; 14(6):299–302.

140. Clinical experience with intracoronary tissue plasminogen activator: results of a multicenter registry. Intracoronary t-PA Registry Investigators. Cathet Cardiovasc Diagn 1995; 34(3):196–201.

141. Belli G, Pezzano A, De Biase AM, Bonacina E, Silva P, Salvade P, et al. Adjunctive thrombus aspiration and mechanical protection from distal embolization in primary percutaneous intervention for acute myocardial infarction. Catheter Cardiovasc Interv 2000; 50(3):362–370.

142. Beran G, Lang I, Schreiber W, Denk S, Stefenelli T, Syeda B, et al. Intracoronary thrombectomy with the X-sizer catheter system improves epicardial flow and accelerates ST-segment resolution in patients with acute coronary syndrome: a prospective, randomized, controlled study. Circulation 2002; 105(20):2355–2360.

143. Rinfret S, Katsiyiannis PT, Ho KK, Cohen DJ, Baim DS, Carrozza JP, et al. Effectiveness of rheolytic coronary thrombectomy with the AngioJet catheter. Am J Cardiol 2002; 90(5):470–476.

144. Nakagawa Y, Matsuo S, Kimura T, Yokoi H, Tamura T, Hamasaki N, et al. Thrombectomy with AngioJet catheter in native coronary arteries for patients with acute or recent myocardial infarction. Am J Cardiol 1999; 83(7):994–999.

145. Murakami T, Mizuno S, Takahashi Y, Ohsato K, Moriuchi I, Arai Y, et al. Intracoronary aspiration thrombectomy for acute myocardial infarction. Am J Cardiol 1998; 82(7):839–844.

146. Yip HK, Wu CJ, Chang HW, Fang CY, Yang CH, Chen SM, et al. Effect of the PercuSurge GuardWire device on the integrity of microvasculature and clinical outcomes during primary transradial coronary intervention in acute myocardial infarction. Am J Cardiol 2003; 92(11):1331–1335.

147. Napodano M, Pasquetto G, Sacca S, Cernetti C, Scarabeo V, Pascotto P, et al. Intracoronary thrombectomy improves myocardial reperfusion in patients undergoing direct angioplasty for acute myocardial infarction. J Am Coll Cardiol 2003; 42(8):1395–1402.

148. van Ommen V, Michels R, Heymen E, van Asseldonk J, Bonnier H, Vainer J, et al. Usefulness of the rescue PT catheter to remove fresh thrombus from coronary arteries and bypass grafts in acute myocardial infarction. Am J Cardiol 2001; 88(3):306–308.

149. Kaplan BM, Larkin T, Safian RD, O'Neill WW, Kramer B, Hoffmann M, et al. Prospective study of extraction atherectomy in patients with acute myocardial infarction. Am J Cardiol 1996; 78(4):383–388.

150. Topaz O, Bernardo NL, Shah R, McQueen RH, Desai P, Janin Y, et al. Effectiveness of excimer laser coronary angioplasty in acute myocardial infarction or in unstable angina pectoris. Am J Cardiol 2001; 87(7):849–855.

151. Rosenschein U, Brosh D, Halkin A. Coronary ultrasound thrombolysis: from acute myocardial infarction to saphenous vein grafts and beyond. Curr Interv Cardiol Rep 2001; 3(1):5–9.

152. Cohen MG, Tuero E, Bluguermann J, Kevorkian R, Berrocal DH, Carlevaro O, et al. Transcutaneous ultrasound-facilitated coronary thrombolysis during acute myocardial infarction. Am J Cardiol 2003; 92(4):454–457.

153. Dixon SR, Bartorelli AL, Marcovitz PA, Spears R, David S, Grinberg I, et al. Initial experience with hyperoxemic reperfusion after primary angioplasty for acute myocardial infarction: results of a pilot study utilizing intracoronary aqueous oxygen therapy. J Am Coll Cardiol 2002; 39(3):387–392.

154. Dixon SR, Whitbourn RJ, Dae MW, Grube E, Sherman W, Schaer GL, et al. Induction of mild systemic hypothermia with endovascular cooling during primary percutaneous coronary intervention for acute myocardial infarction. J Am Coll Cardiol 2002; 40(11):1928–1934.

155. Cohen MG, Ohman EM. The everlasting effect of primary angioplasty—even after transport? Can J Cardiol 2003; 19(10):1119–1122.

17-1

Coronary Radiation Therapy for the Prevention of Restenosis

Christoph Hehrlein and Christoph Bode
University Hospital, Freiburg, Germany

I. INTRODUCTION

Intracoronary radiation therapy, also called intravascular brachytherapy (IVB), is a novel strategy in the early phase of a routine clinical trial for prevention of restenosis after percutanous intracoronary angioplasty (PTCA) in Europe. The results of major randomized studies in particular the SCRIPPS coronary restenosis prevention trial with a 3-year follow-up, have shown efficacy for VBT. Multiple clinical studies have been completed in the United States, and several brachytherapy systems are now under investigation in Europe. However, recent results from clinical trials have demonstrated important deleterious effects, such as late thrombosis and edge effect. Their mechanisms are still poorly understood and require further investigation. After discussing the main pathophysiological mechanisms by which radiation therapy reduces restenosis, this review describes the different delivery systems and radioactive isotopes and summarizes the main results of clinical studies, especially the side effects of IVB.

II. PATHOPHYSIOLOGY OF RESTENOTIC LESION FORMATION

Two major mechanisms, neointimal hyperplasia and negative vascular remodeling ("shrinkage"), explain the development of restenosis after PTCA. The process of restenosis starts with platelet adhesion at site of endothelial lesion, followed by local thrombus formation. Cytokine release from platelets stimulates proliferation and migration of medial smooth muscle cells (SMCs), leading to neointimal hyperplasia (1). The proliferative process begins 2–3 days after PTCA and is maintained for several weeks. After this phase, extracellular matrix synthesis is responsible for 80% of the plaque volume after 3 months. Scott et al. demonstrated the role of adventitial myofibroblasts in neointimal formation (2). However, the mechanisms of negative vascular remodeling after PTCA are not fully understood. One mechanism might be adventitial fibrosis (3,4). Chronic vascular constriction causing negative vascular remodeling after PTCA is prevented by stent implantation. However, the placement of a stent exacerbates neointimal regrowth via excessive inflammatory and proliferative stimuli in the acute phase of PTCA.

III. MECHANISMS OF RESTENOSIS PREVENTION BY IONIZING RADIATION

Irradiation provokes cellular lesions in a number of biologically active molecules. DNA is the major target of irradiation in a process involving reactive oxygen species production. The hydroxyl radical (OH∞) is the most active species, inducing DNA breaks, DNA-DNA crossing, or alteration in DNA base pairs. These reactions are responsible for the induction of cell death by ionizing radiation. Radiation can also induce modulation of the expression and/or activity of various genes, particularly related to pro- and anti-inflammatory cytokines, or cell-signalling molecules. These molecules may exert at least part of the effects of radiation on cell function. In vascular tissue, irradiation inhibits migration of medial SMCs into the intima and synthesis of the extracellular matrix (5,6). This effect is responsible for the inhibition of neointima formation at early and late stages in rabbit arteries (Fig. 1). This effect persists up to 6 months in an experimental restenosis model in swine (7). Endovascular irradiation has demonstrated an inhibitory effect on adventitial fibrosis, modulating unfavorable vascular remodeling (8,9). Verin and coworkers showed that cell death via apoptosis pathway is one of the phenomena implicated in the effects of irradiation on restenosis (10). Furthermore, Rubin et al. have postulated a major influence of monocytes/macrophages on the restenosis process and its inhibition by radiation treatment (11). Inflammatory infiltration of macrophages recruited from the vasa vasorum occurs during the initial phase of vascular injury after PTCA in human. These macrophages may represent the main target of irradiation during the restenosis process, explained by their high radiosensitivity (11).

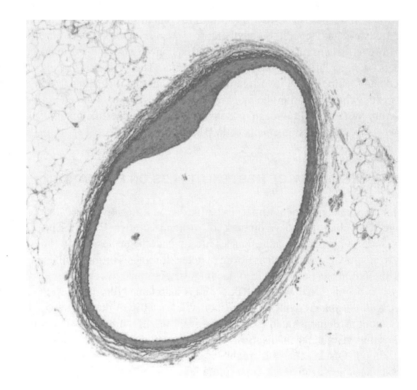

Figure 1. Effects of radiation on neointima formation in rabbit ateries.

IV. RADIOISOTOPES IN USE FOR CORONARY RADIOTHERAPY

Several radioisotopes differing in their physical characteristics and methods of delivery (Table 1) are available.

A. Beta-Radiation

Beta-radiation is characterized by electron production, interacting with other electrons to induce energy transfer to the matter. The weak penetration distance of these electrons within biological media requires only little radioprotection precautions for the staff (radiation can be stopped by a plastic barrier); however β-radiation is inadequate for targeting high-diameter vessels (> 4 mm). The application time is short (approximately 5 minutes). The major concern about b-radiation remains the crucial importance of source centering inside the vessel, particularly in eccentric lesions.

B. Gamma-Radiation

In this type of emitter energy is transmitted to the matter via a photon. ^{192}Ir is the most commonly used radioelement, with a half-life of 74 days. γ-Irradiation penetrates strongly into the biological tissue, rendering the problem of centering less crucial than with b-radiation. Treatment time to deliver an adequate dose is longer compared to β-irradiation: 10–20 minutes. Problems of radiation safety are of greater concern. Total body irradiation absorbed by the patient is higher when compared to b-radiation.

C. Dosimetry

The optimum dose required for IVB is currently not known. Doses may vary from 1 to 2 mm from the source center and are generally in the 12–18 Gy range in most clinical trials, with a minimum dose of 10 Gy and maximum of 30 Gy (12).

V. TECHNIQUES OF INTRACORONARY RADIATION DELIVERY: RADIOACTIVE STENTS

Palmaz-Schatz (PS) or BX stents are most commonly used. They are activated with a pure b-emitter (^{32}P) or a mixture of β- and γ-emitter (^{55}Co, ^{57}Ni). Three methods of activation are used: (a) the metallic stents are bombarded with charged particles (deuterons or protons) derived from a cyclotron, (b) the surface of the stent is covered ("covered stents")

Table 1 Radioactive Elements Used for IVB

Radioactive element	Emitter	Half-life	Mode of delivery
^{32}P	β	13-14 d	Stents
^{90}Y	β	64 h	Catheter
^{90}Sr/^{90}Y	β	28 yr	Catheter
^{192}Ir	γ	74 d	Catheter
^{99}T	β- and χ-ray	6 h	Liquid
^{188}Re	β- and χ-ray	17 h	Catheter + liquid

with the isotope (e.g., ^{32}P), or (c) the isotope is directly implanted into the metallic stent (13). Several experimental studies have shown the efficacy of radioactive stents for neointimal proliferation in restenosis in the vascular walls of rabbit iliac arteries (14,15) or pig coronary arteries (16,17). The first radioactive stent implantation in Europe took place in June 1997 at the University of Heidelberg in Germany. In the European pilot phase of the IRIS (Isostent for Restenosis Intervention Study) trials, 11 patients received Palmaz-Schatz stents impregnated with ^{32}P with activity levels between 1.5 and 3 μCi. The Heidelberg study revealed a high restenosis rate of 54% due to new lumen narrowing at the stent margins. These so-called "edge effects" occurred at the articulation of the radioactive Palmaz-Schatz stent and the distal stent margins. The early Americam IRIS results using radioactive Palmaz-Schatz stents in 22 patients with de novo lesions did not reveal edge effects after 6 months, but within-stent restenosis was not significantly reduced(18). The Italian group of Colombo and coworkers and the Rotterdam group of Serruys et al. implanted the second-generation radioactive stent without an articulation. The so-called candy-wrapper restenosis is a lumen renarrowing or edge effect at the proximal and distal stent margins with in-stent inhibition of restenosis (19).

VI. CATHETER-BASED IRRADIATION-DELIVERY SYSTEMS

A. Gamma-Emitters

Radioactivity is delivered via an afterloader loaded using a 192 Ir wire placed manually (Best Medical) or automatically (Nucletron) at the side of dilatation (e.g., SCRIPPS, WRIST, GAMMA, ARTISTIC, ARREST, SMARTS trials). In the United States the Checkmate' Gamma-Emitter will be approved by the FDA for intracoronary use shortly.

B. Beta-Emitters

Different beta isotopes (^{32}P, ^{90}Sr/Y, or ^{90}Y) with a variety of delivery catheters are available: noncentered systems using source trains (Novoste, Norcross, GA), wire systems centered with either a helical (Guidant, Santa Clara, CA) or segmented balloon (Boston Scientific, Namic, MA), and angioplasty balloons impregreated with radioisotopes (Radiance, Palo Alto, CA).

VII. AAPM RECOMMENDATIONS FOR USE OF CORONARY RADIATION SYSTEMS

In 1999 the American Association of Physics and Medicine (AAPM) and the American Brachytherapy Society (ABS) published recommendations for the use of IVB (20). They recommended that for catheter-based systems the dose specifications be prescribed at 2 mm from source center to cover the advential zone. The presence of a radiation oncologist in the catheterization laboratory is necessary to manage source, storage, transfer, placement, and dose prescription. Finally, the ABS recommends radioprotective precautions, with permanent badges to be worn by the staff exposed to radiation.

The major clinical studies, especially SCRIPPS, have identified consensus areas concerning the potential indications of IVB for restenosis. Suitable patients are limited to those presenting increased risk for restenosis (diffuse restenosis, in-stent restenosis, restenosis in diabetic patients, multifocal or very long lesions). Exclusion criteria include prior irradiation to the vessel site, unprotected left main disease, pregnant women, age < 18 years, totally occluded vessels, left ventricular ejection fraction < 20–30%, and myocardial infarction within 72 hours.

VIII. MILESTONES IN CLINICAL INVESTIGATIONS OF CORONARY RADIATION THERAPY

Major clinical studies on IVB have focused on treatment of in-stent restenosis and less frequently on restenosis prevention on de novo lesions (Table 2) or on radioactive stents.

A. De Novo Lesions

The Venezuelan experience of Condado et al. first reported a feasibility study on 21 patients with 22 de novo lesions, 18 of which received 25 Gy of ^{192}Ir to 1.5 mm from the source center following PTCA. The authors reported a 26% (6/22 lesions) binary restenosis rate at 6-month follow-up (21). These results were stable at 2-year follow-up.

Verin et al. reported the results of a pilot study with a cohort of 15 patients with de novo lesions: 6 patients out of 15 presented with angiographic restenosis. These results can be explained by the low doses used in the study: the dose delivered to the inner surface of the artery was 18 Gy (^{90}Y), which corresponds to a dose of 8 Gy 2 mm from the center of the source (22).

In the BERT (Beta Energy Restenosis Trial) study, 23 patients were treated with a b-emitter in native coronary arteries. After PTCA, doses ranging from 12 to 16 Gy were delivered at 2 mm (23). The rate of restenosis was 15% for the target lesion and 24.3% for the target vessel 6 months after coronary intervention (24).

PREVENT (Proliferation Reduction with Vascular Energy Trial) is a randomized prospective study with 72 patients, 47 (65%) of presented with whom de novo lesions and received 0, 16, 20, or 24 Gy (25). At the lesion site the restenosis rate for the target vessel was 6% in the irradiated group and 33% in the placebo group. At the target vessel, the restenosis rates were similar (25% in the irradiated group and 44% in the placebo group) mainly due to edge effects. More infarctions were found in the treated group (11%) than the control group (6%).

In the European Schneider study, 181 patients native arteries were treated with a b-emitter, with doses of 9, 12, 15, and 18 Gy prescribed at 1 mm. At the lesion site the restenosis rate was 27.5, 15.8, 17.8, and 8.3%, respectively. In contrast, the target vessel revascularization was 13.3, 6.7, 6.5, and 6.7%, respectively.

Table 2 First Pilot Studies with Intravascular Brachytherapy on De Novo Coronary Artery Lesions

Investigator	Study	Isotope	Dose (Gy)	No. of patients	RR (C vs. RA)
Condado	Venezuelin	^{192}I	18–25	22	27%
Verin	GENEVA	^{90}Y	18	15	40%
King	BERT	^{90}Sr/Y	12–16	23	15%
Raizner	PREVENT	^{32}P	16–24	250	6 vs. 33%
Erbel	Schneider	^{90}Y	9–18	181	8.3 vs. 27%

RR = restenosis rate; RA = radiation group; C = control group.

B. Restenosis Lesions

Clinical trials on radiation effects on treated restenotic lesions, particularly intrastent injury, have shown encouraging results (Table 3).

Teirstein et al. reported the results of the first randomized and double-blinded study (SCRIPPS) using ^{192}Ir in 55 patients, who received either PTCA alone or PTCA with stent implantation (26 patients in the treated group, 29 patients in the placebo group) (26). SCRIPPS reports the longest follow-up period (3 years) (27). At 6-month follow-up the restenosis rate was 17% in the treated group compared to 54% in the placebo group. At 3 years the combined criteria of death, myocardial infarction, or revascularization at the lesion site was significantly lower in the irradiated groups as compared to placebo treatment (23 vs. 55%, $p < 0.01$). Three-year follow-up showed an increase in restenosis rate in the irradiated groups from 17% at 6 months to 33%. This radiation effect is associated with a loss of luminal diameter from 2.49 ± 0.81 mm (6 months) to 2.12 ± 0.73 mm (3 years).

The WRIST (Washington Radiation for In-Stent restenosis Trial) study compared the ^{192}Ir wire (15 Gy) with placebo and included 130 patients (28). The rate of lesion revascularization and vessel revascularization in the treated group (14 and 26%, respectively) was significantly lower when compared to the placebo group (63 and 68%, respectively). In addition, the 6-month angiographic restenosis rate decreased to 19% in the irradiated group compared to 58% in the placebo group.

The GAMMA-1 trial was a randomized and double-blind study in 252 patients with 131 irradiated patients (^{192}Ir) and 121 patients who received placebo treatment. The prescribed dose was similar to the dose used in SCRIPPS. At 9-month follow-up the reduction of risk of intrastent restenosis was 58% and the restenosis risk reduction in de novo lesions was 43%. Survival rate without target lesion revascularization was 71% in the treated group versus 57% in the placebo group. However, major cardiac events (4% vs. 1%) or AMI (16% vs. 8%) occurred with higher frequency in the irradiated group and seem to be linked to late thrombosis after repetitive stent implantation and after ticlopidine or clopidogrel medication (28).

Beta-WRIST was the first study to report on the efficacy of b-radiation for the treatment of in-stent restenosis. A group of 50 patients was treated with ^{90}Y. A historical placebo group from the WRIST trial served as the placebo group. At 6 months the rate of

Table 3 Clinical Placebo-Controlled Studies with Intravascular Brachytherapy on Restenotic Coronary Lesions (In-Stent Restenosis)

Investigator	Study	Isotope	Dose (Gy)	No. of patients	RR (RA vs. C)
Teirstein	SCRIPPS	^{192}Ir	8–30	55	17 vs. 54%
Waksman	WRIST	^{192}Ir	15	130	19 vs. 58%
Leon	GAMMA-1	^{192}Ir	8–30	250	21.6 vs. 52%
Waksman	BETA-WRIST	^{90}Y	14–30	50	28 vs. 66%
Waksman	INHIBIT	^{32}P	20	320	28 vs. 54%
Popma	START	^{90}Sr/Y	18–20	476	34 vs. 52%
Serruys	BRIE	^{90}Sr/Y	14–18	150	24 vs. 56%
Waksman	SVG WRIST	^{192}Ir	15	120	38 vs. 64%
Waksman	LONG WRIST	^{192}Ir	15	120	32 vs. 51%

RR = restenosis rate; RA = radiation group; C = control group.

restenosis and the rate of target lesion revascularization were significantly lower in the irradiated group (22 and 26%, respectively) (29).

START is a randomized study with 476 patients who presented with in-stent restenosis. The results showed a reduction in angiographic restenosis of 36% in the radiation-treated group (^{90}Sr/Y) at 8 months. With prolonged antiplatelet treatment, the patients presented similar results for late total occlusion in the treated and the control groups (4%).

The European *BRIE* register is currently being evaluated, enrolling 150 patients treated with either 14 or 18 Gy (^{90}Sr/Y).

C. Clinical Trials with Radioactive Stents

Only a few clinical studies have examined the effect of radioactive stents on restenosis (Table 4). The nonrandomized IRIS study a used stents with very low activity (0.5–1 mCi). Restenosis rate at 6 months was 31% with revascularization level of 21% (30).

The Heidelberg study was a nonrandomised safety and feasibility study using radioactive ^{32}P Palmaz-Schatz stents (1.5–3 mCi). The patients received antiplatelet aggregation therapy (ticlopidine) for 2 months. The restenosis rate was 54% after 6 months.

Albiero and coworkers (Milan Dose Study) reported the results in 91 lesions of 82 patients using the radioactive BX stent with three activity levels. At 6-month follow-up the restenosis rate was favorable, with 0% in the group treated with a radioactive stent in dose of 6–12 μCi (31). However, an edge effect occurred at the injured zone edges in about 50% of the patients. The use of highly radioactive stents (12–21 μCi) diminishes neointimal hyperplasia at 6 months but does not avoid the edge effect (31).

IX. POTENTIAL PROBLEMS OF CORONARY RADIATION THERAPY

A. Late Thrombosis

Late thrombosis is defined as angiographically documented thrombosis that occurs 1 month or later after coronary intervention (32). In the BETA-WRIST study (^{90}Y), late thrombosis level increased to 10% (5 patients of 50, with 2 asymptomatic) at 6-month follow-up (32). At 2 years SCRIPPS (26 irradiated patients vs. 29 placebo patients) showed 1 thrombosis at 18 days in the irradiated group compared to 2 fatal infarctions in the placebo group (33). The patients who died in the radiation group prematurely stopped ticlopidine treatment. The Serruys et al. study (34) found 6 (2 PTCA and 4 stent) patients out of 91 (thrombosis rate: 6.6%) who presented with total occlusion after b-irradiation. These late occlusions underwent thrombotic composition, but their origin remains to be elucidated.

An experimental study in the porcine model demonstrated that the total amount of radiation-induced thrombi (mural and luminal) and platelet recruitment depends on the delivered dose (35). Prolonged antiplatelet treatment combining aspirin and clopidogrel for 6–12 months has been suggested as a potential solution for the problem.

Other studies are necessary to define the long-term outcome and treatment of such complications, especially late late thrombosis (> 6 months) risk.

B. The Edge Effect

This effect is defined by de novo stenosis occurring at the boarder of the treated zone. Recent clinical studies have examined, this effect not yet reported in experimental studies. In 82 patients receiving radioactive ^{32}P-stent, Albiero et al. described a high rate of intralesional restenosis (e.g., edge effect) at 6-month follow-up (52% with 0.75–3 mCi, 41% with 3–6 mCi, and 50% with 6–12 mCi) (37). The edge effect corresponds to a technique-dependent issue in radiotherapy called geographical miss (GM) and is related to inadequate radiation margin. This GM refers to an arterial section that has undergone injury during the interventional procedure but has not received the prescribed dose of radiation. This includes a vessel zone receiving either no radiation or a dose less than prescribed. IVUS imaging showed that the edge effect is mainly due to two mechanisms: increased plaque/media volume at the immediate edge stent (covering 1–3 mm) and negative remodeling ("shrinkage") covering 4–10 mm at stent edges. This effect may occur with radioactive stents or catheter-based techniques (38) or liquid-filled balloons (39). Increased plaque volume in the GM zone might be related to intima and media fibrosis (40). Shrinkage associated with GM is associated with adventitial fibrosis observed with low doses in animal models (41). To reduce this effect, care must be taken as to proper radiation source positioning, meticulous documentation of injury length, and availability of appropriate-length radiation-delivery devices.

C. Nonhealed Coronary Dissections

In humans intracoronary dissection after PTCA without stent placement is angiographically healed at 6 months. Using IVUS imaging, Meerkin et al. examined coronary dissections in 16 of 26 patients without stent but with endovascular brachytherapy (42). Of the 16 dissections, 9 were spontaneously resolved and 7 persisted at 6 months. The authors excluded a correlation between dose and the persistence of dissections. They concluded that dissection may contribute to late thrombosis and indicate delayed healing following radiation treatment. Furthermore, Cottin and coworkers reported unhealed dissections in the radiation group at 14 days in the porcine balloon overstretch model. This study also showed the presence of mural thrombi located between the media layer and external elastic lamina and raised a positive correlation between dissection area and mural thrombus formation ($r^2 = 0.889$, $p < 0.001$) (43).

D. Late Results and Catch-Up Effects

The SCRIPPS trial (27) found unexplained luminal loss between 6 months and 3 years in the irradiated group (from 2.49 ± 0.81 to 2.12 ± 0.73 mm) associated with an increased rate of angiographic restenosis rate from 17 to 33%. Luminal diameter measurements in the control group remained unchanged. The mechanism of this late luminal loss (late catch-up) remains to be elucidated. However, recently published data from Waksman and Teirstein on the long-term effects of β- and γ-radiation therapy show that a benefit for patients is present up to 5 years after the procedure (44–47).

Table 4 Clinical Studies Using Radioactive Stents

Investigator	Study	Stent	No. of patients	Restenosis rate
Fischell	IRIS	Stent P-S 15 mm	32	31%
Moses	IRIS IB	Stent P-S 15 mm	25	>35%
Hehrlein	Heidelberg	Stent P-S 15 mm	11	>35%
Colombo	Milan	Stent P-S and BX 15 mm	122	>50%

REFERENCES

1. Adams PC, Badimon JJ, Badimon L, Chesebro JH, Fuster V. Role of platelets in atherogenesis: relevance to coronary arterial restenosis after angioplasty. Cardiovasc Clin 1987; 18(1):49–71.
2. Scott NA, Cipolla GD, Ross CE, Dunn B, Martin FH, Simonet L, Wilcox JN. Identification of a potential role for the adventitia in vascular lesion formation after balloon overstretch injury of porcine coronary arteries. Circulation 1996; 93:2178–2187.
3. Lafont A, Guzman LA, Whitlow PL, Goormastic M, Cornhill JF, Chisolm GM. Restenosis after experimental angioplasty. Intimal, medial, and adventitial changes associated with constrictive remodeling. Circ Res 1995; 76:996–1002.
4. Kakuta T, Currier JW, Haudenschild CC, Ryan TJ, Faxon DP. Differences in compensatory vessel enlargement, not intimal formation, account for restenosis after angioplasty in the hypercholesterolemic rabbit model. Circulation 1994; 89:2809–2815.
5. Verin V, Popowski Y, Urban P, Belenger J, Redard M, Costa M, Widmer MC, Rouzaud M, Nouet P, Grob E. Intra-arterial beta irradiation prevents neointimal hyperplasia in a hypercholesterolemic rabbit restenosis model. Circulation 1995; 92:2284–2290.
6. Waksman R, Robinson KA, Crocker IR, Gravanis MB, Cipolla GD, King SB3. Endovascular low-dose irradiation inhibits neointima formation after coronary artery balloon injury in swine. A possible role for radiation therapy in restenosis prevention. Circulation 1995; 91:1533–1539.
7. Waksman R, Robinson KA, Crocker IR, Wang C, Gravanis MB, Cipolla GD, Hillstead RA, King SB3. Intracoronary low-dose beta-irradiation inhibits neointima formation after coronary artery balloon injury in the swine restenosis model. Circulation 1995; 92:3025–3031.
8. Wilcox JN, Waksman R, King SB, Scott NA. The role of the adventitia in the arterial response to angioplasty: the effect of intravascular radiation. Int J Radiat Oncol Biol Phys 1996; 36:789–796.
9. Waksman R, Rodriguez JC, Robinson KA, Cipolla GD, Crocker IR, Scott NA, King SB3, Wilcox JN. Effect of intravascular irradiation on cell proliferation, apoptosis, and vascular remodeling after balloon overstretch injury of porcine coronary arteries. Circulation 1997; 96:1944–1952.
10. Verin V, Popowski Y, Bochaton-Piallat ML, Belenger J, Urban P, Neuville P, Redard M, Costa M, Celetta G, Gabbiani G. Intraarterial beta irradiation induces smooth muscle cell apoptosis and reduces medial cellularity in a hypercholesterolemic rabbit restenosis model. Int J Radiat Oncol Biol Phys 2000; 46(3):661–670.
11. Rubin P, Williams JP, Riggs PN, Bartos S, Sarac T, Pomerantz R, Castano J, Schell M, Green RM. Cellular and molecular mechanisms of radiation inhibition of restenosis. Part I: role of the macrophage and platelet-derived growth factor [see comments]. Int J Radiat Oncol Biol Phys 1998; 40:929–941.
12. Amols HI, Reinstein LE, Weinberger J. Dosimetry of a radioactive coronary balloon dilatation catheter for treatment of neointimal hyperplasia. Med Phys 1996; 23:1783–1788.
13. Fischell TA, Carter AJ, Laird JR. The beta-particle-emitting radioisotope stent (isostent): animal studies and planned clinical trials. Am J Cardiol 1996; 78:45–50.
14. Hehrlein C, Gollan C, Donges K, Metz J, Riessen R, Fehsenfeld P, von Hodenberg E, Kubler W. Low-dose radioactive endovascular stents prevent smooth muscle cell proliferation and neointimal hyperplasia in rabbits. Circulation 1995; 92:1570–1575.
15. Fischell TA, Kharma BK, Fischell DR, Loges PG, Coffey CW2, Duggan DM, Naftilan AJ. Low-dose, beta-particle emission from 'stent' wire results in complete, localized inhibition of smooth muscle cell proliferation [see comments]. Circulation 1994; 90:2956–2963.
16. Laird JR, Carter AJ, Kufs WM, Hoopes TG, Farb A, Nott SH, Fischell RE, Fischell DR, Virmani R, Fischell TA. Inhibition of neointimal proliferation with low-dose irradiation from a beta-particle-emitting stent. Circulation 1996; 93:529–536.
17. Carter AJ, Laird JR. Experimental results with endovascular irradiation via a radioactive stent. Int J Radiat Oncol Biol Phys 1996; 36:797–803.

18. Wardeh AJ, Kay IP, Sabate M, Coen VL, Gijzel AL, Ligthart JM, den Boer A, Levendag PC, Der Giessen WJ, Serruys PW. beta-particle-emitting radioactive stent implantation: a safety and feasibility study. Circulation 1999; 100(16):1684–1689.

19. Albiero R, Nishida T, Adamian M, Amato A, Vaghetti M, Corvaja N, Di Mario C, Colombo A. Edge restenosis after implantation of high activity (32)P radioactive beta-emitting stents. Circulation 2000; 101(21):2454–2457.

20. Nath R, Amols H, Coffey C, Duggan D, Jani S, Li Z, Schell M, Soares C, Whiting J, Cole PE, Crocker I, Schwartz R. Intravascular brachytherapy physics: report of the AAPM Radiation Therapy Committee Task Group no. 60. American Association of Physicists in Medicine. Med Phys 1999; 26:119–52.

21. Condado JA, Waksman R, Gurdiel O, Espinosa R, Gonzalez J, Burger B, Villoria G, Acquatella H, Crocker IR, Seung KB, Liprie SF. Long-term angiographic and clinical outcome after percutaneous transluminal coronary angioplasty and intracoronary radiation therapy in humans [see comments]. Circulation 1997; 96:727–732.

22. Verin V, Urban P, Popowski Y, Schwager M, Nouet P, Dorsaz PA, Chatelain P, Kurtz JM, Rutishauser W. Feasibility of intracoronary beta-irradiation to reduce restenosis after balloon angioplasty. A clinical pilot study [see comments]. Circulation 1997; 95:1138–1144.

23. King SB3, Williams DO, Chougule P, Klein JL, Waksman R, Hilstead R, Macdonald J, Anderberg K, Crocker IR. Endovascular beta-radiation to reduce restenosis after coronary balloon angioplasty: results of the Beta Energy Restenosis Trial (BERT). Circulation 1998; 97:2025–2030.

24. Sabate M, Marijnissen JP, Carlier SG, Kay IP, van der Giessen WJ, Coen VL, Ligthart JM, Boersma E, Costa MA, Levendag PC, Serruys PW. Residual plaque burden, delivered dose, and tissue composition predict 6-month outcome after balloon angioplasty and beta-radiation therapy. Circulation 2000; 101(21):2472–2477.

25. Raizner AE, Oesterle SN, Waksman R, Serruys PW, Colombo A, Lim YL, Yeung AC, van der Giessen WJ, Vandertie L, Chiu JK, White LR, Fitzgerald PJ, Kaluza GL, Ali NM. Inhibition of restenosis with beta-emitting radiotherapy: report of the Proliferation Reduction with Vascular Energy Trial (PREVENT). Circulation 2000; 102(9):951–958.

26. Teirstein PS, Massullo V, Jani S, Russo RJ, Cloutier DA, Schatz RA, Guarneri EM, Steuterman S, Sirkin K, Norman S, Tripuraneni P. Two-year follow-up after catheter-based radiotherapy to inhibit coronary restenosis [see comments]. Circulation 1999; 99:243–247.

27. Teirstein PS, Massullo V, Jani S, Popma JJ, Russo RJ, Schatz RA, Guarneri EM, Steuterman S, Sirkin K, Cloutier DA, Leon MB, Tripuraneni P. Three-year clinical and angiographic follow-up after intracoronary radiation: results of a randomized clinical trial [see comments]. Circulation 2000; 101(4):360–365.

28. Waksman R, White RL, Chan RC, Bass BG, Geirlach L, Mintz GS, Satler LF, Mehran R, Serruys PW, Lansky AJ, Fitzgerald P, Bhargava B, Kent KM, Pichard AD, Leon MB. Intracoronary gamma-radiation therapy after angioplasty inhibits recurrence in patients with in-stent restenosis. Circulation 2000; 101(18):2165–2171.

29. Waksman R, Bhargava B, White L, Chan RC, Mehran R, Lansky AJ, Mintz GS, Satler LF, Pichard AD, Leon MB, Kent KK. Intracoronary beta-radiation therapy inhibits recurrence of in-stent restenosis. Circulation 2000; 101(16):1895–1898.

30. Wardeh AJ, Kay IP, Sabate M, Coen VL, Gijzel AL, Ligthart JM, den Boer A, Levendag PC, Der Giessen WJ, Serruys PW. Beta-particle-emitting radioactive stent implantation. A safety and feasibility study. Circulation 1999; 100(16):1684–1689.

31. Albiero R, Adamian M, Kobayashi N, Amato A, Vaghetti M, Di Mario C, Colombo A. Short- and intermediate-term results of (32)P radioactive beta-emitting stent implantation in patients with coronary artery disease: The Milan Dose-Response Study [see comments]. Circulation 2000; 101(1):18–26.

32. Waksman R, Bhargava B, Mintz GS, Mehran R, Lansky AJ, Satler LF, Pichard AD, Kent KM, Leon MB. Late total occlusion after intracoronary brachytherapy for patients with in-stent restenosis. J Am Coll Cardiol 2000; 36(1):65–68.

33. Teirstein PS, Massullo V, Jani S, Russo RJ, Cloutier DA, Schatz RA, Guarneri EM, Steuterman S, Sirkin K, Norman S, Tripuraneni P. Two-year follow-up after catheter-based radiotherapy to inhibit coronary restenosis [see comments]. Circulation 1999; 99(2):243–247.

34. Costa MA, Sabat M, van der Giessen WJ, Kay IP, Cervinka P, Ligthart JM, Serrano P, Coen VL, Levendag PC, Serruys PW. Late coronary occlusion after intracoronary brachytherapy [see comments]. Circulation 1999; 100(8):789–792.

35. Vodovotz Y, Bhargava B, Collins S, Chan R, Waksman R. Intracoronary radiation increases thrombosis rate with decreased luminal thrombi and thrombus area. J Am Coll Cardiol 1999; 33 (Suppl.A):300A.

36. Salame MY, Verheye S, Mulkey SP, Chronos NA, King SB, III, Crocker IR, Robinson KA. The effect of endovascular irradiation on platelet recruitment at sites of balloon angioplasty in pig coronary arteries. Circulation 2000; 101(10):1087–1090.

37. Albiero R, Colombo A. European high-activity (32)P radioactive stent experience. J Invasive Cardiol 2000; 12(8):416–421.

38. Sabate M, Costa MA, Kozuma K, Kay IP, van der Giessen WJ, Coen VL, Ligthart JM, Serrano P, Levendag PC, Serruys PW. Geographic miss: a cause of treatment failure in radio-oncology applied to intracoronary radiation therapy. Circulation 2000; 101(21):2467–2471.

39. Weinberger J. Intracoronary radiation using radioisotope solution-filled balloons. Herz 1998; 23:366–72

40. Weinberger J, Amols H, Ennis RD, Schwartz A, Wiedermann JG, Marboe C. Intracoronary irradiation: dose response for the prevention of restenosis in swine. Int J Radiat Oncol Biol Phys 1996; 36:767–775.

41. Powers BE, Thames HD, Gillette EL. Long-term adverse effects of radiation inhibition of restenosis: radiation injury to the aorta and branch arteries in a canine model. Int J Radiat Oncol Biol Phys 1999; 45(3):753–759.

42. Meerkin D, Tardif JC, Crocker IR, Arsenault A, Joyal M, Lucier G, King SB3, Williams DO, Serruys PW, Bonan R. Effects of intracoronary beta-radiation therapy after coronary angioplasty: an intravascular ultrasound study. Circulation 1999; 99:1660–1665.

43. Cottin Y, Kollum M, Chan R, Bhargava B, Vodovotz Y, Waksman R. Vascular repair after balloon overstretch injury in porcine model effects of intracoronary radiation. J Am Coll Cardiol 2000; 36(4):1389–1395.

44. Waksman R, Ajani AE, White RL, et al. Two-year follow-up after beta and gamma intracoronary radiation therapy for patients with diffuse in-stent restenosis. Am J Cardiol 2001; 88:425–428

45. Waksman R, Raizner AE, Yeung AC, et al. Use of localised intracoronary beta radiation in treatment of in-stent restenosis: the INHIBIT randomised controlled trial. Lancet 2002; 359:551–7

46. Waksman R, Ajani AE, White RL, et al. Intravascular gamma radiation for in-stent restenosis in saphenous-vein bypass grafts. N Engl J Med 2002; 346:1194–9

47. Gries MA, Masullo V, Jani S, et al. Five-year clinical follow-up after intracoronary radiation: results of a randomized clinical trial. Circulation 2002; 2699–2700

18-1

Anticoagulation Monitoring in Cardiovascular Disease

Kamal Gupta, J. Michael Wilson, and James J. Ferguson
St. Luke's Episcopal Hospital, Texas Heart Institute, Baylor College of Medicine, The University of Texas Health Science Center at Houston, Houston, Texas, U.S.A.

I. INTRODUCTION

Inhibition of normal hemostatic mechanisms is the cornerstone of medical therapy for many cardiovascular diseases, especially acute coronary syndromes (ACSs) and percutaneous coronary interventions (PCIs). However, if antithrombotic therapy is to be of value, a delicate balance has to be maintained between the prevention of pathological thrombosis and excess risk of significant hemorrhage. Thus, therapeutic administration of these agents must be guided by appropriate clinical and laboratory tests to assess risk of bleeding or continued thrombosis. Multiple types of assessments are possible, including individual enzyme inhibition (1–3), quantitation of thrombosis byproducts (4,5), and overall measures of clotting efficiency (6–8). This chapter discusses the physiological and clinical basis of the more commonly used laboratory tests for monitoring anticoagulation in patients with cardiovascular diseases. Some of the newer and more promising tests will also be discussed.

II. BASIC PRINCIPLES

Beneath the apparent simplicity of the routine coagulation times lies the incredible complex interplay of enzymes, coenzymes, and inhibitors that combine to produce coagulation (Fig.1). Blood and plasma coagulation tests are a laboratory reproduction of events resulting in fibrin polymer formation, with or without platelet assistance. However, the two processes are not necessarily synonymous. Coagulation tests are inititiated artificially, within the static confines of a test tube, often without the presence of erythrocytes or platelets. In vivo thrombosis is far more complex and may not be adequately represented (or in some cases be misrepresented) by in vitro tests (9). For instance, the presence of lupus anticoagulant, while prolonging in vitro coagulation, confers an increased risk of thrombosis (9). The two principles that govern laboratory measures of coagulation are: the need for activation of an enzyme pathway and the need for a functional cofactor to assist enzyme function (10–12). The characteristics of an individual test are determined by the activator and whether or not there is an excess of the necessary cofactors, such as phospholipid membrane. With the activator supplied in a simplified test tube product, which obviates many of the regulatory and counter regulatory mechanisms, the primary limitation to thrombus initiation and growth is cofactor availability.

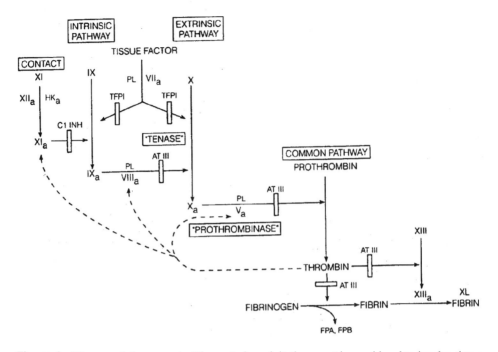

Figure 1 The coagulation cascade. The central precipitating event is considered to involve tissue factor (TF), which under physiological conditions is not exposed to blood. With vascular or endothelial cell injury, TF acts in concert with activated factor $VIIa$ and phospholipids (PL) to convert factor IX to IX_a and X to X_a. The intrinsic pathway includes "contact" activation of factor XI by factor XII_a/activated high molecular weight kininogen (HK_a) complex. It should be noted that the contact system contributes to fibrinolysis and bradykinin formation in vivo. Factor XI_a also converts factor IX to IX_a and factor IX_a in turn converts factor X to X_a, in concert with factor VIII_a and PL (the tenase complex). Factor X_a is the catalytic ingredient of the prothrombinase complex and converts prothrombin to thrombin. Thrombin cleaves the fibrinopeptides (FPA, FPB) from fibrinogen, allowing the resultant fibrin monomers to polymerize, and converts factor XIII to XIII_a, which crosslinks (XL) the fibrin clot. Thrombin accelerates the process (interrupted lines) by its potential to activate factors V and VIII, but continued proteolytic process also dampens the process by activating protein C, which degrades factors V_a and VIII_a. Natural plasma inhibitors retard clotting: C1 inhibitor (C1 INH) neutralizes factor XIIa, tissue factor pathway inhibitor (TFPI) blocks factor VII_a/TF, and antithrombin (AT III) blocks factors IX_a and X_a and thrombin. (Arrows, active enzymes; filled rectangles, sites of inhibitor action; dashed lines., feedback reactions.) (From Ref. 122.)

The endpoint of a test is the time at which sufficient fibrin has been generated to be detectable. Fibrin polymerization may be detected by a variety of methods including, the appearance of a visible fibrin clot, an increase in the optical density of the specimen, or a change in the mechanical resistance (using magnetic field manipulation or electrical conduction) (Fig. 2) (13).

III. SPECIFIC LABORATORY TESTS TO MONITOR ANTICOAGULATION

A. Prothrombin Time

When tissue factor and a suitable phospholipid membrane are added to recalcified, platelet-poor plasma, the extrinsic pathway is activated, producing thrombin and fibrin clot (11,14,15). Devised in the 1930s by A.J. Quick (16), the prothrombin time (PT) test is based

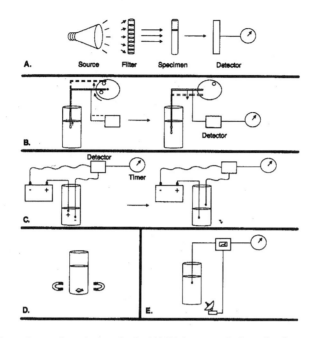

Figure 2 Fibrinopolymer detection methods. (A) Light transmission of a plasma sample increases as fibrinogen leaves the solution in fibrin polymers. A threshold value or percentage of light transmission may be set to stop the timer. (B) As fibrin polymers form, specimen viscosity rises. When a plunger is lifted and then allowed to fall, the rate of fall is a measure of specimen viscosity. (C) Two electrodes may be placed in a specimen and a current established. One of the electrodes may be withdrawn from the specimen at preset intervals. When viscosity rises, contact between the moving electrode and the specimen will not be broken and the timer will stop. (D) If a ferromagnetic specimen is placed in a specimen, motion may be established by an oscillating magnetic field. When motion is restricted to a preset value, timing will stop. (E) A probe may be placed in the specimen and vibrated at a preset frequency. A sensor positioned outside the specimen regulates the output of the probe to maintain a constant value. Fibrin polymerization and increased viscosity decrease sound transmission, increasing the output required of the probe.

on the fact that in the presence of excess tissue factor, the efficiency of fibrin formation depends on the presence and activity of factors VII, X, and V, and of thrombin and fibrinogen. The test is usually performed in a glass tube with an inner coating to prevent the activation of factor XII. Briefly, citrated platelet poor plasma is added to a calcium and thromboplastin suspension and the timer is started. The end of the test is marked by fibrin polymerization, usually detected by change in the optical density of the specimen. The ratio of clotting time of test plasma to that of control plasma gives an estimate of the function of the extrinsic pathway clotting factors. The amount of tissue factor supplied during the test makes the activity of factor VIIa, rather than the tissue factor, the primary determinant of extrinsic pathway activation (17). Therefore, PT, which hinges on factor VII function, can be used to estimate the severity of factor production abnormalities, such as liver dysfunction, warfarin effect, or vitamin K deficiency. Of note, heparin and the specific antithrombins also prolong PT (18,19). However, the plasma activity of heparin required to prolong PT is close to 1.0 U/mL. Because the most commonly used heparin regimens attempt to achieve heparin concentrations near 0.4 U/mL, this is not of much clinical utility.

There may be substantial interlaboratory variation in PT of identical specimens due to the differences in the commercially available thromboplastin preparations (20–22). These preparations differ in their ability to initiate and support coagulation factor activity due to many factors, including the amount and activity of tissue factor supplied and the physical properties of the accompanying phospholipid membrane (23). A particularly powerful tissue factor–phospholipid preparation may overcome a mild deficiency in factor activity, producing a normal PT, whereas a weaker preparation may produce a prolonged PT and differences in the ratio of test to control PT. Although long suspected, the effect of these different thromboplastins was clearly established in a multinational study of the treatment of venous thrombosis, which reported an increased risk of bleeding when drug dosing was guided by prothrombin time ratios in North America (24). A method of controlling variations in thromboplastin sensitivity to the effect of warfarin was established in 1983 (23,25). This standardization method employs the International Normalized Ratio (INR), which is a mathematical computation of the ratio of the activity of the thromboplastin to be used to a reference thromboplastin held by the World Health Organization (25). When prothrombin times using the different reagents are plotted on a logarithmic scale, there is a linear relationship between the different values. The slope of this relationship is a function of an individual thromboplastin's sensitivity to the effects of factor depletion and is known as the International Sensitivity Index (ISI). Reference thromboplastins have an ISI value of 1.0. Less sensitive preparations have a value near 2.0. Using ISI, an INR can be calculated according to the following formula: INR = (PT ratio)^{ISI} (25,26).

B. Whole Blood Clotting Time

Lee and White described the whole blood clotting time (WBCT) in 1913 as a method for evaluating the intrinsic capability of blood to clot (27). WBCT is based on the principle that when blood is placed in a glass tube, the intrinsic pathway to thrombin generation is activated and the initial thrombin generation is limited by the availability of cofactors that augment enzyme function, especially factors VIIa and Va, and calcium and a phospholipids membrane (10,14,28,29). The initial appearance of active thrombin, albeit in low concentrations, leads to the generation of necessary cofactors through its action on factors VIII and V and platelet activation (10,14,28,30,31). A burst of thrombin generation and fibrin polymerization ensues. This test does not utilize exogenous activators, except the glass tube.

The WBCT is primarily of historical interest now because the test methodology and results varied greatly. Among its many derivatives, the activated partial thromboplastin time (aPTT) and the activated clotting time (ACT) are in widespread contemporary use.

1. Activated Partial Thromboplastin Time

In the 1950s a group of investigators developed a variation of the PT that used a lipophilic extract of mammalian (nonhuman) brain for thromboplastin preparation (32). They used platelet-poor plasma and an excess amount of a membrane substitute. They called this test PTT, as they thought that their thromboplastin must be incomplet because, unlike the PT, it gave abnormal results with plasma from hemophiliacs (33). The aPTT is a modification of the above, which avoids variation in the intensity of activation by initiating activation (during a pretest incubation period) with a constant quantity of activator (kaolin, celite, etc.). When citrated, platelet-poor plasma is exposed to strong contact activation, is recalcified, and platelet membrane substitute is supplied, the time required for fibrin clot to form is dependent on the integrity of the intrinsic pathway. The aPTT avoids the extrinsic pathway by excluding tissue factor from its reagents and also separates coagulation from platelet function.

The normal range for aPTT for most laboratories is 20–40 seconds. It is prolonged when any of the factors from contact activation to fibrin polymerization are deficient or are inhibited to <30% of normal activity (34–36).

When heparin is complexed with antithrombin III (AT III), the ability of the heparin–AT III to inhibit thrombin may be increased 1000-fold over that of AT III alone (37). As a result, the initial steps following contact activation proceed slowly through the regulatory points. The small amount of thrombin produced decays at an accelerated rate, and the activation of factor VIII is impaired. Consequently, more time is required to produce thrombin in sufficient concentrations to effectively overcome the rate-limiting steps in the intrinsic pathway. This lag time is the measurable prolongation of clotting times produced by the thrombin inhibitors (e.g., heparin) (10,12,38). Because aPTT has a strong contact activation step, it is intermediately sensitive to the presence of thrombin inhibitors. The aPTT is prolonged at a level of thrombin inhibition that correlates with heparin activity of 0.1–0.6 U/mL, a range known to be clinically effective for medical treatment of venous and some arterial thrombosis (6,39–41). The aPTT is the most widely used test for guiding heparin therapy for venous and arterial thrombosis and for medical management of ACSs, with theusual target range of 1.5–2.5 times the control value (6,37,39,40). However, when heparin is administered to achieve higher concentrations (as in the setting of PCI or cardiopulmonary bypass) (42–44), the aPTT is nonlinear in its response to heparin and may be almost infinitely prolonged; the aPTT in these circumstances is no longer a useful test (7,45–47).

Direct thrombin inhibitors (DTIs), in contrast to heparin, are active against fibrin-bound thrombin, and, like heparin, not only do they inhibit thrombin production and activity, they may also inhibit thrombin-induced platelet activation (48,49). Thus, because DTIs have different mechanisms of action and different dose-effect relationships, the relationship between aPTT prolongation and antithrombotic effect will be different from that of heparin. A given aPTT range for DTI may correspond to an equal or greater antithrombotic effect than for heparin, especially in situations where the thrombosis is platelet dependent (as in ACS) (50,51). Thus, direct comparisons of drug efficacy cannot necessarily be made based on equal prolongation of aPTT (51). Risk/benefit ratios, with respect to measures of antithrombotic effect, must be determined separately for anticoagulants of different classes. Therefore, antithrombotic recommendations using the aPTT must not only specify the reagents but also the type of antithrombotic therapy used.

Conventionally, the aPTT is performed in a central laboratory. This involves a substantial delay in the reporting of results from the time of ordering the test (52). A survey of 79 hospitals that participated in the GUSTO I trial showed that the mean time from blood draw to availability of the aPTT result was 1 hour and 46 minutes (53). Since patients with acute coronary syndromes would benefit from a more rapid turnover time for aPTT, several point-of-care anticoagulation systems have been clinically tested and are now commercially available. There are three commercially available bedside aPTT monitors in the United States designed for use in critical care settings. Each provides a rapid determination of aPTT (typically within 3 min). Table 1 provides a comparison of these point-of-care devices.

2. Activated Clotting Time

The activated clotting time, first described by Hattersley in 1966, (54) is essentially a modified WBCT in which an attempt has been made to standardize contact activation by using a constant amount of kaolin or celite. The ACT is similar to the aPTT in its dependence on the contact activation pathway for thrombin generation, but the ACT does not supply an excess of phospholipid membrane. In the aPTT, the phospholipid area is supplied in excess

Table 1 Point-of-Care Devices for Determination of aPTT

	Instrument		
	Coagucheck Plus	Hemochron Jr.	Thrombolytic Assesment System
Manufacturer	Roche & Boehringer-Mannheim Diagnostics	International Technidyne Corp.	Cardiovascular Diagnostics Inc.
Blood sample	Fresh whole blood	Whole blood or citrated plasma	Citrated whole blood or plasma
Sample volume	1 drop	1 drop	1 drop
Time to result	Minutes	Minutes	Minutes
Setting of clot formation	Capillary flow of unclotted blood	Forced movement of unclotted blood through a narrow channel	Chamber with magnetic particles with oscillating electric field
Clot-detection method	Laser photometry	Optical light transmission	Optical light transmission
Correlation with standard laboratory	$r = 0.78–0.89$	$r = 0.87$	$r = 0.84$
Therapeutic aPTT[a]	60–85 s (GUSTO III)	50–70 s (PARAGON)	Customized to each hospitals standard aPTT range

[a]Corresponding to heparin level of 0.2–0.4 U/mL.

so that it will not interfere with the coagulation enzyme function. The ACT requires that this area be developed through platelet activation during the testing process. This intrtoduces an additional variable to the function of coagulation enzymes. In the ACT following contact activation, the first thrombin to appear must activate platelets, in addition to factors V and VIII, and any alteration in endogenous platelet function may also alter ACT. Thus, rather than being a pure test of coagulation enzyme function, the ACT is also a somewhat imprecise measure of the cooperation between the intrinsic pathway and platelet function. For this reason (as will be detailed in a later section), ACT is useful in monitoring the combined use of heparin and glycoprotein IIb/IIIa. Also, the ACT is less sensitive to low levels of heparin anticoagulation than aPTT. However, it maintains a good correlation with the heparin effect at higher heparin doses (7,55,56) and thus is widely used for guiding heparin therapy in clinical situations needing high-dose heparin, such as cardiopulmonary bypass and PCI (42–46).

Unlike Hattersley's original assay (54), which required manual mixing of a blood sample with the contact activator and visual assessment of the tube for time to visible clot formation, commercial automated ACT monitors are now in routine use. The Hemochron system (International Technidyne, Edison, NJ) uses a celite activator and detects fibrin polymerization using an oscillating magnetic field. The HemoTec (Medtronic HemoTec, Englewood, CO) uses a kaolin activator and measures the rate of plunger fall to detect fibrin polymerization. Thus, system activators and fibrin-detection mechanisms differ, giving different sensitivities to factor depletion and inhibitor therapy. Although there is reasonable correlation, the values of one system cannot be extrapolated to other systems (57). Thus, any recommendations for anticoagulation intensity measured by ACT must be qualified by the specific type of device used (58).

The normal ACT range in general is 90–130 seconds. Due to the range of variation in normal values, effects of low-dose anticoagulants may go unnoticed in individual patients. The ACT may be shortened during ongoing thrombosis, such as in surgical procedures or unstable coronary syndromes, largely as a function of the availability of activated platelets. Contamination of blood samples with activated platelets (as with indwelling catheters) may also shorten ACT. Also, aprotinin inhibits contact activation by celite (diatomaceous earth) (59). If this interaction is not considered, an insufficient dose of heparin may be administered in this setting. Thus, kaolin ACT should be used in patients receiving aprotinin.

Because aPTT and ACT measure similar phenomena, (except for the contribution of activated platelets), there is a fair correlation between the tests when assessing heparin therapy (45). However, DTIs, in addition to impairing the feedback amplification of coagulation enzyme function, also prevent thrombin-induced platelet activation (48,49). The resultant denial of factors VIIIa and Va and a phospholipid surface prolongs ACT. In drug concentration ranges at which the two tests are responsive, antithrombins produce a proportionately greater rise in ACT than aPTT (51). Thus, at drug concentrations producing an equivalent rise in the aPTT, the ACT increase with specific thrombin inhibitors is significantly greater than that with heparin. Powerful antiplatelet drugs like glycoprotein (GP) IIb/IIIa inhibitors may prolong ACT (60). Thus, ACT may be a good tool to assess the intensity of antithrombotic drugs when combined anticoagulants and antiplatelet agents are used in a clinical syndrome that may involve endogenous platelet activation (as in PCI setting).

More recently, another point-of-care ACT monitoring device has become available. The i-STAT system (i-STAT Corp., Princeton, NJ) is modular and consists of a handheld unit into which disposable cartridges are placed. The cartridges are self-contained and need <1 mL of blood. Individual cartridges are available to measure electrolytes, blood gases, and anticoagulation level (ACT) (61,62). Each i-STAT unit can download patient data to a central computer for storage and subsequent retrieval. Unlike traditional ACT, the i-STAT ACT is not based on the formation of a stable thrombus. Instead, a substrate marker releases an electric signal when it is cleaved by active thrombin. The time to generation of the electroactive marker is reported as the ACT (63). Therefore, the i-STAT is less susceptible to fibrinogen levels, temperature, hematocrit, dilution, and the addition of GP IIb/IIIa inhibitors. Because the production of thrombin occurs before the formation of a stable clot, one would expect the value of the i-STAT to be lower than that of the Hemochron ACT. Schusssler et al. compared i-STAT ACT with Hemochron ACT during and after PCI (63). They found a high degree of correlation between the two ACTs at both low and high levels of anticoagulation. Statistically there was no difference between these two devices at lower levels of anticoagulation; at higher levels of anticoagulation there was a statistically significant difference that was not thought to be clinically significant. The use of GP IIb/IIIA inhibitors did not significantly change these relationships. Due to small numbers of patients, no conclusion could be drawn for use with DTI.

C. Dry Reagent Technology

Rather than using separate solutions that must be added to a test tube, the dry reagent technology places the coagulation activator and cofactors on a card. A very small amount of citrated blood is placed in a reaction chamber; the particular reagent preparation used determines the type of clotting time performed. Thus, if the same detection system is used, a single analyzer may be used for a variety of different tests. The Heparin Management Test (HMT) (Cardiovascular Diagnostics, Inc., Raleigh, NC), based on this technology, is a measure of whole blood anticoagulation introduced as an alternative to conventional ACT measurements. It is similar to ACT in principal (i.e., uses celite as activator) but uses a microprocessor-controlled analyzer and disposable test cards. A reaction chamber within each test card contains the paramagnetic iron oxide beads and dry chemical reagents necessary to activate the coagulation cascade in the blood sample (64). After a drop of blood is added, capillary action draws a small portion of this blood into the reaction chamber. An oscillating magnetic field is applied to the blood, chemical reactants, and beads. An infrared light beam passed through the test chamber detects oscillations in the amplitude of transmitted light coincident with the bead movement in the test chamber. As clot formation occurs, the beads become enmeshed within the clot, reducing the amplitude of light oscillations to trigger the end time for the HMT measurement (Fig. 3). The system come as an analyzer (TAS/ Rapidpoint Coag analyzer®) and a variety of test cards that can be used to monitor different aspects of anticoagulation. The low HMT cards are used to monitor low to moderate levels of unfractionated heparin (heparin concentration 0.25–3.0 U/mL) such as during PCI, while the HMT test cards are intended to monitor the effects of higher doses of heparin (1.0–10.0 U/mL). The test system can use both citrated and noncitrated whole blood. Table 2 compares the salient features of some of the available whole blood coagulation analyzers. The TAS HMT has been compared to the Hemochron and HemoTec ACT in prospective studies in the PCI setting. Tsimikas et al. noted that the the TAS-HMT gave significantly higher readings (~ 15% higher) than the HemoTec ACT, but a good correlation was noted between the two methods ($r = 0.77$), and the relation was similar in patients who received GP IIb/IIIa inhibitors (65). However, at ACT values of

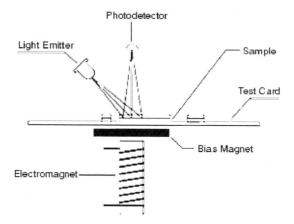

Figure 3   The internal mechanism of the Rapidpoint Coag® heparin management test (dry reagent technology). Above the platform for the test card is a photodetector and a photodiode. Below the platform are the bias and electromagnets, which, during the test procedure, influence the PIOP to move. As a clot begins to form, fibrin strands attach themselves to the particles, impeding their movement. Movement slows until the particles are entrapped in the clot and stop moving. The particle movement is monitored optically as changes in reflected light from the surface of the test card. When the movement stops, no light changes are seen and the test is complete. For fibrinolysis tests the process is reversed. When a sample is added to the test card, a clot is formed immediately and the particles are trapped. The analyzer monitors time for the clot to dissolve and free the particles to begin moving. (From Cardiovascular Diagnostics, INC., Raleigh, NC.)

Table 2 Salient Features of Point-of-Care Whole Blood Coagulation Analyzers

	Hemochron	HemoTec	TAS/HMT
Manufacturer	International Technidyne Corp., Edison, NJ	Medtronic, Inc., Englewood, CO	Cardiovascular Diagnostics, Inc., Raleigh, NC
Amount of blood	2 mL	0.2–0.4 mL	1 drop (35 μL)
Contact activator	Celite	Kaolin	Celite
Testing vehicle	Test tube	Test cartridge	Test card
Sensor method	Electro-mechanical	Electro-mechanical	Electro-optical
Detection system	Magnet in test tube	Plastic flag	Iron oxide particles on test card
Data management/ storage	No	No	Yes

Source: Modified from Ref. 65.

>300seconds the correlation was less strong. When compared to the Hemochron ACT, the two systems gave fairly similar values (HMT 292 ± 33 s and ACT 284 ± 31 s) and there was a reasonable correlation (0.66) (66,67). Also, HMT was shown to have a good correlation with anti-factor Xa activity in patients undergoing cardiovascular surgery (68).

D. Ecarin Clotting Time

In most large clinical trials aPTT has been used to monitor heparins; it is also the assay most commonly used to monitor heparin in clinical practice. The manufacturers of most DTIs recommend aPTT to these agents (69–71). However, unlike heparins that indirectly inhibit factors IIa, Xa, IXa, XIa, and XIIa, DTIs inhibit only thrombin (72). On the other hand, aPTT reflects inhibition of factors IIa, IXa, and Xa (73). Thus, intuitively, aPTT would not be the optimal method of monitoring DTIs because its values are affected by clotting factors not directly influenced by DTIs (74). Data in human studies showed only a moderate correlation of the concentration of these agents to aPTT values (75,76). The ecarin clotting time (ECT), on the other hand, is used specifically to monitor the effect of DTIs. Ecarin, used as a thrombin-generating agent in the ECT, is derived from the venom of a snake (*Echis carinatus*). Ecarin cleaves the arginine 320–isoleucine 321 protein bond of prothrombin, thereby generating meizothrombin. Meizothrombin possesses thrombin-like proteolytic activity. Like thrombin, its active site is inhibited by direct DTIs. The principle behind the ECT is that after the addition of a specific quantity of ecarin to blood containing a DTI, meizothrombin is generated. meizothrombin then reacts with the DTI to neutralize it. Once the inhibitor is neutralized, the remaining free Meizothrombin can activate the clotting process by stimulating the conversion of fibrinogen to fibrin. Since heparins are poor inhibitors of meizothrombin, the ECT is relatively specific for DTIs 77,78).

Clinical use of ECT has been reported. One study examined the precision of ECT compared to aPTT for monitoring lepirudin in 10 patients with a history of heparin-induced thrombocytopenia undergoing open heart surgery (79). These investigators found a strong linear relationship between the ECT values and lepirudin concentrations that ranged from 0.35 to 5.88 μg/mL ($r = 0.94$), whereas the aPTT demonstrated only a weak correlation ($r = 0.61$). Other studies also have shown that ECT correlates better with lepirudin levels and demonstrates less interpatient variability compared with the aPTT (80) or the ACT (78,80).

The thrombin inhibitor management test (TIM) (Pharmanetics, Morrisville, NC), a point-of-care test based on the ECT, has been developed using the dry reagent technology similar to that in the HMT test cards (81). Cho et al. compared the TIM ECT test and ACT [using the Hemochron ACT (International Technidyne, Edison, NJ) and Coagucheck Pro/DM (Roche Diagnostics, Indianapolis, IN) with central laboratory anti-factor IIa assay for monitoring bivalirudin-mediated anticoagulation in the setting of nonemergency PCI (82). All 64 patients received bivalirudin bolus of 0.75 mg/kg followed by a 1.75 mg/kg/h infusion. Fifty-five patients also received concomitant GP IIb/IIIa inhibitors. Samples were drawn at baseline, after administration of bivalirudin, after GP IIb/IIIa inhibitor bolus, and during the procedure and at sheath pull. The results showed that TIM ACT provided more accurate assessment of bivalirudin during PCI than ACT (Fig. 4). After GP IIb/IIIa inhibitor administration, no significant change in bivalirudin concentration or ECT values was noted, although the Hemochron ACT values increased. Thus, serum DTI concentrations correlate with the degree of clotting time prolongation, and the ECT may be an alternative to monitoring patients' DTI levels (83).

E. Viscoelastic Measures of Coagulation

Initially developed in the 1940s, viscoelastic measures of coagulation have undergone a resurgence in popularity. These tests are unique as they can measure the entire spectrum of clot formation from early fibrin strand generation through clot retraction and eventual fibrinolysis. Currently two such devices are in clinical use and will be described.

1. Thromboelastography

Thromboelastography was first described in 1948 by Hartert (84). With the advent of computerization, this has evolved from a research tool into a compact, commercially available point-of-care instrument: the Thrombolestagraph (TEG) (Hemoscope, Morton Grove, IL). It consists of a heated (37°C) cuvette that holds the blood (0.36 mL) as it oscillates through an angle of 4°45′. Each rotation lasts 10 seconds, which includes a 1-second rest period at the end of excursion. A pin, which is suspended freely in the blood by a torsion wire, is monitored for motion (Fig. 5). The torque of the rotating cup is transmitted to the pin once the clot starts to form. Therefore, the strength and rate of these fibrin-platelet bonds affect the magnitude of pin motion. When the clot lyses, the bonds are broken and the transfer of

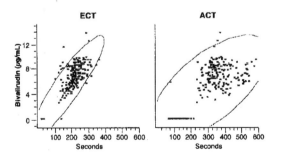

Figure 4   Correlation between ECT, ACT, and bivalirudin levels. Considering samples from all time points, the correlations between clotting time and bivalirudin concentration were $r = 0.90$ for ECT and $r = 0.71$ for Hemochron ACT. The ellipse shown on each graph represents the 90% density contour (confidence curve for the bivariate distribution). The ellipse becomes more circular in shape as the correlation decreases. (From Ref. 82.)

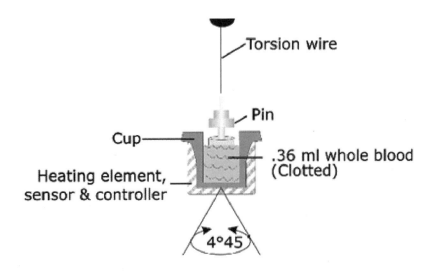

Figure 5 The Thromboelastograph® (Hemoscope, Morton Grove, IL). See text for details.

cup motion is diminished. The rotation of the pin is converted by a mechanical-electrical transducer to an electrical signal that can be monitored and recorded by a computer. Thus, TEG documents initial fibrin formation, clot rate strengthening, and fibrin-platelet bonding via GP IIb/IIIa to eventual clot lysis (Fig. 6).

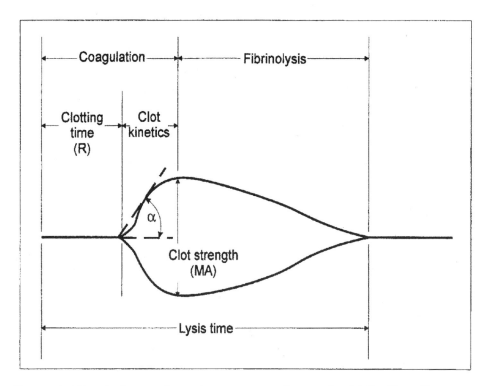

Figure 6 Thromboelastography tracing parameters. See text for details. (From Hemoscope, Skokie, IL)

The strength of a clot is graphically represented over time as a characteristic cigar shaped figure. There are five parameters of the TEG tracings that measure different stages of clot development (85–87) (Fig. 6):

R: The R value or the reaction time is the period of time from initiation of the test to the initial fibrin/clot formation (normal: 7.5–15 min). It is considered comparable to the whole blood clotting time and may be accelerated by adding celite to the sample cuvette. The R value is prolonged by a adeficiency of one or more plasma coagulation factors and shortened in hypercoaguable states.

K: This is measured from R time (i.e., from the beginning of clot formation) until the level of clot firmness reaches 20 mm (divergence of the lines from 2 to 20 mm). Therefore, K is a measure of clot strengthening. It is shortened by an increased fibrinogen level and, to a lesser extent , by increased platelet function and is prolonged by anticoagulants.

α: Alpha angle is formed by the slope of the TEG tracing at R from the horizontal line. It represents the acceleration kinetics of fibrin build-up and cross-linking. Like K, it is also increased by increased fibrinogen levels and, to a lesser extent , by increased platelet function and is decreased by anticoagulants. In hypercoaguable states, in which the clot amplitude never reaches 20 mm (i.e., K is undefined), the angle is more comprehensive than K time.

MA: Maximum amplitude (MA) reflects strength of a clot, which is dependent on the number and function of platelets and its interaction with fibrin. It may be decreased by either qualitative or quantitative platelet dysfunction or decreased fibrinogen concentration. Normal MA is 50–60 mm.

CI: The coagulation index describes the patients overall coagulation status. It is derived from the R, K, MA, and α of native or celite-activated whole blood tracings (CI for celite activated blood = 0.3258R − 0.1886K + 0.1224 MA + 0.0759 α − 7.7922). Normal values range from -3.0 to +3.0, which is equivalent to 3 standard deviations about the mean of zero. Positive values outside the range (CI > 3) indicate that the sample is hypercoaguable, whereas negative values outside this range (CI < 3) indicate that the sample is hypocoaguable.

Ly30/LY60:   These values measure percentage lysis at 30 and 60 minutes, respectively, after the MA is reached. Measurements are based on the reading of the area under the TEG tracing from the time MA is measured until 30 and 60 minutes after the MA. Therefore, when these values are high, the fibrinolytic activity is high.

TEG tracings can be qualitatively and quantitatively analyzed (88). Various patterns can be easily recognized (Fig. 7) as hypocoagulation, normal coagulation, hypercoagulation, and fibrinolysis. However, by using measurements and established normal ranges and indices, the patterns can be quantified as to the degree of abnormality, which allows better monitoring of therapies. Measurements derived from these diagrams have been related to more traditional measures of coagulation, such as ACT (89). TEG monitoring has been used in liver transplant surgery to rapidly analyze and treat the changing coagulation profile of the patients (90). Studies have evaluated the utility of TEG in cardiac surgery after cardiopulmonary bypass (CPB) (91) and to assess blood product transfusion requirements. Shore-Lesserson et al. (91) compared transfusion requirements in a arandomized, prospective trial of high-risk cardiac surgical patients. Patients were randomly assigned to TEG-guided transfusion therapy or standard laboratory based transfusion therapy. Patients in both groups

Normal

Thrombocytopenia

Severe Platelet Dysfunction

Coagulation Factor Deficiency

Fibrinolysis

Hypercoagulable State

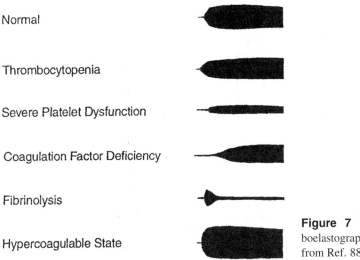

Figure 7 Characteristic thromboelastograph tracings. (Modified from Ref. 88.)

received antifibrinolytic therapy with EACA. They noted that patients in the TEG group received fewer total transfusions and a significantly smaller volume of fresh frozen plasma. The authors concluded that the TEG-based transfusion algorithm reduced transfusion requirements. TEG may also be used to differentiate surgical bleeding from coagulopathy following cardiac surgery (92). TEG has also been used successfully to monitor hirudin therapy during CPB in the setting of heparin-induced thrombocytopenia (87). TEG has been used to assess the coagulation status in obstetrical patients receiving low molecular weight heparins (93) in the peripartum period and in disseminated intravascular coagulation (94,95).

2. Sonoclot Analyzer

The Sonoclot® analyzer (Sienco, Inc.; Morrison, CO) provides an alternative viscoelastic measure of coagulation. Compared with TEG, the Sonoclot immerses a rapidly vibrating probe into a 0.4 ml sample of blood. As the clot formation occurs, impedance to probe movement through the blood increases and generates an electrical and a characteristic "clot signature." The Sonoclot may be used to derive ACT as well as provide information regarding clot strength and clot lysis (96). The Sonoclot generates both a qualitative graph, known as the Sonoclot signature (Fig. 8), and quantitative results on the clot formation time (ACT onset) and the rate of fibrin polymerization (clot rate) for identifying numerous coagulopathies including platelet dysfunction, factor deficiencies, anticoagulation effect, hypercoaguable tendencies, and fibrinolysis. As the blood sample clots, numerous mechanical changes related to the performance of the patients hemostasis system occur that alter the clot signal value (97). The record of clot evolution is saved as a graph of the clot signal versus time. Both celite- and kaolin-activated Sonoclot ACT tests are available (98).

In a Sonoclot signature, the coagulation cascade reactions develop from the beginning and continue throughout the liquid phase (initial horizontal portion of graph in Fig. 8). This phase ends when the viscosity of the sample increases with thrombin generation and resulting intitial fibrin formation and represents the ACT. This is followed by the continued conversion of fibrinogen to fibrin and its polymerization into a gel. This is affected by both the rate of conversion to fibrin and the availability of fibrinogen. This phase is represented by the slope of the graph (clot rate) and by the height of the signature when the gel formation is completed. This information is important in clinical applications including

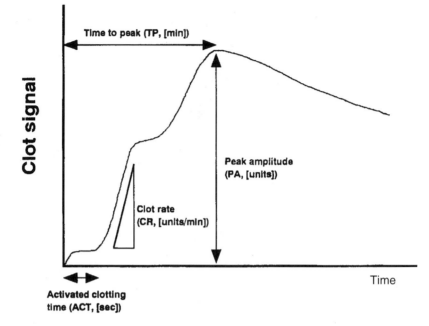

Figure 8   Description of the the Sonoclot Signature and variables. (From Ref. 99.)

monitoring anticoagulants hypercoaguable states, and fibrin hemodilution. Sonoclot also responds to clot retraction occurring within the test sample. As the clot retracts it tightens causing the signature to rise. Eventually, the clot often pulls away from some of the surfaces of the cuvette or probe. This results in a fall in the graph.

The sonoclot has been used to monitor the coagulation status in a multitude of conditions including cardiac surgery (89), hemodialysis patients (99) and malignancy associated. hypercoaguable states (100).

F.   ENOX Test

The ENOX® test (Pharmanetics Inc., Morrisville, NC) measures the combined anti-Xa and anti-IIa activity of the low molecular weight heparin (LMWH) enoxaparin (101). Unlike heparin, which has an anti-Xa/anti-IIa activity ratio of one, the LMWHs have a much higher relative anti-Xa inhibition. This is an important distinction, as the ability to prolong aPTT and ACT is proportional to the anti-IIa activity. The ENOX test was developed for exculsive use with the LMWH enoxaparin. In the ENOX test, factor X is rapidly converted to factor Xa by a specific activator of factor X, initiating the clotting process. Enoxaparin from the patient's blood complexes with antithrombin to inhibit factor Xa and proportionately lengthen the clotting time. Conventional chromogenic anti-Xa assays provide drug concentrations only in dilute, supplement plasma and are not suitable for point-of-care use. ENOX test is commercially available for point-of-care use and is based on dry reagent technology. The ENOX test cards are manufactured to be used with the Rapidpoint® Coag analyzer (Bayer Corp). As with all similar tests, all the components needed to perform the test, with the exception of the patient sample, are included in the reaction chamber of the test card (101). The test uses one drop (35 μL) of citrated venous or arterial blood sample. The ENOX test was designed to measure citrated whole blood clotting times corresponding to enoxaparin concentration of 0.0–3.0 anti-Xa IU/ml in derived plasma (102).

In a clinical trial that included patients undergoing PCI using enoxaparin, the ENOX clotting times correlated well ($r = 0.80$) with chromogenic anti-Xa assay–derived plasma enoxparin concentrations (range <0.1–1.8IU/mL) (103). Based on prior studies, a proposed targeted window for PCI anticoagulation with enoxaparin is 0.8–2.0 IU/mL (104–106). This corresponds to an ENOX clotting time of 250–450 seconds (104–106). The recently completed ELECT (Evaluation of ENOX Clotting Times) trial (107) examined data from 445 patients receiving iv or sc enoxaparin who underwent PCI. Only 33 (7.4%) had actually received sc enoxaparin; the vast majority were treated with enoxaparin in the catheterization laboratory. Most patients (336/445; 75.5% also received concomitant GPIIb/IIIa antagonists. Overall, in ELECT, the incidence of ischemic and hemorrhagic endpoints was low. There was no significant relationship between ENOX times and clinical outcomes, although ischemic events appeared lowest in the midrange of ENOX times. Total bleeding events were noted to increase with increasing ENOX times, although major bleeding events did not. The authors recommended (in light of suggested procedural anti-Xa levels of 0.8–1.8 IU/ml) a range of 350–450 sec on the ENOX test for PCI, and <200–250 seconds for sheath removal. The test itself showed considerable variability; an anti-Xa activity of approximately 0.8 IU/mL could be associated with an ENOX time as low as about 170 sec or a time as high as approximately 600 sec. This degree of variability would conceivably make it difficult to reliably titrate therapy with enoxaparin. Clearly, further studies will be needed to test the optimal ENOX time regarding clinical outcome. The targeted anti-Xa range of 0.8–1.8 IU.mL must also be considered somewhat arbitrary as no prospective study has been performed to validate this range.

G. Monitoring of Platelet Function

The pivotal role of the platelet in arterial thrombosis in general, and in acute coronary syndromes in particular, is well established. It is also clear that inhibition of platelets with an antiplatelet agent (e.g., aspirin, thienopyridines, or platelet glycoprotein GP IIb/IIIa inhibitors) can reduce progression to myocardial infarction in unstable coronary syndromes and reduce the incidence of ischemic complications during PCI. However, despite the effectiveness of these agents, they fail to prevent thrombotic events in all patients. One of the explanations for this is a potential heterogeneous response among individuals to standard dosing regimens. Current clinical practice (and practice guidelines) (107a) do not include any measurement of the effectiveness of platelet inhibitor therapy. Significant variation in the response to aspirin has been demonstrated by various studies (108,109).

However, only since the introduction of GP IIb/IIIa inhibitors has there been an expansion in our capabilities to assess platelet inhibition (110). Platelet function tests measure the capacity of platelets to adhere, activate, aggregate, and secrete. The goal of platelet function testing is to provide information about the platelet contribution to the risk of thrombosis or hemostasis. Important clinical questions in acute coronary syndromes are whether the antiplatelet agent is having the desired effect on platelet inhibition (inhibition) and whether the patient has sufficient platelet function to avoid significant bleeding (safety).

Platelet thrombus formation involves a number of processes, including activation of the platelet, secretion of vasoactive and prothrombotic chemicals, promotion of the clotting cascade, and platelet aggregation; each of these individual platelet functions may be affected by platelet therapy and could form the basis for a functional assay (110). It is not clear which function is most important. A variety of platelet function tests are available for use in the central laboratory, of which the Photo-Optical Tubidometric Aggregometric Assay is considered the gold standard. This test involves addition of a platelet aggregation agonist [e.g., ADP, collagen, epinephrine, or thrombin receptor activating peptide (TRAP)] to platelet-rich plasma. As platelets aggregate, light transmission increases. Maximum transmittance is calibrated using platelet-poor plasma, while minimum transmittance is determined with platelet-rich plasma prior to addition of the agonist.

For rapid clinical use in the critical care/cardiac catheterization laboratory setting, various point-of-care tests have been described, of which the following are more commonly used clinically in cardiovascular settings.

1. Rapid Platelet Function Assay

The Ultegra-RPFA (Accumetrics, San Diego, CA) is an automated, whole blood, cartridge-based optical aggregometer that utilizes fibrinogen-coated polystyrene beads. After addition of an agonist (iso-TRAP), these beads agglutinate in whole blood in proportion to the number of unblocked GP IIb/IIIa inhibitor receptors (111). The light transmittance increases with progressive binding of the platelets to the beads, leading to their agglutination. Current use involves a baseline measurement and repeat tests after drug administration. The results can be reported as a percentage of baseline aggregation or as an absolute rate of aggregation. One of the drawbacks of the test, as is the case with most currently available tests, is that it differs from in vivo conditions in that it is not conducted under flow conditions. The RPFA has been validated versus turbidometric aggregometry (112). At increasing concentrations of abciximab, the percentage inhibition of the RPFA correlated well with the turbidometric assay ($r^2 = 0.95$). This study also showed an excellent correlation with the degree of GP IIb/IIIa inhibitors receptor occupancy (measured using radiolabeled abciximab) ($r^2 = 0.96$).

Initial animal studies with monoclonal antibody 7E3 demonstrated that blockade of $\geq 80\%$ of GP IIb/IIIa inhibitors receptors with suppression of platelet aggregation to $\leq 20\%$ of baseline was necessary to prevent in vivo thrombosis (113). This level of platelet inhibition was used as the basis for the early dosing studies for abciximab (c7E3 Fab, ReoPro, Centocor, Inc., Malvern, PA) (114) and the importance of maintaining this level of platelet inhibition in the clinical setting was not tested directly. Numerous small studies have used RPFA to measure platelet inhibition after administration of glycoprotein GP IIb/IIIa inhibitors (115,116). The multicenter GOLD trial correlated the degree of platelet inhibition (using the RPFA device) to the clinical outcomes in 500 patients undergoing PCI with adjunctive GP IIb/IIIa inhibitor use (117). Major adverse cardiac events (MACEs) were prospectively monitored. One quarter of all patients did not achieve $\geq 95\%$ inhibition 10 minutes after the bolus and experienced a significantly higher incidence of MACEs (14.4% vs. 6.4%; $p = 0.006$). Patients whose platelet function was <70% inhibited at 8 hours after the start of therapy had a MACE rate of 25% versus 8.1% for those $\geq 70\%$ inhibited ($p = 0.009$). By multivariate analysis, platelet function inhibition of $\geq 95\%$ at 10 minutes after start of therapy was associated with a significant decrease in the incidence of a MACE (OR 0.46, 95% CI 0.22–0.96, $p = 0.04$). The authors concluded that there was substantial variability in the level of platelet function inhibition achieved with GP IIb/IIIa inhibitors among patients undergoing PCI. Also, the level of platelet function inhibition as measured by RPFA was an independent predictor for the risk for MACEs after PCI.

2. Platelet Function Analyzer (PFA-100)

The PFA-100 test (Dade Behring, Miami, FL) evaluates primary hemostasis through platelet-platelet interaction as whole blood flows under shear stress conditions through an aperture (118). The instrument uses citrated whole blood, which is drawn by means of a vacuum through a capillary tube producing high shear forces and then through a precisely defined aperture in a membrane that has been coated with either collagen and epinephrine or collagen and ADP. The platelets adhere and aggregate at the aperture until it is occluded, and the results are reported as the closure time (CT). The testing process takes about 10 minutes. The use of whole blood allows for the interaction of platelets with red blood cells and other whole blood components that may play a role in thrombus formation. Also, the addition of shear stress to platelet activation may make this test theoretically more physiologically sound (119). The test is prolonged by platelet counts below 50,000 and hematocrit levels below 25%. The normal range for CT for healthy subjects is 59–120 seconds (120). The maximal CT has been set at 300 seconds, which represents nonclosure of the aperture after 300 seconds. In a study of healthy volunteers treated with different concentrations of Tirofiban, there was found to be a good linear correlation of turbidometric aggregation with PFA with collagen-epinephrine membrane percent maximal CT prolongation ($r^2 = 0.97$) and a strong quadratic correlation of turbidometric aggregation and PFA with collagen-ADP membrane percent maximal CT prolongation ($r^2 = 0.098$).

IV. CONCLUSIONS

A variety of laboratory and point-of-care methods are available to help guide antithrombotic therapy. Depending on the clinical situation at hand, the appropriate test varies. For example, there is substantial evidence and clinical experience supporting the use of the standard aPTT in guiding heparin therapy for the prevention of pulmonary thromboembolism in patients with deep venous thrombosis. In contrast, ACT is used to assess heparenization for angioplasty or bypass surgery. For DTIs conventional methods like aPTT or ACT may not be optimal and newer tests such as the ECT are being investigated. Viscoelastic measures of coagulation are also being investigated in various clinical settings, including during cardiopulmonary bypass. Point-of-care tests are becoming increasingly popular, especially in the acute care setting. In this regard it is important to have stringent rules and guidelines to ensure proper quality measures and calibration to ensure reliability. This is especially true as these devices typically have higher coefficients of variability than standard laboratory tests (121). Finally, it should be remembered that although two tests may measure the same parameter (e.g., ACT), the numerical values may not be (and usually are not) identical. Thus, each coagulation test value should be qualified by the type of device used to measure it.

REFERENCES

1. Hoppensteadt DA, Walenga JM, Fareed J. Validity of serine protease inhibition tests in the evaluation and monitoring of the effect of heparin and its fractions. Semin Thromb Hemost. 1985; 11:112–20.
2. Holm HA, Abildgaard U, Larsen ML, Kalvenes S. Monitoring of heparin therapy: should heparin assays also reflect the patient's antithrombin concentration? Thromb Res. 1987; 46:669–675.
3. van den Besselaar AM, Meeuwisse-Braun J, Bertina RM. Monitoring heparin therapy: relationships between the activated partial thromboplastin time and heparin assays based on ex-vivo heparin samples. Thromb Haemost. 1990; 63:16–23.
4. Mannucci PM, Bottasso B, Tripodi A, Bianchi Bonomi A. Prothrombin fragment 1 + 2 and intensity of treatment with oral anticoagulants. Thromb Haemost. 1991; 66:741.
5. Hoek JA, Nurmohamed MT, ten Cate JW, Buller HR, Knipscheer HC, Hamelynck KJ, Marti RK, Sturk A. Thrombin-antithrombin III complexes in the prediction of deep vein thrombosis following total hip replacement. Thromb Haemost. 1989; 62:1050–1052.

6. Basu D, Gallus A, Hirsh J, Cade J. A prospective study of the value of monitoring heparin treatment with the activated partial thromboplastin time. N Engl J Med. 1972; 287:324–327.

7. Congdon JE, Kardinal CG, Wallin JD. Monitoring heparin therapy in hemodialysis. A report on the activated whole blood coagulation time tests. JAMA. 1973; 226:1529–1533.

8. Bounameaux H, Marbet GA, Lammle B, Eichlisberger R, Duckert F. Monitoring of heparin treatment. Comparison of thrombin time, activated partial thromboplastin time, and plasma heparin concentration, and analysis of the behavior of antithrombin III. Am J Clin Pathol. 1980; 74:68–73.

9. Alving B. Lupus Anticoagulants, Anticardiolipin Antibodies, and the Antiphospholipid Syndrome. Boston: Blackwell Scientific; 1994.

10. Hemker HC, Kessels H. Feedback mechanisms in coagulation. Haemostasis. 1991; 21:189–196.

11. Rapaport SI, Rao LV. Initiation and regulation of tissue factor-dependent blood coagulation. Arterioscler Thromb. 1992; 12:1111–21.

12. Hemker HC BS. The mode of action of heparins in vitro and in vivo. In: Lane, ed. Heparin and Related Polysaccharides. New York: Plenum Press; 1992:221.

13. Alson JD PB. Automated Coagulation Systems. New York: Van Nostrand Reinhold; 1995.

14. Mann KG, Krishnaswamy S, Lawson JH. Surface-dependent hemostasis. Semin Hematol. 1992; 29:213–226.

15. Tracy PB, Eide LL, Mann KG. Human prothrombinase complex assembly and function on isolated peripheral blood cell populations. J Biol Chem. 1985; 260:2119–2124.

16. Quick AJ S-BM, Bancroft FW. A study of the coagulation defect in hemophilia and jaundice. Am J Med Sci. 1935; 190:501.

17. Morrissey JH, Macik BG, Neuenschwander PF, Comp PC. Quantitation of activated factor VII levels in plasma using a tissue factor mutant selectively deficient in promoting factor VII activation. Blood. 1993; 81:734–744.

18. Zoldhelyi P, Webster MW, Fuster V, Grill DE, Gaspar D, Edwards SJ, Cabot CF, Chesebro JH. Recombinant hirudin in patients with chronic, stable coronary artery disease. Safety, half-life, and effect on coagulation parameters. Circulation. 1993; 88:2015–2022.

19. Sharma GV, Lapsley D, Vita JA, Sharma S, Coccio E, Adelman B, Loscalzo J. Usefulness and tolerability of hirulog, a direct thrombin-inhibitor, in unstable angina pectoris. Am J Cardiol. 1993; 72:1357–1360.

20. Hirsh J, Levine M. Confusion over the therapeutic range for monitoring oral anticoagulant therapy in North America. Thromb Haemost. 1988; 59:129–132.

21. Eckman MH, Levine HJ, Pauker SG. Effect of laboratory variation in the prothrombin-time ratio on the results of oral anticoagulant therapy. N Engl J Med. 1993; 329:696–702.

22. Bussey HI, Force RW, Bianco TM, Leonard AD. Reliance on prothrombin time ratios causes significant errors in anticoagulation therapy. Arch Intern Med. 1992; 152:278–282.

23. Kirkwood T. Combination of refernce thromboplastins and satndardization of the pro-thrombin time ratio. Thromb Haemost. 1983; 49:238.

24. Hull R, Hirsh J, Jay R, Carter C, England C, Gent M, Turpie AG, McLoughlin D, Dodd P, Thomas M, Raskob G, Ockelford P. Different intensities of oral anticoagulant therapy in the treatment of proximal-vein thrombosis. N Engl J Med. 1982; 307:1676–1681.

25. Thompson J. The Implementation of International Normalized Ratios for Standardization of the Prothrombin Time in the Oral Anticoagulant Control. New York: Churchill Livingstone; 1991.

26. Poller L, Keown M, Chauhan N, Shiach C, Van Den Besselaar AM, Tripodi A, Jespersen J. European Concerted Action on Anticoagulation (ECAA): international normalized ratio vari-ability of CoaguChek and TAS point-of-care testing whole blood prothrombin time monitors. Thromb Haemost. 2002; 88:992–995.

27. Lee RI Wp. A clinical study of coagulation time of blood. Am J Med Sci. 1913; 145:495.

28. Jesty J. Interaction of feedback control and product inhibition in the activation of factor X by factors IXa and VIII. Haemostasis. 1991; 21:208–218.

29. Willems GM, Lindhout T, Hermens WT, Hemker HC. Simulation model for thrombin gener-ation in plasma. Haemostasis. 1991; 21:197–207.

30. Pieters J, Lindhout T, Hemker HC. In situ-generated thrombin is the only enzyme that effectively activates factor VIII and factor V in thromboplastin-activated plasma. Blood. 1989; 74:1021–1024.

31. Nesheim ME, Taswell JB, Mann KG. The contribution of bovine factor V and Factor Va to the activity of prothrombinase. J Biol Chem. 1979; 254:10952–10962.

32. Langdell RD WR, Brinkhous KM. Effect of hemophillic factor on one stage clotting tests. J Lab Clin Med. 1953; 41:637.

33. Nye SW GJ, Brinkhous KM. The partial thromboplastin time for the detection of late bleeders. Am J Med Sci. 1962; 243:279.

34. Quick A GM. Screening for bleeding states- the partial thromboplastin time. Am J Clin Pathol. 1963; 40:465.

35. Goulian M Bw. The partial thromboplastin time test. Modification of the procedure and a study of the senisivity and optimal conditions. Am J Clin Pathol. 1965; 44:97.

36. Mant M. J HJ, Pineo GF, Luke KH. Prolonged prothrombin time and partial thomboplastin time in disseminated intravascular coagulation not due to the deficiency of factors V and VIII. Br J Haematol. 1973; 24:725.

37. Hirsh J. Heparin. N Engl J Med. 1991; 324:1565–1574.

38. Ofosu FA, Sie P, Modi GJ, Fernandez F, Buchanan MR, Blajchman MA, Boneu B, Hirsh J. The inhibition of thrombin-dependent positive-feedback reactions is critical to the expression of the anticoagulant effect of heparin. Biochem J. 1987; 243:579–588.

39. Hull RD, Raskob GE, Hirsh J, Jay RM, Leclerc JR, Geerts WH, Rosenbloom D, Sackett DL, Anderson C, Harrison L, et al. Continuous intravenous heparin compared with intermittent subcutaneous heparin in the initial treatment of proximal-vein thrombosis. N Engl J Med. 1986; 315:1109–1114.

40. Theroux P, Ouimet H, McCans J, Latour JG, Joly P, Levy G, Pelletier E, Juneau M, Stasiak J, deGuise P, et al. Aspirin, heparin, or both to treat acute unstable angina. N Engl J Med. 1988; 319:1105–1111.

41. Hsia J, Hamilton WP, Kleiman N, Roberts R, Chaitman BR, Ross AM. A comparison between heparin and low-dose aspirin as adjunctive therapy with tissue plasminogen activator for acute myocardial infarction. Heparin-Aspirin Reperfusion Trial (HART) investigators. N Engl J Med. 1990; 323:1433–1437.

42. Mattox KL, Guinn GA, Rubio PA, Beall AC, Jr. Use of the activated coagulation time in intraoperative heparin reversal for cardiopulmonary operations. Ann Thorac Surg. 1975; 19:634–638.

43. Bull BS, Huse WM, Brauer FS, Korpman RA. Heparin therapy during extracorporeal circulation. II. The use of a dose-response curve to individualize heparin and protamine dosage. J Thorac Cardiovasc Surg. 1975; 69:685–689.

44. Young JA, Kisker CT, Doty DB. Adequate anticoagulation during cardiopulmonary bypass determined by activated clotting time and the appearance of fibrin monomer. Ann Thorac Surg. 1978; 26:231–240.

45. Dougherty KG, Gaos CM, Bush HS, Leachman DR, Ferguson JJ. Activated clotting times and activated partial thromboplastin times in patients undergoing coronary angioplasty who receive bolus doses of heparin. Cathet Cardiovasc Diagn. 1992; 26:260–263.

46. Ogilby JD, Kopelman HA, Klein LW, Agarwal JB. Adequate heparinization during PTCA: assessment using activated clotting times. Cathet Cardiovasc Diagn. 1989; 18:206–209.

47. Colman RW, Oxley L, Giannusa P. Statistical comparison of the automated activated partial thromboplastin time and the clotting time in the regulation of heparin therapy. Am J Clin Pathol. 1970; 53:904–907.

48. Green D, Ts'ao C, Reynolds N, Kahn D, Kohl H, Cohen I. In vitro studies of a new synthetic thrombin inhibitor. Thromb Res. 1985; 37:145–53.

49. Jakubowski JA, Maraganore JM. Inhibition of coagulation and thrombin-induced platelet activities by a synthetic dodecapeptide modeled on the carboxy-terminus of hirudin. Blood. 1990; 75:399–406.

50. Jang IK, Gold HK, Ziskind AA, Leinbach RC, Fallon JT, Collen D. Prevention of platelet-rich arterial thrombosis by selective thrombin inhibition. Circulation. 1990; 81:219–225.

51. Carteaux JP, Gast A, Tschopp TB, Roux S. Activated clotting time as an appropriate test to compare heparin and direct thrombin inhibitors such as hirudin or Ro 46–6240 in experimental arterial thrombosis. Circulation. 1995; 91:1568–1574.

52. Granger CB MD. Bedside anticoagulation testing. In: Topol E, ed. Acute Coronary Syndromes. 2nd ed. New York: Marcel Dekker, Inc.; 2001.

53. Gusto Gazzette. 1992; July/August:2.

54. Hattersley PG. Activated coagulation time of whole blood. JAMA. 1966; 196:436–40.

55. Colman RW, Bagdasarian A, Talamo RC, Scott CF, Seavey M, Guimaraes JA, Pierce JV, Kaplan AP. Williams trait. Human kininogen deficiency with diminished levels of plasminogen proactivator and prekallikrein associated with abnormalities of the Hageman factor-dependent pathways. J Clin Invest. 1975; 56:1650–1662.

56. Schriever HG, Epstein SE, Mintz MD. Statistical correlation and heparin sensitivity of activated partial thromboplastin time, whole blood coagulation time, and an automated coagulation time. Am J Clin Pathol. 1973; 60:323–329.

57. Avendano A, Ferguson JJ. Comparison of Hemochron and HemoTec activated coagulation time target values during percutaneous transluminal coronary angioplasty. J Am Coll Cardiol. 1994; 23:907–910.

58. Ferguson J. All ACT's are not the same. Texas Heart Inst J. 1992; 19.

59. Dietrich W JM. Effect of celite and kaolin on activated clotting time in the presence of aprotinin: Activated clotting time is reduced by binding of aprotinin to kaolin. J Thorac Cardiovasc Surg. 1995; 109:177.

60. Moliterno DJ, Califf RM, Aguirre FV, Anderson K, Sigmon KN, Weisman HF, Topol EJ. Effect of platelet glycoprotein IIb/IIIa integrin blockade on activated clotting time during percutaneous transluminal coronary angioplasty or directional atherectomy (the EPIC trial). Evaluation of c7E3 Fab in the Prevention of Ischemic Complications trial. Am J Cardiol. 1995; 75:559–562.

61. Feuillu A, Morel I, Mollard JF. [Evaluation of portable point of care instrument: the i-STAT. Report of 7,000 analyses]. Ann Biol Clin (Paris). 2002; 60:153–164.

62. Papadea C, Foster J, Grant S, Ballard SA, Cate JCt, Southgate WM, Purohit DM. Evaluation of the i-STAT Portable Clinical Analyzer for point-of-care blood testing in the intensive care units of a university children's hospital. Ann Clin Lab Sci. 2002; 32:231–243.

63. Schussler JM, Aguanno JJ, Glover EN, Vish NA, Wissinger LA, Schumacher JR, Wheelan KR. Comparison of the i-STAT handheld activated clotting time with the Hemochron activated clotting time during and after percutaneous coronary intervention. Am J Cardiol. 2003; 91:464–466.

64. Oberhardt BJ, Dermott SC, Taylor M, Alkadi ZY, Abruzzini AF, Gresalfi NJ. Dry reagent technology for rapid, convenient measurements of blood coagulation and fibrinolysis. Clin Chem. 1991; 37:520–526.

65. Tsimikas S, Beyer R, Hassankhani A. Relationship between the heparin management test and the HemoTec activated clotting time in patients undergoing percutaneous coronary intervention. J Thromb Thrombolysis. 2001; 11:217–221.

66. Helft G, Bartolomeo P, Zaman AG, Worthley SG, Chokron S, Le Pailleur C, Beygui F, Le Feuvre C, Metzger JP, Vacheron A, Samama MM. The heparin management test: a new device for monitoring anticoagulation during coronary intervention. Thromb Res. 1999; 96:481–485.

67. Helft G, Choktron S, Beygui F, Le Feuvre C, Elalamy I, Metzger JP, Vacheron A, Samama MM. Comparison of activated clotting times to heparin management test for adequacy of heparin anticoagulation in percutaneous transluminal coronary angioplasty. Cathet Cardiovasc Diagn. 1998; 45:329–331.

68. Fitch JC, Geary KL, Mirto GP, Byrne DW, Hines RL. Heparin management test versus activated coagulation time during cardiovascular surgery: correlation with anti-Xa activity. J Cardiothorac Vasc Anesth. 1999; 13:53–57.

69. Berlex Laboratories W, NJ. Refludan (Lepirudin) package insert. 2001.

70. The Medicines Company C, MA. Angimax (bivalirudin) package insert. 2000.

71. Texas Biotechnology Corporation and GlaxoSmithkline, Houston, TX, and Philadelphia, PA. Argatroban package insert. 2000.

72. Bates SM WJ. The mechanism of action of thrombin inhibitors. J Invasive Cardiol. 2001; 12:27F-32.

73. Simko RJ, Tsung FF, Stanek EJ. Activated clotting time versus activated partial thromboplastin time for therapeutic monitoring of heparin. Ann Pharmacother. 1995; 29:1015–1021; quiz 1061.

74. de Denus S, Spinler SA. Clinical monitoring of direct thrombin inhibitors using the ecarin clotting time. Pharmacotherapy. 2002; 22:433–435.

75. Cannon CP, Maraganore JM, Loscalzo J, McAllister A, Eddings K, George D, Selwyn AP, Adelman B, Fox I, Braunwald E, et al. Anticoagulant effects of hirulog, a novel thrombin inhibitor, in patients with coronary artery disease. Am J Cardiol. 1993; 71:778–782.

76. Herrman JP, Suryapranata H, den Heijer P, Gabriel L, Kutryk MJ, Serruys PW. Argatroban during percutaneous transluminal coronary angioplasty: results of a dose-verification study. J Thromb Thrombolysis. 1996; 3:367–375.

77. Moser M, Ruef J, Peter K, Kohler B, Gulba DC, Paterna N, Nordt T, Kubler W, Bode C. Ecarin clotting time but not aPTT correlates with PEG-hirudin plasma activity. J Thromb Thrombolysis. 2001; 12:165–169.

78. Nowak G BE. Quantitative determination of hirudin in blood and body fluids. Semin Thromb Hemost. 1996; 22:197–202.

79. Potzsch B, Hund S, Madlener K, Unkrig C, Muller-Berghaus G. Monitoring of recombinant hirudin: assessment of a plasma-based ecarin clotting time assay. Thromb Res. 1997; 86:373–383.

80. Potzsch B, Madlener K, Seelig C, Riess CF, Greinacher A, Muller-Berghaus G. Monitoring of r-hirudin anticoagulation during cardiopulmonary bypass—assessment of the whole blood ecarin clotting time. Thromb Haemost. 1997; 77:920–925.

81. Diagnostic. C. TAS ECT test card package insert. In: Raleigh N, ed.; 2000.

82. Cho L, Kottke-Marchant K, Lincoff AM, Roffi M, Reginelli JP, Kaldus T, Moliterno DJ. Correlation of point-of-care ecarin clotting time versus activated clotting time with bivalirudin concentrations. Am J Cardiol. 2003; 91:1110–1113.

83. Nowak G. Clinical monitoring of hirudin and direct thrombin inhibitors. Semin Thromb Hemost. 2001; 27:537–541.

84. Hartert H. Blutgerinnungsstudien mit der Thrombelatographie, einem neuen Untersuchungsverfahren. Klin Wochenscgr. 1948; 26:577–583.

85. Mallett SV, Cox DJ. Thrombelastography. Br J Anaesth. 1992; 69:307–313.

86. Wenker O, Wojciechowski Z, Sheinbaum R, Zisman E. Thrombelastography. Internet J Anesthesiol. 2000; 1.

87. Pivalizza EG. Monitoring of hirudin therapy with the Thrombelastograph. J Clin Anesth. 2002; 14:456–458.

88. Srinivasa V, Gilbertson LI, Bhavani-Shankar K. Thromboelastography: where is it and where is it heading? Int Anesthesiol Clin. 2001; 39:35–49.

89. Tuman KJ, Spiess BD, McCarthy RJ, Ivankovich AD. Comparison of viscoelastic measures of coagulation after cardiopulmonary bypass. Anesth Analg. 1989; 69:69–75.

90. Kang YG, Martin DJ, Marquez J, Lewis JH, Bontempo FA, Shaw BW, Jr., Starzl TE, Winter PM. Intraoperative changes in blood coagulation and thrombelastographic monitoring in liver transplantation. Anesth Analg. 1985; 64:888–896.

91. Shore-Lesserson L, Manspeizer HE, DePerio M, Francis S, Vela-Cantos F, Ergin MA. Thromboelastography-guided transfusion algorithm reduces transfusions in complex cardiac surgery. Anesth Analg. 1999; 88:312–319.

92. Spiess BD, Tuman KJ, McCarthy RJ, DeLaria GA, Schillo R, Ivankovich AD. Thromboelastography as an indicator of post-cardiopulmonary bypass coagulopathies. J Clin Monit. 1987; 3:25–30.

93. Gorton H. Thromboelastography and low molecular weight therapy in pregnancy. Anesthesiology. 1999; 90.

94. Steer PL. Anaesthetic management of a parturient with thrombocytopenia using thrombelastography and sonoclot analysis. Can J Anaesth. 1993; 40:84–85.

95. Steer P, Blumenthal LA. Abruptio placentae and disseminated intravascular coagulation, use of thromboelastography and sonoclot analysis. Int J Obstet Anesth. 1994; 3:229–233.

96. Shenaq SA. Viscoelastic Measurement of Clot Formation: The Sonoclot. Philadelphia: WB Saunders Company; 1988.

97. Hett DA, Walker D, Pilkington SN, Smith DC. Sonoclot analysis. Br J Anaesth. 1995; 75:771–776.

98. Sonoclot coagulation & platelet function analyzer: an overview (Product monograph). In: Sienco, Inc., CO,USA.

99. Furuhashi M, Ura N, Hasegawa K, Yoshida H, Tsuchihashi K, Miura T, Shimamoto K. Sonoclot coagulation analysis: new bedside monitoring for determination of the appropriate heparin dose during haemodialysis. Nephrol Dial Transplant. 2002; 17:1457–1462.

100. Francis JL, Francis DA, Gunathilagan GJ. Assessment of hypercoagulability in patients with cancer using the Sonoclot Analyzer and thromboelastography. Thromb Res. 1994; 74:335–346.

101. Pharmanetics Inc., Morrisville, NC, USA. ENOX test card package insert. 2002.

102. Mize P CG, Oliver J, Stallings P, Leumas J, Mahan D, DeAnglis A. Development of the Rapidpoint™ Coag Enoxaparin Test Card System to Monitor Lovenox® (enoxaparin sodium) in PCI patients. Blood. 2001; 98:185a.

103. Mize P CG, Oliver J, Stallings P, Leumas J, Mahan D, DeAnglis A. Rapidpoint™ Coag Enoxaparin Test: clinical results for a POC method for monitoring Lovenox® (enoxaparin sodium) in Patients Undergoing PCI. Blood. 2001; 98:193a.

104. Kereiakes DJ, Grines C, Fry E, Esente P, Hoppensteadt D, Midei M, Barr L, Matthai W, Todd M, Broderick T, Rubinstein R, Fareed J, Santoian E, Neiderman A, Brodie B, Zidar J, Ferguson JJ, Cohen M. Enoxaparin and abciximab adjunctive pharmacotherapy during percutaneous coronary intervention. J Invasive Cardiol. 2001; 13:272–278.

105. Young JJ, Kereiakes DJ, Grines CL. Low-molecular-weight heparin therapy in percutaneous coronary intervention: the NICE 1 and NICE 4 trials. National Investigators Collaborating on Enoxaparin Investigators. J Invasive Cardiol. 2000; 12 (suppl E): E14–8; discussion E25–28.

106. Collet JP, Montalescot G, Lison L, Choussat R, Ankri A, Drobinski G, Sotirov I, Thomas D. Percutaneous coronary intervention after subcutaneous enoxaparin pretreatment in patients with unstable angina pectoris. Circulation. 2001; 103:658–663.

107. Moliterno, DJ, Hermiller JB, Keriakes DJ, et al. A novel point-of-care enoxaparin monitor for use during percutaneous coronary Intervention: Results of the Evaluating Enoxaparin Clotting Times (ELECT) study. J Am Coll Cardiol 2003; 42:1132–1139.

107a. Braunwald E AE, Beasley JW, Califf RM, Cheitlin MD, Hochman JS, Jones RH, Kereiakes D, Kupersmith J, Levin TN, Pepine CJ, Schaeffer JW, Smith EE 3rd, Steward DE, Theroux P, Gibbons RJ, Alpert JS, Faxon DP, Fuster V, Gregoratos G, Hiratzka LF, Jacobs AK, Smith SC Jr. ACC/AHA guideline update for the management of patients with unstable angina and non-ST-segment elevation myocardial infarction—2002: summary article: a report of the American College of Cardiology/American Heart Association Task Force on Practice Guidelines (Committee on the Management of Patients With Unstable Angina). J Am Coll Cardiol. 2002; 40:1366–1374.

108. Buchanan MR, Brister SJ. Individual variation in the effects of ASA on platelet function: implications for the use of ASA clinically. Can J Cardiol. 1995; 11:221–227.

109. Helgason CM BK, Hoff JA, Winkler SR, Mangat A, Tortorice KL, Brace LD. Development of aspirin resistance in persons with previous ischemic stroke. Stroke. 1994; 25:2331–2336.

110. Thompson CM, Steinhubl SR. Monitoring of platelet function in the setting of glycoprotein IIb/IIIa inhibitor therapy. J Interv Cardiol. 2002; 15:61–70.

111. Coller BS, Lang D, Scudder LE. Rapid and simple platelet function assay to assess glycoprotein IIb/IIIa receptor blockade. Circulation. 1997; 95:860–867.

112. Smith JW, Steinhubl SR, Lincoff AM, Coleman JC, Lee TT, Hillman RS, Coller BS. Rapid platelet-function assay: an automated and quantitative cartridge-based method. Circulation. 1999; 99:620–635.

113. Coller BS, Folts JD, Smith SR, Scudder LE, Jordan R. Abolition of in vivo platelet thrombus formation in primates with monoclonal antibodies to the platelet GPIIb/IIIa receptor. Correlation with bleeding time, platelet aggregation, and blockade of GPIIb/IIIa receptors. Circulation. 1989; 80:1766–1774.

114. Tcheng JE, Ellis SG, George BS, Kereiakes DJ, Kleiman NS, Talley JD, Wang AL, Weisman HF, Califf RM, Topol EJ. Pharmacodynamics of chimeric glycoprotein IIb/IIIa integrin antiplatelet antibody Fab 7E3 in high-risk coronary angioplasty. Circulation. 1994; 90:1757–1764.

115. Casterella P KD, Steinhubl SR, et al. coronary intervention. Use of the rapid platelet function analyzer (RPFA) to evaluate platelet function in patients receiving incremental bolus dosing of abciximab during percutaneous. J Am Coll Cardiol. 1999; 33:39A.

116. Steinhubl SR, Kottke-Marchant K, Moliterno DJ, Rosenthal ML, Godfrey NK, Coller BS, Topol EJ, Lincoff AM. Attainment and maintenance of platelet inhibition through standard dosing of abciximab in diabetic and nondiabetic patients undergoing percutaneous coronary intervention. Circulation. 1999; 100:1977–1982.

117. Steinhubl SR, Talley JD, Braden GA, Tcheng JE, Casterella PJ, Moliterno DJ, Navetta FI, Berger PB, Popma JJ, Dangas G, Gallo R, Sane DC, Saucedo JF, Jia G, Lincoff AM, Theroux P, Holmes DR, Teirstein PS, Kereiakes DJ. Point-of-care measured platelet inhibition correlates with a reduced risk of an adverse cardiac event after percutaneous coronary intervention: results of the GOLD (AU-Assessing Ultegra) multicenter study. Circulation. 2001; 103:2572–2578.

118. Mammen EF, Comp PC, Gosselin R, Greenberg C, Hoots WK, Kessler CM, Larkin EC, Liles D, Nugent DJ. PFA-100 system: a new method for assessment of platelet dysfunction. Semin Thromb Hemost. 1998; 24:195–202.

119. Nicholson NS, Panzer-Knodle SG, Haas NF, Taite BB, Szalony JA, Page JD, Feigen LP, Lansky DM, Salyers AK. Assessment of platelet function assays. Am Heart J. 1998; 135:S170–178.

120. Fressinaud E VA, Truchaud F, Martin I, Boyer-Neumann C, Trossaert M, Meyer D. Screening for von Willebrand disease with a new analyzer using high shear stress: a study of 60 cases. Blood. 1998; 91:1325–1331.

121. Macik BG. Designing a point-of-care program for coagulation testing. Arch Pathol Lab Med. 1995; 119:929–938.

18-2

Anticoagulation Monitoring in the Management of Venous Disease

Kamal Gupta, J. Michael Wilson, and James J. Ferguson
St. Luke's Episcopal Hospital, Texas Heart Institute, Baylor College of Medicine, The University of Texas Health Science Center at Houston, Houston, Texas, U.S.A.

I. INTRODUCTION

Venous thromboembolism (VTE) is common and causes significant morbidity and, in the form of massive pulmonary embolism (PE), can cause sudden death (1,2). It is estimated that more than 250,000 patients are hospitalized with VTE annually in the United States, and as many as 50,000 deaths may be attributed to this disease(3). Mortality from VTE is significant and is substantially higher in patients with symptomatic PE (46% 1 year survival) compared to patients with deep vein thrombosis (DVT) alone (85% 1 year survival). However, both are manifestations of the same process and will be discussed together. More than one third of deaths occur within 24 hours of onset of symptoms (4), thus the need for immediate recognition and treatment. The ideal treatment of VTE is prevention of the initial thrombus formation (5,6). The decision to use prophylaxis and the type of preventive measures used depend on the estimated risk of occurrence of VTE. The pharmacological management of VTE advanced significantly over the last 50 years as warfarin and heparin became more widely used. Cumulative clinical experience with warfarin and heparin for the prevention and treatment of VTE has highlighted a number of efficacy and safety limitations. This prompted accelerated research into newer strategies and incorporation of new agents such as low molecular weight heparins (LMWHs) into standard therapy for VTE. Other newer agents, such as direct thrombin inhibitors and indirect anti-Xa inhibitors (fondaparinux), are also being investigated. This chapter will discuss the various strategies and use of anticoagulation monitoring for the treatment of venous disorders, specifically VTE.

II. ACUTE TREATMENT OF VENOUS THROMBOEMBOLIC DISEASE

Treatment regimens for PE and DVT are generally similar because the two conditions are basically manifestations of the same disease process. When patients with VTE are carefully studied, the majority of those with proximal DVT also have PE and vice versa. Furthermore, clinical trials in DVT alone have validated treatment regimens that are similar to regimens used in patients with both DVT and PE or those with known PE alone. Since more than a third of deaths from VTE occur on the day of presentation(4), early initiation of effective treatment is the key to better outcomes.

A. Heparin

Unfractionated heparin (UFH) is a time-honored and effective antithrombotic agent for VTE. The first study that compared heparin with placebo was completed before the advent of perfusion lung imaging and pulmonary angiography (7). Despite its many flaws, this seminal study was persuasive for the use of anticoagulation in PE, as the untreated group had a much higher mortality (25%), with a large majority of deaths being due to autopsy-proven PE. Subsequent studies (8,9) have attested to the reduced mortality rate in heparin-treated patients, and to the high mortality when patients with PE did not receive heparin (10). Recent randomized trials (11–17) have confirmed the efficacy of continuous intravenous (IV) heparin in the treatment of DVT. Other trials indicate that subcutaneous heparin is also adequate as initial therapy for DVT as long as activated partial troumboplastin time (aPTT) is adequately prolonged or adequate doses are used (18–20). While most patients with symptomatic calf vein thrombosis should receive anticoagulation, asymptomatic thrombosis that is limited to the deep calf veins appears to be associated with a low risk of clinically important PE. Such patients could be followed with serial impedance plethesmography or duplex ultrasonography for 10–14 days to look for proximal extension of the thrombus. Lack of extension is associated with a low risk of clinically significant PE (<1%) or recurrent venous thrombosis (2%) (21).

A minimal level of anticoagulation must be maintained to achieve an effective antithrombotic state (11,12,22,23). Inadequate anticoagulant therapy results in unacceptably high rates of recurrent thromboembolism. The most widely used test for monitoring heparin therapy in VTE is aPTT. A retrospective analysis published almost 3 decades ago suggested that recurrent VTE is infrequent if continuous IV heparin is administered in doses adjusted to prolong the aPTT > 1.5 times the control (24). A randomized prospective trial (11) comparing IV and subcutaneous administration of heparin in patients with proximal vein thrombosis demonstrated that failure to achieve an adequate anticoagulant response (aPTT > 1.5 times control) is associated with a high risk (20–25%) of recurrent VTE. An analysis of three consecutive double-blind trials supported this observation (25). In general, an aPTT of >1.5 times control (or mean normal) corresponded to a blood heparin level of 0.2 IU/mL in these studies. Both animal and human studies have shown that a plasma heparin level in the range of 0.2–0.4 IU/ml (protamine titration method) effectively inhibits thrombus propogation (26–28).

Audits of heparin therapy indicate that the clinical practice of ordering heparin based on fixed doses, with subsequent doses being driven empirically by aPTT values, often results in underanticoagulation, probably because of underdosing secondary to fear of bleeding (29,30). Though several nomograms are available, weight based heparin dosing nomograms are widely employed and have resulted in a decrease in the incidence of recurrent thromboembolism and bleeding (31). It is suggested that heparin be started with a bolus of 80 IU/kg IV followed by an infusion rate of 18 IU/k/h. An aPTT level is checked in 6 hours. The infusion rate is titrated according to the aPTT level with a goal of 1.5–2.5 times the control. An aPTT level of <1.2 times the control is given an additional bolus of 80 IU/kg followed by an increase in infusion rate of 4 IU/kg/h. An aPTT of 1.2–1.5 times control is given a 40 IU/kg bolus followed by an increase in infusion rate of 2 IU/kg/h. If the aPTT level is within the goal (1.5–2.5), no change is made. For an aPTT of 2.5–3.0, the infusion rate is decreased by 2 IU/kg/h. If aPTT is more than 3.0 times the control value, then the infusion is typically held for an hour and then restarted at a rate decreased by 3 IU/kg/h. Monitoring of aPTT is performed every 6 hours until steady state is reached (32). When heparin is given subcutaneously as an initial anticoagulation dose, therapy should begin with a small IV loading dose (3000–5000 IU) followed by 17,500I U (or 250

IU/kg) subcutaneously every 12 hours (19). The dose should then be adjusted to give an aPTT that corresponds to a plasma heparin level of 0.2 IU/mL within 1 hour of the next scheduled subcutaneous dose. Heparin requirements are usually greatest during the first few days after the acute thromboembolic event (33,34); consequently therapy should be monitored most closely then. After that, the monitoring test may be obtained once daily.

Since most patients need longer-term anticoagulation, the general approach after initiation of acute treatment with heparin is to begin concurrent treatment with warfarin and to discontinue heparin between the fourth and the seventh day (after 2–4 days of achieving a therapeutic INR). This approach is effective and seems to avoid an additional 4–5 days of subsequent hospitalization needed to achieve adequate INR.

B. Low Molecular Weight Heparins

LMWHs are now probably used more often in the treatment of VTE than UFH. LMWHs have greater bioavailability, longer half-life, more predictable dose response, and less frequent thrombocytopenia and osteopenia (35). LMWH can be given as the initial treatment for VTE in a fixed dose in most patients without monitoring. If monitoring is deemed necessary in certain clinical situations, then plasma anti-Xa levels are measured 4 hours after subcutaneous injection of a weight-adjusted dose. A therapeutic range of 0.6–1.0 IU/mL should be achieved for twice-daily dosing and 1.9–2.0 IU/mL for once-daily dosing (36). Multiple early randomized clinical trials (37–48) with differing endpoints compared LMWH with UFH for the initial treatment of patients with VTE. Three studies (38,39,42) compared IV LMWH with continuous UFH , one trial (41)compared subcutaneous LMWH with subcutaneous UFH, and another three studies (43,49,50) compared subcutaneous LMWH with continuous IV UFH. The results indicate that LMWH administered subcutaneously is as effective and safe as continuous IV UFH. However, in early studies, conclusions of efficacy were largely based on venographic observations rather than clinical outcomes.

Since then, several studies (13–17,49–52) have evaluated long-term clinical outcomes using LMWH. Most studies (13–16,49–52) showed comparable outcomes when LMWH (dosed subcutaneously without monitoring) was compared with IV UFH (with monitoring and subsequent dose adjustment). One large study (50) showed lower rates of VTE recurrence and bleeding when LMWH was compared to UFH. Several meta-analysis (53,54) have also suggested that LMWH results in fewer episodes of recurrence and bleeding than UFH. A small survival benefit may accrue to patients with malignancy and VTE who receive LMWH (53,54).

Two studies have shown that selected patients with proximal DVT can be treated at home with LMWH (and warfarin therapy could be initiated simultaneously) (13,14). This approach has been reviewed (55) and it has been estimated that an average of 5–6 hospital days could be saved by outpatient administration. Utilization of LMWH with a component of outpatient therapy could save approximately $250 million annually in the United States alone (54,56–60). Of course, proper patient selection is critical to ensure safe outpatient therapy, and recommendations in this regard have been formulated (61). The patients should be clinically stable, without significant renal impairment or additional bleeding risks, and there should be a practical system in place for easy administration of the LMWH and for surveillance for recurrence of VTE and for bleeding complications.

C. Direct Thrombin Inhibitors

Direct thrombin inhibitors (DTIs) are indicated for anticoagulation in patients with heparin-induced thrombocytopenia and other associated thromboembolic disease to prevent further thromboembolic complications (62). In other clinical scenarios, only limited data are available regarding utility of DTIs in VTE. In a phase II trial, Schiele et al. (63) randomized patients with DVT to one of three doses of subcutaneous hirudin (0.75, 1.25, or 2.00 mg/kg twice daily) or continuous IV UFH. All patients underwent venography and ventilation/perfusion scans on days 1 and 5. Thrombus extension occurred more frequently in those given IV UFH compared with the hirudin group (10% vs. 3%, respectively). In addition, new perfusion abnormalities on lung scanning were more frequent in the UFH group (26% compared with less than 10% in each of the hirudin groups). Major bleeding was seen only in the highest dose hirudin and the UFH group and was less than 3% in both. Despite these promising results, no major further work has been done in this area. While not approved for treatment of acute VTE, recombinant hirudin (lepirudin) and argatroban are U.S. FDA approved for the treatment of heparin-induced thrombocytopenia, which often manifests as acute VTE.

Ximelagatran is a novel, oral direct thrombin inhibitor. After administration, it is rapidly absorbed and transformed to its active form, melagatran, which provides competitive, direct inhibition of both free and clot-bound thrombin. Oral administration results in predictable plasma concentrations of melagatran that increase linearly in relation to dose (64,65). Ximelagatran is in the early stages of being investigated for use in treatment of VTE. This is especially attractive as its administration does not require monitoring and its oral administration significantly reduces the complexity of treatment and may lower health care costs. In an open-label study (66), 12 patients with pulmonary embolism received a fixed dose of 48 mg oral ximelagatran twice daily for 6–9 days. Plasma samples were collected for determination of melagatran concentrations and scintigraphic changes and adverse events were recorded. Peak plasma concentrations of melagatran were attained approximately 2 hours after administration of ximelagatran. Melagatran plasma concentration profiles were similar on days 1, 2, and 6–9. All but one patient (with malignancy) showed regressed or unchanged lung scintigraphic findings, and six of these demonstrated no, or only minor, perfusion defects at central evaluation after 6–9 days of ximelagatran treatment. Clinical symptoms were improved in all. Ximelagatran was well tolerated, with no deaths or severe bleeding events reported during treatment. Thus, this early study showed that treatment with a fixed dose of oral ximelagatran, used without routine coagulation monitoring, showed reproducible pharmacokinetics and pharmacodynamics with a rapid onset of action and promising clinical results in patients with pulmonary embolism.

D. Fondaparinux

Fondaparinux, a small synthetic pentasaccharide, is an indirect factor Xa inhibitor and acts as a catalyst, enhancing antithrombin (AT)-mediated inhibitory activity against factor Xa (67,68). By selectively inactivating factor Xa, fondaparinux inhibits thrombin generation without any direct inhibitory effect on thrombin. Thus, unlike direct thrombin inhibitors, its activity is totally dependent on AT. It has 100% bioavailability, exhibits no nonspecific binding to plasma or cellular proteins within its therapeutic range, and because it is produced by total chemical synthesis, it provides batch-to-batch consistency and a very predictable dose-response relationship (67). Given the absence of fondaparinux binding to platelet factor 4, the risk of thrombocytopenia is very low (69). Fondaparinux is rapidly absorbed after subcutaneous administration, reaching its maximal plasma concentration in 1.7 hours and exhibiting a terminal half-life of 17 hours (70). These properties allow for once-daily subcutaneous administration, a rapid onset of action, and a predictable drug effect requiring no monitoring or dose adjustment.

In a dose-ranging trial involving patients with symptomatic proximal deep vein thrombosis, 7.5mg of fondaparinux appeared to have efficacy and safety similar to that of a LMWH (dalteparin) (71). The MATISSE Investigators conducted a randomized, open-label trial involving 2213 patients with acute symptomatic pulmonary embolism to compare the efficacy and safety of fondaparinux with that of unfractionated heparin and to document non-inferiority in terms of efficacy (72). Patients received either fondaparinux (5, 7.5, or 10 mg in patients weighing <50, 50–100, or >100 kg, respectively) subcutaneously once daily or a continuous infusion of unfractionated heparin (ratio of aPTT to control value, 1.5–2.5), both given for at least 5 days and until the use of warfarin resulted an in INR above 2.0. The primary efficacy outcome was the 3-month incidence of the composite endpoint of symptomatic, recurrent pulmonary embolism (fatal or nonfatal), and new or recurrent DVT. In those who received fondaparinux, 3.8% had recurrent thromboembolic events, as compared to 5% in those receiving heparin [absolute difference of-1.2% in favor of fondaparinux (95%CI -3.0–0.5)]. There was no difference in the rates of major bleeding between the two groups (1.3% vs. 1.1%) and mortality rates at 3 months were similar. Of the fondaparinux group, 14.5% received the drug, in part on an outpatient basis. Thus, this study showed that subcutaneous therapy with fondaparinux without monitoring is at least as effective and as safe as adjusted-dose, IV administration of unfractionated heparin in the intitial treatment of hemodynamically stable patients with PE. Again, as of this writing this is not an FDA-approved therapy.

III. PROPHYLAXIS

A. Secondary Prevention

All patients with documented VTE are candidates for several weeks to months of anticoagulation once the acute phase is over. The exact duration of therapy depends on competing risks of recurrent VTE and bleeding. The risk of recurrent thromboembolism when anticoagulant therapy is discontinued depends on whether the VTE was unprovoked (idiopathic), secondary to an underlying prothrombotic state or secondary to a reversible predisposing cause; a longer course of therapy is warranted when thrombosis is idiopathic or associated with a continuing risk factor (73). The reported recurrence in patients with idiopathic proximal vein thrombosis has been reported to be between 10 and 27% when anticoagulants are discontinued after 3 months (74). Extending therapy beyond 6 months seems to reduce the risk of recurrence to 7% during the year after treatment is discontinued (75).

Moderate-intensity anticoagulation (INR 2.0–3.0) with warfarin is as effective as a more intense regimen (INR 3.0–4.0) but is associated with less bleeding (76). Treatment should be longer in patients with proximal DVT than in those with distal thrombosis and in patients with recurrent thrombosis versus those with an isolated episode (74). Laboratory evidence of thrombophilia also may warrant a longer duration of anticoagulation. Oral anticoagulation therapy is indicated for ≥3 months in patients with proximal DVT (77,78) with a reversible predisposing factor, for ≥6 months in those with proximal DVT without an identifiable reversible cause (or one that cannot be eliminated) or those with recurrent venous thrombosis, and for 6–12 weeks in patients with symptomatic calf vein thrombosis (79–81). Indefinite anticoagulation should be considered in patients with more than one 1 episode of idiopathic proximal DVT, thrombosis complicating malignancy, or idiopathic venous thrombosis and homozygous factor V Leiden genotype, the antiphospholipid antibody syndrome, or deficiencies of antithrombin III or protein C or S (74,82–84). Prospective cohort studies indicate that heterozygous factor V Leiden or the

G20210A prothrombin gene mutation in patients with idiopathic venous thrombosis do not increase the risk of recurrence (83,85). These recommendations follow the American Heart Association/American College of Cardiology guidelines (74) and are based on results of randomized trials that demonstrated that oral anticoagulants effectively prevent recurrent venous thrombosis (risk reduction > 90%), that treatment for 6 months is more effective than treatment for 6 weeks (82), and that treatment for 2 years is more effective than treatment for 3 months (84). However, since long-term treatment with warfarin carries an increased risk of bleeding and the inconvenience and expense of prothrombin time/INR monitoring, investigators have evaluated the efficacy of prolonged therapy with low dose warfarin after 3–6 months of treatment with standard-dose warfarin.

It has been suggested that long-term low-dose anticoagulation may be even more protective in patients with idiopathic DVT. In a recently published multicenter, double-blind, randomized, secondary prevention trial, Ridker and associates (86) compared long-term, low-intensity anticoagulation (INR 1.5–2.0) in patients with idiopathic DVT with the more conventional treatment for 3–12 months. The trial was terminated early after 508 patients had been enrolled and had been followed up to 4.3 years. There was a risk reduction of 64% (hazard ratio 0.36, 95% CI 0.19–0.67; $p < 0.001$) in the long-term anticoagulation arm compared with the placebo arm. Thus, long-term, low-intensity anticoagulation seems to be an effective method of preventing recurrent idiopathic DVT. However, whether this degree of anticoagulation will be effective in patients with predispositions like antiphospholipid syndrome is not known.

Another strategy that has been investigated is to use standard dose-adjusted warfarin for 6 months and then-long term therapy with fixed-dose ximelagatran. Schulman et al. in a randomized, double-blind, multicenter trial, enrolled 1233 patients with venous thromboembolism (who had undergone 6 months of standard anticoagulant therapy) to extended secondary prevention with ximelagatran (24 mg) or placebo, taken twice daily, for 18 months without monitoring anticoagulation (87). The primary endpoint of symptomatic recurrent VTE was confirmed in 12 of 612 patients in the ximelagatran group and 71 of 611 patients in the placebo group (hazard ratio 0.16, 95% CI 0.09–0.30]; $p < 0.001$). There was no statistically significant difference in the incidence of death or major bleeding. Thus, the study concluded that oral ximelagatran was superior to placebo for the extended secondary prevention of VTE. As with other studies with ximelagatran, there was a 6.4% incidence of transient elevation of liver enzymes. Thus, though promising, until further data are available this cannot be recommended as routine strategy.

B. Primary Prevention of Venous Thromboembolism

Venous thromboembolism is often clinically silent or presents with atypical signs and symptoms. Therefore, prevention is the most effective means to reduce associated morbidity and mortality (6). Preventive therapy is usually focused on patients at highest risk, such as those who have undergone major surgery or prolonged hospitalization. Preventive interventions have focused either on anticoagulants, such as fixed low-dose subcutaneous UFH, adjusted-dose heparin, LMWH, or warfarin, or mechanical methods such as intermittent pneumatic compression (IPC) of the legs, elastic compression stockings, or inferior vena cava filters (88). Additional benefit can be achieved when more than one preventive strategy is combined, such as LMWHs and compression stockings (89). The choice of a specific preventive strategy is based on an assessment of risk factors for VTE. The American College of Chest Physicians criteria for VTE risk stratification (Table 1) are widely endorsed and categorize patients on the basis of age, type of surgery, and presence or absence of additional thromboembolic factors (88). For nonsurgical patients the need for VTE prophylaxis is based on the estimates of risk, which have been derived from studies that looked at the incidence of VTE in such patients (90). In general surgery patients, the incidence is approximately 25%, with 0.1–0.8% of patients experiencing a fatal PE. In elective total hip replacement, the prevalence of DVT as determined by venography is 51% (91). Several large studies have looked at the various treatment regimens and agents in the different clinical scenarios. Current ACCP recommendations for VTE prophylaxis are detailed in the Appendix.

LMWHs appear to be at least as efficacious in preventing VTE in general surgery patients as fixed-dose UFH. Although drug costs of LMWH may be more expensive than UFH, when all the associated costs are included LMWH can be more cost-effective (92). Mechanical devices such as IPC are effective in reducing DVT in the lower extremities in most general surgery patients. These devices are especially useful in patients who are at high bleeding risk with anticoagulation, such as neurosurgical patients. In patients at higher risk for VTE, these mechanical devices can be used in combination with low-dose subcutaneous UFH or LMWH (88). Low-dose subcutaneous UFH is less effective in patients undergoing total hip replacement or knee replacement surgery. In these types of orthopedic surgery patients, LMWH or adjusted dose warfarin is the better choice. Warfarin can be initiated the evening prior to surgery or soon after surgery (once hemostasis is assured), and the dose is adjusted to keep the INR between 2.0 and 3.0. A delicate balance must be struck between the the effectiveness of VTE prophylaxis (more effective when begun earlier) and concern over bleeding complications (reduced when begun later).

Medical illness may also significantly increase the risk of VTE, and many such patients (in intensive care units or not) are candidates for prophylaxis. The use of low-dose subcutaneous UFH (93–95) or LMWH (96,97) has been shown to be effective in preventing VTE in patients with myocardial infarction and ischemic stroke or other medical

Table 1   Risk Factors for Venous Thromboembolism

Surgery
Trauma (major or lower extremity)
Immobility
Malignancy
Cancer therapy (chemotherapy, radiotherapy or hormonal therapy)
Prior VTE event
Increasing age
Pregnancy and postpartum period
Estrogen-containing oral contraceptives or hormone replacement therapy
Selective estrogen receptor modulators
Acute medical illness
Congestive heart failure
Severe respiratory failure
Inflammatory bowel disease
Nephrotic syndrome
Myeloproliferative disorders
Paroxysmal nocturnal hemoglobinuria
Obesity
Smoking
Varicose veins
Central venous catheterization
Inherited or acquired thrombophilia

illness. Most of the studies that looked at the efficacy of twice-daily UFH in medically ill patients are several decades old. Since then, the acuity of medically ill patients in hospitals has become worse, and thus it is felt that it may not be appropriate to apply these studies to very critically ill patients. Most newer studies that have compared UFH with LMWH have used UFH administered 8-hourly (98–101). In each comparison LMWH was at least as efficacious as UFH and safer to administer. Thus, in critically ill patients either subcutaneous UFH should be given 8-hourly or LMWH should be used.

In cancer patients receiving chemotherapy, low-dose warfarin adjusted to keep the INR 1.5 was found effective (28). Similarly a very low, warfarin dose (1 mg daily) prevented subclavian vein thrombosis in patients with malignancy and an indwelling catheter (102). In contrast, several randomized trials found this dose of warfarin ineffective for preventing postoperative venous thrombosis in patients undergoing major orthopedic surgery (103–105). In general, when warfarin is used to prevent DVT, INR should be maintained between 2.0 and 3.0.

1. Fondaparinux

Fondaparinux, a small synthetic pentasaccharide, is an indirect factor Xa inhibitor. It is rapidly absorbed after subcutaneous administration, reaching maximal plasma concentration in 1.7 hours and exhibiting a terminal half-life of 17 hours (70). These properties allow for once-daily subcutaneous administration, a rapid onset of action, and a predictable drug effect requiring no monitoring or dose adjustment. The drug has shown great promise for prevention of DVT and received FDA approval in 2001 for VTE prevention in hip and knee replacement and hip fracture surgical procedures. Phase II trials in hip replacement surgery (106) and phase III trials in hip replacement (107), hip fracture (108), and major knee surgery (109) have demonstrated the superiority of fondaparinux relative to a LMWH (enoxaparin) in reducing VTE risk following major orthopedic procedures. A recent meta-analysis (110) of these phase III trials indicates an overall significant 55.2% reduction in VTE risk ($p < 0.001$) in favor of fondaparinux, with no difference in clinically relevant bleeding.

2. Ximelagatran

Ximelagatran is a novel, univalent, oral direct thrombin inhibitor. After administration it is rapidly absorbed and transformed to its active form, melagatran, which provides competitive, direct inhibition of both free and clot-bound thrombin. Oral administration results in predictable plasma concentrations of melagatran that increase linearly in relation to dose (64,65). Fixed doses of ximelagatran without coagulation monitoring have been studied in phase II (64,111–114) and phase III (115–117) trials of prophylaxis of venous thromboembolism after total hip or knee arthroplasty. The results of these trials show that ximelagatran is at least as effective as or superior to enoxaparin or warfarin in preventing VTE, with no increase in risk of bleeding (Table 2). Thus, the ease of oral administration favors ximelagatran over LMWHs, and the lack of need of coagulation monitoring and predictable effect favor it over warfarin in thromboprophylaxis in the perioperative setting of major orthopedic surgery. However, as of this writing the drug does not have FDA approval for routine clinical use.

C. Timing of Prophylaxis

In most patients it is appropriate to initiate prophylaxis as soon as the risk of developing thrombosis begins—for trauma patients and those medically ill, this means as soon as they are hospitalized (118). For elective surgery patients, it can be as soon as they are taken to the

Table 2 Melagatran/Ximelagatran vs LMWH or Warfarin in Primary Prevention of VTE

Source/Surgery	Variables	Thrombin inhibitor	LMWH[a] dose	Warfarin dose
Heit et al./TKR	Ximelagatran dose	24 mg bid	30 mg bid	—
(n = 443)	Overall VTE (%)	15.8	22.7	
Note: no statistical	Proximal VTE (%)	3.2	3.1	
difference between	Major bleeding (%)	0	0.8	
the two groups				
Colwell (114) et al/TKR	Ximelagatran dose	24 mg bid	30 mg bid	—
(n = 1838)	Overall VTE (%)	7.9	4.6	
Note: ximelagatran	Proximal VTE (%)	3.6	1.2	
group had higher total	Major bleeding (%)	0.8	0.9	
and proximal VTE				
Eriksson et al./ THR or	Ximelagatran dose[b]	24 mg bid	40 mg qd	—
TKR (n = 2764)	Overall VTE (%)	20.3	26.7	
Note: ximelagatran had	Proximal VTE (%)	2.3	6.3	
significantly lower	Major bleeding (%)	3.3	1.2	
total and proximal				
Francis et al./TKR	Ximelagatran dose	24 mg bid	—	INR 2.5 (1.8–3.0)
(n = 1851)	Overall VTE (%)	24.9		27.6
Note: ximelagatran had	Proximal VTE (%)	2.5		4.1
significantly lower total	Major bleeding (%)	0.8		0.7
and proximal VTE				

[a]Enoxaparin.
[b]Dose of ximelagatran preceded by melagatran 5 mg subcutaneously.
Source: Modified from Ref. 117.

operating room or as soon as adequate hemostasis is assured; for recently immobilized patients it may be prior to admission to the hospital (118). Stockings and IPC devices should be initiated preoperatively as soon as the risk of DVT from immobility increases, then continued through the procedure and through hospitalization. Warfarin can be started at a low dose a few days preoperatively or at a therapeutic dose on the night prior to surgery (118). For LMWH, the options include initiating LMWH 12 hours preoperatively, immediately prior to surgery, or as soon as hemostasis is achieved after the surgery (frequently 12–24 hours postoperatively). As noted above, the closer the initiation of prophylaxis is to surgery, the greater the potential risk of bleeding complications. There are no large studies that have looked at this issue, but in a meta-analysis, Hull et al. found that LMWH initiated preoperatively was associated with lower rates of venographically proven VTE and no significant increase in major bleeding (119). The timing of pharmacological prophylaxis should always be clarified with the surgeons and the anesthesia team, particularly if spinal or epidural anesthesia is planned. Spinal anesthesia should be delayed for 12 hours after the initial dose of LMWH, and LMWH prophylaxis should be delayed for 2 hours after the needle or catheter is removed (88).The use of preprinted orders, computer reminders, or practice guidelines may be an effective method of prompting appropriate VTE prophylaxis (120).

D. Duration of Primary Prophylaxis for Venous Thromboembolism

The optimal duration of thromboprophylaxis is not known. In the 1970s and 1980s when hospitalizations were longer, patients were given thromboprophylaxis for the duration of their stay in the hospital (usually 7–10 days). As the duration of stay has decreased, so has the duration of thromboprophylaxis. Studies looking for asymptomatic VTE after hospital discharge noted a high incidence of asymptomatic DVT (121,122). For general surgery patients, studies that have looked at the value of extended thromboprophylaxis found either no benefit (123) from prophylaxis or a small advantage (124) that on economic analysis did not justify its use on routine basis (125). The only procedure for which there is strong evidence in favor of extended prophylaxis is total hip replacement/arthroplasty (126,127). Though the optimal duration of prophylaxis is not known, 4–6 weeks appears reasonable. Both the use of warfarin to keep an INR of 2.0–3.0 (128,129) and the use of LMWH are acceptable. In all other patients, extended thromboprophylaxis should be individualized depending on the extent of limitation in mobility after hospital discharge and other risk factors for VTE such as obesity, heart failure, underlying malignancy, etc. Continued use of well-fitting stockings is reasonable, although there is not much evidence to support this recommendation (118).

REFERENCES

1. Anderson DR OBB. Cost effectiveness of the prevention and treatment of deep vein thrombosis and pulmonary embolism. Pharmacoeconomics. 1997; 12:17–29.
2. Bick R. Proficient and cost-effective approaches for the prevention and treatment of venous thrombosis and thromboembolism. Drugs. 2000; 60:575–595.
3. Hyers T. State of the art: venous thromboembolism. Am J Respir Crit Care Med. 1999; 159:1–14.
4. Heit JA SM, Mohr DN, Petterson TM, O'Fallon WM, Melton LJ 3rd. Predictors of survival after deep vein thrombosis and pulmonary embolism: a population-based, cohort study. Arch Intern Med. 1999; 159:445–453.
5. Hirsh J. Antithrombotic therapy in deep vein thrombosis and pulmonary embolism. Am Heart J. 1992; 123:1115–1122.
6. Clagett GP, Anderson FA, Jr., Heit J, Levine MN, Wheeler HB. Prevention of venous thromboembolism. Chest. 1995; 108:312S-334S.
7. Barritt DW JS. Anticoagulant drugs in the treatment of pulmonary embolism: a controlled clinical trial. Lancet. 1960; 1:1309–1312.
8. Kernohan RJ, Todd C. Heparin therapy in thromboembolic disease. Lancet. 1966; 1:621–623.
9. Alpert JS, Smith R, Carlson J, Ockene IS, Dexter L, Dalen JE. Mortality in patients treated for pulmonary embolism. Jama. 1976; 236:1477–1480.
10. Kanis JA. Heparin in the treatment of pulmonary thromboembolism. Thromb Diath Haemorrh. 1974; 32:519–527.
11. Hull RD, Raskob GE, Hirsh J, Jay RM, Leclerc JR, Geerts WH, Rosenbloom D, Sackett DL, Anderson C, Harrison L, et al. Continuous intravenous heparin compared with intermittent subcutaneous heparin in the initial treatment of proximal-vein thrombosis. N Engl J Med. 1986; 315:1109–1114.
12. Brandjes DP, Heijboer H, Buller HR, de Rijk M, Jagt H, ten Cate JW. Acenocoumarol and heparin compared with acenocoumarol alone in the initial treatment of proximal-vein thrombosis. N Engl J Med. 1992; 327:1485–1489.
13. Levine M, Gent M, Hirsh J, Leclerc J, Anderson D, Weitz J, Ginsberg J, Turpie AG, Demers C, Kovacs M. A comparison of low-molecular-weight heparin administered primarily at home with unfractionated heparin administered in the hospital for proximal deep-vein thrombosis. N Engl J Med. 1996; 334:677–681.
14. Koopman MM, Prandoni P, Piovella F, Ockelford PA, Brandjes DP, van der Meer J, Gallus AS, Simonneau G, Chesterman CH, Prins MH. Treatment of venous thrombosis with intravenous unfractionated heparin administered in the hospital as compared with subcutaneous low-molecular-weight heparin administered at home. The Tasman Study Group. N Engl J Med. 1996; 334:682–687.

15. Low-molecular-weight heparin in the treatment of patients with venous thromboembolism. The Columbus Investigators. N Engl J Med. 1997; 337:657–662.

16. Simonneau G, Sors H, Charbonnier B, Page Y, Laaban JP, Azarian R, Laurent M, Hirsch JL, Ferrari E, Bosson JL, Mottier D, Beau B. A comparison of low-molecular-weight heparin with unfractionated heparin for acute pulmonary embolism. The THESEE Study Group. Tinzaparine ou Heparine Standard: Evaluations dans l'Embolie Pulmonaire. N Engl J Med. 1997; 337:663–669.

17. Hull RD, Raskob GE, Brant RF, Pineo GF, Elliott G, Stein PD, Gottschalk A, Valentine KA, Mah AF. Low-molecular-weight heparin vs heparin in the treatment of patients with pulmonary embolism. American-Canadian Thrombosis Study Group. Arch Intern Med. 2000; 160:229–236.

18. Doyle DJ, Turpie AG, Hirsh J, Best C, Kinch D, Levine MN, Gent M. Adjusted subcutaneous heparin or continuous intravenous heparin in patients with acute deep vein thrombosis. A randomized trial. Ann Intern Med. 1987; 107:441–445.

19. Pini M, Pattachini C, Quintavalla R, Poli T, Megha A, Tagliaferri A, Manotti C, Dettori AG. Subcutaneous vs intravenous heparin in the treatment of deep venous thrombosis—a randomized clinical trial. Thromb Haemost. 1990; 64:222–226.

20. Andersson G, Fagrell B, Holmgren K, Johnsson H, Ljungberg B, Nilsson E, Wilhelmsson S, Zetterquist S. Subcutaneous administration of heparin. A randomised comparison with intravenous administration of heparin to patients with deep-vein thrombosis. Thromb Res. 1982; 27:631–639.

21. Hyers TM, Agnelli G, Hull RD, Weg JG, Morris TA, Samama M, Tapson V. Antithrombotic therapy for venous thromboembolic disease. Chest. 1998; 114:561S-578S.

22. Wilson JE, 3rd, Bynum LJ, Parkey RW. Heparin therapy in venous thromboembolism. Am J Med. 1981; 70:808–816.

23. Coon WW, Willis PW, 3rd, Symons MJ. Assessment of anticoagulant treatment of venous thromboembolism. Ann Surg. 1969; 170:559–68.

24. Basu D GA, Hirsh J, Cade J. A prospective study of the value of monitoring heparin treatment with the activated partial thromboplastin time. N Engl J Med. 1972; 287:325–327.

25. Hull RD, Raskob GE, Brant RF, Pineo GF, Valentine KA. Relation between the time to achieve the lower limit of the APTT therapeutic range and recurrent venous thromboembolism during heparin treatment for deep vein thrombosis. Arch Intern Med. 1997; 157:2562–2568.

26. Chiu HM, Hirsh J, Yung WL, Regoeczi E, Gent M. Relationship between the anticoagulant and antithrombotic effects of heparin in experimental venous thrombosis. Blood. 1977; 49:171–184.

27. Gitel SN WS. The antithrombotic effects of warfarin and heparin following infusions of tissue thromboplastin in rabbits: clinical implications. J Lab Clin Med. 1979; 94:481–488.

28. Levine M, Hirsh J, Gent M, Arnold A, Warr D, Falanga A, Samosh M, Bramwell V, Pritchard KI, Stewart D, et al. Double-blind randomised trial of a very-low-dose warfarin for prevention of thromboembolism in stage IV breast cancer. Lancet. 1994; 343:886–889.

29. Wheeler AP, Jaquiss RD, Newman JH. Physician practices in the treatment of pulmonary embolism and deep venous thrombosis. Arch Intern Med. 1988; 148:1321–1325.

30. Hull RD, Raskob GE, Rosenbloom D, Lemaire J, Pineo GF, Baylis B, Ginsberg JS, Panju AA, Brill-Edwards P, Brant R. Optimal therapeutic level of heparin therapy in patients with venous thrombosis. Arch Intern Med. 1992; 152:1589–1595.

31. Hyers TM, Agnelli G, Hull RD, Morris TA, Samama M, Tapson V, Weg JG. Antithrombotic therapy for venous thromboembolic disease. Chest. 2001; 119:176S-193S.

32. Raschke RA, Reilly BM, Guidry JR, Fontana JR, Srinivas S. The weight-based heparin dosing nomogram compared with a "standard care" nomogram. A randomized controlled trial. Ann Intern Med. 1993; 119:874–881.

33. Hirsh J, van Aken WG, Gallus AS, Dollery CT, Cade JF, Yung WL. Heparin kinetics in venous thrombosis and pulmonary embolism. Circulation. 1976; 53:691–695.

34. Cipolle RJ, Seifert RD, Neilan BA, Zaske DE, Haus E. Heparin kinetics: variables related to disposition and dosage. Clin Pharmacol Ther. 1981; 29:387–93.

35. Weitz JI. Low-molecular-weight heparins. N Engl J Med. 1997; 337:688–98.

36. Laposta M GK, Elizabeth MVC, et al. College of american pathologists XXXI conference on laboratory monitoring of anticoagulant therapy. The clinical use and laboratory monitoring of low molecular weight heparin, danaparoid, hirudin and related compounds, and argatroban. Arch Pathol Lab Med. 1998; 122:799–807.

37. A randomised trial of subcutaneous low molecular weight heparin (CY 216) compared with intravenous unfractionated heparin in the treatment of deep vein thrombosis. A collaborative European multicentre study. Thromb Haemost. 1991; 65:251–256.

38. Albada J, Nieuwenhuis HK, Sixma JJ. Treatment of acute venous thromboembolism with low molecular weight heparin (Fragmin). Results of a double-blind randomized study. Circulation. 1989; 80:935–940.

39. Bratt G, Aberg W, Johansson M, Tornebohm E, Granqvist S, Lockner D. Two daily subcutaneous injections of fragmin as compared with intravenous standard heparin in the treatment of deep venous thrombosis (DVT). Thromb Haemost. 1990; 64:506–510.

40. Bratt G, Tornebohm E, Granqvist S, Aberg W, Lockner D. A comparison between low molecular weight heparin (KABI 2165) and standard heparin in the intravenous treatment of deep venous thrombosis. Thromb Haemost. 1985; 54:813–817.

41. Holm HA, Ly B, Handeland GF, Abildgaard U, Arnesen KE, Gottschalk P, Hoeg V, Aandahl M, Haugen K, Laerum F, et al. Subcutaneous heparin treatment of deep venous thrombosis: a comparison of unfractionated and low molecular weight heparin. Haemostasis. 1986; 16 (suppl 2):30–37.

42. Lockner D, Bratt G, Tornebohm E, Aberg W, Granqvist S. Intravenous and subcutaneous administration of Fragmin in deep venous thrombosis. Haemostasis. 1986; 16 (suppl 2):25–29.

43. Prandoni P, Vigo M, Cattelan AM, Ruol A. Treatment of deep venous thrombosis by fixed doses of a low-molecular-weight heparin (CY216). Haemostasis. 1990; 20 (suppl 1):220–223.

44. Simonneau G, Charbonnier B, Decousus H, Planchon B, Ninet J, Sie P, Silsiguen M, Combe S. Subcutaneous low-molecular-weight heparin compared with continuous intravenous unfractionated heparin in the treatment of proximal deep vein thrombosis. Arch Intern Med. 1993; 153:1541–1546.

45. Handeland GF, Abildgaard U, Holm HA, Arnesen KE. Dose adjusted heparin treatment of deep venous thrombosis: a comparison of unfractionated and low molecular weight heparin. Eur J Clin Pharmacol. 1990; 39:107–112.

46. Harenberg J, Huck K, Bratsch H, Stehle G, Dempfle CE, Mall K, Blauth M, Usadel KH, Heene DL. Therapeutic application of subcutaneous low-molecular-weight heparin in acute venous thrombosis. Haemostasis. 1990; 20 Suppl 1:205–219.

47. Huet Y, Janvier G, Bendriss PH, Winnock S, Dugrais G, Freyburger G, Boisseras P. Treatment of established venous thromboembolism with enoxaparin: preliminary report. Acta Chir Scand Suppl. 1990; 556:116–20.

48. Janvier G, Winnock S, Dugrais G, Vallet A, Dardel E, Serise JM, Calen S, Vergnes C, Toulemonde F. Treatment of deep venous thrombosis with a very low molecular weight heparin fragment (CY 222). Haemostasis. 1987; 17:49–58.

49. Prandoni P, Lensing AW, Buller HR, Carta M, Cogo A, Vigo M, Casara D, Ruol A, ten Cate JW. Comparison of subcutaneous low-molecular-weight heparin with intravenous standard heparin in proximal deep-vein thrombosis. Lancet. 1992; 339:441–445.

50. Hull RD, Raskob GE, Pineo GF, Green D, Trowbridge AA, Elliott CG, Lerner RG, Hall J, Sparling T, Brettell HR, et al. Subcutaneous low-molecular-weight heparin compared with continuous intravenous heparin in the treatment of proximal-vein thrombosis. N Engl J Med. 1992; 326:975–982.

51. Lindmarker P, Holmstrom M, Granqvist S, Johnsson H, Lockner D. Comparison of once-daily subcutaneous Fragmin with continuous intravenous unfractionated heparin in the treatment of deep vein thrombosis. Thromb Haemost. 1994; 72:186–190.

52. Fiessinger JN, Lopez-Fernandez M, Gatterer E, Granqvist S, Kher A, Olsson CG, Soderberg K. Once-daily subcutaneous dalteparin, a low molecular weight heparin, for the initial treatment of acute deep vein thrombosis. Thromb Haemost. 1996; 76:195–199.

53. Siragusa S, Cosmi B, Piovella F, Hirsh J, Ginsberg JS. Low-molecular-weight heparins and unfractionated heparin in the treatment of patients with acute venous thromboembolism: results of a meta-analysis. Am J Med. 1996; 100:269–277.

54. Gould MK, Dembitzer AD, Doyle RL, Hastie TJ, Garber AM. Low-molecular-weight heparins compared with unfractionated heparin for treatment of acute deep venous thrombosis. A meta-analysis of randomized, controlled trials. Ann Intern Med. 1999; 130:800–809.

55. Hyers TM. Venous thromboembolism. Am J Respir Crit Care Med. 1999; 159:1–14.

56. Hull RD, Raskob GE, Rosenbloom D, Pineo GF, Lerner RG, Gafni A, Trowbridge AA, Elliott CG, Green D, Feinglass J. Treatment of proximal vein thrombosis with subcutaneous low-molecular-weight heparin vs intravenous heparin. An economic perspective. Arch Intern Med. 1997; 157:289–94.

57. van den Belt AG, Bossuyt PM, Prins MH, Gallus AS, Buller HR. Replacing inpatient care by outpatient care in the treatment of deep venous thrombosis—an economic evaluation. TASMAN Study Group. Thromb Haemost. 1998; 79:259–263.

58. O'Brien B, Levine M, Willan A, Goeree R, Haley S, Blackhouse G, Gent M. Economic evaluation of outpatient treatment with low-molecular-weight heparin for proximal vein thrombosis. Arch Intern Med. 1999; 159:2298–304.

59. Dolovich LR, Ginsberg JS, Douketis JD, Holbrook AM, Cheah G. A meta-analysis comparing low-molecular-weight heparins with unfractionated heparin in the treatment of venous thromboembolism: examining some unanswered questions regarding location of treatment, product type, and dosing frequency. Arch Intern Med. 2000; 160:181–188.

60. Rooke TW, Osmundson PJ. Heparin and the in-hospital management of deep venous thrombosis: cost considerations. Mayo Clin Proc. 1986; 61:198–204.

61. Dunn AS, Coller B. Outpatient treatment of deep vein thrombosis: translating clinical trials into practice. Am J Med. 1999; 106:660–669.

62. Weitz JI HJ. New anticoagulant drugs. Chest. 2001; 119:95s-107s.

63. Schiele F, Lindgaerde F, Eriksson H, Bassand JP, Wallmark A, Hansson PO, Grollier G, Sjo M, Moia M, Camez A, Smyth V, Walker M. Subcutaneous recombinant hirudin (HBW 023) versus intravenous sodium heparin in treatment of established acute deep vein thrombosis of the legs: a multicentre prospective dose-ranging randomized trial. International Multicentre Hirudin Study Group. Thromb Haemost. 1997; 77:834–838.

64. Eriksson UG, Bredberg U, Gislen K, Johansson LC, Frison L, Ahnoff M, Gustafsson D. Pharmacokinetics and pharmacodynamics of ximelagatran, a novel oral direct thrombin inhibitor, in young healthy male subjects. Eur J Clin Pharmacol. 2003; 59:35–43.

65. Johansson LC, Frison L, Logren U, Fager G, Gustafsson D, Eriksson UG. Influence of age on the pharmacokinetics and pharmacodynamics of ximelagatran, an oral direct thrombin inhibitor. Clin Pharmacokinet. 2003; 42:381–392.

66. Wahlander K, Lapidus L, Olsson CG, Thuresson A, Eriksson UG, Larson G, Eriksson H. Pharmacokinetics, pharmacodynamics and clinical effects of the oral direct thrombin inhibitor ximelagatran in acute treatment of patients with pulmonary embolism and deep vein thrombosis. Thromb Res. 2002; 107:93–99.

67. Hyers T. Management of venous thromboembolism. Arch Intern Med. 2003; 163:759–768.

68. Choay J PM, Lormeau JC, Sinay P, Casu B, Gatti G. Structure-activity relationship in heparin: a synthetic pentasaccharide with high affinity for antithrombin III and eliciting high anti-factor Xa activity. Biochem Biophys Res Commun. 1983; 116:492–499.

69. Warkentin TE, Levine MN, Hirsh J, Horsewood P, Roberts RS, Gent M, Kelton JG. Heparin-induced thrombocytopenia in patients treated with low-molecular-weight heparin or unfractionated heparin. N Engl J Med. 1995; 332:1330–1335.

70. Donat F DJ, Santoni A, Cariou R, Necciari J, Magnani H, de Greef R. The pharmacokinetics of fondaparinux sodium in healthy volunteers. Clin Pharmacokinet. 2002; 41:1–9.

71. Treatment of proximal deep vein thrombosis with a novel synthetic compound (SR90107A/ORG31540) with pure anti-factor Xa activity: A phase II evaluation. The Rembrandt Investigators. Circulation. 2000; 102:2726–2731.

72. Buller HR, Davidson BL, Decousus H, Gallus A, Gent M, Piovella F, Prins MH, Raskob G, van den Berg-Segers AE, Cariou R, Leeuwenkamp O, Lensing AW. Subcutaneous fondaparinux versus intravenous unfractionated heparin in the initial treatment of pulmonary embolism. N Engl J Med. 2003; 349:1695–1702.

73. Hirsh J. The optimal duration of anticoagulant therapy for venous thrombosis. N Engl J Med. 1995; 332:1710–1.

74. Hirsh J FV, Ansell J, Halperin JL. American Heart Association/American College of Cardiology Foundation guide to warfarin therapy. J Am Coll Cardiol. 2003; 41:1633–1652.

75. Hirsh J, Lee AY. How we diagnose and treat deep vein thrombosis. Blood. 2002; 99:3102–3110.

76. Landefeld CS, Rosenblatt MW, Goldman L. Bleeding in outpatients treated with warfarin: relation to the prothrombin time and important remediable lesions. Am J Med. 1989; 87:153–159.

77. Hull R, Delmore T, Genton E, Hirsh J, Gent M, Sackett D, McLoughlin D, Armstrong P. Warfarin sodium versus low-dose heparin in the long-term treatment of venous thrombosis. N Engl J Med. 1979; 301:855–858.

78. Hull R, Delmore T, Carter C, Hirsh J, Genton E, Gent M, Turpie G, McLaughlin D. Adjusted subcutaneous heparin versus warfarin sodium in the long-term treatment of venous thrombosis. N Engl J Med. 1982; 306:189–194.

79. Lagerstedt CI, Olsson CG, Fagher BO, Oqvist BW, Albrechtsson U. Need for long-term anticoagulant treatment in symptomatic calf-vein thrombosis. Lancet. 1985; 2:515–518.

80. Schulman S, Rhedin AS, Lindmarker P, Carlsson A, Larfars G, Nicol P, Loogna E, Svensson E, Ljungberg B, Walter H. A comparison of six weeks with six months of oral anticoagulant therapy after a first episode of venous thromboembolism. Duration of Anticoagulation Trial Study Group. N Engl J Med. 1995; 332:1661–1665.

81. Schulman S, Granqvist S, Holmstrom M, Carlsson A, Lindmarker P, Nicol P, Eklund SG, Nordlander S, Larfars G, Leijd B, Linder O, Loogna E. The duration of oral anticoagulant therapy after a second episode of venous thromboembolism. The Duration of Anticoagulation Trial Study Group. N Engl J Med. 1997; 336:393–398.

82. Schulman S, Svenungsson E, Granqvist S. Anticardiolipin antibodies predict early recurrence of thromboembolism and death among patients with venous thromboembolism following anticoagulant therapy. Duration of Anticoagulation Study Group. Am J Med. 1998; 104:332–338.

83. Simioni P, Prandoni P, Zanon E, Saracino MA, Scudeller A, Villalta S, Scarano L, Girolami B, Benedetti L, Girolami A. Deep venous thrombosis and lupus anticoagulant. A case-control study. Thromb Haemost. 1996; 76:187–9.

84. Rance A, Emmerich J, Fiessinger JN. Anticardiolipin antibodies and recurrent thromboembolism. Thromb Haemost. 1997; 77:221–222.

85. Kearon C, Gent M, Hirsh J, Weitz J, Kovacs MJ, Anderson DR, Turpie AG, Green D, Ginsberg JS, Wells P, MacKinnon B, Julian JA. A comparison of three months of anticoagulation with extended anticoagulation for a first episode of idiopathic venous thromboembolism. N Engl J Med. 1999; 340:901–907.

86. Ridker PM GS, Danielson E, Rosenberg Y, Eby CS, Deitcher SR, Cushman M, Moll S, Kessler CM, Elliott CG, Paulson R, Wong T, Bauer KA, Schwartz BA, Miletich JP, Bounameaux H, Glynn RJ; PREVENT Investigators. Long-term, low-intensity warfarin therapy for the prevention of recurrent venous thromboembolism. N Engl J Med. 2003; 348:1425–1434.

87. Schulman S, Wahlander K, Lundstrom T, Clason SB, Eriksson H. Secondary prevention of venous thromboembolism with the oral direct thrombin inhibitor ximelagatran. N Engl J Med. 2003; 349:1713–1721.

88. Geerts WH CG, Pineo GF, Heit JA, Borgovist D, Lassen MR, Colwell CW, Ray JG. Prevention of venous thromboembolism: The seventh ACCP conference on antithrombotic and thrombolytic therapy. Chest. 2004; 126:338S–400S..

89. Ramos R, Salem BI, De Pawlikowski MP, Coordes C, Eisenberg S, Leidenfrost R. The efficacy of pneumatic compression stockings in the prevention of pulmonary embolism after cardiac surgery. Chest. 1996; 109:82–85.

90. Michota F. Venous thromboembolism prophylaxis in the medically ill patient. Clin Chest Med. 2003; 24:93–101.

91. Nazario R DL, Maguire AG. Treatment of venous thromboembolism. Cardiol Rev. 2002; 10:249–259.

92. Etchells E MR, Geerts W, Barton P, Detsky AS. Economic analysis of low-dose heparin vs the low-molecular-weight heparin enoxaparin for prevention of venous thromboembolism after colorectal surgery. Arch Intern Med. 1999; 159:1221–1228.

93. McCarthy ST TJ, Robertson D, Hawkey CJ, Macey DJ. Low-dose heparin as a prophylaxis against deep-vein thrombosis after acute stroke. Lancet. 1977; 2:800–801.

94. Belch JJ LG, Ward AG, Forbes CD, Prentice CR. Prevention of deep vein thrombosis in medical patients by low-dose heparin. Scott Med J. 1981; 26:115–117.

95. Halkin H GJ, Modan M, Modan B. Reduction of mortality in general medical in-patients by low-dose heparin prophylaxis. Ann Intern Med. 1982; 96:561–565.

96. Dahan R HD, Caulin C, Cuzin E, Viltart C, Woler M, Segrestaa JM. Prevention of deep vein thrombosis in elderly medical in-patients by a low molecular weight heparin: a randomized double-blind trial. Hemostasis. 1986; 16:159–162.

97. Samama MM, Cohen AT, Darmon JY, Desjardins L, Eldor A, Janbon C, Leizorovicz A, Nguyen H, Olsson CG, Turpie AG, Weisslinger N. A comparison of enoxaparin with placebo for the prevention of venous thromboembolism in acutely ill medical patients. Prophylaxis in Medical Patients with Enoxaparin Study Group. N Engl J Med. 1999; 341:793–800.

98. Harenberg J, Kallenbach B, Martin U, Dempfle CE, Zimmermann R, Kubler W, Heene DL. Randomized controlled study of heparin and low molecular weight heparin for prevention of deep-vein thrombosis in medical patients. Thromb Res. 1990; 59:639–650.

99. Bergmann JF, Neuhart E. A multicenter randomized double-blind study of enoxaparin compared with unfractionated heparin in the prevention of venous thromboembolic disease in elderly in-patients bedridden for an acute medical illness. The Enoxaparin in Medicine Study Group. Thromb Haemost. 1996; 76:529–534.

100. Lechler E, Schramm W, Flosbach CW. The venous thrombotic risk in non-surgical patients: epidemiological data and efficacy/safety profile of a low-molecular-weight heparin (enoxaparin). The Prime Study Group. Haemostasis. 1996; 26 (suppl 2):49–56.

101. Kleber FX, Witt C, Vogel G, Koppenhagen K, Schomaker U, Flosbach CW. Randomized comparison of enoxaparin with unfractionated heparin for the prevention of venous thromboembolism in medical patients with heart failure or severe respiratory disease. Am Heart J. 2003; 145:614–621.

102. Bern MM, Lokich JJ, Wallach SR, Bothe A, Jr., Benotti PN, Arkin CF, Greco FA, Huberman M, Moore C. Very low doses of warfarin can prevent thrombosis in central venous catheters. A randomized prospective trial. Ann Intern Med. 1990; 112:423–428.

103. Dale C, Gallus A, Wycherley A, Langlois S, Howie D. Prevention of venous thrombosis with minidose warfarin after joint replacement. BMJ. 1991; 303:224.

104. Fordyce MJ, Baker AS, Staddon GE. Efficacy of fixed minidose warfarin prophylaxis in total hip replacement. BMJ. 1991; 303:219–220.

105. Poller L, MacCallum PK, Thomson JM, Kerns W. Reduction of factor VII coagulant activity (VIIC), a risk factor for ischaemic heart disease, by fixed dose warfarin: a double blind crossover study. Br Heart J. 1990; 63:231–3.

106. Turpie AG, Gallus AS, Hoek JA. A synthetic pentasaccharide for the prevention of deep-vein thrombosis after total hip replacement. N Engl J Med. 2001; 344:619–625.

107. Lassen MR, Bauer KA, Eriksson BI, Turpie AG. Postoperative fondaparinux versus preoperative enoxaparin for prevention of venous thromboembolism in elective hip-replacement surgery: a randomised double-blind comparison. Lancet. 2002; 359:1715–1720.

108. Eriksson BI, Bauer KA, Lassen MR, Turpie AG. Fondaparinux compared with enoxaparin for the prevention of venous thromboembolism after hip-fracture surgery. N Engl J Med. 2001; 345:1298–1304.

109. Bauer KA, Eriksson BI, Lassen MR, Turpie AG. Fondaparinux compared with enoxaparin for the prevention of venous thromboembolism after elective major knee surgery. N Engl J Med. 2001; 345:1305–1310.

110. Turpie AG. Overview of the clinical results of pentasaccharide in major orthopedic surgery. Haematologica. 2001; 86:59–62.

111. Heit JA, Colwell CW, Francis CW, Ginsberg JS, Berkowitz SD, Whipple J, Peters G. Comparison of the oral direct thrombin inhibitor ximelagatran with enoxaparin as prophylaxis against venous thromboembolism after total knee replacement: a phase 2 dose-finding study. Arch Intern Med. 2001; 161:2215–2221.

112. Eriksson BI, Bergqvist D, Kalebo P, Dahl OE, Lindbratt S, Bylock A, Frison L, Eriksson UG, Welin L, Gustafsson D. Ximelagatran and melagatran compared with dalteparin for prevention of venous thromboembolism after total hip or knee replacement: the METHRO II randomised trial. Lancet. 2002; 360:1441–1447.

113. Eriksson BI, Agnelli G, Cohen AT, Dahl OE, Lassen MR, Mouret P, Rosencher N, Kalebo P, Panfilov S, Eskilson C, Andersson M. The direct thrombin inhibitor melagatran followed by oral ximelagatran compared with enoxaparin for the prevention of venous thromboembolism after total hip or knee replacement: the EXPRESS study. J Thromb Haemost. 2003; 1:2490–2496.

114. Colwell CW, Berkowitz SD, Davidson BL, Lotke PA, Ginsberg JS, Lieberman JR, Neubauer J, McElhattan JL, Peters GR, Francis CW. Comparison of ximelagatran, an oral direct thrombin inhibitor, with enoxaparin for the prevention of venous thromboembolism following total hip replacement. A randomized, double-blind study. J Thromb Haemost. 2003; 1:2119–2130.

115. Francis CW, Davidson BL, Berkowitz SD, Lotke PA, Ginsberg JS, Lieberman JR, Webster AK, Whipple JP, Peters GR, Colwell CW, Jr. Ximelagatran versus warfarin for the prevention of venous thromboembolism after total knee arthroplasty. A randomized, double-blind trial. Ann Intern Med. 2002; 137:648–655.

116. Eriksson BI, Agnelli G, Cohen AT, Dahl OE, Mouret P, Rosencher N, Eskilson C, Nylander I, Frison L, Ogren M. Direct thrombin inhibitor melagatran followed by oral ximelagatran in comparison with enoxaparin for prevention of venous thromboembolism after total hip or knee replacement. Thromb Haemost. 2003; 89:288–296.

117. Francis CW, Berkowitz SD, Comp PC, Lieberman JR, Ginsberg JS, Paiement G, Peters GR, Roth AW, McElhattan J, Colwell CW, Jr. Comparison of ximelagatran with warfarin for the prevention of venous thromboembolism after total knee replacement. N Engl J Med. 2003; 349:1703–1712.

118. Kaboli P HM, White RH. DVT prophylaxis and anticoagulation in the surgical patient. Med Clin North Am. 2003; 87:77–110, viii.

119. Hull RD BR, Pineo GF, Stein PD, Raskob GE, Valentine KA. Preoperative vs postoperative initiation of low-molecular-weight heparin prophylaxis against venous thromboembolism in patients undergoing elective hip replacement. Arch Intern Med. 1999; 159:137–141.

120. Goldstein WM JM, Bailie DS, Wall R, Branson J. Safety of a clinical surveillance protocol with 3– and 6–week warfarin prophylaxis after total joint arthroplasty. Orthopedics. 2001; 24:651–654.

121. Scurr JH C-SP, Hasty JH. Deep venous thrombosis: a continuing problem. BMJ. 1988; 297:28.

122. Berqvist D. Prolonged prophylaxis in post opertaive medicine. Semin Thromb Hemost. 1997; 23:149–154.

123. Lausen I, Jensen R, Jorgensen LN, Rasmussen MS, Lyng KM, Andersen M, Raaschou HO, Wille-Jorgensen P. Incidence and prevention of deep venous thrombosis occurring late after

general surgery: randomised controlled study of prolonged thromboprophylaxis. Eur J Surg. 1998; 164:657–663.

124. Bergqvist D, Agnelli G, Cohen AT, Eldor A, Nilsson PE, Le Moigne-Amrani A, Dietrich-Neto F. Duration of prophylaxis against venous thromboembolism with enoxaparin after surgery for cancer. N Engl J Med. 2002; 346:975–980.

125. Sarasin FP, Bounameaux H. Cost-effectiveness of prophylactic anticoagulation prolonged after hospital discharge following general surgery. Arch Surg. 1996; 131:694–698.

126. Eikelboom JW, Quinlan DJ, Douketis JD. Extended-duration prophylaxis against venous thromboembolism after total hip or knee replacement: a meta-analysis of the randomised trials. Lancet. 2001; 358:9–15.

127. White RH, Romano PS, Zhou H, Rodrigo J, Bargar W. Incidence and time course of thromboembolic outcomes following total hip or knee arthroplasty. Arch Intern Med. 1998; 158:1525–1531.

128. Francis CW, Marder VJ, Evarts CM, Yaukoolbodi S. Two-step warfarin therapy. Prevention of postoperative venous thrombosis without excessive bleeding. JAMA. 1983; 249:374–378.

129. Powers PJ, Gent M, Jay RM, Julian DH, Turpie AG, Levine M, Hirsh J. A randomized trial of less intense postoperative warfarin or aspirin therapy in the prevention of venous thromboembolism after surgery for fractured hip. Arch Intern Med. 1989; 149:771–774.

Appendix   Prophylaxis of Venous Thromboembolism

General recommendations:
- Mechanical methods are to be used primarily in patients who are at high risk of bleeding or as an adjunct to anticoagulant-based prophylaxis.
- Aspirin alone is NOT recommended for prophylaxis in any patient group.
- Consider renal impairment when selecting dose of anticoagulant.
- Special caution is needed with anticoagulants in patients undergoing neuraxial anesthesia.

General surgery:
- *Low risk*:
  (Minor procedure, age < 40 years and no additional risk factors)
  —No specific prophylaxis
  —Early and persistent mobilization
- *Moderate risk*:
  (Non-major procedure, 40–60 years or additional risk factors)
  (Major procedure, < 40 years, no additional risk factors)
  —LDUH 5000 U bid or
  —LMWH ≤ 3400 U once daily
- *High risk*:
  (Non-major surgery, >60 years or additional risk factors)
  (Major surgery, >40 years or additional risk factors)
  —LDUH 5000 U tid or
  —LMWH >3400 U once daily
  In high risk general surgery patients with multiple risk factors, pharmacologic agents should be combined with CGS and/or IPC.

Vascular surgery:
- For patients undergoing vascular surgery who do not have additional risk factors, clinicians should NOT routinely use prophylaxis.
- For patients undergoing major vascular surgery who have additional thromboembolic risk factors
  —LDUH or
  —LMWH

Gynecologic surgery:
- For patients undergoing brief procedures of < 30 min for benign disease
  —No specific prophylaxis
  —Early and persistent mobilization
- Laparascopic procedures
  —One or more of the following: LDUH, LMWH, IPC, CGS
- Major gynecologici surgery (benign disease, no additional risk factors)
  —LDUH 5000 U bid or
  —LMWH <3400 U once daily or
  —IPC started just before surgery and used continuously while the patient is not ambulating.
- Extensive gynecologic surgery for malignancy, or additional risk factors
  —LDUH 5000 tid or
  —LMWH >3400 U once daily or
  —A combination of LDUH or LMWH plus CGS or IPC

Urologic surgery:
- For patients undergoing transurethral or other low-risk procedures
  —No specific prophylaxis
  —Early and persistent mobilization
- Major open urologic procedures
  —LDUH 5000 U bid or tid or

—IPC or CGS
- Patients with multiple risk factors
  —A combination of LDUH or LMWH plus IPC or CGS

Laparascopic surery:
- For patients without additional risk factors
  —No specific prophylaxis
  —Early and persistent mobilization
- Patients with additional risk factors
  —One or more of the following: LDUH, LMWH, IPC, CGS

Elective hip arthroplasty:
- Elective THR (equal alternatives)
  —LMWH >3400 U daily beginning:
    12 hr before surgery
    12–24 hr after surgery
    4–6 hr after surgery (1/2 dose, moving to full dose the next day)
  —Fondaparinux 2.5 mg started 6–8 hours after surgery
  —Adjusted dose warfarin (INR target 2.5, range 2–3) begun preoperatively or the evening after surgery
- The use of ASA, dextran, LDUH, CGS, IPC or VPB as the only method of thromboprophyaxis is NOT recommended.

Elective knee arthroplasy:
- Elective TKA (equal alternatives)
  —LMWH >3400 U daily beginning:
    12 hr before surgery
    12–24 hr after surgery
    4–6 hr after surgery (1/2 dose, moving to full dose the next day)
  —Fondaparinux 2.5 mg started 6–8 hr after surgery
  —Adjusted dose warfarin (INR target 2.5, range 2–3) begun preoperatively or the evening after surgery
  —Optimal IPC is an alternative to anticoagulant prophylaxis
- The use of ASA, LDUH, or VPB as the only method of thromboprophyaxis is NOT recommended.

Knee arthroscopy:
- Patients with no additional risk factors
  —No specific prophylaxis
  —Early and persistent mobilization
- Patients undergoing arthroscopic knee surgery who are at higher than usual risk
  —LMWH >3400 U once daily

Hip fracture surgery:
  —Fondaparinux or LMWH >3400 U once daily
  —Adjusted dose warfarin (INR target 2.5, range 2–3)
  —LDUH
  —ASA alone is NOT recommended.
  —If surgery is going to be delayed, prophylaxis with either LMWH or LDUH should be initiated during the time between admission and surgery.

Elective spine surgery:
- Patients with no additional risk factors
  —No specific prophylaxis
  —Early and persistent mobilization
- Patients with additional risk factors

—Postoperative LDUH alone
—Postoperative LMWH alone
—Perioperative IPC and/or CGS
- Patients with multiple additional risk factors
  —A combination of LDUH or LMWH plus IPC or CGS

Neurosurgery:
- Intracranial neurosurgery
  —IPC with or without CGS
  —Acceptable alternatives: LDUH or postoperative LMWH
- High-risk neurosurgery
  —A combination of LDUH or LMWH plus IPC or CGS

Trauma:
- All patients with at least one risk factor (in the absence of contraindications)
  —LMWH >3400 U daily, starting as soon as it is considered safe

Spinal cord injury:
- All patients
  —LMWH >3400 U daily (with or without IPC) once primary hemostasis is evident
  —LDUH plus IPC is an alternative

Burn patients:
- All patients with additional risk factors (if no contraindications)
  —LMWH or LDUH starting as soon as possible

Medical illness:
- CHF, severe respiratory disease, or bedridden
  —LMWH or LDUH

Cancer:
- Surgical prophylaxis as appropriate for procedure
- Medical illness prophylaxis as appropriate

ICU patients:
- Assess for VTE risk at admission
- Moderate risk patients
  —LMWH or LDUH
- Higher risk patients
  —LMWH

18-3

Monitoring Chronic Oral Anticoagulant Therapy in Cardiac Disease

Kamal Gupta, J. Michael Wilson, and James J. Ferguson
St. Luke's Episcopal Hospital, Texas Heart Institute, Baylor College of Medicine, The University of Texas Health Science Center at Houston, Houston, Texas, U.S.A.

I. INTRODUCTION

The efficacy of oral anticoagulant therapy with warfarin is well established for preventing and treating venous and arterial thromboembolism in varied clinical settings. In this chapter we discuss the guidelines for use of oral anticoagulants (warfarin and derivatives) in various cardiac diseases. Standardized laboratory monitoring and point-of-care testing have dramatically improved the safety and ease of administration of these drugs. Self-management of chronic warfarin therapy is a rapidly evolving topic, and we have highlighted the major points in this field. We also briefly discuss the recent data on use of ximelagatran as an alternative to warfarin in long-term oral anticoagulation.

II. CHRONIC ANTICOAGULATION IN CARDIAC DISEASE

A. Prosthetic Heart Valves

There is convincing evidence from many trials that oral anticoagulants significantly reduce the risk of thromboembolism in patients with both mechanical and biological prosthetic valves (1–6). Various studies have also tested the optimal degree of anticoagulation and determined that the intensity needed depends on the type of prosthesis (2,4,6) and the position of the valve in the heart. Almost all studies have showed that risk of embolism is greater with a valve at the mitral position (mechanical or biological) than with a valve at the aortic position (7–9). With either type of prosthesis or valve location, the risk of thromboembolism is probably higher in the first few days and months after valve insertion (10), before the valve is fully endothelialized. Furthermore, addition of aspirin to warfarin therapy may be of additional benefit. In a recent trial, addition of aspirin (100 mg) to warfarin (INR 3.0–4.5) improved the efficacy of the regimen compared to warfarin alone (11). This combination of low-dose aspirin and high-dose warfarin was associated with a reduction in all-cause mortality, cardiovascular mortality, and stroke at the expense of increased minor bleeding; the difference in major bleeding, including intracranial hemorrhage, did not reach statistical significance. Guidelines developed by the American College of Cardiology and the American Heart Association for management of patients with valvular heart diseases provide recommendations regarding optimal anticoagulation in patients with prosthetic valves (12). Table 1 highlights these recommendations, which have incorporated many of the previously mentioned trials.

B. Atrial Fibrillation

Five large randomized trials published between 1989 and 1992 evaluated oral anticoagulation, and two trials tested aspirin for the primary prevention of thromboembolism in patients with nonvalvular atrial fibrillation (AF) (13–16). Another trial focused on secondary prevention among survivors of a nondisabling stroke or a transient ischemic attack (17). This trial compared warfarin therapy, aspirin, and placebo. Compared with placebo, there was a 68% reduction in stroke with warfarin and an insignificant 16% reduction with aspirin. A meta-analysis showed that adjusted-dose oral anticoagulation is highly efficacious for prevention of all strokes, with a risk reduction of 61% (95% CI 47–71%) versus placebo (18) (Fig. 1). This reduction was similar for both primary and secondary prevention. Patient age and intensity of anticoagulation are the most powerful predictors of major bleeding (19,20). Trial participants had a mean age of 69 years, and the trials were done in a closely monitored setting . It is thus unclear whether the relatively low rates of hemorrhage are valid for AF patients in clinical practice who are older (mean age 75 years) and less well monitored (21,22). It is important to strike a balance between adequate protection from thromboembolism and risk of bleeding. Maximum protection against ischemic strokes in AF is probably achieved with an INR of 2–3 (23–25), whereas an INR of 1.6–2.5 appears to be associated with incomplete efficacy, estimated at approximately 80% of that achieved with higher levels of anticoagulation (24,26) (Fig. 2).

The SPAF II trial (13) compared efficacy and safety of warfarin with aspirin in patients with AF. Warfarin was more effective than aspirin for preventing ischemic stroke,

Table 1 Recommendations for Antithrombotic Therapy in Patients with Prosthetic Heart Valves

Indication	Class
1. First 3 months after valve replacement: warfarin, INR 2.5–3.5	I
2. ≥3 months after valve replacement:	
A. Mechanical valve	
AVR and no risk factor[a]	
Bileaflet valve or Medtronic Hall valve: warfarin, INR 2–3	I
Other disk valves or Starr-Edwards valve: warfarin, INR 2.5–3.5	I
AVR plus risk factor[a]: warfarin, INR 2.5–3.5	I
MVR: Warfarin, INR 2.5–3.5	I
B. Bioprosthesis	
AVR plus no risk factor[a]: aspirin, 80–100 mg/d	I
AVR plus risk factor[a]: warfarin, INR 2–3	I
MVR plus no risk factor[a]: aspirin, 80–100 mg/d	I
MVR plus risk factor[a]: warfarin, INR 2.5–3.5	I
3. Addition of aspirin, 80–100 mg once daily, if not on aspirin	IIa
4. Warfarin, INR 3.5–4.5, in high-risk patients when aspirin cannot be used	IIa
5. Warfarin, INR 2.0–3.0, in patients with Starr-Edwards AVR and no risk factor	IIb
6. Mechanical valve, no warfarin therapy	III
7. Mechanical valve, aspirin therapy only	III
8. Bioprosthesis, no warfarin and no aspirin therapy	III

[a]Risk factors: atrial fibrillation, LV dysfunction, previous thromboembolism, and hypercoagulable condition.
Source: From Ref. 12.

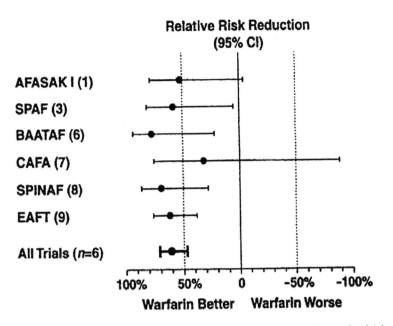

Figure 1 Antithrombotic therapy for prevention of stroke (ischemic and hemorrhagic) in patients with nonvalvular AF: adjusted-dose warfarin compared with placebo. (From Ref. 30.)

but this difference was almost entirely offset by a higher rate of intracranial bleeding with warfarin, particularly among patients older than 75 years age. The intensity of anticoagulation in SPAF trials was greater than in several other primary prevention studies; in addition, the majority of hemorrhages occurred when the estimated INR was >3.0. In the SPAF III study (23), warfarin (INR 2.0–3.0) was much more effective than a fixed-dose combination of warfarin (1–3 mg/d; INR 1.2–1.5) plus aspirin (325 mg) in high-risk patients

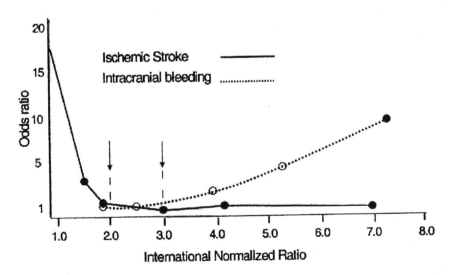

Figure 2 Adjusted odds ratios for ischemic stroke and intracranial bleeding in relation to intensity of anticoagulation in randomized trials of antithrombotic therapy for patients with AF. (Adapted from Refs. 24,27,73.)

with AF, whereas aspirin alone was sufficient for patients with low intrinsic risk of thromboembolism. Table 2 presents the recommendations of the ACC/AHA task force for management of antithrombotic therapy in patients with atrial fibrillation (27).

In view of the many problems associated with the use of warfarin, including frequent monitoring of INR, need for dose adjustments, and its many drug interactions, there has been a lot of interest in use of fixed-dose ximelagatran as a possible replacement for warfarin. Two recent trials (28) (SPORTIF III and V) have explored this area. SPORTIF III was a randomized, multicenter, open-labeled, parallel-group trial comparing oral ximelagatran with adjusted-dose warfarin for prevention of stroke and systemic embolism in high-risk patients (one or more risk factors: hypertension, age >75 years, previous stroke, transient ischemic attack or systemic embolism, age and coronary artery disease or diabetes mellitus) with paroxysmal AF (29). The study randomized 3410 such patients to open-label dose-adjusted warfarin (INR 2.0–3.0) or oral fixed-dose ximelagatran (36 mg twice a day). The primary endpoint was stroke or systemic embolism. During 4941 patient-years of exposure (mean 17.4 months, SD 4.1), 96 patients had primary events (56 in warfarin group and 40 in ximelagatran group). The primary event rate by intention-to-treat analysis 2.3% per year with warfarin and 1.6% per year with ximelagatran (absolute risk reduction 0.7%, 95% CI 0.1–1.4; $p = 0.10$; relative risk reduction 29%, 95% C 6.5–52). Rates of disabling or fatal stroke, mortality, and major bleeding were similar between groups, but combined major and minor hemorrhages were lower with ximelagatran than with warfarin (29.8% vs. 25.8% per year; relative risk reduction 14%, 95% CI 4–22; $p = 0.007$).

The almost identical but double-blind SPORTIF V trial enrolled 3922 high risk patients with nonvalvular (unlike SPORTIF III, this trial was done only in United States

Table 2 Recommendations for Antithrombotic Therapy in Patients with Atrial Fibrillation Based on Thromboembolic Risk Stratification

Patient features	Antithrombotic therapy	Grade of recommendation
Age less than 60 years; no heart disease (lone AF)	Aspirin (325 mg daily) or no therapy	I
Age less than 60 years; heart disease but no risk factors[a]	Aspirin (325 mg daily)	I
Age greater than or equal to 60 years; no risk factors[a]	Aspirin (325 mg daily)	I
Age greater than or equal to 60 years; with diabetes mellitus or CAD	Oral anticoagulation (INR 2.0–3.0)	I
Addition of aspirin, 81–162 mg daily is optional	IIb	
Age greater than or equal to 75 years, especially women	Oral anticoagulation (INR 2.0)	I
HF LV ejection fraction less than or equal to 0.35; thyrotoxicosis; hypertension	Oral anticoagulation (INR 2.0–3.0)	I
Rheumatic heart disease (mitral stenosis); prosthetic heart valves; prior thromboembolism; persistent atrial thrombus on TEE	Oral anticoagulation (INR 2.5–3.5 or higher may be appropriate)	I

[a]Risk factors for thromboembolism include HF, LV ejection fraction less than 0.35, and history of hypertension.
AF, atrial fibrillation; CAD, coronary artery disease; HF, heart failure; INR, international normalized ratio; LV, left ventricular; TEE, transesophageal echo.

and Canada) and randomized them to dose-adjusted warfarin (INR 2.0–3.0) or ximelaga-tran 36 mg twice daily (30). At one year there were no significant differences in primary event rates for ximelagatran (1.6%) and warfarin (1.2%). This was true even though patients in the warfarin arm were tightly controlled, with 68% maintaining, INR of 2–3 and 83% of 1.8–3.2. There was no difference in the incidence of intracranial and major bleeding in the two groups, although the rate of all bleeding (major and minor) was sig-nificantly lower in the ximelagatran group compared with warfarin (37% vs. 47%; $p <$ 0.0001) over a follow-up of about 20 months.

Thus, both SPORTIF III and V concluded that in high-risk patients with nonvalvular AF, fixed-dose oral ximelagatran was at least as effective as well-controlled warfarin for prevention of stroke and systemic embolism. However, the drug is not approved for use in the United States at the time of this writing. Also, there are some concerns regarding the hepatotoxicity of ximelagatran. In both SPORTIF III and V, about 6% of patients had ele-vation of liver enzymes more than three times normal, and this was statistically higher than with warfarin. Though most were transient, this issue needs further study, and the authors recommended that liver function function tests be performed every 6 months.

The platelet-ADP-receptor antagonist clopidogrel, which has a good track record in the invasive and noninvasive treatment of coronary artery disease, is also being tested (combined with aspirin) in comparison to dose-adjusted warfarin in patients with AF in the ACTIVE study of 6500 patients. However, currently no recommendations can be made for its use in patients with AF.

C. Dilated Cardiomyopathy

Both pulmonary embolism and peripheral arterial embolism contribute in part to the high morbidity and mortality of congestive heart failure (31–33). Compared to the annual stroke risk of <0.5% in the general population, the risk is almost 4% in patients with severe heart failure (33,34). Even mild-moderate heart failure is associated with an annual stroke risk of approximately 1.5% (35–38). The SAVE study reported an inverse rela-tionship between stroke risk and ejection fraction (EF), with an 18% increase in stroke risk for every 5% reduction in EF. In spite of this increased risk, the use of anticoagula-tion in the setting of systolic dysfunction is still controversial. No large randomized trials have addressed this issue directly. Fuster et al. reported 19 embolic events during 624 patient-years in 103 patients who did not receive anticoagulants (3.5 events/100 patient-years); none of 32 patients (101 patient-years) receiving warfarin had an embolic event ($p <$ 0.05). However, post-hoc analysis of most large CHF trials failed to show a protec-tive effect of anticoagulation. These trials did not randomize patients to anticoagulant therapy (physician discretion) or set strict guidelines for INR (35–37,39). In the V-HeFT I trial the embolic rate in anticoagulated patients was similar to those not on anticoagula-tion (2.9 vs. 2.7 events/100 patient-years); V-HeFT II showed similar findings (37,38). A recent analysis of the SOLVD database did not show a reduction in embolic events among either men or women receiving warfarin (40). However, the SAVE trial reported an 81% risk reduction of stroke among anticoagulated patients (39). One retrospective analysis of limited data from the PROMISE trial found that use of warfarin in 324 patients was asso-ciated with a significant reduction in stroke (0.6% vs. 3.3% in controls; $p <$ 0.05) only in those with severe systolic impairment (EF $\leq$ 20% (41). The only prospective study that has directly addressed this issue is a pilot study: the WASH (Warfarin Aspirin Study in Heart Failure) trial (42). WASH reported preliminary data on 279 patients randomized to receive oral anticoagulation with warfarin (INR 2.5) vs. aspirin (325 mg) versus no antithrombotic therapy. There was no significant difference in the composite endpoint of death/nonfatal MI or stroke in the aspirin, warfarin, and no antithrombotic groups (32, 24, and 27%, respectively).

Thus, routine use of anticoagulant therapy for all patients with systolic heart failure currently cannot be recommended (33), though patients with very severe systolic dysfunction and very dilated left ventricles is a subgroup that may derive the most benefit. The Veterans Administration is currently conducting the WATCH (Warfarin Antiplatelet Trial in Chronic Heart Failure) trial. This trial, which plans to randomize 4500 patients with NYHA class III–IV CHF and EF < 30% to warfarin or antiplatelet therapy (blinded aspirin or clopidogrel), should help resolve this conflict to some extent. Presently the only supported indications for routine anticoagulation in CHF are atrial fibrillation, prior thromboembolic event, and presence of LV thrombus.

D. Chronic Left Ventricular Aneurysm

In contrast to the prevalence of thromboembolism in acute MI, the incidence of embolism in chronic LV aneurysm (occurring ≥3 months after a MI) is very low (0.35% per year (43). Thrombi formed immediately after an acute MI are friable, mobile, and protrude into the ventricular cavity compared to the organized, laminated ones formed within a chronic aneurismal sac (44). Despite the higher prevalence of thrombi in the LV aneurysms, these rarely embolize, and anticoagulant treatment does not seem to effect the development of or embolization of the thrombus (45–47). Therefore, the current recommendation is that routine anticoagulation for chronic LV aneurysms is not indicated. Whether these drugs should be given in the presence of an associated thrombus is also controversial (48).

III. PATIENT SELF-MANAGEMENT OF ORAL ANTICOAGULATION

Warfarin is the mainstay of therapy for the prevention and treatment of thromboembolic diseases. However, the management of warfarin anticoagulation is complicated because of a narrow therapeutic index and the many variables that affect the INR. This requires regular and frequent monitoring, conventionally done by the physician's office or at specialized "coumadin clinics." These traditional methods are both cumbersome and inconvenient (49), and there is a potential for dosing errors due to misinterpretation of information conveyed by the physician or delays in conveying the information. Only 30–60% of the INRs are in the therapeutic range in the traditional physician-managed model (50–54). Anticoagulation clinics improve on the physician-managed model (55–58) but still leave a lot to be desired. Patient self-management of oral anticoagulation refers to a system wherein the patients measure their own INRs and interpret the results themselves, as opposed to self-testing, in which patients measure their own INRs but have to contact their health professional for interpretation of the results. This is analogous to diabetic patients managing their glucose on their own. This method can empower the patient and has the potential of improved coagulation control by improving patient compliance.

A. Point-of-Care Prothrombin Time/INR Instruments

Accurate, reliable, and user-friendly point-of-care (POC) instruments are critical for the success of any self-management anticoagulation program. Two of the more popular and widely available monitors are the ProTime (International Technidyne Corporation) and CoaguCheck S (Roche Diagnostics) and both have been shown acceptable correlation, precision, and clinical agreement when tested against laboratory standards (56,59–61). Both are hand-held devices that use whole blood from finger puncture. The clotting time is then converted to a plasma PT equivalent and reported as a PT or an INR within minutes (56). Of these studies, two compared the performance of the ProTime device not just with local laboratories but also with a national reference laboratory (60,61). There was a good correlation, with more than two thirds of the POC and laboratory INR results matching those of the reference laboratory (60). As previously seen with the CoaguCheck sytem (62), the variability of the ProTime INRs increased at higher INR values exceeding 4.5 (60). The results also demonstrated that almost 80% of the hospital laboratory INRs and ProTime results were within 0.4 INR of the refernce laboratory values and 93% were within 0.7 INR (61).

Quality control of these home monitoring devices is an important issue. The ProTime monitor and CoaguCheck S both have built-in internal quality controls supplied by the manufacturer (63). The British Society of Hematology Task Force for Hemostasis and Thrombosis has recently published recommendations for self-management of oral anticoagulation (64). The report recommends that patients should have their INRs on the POC monitor assessed with a concurrent laboratory every 6 months. A difference of <0.5 INR between the paired results would be considered satisfactory (64).

B. Anticoagulation Self-Management: Evidence-Based Practice

Apart from some small nonrandomized and pilot studies (63,65,66), the support for this management strategy comes from several randomized trials directly comparing it with conventional strategies (53,54,67–69). All of these studies showed either superior or equivalent anticoagulation control with self management. Koertke et al. (70) compared self-management of INR early after valve-replacement surgery with conventional management [The Early Self Controlled Anticoagulation Trial (ESCAT I)]. Data were collected from the first 600 surviving patients (from a total study sample of 1200 patients) who completed follow-up of at least 2 years. Patients were randomly divided into a self-management group and a control group. INR self-management reduced severe hemorrhagic and thromboembolic complications ($p = 0.018$). Nearly 80% of the INR values recorded by patients themselves, regardless of educational level, were within the target therapeutic range of INR 2.5–4.5, compared with 62% of INR values monitored by family practitioners. Only 8.3% of patients trained in self-management immediately after surgery were unable to continue with INR self-management.

The same group then conducted the ESCAT II trial to investigate whether lowering the target range for INR self-management would further reduce complications. ESCAT II was a prospective controlled randomized (valves: St. Jude Medical Standard or Medtronic Hall; treatment: conventional/low-dose) multicenter study with 3300 patients. The interim results of 1 818 patients were recently published (54); 908 patients were categorized as having a low-dose target range, which was INR 1.8–2.8 for prostheses in the aortic position and 2.5–3.5 for prostheses in the mitral position or in combined valve replacement. The control group (conventional group) with 910 patients aimed at an INR of 2.5–4.5 for all valve positions. In the conventional group, 74% of INR values measured were within the therapeutic range. In the low-dose group, 72% of the values were within that range. The linearized thromboembolism rate (% per patient-year) was 0.21% for both groups. The bleeding complication rate was 0.56% in the low-dose regimen group versus 0.91% in the conventional group. The authors concluded that early-onset INR self-management under oral anticoagulation after mechanical heart valve replacement enables patients to stay within a lower and smaller INR target range. The reduced anticoagulation level resulted in fewer grade III bleeding complications without increasing thromboembolic event rates. Several trials of anticoagulation self-management are ongoing (64,71), and these will shed further light on the clinical and economic aspects of this evolving strategy of anticoagulant management.

REFERENCES

1. Mok CK, Boey J, Wang R, Chan TK, Cheung KL, Lee PK, Chow J, Ng RP, Tse TF. Warfarin versus dipyridamole-aspirin and pentoxifylline-aspirin for the prevention of prosthetic heart valve thromboembolism: a prospective randomized clinical trial. Circulation. 1985; 72:1059–1063.
2. Cannegieter SC, Rosendaal FR, Wintzen AR, van der Meer FJ, Vandenbroucke JP, Briet E. Optimal oral anticoagulant therapy in patients with mechanical heart valves. N Engl J Med. 1995; 333:11–17.
3. Saour JN, Sieck JO, Mamo LA, Gallus AS. Trial of different intensities of anticoagulation in patients with prosthetic heart valves. N Engl J Med. 1990; 322:428–432.
4. Butchart EG, Lewis PA, Bethel JA, Breckenridge IM. Adjusting anticoagulation to prosthesis thrombogenicity and patient risk factors. Recommendations for the Medtronic Hall valve. Circulation. 1991; 84:III61–69.
5. Acar J, Iung B, Boissel JP, Samama MM, Michel PL, Teppe JP, Pony JC, Breton HL, Thomas D, Isnard R, de Gevigney G, Viguier E, Sfihi A, Hanania G, Ghannem M, Mirode A, Nemoz C. AREVA: multicenter randomized comparison of low-dose versus standard-dose anticoagulation in patients with mechanical prosthetic heart valves. Circulation. 1996; 94:2107–2112.
6. Altman R, Rouvier J, Gurfinkel E, D'Ortencio O, Manzanel R, de La Fuente L, Favaloro RG. Comparison of two levels of anticoagulant therapy in patients with substitute heart valves. J Thorac Cardiovasc Surg. 1991; 101:427–431.
7. Grunkemeier GL, Starr A, Rahimtoola SH. Prosthetic heart valve performance: long-term follow-up. Curr Probl Cardiol. 1992; 17:329–406.
8. Cannegieter SC, Rosendaal FR, Briet E. Thromboembolic and bleeding complications in patients with mechanical heart valve prostheses. Circulation. 1994; 89:635–641.
9. Bloomfield P, Wheatley DJ, Prescott RJ, Miller HC. Twelve-year comparison of a Bjork-Shiley mechanical heart valve with porcine bioprostheses. N Engl J Med. 1991; 324:573–579.
10. Heras M, Chesebro JH, Fuster V, Penny WJ, Grill DE, Bailey KR, Danielson GK, Orszulak TA, Pluth JR, Puga FJ, et al. High risk of thromboemboli early after bioprosthetic cardiac valve replacement. J Am Coll Cardiol. 1995; 25:1111–1119.
11. Turpie AG GM, Laupacis A, Latour Y, Gunstensen J, Basile F, Klimek M, Hirsh J. A comparison of aspirin with placebo in patients treated with warfarin after heart-valve replacement. N Engl J Med. 1993; 329:524–529.
12. ACC/AHA guidelines for the management of patients with valvular heart disease. A report of the American College of Cardiology/American Heart Association. Task Force on Practice Guidelines (Committee on Management of Patients with Valvular Heart Disease). J Am Coll Cardiol. 1998; 32:1486–1588.
13. Stroke Prevention in Atrial Fibrillation Study. Final results. Circulation. 1991; 84:527–539.
14. Petersen P, Boysen G, Godtfredsen J, Andersen ED, Andersen B. Placebo-controlled, randomised trial of warfarin and aspirin for prevention of thromboembolic complications in chronic atrial fibrillation. The Copenhagen AFASAK study. Lancet. 1989; 1:175–179.
15. Ezekowitz MD, Bridgers SL, James KE, Carliner NH, Colling CL, Gornick CC, Krause-Steinrauf H, Kurtzke JF, Nazarian SM, Radford MJ, et al. Warfarin in the prevention of stroke associated with nonrheumatic atrial fibrillation. Veterans Affairs Stroke Prevention in Nonrheumatic Atrial Fibrillation Investigators. N Engl J Med. 1992; 327:1406–1412.
16. The effect of low-dose warfarin on the risk of stroke in patients with nonrheumatic atrial fibrillation. The Boston Area Anticoagulation Trial for Atrial Fibrillation Investigators. N Engl J Med. 1990; 323:1505–1511.
17. Secondary prevention in non-rheumatic atrial fibrillation after transient ischaemic attack or minor stroke. EAFT (European Atrial Fibrillation Trial) Study Group. Lancet. 1993; 342:1255–1262.

18. Hart RG, Benavente O, McBride R, Pearce LA. Antithrombotic therapy to prevent stroke in patients with atrial fibrillation: a meta-analysis. Ann Intern Med. 1999; 131:492–501.

19. Bleeding during antithrombotic therapy in patients with atrial fibrillation. The Stroke Prevention in Atrial Fibrillation Investigators. Arch Intern Med. 1996; 156:409–416.

20. Gorter JW. Major bleeding during anticoagulation after cerebral ischemia: patterns and risk factors. Stroke Prevention In Reversible Ischemia Trial (SPIRIT). European Atrial Fibrillation Trial (EAFT) study groups. Neurology. 1999; 53:1319–1327.

21. Feinberg WM, Blackshear JL, Laupacis A, Kronmal R, Hart RG. Prevalence, age distribution, and gender of patients with atrial fibrillation. Analysis and implications. Arch Intern Med. 1995; 155:469–473.

22. Sudlow M, Thomson R, Thwaites B, Rodgers H, Kenny RA. Prevalence of atrial fibrillation and eligibility for anticoagulants in the community. Lancet. 1998; 352:1167–1171.

23. Adjusted-dose warfarin versus low-intensity, fixed-dose warfarin plus aspirin for high-risk patients with atrial fibrillation: Stroke Prevention in Atrial Fibrillation III randomised clinical trial. Lancet. 1996; 348:633–638.

24. Hylek EM, Skates SJ, Sheehan MA, Singer DE. An analysis of the lowest effective intensity of prophylactic anticoagulation for patients with nonrheumatic atrial fibrillation. N Engl J Med. 1996; 335:540–546.

25. Optimal oral anticoagulant therapy in patients with nonrheumatic atrial fibrillation and recent cerebral ischemia. The European Atrial Fibrillation Trial Study Group. N Engl J Med. 1995; 333:5–10.

26. Hart RG. Intensity of anticoagulation to prevent stroke in patients with atrial fibrillation. Ann Intern Med. 1998; 128:408.

27. Fuster V, Ryden LE, Asinger RW, Cannom DS, Crijns HJ, Frye RL, Halperin JL, Kay GN, Klein WW, Levy S, McNamara RL, Prystowsky EN, Wann LS, Wyse DG, Gibbons RJ, Antman EM, Alpert JS, Faxon DP, Gregoratos G, Hiratzka LF, Jacobs AK, Russell RO, Smith SC, Alonso-Garcia A, Blomstrom-Lundqvist C, De Backer G, Flather M, Hradec J, Oto A, Parkhomenko A, Silber S, Torbicki A. ACC/AHA/ESC guidelines for the management of patients with atrial fibrillation: executive summary. A Report of the American College of Cardiology/ American Heart Association Task Force on Practice Guidelines and the European Society of Cardiology Committee for Practice Guidelines and Policy Conferences (Committee to Develop Guidelines for the Management of Patients With Atrial Fibrillation): developed in Collaboration With the North American Society of Pacing and Electrophysiology. J Am Coll Cardiol. 2001; 38:1231–166.

28. Halperin JL. Ximelagatran compared with warfarin for prevention of thromboembolism in patients with nonvalvular atrial fibrillation: Rationale, objectives, and design of a pair of clinical studies and baseline patient characteristics (SPORTIF III and V). Am Heart J. 2003; 146:431–438.

29. Olsson SB. Stroke prevention with the oral direct thrombin inhibitor ximelagatran compared with warfarin in patients with non-valvular atrial fibrillation (SPORTIF III): randomised controlled trial. Lancet. 2003; 362:1691–1698.

30. Halperin JL. Efficay and safety study of oral direct thrombin inhibitor ximelagatran compared with dose-adjusted warfarin in the prevention of stroke and systemic embolic events in patients with atrial fibrillation: SPORTIFF V. American Heart Association Scientific Sessions, Orlando, FL, November 2003.

31. Fuster V, Gersh BJ, Giuliani ER, Tajik AJ, Brandenburg RO, Frye RL. The natural history of idiopathic dilated cardiomyopathy. Am J Cardiol. 1981; 47:525–531.

32. Kyrle PA, Korninger C, Gossinger H, Glogar D, Lechner K, Niessner H, Pabinger I. Prevention of arterial and pulmonary embolism by oral anticoagulants in patients with dilated cardiomyopathy. Thromb Haemost. 1985; 54:521–523.

33. Lip GY, Gibbs CR. Antiplatelet agents versus control or anticoagulation for heart failure in sinus rhythm: a Cochrane systematic review. Qjm. 2002; 95:461–468.

34. Packer M, Carver JR, Rodeheffer RJ, Ivanhoe RJ, DiBianco R, Zeldis SM, Hendrix GH, Bommer WJ, Elkayam U, Kukin ML, et al. Effect of oral milrinone on mortality in severe chronic heart failure. The PROMISE Study Research Group. N Engl J Med. 1991; 325:1468–1475.

35. Effect of enalapril on survival in patients with reduced left ventricular ejection fractions and congestive heart failure. The SOLVD Investigators. N Engl J Med. 1991; 325:293–302.

36. Effect of enalapril on mortality and the development of heart failure in asymptomatic patients with reduced left ventricular ejection fractions. The SOLVD Investigators. N Engl J Med. 1992; 327:685–691.

37. Dunkman WB, Johnson GR, Carson PE, Bhat G, Farrell L, Cohn JN. Incidence of thromboembolic events in congestive heart failure. The V-HeFT VA Cooperative Studies Group. Circulation. 1993; 87:VI94–101.

38. Cohn JN, Archibald DG, Ziesche S, Franciosa JA, Harston WE, Tristani FE, Dunkman WB, Jacobs W, Francis GS, Flohr KH, et al. Effect of vasodilator therapy on mortality in chronic congestive heart failure. Results of a Veterans Administration Cooperative Study. N Engl J Med. 1986; 314:1547–1552.

39. Loh E SM, Wun CC, Rouleau JL, Flaker GC, Gottlieb SS, Lamas GA, Moye LA, Goldhaber SZ, Pfeffer MA. Ventricular dysfunction and the risk of stroke after myocardial infarction. N Engl J Med. 1997; 336:251–257.

40. Dries DL, Rosenberg YD, Waclawiw MA, Domanski MJ. Ejection fraction and risk of thromboembolic events in patients with systolic dysfunction and sinus rhythm: evidence for gender differences in the studies of left ventricular dysfunction trials. J Am Coll Cardiol. 1997; 29:1074–1080.

41. Falk RH PA, Tandon PK, Packer M. The effect of warfarin on prevalence of stroke in patients with heart failure. J Am Coll Cardiol. 1993; 21:218A.

42. Jones CG, Cleland JG. Meeting report—the LIDO, HOPE, MOXCON and WASH studies. Heart Outcomes Prevention Evaluation. The Warfarin/Aspirin Study of Heart Failure. Eur J Heart Fail. 1999; 1:425–431.

43. Lapeyre AC, 3rd, Steele PM, Kazmier FJ, Chesebro JH, Vlietstra RE, Fuster V. Systemic embolism in chronic left ventricular aneurysm: incidence and the role of anticoagulation. J Am Coll Cardiol. 1985; 6:534–538.

44. Meltzer RS, Visser CA, Fuster V. Intracardiac thrombi and systemic embolization. Ann Intern Med. 1986; 104:689–698.

45. Hamby RI, Wisoff BG, Davison ET, Hartstein ML. Coronary artery disease and left ventricular mural thrombi: clinical, hemodynamic and angiocardiographic aspects. Chest. 1974; 66:488–494.

46. Simpson MT, Oberman A, Kouchoukos NT, Rogers WJ. Prevalence of mural thrombi and systemic embolization with left ventricular aneurysm. Effect of anticoagulation therapy. Chest. 1980; 77:463–469.

47. Reeder GS, Lengyel M, Tajik AJ, Seward JB, Smith HC, Danielson GK. Mural thrombus in left ventricular aneurysm: incidence, role of angiography, and relation between anticoagulation and embolization. Mayo Clin Proc. 1981; 56:77–81.

48. Fuster V IJ, Jang IK, Fay W, Chesebro J. Antithrombotic therapy in cardiac disease. Philadelphia: Lippincott; 1995.

49. Ansell JE, Patel N, Ostrovsky D, Nozzolillo E, Peterson AM, Fish L. Long-term patient self-management of oral anticoagulation. Arch Intern Med. 1995; 155:2185–2189.

50. Pell JP, McIver B, Stuart P, Malone DN, Alcock J. Comparison of anticoagulant control among patients attending general practice and a hospital anticoagulant clinic. Br J Gen Pract. 1993; 43:152–154.

51. Hasenkam JM, Kimose HH, Knudsen L, Gronnesby H, Halborg J, Christensen TD, Attermann J, Pilegaard HK. Self management of oral anticoagulant therapy after heart valve replacement. Eur J Cardiothorac Surg. 1997; 11:935–942.

52. Chiquette E, Amato MG, Bussey HI. Comparison of an anticoagulation clinic with usual medical care: anticoagulation control, patient outcomes, and health care costs. Arch Intern Med. 1998; 158:1641–1647.

53. Horstkotte D, Piper C, Wiemer M. Optimal frequency of patient monitoring and intensity of oral anticoagulation therapy in valvular heart disease. J Thromb Thrombolysis. 1998; 5 (suppl 1):19–24.

54. Koertke H, Minami K, Boethig D, Breymann T, Seifert D, Wagner O, Atmacha N, Krian A, Ennker J, Taborski U, Klovekorn WP, Moosdorf R, Saggau W, Koerfer R. INR self-manage-

ment permits lower anticoagulation levels after mechanical heart valve replacement. Circulation. 2003; 108 (suppl 1):II75–78.

55. Garabedian-Ruffalo SM, Gray DR, Sax MJ, Ruffalo RL. Retrospective evaluation of a pharmacist-managed warfarin anticoagulation clinic. Am J Hosp Pharm. 1985; 42:304–308.

56. Ansell J, Hirsh J, Dalen J, Bussey H, Anderson D, Poller L, Jacobson A, Deykin D, Matchar D. Managing oral anticoagulant therapy. Chest. 2001; 119:22S-38S.

57. Norton JL, Gibson DL. Establishing an outpatient anticoagulation clinic in a community hospital. Am J Health Syst Pharm. 1996; 53:1151–7.

58. Wilt VM, Gums JG, Ahmed OI, Moore LM. Outcome analysis of a pharmacist-managed anticoagulation service. Pharmacotherapy. 1995; 15:732–39.

59. Pierce MT, Crain L, Smith J, Mehta V. Point-of-care versus laboratory measurement of the International Normalized Ratio. Am J Health Syst Pharm. 2000; 57:2271–2274.

60. Prothrombin measurement using a patient self-testing system. Oral Anticoagulation Monitoring Study Group. Am J Clin Pathol. 2001; 115:280–287.

61. Point-of-care prothrombin time measurement for professional and patient self-testing use. A multicenter clinical experience. Oral Anticoagulation Monitoring Study Group. Am J Clin Pathol. 2001; 115:288–296.

62. Douketis JD, Lane A, Milne J, Ginsberg JS. Accuracy of a portable International Normalization Ratio monitor in outpatients receiving long-term oral anticoagulant therapy: comparison with a laboratory reference standard using clinically relevant criteria for agreement. Thromb Res. 1998; 92:11–17.

63. Sunderji R, Campbell L, Shalansky K, Fung A, Carter C, Gin K. Outpatient self-management of warfarin therapy: a pilot study. Pharmacotherapy. 1999; 19:787–793.

64. Fitzmaurice DA, Machin SJ. Recommendations for patients undertaking self management of oral anticoagulation. BMJ. 2001; 323:985–989.

65. Watzke HH, Forberg E, Svolba G, Jimenez-Boj E, Krinninger B. A prospective controlled trial comparing weekly self-testing and self-dosing with the standard management of patients on stable oral anticoagulation. Thromb Haemost. 2000; 83:661–665.

66. Ansell J, Holden A, Knapic N. Patient self-management of oral anticoagulation guided by capillary (fingerstick) whole blood prothrombin times. Arch Intern Med. 1989; 149:2509–2511.

67. Sawicki PT. A structured teaching and self-management program for patients receiving oral anticoagulation: a randomized controlled trial. Working Group for the Study of Patient Self-Management of Oral Anticoagulation. JAMA. 1999; 281:145–150.

68. Cromheecke ME, Levi M, Colly LP, de Mol BJ, Prins MH, Hutten BA, Mak R, Keyzers KC, Buller HR. Oral anticoagulation self-management and management by a specialist anticoagulation clinic: a randomised cross-over comparison. Lancet. 2000; 356:97–102.

69. Gadisseur AP, Breukink-Engbers WG, van der Meer FJ, van den Besselaar AM, Sturk A, Rosendaal FR. Comparison of the quality of oral anticoagulant therapy through patient self-management and management by specialized anticoagulation clinics in the Netherlands: a randomized clinical trial. Arch Intern Med. 2003; 163:2639–2646.

70. Koertke H, Minami K, Bairaktaris A, Wagner O, Koerfer R. INR self-management following mechanical heart valve replacement. J Thromb Thrombolysis. 2000; 9 Suppl 1:S41–45.

71. Voller H, Glatz J, Taborski U, Bernardo A, Dovifat C, Burkard G, Heidinger K. [Background and evaluation plan of a study on self-management of anticoagulation in patients with non-valvular atrial fibrillation (SMAAF study)]. Z Kardiol. 2000; 89:284–288.

72. Sunderji R, Fung A, Gin K, Shalansky K, Carter C. Patient self-management of oral anticoagulation: a review. Can J Cardiol. 2003; 19:931–935.

73. Hylek EM, Singer DE. Risk factors for intracranial hemorrhage in outpatients taking warfarin. Ann Intern Med. 1994; 120:897–902.

18-4

Clinical Application of Anticoagulation Monitoring for Arterial Disease

James J. Ferguson, Kamal Gupta, and J. Michael Wilson
Texas Heart Institute at St. Luke's Episcopal Hospital, Baylor College of Medicine, The University of Texas Health Science Center at Houston, Houston, Texas, U.S.A.

I. INTRODUCTION

This chapter focuses on the clinical application of coagulation monitoring for a variety of indications in patients with arterial disease. The individual agents themselves and the specific clinical indications for the use of these agents are covered elsewhere in the text. Both acute and long-term aspects of monitoring and adjusting therapy will be considered.

II. ACUTE APPLICATIONS

A. Percutaneous Coronary Interventions

1. Anticoagulation and Percutaneous Coronary Intervention (PCI)

Procedural anticoagulation is an important adjunctive therapy for percutaneous coronary intervention (PCI). Traditionally, the presence of thrombus has been viewed as a major risk factor for adverse outcome following interventional procedures (1–11). Multiple studies have demonstrated that angiographic evidence of pre-existing thrombus prior to PTCA, although infrequent (<4%), may double or triple the likelihood of procedural failure (9–12). Patients with unstable angina undergoing PCI in the setting of angiographically demonstrable thrombus were also at higher risk of abrupt vessel closure and had worse in-hospital clinical outcomes (11). In the early days of coronary stenting, preexisting thrombus was a relative contraindication to stent implantation because of a higher associated degree of stent thrombosis.

The development of thrombus during a procedure (as a manifestation of inadequate procedural anticoagulation) is an even more powerful predictor of procedural failure (13–14). The development of new thrombus during PCI was independently associated with lower procedural success and higher rates of abrupt vessel closure and major complications. Thrombus is also a significant risk factor for restenosis following interventional procedures due primarily to a higher incidence of target lesion occlusion at follow-up (Fig. 1) (15).

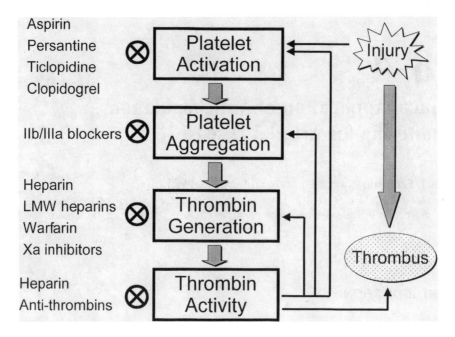

Figure 1   Site of action of currently available antithrombotic agents.

2.   *Unfractionated Heparin for PCI*

Intravenous unfractionated heparin is presently the most frequently utilized form of procedural anticoagulation during PCI and significantly reduces the risk of abrupt coronary closure (14). During PCI heparin effect is measured by the activated clotting time (ACT), which is the time required for whole blood to clot in response to a potent procoagulant (usually kaolin or diatomaceous earth) (16). No prospectively defined objective standards exist to identify a "therapeutic" level of anticoagulation during PCI. Therapeutic values during PCI have been empirically derived from the early cardiac surgery experience (i.e., ACT required to prevent microemboli in the bypass circuit) (17), from small and contradictory clinical trials (18,19), and from empirical observations (20–28) (Fig. 2). Ischemic complications following PCI were increased in patients with an ACT of <250 seconds (HemoTec) (24), but were rare (0.3%) when the final ACT was greater than 300 seconds. The average heparin dose required to achieve an ACT >300 seconds has been shown to vary directly with the acuity of anginal syndrome (29) However, higher heparin doses are also associated with a greater degree of platelet activation (30). Additionally, a significant variability exists from patient to patient, even within closely matched anginal syndromes, presumably due to the underlying limitations and unreliability of unfractionated heparin, with a high degree of protein binding (31), heparin-induced platelet activation (30), and heparin-resistant thrombin activity (32) (Fig. 3).

In the early days of PCI heparin was empirically administered in large bolus doses (10,000–15,000 U) without monitoring. Additional bolus doses were used if the procedure was prolonged. Later, the initial dose of heparin for PCI remained approximately 10,000 U (or 100 U/kg), but the degree of anticoagulation was titrated to the ACT, with supplemental heparin administered to achieve ACTs of >300 seconds. In recent years, with more widespread use of stenting [along with adjunctive use of thienopyridines and glycoprotein

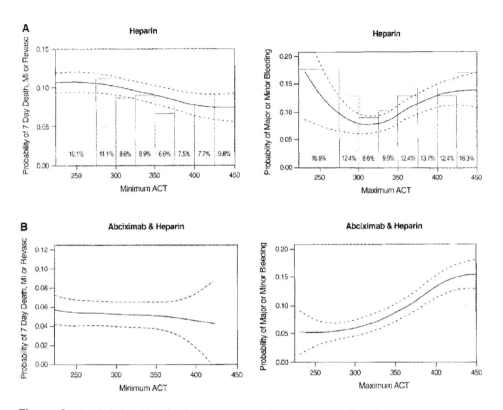

Figure 2 (a) Relationship of minimum and maximum ACT to clinical outcomes in patients receiving UFH for PCI (b) Relationship of minimum and maximum ACT to clinical outcomes in patients receiving concomitant abciximab and UFH for PCI. (From Ref. 26.)

(GP) IIb/IIIa antagonists], lower heparin doses and lower ACT targets (> 275 s) are frequently employed. This comes as a result of better postprocedural coronary flow (stenting) and reduced likelihood of procedure-associated thrombosis in the setting of a widely patent lumen. If adjunctive IIb/IIIa antagonists are employed, the heparin dose is generally reduced to 50–70 U/kg (with a target ACT of approximately 200 sec). Several reports have suggested that even lower doses of heparin (a single 5000 U bolus) may be safe and effective in lower-risk patients, even in the absence of a GP IIb/IIIa antagonist (18,19,33). Other recent reports (34) have advocated very-low-dose heparin (1000–3000 U bolus) in conjunction with a GP IIb/IIIa antagonist; there are even anecdotal reports of cases where no heparin was used, only a GP IIb/IIIa antagonist.

Narins et al. (25) demonstrated that the degree of heparin anticoagulation during coronary angioplasty (as measured by the activated clotting time) is strongly related to the risk of abrupt vessel closure. A strong inverse linear relationship existed between the activated clotting time and the probability of abrupt closure. A minimum target-activated clotting time could not be identified; rather, the higher the intensity of anticoagulation, the lower the risk of abrupt closure.

The ACT and all similar tests must be viewed as surrogate measures of antithrombotic treatment efficacy. Elevated fibrinopeptide A (FPA) levels reflecting thrombin activity (conversion of fibrinogen to fibrin) may be seen in approximately one third of patients undergoing intervention, despite "therapeutic" ACTs and high heparin levels (32). Weight-adjusted heparin doses appear to be more effective in achieving adequate (ACT >

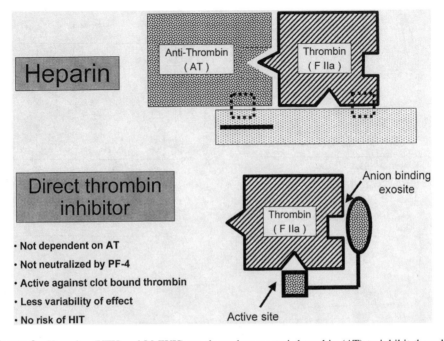

Figure 3 Heparins (UFH and LMWH) are dependent on anti-thrombin (AT) to inhibit thrombin (F IIa). In contrast, direct thrombin inhibitors do not require the intermediary of AT, and act directly on the thrombin molecule.

300 sec) anticoagulation (35), but this has not been tested in the modern era of lower anti-coagulation levels for stents and with adjuncture GP IIb/IIIa antagonests and thieno-phyridines. Unfortunately, there are at present no readily available bedside assays to provide the sophisticated analyses of coagulation activation necessary to identify patients at risk for future adverse events.

Much of the ambiguity relating to "adequate" anticoagulation as assessed by the ACT may relate to the fact that the ACT is not a "threshold" test. It is not the ACT *level* that relates to heparin concentration, but instead the *change* in ACT from baseline that best reflects heparin concentration—this is how the test was designed (36). In other words, the magnitude of response to a given dose of heparin may be more important than the abso-lute level achieved. Unfortunately, the response to sequential doses of heparin in the catheterization laboratory is frequently not uniform (37). Add to this the further con-founding issues of heterogeneous populations, multiple adjunctive therapies, and differ-ences among the various ACT tests themselves (i.e., Hemochron vs. Hemotec) (38,39), and it quickly becomes clear why we have so little definitive data.

Although most retrospective studies have suggested an inverse relation between ACT and ischemic complications (at least for balloon angioplasty), some studies (40) have suggested that adverse outcomes may be more frequent with higher ACT levels, while other recent studies suggest no relationship (41). Bittl et al. (21) have suggested that there may in fact be a group of patients who respond well to the initial dose of heparin, and a separate group (non-responders) who require substantially higher doses of heparin. Higher ACTs are strongly correlated with a higher risk of bleeding complications (26). A pooled analysis of multiple trials identified an "optimal zone" for ACT levels of 350–375 sec in patients who were not receiving adjunctive platelet GP IIb/IIIa blockade (26). A recent analysis of the ESPRIT study (41) has pointed out that the doses of UFH and the ACT targets are both lower in the modern world of stents, even in the absence of GP IIb/IIIa antagonists. In the 2064 patients in the ESPRIT study, using modern-day stents and thienopyridines, the authors noted no relationship between decreasing ACT levels (at least down to 200 sec) and adverse outcomes. Major bleeding rates were noted to increase as the ACT increased in eptifibatide-treated patients.

In recent years the use of postprocedure heparin has declined dramatically, particularly with more sophisticated stent technology and improved adjunctive therapy. A number of studies (42–45) have suggested no advantage to routine post-procedure heparin and, in fact, both cost and bleeding complication rates appear significantly increased with this strategy. Some concerns remain related to the abrupt cessation of UFH and potental rebound effects, particularly in higher-risk circumstances (59,60). When anticoagulation for longer periods of time postprocedure is required [as may be necessary with low molecular weight heparins (LMWH) to "bridge" patients back to chronic warfarin therapy for prosthetic valves or atrial fibrillation], there is an increased risk of access site complications (48).

3. Low Molecular Weight Heparins for PCI

Early studies LMWHs during PCI in the context of restenosis trials demonstrated no clear advantage or disadvantage over UFH (49,50). The use of LMWH as an alternative to UFH for procedural anticoagulation has subsequently been investigated in a number of more recent studies (Table 1). In a preliminary report by Rabah et al. (51), 60 patients undergoing elective coronary angioplasty were randomized to LMWH (1 mg/kg of enoxaparin i.v.) or UFH. All patients in the LMWH group had "adequate" anticoagulation as indicated by a degree of Xa inhibition comparable to that seen with UFH (Fig. 3). PCI success rates and adverse events were similar between groups.

Diez et al. (52), in a nonrandomized study, compared UFH to LMWH (1.5 mg/kg of enoxaparin i.v.; dose decreased to 1.25 mg/kg in patients <70 kg) in 70 patients undergoing coronary intervention. Again, no differences in clinical outcomes were noted between groups.

The National Investigators Collaborating on Enoxaparin (NICE) investigators initiated a series of trials that examined the use of the enoxaparin (± GP IIb/IIIa antagonists) in patients undergoing coronary intervention (53) and managed medically prior to PCI (54). In NICE 1, 828 patients undergoing PCI (85% of whom received stents) were treated with intravenous enoxaparin (1 mg/kg bolus) at the time of procedure. At 30 days the incidence of major bleeding was 1.1% and the incidence of non-CABG major bleeding was 0.5%. In NICE 4, 818 patients undergoing elective or urgent PCI received a reduced dose of enoxaparin (0.75 mg/kg bolus) intravenously in combination with abciximab. At 30 days the incidence of major bleeding was 0.4%, and the incidence of non-CABG bleeding was 0.2% (53). These rates are at least as good as those in similarly designed historical intervention trials that used UFH in the setting of PCI and stenting, such as EPISTENT (55) and ESPRIT (56). The anti-Xa and anti-IIa levels from NICE 1 and NICE 4 are shown in Table 1. The incidence of clinical outcome events such as death, MI, or urgent revascularization in NICE 1 and 4 also compared favorably to historical rates in prior trials.

In the Coronary Revascularization Utilizing Integrilin and Single-Bolus Enoxaparin (CRUISE) trial, 250 patients undergoing PCI were treated with the GP IIb/IIIa antagonist

Table 1 Outcomes in Recent Studies of LMW Heparins in PCI

Trial	Study Drug	Early Time Point	Major Bleeding	Early Death	Early MI	Early (CABG)	Early Revasc. Point	Late Time Death	Late MI	Late Revasc.
REDUCE (PCI) n = 612	UFH 10,000 U bolus 24,000 U over 16 hr inf	3 days	2.6%	0	1.0%	7.2%	N/A	N/A	N/A	N/A
	Reviparin 7000 IU bolus 10,500 IU/16 hr inf 3500 sc BID x 28 days		2.3%	0	1.3%	2.7%				
NICE 1 N = 282	Enoxaparin 1 mg/kg iv	In hospital	1.1% (0.5% non-cabg)	0.5%	5.2%	1.3%	30 day	0.8%	5.4%	2.5%
NICE 4 N = 818	Enoxaparin 1 mg/kg iv abciximab	In hospital	0.4% (non-cabg 0.2%)	0.2%	6.0%	0.5%	30 day	0.4%	6.2%	0.6%
NICE 3 (PCI subset) N=283	Enoxapain (1 mg/kg sq; iv bolus 0.3 mg/kg if necessary) GP IIb/IIIa antagonis (abciximab, eptifibatide, tirofiban)	In hotpital	1.4% (non-cabg 1.4%)	0.7%	4.6%	2.1%	30 day	1.1%	4.9%	6.7%
Dalteparin Pilot	Dalteparin 40 IU/kg Abciximab (discontinued)	In hospital	3.7%	0	11.1%	0	N/A	N/A	N/A	N/A
N = 103	Dalteparin 40 IU/kg		2.6%	1.3%	15.8%	1.3%				
Collet et al. (PCI subset) N = 132	Enoxaparin 1 mg/kg sc ± abciximab	In hospital	3.0%	N/A	N/A	N/A	30 days	0	<1%	0

eptifibatide and subsequently randomized to either standard i.v. UFH or i.v. enoxaparin (0.75 mg/kg bolus) at the time of intervention (57). Clinical outcomes in the enoxaparin/eptifibatide arm were similar to those of UFH/eptifibatide. There was a trend toward less bleeding events in the group receiving enoxaparin plus eptifibatide (4.1% vs. 10.5%), but this difference did not reach significance.

Choussat and coworkers (58) recently reported on the use of very-low-dose intravenous enoxaparin (0.5 mg/kg) in 242 patients undergoing elective PCI, 64 (26%) of whom also received eptifibatide. Sheaths were removed immediately after the procedure in patients receiving enoxaparin and 4 hours after the procedure in patients who received both enoxaparin and eptifibatide. Peak anti-Xa levels were >0.5 U/mL in 97.5% of the patients. At 30 days the composite incidence of death, MI, and urgent revascularization was 2.5%. There was only one major bleeding event and three minor bleeding events; none were associated with excessive anticoagulation levels.

Kereiakes et al. (59) investigated the use of the LMWH dalteparin in patients undergoing PCI. All patients received adjunctive abciximab, aspirin, and clopidogrel. Four patients out of of 107 had received prior subcutaneous dalteparin and were treated with a modified dosing regimen. Patients not on prior dalteparin were randomized in the catheterization laboratory to either 40 or 60 IU/kg intravenously. It was noted after 56 patients had been enrolled in the randomized portion that there were 3 patients in whom new thrombus development was observed, all in the lower-dose group. Subsequent enrollment in the lower dose was halted, and an additional 48 patients enrolled in an open-label fashion in the 60 IU/kg arm. In the total of 76 patients in this group, outcome events included death, 1.3%; Q-wave MI, 3.9%; urgent PC, 0; urgent CABG, 1.3%; CKMB>3x ULN, 15.8%; and major bleeding, 2.6%. Mean anti-Xa activity in the 60 IU/kg group was 0.9 ± 0.3 U/mL at 30 minutes and 0.2 ± 0.14 U/mL at 4 hours.

Recent ACC/AHA guidelines (60) have more strongly advocated the use of LMWH over UFH in patients with acute coronary syndromes (ACS); i.e., unstable angina and non ST-segment elevation acute myocardial infarction. However, a major remaining issue is the appropriate management of patients who may come forward to the catheterization laboratory after treatment with LMWH.

In early ACS trials utilizing LMWH in which most patients were treated conservatively [such as ESSENCE (61,62) and TIMI 11B (63)], coronary interventions, if necessary, were performed using full-dose UFH, titrated to ACTs >300 sec, as per clinical routine. Subsequently, Collet et al. examined 132 patients undergoing PCI within 8 hr of SC enoxaparin administration (1 mg/kg q12h) (64). These patients were part of a larger group of 451 ACS patients who had been pre-treated with enoxaparin and other standard-of-care therapies for a minimum of 48 hours. PCI was performed without any additional anti-coagulation or monitoring. Anti-Xa activity was measured in all patients and was found to be adequate (> 0.5 IU/ml), regardless of the exact timing of last dose of enoxaparin within the previous 8 hr. The incidences of death/MI and major bleeding in the PCI group at 30 days were low (3.0% and <1%, respectively). The Pharmacokinetic Study of Enoxaparin in Patients Undergoing Percutaneous Coronary Intervention (PEPCI) study (65) examined the pharmacodynamics of supplemental intravenous enoxaparin doses on a background of subcutaneous medical management, and found that anti-Xa activity was within an acceptable range following 0.3 mg/kg IV boluses in the 8–12 hour window following subcutaneous enoxaparin injections of 1 mg/kg.

While the NICE-1 and NICE-4 trials focused on the use of intravenous enoxaparin in the catheterization laboratory as a procedural anticoagulant, NICE-3 sought to examine the safety of subcutaneously administered enoxaparin and a GP IIb/IIIa antagonist (abciximab, eptifibatide, or tirofiban) in ACS patients, including those coming to the catheterization laboratory, without the use of supplemental UFH. In NICE-3 (54), 628 ACS patients were treated with SC enoxaparin (1 mg/kg q12h) and a IIb/IIIa antagonist; 283 of them subsequently underwent coronary intervention without the use of UFH. Patients who underwent angioplasty within 8 hr of their last subcutaneous dose of enoxaparin received no additional anticoagulation. Patients brought to the catheterization laboratory 8-12 hr after their last subcutaneous dose of enoxaparin received an additional 0.3 mg/kg IV enoxaparin at the time of PCI. The overall incidence of non-surgical related major bleeding was 1.9%, and 1.4% in patients undergoing percutaneous coronary intervention, with acceptably low rates of death, myocardial infarction, and urgent revascularization.

INTERACT was a randomized study of 746 ACS patients treated with eptifibatide and aspirin and randomized to receive either enoxaparin 1mg/kg SC q12h (using a transition strategy similar to NICE-3) or standard dose UFH. (66). As an invasive management strategy was not precluded, approximately 63% of the patients came to coronary angiography and about half of those coming to angiography underwent PCI. In the overall population the enoxaparin group had a significantly lower incidence of major bleeding at 48 and 96 hr, a lower incidence of recurrent ischemia within the first 96 hr, and a lower composite of death and re-infarction at 30 days.

Additional preliminary data on handling invasively managed patients receiving subcutaneous enoxaparin have come from ENTIRE/TIMI-23 (67), an acute myocardial infarction study that used a transition strategy for enoxaparin patients (who also received a 30 mg IV bolus dose to initiate therapy) similar to NICE-3; RITA-3 (68) (a trial of medium-risk ACS patients in which enoxaparin-treated patients had their morning dose held and were transitioned to UFH in the catheterization laboratory); ASSENT-3 (69) (an acute myocardial infarction study comparing TNK plus UFH, TNK plus enoxaparin, and half-dose TNK plus the GP IIb/IIIa antagonist abciximab with low-dose UFH; a recently presented subset analysis examined the outcomes of patients undergoing elective PCI following thrombolysis (70), (although a precise transition strategy to the catheterization laboratory was not specified); and PARAGON-B [an unstable angina study comparing the GP IIb/IIIa antagonist lamifiban with placebo; a subset of patients (approx. 20%) received LMWH; again, a precise transition strategy was not specified] (71). In all three of these studies the incidence of major bleeding in invasively managed patients was as low (if not lower) with enoxaparin than with UFH.

In the A phase of the Aggrastat to Zocor (A to Z) trial, 72 3,987 patients with acute coronary syndromes were treated with aspirin and upstream tirofiban, and randomized to weight adjusted unfractionated heparin vs. unfractionated heparin. Catheterization was performed in approximately 60% of patients, at a mean time of 4.5 days. The primary endpoint of death, myocardial infarction or refractory ischemia at 7 days was not significantly lower in the enoxaparin treated patients (8.4% vs. 9.4% with UFH, $p = 0.23$), and met prespecified criteria for noninferiority. This trend was consistent by intention-to-treat or per-protocol analysis, and in patients treated conservatively or with an invasive strategy. Trends were present toward greater rates of TIMI major or TIMI major plus minor bleeding with enoxaparin, though there was no difference in the rate of transfusions.

The SYNERGY study (Superior Yield of the New Strategy of Enoxaparin, Revascularization and Glycoprotein IIb/IIIa inhibitors) randomized high-risk NSTEMI ACS patients destined for an early invasive management strategy to either enoxaparin (1 mg/kg sc q 12h) or intravenous aPTT-guided UFH (73). The transition to the catheterization laboratory was again handled similar to NICE-3. The primary endpoint (death or myocardial infarction at 30 days) was not significantly different between groups (14.0% with enoxaparin, 14.5% with UFH), but also met prespecified statistical criteria for noninferiority. The use of enoxaparin was not associated with higher rates of ischemic events during PCI (abrupt closure, threatened closure, unsuccessful PCI, emergency CABG).

There was slightly more TIMI major bleeding with enoxaparin, but no significant difference in GUSTO severe bleeding or transfusion.

4. Monitoring LMWH Therapy for PCI

One major difficulty with the use of LMWHs in the catheterization laboratory is the concern that unlike unfractionated heparin (where ACTs and aPTTs are in common usage), bedside assays have not been felt to be useful in assessing the anticoagulant effect of LMWHs. Although LMWHs may have a more predictable anticoagulant dose response, which may obviate the need for monitoring in the majority of cases, a rapid point of care monitoring system could improve the safety and/or efficacy of LMWH administration in cases of weight extreme, renal insufficiency, access hemostasis following subcutaneous administration (to determine the timing and safety of vascular sheath removal), and to guide protamine reversal of LMWHs in the context of clinical bleeding.

A card-based technology has been developed which incorporates a dry reagent in which is embedded paramagnetic iron oxide particles. A drop of whole blood is placed on the card, and an oscillating magnetic field is activated and light reflection off the card measured by sensor. Thus, a LMWH "clotting time" is determined, which may be analogous to the ACT measured following UFH administration. The LMWH clotting time appears to most closely reflect the antifactor Xa activity. This rapid point-of-care monitoring technology could obviate the need for arbitrary and empirical dose reduction in cases of renal insufficiency or low body mass.

The recently completed ELECT (EvaLuating Enox Clotting Times) study highlights the potential utility of just such a bedside device (ENOX clotting time, Pharmanetics) for assessing anti-Xa activity (74). The ELECT study was a non-randomized, multicenter, observational trial assessing the predictive value of the ENOX test in 445 patients undergoing elective PCI. In ELECT, Moliterno et al. have proposed an ENOX time range of 250–450 seconds as a recommended target for PCI. Event rates in patients with ENOX times in this range were 4.0%, as opposed to 7.2% for those outside this range ($p = 0.134$). The lower cut-off of 250 seconds appears to reliably predict an anti-Xa activity of >1.0 IU/mL (a level felt to adequate for PCI). The exact clinical utility of this test remains to be demonstrated in prospective studies.

Other bedside devices have been investigated for monitoring the efficacy of LMWHs heparins. Henry et al. (75) retrospectively examined ACTs in 26 patients from 2 institutions who had been enrolled in the TIMI 11A study comparing subcutaneous enoxaparin to UFH in patients with ACS. They noted no significant change in HemoTec ACTs and minor changes in Hemochron ACTs, although the exact measurement cartridges or tubes used in the study were not specified. Rabah et al. (51) reported moderate increases in Hemochron ACTs (130 ± 19 seconds to 188 ± 29 seconds) in 30 patients receiving intravenous enoxaparin (1 mg/kg) for PCI. Other investigators have also noted changes in ACTs and aPTTs (using special cartridges) that correlate relatively well with anti-Xa activity in patients receiving intravenous LMWH (76).

Marmur et al. (77) examined the utility of ACTs (Hemochron, CA510 tubes) in blood samples from 10 volunteers spiked with increasing concentrations of dalteparin or UFH, in 15 patients sequentially treated with intravenous dalteparin and then UFH, and in 110 patients undergoing PCI who received either 60 or 80 IU/kg dalteparin intravenously, with and without abciximab (dosing was modified in a small number of patients on prior dalteparin). The ACT appeared to be sensitive to increasing concentrations of dalteparin, albeit in a different range than that seen with UFH. There were no deaths or urgent repeat revascularizations in the PCI population; 2 patients had procedural MIs.

A recent similar study examined the effect of intravenous procedural enoxaparin in 48 patients undergoing PCI (78). A total of 36 patients were treated with enoxaparin alone (1 mg/kg iv); 9 received a reduced dose of enoxaparin (0.75 mg/kg iv) with eptifibatide. The mean postenoxaprin ACT was 207 seconds in the 0.75 mg/kg group (mean increase of 74 ± 20 sec) and 212 sec in the 1.0 mg/kg group (mean increase 92 ± 28 sec).

Another recent study randomized 321 patients undergoing elective or ad-hoc PCI to either dalteparin (100U/kg iv if used alone or 70 U/kg with a GP IIb/IIIa antagonist) or UFH (79). The primary endpoint was the incidence of death, MI, urgent revascularization or need for bailout GP IIb/IIIa. There was no significant difference between groups in the primary endpoint (13.1% with dalteparin, 13.7% with UFH) . The mean ACT at 30 min was 239 sec in the dalteparin group and 345 sec in the UFH group. This corresponded to anti-Xa levels at 30 min of 1.1 μg/mL and 0.8 μg/mL, respectively.

As far as future studies of LMWH in the catheterization laboratory, STEEPLE is a recently initiated, controlled study of approximately 2000 patients undergoing PCI who are randomized to either standard UFH doses or to one of two doses of intravenous enoxaparin (0.5 or 0.75 mg/kg IV, with or without a GP IIb/IIIa antagonist) for procedural anticoagulation. This is primarily designed as a safety study, with bleeding as the primary endpoint.

5. Direct Thrombin Inhibitors for PCI

Hirudin, a molecule originally derived from leech saliva, is a direct-acting thrombin inhibitor that prevents thrombin-catalyzed activation of factors V, VIII and XIII, and thrombin-induced platelet activation (80,81). HELVETICA was an early randomized study comparing heparin with hirudin in the prevention of thrombotic complications related to PCI, hirudin significantly reduced the incidence of postprocedural ischemic events. There was also a significant benefit of hirudin over heparin at 96 hours postprocedure in patients with unstable angina. This initial benefit was not sustained, and at 6–month follow-up there were no differences in event rates between groups. In this study, fixed-dose boluses of heparin (10,000 U) were given in the control group, without titration to ACTs.

Hirulog, also now known as bivalirudin, is a 20-amino-acid synthetic peptide that, like hirudin, binds to thrombin at both the fibrinogen-binding exosite and the active site and acts to inhibit both free and clot-bound thrombin. The initial large report of bivalirudin for PCI was a multicenter dose-ranging study (84); a total of 291 patients undergoing elective PCI were enrolled in one of five ascending dose groups. The abrupt closure rate in the three lowest-dose groups was 11.3%, compared with 3.9% in the two highest-dose groups. There was a reproducible dose-response curve of both ACTs and aPTT to hirulog, and there were no thrombotic closures in patients with ACTs of >300 seconds. Hirulog was associated with a rapid-onset dose-dependent anticoagulant effect and in higher doses appeared to provide safe and adequate anticoagulation for PCI.

In the Hirulog Angioplasty Study (subsequently renamed the Bivalirudin 4098 patients undergoing angioplasty for unstable or postinfarction angina were randomized to procedural anticoagulation with either heparin [175 U/kg bolus and 18- to 24-h infusion of 15 U/kg; with procedural ACTs (Hemochron) titrated to >350 sec] or hirulog (1 mg/kg bolus, a 4–h infusion of 2.5 mg/kg/h and a 14- to 20-h infusion of 0.2 mg/kg/h; no titration of procedural anticoagulation ACT levels). The primary endpoint was the in-hospital incidence of death, MI, abrupt vessel closure, or rapid clinical deterioration of cardiac origin. In the total study group (n = 4098), hirulog did not significantly reduce the incidence of the primary endpoint (11.4% vs. 12.2% for heparin) but did result in a lower incidence of bleeding (3.8% vs. 9.8%, $p < 0.001$). Patients in the hirulog group had slightly lower ACTs after the initial study drug bolus; 37% of the heparin group received additional boluses. In the subgroup of 704 patients with postinfarction angina, hirulog therapy resulted in a lower incidence of the primary endpoint; there was, however, no difference in the primary endpoint or 6–month outcome of the 3194–patient unstable angina subgroup or the total study population.

Later, after The Medicines Company acquired the subsequent commercialization of bivalirudin from Biogen (the original developer and sponsor), a re-analysis of the original data was performed, in which previously missing data were included and endpoints were fully adjudicated, and a primary composite endpoint re-defined (death, MI, urgent revascularization) that was more in line with other similar studies. The complete intention-to-treat data on all 4312 patients enrolled in the trial were then re-analyzed and re-published (85). This analysis showed that the bivalirudin group had a significant reduction in the composite of death, MI, and urgent revascularization at 7 days (6.2% vs 7.9% with UFH, $p = 0.039$). Similar to the original analysis, the bivalirudin group had a significant reduction in bleeding (3.5% vs. 9.3% with UFH, $p < 0.001$). These clinical benefits were sustained out to 90 days, and, again, were more prominent in patients with post-infarction angina.

The stardard of care for coronary intervention has changed substantially from the original technique of balloon angioplasty, with the use of balloon-expandable stents and widespread use of adjunctive therapies such as thienopyridines and GP IIb/IIIa antagonists. CACHET (Comparison of Abciximab Complications with Hirulog for ischemic Events Trial) (86) was a pilot study evaluating the use of bivalirudin in more contemporaneous interventional circumstances. A total of 268 patients undergoing elective PCI were randomized to bivalirudin (with three different dosing arms), or UFH (70 U/kg bolus). Abciximab was used in all of the UFH patients, and "provisionally" in the bivalirudin patients (24% of the time). The composite of death, MI, urgent revascularization and bleeding were significantly lower in the pooled bivalirudin groups, driven mainly by reductions in urgent revascularization, and bleeding (and not death or MI). The REPLACE I (Randomized Evaluation in PCI Linking Angiomax to reduced Clinical Events) trial (87) randomized 1056 patients undergoing PCI to either bivalirudin or UFH. GP IIb/III inhibitors were permitted in both arms of the study, and utilized in 72% of patients. Clinical outcomes at 48 hr were lower in bivalirudin-treated patients, both in the total population and those treated with GP IIb/IIIa antagonists; bleeding events tended to be lowere with bivalirudin in both the total cohort and the IIb/IIIa-treated subset.

Bittl et al. (21) retrospectively examined the relationship between degree of anticoagulation in the Hirulog Angioplasty Study and outcome. With heparin there were decreasing event rates at higher ACT values, but no such relationship existed for bivalirudin. The authors speculated that high doses of heparin may overcome local resistance to heparin, but that direct-acting thrombin inhibitors (which are not subject to local resistance) may be effective at a lower intensity of systemic anticoagulation.

Argatroban is an arginine derivative that also directly blocks the action of thrombin. In contrast to hirudin and hirulog, which irreversibly inhibit thrombin binding to both the active site and the fibrinogen-binding exosite, argatroban is a competitive inhibitor that binds only to the active site of thrombin. It is a much smaller molecule than hirudin or hirulog and is also being evaluated as an alternative to heparin in a variety of clinical circumstances (91).

A number of studies have suggested that ACTs and aPTTs do not show parallel changes in patients treated with direct thrombin inhibitors and heparin. This suggests that there may be fundamental problems in assessing anticoagulation with these new agents, and that comparisons with heparin at similar levels of ACT or aPTT are not necessarily meaningful. Carteaux et al. (92) have suggested that the antithrombotic effect of a direct thrombin inhibitor is more properly assessed by the ACT than the aPTT. Others have advocated the ecarin clotting time (ECT) (93). No comparison data are available at present for all four of the commercially available direct thrombin inhibitors, and whether there are differences *among* the agents is, at present, not known.

The most recent data on thrombin inhibitors in PCI come from REPLACE II, a randomized, blinded parallel group study of 6010 patients undergoing urgent or elective PCI who were randomly assigned to receive either UFH (65 U/kg initial intravenous bolus, target ACT > 225) with planned GP IIb/IIIa antagonist administration (either abciximab or eptifibatide) or bivalirudin (0.75 mg/kg bolus with 1.75 mg/kg/h intravenous infusion during PCI, target ACT > 225) with provisional GP IIb/IIIa antagonist use (utilized in 7.2% of cases). The primary endpoint was a 30–day quadruple composite of death, MI, urgent revascularization, or major in-hospital hemorrhage (94). Secondary endpoints included the triple composite of death, MI, or need for urgent revascularization to 30 days and the triple composite of death, MI, or target vessel revascularization at 6 months, and one-year mortality. The primary analysis tested a "noninferiority" hypothesis, that bivalirudin plus provisional GP IIb/IIIa inhibition would be clinically equivalent or "noninferior" to UFH plus routine GP IIb/IIIa use. The noninferiority standard utilized was that bivalirudin therapy needed to have at least 50% of the established benefit of the addition of IIb/IIIa inhibition to heparin monotherapy—as determined from the EPISTENT and ESPRIT trials. The pre-specified boundary for noninferiority in comparison to the benefit of adding a GP IIb/IIIa antagonist to UFH was determined to be 0.92.

The incidence of the primary quadruple composite endpoint was 9.2% in the bivalirudin group ($n = 3008$) and 10.0% in the UFH + IIb/IIIa group ($n = 2994$; $p = 0.31$ via direct comparison). The test for noninferiority of bivalirudin-based therapy in comparison to heparin-based therapy was achieved with the upper limit of the 95% confidence interval for bivalirudin not exceeding the prespecified non-inferiority threshold. Similarly, there was no significant difference between bivalirudin (7.6%) and UFH (7.1%) in the secondary triple endpoint at 30 days. There was a significant difference in major bleeding events (2.4% of the bivalirudin group vs. 4.1% of the UFH + GP IIb/IIIa group; $p < 0.001$). There was no significant difference in the rate of death (0.2% vs. 0.4%) or urgent revascularization (1.2% vs. 1.4%) between the bivalirudin and UFH groups. There was, however, a non-significant trend toward a slightly increased rate of myocardial infarction (mainly non–Q-wave MI) in the bivalirudin group (7.0%) when compared with the UFH group (6.2%). In REPLACE II, the median ACT at 5 minutes was 317 seconds in the heparin + IIb/IIIa group and 358 seconds in the bivalirudin group, and at 30 minutes was 276 seconds and 344 seconds, respectively. There was significantly less variability in the ACT response in the bivalirudin group; only 3% required additional bolus doses of study drug, compared with 12% of the heparin + IIb/IIIa group.

There was a significant difference in major bleeding events (2.4% of the bivalirudin group vs 4.1% of the UFH + GP IIb/IIIa group; $p < 0.001$). There was no significant difference in the rate of death (0.2% vs. 0.4%) or urgent revascularization (1.2% vs. 1.4%) between the bivalirudin and UFH groups. There was, however, a non-significant trend toward a slightly increased rate of myocardial infarction (mainly non-Q-wave MI) in the bivalirudin group (7.0%) when compared with the UFH group (6.2%). In REPLACE II, the median ACT at 5 min was 317 sec in the heparin+IIb/IIIa group, and 358 seconds in the bivalirudin group, and at 30 minutes was 276 seconds and 344 seconds, respectively. There was significantly less variability in the ACT response in the bivalirudin group; only

3% required additional bolus doses of study drug, compared with 12% of the heparin+IIb/IIIa group. Benefits were sustained out to 6 months; at 1 year there was no significant difference in mortality (2.5% in patients treated with UFH and a GP IIb/IIIa antagonist, 1.9% with bivalirudin) (95). Analysis showed that, compared to heparin and routine GP IIb/IIIa use, bivalirudin resulted in similar clinical outcomes and \$375–\$400 savings (96). Bivalirudin has also recently been shown to be of benefit in patients with HIT undergoing PCI [the AT-BAT trial (97)].

6. Warfarin and PCI

One large-scale study (the BAAS trial) has evaluated the efficacy of coumarins, administered pre and postprocedure, in reducing acute procedural and long-term events following PCI. A total of 1058 patients were randomized to aspirin plus coumarins (n = 530) or aspirin alone (n = 528). Therapy was initiated prior to the procedure and continued for 6 months, with a target INR of 2.1–4.8. The mean time from randomization to the procedure was approximately 12 days. The mean INR in the coumarin group was 2.7 + 1.1 at the time of the procedure, and 3.0 + 1.1 during follow-up. At 30 days, the composite of death, MI, TVR, and stroke occurred in 3.4% of the aspirin plus coumarin group and 6.4% of the aspirin-alone group. At 1 year, composite events had occurred in 14.3% of the aspirin plus coumarin group, and 20.3% of the aspirin alone group. Major bleeding and pseudoaneurysm formation occurred in 3.2% of the aspirin plus coumarin group and in 1.0% of the aspirin-alone group.

7. Antiplatelet Agents/Monitoring for PCI

Percutaneous coronary interventions such as percutaneous transluminal coronary angioplasty (PCI) or coronary stenting involve mechanical disruption of atherosclerotic plaques. At this site of iatrogenic vessel injury, as noted above, there is a risk of thrombus formation, and given the key role that platelets play in acute thrombotic processes, antiplatelet therapy is a mainstay of adjunctive therapy for PCI. Aspirin (for PCI) and aspirin/clopidogrel (for stents) are part of standard interventional practice, although the appropriate duration of post-procedure clopidogrel therapy is hotly debated, as discussed below.

Over the last decade, more potent antiplatelet therapy, in the form of GP IIb/IIIa antagonists, has also become available. During platelet aggregation, GP IIb/IIIa receptors bind fibrinogen and vWF, which act to cross-link adjacent activated platlets and generate a critical mass of activated platelet membrane, and serve as the final common pathway of platelet aggregation. Since acute thrombotic processes are intensely dependent on the presence of the activated platelet membrane as a necessary cofactor, blocking GP IIb/IIa has profound effects on acute thrombus formation. A variety of antibody, peptide, and peptidomimetic compounds that interfere with the GPIIb/IIIa receptor have been developed (Fig. 4).

The ESPRIT trial (56) highlighted the benefit of GP IIb/IIIa antagoinists in moderate-risk patients, and demonstrated the importance of a double bolus regimen of eptifibatide for coronary intervention. The role of IIb/IIIa antagonists has been questioned somewhat by studies such as REPLACE II (94), but nevertheless, they are, at present, an integral part of the care of higher-risk patients undergoing PCI. The necessity for high levels of platelet inhibition has also recently been questioned for low risk patients, as evidenced by the fact that in ISAR-REACT (99) there was no incremental benefit of abciximab on a background of aspirin and clopidogrel (given as a 600 mg load at least 2 hr prior to the procedure. However there is also evidence of incremental effects of GP IIb/IIIa antagonists on laboratory markers of platelet inhibition (PEACE) (100), and clinical outcomes (101). Other recent studies have investigated a modified dosing regimen for tirofiban, using a larger initial bolus (102,103).

	ISAR-REACT Abciximab	REPLACE 2 Abciximab	ESPRIT Eptifibatide	ISAR-REACT Placebo	REPLACE 2 Bivalirudin	ESPRIT Placebo
Death	0.3 %	0.4 %	0.1 %	0.3 %	0.2 %	0.2 %
MI	3.7 %	6.2 %	5.4 %	3.8 %	7.0 %	9.0 %
D/MI/uTVR	4.2 %	7.1 %	6.0 %	4.0 %	7.6 %	9.3 %
Major bleed (TIMI)	1.1 %	0.9 %	1.0 %	0.7 %	0.6 %	0.4 %
Minor bleed (TIMI)	2.5 %	3.0 %	2.8 %	1.9 %	1.3 %	1.7 %
Transfusion	2.4 %	2.5 %	1.0 %	0.9 %	1.7 %	1.0 %

Figure 4 30-day Events in Recent Major PCI Studies

With the emergence of coronary stenting as the dominant coronary interventional technique, early anticoagulation strategies included aspirin, dipyridamole, LMW dextran, and warfarin. These early regimens were supplanted with the use of aspirin plus thienopyridines (described below under chronic therapy). One problem with thienopyridines was that they required time to achieve steady-state concentrations; hence, a strategy of oral loading—first with ticlopidine, and then with clopidogrel as it became the preferred agent—was adopted. Oral loading does not appear to achieve a greater degree of inhibition, but faster arrival at steady-state equilibrium levels. However, the early results of CREDO (104) showed no significant benefit (though there was a favorable trend) in death, MI or urgent revascularization associated with a 300 mg oral loading dose of clopidogrel prior to the procedure. Nevertheless, oral loading is widely practiced, and there appears to also be significant benefit to loading earlier, in advance of the procedure (as was done in ISAR-REACT), since even with a 600 mg oral load it still takes a few hours to achieve therapeutic levels of platelet inhibition. However, a small study by van der Heijden (105) showed no benefit of three days of pretreatment with clopidogrel in reducing the incidence of Troponin I or CK-MB elevations in 203 patients undergoing elective stenting (Fig. 5).

As noted in Chapter 18-1, there are also techniques currently available for monitoring the intensity of anti-platelet therapy. In the GOLD study (106), 500 patients undergoing PCI with planned use of a GP IIb/IIIa antagonist had their extent of platelet inhibition measured with the Ultegra Rapid Platelet Function Assay (Accumetrics). Platelet function was determined at baseline (prior to GP IIb/IIIa antagonist administration), at 10 min, 1 hr, 8 hr, and 24 hr after the GP IIb/IIIa antagonist bolus. Approximately 1/4 of patients did not achieve $\geq 95\%$ inhibition by 10 min after the bolus; these patients had a significantly higher incidence of major adverse clinical events (14.4% vs. 6.4%). Patients with $< 70\%$ inhibition at 8 hr also had significantly higher event rates (25% vs. 8.1%). Having $\geq 95\%$ inhibition after the bolus was an independent predictor of a favorable outcome. However, there is, as yet, no widely accepted "therapeutic range" for procedural platelet inhibition. The problem is further compounded by the fact that multiple devices are used to monitor anti-platelet efficacy.

	Experience	Outcomes	Bleeding	Monitoring	Cost
UFH / ASA	++++	++	++	ACT (275-300)	$
UFH / ASA / Clopidogrel	++++	+++ ++++	++	ACT (275-300)	$
UFH / ASA / IIb/IIIa antag	++++	++++	+++	ACT (> 200)	$$$ $$$$
UFH / ASA /Clopidogrel / IIb/IIIa antag	++++	++++	++++	ACT (> 200)	$$$ $$$$
LMWH / ASA	+	?	+	? Necessary	$
LMWH / ASA / Clopidogrel	++	+++ ++++	+ ++	? Necessary	$
LMWH / ASA / IIb/IIIa antag	++	+++	++ +++	? Necessary	$$$ $$$$
LMWH / ASA /Clopidogrel / IIb/IIIa antag	+++	++++	+++ ++++	? Necessary	$$$ $$$$
DTI / ASA	++	+++	+	ACT (>300)	$$$
DTI / ASA / Clopidogrel	++	+++	+	ACT (> 300)	$$$
DTI / ASA / IIb/IIIa antag	++	+++ ++++	++	ACT (?)	$$$$
DTI / ASA / Clopidogrel /IIb/IIIa antag	++	++++	+++	ACT (?)	$$$$

Figure 5 Comparison of current alternative antithrombotic regiments for PCI

It has been suggested that aspirin resistance (discussed below under Chronic Therapy), at least as assessed with the Ultegra Rapid Platelet Function Assay, may be one way of identifying patients at increased risk for post-procedure myonecrosis, even in the setting of concomitant clopidogrel (107). Another study (108) has suggested that clopidogrel may not be necessary—that aspirin alone may be sufficient—in selected patients treated with a heparin-coated stent.

B. Acute Coronary Syndromes

1. UFH in ACS

The aPTT has traditionally been used to monitor and adjust the degree of anticoagulation with UFH. However, the so-called therapeutic range for UFH is largely derived from studies in patients with venous thromboembolism (109,110). The general approach has been to reduce the risk of recurrent thrombosis by establishing a lower limit of what is felt to be therapeutic, while minimizing the risk of bleeding by establishing an upper limit to the therapeutic range. Surprisingly few studies have critically examined the relationship between the degree of anticoagulation and subsequent clinical outcomes in patients with manifest coronary artery disease. Previous studies (111,112) have suggested that in acute MI patients treated with thrombolytic therapy, there is a strong association between the risk of bleeding and higher aPTTs. Somewhat paradoxically, Granger et al. (112) noted that in GUSTO I, higher aPTTs were associated with an increased likelihood of recurrent ischemia and death. Preliminary retrospective analyses of the OASIS data confirm that in ACS patients, higher aPTT values are associated with more major bleeding episodes, even in patients whose aPTTs are still in the therapeutic range (113) (Fig. 6). In general, the use of UFH has not resulted in "reliable" degrees of anticoagulation.

With unfractionated heparin there are also issues related to the ability to achieve and sustain therapeutic levels of anticoagulation. In TIMI 9B (114) acute MI patients treated

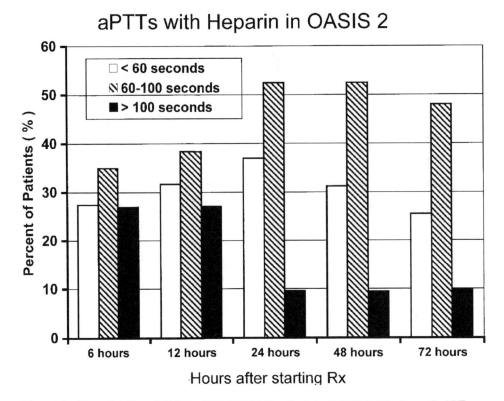

Figure 6 The reliability of UFH in 5058 NSTEMI patients in OASIS 2. The "target" aPPT was defined as 60–100 seconds. (Adapted from Ref. 113.)

with either t-PA or streptokinase were randomized to receive UFH (5000 U bolus; 1000 U/h infusion) or hirudin (0.1 mg/kg bolus; 0.1 mg/kg/h infusion). The target aPTT was 55–85 seconds. Within the first 6–12 hours only 23% of the heparin patients were in the therapeutic range, compared with 49% of the hirudin patients. Within 12–24 hs, 24–48 hs, and 48–72 hours, only 31, 33, and 33% of the heparin patients, respectively, were in the therapeutic range, compared with 55, 65, and 69% of the hirudin patients (Fig. 7). A recent review of 5028 ACS patients from OASIS 2 who received UFH (and no lytic therapy) showed that at 6, 12, 24, 48, and 72 hours, only 34.8, 38.2, 52.3, 52.4, and 48% of UFH patients, respectively, were in the target therapeutic aPPT range of 60–100 sec (113).

2. LMWH in ACS

Multiple studies (Table 2) have demonstrated the superiority or non-inferiority of low molecular weight heparins in comparison to UFH in ACS patients. 61-63,72,73,115-118 There are, however, only limited data on the appropriate or optimal degree of anticoagulation with LMWH in ACS.

TIMI 11A was a dose-ranging trial of enoxaparin in patients with unstable angina (119). In the first dose tier ($n = 321$) the dose was 1.25 mg/kg sc q 12h; peak and trough anti-Xa levels were 1.5 and 0.6 IU/mL, respectively, and the incidence of major bleeding was 6.5% (priomarily at instrumented sites). In the second dose tier ($n = 309$) the dose was 1 mg/kg sc q 12h; peak and trough anti-Xa levels were 1.0 and 0.5 IU/mL, respectively, and the incidence of major bleeding was reduced to 1.9%. The incidence of death,

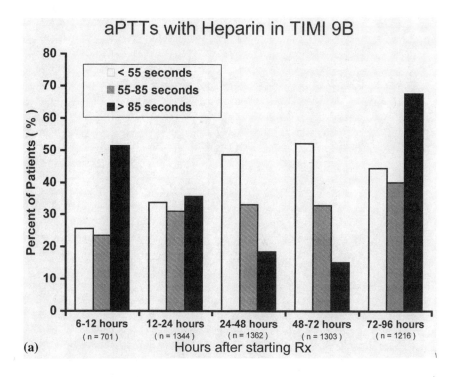

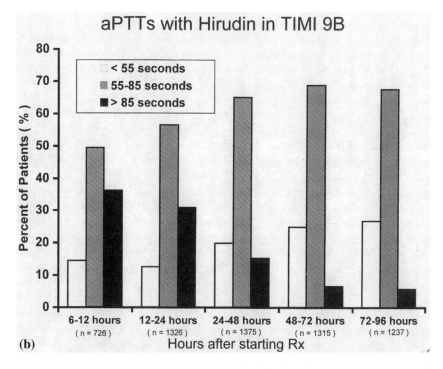

Figure 7 (a) The reliability of UFH in STEMI patients in TIMI 9B. (b) The reliability of hirudin in STEMI patients in TIMI 9B. Adapted from reference 114.

Table 2 Clinical Outcomes in Randomized Trials of LMWH vs UFH in Unstable Angina

Trial	Population	Study drugs	Follow-up	Endpoint	UFH	LMWH	P-value
FRIC	UA or NQMI (n = 1482)	*Dalteparin:* 120 IU/kg SC BID (median duration not reported) **vs.** *UFH:* 5000 U bolus, infusion titrated to aPPT 1.5–2.5 x control IV Rx for at least 48 hrs, then could switch to SC Rx (median duration 2.3 days)	6 days	Death MI Rec angina D/MI/rec angina	0.4% 3.2% 5.4% 7.6%	1.5% 2.6% 6.0% 9.3%	NS NS NS NS
ESSENCE	UA or NQMI (n = 3171)	*Enoxcparin:* 100 IU/kg SC BID (median duration 2–6 days) **vs.** *UFH:* 5000 U bolus infusion titrated to aPPT 55-85 sec (median duration 2.6 days)	14 days	Death MI Rec angina D/MI/rec angina	2.3% 4.5% 15.5% 19.8%	2.2% 3.2% 12.9% 16.6%	MS .06 .03 .019
TIMI 11B	UA or NQMI (n = 3910)	*Enoxapain:* 300 IU bolus 100 IU/kg SC BID (median duration 4.6 days) **vs.** *UFH:* 70 U/kg IV, 150/kg/hr infusicn titrated to aPTT 15–25 x control (median duration	614 days	Death MI Rec angina D/MI/rec angina	2.8% 5.4% 11.1% 16.7	2.2% 4.2% 9.6% . 14.2%	NS NS NS .029%
FRAXIS	UA or NQMI n = 3468	*Nadroparin:* 87 IU/kg bolus 3 days; 87 IU/kg(Rx 6 days or 14 days) **vs.** *UFH* 5000 U bolus titrated to aPTT per center	6 days 14 days	D/MI/rec angina D/MI/rec angina	14.9% 18.1%	13.8% NR (6d) (14d) 17.8% 20% (6d) (14d)	NS NS

recurrent MI, or recurrent ischemia requiring revascularization was 5.6% in dose tier 1 and 5.2% in dose tier 2.

As previously noted, Collet et al. (64) examined 132 patients undergoing PCI within 8 hours of sc enoxaparin administration (1 mg/kg q 12h) (82). These patients were part of a larger group of 451 ACS patients who had been pretreated with enoxaparin and other standard-of-care therapies for a minimum of 48 hours. PCI was performed without any additional anticoagulation or monitoring. Anti-Xa activity was measured in all patients and was found to be adequate (>0.5 IU/mL), regardless of the exact timing of the last dose of enoxaparin within the previous 8 hours.

The previously mentioned PEPCI study (65) examined the pharmacodynamics of supplemental intravenous enoxaparin doses on a background of subcutaneous medical management, and found that anti-Xa activity was within an acceptable range.

Recent data has also suggested that the level of anti-Xa activity in ACS patients treated with subcutaneous enoxaparin and brought forward to the cathterization laboratory is stable after as few as 2 subcutaneous doses of enoxaparin (120). A major problem with all of the foregoing analyses is that the "therapeutic range" for anti-Xa activity is still incompletely understood on the arterial side, and largely extrapolated from prior venous literature.

On the MI side of things (Table 3), although enoxaparin was superior to UFH in ASSENT 3 (69) when given in conjuction with fibrinolytic therapy (TNK) in acute MI, there was also a non-significant trend toward more bleeding with enoxaparin (although this was not as prominent as that observed with the combination of the GP IIb/IIIa antagoinist abciximab and TNK). In the subsequent ASSENT 3 PLUS study (121), there was significantly more bleeding with enoxaparin (in comparison to UFH) in MI patients receiving pre-hospital thrombolysis. This excess in bleeding was primarily restricted to elderly patients, and there was a significantly higher rate of ICH with enoxaparin in elderly patients in ASSENT 3 PLUS. In the ongoing ExTRACT/TIMI 25 study the dose of enoxaparin has been reduced in elderly patients.

Another difference in the dosing of LMWH in the MI studies has been the use of an intravenous bouls dose of enoxaparin when therapy is initiated. Among prior unstable angina trials, the TIMI 11B study (63) did use an iv bolus of enoxapari, while the ESSENCE study (61) did not. The primary theoretical benefit of an iv bolus is the rapid achievement of therapeutic levels—this has been confirmed with measurement of anti-Xa activity in ENTIRE/ TIMI 23 (67) and another smaller unstable angina study (122). However, given the bleeding problems observed, particularly in the elderly in ASSENT 3 PLUS with pre-hospital thrombolysis, an iv bolus is not being used in elderly patients in ExTRACT/TIMI 25. As noted above, one of the advantages of LMWHs over UFH is that they do not require routine monitoring and adjustment in order to achieve a reliable therapeutic effect. They are recommended as the preferred agents in medically managed unstable angina patients (60) Given the results of SYNERGY (94), A to Z (93) and a recent overview of recent enoxaparin unstable angina studies (123), the utility of LMWH in invasively managed patients appears to be confirmed, and monitoring of antithrombotic efficacy even in rapidly invasively managed patients may not be necessary (though it is still possible) if a LMWH is used for the initial therapy. Additional data on appropriate LMWH dosing in renally impaired and obese ACS patients is also available (124).

3. Direct Thrombin Inhibitors in ACS

A recent meta-analysis examined 11 randomized trials comparing direct thrombin inhibitors with unfractionated heparin (125); 9 of these trials included patients with ACS,

Table 3 Clinical Trials of LMWH for Acute MI

Trial	n	Study agents	Study population	Endpoints	Findings
FRAMI	776	Dalteparin Placebo	Acute anterior MI Rx sreptokinase	Thrombus formation Embolism	↑ Risk thrombus formation (14% vs. 22%) ↑ Risk bleeding
BIOMACS II	101	Dalteparin Placebo	Acute MI Rx streptokinase	Argiography after 20–28 hr Continuous ECG	Trend toward ↑ TIMI III flow with dalteparin (68% vs. 57%) More reinfarction with dalteparin Low incidence bleeding
HART II	400	Enoxaparin Placebo	Acute MI Rx rt-PA	Angiography prior to discharge	Trend toward ↑ patency with enoxaparin TIMI II/III—80% vs. 75% TIMI III—53% vs. 48% No difference in major bleeding
AMI-SK	496	Enoxaparin Placebo	Acute MI Rx streptokinase	Angiography at 5–10 days ST-segment monitoring	Better patency with enoxaparin TIMI II/III—88% vs. 72% TIMI III—70% vs. 58% Better ST-segment resolution with enoxaparin Slightly (but significantly) ↑ Higher bleeding
ASSENT-Plus	439	Dalteparin UFH	Acute MI Rx rt-PA	Angiography prior to discharge	TIMI III flow slightly (but not significantly) better with dalteparin (69% vs. 62.5%) TIMI 0/I, TIMI 0/I + thrombus less frequent with dalteparin reinfarction with dalteparin
ASSENT III	6095	TNK + UFH TNK + enoxaparin _dose TNK + abciximab + UFH	Acute MI	Composite (30 days mortality, in- hospital reinfarction)	Composite significantly reduced in enoxaparin and abciximab groups Enoxaparin—114% Abciximab—11.1% TNK + UFH—15.4% Slight increase in major bleeding
ENTIRE/TIMI	456 23	TNK + UFH TNK + enoxaparin _dose TNK + abciximab + UFH 1/2 dose TNK + abciximab + enoxaparin	Acute MI	Angiography (60 min) Clinical events	TIMI flow slightly better with LMWH ST-segment resolution, clinical outcomes better with enoxaparin Bleeding not increased

and 2 involved PCI patients. This analysis did not include data from the REPLACE 2 study (discussed above) or the HERO 2 study (discussed below). The degree of anticoagulation targeted in these studies was generally similar with thrombin inhibitors as with UFH, at least as assessed by ACTs or aPTTs. The analysis concluded that in ACS patients the use of direct thrombin inhibitors did not provide mortality benefit, but did result in a consistently lower incidence of recurrent MI. Similar observations were made in TIMI9B (114). Despite these findings, as yet no direct thrombin inhibitors have been approved by the U.S. FDA for use in the medical management of acute coronary syndromes.

The HERO 2 trial (126) was a large-scale study evaluating the use of the direct thrombin inhibitor bivalirudin versus UFH in 17,073 STEMI patients treated with streptokinase. The primary endpoint, 30-day mortality, was not significantly different between groups (10.8% with bivalirudin, 10.9% with UFH). There were significantly fewer reinfarctions in the first 96 hours in the bivalirudin group, but this came at the price of a significant increase in moderate or mild bleeding, with no significant difference between groups in the incidence of major bleeding, intracranial hemorrhage, or transfusion.

In contrast to prior studies, in HERO 2 the dose of bivalirudin was adjusted differently than with UFH. In the bivalirudin group, aPTTs were measured at 12 and 24 hours, but reduction of the dose at 12 hours was not permitted unless there was major bleeding. If the aPTT was greater than 150 seconds (without major bleeding), it was measured again at 18 hours, and the dose could then be reduced only if it was still >150 seconds. At the 24-hour time point, the dose could be reduced by a third if there was major bleeding or if the aPTT was >120 seconds. In contrast, the UFH infusion was titrated to maintain aPTTs of 50–75 seconds after 12 hours. Not surprisingly, aPTTs were significantly higher in the bivalirudin group. Also not surprisingly, bleeding rates increased in association with 12- and 24-hour aPTTs. In a nonprespecified analysis, when post–12-hour bleeding rates were adjusted for differences between groups in the 12-hour aPTTs, the differences in bleeding complications between groups were no longer significant. Thus, the optimal target range for aPTTs with bivalirudin has yet to be defined, but some degree of dose adjustment and titration would appear to be warranted to reduce the risk of bleeding.

C. Acute Stroke

The utility of emergent anticoagulation in patients with acute stroke has been the subject of considerable recent debate. There is no general agreement on the best agent (if any) to use, the proper level of anticoagulation, the duration of therapy, or whether initial bolus doses should be used. Association guidelines (127) do not recommend urgent routine anticoagulation to improve neurological outcomes or to prevent early recurrent stroke in patients with acute ischemic stroke, primarily because of the high risk of serious intracranial bleeding complications. Anticoagulant therapy is not recommended within 24 hours of treatment with intravenous t-PA. Parenteral anticoagulants should not be utilized until an imaging study has excluded the possibility of intracranial hemorrhage. If a patient does receive parenteral anticoagulants, the guidelines recommend that the level of anticoagulation should be closely monitored and adjustment of the dosage of medication should be done if the level of anticoagulation is outside the desired range, although the guidelines do not specify what that range should be.

Recent guidelines specifically focusing on anticoagulants and antiplatelet agents in stroke (128) also noted that UFH, LMWH, and heparinoids did not reduce mortality, stroke-related morbidity, or stroke recurrence when used within 48 hours of onset of symptoms. The authors did note, however, that the frequency of DVT in acute stroke is reduced by anticoagulant therapy, but again, they do not a specific desired therapeutic range other than that used for routine DVT prophylaxis. This benefit must be balanced against the increased risk of bleeding in the acute setting.

While there are good data favoring the use of aspirin in acute stroke and emerging data [the AbBEST trial (129)] regarding the efficacy of abciximab in reducing the subsequent neurological deficit, there are at present no data regarding monitoring antiplatelet therapy in patients with acute stroke.

III. CHRONIC APPLICATIONS

A. Atherosclerosis

1. *Warfarin*

The Thrombosis Prevention Trial compared low-intensity warfarin (target INR 1.3–1.8), aspirin (75 mg/day), both, or neither in 5499 men, aged 45–69 years who were at risk for a first MI but had not yet had an event (130). The trial was initiated in 1984, initially as a trial of warfarin versus placebo. A total of 1427 men entered the first nonfactorial portion of the study between 1984 and 1989; the median follow-up was 1.1 years. In 1989 the trial was changed to a factorial comparison of warfarin/placebo and aspirin/placebo; the overall mean follow-up was 6.8 years. The primary endpoint was all ischemic heart disease events, defined as coronary death and fatal and nonfatal MI. In the overall trial there were a total of 410 primary outcome events. The total primary event rate over the course of the study was 8.4% in the placebo group (1.3% per year). Neither warfarin alone nor aspirin alone significantly reduced outcome events; the primary event rates were similar in both groups: 6.5% overall, or 1.0% per year. Primary outcome events were significantly lower with combination therapy: 5.6% overall or 0.9% per year, although combination therapy was also associated with a small but significant increase in incidence of hemorrhagic stroke (0.1%).

The initial data regarding the role of oral anticoagulants in patients with myocardial infarction come from three randomized trials using moderate-intensity anticoagulation (estimated INR 1.5–2.5). Two of these studies, the Medical Research Council Study (131) and the Veterans Administration Cooperative Study (132) showed a significant reduction with anticoagulant therapy in the incidence of stroke, but no effect on mortality. The third study, the Bronx Municipal Study (133), showed a significant reduction in mortality with anticoagulant therapy and a nonsignificant trend toward fewer strokes. All three studies showed a reduction in the incidence of pulmonary embolism.

A pooled analysis of data from seven randomized trials published between 1964 and 1980 showed that chronic oral anticoagulant therapy after MI reduced the combined endpoints of mortality and nonfatal reinfarction by approximately 20% over a 1- to 6-year treatment period (134–136). A subsequent comprehensive review of 32 trials also suggested that anticoagulant treatment significantly reduced mortality (137).

Regarding the optimal degree of chronic anticoagulation in patients with cornary artery disease, a review of 19 trials of oral anticoagulants (138) found that in trials with an INR target range of 2.5–5, mortality was reduced by approximately 40%, and the risk of nonfatal MI was reduced by approximately two thirds. In contrast, studies with inadequate or poor documentation of degree of anticoagulation showed no difference in mortality, but did identify a trend in favor of anticoagulant therapy in prevention of reinfarction.

The beneficial effects of more intense anticoagulant therapy in the postinfarction period have been examined in a number of subsequent studies. The Sixty-Plus Reinfarction Study was limited to patients older than 60 years following an MI who had been treated with oral anticoagulants for at least 6 months prior to enrollment; qualifying patients were then randomized to continue on oral anticoagulant therapy or to have it withdrawn (139). There was a significant reduction in the incidence of reinfarction and stroke in patients randomized to continue warfarin therapy. The Warfarin Reinfarction Study (WARIS) was a study in which 1214 post-MI patients (with no age restriction) were randomized to warfarin (target INR 2.8–4.8) or placebo, and followed for an average of 37 months (140). There was a highly significant reduction in mortality in the warfarin group (24% relative reduction in the intention-to-treat cohort, and 35% relative reduction in the on-treatment cohort), along with a 50% relative reduction in the incidence of nonfatal reinfarction and a 55% reduction in the incidence of fatal CVA. There was a slightly increased risk of intracranial hemorrhage with warfarin, but this risk was far outweighed by the significant reduction in overall cerebrovascular events. The Anticoagualants in the Secondary Prevention of Events on Coronary Thrombosis (ASPECT) study (141) also had no age restrictions and randomized patients to higher-intensity warfarin therapy (INR 2.8–4.8) or placebo. ASPECT demonstrated that warfarin was associated with a 40% relative reduction in the incidence of stroke and a >50% relative reduction in the incidence of reinfarction.

More recently, a number of studies have evaluated a variety of intensities of anticoagulation, either alone or in combination with aspirin in patients with acute coronary syndromes. The ASPECT II study compared longer-term therapy with warfarin alone (target INR 3.0–4.0), aspirin (80 mg/day), and the combination of warfarin (INR 2.0–2.5) plus aspirin in 993 patients following an acute coronary syndrome (142). The study was stopped early by the sponsor because of slow recruitment. The composite end-point of death, MI, and stroke occurred in 9.0% of patients on aspirin alone, 5.0% of those on warfarin alone, and 5.0% of those on warfarin and aspirin. There were slightly higher rates of minor bleeding in the group on combination therapy. The Antithrombotics in the Prevention of Reocclusion in Coronary Thrombolysis (APRICOT) II study (142) involved 308 patients with TIMI grade 3 coronary flow after thrombolysis for ST segment elevation MI who were randomized to aspirin (160 mg initially followed by 80 mg daily) or to aspirin plus warfarin (INR 2.0 to 3.0) The primary endpoint was the rate of angiographic reocclusion at 3 months. Reocclusion occurred in 30% of the group given aspirin alone compared with 18% in those given aspirin plus warfarin (a 40% relative reduction). There was an increase in minor but not major bleeding events in the combination therapy group.

The WARIS II trial compared warfarin alone (mean INR 2.8), aspirin alone (160 mg/d), or both (mean INR 2.2; aspirin 75 mg/d) in 3630 patients <75 years of age with AMI randomized at the time of hospital discharge and followed up for 2 years (143). The primary endpoint was the first occurrence of the composite of all-cause death, nonfatal reinfarction, or thromboembolic stroke; this occurred in 20% of the patients on aspirin alone, 16.7% of those on warfarin alone, and 15% of those on the combination of both drugs. Combination therapy was significantly superior to aspirin alone ($p = 0.0005$), but there was no significant difference between the two warfarin groups. The incidence of major bleeding was 0.15% per year in the aspirin-alone group, 0.58% per year in the warfarin-alone group, and 0.52% per year in the combination group.

Two other recent studies, CARS and the Combined Hemotherapy And Mortality Prevention Study (CHAMP), compared aspirin alone with the combination of aspirin and low-intensity warfarin (lower limit of targeted INR <2.0). The CARS study involving 8803 patients with AMI demonstrated that low fixed-dose warfarin (1 or 3 mg/d) plus aspirin (80 mg) was no more effective than aspirin alone (160 mg) for long-term treatment (144). The incidence of death, recurrent MI, or stroke was 8.6% in the aspirin-alone group and 8.4% in the aspirin plus warfarin group after a mean of 14 months of follow-up. The aspirin plus warfarin group also was noted to have a significant increase in major bleeding events. The CHAMP study evaluated the relative efficacy and safety of aspirin alone (160 mg/d) and the combination of warfarin (INR 1.5–2.5) and aspirin (81 mg/d) in 5059 patients following MI in an open-label trial (145). There were no differences between the two groups in total mortality (17.3% vs. 17.3%), nonfatal MI (13.1% vs. 13.3%), or nonfatal stroke (4.7% vs. 4.2%). Again, major bleeding was more common in the combination group.

The recent ACC/AHA guidelines for warfarin therapy (146) cited a recent meta-analysis of 31 randomized trials of oral anticoagulant therapy published between 1960 and 1999 (147). These studies all involve patients with coronary artery disease treated for ≥3 months. When the results are stratified by the intensity of anticoagulation therapy, high-intensity (INR 2.8–4.8) and moderate-intensity (INR 2–3) oral anticoagulation regimens reduced the rates of MI and stroke but increased the risk of bleeding 6.0– to 7.7–fold. In combination with aspirin, low-intensity anticoagulation (INR < 2.0) was not superior to aspirin alone, whereas moderate- to high-intensity oral anticoagulation and aspirin versus aspirin alone at least showed encouraging trends. There was a modest increase in the bleeding risk associated with the combination.

Three other contemporary studies have evaluated oral anticoagulant therapy to prevent reinfarction in unstable angina patients over shorter time periods. The Organization to Assess Strategies for Ischemic Syndromes (OASIS) pilot study (148), the Antithrombotic Therapy in Acute Coronary Syndromes (ATACS) trial (149), and the OASIS 2 study (150) all suggested that in the short term, oral anticoagulation therapy could reduce the incidence of adverse events in the first 30 days if given in an intermediate INR range (2–3), but that the benefits of extended therapy were less well established.

Some preliminary data are also available regarding the use of ximelagatran (an oral direct thrombin inhibitor) in secondary prevention after acute MI. The ESTEEM trial (151) was a dose-finding randomized, double-blind, multicenter, multinational, placebo-controlled trial that randomized 1883 patients within 14 days of a ST elevation or non–ST elevation MI in proportions 1/1/1/1/2 to oral ximelagatran at doses of 24, 36, 48, or 60 mg twice daily or placebo, respectively, for 6 months. All patients received acetylsalicylic acid 160 mg once daily. The primary efficacy outcome was the dose response of ximelagatran by comparison to placebo for the occurrence of all-cause mortality, nonfatal MI, and severe recurrent ischemia. Results showed that oral ximelagatran reduced the risk for primary endpoint compared with placebo from 16.3% to 12.7% (hazard ratio 0.76, 95% C.I. 0.59–0.98) for the combined ximelagatran groups versus placebo. There was no indication of a dose response between the ximelagatran groups, and the major bleeding rates were rare, 1.8% and 0.9% (hazard ratio 1.97, 95% CI 0.80–4.84), in the combined ximelagatran groups and placebo, respectively. The authors concluded that oral ximelagatran combined with daily aspirin is more effective than aspirin alone in preventing major cardiovascular adverse events during 6 months of treatment after a recent cute MI. However, more data is needed before this agent can be recommended for clinical use in secondary prevention after acute MI.

There are relatively few randomized trials of oral anticoagulant therapy in patients with peripheral arterial disease. In a population of patients following surgical revascualrization, a relatively high-intensity oral anticoagulant regimen (INR 2.6–4.5) was associated with a significant 51% reduction in mortality (from 6.8% to 3.3% per year) compared with an untreated control group (p < 0.023) (152). ADMIT was an NIH-sponsored pilot trial evaluating the use of warfarin, niacin, and an antioxidant "cocktail" in patients with peripheral arterial disease. It was not designed to look at clinical outcomes; instead, it focused on how effective therapy was in affecting laboratory parameters related to treatment; it was designed as a pilot for a later, larger, definitive, efficacy-powered trial (153). However, the larger-scale subsequent NIH-sponsored outcomes-powered trial was never performed.

2. ASA

Much of the support for the routine use of aspirin in patients with atherosclerotic disease comes from the Antithrombotic Trialists meta-analyses. The first meta-analysis (The Antiplatelet Trialists Collaboration), published in 1994, and including clinical trials up through 1990, demonstrated that oral antiplatelet therapy (primary aspirin) was effective in preventing recurrent events across a wide range of atherosclerotic vascular disease, primarily coronary and cerebrovascular (67–69). It did deal with poststroke therapy (where aspirin was effective) but did not examine other peripheral arterial disease. A more recent and more comprehensive analysis was undertaken, involving trials up through 1997, with additional focus on stroke and peripheral arterial disease, and published in 2002 (157). The analysis included 287 studies, which involved 135,000 patients in whom antiplatelet therapy was compared with control and 77,000 patients in whom different antiplatelet regimens were compared.

Overall, antiplatelet therapy (primarily aspirin) reduced the incidence of any serious vascular event by one quarter, of nonfatal MI by one third, of nonfatal stroke by one quarter, and vascular mortality by one sixth. The absolute reduction in serious vascular events was 36 per 1000 treated for 2 years with previous stroke or transient ischemic attack (TIA). In 21 trials of patients with stroke or TIA, antiplatelet therapy reduced vascular events from 21.4% with control to 17.8%. Overall, among 9214 patients with PAD in 42 trials, there was a relative reduction of 23% in total vascular events (from 7.1% to 5.8%). In 26 trials of patients with intermittent claudication, antiplatelet therapy reduced vascular event from 7.9% with control to 6.4%. Similarly, in 12 trials of patients following surgical grafting of peripheral lesions, antiplatelet therapy reduced events from 6.5% to 5.4%, and from 3.6% to 2.5% in four trials of patients undergoing peripheral angioplasty. In six trials in patients with carotid disease, antiplatelet therapy reduced events from 12.8% to 10.6%.

In the meta-analyses, aspirin doses of 75–150 mg daily were at least as effective as higher doses. The effect of doses <75 mg were less certain. There was no good evidence to support the hypothesis that doses of aspirin ≥ 1000 mg daily might be preferable in patients at higher risk of stroke. A more recent trial (not included in the meta-analysis) supports this. The Aspirin and Carotid Endarterectomy trial showed that in 2849 patients undergoing carotid endarterectomy, the composite outcome of MI, stroke, or death was significantly lower among patients taking 81 or 325 mg of aspirin versus those taking 625–1300 mg (158).

The addition of additional oral antiplatelet therapy to aspirin generally appeared to provide some incremental benefit (157). In 25 trials comparing dipyridamole plus aspirin with aspirin alone (involving 10,404 patients), combination therapy was associated with a nonsignificant 6% relative reduction in events (from 12.4% with aspirin to 11.8% with aspirin plus dipyridamole). Only one trial, ESPS 2 (159), showed benefit in poststroke patients, but that benefit was in recurrent stroke, not MI or vascular death. Stronger data support the addition of ticlopidine or clopidogrel, as noted below.

A recent study (160) examined the efficacy of low (<150 mg) and intermediate (≥150 mg) doses of aspirin on 6 month outcomes (death, MI, and stroke) in 20,521 patients from the GUSTO IIb and PURSUIT studies. Initial unadjusted data and multivariate-adjusted data showed no difference between low and intermediate doses of aspirin on composite events at 6 months. However, the higher aspirin dose ($\geq$150 mg) was associated with a reduction in MI at 6 months. Another recent study by Patel et al. (161) suggested that the addition of ibuprofen to aspirin does not adversely affect the risk of myocardial infarction, contrary to prior in-vitro (162,163) and clinical studies (164) that had suggested that NSAIDs may blunt the therapeutic efficacy of aspirin.

Aspirin alone has also been shown to potentially alter the need for revascularization in patients with PAD. The Physicians Health Study (165–167) evaluated the effects of low-dose aspirin (325 mg/day) compared to placebo in 22,071 male physicians who did not have a history of MI or cerebrovascular disease at baseline; the average treatment period was approximately 5 years. The aspirin group had a 46% reduction in the need for surgical limb revascularization, but there was no difference between groups in the incidence of intermittent claudication (165). From the perspective of coronary events, there was a substantial reduction (44%) in the risk of myocardial infarction, but no reduction in the incidence of stroke, all-cause cardiovascular mortality, or the incidence of new angina (167). Thus, long-term aspirin therapy appears to be effective in reducing the incidence of acute thrombotic events, but may not affect the progress of the underlying atherosclerotic disease.

In the recently reported African-American Antiplatelet Stroke Prevention Study (AAASPS), aspirin alone (650 mg/day) appeared just as good as ticlopidine (250 mg bid) in the treatment of 1809 African-American patients with a recent (7–90 days) noncardioembolic ischemic stroke (168). The trial was halted prematurely by the DSMC on the basis of a futility analysis. The primary outcome of recurrent stroke, MI, or vascular death occurred in 12.3% of the aspirin group and 14.7% of the ticlopidine group (p = NS). Adverse events were slightly but not significantly higher with ticlopidine.

The phenomenon of aspirin "resistance" has become the focus of recent attention in the literature (169,170 . "Resistance" is, of course, a relative term, and becomes a function of exactly *what* you are measuring and exactly *how* you are measuring it. It generally refers to patients who, despite taking aspirin, have less platelet inhibition than would be expected, or even no impairment of platelet function at all. Eikelboom (171) measured urinary 11-dehydro thromboxane B_2 levels (a marker of urinary thromboxane generation) in patients taking aspirin in the HOPE study, and examined the relationship between urinary thromboxane generation and subsequent clinical events. The highest quartile of thromboxane generation had two times the risk of MI in comparison to the lowest quartile. A subsequent study by Gum and co-workers (172) using platelet aggregometry identified 5.2% of 326 patients with stable cardiovascular disease as being aspirin resistant (defined as a mean aggregation $\geq$70% with 10 μM ADP and $\geq$20% with 0.5 mg/ml AA); these patients were three times as likely to have subsequent adverse clinical events (death, MI, or stroke) as non-resistant patients.

Another recent study assessed aspirin responsiveness (using a bedside device) in patients undergoing PCI, and further examined the relationship between aspirin sensitivity/resistance and post-procedure myonecrosis (106). Using this bedside test (Ultegra Rapid Platelet Function Assay—Accumetrics), 19.2% of patients were described as being aspirin resistant; these patients were twice as likely to have post-PCI myonecrosis. This was true whether or not the patients received clopidogrel; patients receiving GP IIb/IIIa antagonists were excluded from the study. Pulcinelli et al. (173) have demonstrated that long-term treatment with aspirin is associated with a progressive decline in the degree of platelet inhibition with aspirin, although the platelet inhibition induced by ticlopidine remained constant over time.

3. Thienopyridines

Two large studies have examined the utility of ticlopidine in patients with cerebrovascular disease. The CATS trial, performed in 1982–86, compared ticlopidine (250 mg bid) with placebo in 1072 patients with a history of recent stroke (1 week to 4 months) (174). Patients were followed for a mean of 2 years following enrollment; the primary endpoint was the composite of ischemic stroke, MI, or vascular death. The placebo group had a primary event rate of 15.3% per year, while the ticlopidine group had a primary event rate of 10.8% per year (RRR 23.3%; $p = 0.02$). The TASS trial, performed in 1982–87, compared ticlopidine (250 mg bid) with aspirin (650 mg bid) in 3069 patients with a history of a recent stroke precursor or minor stroke within the past 3 months (175). Patients were followed for a mean of 3.4 years following enrollment; the primary endpoint was the composite of nonfatal stroke and all-cause mortality. The aspirin group had a primary event rate of 19% over 3 years, while the ticlopidine group had a primary event rate of 17% over 3 years (RRR 12%; $p = 0.048$).

A single trial has evaluated ticlopidine in unstable angina (176). In an open-label trial, 652 patients with unstable angina were randomized to conventional therapy (excluding ASA) with or without ticlopidine. At 6 months there was a 46% RRR for the endpoints of death or nonfatal MI (from 13.6% to 7.3%; $p = 0.009$). No study to date has compared ticlopidine to ASA in acute coronary syndromes.

The CAPRIE trial (Clopidogrel versus Aspirin in Patients at Risk of Ischemic Events) was a large-scale randomized trial of the safety and efficacy of clopidogrel (75 mg/day) versus aspirin (325 mg/day) in 19,185 patients with atherosclerotic vascular disease followed for up to 3 years (177). The study population included patients with recent ischemic stroke (within 6 months), recent myocardial infarction (within 35 days), or symptomatic peripheral arterial disease. The primary endpoint was the composite incidence of stroke (fatal and nonfatal), myocardial infarction (fatal and nonfatal), and other vascular death. At a mean follow-up of 1.9 years, the clopidogrel group had significantly fewer composite first events (5.32% per year risk vs. 5.83% per year with aspirin; RRR 8.7%; $p = 0.043$). The outcome event most dramatically reduced by clopidogrel therapy was myocardial infarction. The greatest relative risk reduction (23.8%) was noted in patients with peripheral arterial disease, in whom the annual event rate was reduced from 4.86% with aspirin to 3.71% with clopidogrel ($p = 0.0028$). There were no major differences between the aspirin and clopidogrel groups in terms of safety. The incidence of significant neutropenia was 0.10% in the clopidogrel group and 0.17% in the aspirin group. When patients with coronary disease and either concomitant cerebrovascular disease or peripheral vascular disease were examined, there was striking superiority of clopidogrel in reducing outcome events in this population (RRR 22.7%). Mechanistically, an important factor may be the key role that ADP plays in shear-induced platelet aggregation. In peripheral vascular disease and coronary artery disease plus disease in other vascular beds, there is a greater atherosclerotic burden, more shear forces, and, probably, a more important role for ADP-induced platelet activation/aggregation. Recent additional analyses of the CAPRIE cohort have documented the significant benefit of clopidogrel over aspirin in patients with a prior history of CABG (178), patients with diabetes (179), and the benefits of clopidogrel over aspirin in preventing not only initial events (the primary CAPRIE analysis), but recurrent and total vascular events as well (180).

The CURE (Clopidogrel in Unstable angina to Prevent Recurrent ischemic Events) trial was a multicenter, randomized, double-blind, placebo-controlled study comparing combination therapy with aspirin and clopidogrel versus aspirin alone in patients with acute coronary syndromes (181). A total of 12,562 patients with unstable angina or non–Q-wave MI (within 24 hours of their last episode of pain) received ASA 75–325 mg and then were randomized to clopidogrel (300 mg load followed by 75 mg daily) or placebo for 3 months to 1 year. The primary endpoint was a composite of cardiovascular (CV) death, MI, or stroke. The main safety endpoints were major bleeding (disabling or symptomatic intracranial or intraocular bleeding; or transfusion >2 units) and life-threatening bleeding (Hgb decrease of >5 g/dL, hypotension requiring inotropes, bleeding requiring surgery or transfusion of >4 units of blood, or intracranial bleeding).

Seventy-five percent of the patients enrolled in CURE had unstable angina, 25% had an elevated enzyme or troponin level, 94% had an abnormal ECG, and half had ST-segment deviation. Approximately 30% of the patients underwent revascularization; the mean follow-up was 9 months. Treatment with clopidogrel and ASA was associated with a 20% relative reduction in the primary endpoint of CV death, MI or stroke, largely driven by a 23% relative reduction in the incidence of MI. Differences in the other components of the primary endpoint (CV death, stroke, non-CV death) failed to reach statistical significance. There was a 31% reduction in in-hospital refractory ischemia (2.06% to 1.42%; $p = 0.001$) and a 25% reduction in severe ischemia (5.03% to 3.83%; $p = 0.001$). The curves for the primary endpoint began to diverge very early favoring clopidogrel (within the first few hours). At 24 hours, a 20% relative reduction in the composite death, MI, and stroke was also noted. The benefits of clopidogrel were present across all major subgroups: patients with and without major ST segment deviation, enzyme or troponin elevation, and prior and subsequent revascularization, and in the subset undergoing PCI (182). Benefits were also noted in composite events with long-term therapy in addition to in-hospital benefit. Although there was a 34% excess of major bleeding in the clopidogrel arm, there was no significant excess of life-threatening bleeding with combination therapy.

Peters et al. (183) examined in more detail issues surrounding the addition of clopidogrel to aspirin in CURE. They found that adding clopidogrel to aspirin was beneficial across a range of aspirin doses, and that the risk of bleeding increased as a function of aspirin dose, with or without clopidogrel.

The CREDO trial demonstrated that long-term therapy following percutaneous coronary intervention with aspirin and clopidogrel was superior to aspirin alone in reducing the 1–year incidence of death, MI, and stroke (104). This reinforces and extends the potential benefits of secondary prevention with more intense oral antiplatelet therapy beyond the acute coronary syndrome population to a larger population of patients with manifest coronary atherosclerotic disease.

The CHARISMA trial is a currently ongoing prospective, randomized study comparing aspirin alone with aspirin plus clopidogrel (75 mg/day) in patients at risk for vascular events [documented cerebrovascular disease, documented coronary artery disease, symptomatic PAD, or multiple risk factors (2 major, 1 major + 2 minor, or 3 minor)]. A total of at least 15,200 patients are to be randomized; it is an event-driven trial (1040 primary events of stroke, MI, or cardiovascular death)—the estimated duration of follow-up is approximately 42 months. Another trial, MATCH (Management of Atherothrombosis with Clopidogrel in High risk patients with recent TIA or ischemic stroke), is examining the utility of clopidogrel in a high-risk stroke/TIA population of approximately 7600 patients treated and followed for 18 months.

The MATCH TRIAL (Management of Atherothrombosis with clopidogrel in high-risk patients with recent TIA or ischemic stroke) compared clopidogrel alone to clopidogrel plus aspirin, given over 18 months in 7599 patients with a TIA or ischemic stroke within the past 3 months (184). The primary endpoint of the study, first occurrence of MI, vascular death, ischemic stroke, or hospitalization for an acute ischemic event, was not significantly different between groups (16.7% with clopidogrel, 15.7% with clopidogrel plus aspirin). From a safety standpoint, life-threatening bleeding tended to be more frequent with combination thereapy (1.3% with clopidogrel, 2.5% with clopidogrel plus aspirin). These results have altered the already-in-progress 15,000 patient PROFESS trial (Prevention Regimen for effectively avoiding second strokes) which initially was supposed to compare dipyridamole plus aspirin versus clopidogrel plus aspirin; the latter arm has now been changed to clopidogrel alone.

Another issues that has recently come under scrutiny is the issue of clopidogrel "resistance," analogous to aspirin resistance (described above). In a study of 96 patients undergoing coronary stenting, Gurbel et al. (185) found clopidogrel resistance (defined as <10% reduction in platelet aggregation on response to 5 mmol/L ADP, in comparison to pretreatment values) in 63% of patients at 2 hours, 31% at 24 hours, 31% at 5 days, and 15% at 30 days. Matetzky and co-workers (186) described 60 consecutive patients undergoing primary PCI with stenting for acute MI. They found that up to 25% of these patients were "resistant" as defined by ADP-induced platelet aggregation studies, and that the majority of recurrent cardiovascular events occurred in the most clopidogrel-resistant patients. Additional recent work has focused on the antiplatelet effects of clopidogrel loading, and the variability of the antiplatelet response (187,188).

Despite the fact that the combination of aspirin plus clopidogrel has been advocated for 9-12 months following an ACS episode or PCI (60,104,181,189,190), a number of recent articles have questioned whether the long-trm benefits are truly important, or perhaps much less prominent that the acute or early benefit (191,192), particularly since most of the benefit with combination therapy appears early, or in the first few months, and the risk of recurrent events declines rapidly after the initial early at-risk period.

4.   Oral IIb/IIIa Antagonists

There have been five large randomized trials of oral IIb/IIIa antagonists in patients with atherosclerotic disease: EXCITE [7232 patients undergoing coronary intervention (193)], OPUS/TIMI 16 [10,288 patients following acute coronary syndromes (194)], SYM-PHONY [9169 patients following acute coronary syndromes (195)], 2nd SYMPHONY [6637 patients following acute coronary syndromes (196)], and BRAVO [9190 high-risk patients following coronary event, cerebrovascular events, or with multibed vascular disease (197)]. Despite the fact that these studies all used very powerful antiplatelet agents, all five trials demonstrated a trend toward higher mortality in the IIb/IIIa groups. A recent meta-analysis (198) of four of these studies demonstrated a 37% increase in mortality (p = 0.001), and a 40% increase in MI at 30 days ($p = 0.002$) with active therapy. Only one of the five trials, BRAVO, included patients with noncoronary vascular disease as a primary inclusion criteria (197). Of the 9190 patients enrolled in BRAVO, 3319 had had a recent cerebrovascular event (within the prior 5–30 days), and 1481 had other peripheral vascular disease, with either concomitant coronary or cerebrovascular disease. Similar to the overall population, these subgroups showed a trend toward increased mortality with no significant clinical benefit with lotrafiban, although in all patients with cerebrovascular disease there was a nonsignificant thrend favoring lotrafiban. A recent trial of the oral GP IIb/IIIa antagonist chromafiban in patients with peripheral vascular disease was also halted prematurely because of safety concerns.

B. Percutaneous Coronary Interventions

Longer-term antithrombotic therapy following percutaneous coronary intervention has changed radically over the last decade and a half with the advent of coronary stenting and the rapidly evolving therapeutic alternatives for postprocedural anticoagulation (23,28). However, with these alternatives, relatively little attention has been directed at adjusting the degree or intensity of anticoagulation or antiplatelet therapy.

Initially, in the early days of balloon angioplasty, patients were treated with a number of prolonged antiplatelet regimens (aspirin, aspirin plus dipyridamole, aspirin plus ticlopidine, and, in some cases, warfarin) for a period of 4–6 weeks following intervention. This practice persisted with the development of alternative ablative techniques such as laser angioplasty, directional atherectomy, and rotational atherectomy. With the arrival of coronary stents, because of concerns about subacute stent thrombosis, much more aggressive anticoagulant regimens were employed. It was felt (for no particularly good reasons other than empirical) to be necessary to transition stent patients over to oral anticoagulation with warfarin, and most early stent regimens involved a rapid switch-over from postprocedural intravenous unfractionated heparin (titrated to aPTTs of 1.5–2 times control) to warfarin (INR 2–3). Frequently, however, this transition was too abrupt to fully account for the early pro-thrombotic consequences of initiating warfarin therapy, and subacute thrombosis continued to be a problem. It was only with the data from trials such as STARS (199), ISAR (200) MATTIS (201), and FANTASTIC (202) that it was shown that antiplatelet therapy with aspirin and ticlopidine for 4 weeks following stent implantation was superior to the postprocedure use of warfarin. The degree of platelet inhibition was not titrated or adjusted in any way. Additionally, in the face of suboptimally deployed stents, preliminary data from ENTICES (203) suggested that more prolonged and intense antithrombotic thereapy with subcutaneous LMWH for an extended period of time might be beneficial. However, in the larger-scale ATLAST trial, the event rates with modern-generation stents and adjunctive thienopyridines were so low that the trial had to be abandoned (204).

While the intensity of antithrombotic therapy was never really investigated, there was considerable debate about the duration of therapy. While 4 weeks was standard, a number of studies suggested that shorter periods (such as 2 weeks) were equally beneficial and that shortening the duration of therapy with ticlopidine reduced the risk of neutropenia or drug-induced TTP (205,206). This became moot with the advent of clopidogrel, an alternative thienopyridine that had a substantially lower incidence of hematopoeitic side effects. With the widespread conversion to clopidogrel, standard therapy again became 4–6 weeks following intervention (207). More recent data from PCI-CURE (180) and CREDO (104) have also suggested that there may be significant benefits to more prolonged treatment with aspirin and clopidogrel. In CREDO, post-PCI aspirin/clopidogrel continued for 1 year instead of 30 days was associated with a significantly lower incidence of the composite of death, MI, and stroke (104). Another area where prolonged combination therapy is beneficial is following coronary brachytherapy, where prolonged derangements of endothelial function are associated with an extended period of risk for subacute thrombosis; this period may last as long as 12 months (208,209). Another area in evolution is that of drug-eluting stents, which may also be associated with an extended risk for subacute thrombosis and which may require more intense antiplatelet therapy, and generally the combination of aspirin plus colpidogrel is recommended for 3–6 months following implantation of a drug-eluting stent (210,211). Whether the intensity of therapy can be reduced at a later time, and exactly how long therapy should be maintained remains uncertain.

Similar to secondary prevention in ACS patients, little attention has been paid to the intensity of therapy. More potent antiplatelet agents such as the GP IIb/IIIa antagonists have also been investigated following coronary intervention (ORBIT), and similar to the ACS trial (SYMPHONY, OPUS, etc.), they were not beneficial in preventing subsequent events and were associated with an increase in bleeding complications. At present the "optimal" degree or duration of antiplatelet therapy following PCI remains poorly understood.

IV. SUMMARY

The application of coagulation monitoring for arterial disease has evolved substantially over the last few decades. The underlying assumption, of course, is that the degree of coagulation inhibition or platelet inhibition matters; if the *degree* of inhibition matters, then achieving a given threshold (if it can be defined) or adjusting therapy to an accepted target range is of paramount importance if therapy is going to be truly optimized. The problem arises, however, that establishing a "threshold" or "target range" becomes problematic because there are very few prospective, randomized studies that examine this issue directly. Moreover, our monitoring techniques generally examine or describe only one aspect of the thrombotic process, and do not provide a global assessment of the effect of therapy on coagulation as a whole. Finally, different agents (such as UFH, LMWH, or direct thrombin inhibitors—or aspirin and thienopyridines) may not have comparable effects on a given monitoring test (such as the ACT or aPTT—or ADP- or thromboxane-induced aggregation), and valid cross agent comparisons may simply not be possible, especially if therapy is being titrated or adjusted on the basis of a given test. Nevertheless, numerous clinical areas exist where coagulation monitoring may be of benefit in arterial disease. Acutely, for PCI, for acute coronary syndromes, and acute stroke; long-term, for atherosclerotic disease and following PCI. Future work will help expand our physiologic understanding, and will hopefully provide us with better, more reliable and more uniform monitoring capabilities. Ultimately, the question is not whether the degree of coagulation matters—we believe it does—but how we can best define "optimal" therapy, and how we can best achieve it, both with our current arsenal of antithrombotic and antiplatelet weapons, and with our ever-expanding armamentarium.

REFERENCES

1. Mabin TA, Holmes DR, Jr., Smith HC, et al. Intracoronary thrombus: role in coronary occlusion complicating percutaneous transluminal coronary angioplasty. J Am Coll Cardiol 1985; 5:198–202.
2. Sugrue DD, Holmes DR, Jr., Smith HC, et al. Coronary artery thrombus as a risk factor for acute vessel occlusion during percutaneous transluminal coronary angioplasty: improving results. Br Heart J 1986; 56:62–6.
3. de Feyter PJ, van den Brand M, Laarman GJ, et al. Acute coronary artery occlusion during and after percutaneous transluminal coronary angioplasty. Frequency, prediction, clinical course, management, and follow-up. Circulation 1991; 83:927–36.
4. Vaitkus PT, Herrmann HC, Laskey WK. Management and immediate outcome of patients with intracoronary thrombus during percutaneous transluminal coronary angioplasty. Am Heart J 1992; 124:1–8.
5. Bergelson BA, Jacobs AK, Cupples LA, et al. Prediction of risk for hemodynamic compromise during percutaneous transluminal coronary angioplasty. Am J Cardiol 1992; 70:1540–5.

6. Hermans WR, Foley DP, Rensing BJ, et al. Usefulness of quantitative and qualitative angiographic lesion morphology, and clinical characteristics in predicting major adverse cardiac events during and after native coronary balloon angioplasty. CARPORT and MERCATOR Study Groups. Am J Cardiol 1993; 72:14–20.

7. Myler RK, Shaw RE, Stertzer SH, et al. Unstable angina and coronary angioplasty. Circulation 1990; 82:II88–95.

8. Mooney MR, Mooney JF, Goldenberg IF, Almquist AK, Van Tassel RA. Percutaneous transluminal coronary angioplasty in the setting of large intracoronary thrombi. Am J Cardiol 1990; 65:427–31.

9. Ellis SG, Roubin GS, King SB, 3rd, et al. Angiographic and clinical predictors of acute closure after native vessel coronary angioplasty. Circulation 1988; 77:372–9.

10. Detre KM, Holmes DR, Jr., Holubkov R, et al. Incidence and consequences of periprocedural occlusion. The 1985–1986 National Heart, Lung, and Blood Institute Percutaneous Transluminal Coronary Angioplasty Registry. Circulation 1990; 82:739–50.

11. Reeder GS, Bryant SC, Suman VJ, Holmes DR, Jr. Intracoronary thrombus: still a risk factor for PCI failure? Cathet Cardiovasc Diagn 1995; 34:191–5.

12. Zhao XQ, Theroux P, Snapinn SM, Sax FL. Intracoronary thrombus and platelet glycoprotein IIb/IIIa receptor blockade with tirofiban in unstable angina or non-Q-wave myocardial infarction. Angiographic results from the PRISM-PLUS trial (Platelet receptor inhibition for ischemic syndrome management in patients limited by unstable signs and symptoms). PRISM-PLUS Investigators. Circulation 1999; 100:1609–15.

13. Ferguson JJ, Barasch E, Wilson JM, et al. The relation of clinical outcome to dissection and thrombus formation during coronary angioplasty. Heparin Registry Investigators. J Invasive Cardiol 1995; 7:2–10.

14. Laskey MA, Deutsch E, Hirshfeld JW, Jr., Kussmaul WG, Barnathan E, Laskey WK. Influence of heparin therapy on percutaneous transluminal coronary angioplasty outcome in patients with coronary arterial thrombus. Am J Cardiol 1990; 65:179–82.

15. Violaris AG, Melkert R, Herrman JP, Serruys PW. Role of angiographically identifiable thrombus on long-term luminal renarrowing after coronary angioplasty: a quantitative angiographic analysis. Circulation 1996; 93:889–97.

16. Hattersley PG. Activated coagulation time of whole blood. JAMA 1966; 196:436–40.

17. Young JA, Kisker CT, Doty DB. Adequate anticoagulation during cardiopulmonary bypass determined by activated clotting time and the appearance of fibrin monomer. Ann Thorac Surg 1978; 26:231–40.

18. Boccara A, Benamer H, Juliard JM, et al. A randomized trial of a fixed high dose vs a weight-adjusted low dose of intravenous heparin during coronary angioplasty. Eur Heart J 1997; 18:631–5.

19. Vainer J, Fleisch M, Gunnes P, et al. Low-dose heparin for routine coronary angioplasty and stenting. Am J Cardiol 1996; 78:964–6.

20. McGarry TF, Jr., Gottlieb RS, Morganroth J, et al. The relationship of anticoagulation level and complications after successful percutaneous transluminal coronary angioplasty. Am Heart J 1992; 123:1445–51.

21. Bittl JA, Ahmed WH. Relation between abrupt vessel closure and the anticoagulant response to heparin or bivalirudin during coronary angioplasty. Am J Cardiol 1998; 82:50P-56P.

22. Bittl JA, Strony J, Brinker JA, et al. Treatment with bivalirudin (Hirulog) as compared with heparin during coronary angioplasty for unstable or postinfarction angina. Hirulog Angioplasty Study Investigators. N Engl J Med 1995; 333:764–9.

23. Kleiman NS, Weitz JI. Putting heparin into perspective: its history and the evolution of its use during percutaneous coronary interventions. J Invasive Cardiol 2000; 12 Suppl F:20F-6.

24. Ferguson JJ, Dougherty KG, Gaos CM, Bush HS, Marsh KC, Leachman DR. Relation between procedural activated coagulation time and outcome after percutaneous transluminal coronary angioplasty. J Am Coll Cardiol 1994; 23:1061–5.

25. Narins CR, Hillegass WB, Jr., Nelson CL, et al. Relation between activated clotting time during angioplasty and abrupt closure. Circulation 1996; 93:667–71.

26. Chew DP, Bhatt DL, Lincoff AM, et al. Defining the optimal activated clotting time during percutaneous coronary intervention: aggregate results from 6 randomized, controlled trials. Circulation 2001; 103:961–6.

27. Lincoff AM, Tcheng JE, Califf RM, et al. Standard versus low-dose weight-adjusted heparin in patients treated with the platelet glycoprotein IIb/IIIa receptor antibody fragment abciximab (c7E3 Fab) during percutaneous coronary revascularization. PROLOG Investigators. Am J Cardiol 1997; 79:286–91.

28. Popma JJ, Ohman EM, Weitz J, Lincoff AM, Harrington RA, Berger P. Antithrombotic therapy in patients undergoing percutaneous coronary intervention. Chest 2001; 119:321S-336S.

29. Wilson JM, Dougherty KG, Ellis KO, Ferguson JJ. Activated clotting times in acute coronary syndromes and percutaneous transluminal coronary angioplasty. Cathet Cardiovasc Diagn 1995; 34:1–5.

30. Mascelli MA, Kleiman NS, Marciniak SJ, Jr., Damaraju L, Weisman HF, Jordan RE. Therapeutic heparin concentrations augment platelet reactivity: implications for the pharmacologic assessment of the glycoprotein IIb/IIIa antagonist abciximab. Am Heart J 2000; 139:696–703.

31. Young E, Prins M, Levine MN, Hirsh J. Heparin binding to plasma proteins, an important mechanism for heparin resistance. Thromb Haemost 1992; 67:639–43.

32. Oltrona L, Eisenberg PR, Lasala JM, Sewall DJ, Shelton ME, Winters KJ. Association of heparin-resistant thrombin activity with acute ischemic complications of coronary interventions. Circulation 1996; 94:2064–71.

33. Kaluski E, Krakover R, Cotter G, et al. Minimal heparinization in coronary angioplasty—how much heparin is really warranted? Am J Cardiol 2000; 85:953–6.

34. Denardo SJ, Davis KE, Reid PR, Tcheng JE. Efficacy and safety of minimal dose (< or =1,000 units) unfractionated heparin with abciximab in percutaneous coronary intervention. Am J Cardiol 2003; 91:1–5.

35. Snitzer R, Miremath Y, Lee J, Lasala JM, Eisenberg PR, Winters KJ. Suppression of intracoronary thrombin activity by weight-adjusted heparin administration during coronary interventions. Circulation 1995; 92(Suppl. I):1609.

36. Bowers J, Ferguson JJ. Use of the activated clotting time in anticoagulation monitoring of intravascular procedures. Tex Heart Inst J 1993; 20:258–63.

37. Wilson JM, Koshnevis R, Le D, et al. Are weight-based heparin boluses more predictable? J Invasive Cardiol 1996; 8:66.

38. Ferguson J. All ACTs are not created equal. Tex Heart Inst J 1992; 19:1–3.

39. Avendano A, Ferguson JJ. Comparison of Hemochron and HemoTec activated coagulation time target values during percutaneous transluminal coronary angioplasty. J Am Coll Cardiol 1994; 23:907–10.

40. Aguirre FV, Ferguson JJ, Blankenship JC, et al. Association of pre-intervention activated clotting times (ACT) and clinical outcomes following percutaneous coronary revascularization: Results from the IMPACT-II trial. J Am Coll Cardiol 1996; 27:83A.

41. Tolleson TR, O'Shea JC, Bittl JA, et al. Relationship between heparin anticoagulation and clinical outcomes in coronary stent intervention: observations from the ESPRIT trial. J Am Coll Cardiol 2003; 41:386–93.

42. Walford CD, Midei M, Aversano TR, et al. Heparin after PCI: Increased early complications and no clinical benefit. Circulation 1991; 84 (Suppl II):II-592.

43. Tanjura L, Pinto I, Centemero M, et al. Use of heparin in coronary angioplasty: Randomized trial for prevention of abrupt closure. Eur Heart J 1993; 14:179.

44. Friedman HZ, Cragg DR, Glazier SM, et al. Randomized prospective evaluation of prolonged versus abbreviated intravenous heparin therapy after coronary angioplasty. J Am Coll Cardiol 1994; 24:1214–9.

45. Pizzuli L, Zirbes M, Fehske W, Pfeiffer D. Omission of intraveneous heparin and nitroglycerin following uncomplicated coronary angioplasty: A Prospective study. Circulation 1995; 92:174.

46. Gabliani G, Deligonul U, Kern MJ, Vandormael M. Acute coronary occlusion occurring after successful percutaneous transluminal coronary angioplasty: temporal relationship to discontinuation of anticoagulation. Am Heart J 1988; 116:696–700.

47. Granger CB, Miller JM, Bovill EG, et al. Rebound increase in thrombin generation and activity after cessation of intravenous heparin in patients with acute coronary syndromes. Circulation 1995; 91:1929–35.

48. MacDonald LA, Meyers S, Bennett CL, et al. Post-cardiac catheterization access site complications and low-molecular -weight heparin following cardiac catheterization. J Invasive Cardiol 2003; 15:60–2.

49. Faxon DP, Spiro TE, Minor S, et al. Low molecular weight heparin in prevention of restenosis after angioplasty. Results of Enoxaparin Restenosis (ERA) Trial. Circulation 1994; 90:908–14.

50. Karsch KR, Preisack MB, Baildon R, et al. Low molecular weight heparin (reviparin) in percutaneous transluminal coronary angioplasty. Results of a randomized, double-blind, unfractionated heparin and placebo-controlled, multicenter trial (REDUCE trial). Reduction of Restenosis After PCI, Early Administration of Reviparin in a Double-Blind Unfractionated Heparin and Placebo-Controlled Evaluation. J Am Coll Cardiol 1996; 28:1437–43.

51. Rabah MM, Premmereur J, Graham M, et al. Usefulness of intravenous enoxaparin for percutaneous coronary intervention in stable angina pectoris. Am J Cardiol 1999; 84:1391–5.

52. Diez JG, Lievano MJ, Croitoru M, Olaya CA, Ferguson J. Enoxaparin anticoagulation for percutaneous coronary interventions: A pilot safety study. Circulation 1999; 100(18) (Suppl I):I-188.

53. Kereiakes DJ, Grines C, Fry E, et al. Enoxaparin and abciximab adjunctive pharmacotherapy during percutaneous coronary intervention. J Invasive Cardiol 2001; 13:272–8.

54. Ferguson JJ, Antman EM, Bates ER, et al. Combining enoxaparin and glycoprotein IIb/IIIa antagonists for the treatment of acute coronary syndromes: final results of the National Investigators Collaborating on Enoxaparin-3 (NICE-3) study. Am Heart J 2003; 146:628–34.

55. The Evaluation of Platelet IIb/IIIa Inhibitor for Stenting (EPISTENT) Investigators. Randomised placebo-controlled and balloon-angioplasty-controlled trial to assess safety of coronary stenting with use of platelet glycoprotein-IIb/IIIa blockade. Lancet 1998; 352:87–92.

56. ESPRIT Investigators. Novel dosing regimen of eptifibatide in planned coronary stent implantation (ESPRIT): a randomised, placebo-controlled trial. Lancet 2000; 356:2037–44.

57. Bhatt DL, Lee BI, Casterella PJ, et al. Safety of concomitant therapy with eptifibatide and enoxaparin in patients undergoing percutaneous coronary intervention: results of the Coronary Revascularization Using Integrilin and Single bolus Enoxaparin Study. J Am Coll Cardiol 2003; 41:20–5.

58. Choussat R, Montalescot G, Collet JP, et al. A unique, low dose of intravenous enoxaparin in elective percutaneous coronary intervention. J Am Coll Cardiol 2002; 40:1943–50.

59. Kereiakes DJ, Kleiman NS, Fry E, et al. Dalteparin in combination with abciximab during percutaneous coronary intervention. Am Heart J 2001; 141:348–52.

60. Braunwald E, Antman EM, Beasley JW, et al. ACC/AHA 2002 guideline update for the management of patients with unstable angina and non-ST-segment elevation myocardial infarction—summary article: a report of the American College of Cardiology/American Heart Association task force on practice guidelines (Committee on the Management of Patients With Unstable Angina). J Am Coll Cardiol 2002; 40:1366–74.

61. Cohen M, Demers C, Gurfinkel EP, et al. A comparison of low-molecular-weight heparin with unfractionated heparin for unstable coronary artery disease. Efficacy and Safety of Subcutaneous Enoxaparin in Non-Q-Wave Coronary Events Study Group. N Engl J Med 1997; 337:447–52.

62. Antman EM, Cohen M, Radley D, et al. Assessment of the treatment effect of enoxaparin for unstable angina/non-Q-wave myocardial infarction. TIMI 11B-ESSENCE meta-analysis. Circulation 1999; 100:1602–8.

63. Antman EM, McCabe CH, Gurfinkel EP, et al. Enoxaparin prevents death and cardiac ischemic events in unstable angina/non-Q-wave myocardial infarction. Results of the thrombolysis in myocardial infarction (TIMI) 11B trial. Circulation 1999; 100:1593–601.

64. Collet JP, Montalescot G, Lison L, et al. Percutaneous coronary intervention after subcutaneous enoxaparin pretreatment in patients with unstable angina pectoris. Circulation 2001; 103:658–63.

65. Martin JL, Fry ET, Sanderink GJ, et al. Reliable anticoagulation with enoxaparin in patients undergoing percutaneous coronary intervention: The pharmacokinetics of enoxaparin in PCI (PEPCI) study. Catheter Cardiovasc Interv 2004; 61:163–70.

66. Goodman SG, Cohen M, Bigonzi F, et al. Randomized trial of low molecular weight heparin (enoxaparin) versus unfractionated heparin for unstable coronary artery disease: one-year results of the ESSENCE Study. Efficacy and Safety of Subcutaneous Enoxaparin in Non-Q Wave Coronary Events. J Am Coll Cardiol 2000; 36:693–8.

67. Antman EM, Louwerenburg HW, Baars HF, et al. Enoxaparin as adjunctive antithrombin therapy for ST-elevation myocardial infarction: results of the ENTIRE-Thrombolysis in Myocardial Infarction (TIMI) 23 Trial. Circulation 2002; 105:1642–9.

68. Fox KA, Poole-Wilson PA, Henderson RA, et al. Interventional versus conservative treatment for patients with unstable angina or non-ST-elevation myocardial infarction: the British Heart Foundation RITA 3 randomised trial. Randomized Intervention Trial of unstable Angina. Lancet 2002; 360:743–51.

69. ASSENT-3 Investigators. Efficacy and safety of tenecteplase in combination with enoxaparin, abciximab, or unfractionated heparin: the ASSENT-3 randomised trial in acute myocardial infarction. Lancet 2001; 358:605–13.

70. Dubois CL, Belmans A, Granger CB, et al. Outcome of urgent and elective percutaneous coronary interventions after pharmacologic reperfusion with tenecteplase combined with unfractionated heparin, enoxaparin, or abciximab. J Am Coll Cardiol 2003; 42:1178–85.

71. Mukherjee D, Mahaffey KW, Moliterno DJ, et al. Promise of combined low-molecular-weight heparin and platelet glycoprotein IIb/IIIa inhibition: results from Platelet IIb/IIIa Antagonist for the Reduction of Acute coronary syndrome events in a Global Organization Network B (PARAGON B). Am Heart J 2002; 144:995–1002.

72. Blazing MA, de Lemos JA, White HD, et al. Safety and efficacy of enoxaparin vs unfractionated heparin in patients with non-ST-segment elevation acute coronary syndromes who receive tirofiban and aspirin: a randomized controlled trial. JAMA 2004; 292:55–64.

73. SYNERGY Investigators. Enoxaparin vs unfractionated heparin in high-risk patients with non-ST-segment elevation acute coronary syndromes managed with an intended early invasive strategy: primary results of the SYNERGY randomized trial. JAMA 2004; 292:45–54.

74. Moliterno DJ, Hermiller JB, Kereiakes DJ, et al. A novel point-of-care enoxaparin monitor for use during percutaneous coronary intervention. Results of the Evaluating Enoxaparin Clotting Times (ELECT) Study. J Am Coll Cardiol 2003; 42:1132–9.

75. Henry TD, Satran D, Knox LL, Iacarella CL, Laxson DD, Antman EM. Are activated clotting times helpful in the management of anticoagulation with subcutaneous low-molecular-weight heparin? Am Heart J 2001; 142:590–3.

76. Schooley CC, Gilbert JH, Harlan M, Bracey A, Coulter S, Wilson JM. Kinetics of Intravenously administered dalteparin. J Am Coll Cardiol 2003; 41 (Suppl A):25A.

77. Marmur JD, Anand SX, Bagga RS, et al. The activated clotting time can be used to monitor the low molecular weight heparin dalteparin after intravenous administration. J Am Coll Cardiol 2003; 41:394–402.

78. Lawrence M, Mixon T, Cross D, al. e. Assessment of anticoagulation using activated clotting times in patients receiving intravenous enoxaparin during percutaneous coronary intervention. J Am Coll Cardiol 2003; 41:68A.

79. Natarjan MK, Turpie GA, Raco DL, al. e. A randomized comparison of dalteparin versus unfractionated heparin during percutaneous coronary interventions. J Am Coll Cardiol 2003; 41:68A-69A.

80. Becker RC, Cannon CP. Hirudin: Its Biology and Clinical Use. J Thromb Thrombolysis 1994; 1:7–16.

81. Lefkovits J, Topol EJ. Direct thrombin inhibitors in cardiovascular medicine. Circulation 1994; 90:1522–36.

82. Serruys PW, Herrman JP, Simon R, et al. A comparison of hirudin with heparin in the prevention of restenosis after coronary angioplasty. Helvetica Investigators. N Engl J Med 1995; 333:757–63.

83. Lidon RM, Theroux P, Juneau M, Adelman B, Maraganore J. Initial experience with a direct antithrombin, Hirulog, in unstable angina. Anticoagulant, antithrombotic, and clinical effects. Circulation 1993; 88:1495–501.

84. Topol EJ, Bonan R, Jewitt D, et al. Use of a direct antithrombin, hirulog, in place of heparin during coronary angioplasty. Circulation 1993; 87:1622–9.

85. Bittl JA, Chaitman BR, Feit F, Kimball W, Topol EJ. Bivalirudin versus heparin during coronary angioplasty for unstable or postinfarction angina: Final report reanalysis of the Bivalirudin Angioplasty Study. Am Heart J 2001; 142:952–9.

86. Lincoff AM, Kleiman NS, Kottke-Marchant K, et al. Bivalirudin with planned or provisional abciximab versus low-dose heparin and abciximab during percutaneous coronary revascularization: results of the Comparison of Abciximab Complications with Hirulog for Ischemic Events Trial (CACHET). Am Heart J 2002; 143:847–53.

87. Lincoff AM, Bittl JA, Kleiman NS, et al. Comparison of bivalirudin versus heparin during percutaneous coronary intervention (the Randomized Evaluation of PCI Linking Angiomax to Reduced Clinical Events [REPLACE]-1 trial). Am J Cardiol 2004; 93:1092–6.

88. Chen JL. Argatroban: a direct thrombin inhibitor for heparin-induced thrombocytopenia and other clinical applications. Heart Dis 2001; 3:189–98.

89. Walenga JM. An overview of the direct thrombin inhibitor argatroban. Pathophysiol Haemost Thromb 2002; 32 Suppl 3:9–14.

90. Fareed J, Hoppensteadt D, Iqbal O, Tobu M, Lewis BE. Practical issues in the development of argatroban: a perspective. Pathophysiol Haemost Thromb 2002; 32 Suppl 3:56–65.

91. Matthai WH, Jr. Use of argatroban during percutaneous coronary interventions in patients with heparin-induced thrombocytopenia. Semin Thromb Hemost 1999; 25 Suppl 1:57–60.

92. Carteaux JP, Gast A, Tschopp TB, Roux S. Activated clotting time as an appropriate test to compare heparin and direct thrombin inhibitors such as hirudin or Ro 46–6240 in experimental arterial thrombosis. Circulation 1995; 91:1568–74.

93. Fenyvesi T, Jorg I, Harenberg J. Monitoring of anticoagulant effects of direct thrombin inhibitors. Semin Thromb Hemost 2002; 28:361–8.

94. Lincoff AM, Bittl JA, Harrington RA, et al. Bivalirudin and provisional glycoprotein IIb/IIIa blockade compared with heparin and planned glycoprotein IIb/IIIa blockade during percutaneous coronary intervention: REPLACE-2 randomized trial. JAMA 2003; 289:853–63.

95. Lincoff AM, Kleiman NS, Kereiakes DJ, et al. Long-term efficacy of bivalirudin and provisional glycoprotein IIb/IIIa blockade vs. heparin and planned glycoprotein IIb/IIIa blockade during percutaneous coronary revascularization: REPLACE-2 randomized trial. JAMA 2004; 292:696–703.

96. Cohen DJ, Lincoff AM, Lavelle TA, et al. Economic evaluation of bivalirudin with provisional glycoprotein IIb/IIIa inhibition vs. heparin with routine glycoprotein IIb/IIIa inhibition for percutaneous coronary intervention: results from the REPLACE-2 trial. J Am Coll Cardiol 2004; 44:172–1800.

97. Mahaffey KW, Lewis BE, Wildermann NM, et al. The anticoagulant therapy with bivalirudin to assist in the performance of percutaneous coronary intervention in patients with heparin-induced thrombocytopenia (ATBAT) study: main results. J Invasive Cardiol 2003; 15:611–6.

98. ten Berg JM, Kelder JC, Suttorp MJ, Verheugt FW, Plokker HW. A randomized trial assessing the effect of coumarins started before coronary angioplasty on restenosis: results of the 6–month angiographic substudy of the Balloon Angioplasty and Anticoagulation Study (BAAS). Am Heart J 2003; 145:58–65.

99. Kastrati A, Mehilli J, Schuhlen H, et al. A clinical trial of abciximab in elective percutaneous coronary intervention after pretreatment with clopidogrel. N Engl J Med 2004; 350:232–8.

100. Dalby M, Montalescot G, Bal dit Sollier C, et al. Eptifibatide provides additional platelet inhibition in non-ST-elevation myocardial infarction patients already treated with aspirin and clopidogrel. Results of the platelet activity extinction in non-Q-wave myocardial infarction with aspirin, clopidogrel, and eptifibatide (PEACE) study. J Am Coll Cardiol 2004; 43:162–8.

101. Chan AW, Moliterno DJ, Berger PB, et al. Triple antiplatelet therapy during percutaneous coronary intervention is associated with improved outcomes including one-year survival: results from the Do Tirofiban and ReoProGive Similar Efficacy Outcome Trial (TARGET). J Am Coll Cardiol 2003; 42:1188–95.

102. Danzi GB, Sesana M, Capuano C, Mauri L, Berra Centurini P, Baglini R. Comparison in patients having primary coronary angioplasty of abciximab versus tirofiban on recovery of left ventricular function. Am J Cardiol 2004; 94:35–9.

103. Valgimigli M, Percoco G, Barbieri D, et al. The additive value of tirofiban administered with the high-dose bolus in the prevention of ischemic complications during high-risk coronary angioplasty; The advance trial. J Am Coll Cardiol 2004; 44:14–9.

104. Steinhubl SR, Berger PB, Mann JT, 3rd, et al. Early and sustained dual oral antiplatelet therapy following percutaneous coronary intervention: a randomized controlled trial. JAMA 2002; 288:2411–20.

105. Van Der Heijden DJ, Westendorp IC, Riezebos RK, et al. Lack of efficacy of clopidogrel pre-treatment in the prevention of myocardial damage after elective stent implantation. J Am Coll Cardiol 2004; 44:20–4.

106. Steinhubl SR, Talley JD, Braden GA, et al. Point-of-care measured platelet inhibition corre-lates with a reduced risk of an adverse cardiac event after percutaneous coronary intervention: results of the GOLD (AU-Assessing Ultegra) multicenter study. Circulation 2001; 103:2572–8.

107. Chen WH, Lee PY, Ng W, Tse HF, Lau CP. Aspirin resistance is associated with a high inci-dence of myonecrosis after non-urgent percutaneous coronary intervention despite clopido-grel pretreatment. J Am Coll Cardiol 2004; 43:1122–6.

108. Mehran R, Aymong ED, Ashby DT, et al. Safety of an aspirin-alone regimen after intracoro-nary stenting with a heparin-coated stent: final results of the HOPE (HEPACOAT and an Antithrombotic Regimen of Aspirin Alone) study. Circulation 2003; 108:1078–83.

109. Hirsh J, Warkentin TE, Raschke R, Granger C, Ohman EM, Dalen JE. Heparin and low-molecular-weight heparin: mechanisms of action, pharmacokinetics, dosing considerations, monitoring, efficacy, and safety. Chest 1998; 114:489S-510S.

110. Brill-Edwards P, Ginsberg JS, Johnston M, Hirsh J. Establishing a therapeutic range for hep-arin therapy. Ann Intern Med 1993; 119:104–9.

111. Menon V, Berkowitz SD, Antman EM, Fuchs RM, Hochman JS. New heparin dosing recom-mendations for patients with acute coronary syndromes. Am J Med 2001; 110:641–50.

112. Granger CB, Hirsh J, Califf RM, et al. Activated partial thromboplastin time and outcome after thrombolytic therapy for acute myocardial infarction: results from the GUSTO-I trial. Circulation 1996; 93:870–8.

113. Anand SS, Yusuf S, Pogue J, Ginsberg JS, Hirsh J. Relationship of activated partial thrombo-plastin time to coronary events and bleeding in patients with acute coronary syndromes who receive heparin. Circulation 2003; 107:2884–8.

114. Antman EM. Hirudin in acute myocardial infarction. Thrombolysis and Thrombin Inhibition in Myocardial Infarction (TIMI) 9B trial. Circulation 1996; 94:911–21.

115. Eikelboom JW, Anand SS, Malmberg K, Weitz JI, Ginsberg JS, Yusuf S. Unfractionated hep-arin and low-molecular-weight heparin in acute coronary syndrome without ST elevation: a meta-analysis. Lancet 2000; 355:1936–42.

116. Kaul S, Shah PK. Low molecular weight heparin in acute coronary syndrome: evidence for superior or equivalent efficacy compared with unfractionated heparin? J Am Coll Cardiol 2000; 35:1699–712.

117. Klein W, Buchwald A, Hillis WS, et al. Fragmin in unstable angina pectoris or in non-Q-wave acute myocardial infarction (the FRIC study). Fragmin in Unstable Coronary Artery Disease. Am J Cardiol 1997; 80:30E-34E.

118. FRAXIS Investigators. Comparison of two treatment durations (6 days and 14 days) of a low molecular weight heparin with a 6–day treatment of unfractionated heparin in the initial man-agement of unstable angina or non-Q wave myocardial infarction: FRAX.I.S. (FRAxiparine in Ischaemic Syndrome). Eur Heart J 1999; 20:1553–62.

119. The Thrombolysis in Myocardial Infarction (TIMI) 11A Trial Investigators. Dose-ranging trial of enoxaparin for unstable angina: results of TIMI 11A. J Am Coll Cardiol 1997; 29:1474–82.

120. Collet JP, Montalescot G, Golmard JL, al. e. Safety and efficacy of subcutaneous enoxaparin in early invasive strategy of unstable angina. J Am Coll Cardiol 2003; 41 (suppl A):68A.

121. Wallentin L, Goldstein P, Armstrong PW, et al. Efficacy and safety of tenecteplase in combination with the low-molecular-weight heparin enoxaparin or unfractionated heparin in the prehospital setting: the Assessment of the Safety and Efficacy of a New Thrombolytic Regimen (ASSENT)-3 PLUS randomized trial in acute myocardial infarction. Circulation 2003; 108:135–42.

122. Bijsterveld NR, Moons AH, Meijers JC, Levi M, Buller HR, Peters RJ. The impact on coagulation of an intravenous loading dose in addition to a subcutaneous regimen of low-molecular-weight heparin in the initial treatment of acute coronary syndromes. J Am Coll Cardiol 2003; 42:424–7.

123. Petersen JL, Mahaffey KW, Hasselblad V, et al. Efficacy and bleeding complications among patients randomized to enoxaparin or unfractionated heparin for antithrombin therapy in non-ST-Segment elevation acute coronary syndromes: a systematic overview. JAMA 2004; 292:89–96.

124. Spinler SA, Inverso SM, Cohen M, Goodman SG, Stringer KA, Antman EM. Safety and efficacy of unfractionated heparin versus enoxaparin in patients who are obese and patients with severe renal impairment: analysis from the ESSENCE and TIMI 11B studies. Am Heart J 2003; 146:33–41.

125. The Direct Thrombin Inhibitor Trialists' Collaborative Group. Direct thrombin inhibitors in acute coronary syndromes: principal results of a meta-analysis based on individual patients' data. Lancet 2002; 359:294–302.

126. White H. Thrombin-specific anticoagulation with bivalirudin versus heparin in patients receiving fibrinolytic therapy for acute myocardial infarction: the HERO-2 randomised trial. Lancet 2001; 358:1855–63.

127. Adams HP, Jr., Adams RJ, Brott T, et al. Guidelines for the early management of patients with ischemic stroke: A scientific statement from the Stroke Council of the American Stroke Association. Stroke 2003; 34:1056–83.

128. Coull BM, Williams LS, Goldstein LB, et al. Anticoagulants and antiplatelet agents in acute ischemic stroke: report of the Joint Stroke Guideline Development Committee of the American Academy of Neurology and the American Stroke Association (a division of the American Heart Association). Stroke 2002; 33:1934–42.

129. Lapchak PA, Araujo DM. Therapeutic Potential of Platelet Glycoprotein IIb/IIIa Receptor Antagonists in the Management of Ischemic Stroke. Am J Cardiovasc Drugs 2003; 3:87–94.

130. Medical Research Council . Thrombosis prevention trial: randomised trial of low-intensity oral anticoagulation with warfarin and low-dose aspirin in the primary prevention of ischaemic heart disease in men at increased risk. The Medical Research Council's General Practice Research Framework. Lancet 1998; 351:233–41.

131. Medical Research Council Group. Assessment of short-anticoagulant administration after cardiac infarction. Report of the Working Party on Anticoagulant Therapy in Coronary Thrombosis to the Medical Research Council. BMJ 1969; 1:335–42.

132. Ebert RV. Long-term anticoagulant therapy after myocardial infarction. Final report of the Veterans Administration cooperative study. JAMA 1969; 207:2263–7.

133. Drapkin A, Merskey C. Anticoagulant therapy after acute myocardial infarction. Relation of therapeutic benefit to patient's age, sex, and severity of infarction. JAMA 1972; 222:541–8.

134. Cairns JA, Hirsh J, Lewis HD, Jr., Resnekov L, Theroux P. Antithrombotic agents in coronary artery disease. Chest 1992; 102:456S-481S.

135. Goldberg RJ, Gore JM, Dalen JE, Alpert JS. Long-term anticoagulant therapy after acute myocardial infarction. Am Heart J 1985; 109:616–22.

136. Leizorovicz A, Boissel JP. Oral anticoagulant in patients surviving myocardial infarction. A new approach to old data. Eur J Clin Pharmacol 1983; 24:333–6.

137. Chalmers TC, Matta RJ, Smith H, Jr., Kunzler AM. Evidence favoring the use of anticoagulants in the hospital phase of acute myocardial infarction. N Engl J Med 1977; 297:1091–6.
138. Loeliger EA. Oral anticoagulation in patients surviving myocardial infarction. A new approach to old data. Eur J Clin Pharmacol 1984; 26:137–41.
139. Sixty Plus Reinfarction Study Group. A double-blind trial to assess long-term oral anticoagulant therapy in elderly patients after myocardial infarction. Report of the Sixty Plus Reinfarction Study Research Group. Lancet 1980; 2:989–94.
140. Smith P, Arnesen H, Holme I. The effect of warfarin on mortality and reinfarction after myocardial infarction. N Engl J Med 1990; 323:147–52.
141. ASPECT Research Group. Effect of long-term oral anticoagulant treatment on mortality and cardiovascular morbidity after myocardial infarction. Anticoagulants in the Secondary Prevention of Events in Coronary Thrombosis (ASPECT) Research Group. Lancet 1994; 343:499–503.
142. Witte K, Thackray S, Clark AL, Cooklin M, Cleland JG. Clinical trials update: IMPROVEMENT-HF, COPERNICUS, MUSTIC, ASPECT-II, APRICOT and HEART. Eur J Heart Fail 2000; 2:455–60.
143. Coletta AP, Cleland JG. Clinical trials update: highlights of the scientific sessions of the XXIII Congress of the European Society of Cardiology—WARIS II, ESCAMI, PAFAC, RITZ-1 and TIME. Eur J Heart Fail 2001; 3:747–50.
144. Coumadin Aspirin reinfaction Study (CARS) Investigators. Randomised double-blind trial of fixed low-dose warfarin with aspirin after myocardial infarction. Lancet 1997; 350:389–96.
145. Fiore LD, Ezekowitz MD, Brophy MT, Lu D, Sacco J, Peduzzi P. Department of Veterans Affairs Cooperative Studies Program Clinical Trial comparing combined warfarin and aspirin with aspirin alone in survivors of acute myocardial infarction: primary results of the CHAMP study. Circulation 2002; 105:557–63.
146. Hirsh J, Fuster V, Ansell J, Halperin JL. American Heart Association/American College of Cardiology Foundation guide to warfarin therapy. Circulation 2003; 107:1692–711.
147. Anand SS, Yusuf S. Oral anticoagulants in patients with coronary artery disease. J Am Coll Cardiol 2003; 41:62S-69S.
148. Anand SS, Yusuf S, Pogue J, Weitz JI, Flather M. Long-term oral anticoagulant therapy in patients with unstable angina or suspected non-Q-wave myocardial infarction: organization to assess strategies for ischemic syndromes (OASIS) pilot study results. Circulation 1998; 98:1064–70.
149. Cohen M, Adams PC, Parry G, et al. Combination antithrombotic therapy in unstable rest angina and non-Q-wave infarction in nonprior aspirin users. Primary end points analysis from the ATACS trial. Antithrombotic Therapy in Acute Coronary Syndromes Research Group. Circulation 1994; 89:81–8.
150. The Organization to Assess Strategies for Ischemic Syndromes (OASIS) Investigators. Effects of long-term, moderate-intensity oral anticoagulation in addition to aspirin in unstable angina. J Am Coll Cardiol 2001; 37:475–84.
151. Wallentin L, Wilcox RG, Weaver WD, et al. Oral ximelagatran for secondary prophylaxis after myocardial infarction: the ESTEEM randomised controlled trial. Lancet 2003; 362:789–97.
152. Kretschmer G, Wenzl E, Schemper M, et al. Influence of postoperative anticoagulant treatment on patient survival after femoropopliteal vein bypass surgery. Lancet 1988; 1:797–9.
153. Chesney CM, Elam MB, Herd JA, et al. Effect of niacin, warfarin, and antioxidant therapy on coagulation parameters in patients with peripheral arterial disease in the Arterial Disease Multiple Intervention Trial (ADMIT). Am Heart J 2000; 140:631–6.
154. Antiplatelet Trialists' Collaboration. Collaborative overview of randomised trials of antiplatelet therapy—I: Prevention of death, myocardial infarction, and stroke by prolonged antiplatelet therapy in various categories of patients. BMJ 1994; 308:81–106.

155. Antiplatelet Trialists' Collaboration. Collaborative overview of randomised trials of antiplatelet therapy—II: Maintenance of vascular graft or arterial patency by antiplatelet therapy. BMJ 1994; 308:159–68.

156. Antiplatelet Trialists' Collaboration. Collaborative overview of randomised trials of antiplatelet therapy—III: Reduction in venous thrombosis and pulmonary embolism by antiplatelet prophylaxis among surgical and medical patients. BMJ 1994; 308:235–46.

157. Antithrombotic Trialists' Collaboration. Collaborative meta-analysis of randomised trials of antiplatelet therapy for prevention of death, myocardial infarction, and stroke in high risk patients. BMJ 2002; 324:71–86.

158. Taylor DW, Barnett HJ, Haynes RB, et al. Low-dose and high-dose acetylsalicylic acid for patients undergoing carotid endarterectomy: a randomised controlled trial. ASA and Carotid Endarterectomy (ACE) Trial Collaborators. Lancet 1999; 353:2179–84.

159. Diener HC, Cunha L, Forbes C, Sivenius J, Smets P, Lowenthal A. European Stroke Prevention Study. 2. Dipyridamole and acetylsalicylic acid in the secondary prevention of stroke. J Neurol Sci 1996; 143:1–13.

160. Quinn MJ, Aronow HD, Califf RM, et al. Aspirin dose and six-month outcome after an acute coronary syndrome. J Am Coll Cardiol 2004; 43:972–8.

161. Patel TN, Goldberg KC. Use of aspirin and ibuprofen compared with aspirin alone and the risk of myocardial infarction. Arch Intern Med 2004; 164:852–6.

162. Rao GH, Johnson GG, Reddy KR, White JG. Ibuprofen protects platelet cyclooxygenase from irreversible inhibition by aspirin. Arteriosclerosis 1983; 3:383–8.

163. Dejana E, Cerletti C, de Gaetano G. Interaction of salicylate and other non-steroidal anti-inflammatory drugs with aspirin on platelet and vascular cyclo-oxygenase activity. Thromb Res Suppl 1983; 4:153–9.

164. Catella-Lawson F, Reilly MP, Kapoor SC, et al. Cyclooxygenase inhibitors and the antiplatelet effects of aspirin. N Engl J Med 2001; 345:1809–17.

165. Goldhaber SZ, Manson JE, Stampfer MJ, et al. Low-dose aspirin and subsequent peripheral arterial surgery in the Physicians' Health Study. Lancet 1992; 340:143–5.

166. Physicians' Health Study Research Group. Final report on the aspirin component of the ongoing Physicians' Health Study. Steering Committee of the Physicians' Health Study Research Group. N Engl J Med 1989; 321:129–35.

167. Ridker PM, Manson JE, Buring JE, Goldhaber SZ, Hennekens CH. The effect of chronic platelet inhibition with low-dose aspirin on atherosclerotic progression and acute thrombosis: clinical evidence from the Physicians' Health Study. Am Heart J 1991; 122:1588–92.

168. Gorelick PB, Richardson D, Kelly M, et al. Aspirin and ticlopidine for prevention of recurrent stroke in black patients: a randomized trial. JAMA 2003; 289:2947–57.

169. Eikelboom JW, Hankey GJ. Aspirin resistance: a new independent predictor of vascular events? J Am Coll Cardiol 2003; 41:966–8.

170. Patrono C. Aspirin resistance: definition, mechanisms and clinical read-outs. J Thromb Haemost 2003; 1:1710–3.

171. Eikelboom JW, Hirsh J, Weitz JI, Johnston M, Yi Q, Yusuf S. Aspirin-resistant thromboxane biosynthesis and the risk of myocardial infarction, stroke, or cardiovascular death in patients at high risk for cardiovascular events. Circulation 2002; 105:1650–5.

172. Gum PA, Kottke-Marchant K, Welsh PA, White J, Topol EJ. A prospective, blinded determination of the natural history of aspirin resistance among stable patients with cardiovascular disease. J Am Coll Cardiol 2003; 41:961–5.

173. Pulcinelli FM, Pignatelli P, Celestini A, Riondino S, Gazzaniga PP, Violi F. Inhibition of platelet aggregation by aspirin progressively decreases in long-term treated patients. J Am Coll Cardiol 2004; 43:979–84.

174. Gent M, Blakely JA, Easton JD, et al. The Canadian American Ticlopidine Study (CATS) in thromboembolic stroke. Lancet 1989; 1:1215–20.

175. Hass WK, Easton JD, Adams HP, Jr., et al. A randomized trial comparing ticlopidine hydrochloride with aspirin for the prevention of stroke in high-risk patients. Ticlopidine Aspirin Stroke Study Group. N Engl J Med 1989; 321:501–7.

176. Balsano F, Rizzon P, Violi F, et al. Antiplatelet treatment with ticlopidine in unstable angina. A controlled multicenter clinical trial. The Studio della Ticlopidina nell'Angina Instabile Group. Circulation 1990; 82:17–26.

177. CAPRIE Steering Committee. A randomised, blinded, trial of clopidogrel versus aspirin in patients at risk of ischaemic events (CAPRIE). Lancet 1996; 348:1329–39.

178. Bhatt DL, Chew DP, Hirsch AT, Ringleb PA, Hacke W, Topol EJ. Superiority of clopidogrel versus aspirin in patients with prior cardiac surgery. Circulation 2001; 103:363–8.

179. Bhatt DL, Marso SP, Hirsch AT, Ringleb PA, Hacke W, Topol EJ. Amplified benefit of clopidogrel versus aspirin in patients with diabetes 67) Becker RC, Cannon CP. Hirudin: Its Biology and Clinical Use. J Thromb Thrombolysis 1994; 1:7–16.

180. Ferguson J, Villareal RP, Massin EK. The effect of clopidogrel vs aspirin on recurrent clinical events and total vascular mortality: results from the CAPRIE study. J Am Coll Cardiol 2001; 37(2) Suppl A:336A.

181. CURE Study Investigators. Effects of clopidogrel in addition to aspirin in patients with non-ST segment elevation acute coronary syndromes. N Engl J Med 2001; 345:494–502.

182. Mehta SR, Yusuf S, Peters RJ, et al. Effects of pretreatment with clopidogrel and aspirin followed by long-term therapy in patients undergoing percutaneous coronary intervention: the PCI-CURE study. Lancet 2001; 358:527–33.

183. Peters RJ, Mehta SR, Fox KA, et al. Effects of aspirin dose when used alone or in combination with clopidogrel in patients with acute coronary syndromes: observations from the Clopidogrel in Unstable angina to prevent Recurrent Events (CURE) study. Circulation 2003; 108:1682–7.

184. Diener HC. Oral Presentation. 13th European Stroke Conference, Mannheim, Germany, 2004

185. Gurbel PA, Bliden KP, Hiatt BL, O'Connor CM. Clopidogrel for coronary stenting: response variability, drug resistance, and the effect of pretreatment platelet reactivity. Circulation 2003; 107:2908–13.

186. Matetzky S, Shenkman B, Guetta V, et al. Clopidogrel resistance is associated with increased risk of recurrent atherothrombotic events in patients with acute myocardial infarction. Circulation 2004; 109:3171–5.

187. Gurbel PA, Bliden KP, Hiatt BL. The early antiplatelet effects of clopidogrel loading for coronary stenting and the long-term stability of inhibition. J Thromb Haemost 2003; 1:1319–21.

188. Gurbel PA, Cummings CC, Bell CR, Alford AB, Meister AF, Serebruany VL. Onset and extent of platelet inhibition by clopidogrel loading in patients undergoing elective coronary stenting: the Plavix Reduction Of New Thrombus Occurrence (PRONTO) trial. Am Heart J 2003; 145:239–47.

189. Tcheng JE, Campbell ME. Platelet inhibition strategies in percutaneous coronary intervention: competition or coopetition? J Am Coll Cardiol 2003; 42:1196–8.

190. Lange RA, Hillis LD. Antiplatelet therapy for ischemic heart disease. N Engl J Med 2004; 350:277–80.

191. Khot UN, Nissen SE. Is CURE a cure for acute coronary syndromes? Statistical versus clinical significance. J Am Coll Cardiol 2002; 40:218–9.

192. Eriksson P. Long-term clopidogrel therapy after percutaneous coronary intervention in PCI-CURE and CREDO: the "Emperor's New Clothes" revisited. Eur Heart J 2004; 25:720–2.

193. O'Neill WW, Serruys P, Knudtson M, et al. Long-term treatment with a platelet glycoprotein-receptor antagonist after percutaneous coronary revascularization. EXCITE Trial Investigators. Evaluation of Oral Xemilofiban in Controlling Thrombotic Events. N Engl J Med 2000; 342:1316–24.

194. Cannon CP, McCabe CH, Wilcox RG, et al. Oral glycoprotein IIb/IIIa inhibition with orbofiban in patients with unstable coronary syndromes (OPUS-TIMI 16) trial. Circulation 2000; 102:149–56.

195. SYMPHONY Investigators. Comparison of sibrafiban with aspirin for prevention of cardiovascular events after acute coronary syndromes: a randomised trial. The SYMPHONY Investigators. Sibrafiban versus Aspirin to Yield Maximum Protection from Ischemic Heart Events Post-acute Coronary Syndromes. Lancet 2000; 355:337–45.

196. 2nd SYMPHONY Investigators. Randomized trial of aspirin, sibrafiban, or both for secondary prevention after acute coronary syndromes. Circulation 2001; 103:1727–33.

197. Topol EJ, Easton D, Harrington RA, et al. Randomized, double-blind, placebo-controlled, international trial of the oral IIb/IIIa antagonist lotrafiban in coronary and cerebrovascular disease. Circulation 2003; 108:399–406.

198. Chew DP, Bhatt DL, Sapp S, Topol EJ. Increased Mortality With Oral Platelet Glycoprotein IIb/IIIa Antagonists : A Meta-Analysis of Phase III Multicenter Randomized Trials. Circulation 2001; 103:201–206.

199. Leon MB, Baim DS, Popma JJ, et al. A clinical trial comparing three antithrombotic-drug regimens after coronary-artery stenting. Stent Anticoagulation Restenosis Study Investigators. N Engl J Med 1998; 339:1665–71.

200. Kastrati A, Schuhlen H, Hausleiter J, et al. Restenosis after coronary stent placement and randomization to a 4–week combined antiplatelet or anticoagulant therapy: six-month angiographic follow-up of the Intracoronary Stenting and Antithrombotic Regimen (ISAR) Trial. Circulation 1997; 96:462–7.

201. Urban P, Macaya C, Rupprecht HJ, et al. Randomized evaluation of anticoagulation versus antiplatelet therapy after coronary stent implantation in high-risk patients: the multicenter aspirin and ticlopidine trial after intracoronary stenting (MATTIS). Circulation 1998; 98:2126–32.

202. Bertrand ME, Legrand V, Boland J, et al. Randomized multicenter comparison of conventional anticoagulation versus antiplatelet therapy in unplanned and elective coronary stenting. The full anticoagulation versus aspirin and ticlopidine (FANTASTIC) study. Circulation 1998; 98:1597–603.

203. Zidar JP. Low-molecular-weight heparins in coronary stenting (the ENTICES trial). ENoxaparin and TIClopidine after Elective Stenting. Am J Cardiol 1998; 82:29L-32L.

204. Batchelor WB, Mahaffey KW, Berger PB, et al. A randomized, placebo-controlled trial of enoxaparin after high-risk coronary stenting: the ATLAST trial. J Am Coll Cardiol 2001; 38:1608–13.

205. Berger PB, Bell MR, Hasdai D, Grill DE, Melby S, Holmes DR, Jr. Safety and efficacy of ticlopidine for only 2 weeks after successful intracoronary stent placement. Circulation 1999; 99:248–53.

206. Berger PB, Mahaffey KW, Meier SJ, et al. Safety and efficacy of only 2 weeks of ticlopidine therapy in patients at increased risk of coronary stent thrombosis: results from the Antiplatelet Therapy alone versus Lovenox plus Antiplatelet therapy in patients at increased risk of Stent Thrombosis (ATLAST) trial. Am Heart J 2002; 143:841–6.

207. Bertrand ME, Rupprecht HJ, Urban P, Gershlick AH, Investigators FT. Double-blind study of the safety of clopidogrel with and without a loading dose in combination with aspirin compared with ticlopidine in combination with aspirin after coronary stenting : the clopidogrel aspirin stent international cooperative study (CLASSICS). Circulation 2000; 102:624–9.

208. Waksman R, Ajani AE, White RL, et al. Prolonged antiplatelet therapy to prevent late thrombosis after intracoronary gamma-radiation in patients with in-stent restenosis: Washington Radiation for In-Stent Restenosis Trial plus 6 months of clopidogrel (WRIST PLUS). Circulation 2001; 103:2332–5.

209. Waksman R, Ajani AE, Pinnow E, et al. Twelve versus six months of clopidogrel to reduce major cardiac events in patients undergoing gamma-radiation therapy for in-stent restenosis: Washington Radiation for In-Stent restenosis Trial (WRIST) 12 versus WRIST PLUS. Circulation 2002; 106:776–8.

210. CYPHER Stent (Johnson and Johnson) Package Insert.

211. TAXUS Stent (Boston Scientific) Package Insert.

19-1

Large Simple Trials in Thrombocardiology

Michael E. Farkouh and Eve Aymong
New York University School of Medicine and the Cardiovascular Research Foundation, New York, New York, U.S.A.
Marcus Flather
The Royal Brompton Hospital, London, England

I. INTRODUCTION

The advent of the megatrial in cardiology has led to the development of important therapies to reduce mortality and morbidity from myocardial infarction and other acute coronary syndromes. This chapter summarizes the methodology that has laid the groundwork for the landmark trials in the field. The most important developments in the field of ACS have emerged from large simple trials (LSTs) that were specifically designed and powered to assess moderate differences in mortality (1).

II. HISTORY OF THE LARGE SIMPLE TRIAL CONCEPT IN THROMBOCARDIOLOGY

The advent of the LST in thrombocardiology has its roots at Oxford University. When the question of beta-blockers in the early treatment of acute Ml arose in the ISIS 1 trial, Salim Yusuf, Richard Peto, and Peter Sleight devised a methodology that gave birth to the multicenter LST in the field of acute myocardial infarction (M). This allowed for a trial that was adequately powered to detect moderate differences in mortality between treatment strategies. From ISIS 1 forward, the LST, or megatrial concept, became the gold standard for evaluating therapies in thrombocardiology.

III. ADVANTAGES OF LSTs OVER META-ANALYSIS OF MULTIPLE SMALLER TRIALS

Many have argued that a meta-analysis of multiple smaller randomized controlled trials (RCTs) may provide robust evidence for addressing a given question when compared to expensive LSTs, which may take many years to perform reliably. When results of trials are inconsistent, or inadequately powered, meta-analysis is a technique that helps to summarize the totality of the evidence. Over the past decade or so, we have seen examples where the results of meta-analysis disagree with the findings of subsequent LSTs (2–17).

What we have learned is that when meta-analyses are conducted as systematic overviews where the meta-analyst has complete data sets on all patients studied in all trials, the data appear to be reliable. Like LSTs, meta-analyses need to be sufficiently powered to be able to detect important differences between the experimental and control groups.

LeLorier et al. searched the leading general medical journals for instances in which there were both a meta-analysis and a LST of >1000 patients (18). What they found was that for 12 LSTs and 19 meta-analyses, there were no examples where the direction of treatment effect differed; however, the agreement on the degree of benefit was classified as only fair.

The credibility of meta-analyses of smaller RCTs has come into question. There are numerous examples in acute (AMI) where the efficacy of a therapy has been first addressed by a meta-analysis of multiple small trials followed by a LST. This arises from the inability of a meta-analysis to give a single value of benefit complete with confidence intervals around the estimate. At best it can estimate the direction of treatment effect and reconcile differences between trials when the results are disparate. The meta-analysis can generate a hypothesis, but alone it does not lead to changes in policy or practice.

IV. ADVANTAGES OF LSTs OVER META-ANALYSIS OF MULTIPLE SMALLER RCTs

The advantages of LSTs include:

1. Reduced likelihood of publication bias
2. Elimination of meta-analyst bias
3. Single protocol versus multiple protocols—reduction in heterogeneity
4. Reliable estimate of degree of benefit—can determine relative risk reduction and number needed to treat

Pogue and Yusuf formulated an organizational strategy that would help to maximize the utility of the LST concept (19). They suggested that in conducting meta-analyses, investigators should strive for the same methodological standards applied to LSTs (e.g., a prespecified protocol, sample size estimates, and formal interim monitoring).

V. LARGE SIMPLE TRIAL CONCEPTS

A. LST Organization

LSTs are sponsored either by industry, government/charitable funds, or both. Traditionally the structure revolves around a steering committee, which is composed of leaders in the field. The study chair oversees the meetings of the steering committee and is the individual most likely to present the prinicipal findings and final results to the scientific community.

The following section summarize the roles of all study personnel (see Fig. 2).

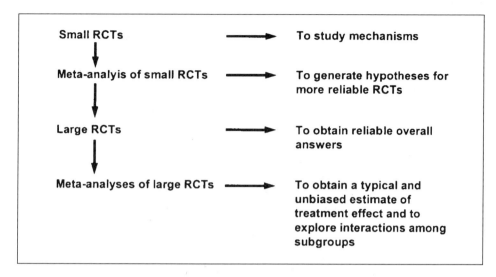

Figure 1 Complementary roles of RCIs and meta-analyses.

1. Principal Investigator/Study Chairman

The principal investigator has overall responsibility to insure that the trial is conducted successfully and with integrity. He or she oversees all study administration committees and specifically chairs the steering committee and the executive committee.

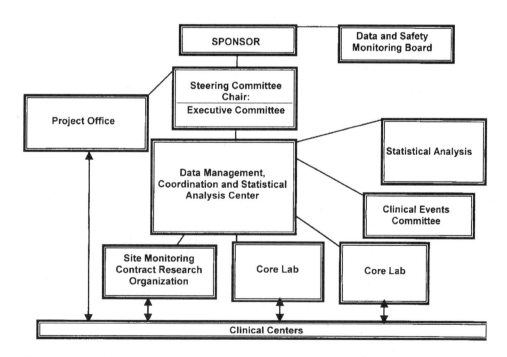

Figure 2 Administrative structure of the trial study group.

2. Sponsor

The sponsor has observer representation on the steering committee (one ex officio member without voting rights). Sponsors usually have no role on any other committee and do not have access to study data. Traditionally they do not participate in any aspect of data analysis or manuscript publications.

3. Steering Committee

This is the governing body of the study and will be composed of academic leaders from the international cardiovascular community. The sponsor will have one ex officio representative with or without voting rights. The steering committee meets frequently during start-up and at least twice annually thereafter. The chairman or one third of the members may call a steering committee meeting. The committee convenes when half of the appointed members are present, and decisions are taken by simple majority of the present members.

   The publications committee is appointed by the Steering Committee and will formulate publication policy for this collaborative research trial and review all abstracts, papers, and scientific presentations utilizing study data. This committee will be responsible for identifying topics for publication, making writing group assignments, as well as reviewing and recommending approval or disapproval of all scientific abstracts, papers, or presentations using unpublished study data, as well as every paper using published data that purports to represent official study views or policy. Another major responsibility of this committee is the development of plans for the dissemination of trial findings and incorporation of the findings into medical care policy. This will involve not only reports in medical journals but consideration of continuing education courses, conferences and seminars, and special efforts such as press conferences, editorials, physician newsletters, and presentations at local medical association meetings.

4. Executive Committee

This committee is usually comprised of about five steering committee members, including the study chairman, who meet on a weekly basis to discuss operational issues of the study. Members of the executive committee are called upon by the project officer to address questions related to the clinical protocol in the areas of their expertise. The executive committee reports directly to the steering committee.

5. Data Safety Monitoring Board

The data safety and monitoring board (DSMB) is usually composed of nine members (eight physicians and one biostatistician), appointed by the study sponsor (as in the case of the NHLBI) or the steering committee, who are not involved in the conduct of the trial and have no affiliation with the sponsor. The DSMB ensures the integrity of the study and the data generated as well as the safety of all patients. The DSMB meets before trial initiation and determines how often to meet. Often it will meet twice annually through study enrollment and primary endpoint follow-up and annually thereafter until study completion. The DSMB is informed immediately of all serious adverse events by the data management, coordination, and statistical analysis center. The DSMB periodically reviews clinical events and may request additional information, as needed. In many cases, scheduled interim analysis is performed according to the wishes of the DSMB, often when about one half of the enrollment is completed; such analysis is then supplied to the DSMB for review. The DSMB is supplied major endpoint data blinded to the treatment group. Based on interim analysis or safety data, the DSMB may recommend that the steering Committee modify or stop the trial. All final decisions regarding trial modifications reside within the study sponsor or the steering committee, depending on whether it is an NHLBI study.

6. *Clinical Events Committee*

The steering committee and the DSMB work together to determine the adverse events that need to be reviewed by the clinical events committee (CEC). All major adverse events are adjudicated by the (CEC). The CEC will often consist of up to seven physicians who are not directly involved in the conduct of the trial and have no affiliation with the sponsor. CEC members must have clinical expertise in clinical cardiology and its associated subspecialties, according to the nature of the trial. The CEC meets twice annually during study enrollment and primary endpoint follow-up and annually thereafter until study completion, or more frequently if deemed necessary by the DSMB. The CEC must establish and enforce explicit rules outlining the minimum amount of data required and the definitions followed in order to classify a clinical event. CEC members agree to preserve confidentiality of study information and recognize that only the DSMB may draw conclusions regarding the results of their adjudication. The CEC is responsible for determining whether reported adverse events meet the criteria for primary or secondary safety and efficacy endpoints.

7. *Project Office*

All clinical queries are directed to a central project office. The project office functions as the liaison between the clinical sites and the executive committee and is directed by a project officer.

The project officer oversees the daily conduct of the trial and reports directly to the executive committee. The project officer is assisted by one or two main study coordinators, who are in direct contact with the local study coordinators at the clinical centers. The project office coordinators advise and guide the local study coordinators and answer study-related and protocol questions. The project officer answers all questions related to medical issues and coordinates communication between the clinical investigators and the executive committee.

8. *Data Management Center*

The data management center (DMC) performs all data management functions for the trial. It will employ a combination of clinical, analytical, and information systems personnel with expertise in the coordination of large-scale, multicenter trials. It uses a centralized data management system to assure data integrity, confidentiality, and validity. Case report form data are mailed, faxed, and/or electronically transferred to the DMC from the clinical centers and transformed into an electronic database using highly trained data entry and data management personnel. Statistical analyses are performed only at the DMC.

B. Interpretation of LST Results

The measures of clinical benefit are:

Absolute risk reduction (ARR) is the difference in the event rate between the control group (CER) and the treated group (ER): ARR = CER − ER

Relative risk reduction (RRR) is the percent reduction in events in the treated group event rate (ER) compared to the control group event rate (CER): RRR = (CER − ER)/CER × 100

Number needed to treat (NNT) is the number of patients who need to be treated to prevent one bad outcome. It is the inverse of the ARR: NNT = 1/ARR.

In each of the examples in Table 1, the relative risk reduction (RRR) is 20%. However, the number needed to treat varies greatly, from 10 to 330, based on the mortality rates and absolute risk reductions. This emphasizes the important difference in RRR and ARR and its clinical impact (measured as NNT) on intervention. This is discussed in further detail below.

C. Hypothesis Testing

In the current era of active controlled trials, the analysis may be unique in that superiority and "clinical equivalence" (including noninferiority comparisons) are both possible important conclusions of any study. Thus, after stating the primary hypothesis test, the interpretation of the findings under different possible outcomes may be described. A hypothetical study assesses the effectiveness of antithrombotic regimen A (a new compound) versus antithrombotic regimen B (the usual care agent). The following hypothesis will be tested for the 30-day survival rate:

Ho: pA = pB

H1: pA π pB

where pA is the 30-day mortality rate (percentage) for antithrombotic regimen A and pB is the 30-day mortality rate for the antithrombotic regimen B patients.

This is tested at the usual 0.05 significance level with a two-sided test. The outcome is presented as a two-sided 95% confidence interval (CI) for the treatment difference, here defined in the order pA – pB. A priori the investigators declared that if the two rates were within 2.5% of each other they were clinically close enough that other factors might be determinative in the choice of therapy; the other factors might include patient preference for one or the other agent, presumed trade-offs in other endpoints, and costs. For this reason if the difference was £2.5%, the two will here be called clinically equivalent. While recognizing the arbitrariness of this equivalence margin, the data will be presented so that others may assess results according to their own clinical equivalence standards. The importance of prespecifying such a margin is clear.

The 30-day survival difference is represented by the difference in the point estimates for the two mortality proportions as well as a 95% CI for the difference. The range of possible values with 95% confidence for this difference is denoted by D; that is, D is the 95% CI for the difference. If D is less than –2.5%, then antithrombotic regimen A would be

Table 1 Measures of Clinical Benefit

30-day Mortality	Control Antithrombotic Regimen B	Treatment Antithrombotic Regimen A	Relative Risk Reduction (RRR)	Number Needed to Treat (NNT)
In actual trial	15%	12%	15–12/15 = 20%	100/3 = 33
High, mortality, hypothetical	50%	40%	50–40/50= 20%	100/10 = 10
Low, mortality, hypothetical	1.5%	1.2%	1.5–1.2/1.5 = 20%	100/0.3 = 330

superior in a clinically important manner. If D has values greater than or equal to -2.5% but all values are less than 0, then antithrombotic regimen A would be superior but not necessarily in a clinically important manner (i.e., it is declared clinically equivalent). If D contains zero, then the two treatments have not been shown to differ in outcome (for detailed discussion, see Fig. 3). If D is entirely greater than zero but has some values less than or equal to 2.5%, then antithrombotic regimen B is superior but not in a clinically important manner. If D is entirely greater than 2.5%, then antithrombotic regimen B is clinically superior to antithrombotic regimen A. From this logic there are 10 possible outcomes (ignoring an exact value of zero for brevity) for the 95% CI of the difference.

D. Sample Size Calculation

Because Antithrombotic Regimen A may be preferable if there is clinical equivalence, the trial is powered for a 2.5% increase in mortality from the Antithrombotic Regimen B rate when using Antithrombotic Regimen A. If the 30-day mortality rate for the usual care arm, antithrombotic regimen B, is 15%, various combinations of event rates per group and the respective power calculations are as shown in Table 2.

Thus, the precision of the estimated differences should allow reasonable evaluation of the possibility of clinical equivalence if the two therapies are identical for the primary 30-day survival outcome of this trial.

E. Intent-to-Treat Analysis

The primary analysis is almost always based on the intent-to-treat principle. All randomized patients are included in the intent-to-treat population. All patients are analyzed in the treatment group to which they were randomized, regardless of whether they actually

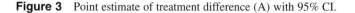

Figure 3 Point estimate of treatment difference (A) with 95% CI.

Table 2 Sample Size Estimates of Acute MI Trial Comparing Antithrombotic Regimen B with Antithrombotic Regimen A

Power (%)	α	Antithrombotic regimen B, 30-day mortality (%)	Antithrombotic regimen A, 30-day mortality (%)	Dikfference (%)	N/Gropup N/Group	Total sample size
80	0.05	12.00	14.50	2.50	2965	5930
80	0.05	13.00	15.50	2.50	3147	6294
80	0.05	14.00	16.50	2.50	3324	6648
80	0.05	15.00	17.50	2.50	3496	6992
80	0.05	16.00	18.50	2.50	3664	7328
80	0.05	17.00	19.50	2.50	3826	7652
80	0.05	18.00	20.50	2.50	3983	7966
80	0.05	19.00	21.50	2.50	4134	8268
80	0.05	20.00	22.50	2.50	4281	8562

received the treatment. Secondary analyses may be used to check whether results may have been biased by failure to perform the allocated treatment.

F. Primary Endpoint

The primary endpoint for this study is the differencc in the 30-day survival rate. The 30-day survival rates for the antithrombotic regimen A and B arms will be presented along with the estimated treatment difference and the two-sided 95% CI of the treatment difference. If a proportional hazards model is clearly violated, which would imply that the therapies differ over time in a nonproportional manner, then the interpretation is complex, and this will be commented upon in the analysis.

VI. EXAMPLES OF LSTS

Tables 3 and 4 summarize the important trials in an evidence-based approach, with summary statistics including number needed to treat.

A. Mortality-Powered Trials in Acute MI–Fibrinolytic Therapy

The management of AMI was altered dramatically with the ISIS-2 trial. A total of 17,187 patients were randomly assigned within 24 hours after the onset of suspected acute myocardial infarction to one of four regimens: placebo infusion and placebo tablets (i.e., routine hospital care); placebo infusion and 162.5 mg of aspirin daily for one month (aspirin only); an infusion of 1.5 million units of streptokinase over a one-hour period and placebo tablets (streptokinase only); or both streptokinase and aspirin (1).

The major issue revolving around the results of LSTs is the distinction between relative and absolute measures of clinical benefit. RRR can be misleading; if both the ARR and the CER are reduced 100-fold between two subgroups (high risk vs. low risk) (see Table 1), the RRR would theoretically remain unchanged. When comparing therapeutic efficacy in mortality: powered trials it is essential to understand this limitation since the absolute and not the relative benefit will be largely used to decide upon whether to change

Table 3 Acute MI LSTs

Trial (Ref.)	Outcome	Treatment	Control	NNT
ISIS 2, 1988 (21) Aspirin and streptoki-nase vs. usual care	35-day vascular mortality	343/4292 8%	568/4300 13%	20
ISIS 3, 1992 (24) Alteplase vs. streptoki-nase	35-day vascular mortality	1418/13,746 10.3%	1455/13,780 10.6%	NS
GUSTO 1, 1993 (25) Alteplase vs. streptok-inase	Mortality at 30 days	/10,344 6.3%	/20,173 7.3%	100
GUSTO 3, 1997 (26) Reteplase vs. alteplase	Mortality at 30 days	/10138 7.47%	/4921 7.24% P = NS	NS
GUSTO 5, 2001 (27) Abciximab and reteplase reteplase alone	Mortality at 30 days	468/8328 (5.6%)	488/8260 (5.9%)	NS

NS = differences not statistically significant.

therapy. In ISIS-2 there was a consistent relative benefit of aspirin and streptokinase across various prespecified subgroups, but the NNTs to prevent one death were lowest in patients at highest baseline risk (21).

B. Multiple Endpoint LSTs in ACS–Antithrombotic Therapy

The CURE trial evaluated the role of adding clopidogrel to aspirin in the short and long term for high-risk patients and followed patients for 1 year.

Table 4 ACS LSTs

Trial (Ref.)	Outcome	Treatment	Control	NNT
Cure, 2001 (28) N = 12,562 Clopidogrel vs. placebo	CV death, stroke, and nonfatal MI at 1 year Major bleeding at 1 year	582/6259 (9.3%) 3.7%	719/6303 (11.4%) P = S 2.7% P = S	48 100
ESSENCE, 1997 (29) N = 3171 Enoxaparin vs. unfrac-tionated heparin	Death/MI at 30 days Major bleeding at 30 days	6.2% 102/1607 (6.5%)	7.7% P = 0.08 107/1564 (7.0%) P = NS	NS
PRISM-PLUS, 1998 (30) Tirofiban vs. Placebo	Death or MI at 30 days	67/73 8.7%	95/797 11.9% P = S	31
PURSUIT, 1998 (31)	Death or MI at 30 days	/4722 14.2%	/4739 15.7%	67
GUSTO IV, 2001 (32)	Death or MI at 30 days	450/5202 9.1%	209/2598 8.0% P = NS	NS

NS = differences not statistically significant.

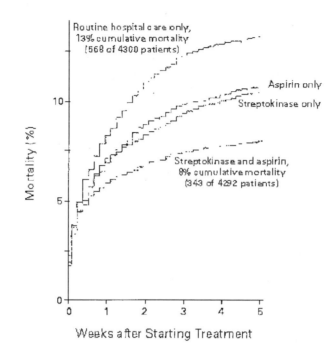

Figure 4   Cumulative mortality from vascular causes up to day 35 in the ISIS-2 trial.

The results of these ACS studies demonstrate differences in MI rates with little or no change in short-term mortality with the newer antiplatelet and antithrombotic regimens. It is important to emphasize the importance of including reliable measures of morbidity in LSTs since mortality-powered trials in ACS may not be feasible given the relatively low observed mortality.

The advent of the LST has led to many important advances in thrombocardiology by providing robust estimates of the efficacy of new therapies in AMI, and new questions have emerged from analysis of the data. An approach to interpreting LSTs is essential for cardiovascular specialists who rely on the findings of LSTs to guide their clinical decision making.

REFERENCES

1. Yusuf S, Collins R, Peto R. Why do we need some large, simple randomized trials? Stat Med 1984; 3:971–980.
2. DerSimonian, R., Levine, R. J. (1999). Resolving discrepancies between a meta-analysis and a subsequent large controlled trial. JAMA 282: 664–670.
3. LeLorier, J., Gregoire, G., Ioannidis, J. P. A., Cappelleri, J. C., Lau, J. (1998). Comparing results from meta-analyses vs large trials. JAMA 280: 518–519.
4. Ioannidis, J. P. A., Cappelleri, J. C., Lau, J. (1998). Issues in comparisons between meta-analyses and large trials. JAMA 279: 1089–1093.
5. Bailar, J. C. (1997). The promise and problems of meta-analysis. N Engl J Med 337: 559–561.
6. Ioannidis, J. P. A., Cappelleri, J. C., Lau, J., Bent, S., Kerlikowske, K., Grady, D., Song, F.-J., Sheldon, T. A., Khan, S., Williamson, P., Sutton, R., Stewart, L. A., Parmar, M. K. B., Tierney, J. F., Sim, I., Lavori, P., Imperiale, T. F., LeLorier, J., Gregoire, G., Bailar, J. C. (1998). Meta-analyses and large randomized, controlled trials. N Engl J Med 338: 59–62.

7. Hennekens CH, Albert CM, Godfried SL, Gaziano JM, Buring JE. Adjunctive drug therapy of acute myocardial infarction: evidence from clinical trials. N Engl J Med. 1996; 335:1660–1667.

8. Antman EM, Lau J, Kupelnick B, Mosteller F, Chalmers TC. A comparison of results of meta-analyses of randomized control trials and recommendations of clinical experts: treatments for myocardial infarction. JAMA. 1992; 268:240–248.

9. Greenland S. A meta-analysis of coffee, myocardial infarction, and coronory death. Epidemiology. 1993; 4:366–374.

10. Thompson SG, Pocock SJ. Can meta-analyses be trusted? Lancet. 1991; 338:1127–1130.

11. Mosteller F, Chalmers TC. Some progress and problems in meta-analysis of clinical trials. Stat Sci. 1992; 7:227–236.

12. Hasselblad V, Mosteller F, Littenberg B, et al. A survey of current problems in meta-analysis: discussion from the Agency for Health Care Policy and Research inter-PORT Work Group on Literature Review/Meta-Analysis. Med Care. 1995; 33:202–220.

13. Cappelleri JC, Ioannidis JP, Schmid CH, et al. Large trials vs meta-analysis of smaller trials: how do their results compare? JAMA. 1996; 276:1332–1338.

14. Woods KL, Fletcher S. Long-term outcome after intravenous magnesium sulphate in suspected acute myocardial infarction: the second Leicester Intravenous Magnesium Intervention Trial (LIMIT-2). Lancet. 1994; 343:816–819.

15. Imperiale TF, Petrulis AS. A meta-analysis of low-dose aspirin for the prevention of pregnancy-induced hypertensive disease. JAMA. 1991; 266:260–264.

16. Bailar JC. Meta-analyses and large randomized, controlled clinical trials. N Engl J Med. 1998; 338:62.

17. Cappelleri JC, Lau J. Issues in comparisons between meta-analyses and large trials. JAMA. 1998; 279:1089–1093.

18. LeLorier J, Gregoire G, Benhaddad A, Lapierre J, Derderian F. Discrepancies between meta-analyses and subsequent large randomized, controlled trials. N Engl J Med. 1997; 337:536–542.

19. Pogue J, Yusuf S. Overcoming the limitations of current meta-analysis of randomised controlled trials. Lancet 1998; 351:47–52.

20. Gruppo Italiano per lo Studio della Streptochinasi nell'infarcto miocardico (GISSI). Effectiveness of intravenous thrombolytic treatment in acute myocardial infarction. Lancet 1986; i:397–402.

21. ISIS-2 Collaborative Group. Randomised trial of intravenous streptokinase, oral aspirin, both, or neither among 17187 cases of suspected acute myocardial infarction: ISIS-2. Lancet 1988; ii:349–360.

22. Fibrinolytic Therapy Trialist (FTT) Collaborative Group. Indications for fibrinolytic therapy in suspected myocardial infarction: collaborative overview of early mortality and major morbidity results from all randomised trials of more than 1000 patients. Lancet 1994; 343:311–322.

23. Gruppo Italiano per Io Studio della Sopravvivenza nell'Infarto Miocardico. GISSI-2: a factorial randomised trial of alteplase versus streptokinase and heparin versus no heparin among 12 490 patients with acute myocardial infarction. Lancet 1990; 336:65–71.

24. ISIS-3 (Third International Study of Infarct Survival) Collaborative Group. ISIS-3: a randomised comparison of streptokinase vs tissue plasminogen activator vs anistreplase and of aspirin plus heparin vs aspirin alone among 41 299 cases of suspected acute myocardial infarction. Lancet 1992;339:753–770.

25. The GUSTO Investigators. An international randomized trial comparing four thrombolytic strategies for acute myocardial infarction. N Engl J Med 1993; 329:673–682.

26. The GUSTO-III Investigators. An international, multicenter, randomized comparison of reteplase with alteplase for acute myocardial infarction. N Engl J Med 1997; 337:1118–1123.

27. The GUSTO V Investigators. Reperfusion therapy for acute myocardial infarction with fibrinolytic therapy or combination reduced fibrinolytic therapy and platelet glycoprotein IIb/IIIa inhibition: the GUSTO V randomized trial. Lancet 2001; 357:1905–1914.

28. The Clopidogrel in Unstable Angina to Prevent Recurrent Events Trial Investigators. Effects of clopidogrel in addition to aspirin in patients with acute coronary syndromes without ST-segment elevation. N Engl J Med. 2001; 345:494–502.

29. Cohen M, Demers C, Gurfinkel EP et al. for the The Efficacy and Safety of Subcutaneous Enoxaparin in Non-Q-Wave Coronary Events Study Group. A comparison of low-molecular-weight heparin with unfractionated heparin for unstable coronary artery disease. N Engl J Med 1997; 337:447–452.

30. PRISM-PLUS Study Investigators. Inhibition of the platelet glycoprotein IIb/IIIa receptor with tirofiban in unstable angina and non-Q-wave myocardial infarction: Platelet Receptor Inhibition in Ischemic Syndrome Management in Patients Limited by Unstable Signs and Symptoms (PRISM-PLUS) Study Investigators. N Engl J Med. 1998; 338:1488–1497.

31. PURSUIT Trial Investigators. Inhibition of platelet glycoprotein IIb/IIIa with eptifibatide in patients with acute coronary syndromes. N Engl J Med. 1998; 339:436–443.

32. GUSTO IV-ACS Investigators. Effect of glycoprotein IIb/IIIa receptor blocker abciximab on outcome in patients with acute coronary syndromes without early coronary revascularisation: the GUSTO IV-ACS randomised trial. Lancet. 2001; 357:1899–1900.

19-2

Clinical Research Design: From Observational Research to Clinical Trials

Eve Aymong, George Danges, Dale Ashby, and Roxana Mehran
New York University School of Medicine and the Cardiovascular Research Foundation, New York, New York, U.S.A.

Clinical research is performed in an attempt to learn about the effects of a phenomenon in a specific population under study and extrapolate that knowledge to the truth of its effect in nature. For practical reasons, a sample of the entire population is chosen to represent the larger population of interest. In other words, the sample is chosen in a way that the results can be generalized to the larger population. This goal can be accomplished with techniques such as observational studies (cohort and crossover designs) as well as clinical trials involving an intervention, especially randomized trials with their variations and complexities.

I. OBSERVATIONAL STUDIES

In general, observational studies are conducted "passively", i.e., patients do not receive intervention of any sort, be it a screening test or investigational treatment. They can be used to describe the incidence and/or prevalence of various prognostic indicators, risk factors, and outcomes as well as to analyze associations between predictors and outcomes. They can also be used to describe the natural history of the disease. Often they are used to explore the lay of the land and provide the basis for more rigorous investigations, i.e., they are hypothesis generating.

A. The Cohort Study

Cohort studies are conducted by selecting a group of subjects, measuring baseline characteristics, and following them over time to establish the occurrence of subsequent outcomes (1,2) (Table 1). They can be either prospective or retrospective in timing. In prospective studies, in which patients are identified before the study starts, baseline measures are obtained before any outcomes have occurred. In retrospective studies the study subjects are identified at a past time point, after which the investigator records the desired predictors and outcomes as they occurred in the past.

1. Prospective Cohort Studies

This is an excellent strategy for defining the incidence and potential causes of a condition or event. Because of the prospective nature, risk factors are measured before an event; this time sequence can strengthen the inference that a factor may cause an outcome (3). It is

Table 1   Important Characteristics of Cohort Studies

Study sample
   Appropriate for question
   Available for follow-up—minimize loss of subjects by collecting detailed, extensive contact
   information
   Generalizable to the population of interest
Measurements
   Standardize assessments (minimize measurement bias)
   Blink assessment of outcomes
   Precise, accurate, and complete measurement of:
      Baseline demographics
      Clinical characteristics
      Outcomes
      Potential confounders
Time sequence
   Prospective design may be stronger than retrospective
      Better able to establish timing
      Suggest causality
      Less able to identify confounders
      Less efficient

essential that the factors of interest as well as possible confounders be measured accurately. They are ideally used to assess outcomes that are adequately frequent.

The Framingham Study is perhaps the classic example of a prospective observational cohort study that has been used to identify many important risk factors for the development of coronary artery disease (4). Over 50 years, this geographically defined cohort has been used to develop insights into some of the seminal associations of cardiovascular disease with diabetes, high cholesterol, and hypertension and also to develop and validate clinical risk factor profiles for the above conditions (Fig. 1).

This design is also used for the evaluation of *future* outcomes after an event, e.g., post–myocardial infarction, or after an intervention, e.g., post–coronary revascularization. An interesting example of this is the inverse relationship of alcohol consumption and cardiovascular mortality. Multiple studies have observed an inverse or U-shaped association between wine consumption and overall morbidity and mortality (5–7). However, alcohol may have myocardial depressant features in patients with existing cardiovascular disease and could be considered potentially harmful for patients with decreased heart function. In order to study this possible deleterious effect, deLorgeril and colleagues in France identified a group of patients with acute myocardial infarction and studied them prospectively (8). In this cohort with recent myocardial infarction, they demonstrated a persistent protective effect of moderate alcohol consumption.

2. Retrospective Cohort Studies

This study design takes a cohort of subjects and looks to the past to obtain measurements of predictors and subsequent outcomes. In the year 2000, the European Society of Cardiology and the American College of Cardiology recommended the adoption of new diagnostic criteria for acute myocardial infarction (MI) using specific serum markers of myocardial damage, specifically serum troponin. In order to examine the impact of this change on incidence, management, and outcome, Pell et al. retrospectively identified a cohort of 2637 patients admitted between 1997 and 2000 with a diag-

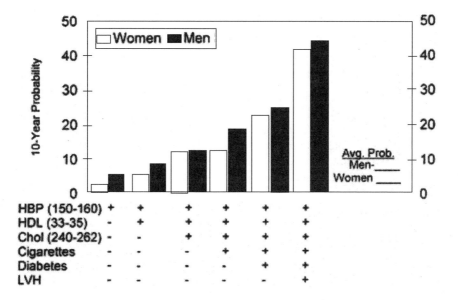

Figure 1 Risk factors for cardiovascular disease among patients with other conditions from the Framingham Study.

nosis of acute MI or chest pain with elevated troponin; 966 of these patients did not meet previous criteria for acute MI (9). They demonstrated significantly worse early and 1-year survival in these newly defined patients with acute MI when their outcomes were compared with the original cohort. This is an important observation, especially given that mortality rates are often used to assess the impact of treatment over time. In this case, the inclusion of patients who meet the new definition for acute MI may make the overall mortality rate of acute MI patients increase, and it may appear that the overall treatment of MI is less effective.

The biggest advantage of the retrospective design is that it is relatively inexpensive and much less time consuming than a prospective design. The obvious disadvantages of such a design are the difficulty in choosing a representative cohort to study and the potential for incomplete measurement of important data—in the preceding example, incomplete measurement of serum troponin. Using this design, the outcomes may already be recorded in a file or ongoing database system that is independent of the study. Alternatively, they may be tracked down by review of records or patient/family contact specifically organized by the investigators.

B. Case-Control Studies

Case-control studies identify one group of subjects with the outcome of interest and attempt to select an appropriate group for comparison without it. They then look back in time to identify the incidence of one or more specific predictors that may be different between the two groups. They are especially efficient in looking at outcomes that are relatively rare. They are also relatively inexpensive and fast to perform. The biggest problem is the large likelihood of sampling bias, i.e., for not having a representative sample of the larger population of interest. This means that it can be very hard to identify a suitable sample of subjects to use as a control. In addition, because the groups are selected based on the occurrence of an outcome, they do not provide information related to the incidence and/or prevalence of the outcome.

C. Variations: The Nested Case-Control Study

Within any cohort study or clinical trial, a smaller case-control study can be performed. All cases of an outcome can be compared to a control group generated from the same cohort as a random sample or using matching techniques. The predictor of interest can then be measured in the subjects in the nested study. This is particularly attractive if the predictor is expensive or difficult to measure. However, it requires the foresight on the investigators part to obtain and preserve biological samples for later analysis (e.g., frozen blood, angiograms for QCA).

The association between C-reactive protein and manifestations of cardiovascular disease has been explored extensively using this design. In the Physician's Health Study, 1096 healthy subjects had baseline plasma samples analyzed for C-reactive protein (10). All subjects with documented myocardial infarction and stroke were matched on the basis of age, smoking status, and time from randomization from randomly selected study participants. This nested study analysis documented that baseline C-reactive protein could predict first myocardial infarction and ischemic stroke. The nested case-control method has been used to extend and validate the C-reactive protein observations to coronary heart disease mortality in the Multiple Risk Factor Intervention Trial (11) and sudden cardiac death in initially healthy individuals (12).

II. CLINICAL TRIALS

In clinical trials the investigator applies an intervention and observes its effect on an outcome of interest. These trials are better able to demonstrate causality and evaluate the effectiveness of the interventions under study than their observational counterparts. The gold standard for clinical research is the randomized trial, which will be discussed in detail (13,14). The properly designed and conducted randomized trial represents the definitive method for assessing clinical efficacy. Issues will include definition of endpoints, choice of controls, superiority vs. equivalence/noninferiority, subgroup analyses, and assessment of outcomes. We will also describe nonrandomized concurrent control studies.

A. The Randomized Clinical Trial

A clinical trial studies patients prospectively and measures the effect of an intervention, prophylactic, diagnostic, or therapeutic on a prespecified outcome. The strongest clinical trials have clear and precise objectives that are specified before the beginning of the trial.

Bias is one of the most troublesome problems in trial interpretation (15). Bias refers to the tendency of factors associated with the design, conduct, analysis, and interpretation of the trial to make the estimate of treatment effect deviate from its true value. In order to reduce bias, two techniques are used in trial design: blinding and randomization.

I. Blinding

Blinding is intended to eliminate the possibility for trial participants and personnel to consciously or unconsciously influence the conduct of the trial in a way that might alter the subsequent findings. The double-blind trial is ideal, in that neither the investigator nor the subject knows the treatment that is given. There are many difficulties with this approach, especially in a field in which the intervention is invasive or surgical. Sometimes there is an institution-based "unblinded investigator," who monitors certain (usually safety) outcomes. The other investigators and the specific institution remain blinded, as are the patients themselves.

The next best thing is the single-blind approach, in which most commonly the investigator knows the study group allocation but the patient does not. Of course, in some cases only an open-label design is sufficient or feasible. In all cases, the research personnel and patient should be blinded to as much of the study content as possible. For example, a patient who undergoes therapy with a device can be treated by research personnel post procedure who are not aware of the allocated treatment performed in the interventional (or surgical) suite. Future assessment of outcomes should be done by personnel who are blinded to assigned treatment group, even if the study was single-blinded. This is readily achieved by using centralized core laboratories to perform laboratory and image assessment of outcomes.

2. Randomization

Randomization introduces a deliberate element of chance into the assignment of treatments in a clinical trial. It tends to produce treatment groups in which the distribution of important prognostic factors and potential confounders are similar. This is especially valuable in eliminating the bias that cannot be adjusted for from unknown and unmeasured variables. If differences are observed in any of the prognostic factors, randomization ensures that the differences arose by chance, and not systematic error.

The primary outcome is often associated with other predictors, distinct from the study treatment. In such cases it can be useful to stratify the randomization a priori. For example, female sex has been shown to be an independent predictor of poor outcome in certain cardiovascular situations. It can be very useful to decide in advance that the males and females in the study will be randomized in separately, i.e., in two strata. This will increase the chance that sex, an important possible confounder, will be distributed evenly between the study groups. This technique is often used to help in the design of multicenter trials in order to control for the impact of treatment effect by center, for example.

Another technique to ensure relatively equal numbers in the randomization groups is the use of blocks. In this case, a block size is chosen, (e.g., 4, 6, 8), and within that block half of the patients will receive each treatment. For example, with a block size of 4, treatments A and B may be given as follows: AABB, BAAB, BABA, etc. With this strategy, there is little chance of a large imbalance at the end of the trial. In the example above with a block size of 4, the groups can only be off by 2. Consider a trial that is enrolling 100 patients into two groups without the use of blocks. The chance of having an imbalance of 10 patients at the end (groups of 45 and 55) is 14%; in two groups of 40 and 60 is 2%! This could lead to significant problems in interpretation.

Another advantage of blocking is demonstrated in trials that enroll subjects over a relatively long period of time. As time passes, patient characteristics may change, for example, from changes to the inclusion/exclusion criteria or current standards of practice. By using blocked randomization, the number of patients entering each group will be relatively close during each time period, or will at least not be off by more than half of the block size.

3. Specific Design Considerations

Parallel Design. The simplest type of design is the parallel group design. In this case patients are allocated to one of two or more treatment arms and followed to the end of the trial. This is the simplest and easiest to analyze and interpret and is by far the most common. The First International Study of Infarct Survival (ISIS-1) was a simple parallel design trial in which over 16,000 patients were randomized to receive a beta-blocker ($n =$ 8037) or placebo ($n =$ 7990) after acute myocardial infarction (16). At one week there was significantly lower mortality in the beta-blocker group (relative risk reduction of 15%, $p <$ 0.04), which was sustained at one-year. (Fig. 2). This simple trial clarified the important role of beta-blockers in acute myocardial infarction.

Cross-Over Design. Another design is the cross-over design. In this case each patient is randomized to receive a sequence of two or more treatments. The benefit of this approach is that each patient acts as its own control. Therefore, it usually reduces the number of subjects needed to adequately power the study. There are limitations, however. One of the most significant is the possibility for carryover and the necessity of a washout period. This means that the effect of one treatment influences the occurrence of the outcome in the second (or later) treatment. This is most likely to bias the interpretation of the results to be too conservative, i.e., a smaller treatment difference will be detected than would be in reality. In order to reduce this effect, the disease should ideally be chronic and relatively stable. Also, adequate time (wash-out period) must be given in between treatments in order to completely reverse the effect of the first therapy. Nonetheless, the effect of the washout period itself after one type of therapy may be different than after another and thus may add bias to the design. Consider a comparison of unfractionated heparin to a direct thrombin inhibitor. The wash-out period may lead to clinical events with the withdrawal of heparin, whereas such an effect may not be present during the wash-out period after a direct thrombin inhibitor (17). On the other hand, a shortened (or eliminated) wash-out period may abolish the aforementioned problem but lead to toxic (bleeding) complications due to a "carry-over" effect of the first therapy (which will essentially be dependent on the half-life of the two drugs used in this example). Finally,

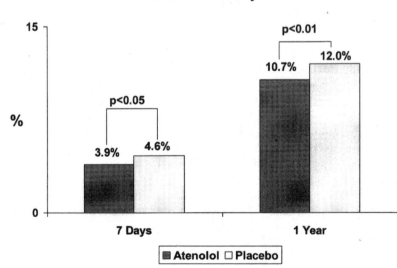

Figure 2   Beta-blocker vs. placebo results from the ISIS-1 trial

repeated measurements require more complex analysis plans for the final interpretation of the data.

Factorial Design. Another important and frequently used variation of the randomized trial uses a factorial design in which two or more *factors* (therapies) are evaluated at the same time (18). In this case, two or more different interventions are evaluated in the same study sample. The simplest example is the 2 ¥ 2 factorial design, in which subjects are randomly allocated to one of the four possible combinations of treatments, say A and B. The subjects can then receive A alone, B alone, both A and B, or neither A nor B. This design can have specific applications. The first is to evaluate the efficacy of *two* therapies instead of *one* in a large number of patients. This is particularly important in trials assessing endpoints, such as mortality, that require very large sample sizes and allows for a more efficient use of patients. From the example above, all of the patients who receive A (A alone and both A and B) will be compared to all of the patients who did not receive A (B alone and neither A nor B); a similar test will be done for B.

The chief limitation of the factorial design is the possibility of interaction of therapies. It may be difficult to ascertain the isolated effect of either treatment, leading to inappropriate interpretations. For this reason, this design is best used for evaluating relatively unrelated research questions.

This limitation can also be a benefit. Another situation in which to use the factorial design is to assess the benefit of two therapies that will likely be used together in order to look for an interaction between treatments. In this case the study should be powered in advance to look for this, as statistical tests for interaction require a larger patient sample.

The CADILLAC trial studied the effects of two factors: (a) intracoronary stent implantation compared to plain old balloon angioplasty (POBA) and (b) concomitant abciximab administration compared to placebo in patients undergoing percutaneous coronary intervention (PCI) for acute myocardial infarction (19). Patients were randomized in a 2 ¥ 2 factorial manner to one of four groups: POBA alone (neither A nor B), POBA plus abciximab (B alone), stent alone (A alone), and stent plus abciximab (A and B). This design enabled the investigators to study the therapeutic effects of these two commonly used treatments in a setting in which they are frequently used together. They concluded that routine stent implantation (mechanical intervention) resulted in higher event-free survival rates at 6 months, independent of abciximab use (pharmacological intervention). A similar result was not observed for abciximab, and there was no significant interaction.

Endpoints. The ideal primary endpoint should be a clinically important, easily assessed variable that is the most clinically relevant outcome for the research question. This is most often used to establish necessary sample size and usually a clinical outcome (as opposed to a safety measure). It may be single or a composite, directly assessable or an indirect, surrogate assessment of clinical activity.

Composite Endpoints. The simplest and easiest-to-interpret design involves a single endpoint, for example, all-cause mortality. However, composite endpoints are often used. A key practical reason for this is to reduce the required sample sizes needed to demonstrate efficacy. Sample size calculations are based on event rates, and by increasing the projected event rate, sample size decreases, all else being held equal. By combining endpoints, a larger event rate is usually observed, leading to a smaller sample of subjects needed. Clinically, this can also provide valuable information about the overall burden of disease. The commonly used composite endpoint of mortality, nonfatal myocardial infarction, and hospitalization for unstable angina is a well-recognized and accepted measure of the activity of coronary artery disease because these three outcomes are considered interrelated based on our knowledge of the pathogenesis of cardiovascular disease.

The TACTICS-TIMI 18 trial used this endpoint to investigate the optimal revascularization strategy, early invasive versus conservative, in patients presenting with unstable coronary syndromes on optimal, aggressive medical therapy (20). The sample size was based on a predicted composite event rate of 22% in the conservative arm and a 25% relative reduction with early invasive therapy, resulting in a sample size of 1720 patients (21). The study demonstrated a significant decrease in the occurrence of the combined endpoint at 6 months in patients treated with the early invasive strategy (odds ratio 0.78 with 95% CI 0.62,0.97; $p = 0.025$). A similar trial using only mortality as the endpoint at 6 months would require over 250,000 patients to definitively demonstrate a significant difference at the mortality rates observed.

Problems arise when a trial observes a significant difference in a composite endpoint, but the components are of unclear importance. For instance, small creatine kinase elevations post-PCI are not as clinically important as mortality but, when included in a composite variable, may be more common and sufficient to influence the statistical significance of a trial. Subsequent studies may be needed to clarify the electrocardiographic versus enzymological evidence of MI (22) and the pathogenesis of CK-MB elevation alone (23). Obviously, this debate complicates the interpretation and generalizability of studies that used the controversial endpoint. Another potential problem in interpretation arises when the effects on individual components of the endpoint go in different directions.

Multiple Endpoints. Another approach to making the most efficient use of the patients in a trial is to include multiple primary endpoints. This is especially true in situations where more than one clinical endpoint is important enough to change therapy. In this situation, a clear plan for accounting for the statistical problems associated with multiple comparisons must be planned in advance. Why are multiple comparisons a problem? As more hypotheses are tested, the likelihood of concluding that one is statistically significant *by chance alone* increases. For example, consider the most commonly used cutoff for statistical significance, $a = 0.05$, and consider testing multiple hypotheses. If we test five multiple hypotheses, the chance is 23% that we will find a significant difference $(1–0.95^5)$; 10 hypotheses and the chance is 40% $(1–0.95^{10})$; 20 hypotheses and the chance is 64% $(1–0.95^{20})$. Statistical adjustments and techniques can be used for multiple comparisons, but a good rule is to have one primary hypothesis on which the trial is judged. Other compelling hypotheses can be assessed secondarily, without statistical penalities if the study has enough patients.

Surrogate Endpoints. In some situations, it may not be possible to measure clinical endpoints directly, and surrogate markers are used to assess clinical and therapeutic benefit. This is especially true when outcomes are relatively infrequent, making trials prohibitively large. Surrogate markers are a reliable predictor of outcome but usually are easier to measure (24). Surrogate markers should have the following characteristics:

Biologically plausible relationship with outcome
Epidemiological evidence of the prognostic value of the surrogate on
clinical outcome—will be accepted by the scientific community
Can be accurately and precisely measured
Will be accessible to people who may want to apply the intervention in clinical
practice

However, there are certainly examples of effective treatment of surrogate markers ultimately having a detrimental impact on clinical outcomes. One of the classic examples was in the treatment of ventricular arrhythmias in patients with coronary artery disease.

Ventricular arrhythmias had been shown to be a predictor of sudden death and all-cause mortality in patients with coronary artery disease. It made sense that suppression of arrhythmias would lead to a reduction in mortality. Unfortunately, in the Cardiac Arrhythmia Suppression Trial, class Ic antiarrhythmics were effective in suppressing the surrogate marker of ventricular arrhythmias but paradoxically increased mortality and sudden death (25).

Treatment of acute coronary syndromes with more potent antiplatelet regimens is also very attractive. Three large randomized trials have assessed the efficacy of three different oral glycoprotein IIb/IIIa inhibitors (26–28). Despite excellent effect on the surrogate, platelet aggregation, these agents had either no effect or a deleterious effect on mortality. In addition, bleeding events were also increased.

Angiographic assessment of coronary perfusion in patients with acute MI treated with varying thrombolytic regimens was the surrogate endpoint used in the TIMI-14 trial (29). This trial used the achievement of complete reperfusion, TIMI grade 3 flow, as its endpoint. Previous trials have shown in post-hoc analyses that the absence of TIMI-3 flow after reperfusion therapy is a predictor of poor outcome (30,31). In this trial the addition of abciximab resulted in earlier and more complete TIMI-3 flow in comparison to patients who received other thrombolytic regimens. This provided powerful evidence of a hypothetical benefit of therapy with abciximab, but without confirmation of a phase 3 clinical trial, the direct clinical benefit cannot be known or potential harm cannot be excluded.

5. Subgroup Analyses

In many trials, specific subsets of patients are compared in a separate analysis from the primary trial analysis. This method can provide valuable ancillary observations (e.g., efficacy of therapy in minorities, diabetics, women) but can be misused and lead to erroneous conclusions.

For a number of reasons, such trials can lead to misleading results (32). They are not often powered to have a large enough sample in order to answer the question from a substudy. This means that a nonsignificant result may be the result of not enough patients (not enough power). An example of this was the initial conclusion that thrombolytic therapy with streptokinase was only effective in patients with anterior, and not inferior, myocardial infarction (33,34). With increased evidence in this lower-risk subset, it became apparent that thrombolysis was of benefit in inferior myocardial infarctions as well (35).

Another potential problem arises as the number of subgroup analyses increases. As the number of comparisons increases, the potential for a positive finding goes up by chance alone. Optimally, they should be planned before trial initiation in order to increase the robustness of the conclusions. In general, the effect of therapy found in the primary analysis is the best estimate of its effect in a subgroup (23). In fact, overviews of various cardiovascular therapies have shown that most subgroup analyses are in the same direction of the primary effect, but different in size (36). At best, they are hypothesis generating and should be confirmed independently and compared with existing evidence.

6. Types of Comparisons

Superiority Trials.   This is the simplest, and most convincing, trial design with the objective of showing that the investigational intervention is superior to a comparative one. Careful choice of control is imperative. The ideal is the use of a placebo control. However, in many situations, another therapy may be shown to be of benefit in the population to be studied. In this case, it may be considered unethical to use a placebo and an active control is used. The active control should represent the current standard of care.

Equivalence and Noninferiority Trials. The term equivalence is often used to describe noninferiority trials. Strictly speaking, equivalence trials are designed to show that the effects of two treatments, one under investigation, differ by less than a clinically important amount in any direction (positive or negative). These are most commonly used to assess bioequivalence of new agents, e.g., generic agents, compared to their predecessors. It is uncommon for new treatments and/or interventions to want only to show clinical equivalence—they would like to be deemed superior to standard therapy if possible. Technically speaking, such an "equivalence" trial is really conducted to demonstrate noninferiority. Non-inferiority trials are designed to show that the efficacy of an investigational product is no worse than that of the active comparator. In other words, they are used to test whether a drug (or device) is as *effective and no worse* than a competitor.

In general, noninferiority trials need fewer patients than superiority trials. For example, a superiority trial designed to detect an absolute difference of 10% between two treatments will require more patients than a noninferiority trial in which a difference of up to 10% is considered acceptable. However, a noninferiority trial of two active treatments will often be much larger than a superiority trial of an active control versus placebo because the effect of treatment is usually greater in a placebo-controlled trial.

A number of issues make equivalence trials more complicated to design appropriately. An important first step is the appropriate choice of active control. A basic knowledge of statistical analysis is also important to understand the differences between superiority and noninferiority trials. Discussions of these fundamental issues follow.

7. Active Controls

A placebo is not an appropriate control for ethical reasons in cases where another well-accepted treatment has demonstrated clinical efficacy. In this situation, the control group should receive the recommended standard-of-care therapy as an active control. An active control must be chosen carefully. It should be a widely used therapy whose efficacy for the indication has been clearly documented in a sound clinical trial. It only makes sense that the proposed trial should be planned for a setting with similar patients, primary endpoints, and doses that have been used to document the active control's efficacy. Of course, little will be learned if an active control is used in a situation where it is of dubious clinical value. To show that an investigational agent is equivalent, or at least not inferior, to something of no intrinsic benefit is of little use.

8. Analysis Issues Related to Equivalence Trials

In order to fully understand some of the intricacies of equivalence trial designs, a basic knowledge of statistical testing is needed. In simple superiority trials, the statistical tests are designed to evaluate size of the treatment effect, i.e., by how much treatment A differs from the control. They are based on testing the null hypothesis (H_0) and the alternative hypothesis (H_A), designated as follows for two-sided tests:

H_0: treatment A has no effect
H_A: treatment A has an effect

Statistical significance testing (e.g., the ubiquitous *p*-value) is designed to test whether H_0, the null hypothesis, is true or not. The basis of statistical testing is that there is no effect, i.e., the null hypothesis is true. This is the most conservative approach in most cases; the burden is on the research to show that the null hypothesis is not true. The investigator uses the data from the study to decide whether there is sufficient evidence from the patients studied to reject the null hypothesis, i.e., discard the idea that there is no effect of treatment. The statistical test gives a p-value based on the study sample; the p-value is the probability of observing an effect at least as large as was seen by chance alone when in reality there is no effect of treatment. This would lead to erroneously concluding that an effect exists (reject the null hypothesis) when there really is no effect.

The above mathematical tests are all based on the assumption that there is no difference between therapies for two-sided tests. In fact, it is very difficult to prove that two things are equivalent. Using conventional sample size techniques, it would require an infinite number of people to prove that two treatments are identical. Therein lies one of the difficulties in designing equivalence trials. In general, most problems and errors in trial design and implementation tend to bias the trial not to reject H_0, i.e., to conclude there was no difference. However, it is not appropriate to conclude that two interventions are the same based on the fact that the standard statistical testing is not significant.

Therefore, there are some important differences in the ways that equivalence trials are designed, implemented, and analyzed. The first step in designing an equivalence trial is to specify an equivalence margin (37). This is the largest difference, d, between the treatment and control that can be considered clinically acceptable to declare equivalence. This margin, or difference, should be justified clinically and is generally less than the differences observed between the active control and placebo in superiority trials. For an equivalence trial (in the strict definition of equivalence), the observed difference must be less than d in both directions. For a noninferiority trial, the intervention must not be worse than the control by d, i.e., it is essentially a one-way equivalence trial (Fig. 3).

In general, these trials are not conservative in nature, that is, most sources of bias tend to lead to the conclusion that the treatments are noninferior (38–41). There is a greater need for rigorous methods and care in their design and conduct. Special attention must be paid to ensure strict adherence to entry criteria, noncompliance, withdrawals, loss to follow-up, and other protocol violations.

Facets of the noninferiority design are demonstrated in the TARGET trial (Do Tirofiban and ReoPro Give Similar Efficacy Trial) (42). Two glycoprotein IIb/IIIa inhibitors, tirofiban and abciximab, were compared in the setting of nonemergent percutaneous coronary revascularization. In this trial, the active control was abciximab. The details of the analysis plan were based on the Evaluation of Glycoprotein IIb/IIIa Platelet Inhibitor for Stenting (EPISTENT) trial, which was felt to have a similar design and cohort of patients (43). The largest acceptable difference for tirofiban, d, was designed to preserve the EPISTENT trial's observed benefit of abciximab compared to placebo (44). In TARGET, the upper bound of the one-sided 95% confidence interval for the relative benefit of tirofiban compared to abciximab had to be less than 1.47 in order to declare equivalence. In fact, the trial resulted in an upper bound of 1.51 for tirofiban, and so non-inferiority was not found. In this well-powered trial, superiority testing went on to show that abciximab was actually superior to tirofiban in this setting.

The TARGET trial also highlights the ability to test noninferiority and superiority in one trial, without statistical penalty. It is generally accepted that after testing for noninferiority, superiority can be tested secondarily. However, non- inferiority testing must be specified as a hypothesis a priori for it to be valid, i.e., it is not acceptable to test for superiority and when it is not found proceed with noninferiority testing (32).

B. Alternatives to the Randomized Design: Nonrandomized Concurrent Control Studies

In general, studies with nonrandomized controls are less satisfactory and are more difficult to interpret. This is because of the concern of confounding variables that may influence the clinical findings and inferences from the investigation. By definition, the participants are allocated to treatment by a nonrandom process. This introduces the possibility of selection bias, i.e., the very likely possibility that the investigator chooses, consciously or unconsciously, a certain subset of patients to receive either treatment based on a characteristic. Despite this, it may be easier in some situations for investigators (*and participants*) to accept a research proposal if the designation of treatment is not by chance alone. In the other hand, the easier acceptance of participants who consent to a nonrandomized design is usually accompanied by a higher rate of non-compliance, drop-out, and cross-over in the control group, leading to serious study imbalances.

III. APPLICATION OF RESEARCH DESIGN PRINCIPLES

When investigating a clinical question using either of the research designs—the randomized controlled trial or observational studies—The first step is to define a question: What is the best approach for coronary revascularization in diabetic patients with multivessel coronary artery disease—percutaneous coronary intervention (PCI) or coronary artery bypass grafting (CABG)?

In 1987, the National Heart, Lung and Blood Institute initiated a randomized clinical trial comparing coronary revascularization strategies in patients with multivessel coronary artery disease, the Bypass Angioplasty Revascularization Investigation (BARI) (45). They designed a simple randomized tria—all patients with multivessel coronary artery disease eligible for either balloon angioplasty or CABG were randomized to one of the revascularization strategies and followed to assess the occurrence of all-cause mortality. They found a nonstatistically significant difference in mortality between the two groups, similar to multiple other randomized trials. However, when the subgroup of patients with diabetes was looked at, there was a striking increase in mortality at 5 years with balloon angioplasty compared with CABG (35% vs. 19%; $p = 0.003$) (46).

This surprising and significant difference led investigators to examine the results from smaller similar randomized trials. In CABRI, RITA, and EAST, the 5-year mortality rates in the PCI and CABG groups were 15% and 12%, respectively (47). Some critics questioned the generalizability of the BARI trial patients. Also, the fact that the diabetic subgroup was not specified a priori made people question the validity of the finding.

At the same time that patients were being randomized into the BARI study, patients who were otherwise eligible for inclusion but were choosing their mode of revascularization were followed in a separate registry (48). The patients were not significantly different than the randomized patients in the majority of their baseline characteristics. However, at 5 years the mortality rates for balloon angioplasty and CABG were 14.4% and 14.9%, not statistically different.

The BARI example provides an excellent basis for comparing the two strategies of research. One of the primary advantages of randomization is the premise that all important confounders, measured, unmeasured, and unknown, should be distributed evenly between the two groups. After adjusting for baseline differences in the two treatment modalities in the registry, CABG was found to be superior to balloon angioplasty in diabetics, although not statistically significantly and to a lesser magnitude than in the randomized cohort.

However, the registry findings demonstrated that the strong benefit of CABG may not be generalizable to all diabetics.

One proposed criticism of randomized trials is that in rapidly moving fields, like cardiology, it is difficult for trial design to keep up with the latest therapies and devices. By the end of a well-designed trial, the results may no longer reflect clinical practice. In the field of coronary revascularization, the evolution of coronary intervention technology has shown that balloon angioplasty, as performed in the BARI trial, is indeed inferior to coronary stent implantation (49). As the field continued to evolve, bare-metal stents were found to be inferior to drug-eluting stents (50,51), especially in diabetics. In the meantime, CABG techniques without cardiopulmonary bypass may decrease the perioperative morbidity and mortality (52–55), especially in high-risk patient subsets.

IV. CONCLUSIONS

An understanding of clinical research methods is an important facet of clinical practice, from interpretation and critical review of clinical trials to implementation of evidence-based medical practice. The impetus is on the clinical researcher's shoulders to design and carry out thoughtful, rigorous, and valid protocols, whether they are observational or interventional.

REFERENCES

1. Gordis L. Epidemiology. 2nd ed. Philadelphia: WB Saunders Company, 2000:131–139.
2. Hulley SB, Cummings SR, Browner WS, Grady D, Hearst N, Newman TB.Designing Clinical Research. 2nd ed. Philadelphia. Lippincott Williams and Wilkins, 2001; 95–105.
3. Kelsey JL, Whittemore AS, Evans AS, Thompson WD. Methods in Observational Epidemiology. 2nd ed. New York: Oxford University Press, 996:86–109.
4. Kannel WB. Clinical misconceptions dispelled by epidemiological research. Circulation 1995; 92:3350–3360.
5. Gronbaek M, Deis A, Sorenson TI, Becker U, Schnohr P, Jensen G. Mortality associated with the moderate intakes of wine, beer, or spirits. BMJ 1995; 310(6988): 1165–1169.
6. Rimm EB, Giovannucci EL, Willett WC, Colditz GA, Ascherio A, Rosner B, Stampfer MJ. Prospective study of alcohol consumption and risk of coronary disease in men. Lancet 1991; 338(8765):464–468.
7. Thun MJ, Peto R, Lopez AD, Monaco JH, Henley J, Heath CW, Doll R. Alcohol consumption and mortality among middle-aged and elderly U.S. adults. N Engl J Med 1997;337:1705–1714.
8. deLogeril M, Salen P, Martin JL, Boucher F, Paillard F, deLeiris J. Wine drinking and risks of cardiovascular complications after recent acute myocardial infarction. Circulation 2002; 106:1465–1469.
9. Pell JP, Simpson E, Rodger JC, Finlayson A, Clark D, Anderson J, Pell ACH. Impact of changing diagnostic criteria on incidence, management, and outcome of acute myocardial infarction: retrospective cohort study. BMJ 2003; 326:134–135.
10. Ridker PM, Cushman M, Stampfer MJ, Tracy RP, Hennekens CH. Inflammation, aspirin, and the risk of cardiovascular disease in apparently healthy men. N Engl J Med 1997;336:973–997.
11. Kuller LH, Tracy RP, Shaten J, Meilahn EN. Relation of C-reactive protein and coronary heart disease in the MRFIT nested case-control study. Multiple Risk Factor Intervention Trial. Am J Epidemiol 1996; 144:537–547.
12. Albert CM, Ma J, Rifai N, Stampfer MJ, Ridker PM. Prospective study of C-reactive protein, homocysteine, and plasma lipid levels as predictors of sudden cardiac death. Circulation 2002; 105(22):2595–2599.

13. Friedman LM, Furberg CD, DeMets DL. Fundamentals of Clinical Trials. 3rd ed. Springer-Verlag, New York 1998.

14. Pocock SJ. Clinical Trials. A Practical Approach. John Wiley & Sons Ltd, 1983.

15. International Conference on Harmonization of Technical Requirements for Registration of Pharmaceuticals for Human Use (ICH). E-9: statistical principles for clinical trials. *Fed Reg* 1998; 63:49583–49598.

16. Randomised trial of intravenous atenolol among 16 027 cases of suspected acute myocardial infarction: ISIS-1. First International Study of Infarct Survival Collaborative Group. *Lancet* 1986; 2(8498):57–66.

17. Granger CB, Miller JM, Bovill EG, Gruber A, Tracy RP, Krucoff MW, Green C, Berrios E, Harrington RA, Ohman EM, et al. Rebound increase in thrombin generation and activity after cessation of intravenous heparin in patients with acute coronary syndromes. *Circulation* 1995; 91(7):1929–1935.

18. Simon R, Freedman LS. Bayesian design and analysis of two ¥ two factorial clinical trials. *Biometrics* 1997; 53:456–464.

19. Stone GW, Grines CL, Cox DA, Garcia E, Tcheng JE, Griffin JJ, Guagliumi G, Stuckey T, Turco M, Carroll JD, Rutherford BD, Lansky AJ; Controlled Abciximab and Device Investigation to Lower Late Angioplasty Complications (CADILLAC) Investigators. Comparison of angioplasty with stenting, with or without abciximab, in acute myocardial infarction. *N Engl J Med* 2002 Mar 28; 346(13):957–966

20. Cannon CP, Weintraub WS, Demopoulos LA, Vicari R, Frey MJ, Lakkis N, Neumann FJ, Robertson DH, DeLucca PT, DiBattiste PM, Gibson CM, Braunwald E; TACTICS (Treat Angina with Aggrastat and Determine Cost of Therapy with an Invasive or Conservative Strategy)—Thrombolysis In Myocardial Infarction 18 Investigators. Comparison of early invasive and conservative strategies in patients with unstable coronary syndromes treated with the glycoprotein IIb/IIIa inhibitor tirofiban. *N Engl J Med* 2001; 344(25):1879–1887

21. Cannon CP, Weintraub WS, Demopoulos LA, Robertson DH, Gormley GJ, Braunwald E. Invasive versus conservative strategies in unstable angina and non-Q-wave myocardial infarction following treatment with tirofiban: rationale and study design of the international TACTICS-TIMI 18 Trial. Treat Angina with Aggrastat and determine Cost of Therapy with an Invasive or Conservative Strategy. Thrombolysis In Myocardial Infarction. *Am J Cardiol* 1998; 82(6):731–736

22. Stone GW, Mehran R, Dangas G, Lansky AJ, Kornowski R, Leon MB. Differential impact on survival of electrocardiographic Q-wave versus enzymatic myocardial infarction after percutaneous intervention: a device-specific analysis of 7147 patients. *Circulation* 2001; 104(6):642–647

23. Mehran R, Dangas G, Mintz GS, Lansky AJ, Pichard AD, Satler LF, Kent KM, Stone GW, Leon MB. Atherosclerotic plaque burden and CK-MB enzyme elevation after coronary interventions: intravascular ultrasound study of 2256 patients. *Circulation* 2000; 101(6):604–610

24. Psaty BM, Weiss NS, Furberg CD, Koepsall TD, Siscovick DS, Rosendaal FR, Smith NL, Heckbert SR, Kaplan RC, Lin D, Fleming TR, Wagner EH. Surrogate endpoints, health outcomes, and the drug-approval process for the treatment of risk factors for cardiovascular disease. *JAMA* 1999; 282:786–790.

25. The Cardiac Arrhythmia Suppression Trial (CAST) Investigators. Preliminary report: effect of encainide and flecanide on mortality in a randomized trial of arrhythmia suppression after myocardial infarction. *N Engl J Med* 1989; 321:406–412.

26. The SYMPHONY Investigators. Comparison of sibrafiban with aspirin for prevention of cardiovascular events after acute coronary syndromes: a randomized trial. *Lancet* 2000; 355:337–345.

27. Cannon CP. Orbofiban in Patients with Unstable coronary Syndromes (TIMI-16) preliminary results. Presented at the 48th Scientific Sessions of the American College of Cardiology, New Orleans, LA, March 1999.

28. O'Neill WW. The Evaluation of Xemilofiban in Controlling Thrombotic Events (EXCITE) trial: 30-day and six-month results. Presented at the 48th Scientific Sessions of the American College of Cardiology, New Orleans, LA, March 1999.

29. Antman EM, Guigliano RP, Gibson CM, McCabe CH, Coussement P, Kleiman NS, Vahanian A, Adgey AA, Menown I, Rupprecht HJ, Van der Weiken R, Ducas J, Scherer J, Anderson K, Van de Werf F, Braunwald E. Abciximab facilitates the rate and extent of thrombolysis: results of the thrombolysis in myocardial infarction (TIMI) 14 trial. The TIMI 14 Investigators. *Circulation* 1999; 99:2720–2732.

30. Gibson CM, Cannon CP, Murphy SA, Marble SJ, Barron HV, Braunwald E; TIMI Study Group. Relationship of the TIMI myocardial perfusion grades, flow grades, frame count, and percutaneous coronary intervention to long-term outcomes after thrombolytic administration in acute myocardial infarction. *Circulation* 2002; 105(16):1909–1913

31. Stone GW, Cox D, Garcia E, Brodie BR, Morice MC, Griffin J, Mattos L, Lansky AJ, O'Neill WW, Grines CL. Normal flow (TIMI-3) before mechanical reperfusion therapy is an independent determinant of survival in acute myocardial infarction: analysis from the primary angioplasty in myocardial infarction trials. *Circulation* 2001; 104(6):636–641

32. Sleight JR. Debate: Subgroup analyses in clinical trials—fun to look at, but don't believe them! *Curr Conrol Trials Cardiovasc Med* 2000; 1:25–27.

33. Randomized trial of intravenous streptokinase, oral aspirin, both, or neither among 17,187 cases of suspected acute myocardial infarction: ISIS-2 (Second International Study of Infarct Survival) Collaborative Group. *J Am Coll Cardiol* 1988; 12(6 suppl A):3A–13A

34. Bates ER. Reperfusion therapy in inferior myocardial infarction. *J Am Coll Cardiol* 1988; 12(6 suppl A):44A–51A

35. Indications for fibrinolytic therapy in suspected acute myocardial infarction: collaborative overview of early mortality and major morbidity results from all randomised trials of more than 1000 patients. Fibrinolytic Therapy Trialists' (FTT) Collaborative Group. *Lancet* 1994; 343(8893):311–322

36. DeMets DL, Califf RM. Lessons learned from recent cardiovascular clinical trials: Part I. *Circulation* 2002; 106:746–751.

37. International Conference on Harmonization of Technical Requirements for Registration of Pharmaceuticals for Human Use (ICH). E-10: guidance on choice of control group in clinical trials. *Fed Reg* 2001; 64:51767–51780.

38. Snapinn S. Noninferiority trials. Curr Control Trials Cardiovasc Med 2000; 1:19–21.

39. Jones B, Jarvis P, Lewis JA, Ebbutt AF. Trials to assess equivalence: the importance of rigorous methods. *Br Med J* 1996; 313:36–39.

40. Hauck WW Anderson S. Some issues in the design and analysis of equivalence trials. *Drug Information J* 1999; 33:109–118.

41. Ware JH, Antman EM. Equivalence trials. *N Engl J Med* 1997; 337:1159–1161.

42. Topol EJ, Moliterno DJ, Herrmann HC, Powers ER, Grines CL, Cohen DJ, Cohen EA, Bertrand M, Neumann FJ, Stone GW, DiBattiste PM, Demopoulos L. Comparison of two platelet glycoprotein IIb/IIIa inhibitors, tirofiban and abciximab, for the prevention of ischemic events with percutaneous coronary revascularization. *N Engl J Med* 2001; 344:1888–1894.

43. David J. Moliterno, MD, Eric J. Topol, MD. A direct comparison of tirofiban and abciximab during percutaneous coronary revascularization and stent placement: Rationale and design of the TARGET study. *Am Heart J* 2000; 140:722–726

44. The EPISTENT investigators. Randomised placebo-controlled and balloon-angioplasty-controlled trial to assess safety of coronary stenting with use of platelet glycoprotein-IIb/IIIa blockade. *Lancet* 1998; 352:87–92.

45. BARI Investigators. Comparison of coronary bypass surgery with angioplasty in patients with multivessel disease. *N Engl J Med* 1996; 335:217–225.

46. The BARI Investigators. Influence of diabetes on 5-Year mortality and morbidity in a randomized trial comparing CABG and PTCA in patients with multivessel disease. *Circulation* 1997; 96:1761–1769.

47. Ellis SG, Narins CR. Problem of angioplasty in diabetics. *Circulation* 1997; 96:1707–1710.

48. Katherine M. Detre, Ping Guo, Richard Holubkov, Robert M. Califf, George Sopko, Richard Bach, Maria Mori Brooks, Martial G. Bourassa, Richard J. Shemin, Allan D. Rosen, Ronald J. Krone, Robert L. Frye, and Frederick Feit. Coronary revascularization in diabetic patients: a

comparison of the randomized and observational components of the Bypass Angioplasty Revascularization Investigation (BARI). *Circulation* 99:633–640.

49. Fischman D. L., Leon M. B., Baim D. S., Schatz R. A., Savage M. P., Penn I., Detre K., Veltri L., Ricci D., Nobuyoshi M., Cleman M., Heuser R., Almond D., Teirstein P. S., Fish R. D., Colombo A., Brinker J., Moses J., Shaknovich A., Hirshfeld J., Bailey S., Ellis S., Rake R., Goldberg S., The Stent Restenosis Study Investigators. A randomized comparison of coronary-stent placement and balloon angioplasty in the treatment of coronary artery disease. *N Engl J Med.* 1994; 331:496–501.

50. Morice MC, Serruys PW, Sousa EJ et al. for the RAVEL Study Group. A randomized comparison of a sirolimus eluting stent with a standard stent for coronary revascularization. *N Engl J Med.* 2002; 346:1773–1780.

51. SIRIUS trial results, presented at TCT 2002, Washington, D.C.

52. Verkkala K, Voutilainen S, Jarvinen A, Keto P, Voutilainen P, Salmenpera M. Minimally invasive coronary artery bypass grafting: one-year follow-up. *J Card Surg* 1999; 14(4):231–239.

53. Stamou SC, Hill PC, Dangas G, Pfister AJ, Boyce SW, Dullum MK, Bafi AS, Corso PJ. Stroke after coronary artery bypass: incidence, predictors, and clinical outcome. *Stroke* 2001; 32(7):1508–1513.

54. Stamou SC, Pfister AJ, Dangas G, Dullum MK, Boyce SW, Bafi AS, Garcia JM, Corso PJ. Beating heart versus conventional single-vessel reoperative coronary artery bypass. *Ann Thorac Surg* 2000; 69(5):1383–1387.

55. Mehran R, Dangas G, Stamou SC, Pfister AJ, Dullum MK, Leon MB, Corso PJ. One-year clinical outcome after minimally invasive direct coronary artery bypass. *Circulation* 2000; 102(23):2799–2802.

20-1

Antithrombotic Drugs and the Pharmaceutical Industry

Clive A. Meanwell
The Medicines Company, Parsippany, New Jersey, U.S.A.

I. INTRODUCTION

A. Antithrombotic Drugs in Bite Size Pieces

The class of antithrombotic drugs includes a wide range of oral and parenteral agents used to prevent and/or treat unwanted intravascular coagulation. Generally these drugs are sub-classified by mode of action and/or indication in venous or arterial thrombotic conditions. Most classification schemes for antithrombotic drugs rely on outmoded models of the coagulation cascade (1), or simplified models of platelet action. These schemes classify drugs according to beliefs about their primary target enzyme or substrate. Hence, "antico-agulants" are supposed to act on cascade substrates or enzymes such as thrombin or factor Xa, whereas "antiplatelet agents" act on platelet receptors and "thrombolytics" act on fibrinogen.

Unfortunately life is not that simple. For example, abciximab (c7E3 Fab—ReoPro®—Johnson and Johnson and Eli Lilly), the prototypical platelet glycoprotein (GP) IIb/IIIa inhibitor, is known to prolong the activated clotting time, raising the possibility that in vivo c7E3 Fab functions not only as an antiplatelet agent, but also as an anticoagulant (2). Abciximab also binds to the vitronectin receptor found on platelets and vessel wall endothelial and smooth muscle cells, raising the possibility of anti-inflammatory effects (3). Bivalirudin (Angiomax®—The Medicines Company), a thrombin-specific serine protease inhibitor, is known to prevent protease-activated receptor (PAR)–mediated platelet activation (4). And finally, drotrecogin alfa (Xigris®—Eli Lilly), a serine protease with the same amino acid sequence as human plasma–derived activated protein C, exerts an antithrombotic effect by inhibiting factors Va and VIIIa and exerts indirect profibrinolytic activity through plasminogen activator inhibitor-1 (PAI-1) and by limiting generation of activated thrombin-activatable fibrinolysis inhibitor.

Each of these examples is a drug usually classified as an antithrombotic. Two of them (abciximab and bivalirudin) are indicated to prevent complications of angioplasty, and one (drotrecogin alfa) is indicated for treatment of sepsis. As the complex, dynamic interdependencies of thrombosis and inflammation are unraveled (5), more logical classification schemes may emerge based on an understanding of the molecular mechanisms. Such classifications would be more informative, more accurate, and perhaps further rationalize drug choices and improve patient care.

This sounds appealing, but is unlikely to happen. The reason? Current classifications of antithrombotics are promulgated by the pharmaceutical industry as part of a massive program of investment in research, development, and marketing ("education"). The industry positions products distinctly, attempts to differentiate them clearly, and to tell their story in bite-size pieces that areeasily understood and recalled by busy caregivers.

B.   Antithrombin Drugs—Big Business

Worldwide, prescription and over-the-counter drug revenues will exceed $400 billion in 2003. North America, Europe, Japan, and Latin America account for 85% of this total. Antithrombotic drugs represent a substantial franchise within the global market, accounting for more than $10 billion in 2003 revenue. The antithrombotic franchise has grown rapidly since 1980, when the available drugs—aspirin, unfractionated heparin, and warfarin—sold no more than $1 billion combined. Average annual growth rates of 12% in recent years have driven total antithrombotic drug revenues from $6.08 billion in 1998 to $9.96 billion in 2002 (6). Revenues are expected to exceed $14 billion by 2010 (7).

Plavix® (clopidogrel), with 2002 revenues of $2.6 billion, and Lovenox®/Clexane® (enoxaparin), with $1.7 billion, dominate today's market. By way of context, Plavix and Lovenox are the sixth and seventh highest revenue cardiovascular drugs in the world. Lipitor® (atorvastatin calcium), the highest, garnered $7.97 billion in 2002 (6). Aspirin (acetylsalicylic acid) and warfarin sodium account for another large proportion of antithrombotic sales, but these products are not growing. Significant changes are likely in the next decade as oral and injectable thrombin-specific agents compete with heparins and warfarin and second-generation P2Y12 platelet inhibitors compete with Plavix in an increasingly complex, globalized market.

II.   INDUSTRIAL HISTORY: ASPIRIN, HEPARIN, AND COUMADIN

An overview of industrial milestones for aspirin, heparin, and Coumadin® (warfarin sodium) is shown in Figure 1.

A.   Aspirin

Salicylate-containing plants such as willow bark were known as cures for fever and pain by ancient Egyptian and Greek physicians (8). Aspirin was industrialized by Bayer, which began in 1863 as Friedrich Bayer & Co., a dye-manufacturing concern in Germany. Seeking growth in the late 1880s, Bayer took on pharmaceuticals and developed phenacetin (acetophenetidin). Building on an established dyestuffs business, Bayer sponsored clinical studies, advertised their drugs in trade journals and employed pharmaceutical sales representatives to promote their products to physicians. Nothing, it seems, is new.

The discovery of aspirin is usually credited to Felix Hoffman, who joined Bayer in 1894. Apparently Hoffman's father was taking salicylic acid, already mass-produced, widely used, and highly profitable by the end of the 1870s, to treat a rheumatic condition. Salicylic acid had an unpleasant taste and was associated with severe gastrointestinal side effects. Hoffman decided to develop a less toxic alternative for his father, but his "discovery" may have been preempted by the French chemist Charles Frédéric Gerhardt in 1853. Furthermore, the active ingredient of aspirin had been synthesized by Johann Kraut

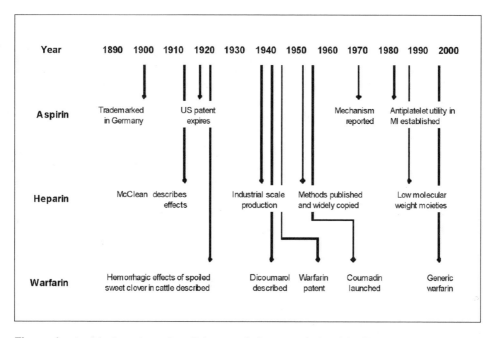

Figure 1 Aspirin, heparin, and warfarin: twentieth-century industrial milestones.

in 1869 and was already being manufactured by the Chemische Fabrik von Heyden Company in 1897, though without a brand name (8,9).

Shortly after making his discovery, Hoffman left Bayer's chemical sciences laboratory to become head of the commercial pharmaceutical department. By some accounts, Bayer was not a happy place to work in 1897. Disagreements between senior executives Arthur Eichengrün, who ran the pharmaceutical division where Hoffmann worked, and Heinrich Dreser, who was in charge of testing and standardization in pharmacology, forced Eichengrün to run clinical trials without approval.

Nevertheless, it was Dreser who published the first article on the pharmacology of aspirin in 1899. Dreser's incentive was a lucrative royalty on the product, once introduced. By contrast, Hoffman and Eichengrün received nothing, since the active ingredient in aspirin was not patentable, even though the trademark was registered on March 6, 1899, in Berlin.

Industrial-scale production of aspirin was quickly established at a plant in Elberfeld, a district of the city of Wuppertal (10). Shortly thereafter, attention switched to the young U.S. market, where Bayer was granted a Method of Manufacture patent for aspirin on February 27, 1900. An industrial plant in Rensselaer, near Albany, New York, began producing aspirin in 1905.

In the early 1900s Bayer began to emphasize the analgesic properties of aspirin now that the mysteries of fever, a prior indication for aspirin use, were being largely solved by Koch and others. The new positioning was effective. Aspirin accounted for nearly one third of Bayer's sales in the United States by 1909. Despite successful prior defense of Bayer's patent position on several occasions, the aspirin manufacturing patents ran out in 1917, just as the United States entered World War I. The U.S. Government Alien Property Custodian seized Bayer's U.S. assets. Trademarks were sold at auction to the Sterling Products Company (later to become Sterling Winthrop) for $5.3 million in 1919, and 75 years of further research began.

Aspirin's mode of action as an anti-inflammatory analgesic with effects on platelets was described in the 1970s (11,12). In the 1980s, aspirin was shown to prevent myocardial infarction after unstable angina (13,14) or after a prior myocardial infarction (15); and to reduce the risk of venous thromboembolic disease (16), first myocardial infarction (17), and colon cancer (18). Eventually, Bayer regained the North American rights to the aspirin brand name by buying Sterling Winthrop in November 1994. The $2.9 billion acquisition also allowed the company to regain the rights to the "Bayer" company name in the United States.

B. Heparin

In 1914 Jay McLean, a medical student at Johns Hopkins, was assigned by Professor of Physiology William Howell to investigate the effects of brain tissue extracts on blood clotting. Howell believed the extracts were procoagulant, but by December 1915, McLean had established the anticoagulant effects of brain, liver, and heart extracts and demonstrated these to a skeptical Howell. Legend has it that McLean placed a beaker of cat's blood with extracted "antithrombin" on Howell's desk and asked his professor to call him when it clotted. Perhaps influenced by a medical student's impertinence, Howell never called McLean, but went on to extract "antithrombin" from liver himself, naming it heparin in 1918.

Dr. Charles H. Best, who also discovered insulin, became involved with heparin in 1928. At the time Best was head of the University of Toronto's Physiology Department and an associate director of Connaught Laboratories, a semi-commercial department of the university. In 1928, Best resolved to produce large amounts of pure heparin and study its effects. Best recruited Drs. Arthur F. Charles, an organic chemist, and David A. Scott, who was closely involved in insulin production at Connaught. Soon after Charles and Scott began their work, Dr. Gordon Murray, a surgeon at Toronto General Hospital, joined the team to conduct experimental surgery using heparin.

Charles and Scott initially used beef liver, readily available from local slaughterhouses, to extract heparin. However, a growing pet food industry drove up the price of beef liver, forcing Charles and Scott to try beef lung and intestines. The work with autolyzed offal gave off a foul stench and was soon moved from the School of Hygiene downtown to a farm outside Toronto. By 1936 Charles and Scott had purified and crystallized heparin in a standard dry form that could be administered in a salt solution. Meanwhile, Murray began the first human trials in May 1935 and by 1937 Connaught's bovine heparin was widely available for surgical procedures such as arterial repair and vein grafting and for the postoperative prevention of thrombosis. In 1949 Drs. Peter Moloney and Edith Taylor published and patented improved methods of heparin production at Connaught. The methods were quickly adapted by pharmaceutical producers to get around patent constraints, and heparin became a commodity. Connaught ended production in the 1950s (19).

Ironically, Connaught was sold in 1989 to Institut Mérieux of Lyon, France, which became part of Pasteur Mérieux Connaught, a subsidiary of Rhone Poulenc of France. Rhone Poulenc developed Lovenox/Clexane, today the most successful heparin product on the market.

C. Warfarin

Early in the twentieth century, American and Canadian farmers imported sweet clover plants from Europe as cattle fodder. Although nutritious when fresh, spoiled sweet clover caused a fatal hemorrhagic disease first described by Schofield, a veterinary pathologist from Alberta in 1921 (20). In February 1933, Ed Carlson, a farmer, visited the University of Wisconsin laboratory of Dr. Karl Paul Link. Carlson took with him a milk can full of blood that refused to clot, a small heap of spoiled sweet clover hay, and a heifer that had died of hemorrhage. Link, who was already investigating the puzzling syndrome, intensified his work. He went on to discover that coumarin, a harmless chemical found in fresh sweet clover, oxidized in spoiled plants to 4–hydroxycoumarin, then coupled with formaldehyde and another coumarin moiety to form dicoumarol, an anticoagulant (19).

Dicoumarol was isolated, then patented for human use in 1941. In 1946 Link and others discovered that a related compound, 3–(2–acetyl-1–phenylethyl)-4–hydroxy-coumarin, was a potent rodenticide. Link gave patent rights for this compound to his research backers, the Wisconsin Alumni Research Foundation (WARF), and named the compound WARF-arin. In 1948 warfarin was launched as a rat poison. Interest in warfarin as a drug was sparked in 1951 when a navy recruit attempted suicide by taking 567 mg of the substance. His surprising full recovery indicated reversible effects in humans. Clinical studies confirmed an acceptable risk-benefit ratio. The compound was licensed by WARF to Endo Pharmaceuticals, a family company formed in Manhattan in 1920 with links to Wisconsin. Endo introduced warfarin sodium to the U.S. market in 1954, branded as Coumadin®. In September of the following year, President Eisenhower suffered a left anterior myocardial infarction while on vacation at his in-laws' house in Denver and was put on long-term treatment that included Coumadin 35 mg/wk (21).

Perhaps encouraged by the presidential endorsement, Endo Pharmaceuticals made a great success of Coumadin, So much so that DuPont, which had been struggling to develop a drug business since the late 1950s, acquired Endo in 1969. Unfortunately, DuPont was unable to expand the business effectively, and in anticipation of further restructuring, Endo was renamed DuPont Pharmaceuticals in 1982. Eight years later, DuPont Pharmaceuticals and drug giant Merck & Company formed a joint venture. Endo was restructured in 1994 to become the generics division of DuPont-Merck, and just 3 years later Endo was spun out as Endo Pharmaceuticals, independent once more. Coumadin, now selling $500 a year in the United States alone, was left behind with DuPont-Merck.

At around the same time, in March 1997, the U.S. Food and Drug Administration (FDA) approved an application by Barr Laboratories to market warfarin sodium tablets as the generic equivalent of Coumadin®. At the time, Coumadin was the eleventh most prescribed product in the United States. For the next 3 years, Barr and DuPont-Merck engaged in legal battles over the sale of generic warfarin. Barr sold the drug throughout. The battle ended in March 2000, when the companies agreed to collaborate in several fields unrelated to Coumadin® Pont was granted the right to purchase 1 million shares of Barr stock. Barr—and later others—continued to sell generic warfarin.

In 1998 DuPont bought out Merck's participation in the joint venture for $2.6 billion and thereby reacquired all rights to Coumadin. Still hesitant about the future of its pharmaceuticals business, DuPont sold its entire pharmaceutical business to Bristol-Myers Squibb for $7.8 billion in October 2001. Bristol-Myers Squibb now market and sell Coumadin tablets. The company reported $300 million in branded Coumadin sales in 2002. Generic forms of warfarin sodium accounted for another $385 million worldwide.

III. DEVELOPING ANTITHROMBOTIC DRUGS

Modern drug developers and regulators aim for a logical progression of chemical, molecular, cellular, tissue, organ, animal, and human studies to establish the effect, safety, dose, quality, and value of a new prescription drug. An ideal process for drug development is mapped in Figure 2.

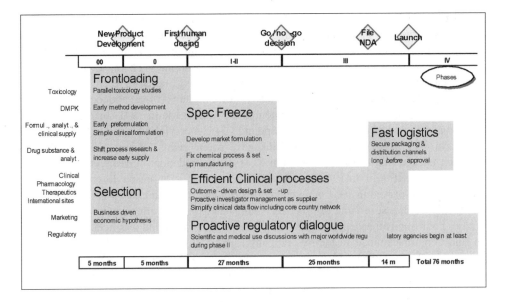

Figure 2 Time-optimized process of drug development. Disciplines (toxicology to regulatory affairs) within the industrial sponsor work as a multifunctional team to orchestrate interdependent tasks from first controlled synthesis and formal (GLP) toxicology studies to launch. This approach is designed to deliver products from 4-week GLP toxicology programs to market within 80 months.

A. Frontloading Product Development

Once a molecule with the desired specificity and potency has been identified and proven in animal models of thrombosis, product development may begin. To shorten the process, significant quantities of the compound may be manufactured before formal toxicology testing gets underway. Such frontloading ensures that manufacturing does not fall on the critical path. Development of methods for estimation of the drug and its metabolites in plasma may also be accelerated, and toxicology programs including acute (1-dose) and subacute (4- and 13-week) studies performed in two mammalian species may be performed in parallel. Antithrombotic agents are typically tested in one small (e.g. rat or rabbit) and one large (e.g., pig or monkey) mammalian model.

B. Early Commitment to the Final Product Manufacturing and Control Methods

Preformulation of the human dosage form should begin almost immediately. For oral agents, a simple drinking solution may expedite the start of phase I clinical studies. However, soon after material for phase I human trials has been manufactured, the process for active ingredient and formulation should be finalized. This manufacturing development work (together with associated quality management procedures) proceeds in parallel to phase II clinical testing, so that product manufactured using the final industrial scale method is available for phase III trials.

C. Focused Clinical Trials

Clinical studies can be classified according to objectives (Table 1). Phase II clinical studies should be directed, rather than exploratory. Dose-finding studies are best designed as blinded parallel-group comparisons of safety and effect in patients with conditions similar to the expected indication. A minimum of five dosage groups should be tested, and particular attention is needed with antithrombotic agents to explore no effect and maximum tolerated doses. In view of the clinical risks of bleeding, maximum tolerated doses may have to be defined using measures of anticoagulant effect as surrogates for clinical risk.

During phase II trials, the key data required to establish effect and safety should be honed. Case report form design is a critical yet often underestimated task. Data collection decisions made at the start of phase II trials will govern the specific fields, descriptions, and frequency of measurement for future trials and potentially dictate labeling. The methods of measurement and definitions of clinical outcomes (e.g., use of CKMB levels to detect myocardial ischemia or ultrasound to detect subclinical venous thrombosis), bleeding (e.g., definition of major versus minor bleeding), and other adverse events (e.g. threshold for thrombocytopenia) devised at this time will shape the profile of the product for many years to come.

Table 1   Classifying Clinical Studies According to Objective

Type of study	Objective	Examples in antithrombotic development
Human pharmacology (phase I)	Assess tolerance Describe PK and PD Explore drug metabolism Estimate activity	Single- and multiple-dose group studies measuring coagulation parameters, duration of action and risk of bleeding, e.g., Frydman et al., Cannon et al. (22,23). typically <100 patients, follow-up 30 days
Therapeutic directive (phase II)	Use in targeted indication Estimate dosage for further studies Provide basis for confirmatory trials	Trials of short duration in well defined populations using surrogate endpoints, such as multidose studies measuring TIMI angiographic blood flow for thrombolysis, e.g., HERO-1 (24); typically 100–1000 patients; follow-up 30–180 days
Therapeutic confirmatory (phase III)	Demonstrate or confirm effectiveness Establish safety profiles Provide an adequate basis for assessing the risk-benefit relationship to support drug licensing Establish dose-response relationship	Double-blind randomized controlled trials with sufficient patients to test clinical hypotheses, e.g., reduction in death, MI, or revascularization after percutaneous coronary intervention; may use more than one dosage, e.g., EPIC (25); typically >1000 patients; follow-up 1 year
Therapeutic use (phase IIIb–IV)	Refine understanding of risk-benefit relationship in general or special populations Identify less common adverse reactions Refine dosing recommendation Position the product	Comparative effectiveness and safety studies often in large populations (e.g., GUSTO-I, GUSTO-II, GUSTO-III (26–28), REPLACE-2 (29)]; these studies may be performed after a drug has been approved for marketing; typically 5,000–40,000 patients; follow-up 1–5 years

Source: Adapted from The International Conference on Harmonisation of Technical Requirements for Registration of Pharmaceuticals for Human Use (ICH) E8: General Considerations for Clinical Trials. ICH Harmonised Tripartite Guideline, July 1997. http://www.ich.org/MediaServer.jser?@_ID=484&@_MODE=GLB.

Data structures and analysis methods should be set up to enable rapid analysis and conclusions from phase II data. These create a basis for phase III trial designs. Key questions to answer with phase II studies include: What is the optimal dosage for phase III (and, hence, for labeling)? What is the expected event rate for thrombosis or bleeding? What is the expected effect size for the drug versus comparator? How many patients are required to establish effect and safety? What inclusion and exclusion criteria should apply?

From the outset, phase III trials must be designed with market entry in mind and include health economic as well as safety and effectiveness variables. In today's crowded marketplace, differentiation on clinical criteria alone may be insufficient to persuade payors to spend more than they do on aspirin, warfarin, or heparin. Ease of product use may be an important consideration in the hospital setting (where, for example, subcutaneous dosing of Lovenox is an important advantage over intravenous heparin) or in the outpatient setting [where, for example, regular monitoring of the International Normalized Ratio (INR) for warfarin is a major cost burden]. Given narrow differences of clinical performance among competitive drugs, apparently modest practical advantages may drive significant market share.

D. Industry Collaboration with Academic Research Organizations

Phase III clinical trials for antithrombotic drugs are often collaborations between pharmaceutical companies, contract research organizations, academic research organizations, and investigators. The interdependency of these parties is complex and demands careful planning, with explicit up-front agreement on roles, accountabilities, and responsibilities. Usually the pharmaceutical company provides trial funding and test medication in kits. The protocol is usually written collaboratively by representatives of the company and lead investigators. For larger trials, steering committees, data safety monitoring boards, blinded endpoint adjudication committees, statistical advisory groups, and other oversight functions may need to be established (30,31).

Most recent phase III antithrombotic trials have been implemented by the industry in partnership with expert groups such as the GUSTO (Global Utilization of Strategies to Open Occluded Coronary Arteries) organization, the TIMI (Thrombolysis in Myocardial Infarction) Group, ISIS (International Study of Infarct Survival), and GISSI (Gruppo Italiano per lo Studio della Sopravvivenza nell'Infarto Miocardico). The VIGOUR (Virtual Co-ordinating Center for Global Collaborative Cardiovascular Research) group (32) has made efforts to coordinate trial activities across these potentially competing organizations on a global basis. Collaborative groups provide an important lever for the pharmaceutical industry and a formidable partner for clinical trials.

IV. MEASURING DRUG DEVELOPMENT

A. How Long Does It Take?

The time required for drug development—from discovery of a new molecular entity to launch in major markets—has become shorter: about 140 months in the 1980s versus 110 months in recent years (Fig. 3). While some objective improvement in FDA review times has been reported (33), and pharmaceutical companies have improved their preclinical programs and phase transition times, there is no consistent evidence that pharmaceutical companies and academic investigators are moving more quickly through clinical trials.

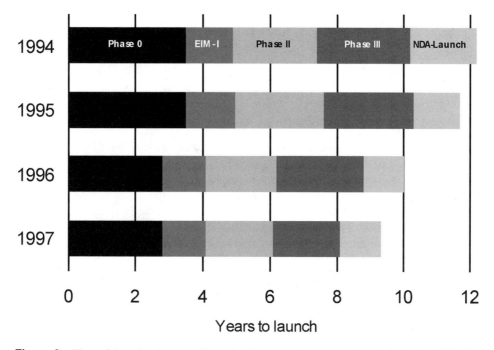

Figure 3 Time of drug development. Drug-development times were reduced during the 1990s but are still above the optimized process target of 7–8 years. Phase 0 includes discovery, preclinical pharmacology and toxicology studies. EIM, entry-into-man. (From Center for Medicines Research (http://www.cmr.org.)

Therefore, the ideal 76–month time period shown in Figure 2 remains—for most drugs, in most companies, at most times—elusive.

B. How Much Does It Cost?

Costs of drug development include the costs of a compound making its way to market the costs associated with compounds that fail along the way. Typically, development programs spend $5–20 million per molecule prior to clinical testing. Clinical trial costs have increased during the last decade. DiMasi et al. (33) estimated total mean clinical trial costs of $28.6 million in 1989 and $125 million in 2000 for each product tested to the end of phase III trials. Adding the cost of long-term animal carcinogenicity studies (around $5 million) results in a total of $145 million per drug. These costs include manufacturing development, but exclude the cost of building new equipment or factories, manufacturing commercial goods for launch, or pursuing further trials (so-called phase IIIb-IV).

C. What Is the Likelihood of Successful Product Commercialization?

Most drugs entering the drug-development process do not reach the market. Less than 1% of newly discovered drug candidates are launched, but the odds improve with each successive stage of product development. Among all drug candidates, 5–10, 20–30, and 65–80% of clinical phase I, II, and III drugs, respectively, reach the market. Failure is usually the result of unexpected safety findings or inadequate effectiveness (70% of cases), but sometimes the high cost of manufacturing (15%) or changing market conditions (15%) may lead to project termination. Decisions to kill development projects are rarely black and white. Usually a combination of problems convinces the sponsor to quit, at least for a period of time.

Risk- and Time-Adjusted Total Costs of Drug Development

Aggregating across phases of drug development and taking into account the costs of failed compounds, DiMasi et al. (33) estimated the total out-of-pocket cost for each new drug approval to be $403 million, while the fully capitalized total cost estimate (taking into account the time-value of money) is $802 million. The inflation-adjusted, total capitalized cost per approved new drug in 2003 was 2.5 times higher than the 1991 estimate (34)—an annual growth in costs of around 7%.

For antithrombotic drugs, the capitalized cost of development is likely to be above the average for all products. Antithrombotic drug development requires stepwise (and sometimes slow) dose exploration, large sample sizes in comparative trials to detect effects on infrequent clinical events such as myocardial infarction or pulmonary embolism, and long-term follow-up. Naturally, there is little tolerance for clinical risk, and safety hurdles are set high.

Clinical trials of antithrombotic agents may therefore be slower, more costly, and higher-risk than typical studies. A phase III trial of 10,000 patients may cost $2,500 per patient in investigator or institutional fees (total $25 million). An additional $20–60 million may be incurred in infrastructure costs, including data management, quality assurance, project management, site coordination and monitoring, endpoint adjudication, statistical analysis, study report preparation, documentation, quality control, clinical audit, and publication. Recruitment over 12–24 months is typical.

Antithrombotic drugs have a patchy record of success in late-stage clinical trials designed to lead to regulatory approval and subsequent commercialization. For example, the entire class of oral GP IIb/IIIa inhibitors was wiped out after phase III trials in 33,326 patients followed for more than 30 days showed a consistent and statistically significant increase in mortality with oral GP IIb/IIIa therapy (OR 1.37; 95% CI 1.13–1.66; $p = 0.001$). This effect was evident regardless of aspirin coadministration and treatment with either low-dose or high-dose therapy (35).

Even when clinical results are positive, regulatory and commercial success may not be automatic. Despite 11 randomized trials in 35,970 patients with acute coronary syndromes showing that compared to heparin, thrombin-specific inhibitors lower the risk of death or myocardial infarction significantly (OR 0.85; 95% CI 0.77–0.94; $p = 0.001$) (36), only one direct thrombin-specific inhibitor, Angiomax (bivalirudin) has so far been approved for use in patients with unstable angina undergoing coronary intervention. Similarly, despite increasing evidence of lower mortality following PCI with intravenous GP IIb/IIIa inhibitors (37,38), tirofiban (Aggrastat®, Merck and Co. and, more recently, Guildford Pharmaceuticals) is not approved for elective PCI in the United States, while eptifibatide (Integrilin®, Millennium and Schering-Plough Corporation) is not approved for PCI in Europe. Both drugs are approved in the United States and Europe for treatment of patients with acute coronary syndromes.

Conversely, abciximab (ReoPro) was approved and very successfully commercialized for use in patients undergoing PCI. Despite this initial progress, the product then failed to demonstrate 30–day clinical advantages over placebo in a trial of more than 7000 patients with ACS without ST elevation who were not scheduled for coronary intervention

(39), and was associated with excess 1–year mortality in subgroups of patients with low cardiac troponin or elevated C-reactive protein (40). Next came the 30–day results of the 16,588–patient GUSTO-V trial, first reported in the summer of 2001, which showed no difference in the primary endpoint of 30–day mortality (or 1–year mortality) and more bleeding complications among patients given ReoPro with Retavase®. Despite a promising reduction in reinfarction, recurrent ischemia, and need for early urgent revascularization in the combination group in this trial, the data have not so far been submitted for extension of the ReoPro label (41).

These clinical programs illustrate the magnitude of investment, clinical endeavor, and risk undertaken with antithrombotic drugs by the pharmaceutical industry. In ACS and PCI, the patient numbers in phase III trials are staggering—a total of 48,000 treated in thrombin-specific inhibitor studies (29,36,42), 33,000 in oral GP IIb/IIIa studies (35), 31,000 in intravenous GP IIb/IIIa studies (43), with an additional 20,000 in PCI studies (37,38). The total—around 132,000 patients—can be multiplied by an average per-patient study fee of $2,000 to estimate funds sent to investigating centers of $264 million for this part of drug development. An industry rule-of-thumb suggests that such fees represent about half the total cost of trials.

Therefore, well over half a billion dollars has been spent on these phase III programs alone in the areas of non-ST elevation ACS and PCI. Even assuming $5.5 billion in sales over the next 10 years for these products in these indications, the phase III investments (which exclude all other development, manufacturing, marketing and sales costs) will not achieve internal rates of return much in excess of industry investment hurdle rates of 10–15%.

V. REGULATORY CONSIDERATIONS

A triangle of academia, industry and regulatory agencies creates the fulcrum for progress with antithrombotic agents. Yet regulators have the final say on safety, effectiveness, dosage, and quality of a new product. Their role in antithrombotic drug development is therefore pivotal.

The U.S. Food and Drug Administration (FDA) is the most adequately resourced of the worldwide drug review agencies. FDA has the authority, capacity and capability, to shape research plans, monitor progress, analyze data, dictate drug positioning in the marketplace, and suspend sales. For the most part, FDA's track record on antithrombotics is unblemished, except perhaps by the agency dragging its feet in the matter of aspirin and Reye's syndrome in the early 1980s (44).

For obscure organizational reasons, FDA divided the task of antithrombotic product assessment among three major groups. The Cardiac and Renal Drug Division oversees antiplatelet agent drug development and review within the Center for Drug Evaluation and Research. The Gastrointestinal and Coagulation Division oversees antithrombin agents. Until recently, biologicals, such as Activase® (t-PA) and Retavase® (reteplase)— but not, for some reason, ReoPro (abciximab), were overseen by the Center for Biologicals Evaluation and Research (CBER). These mixed assignments have sometimes yielded inconsistent approaches within the agency. Occasionally, reinterpretation, integration and guidance by FDA senior management are required and provided. In Europe, the European Medicines Evaluation Agency has taken a decentralized approach to resourcing drug evaluations. Antithrombotic drug applications may be assessed by Rapporteur member states on behalf of the Agency and the Committee on Proprietary Medicinal Products, which oversees drug approvals (45). In Japan, the Ministry of

Health and Welfare has developed a growing resource base with an increasing acceptance of and interest in non-Japanese clinical data. Drug-approval processes in Japan do, however, remain quite different from those followed in the European Union and the United States (46).

A. International Conference on Harmonization

The participation of all three major agencies, alongside academic and industry experts, in the International Conference on Harmonization (ICH) has improved the efficiency and effectiveness of drug development and evaluation worldwide (47). Nowadays, most products are developed for worldwide markets simultaneously—a dramatic shift compared to the 1980s when pharmaceutical development was regionalized. An important early step by the ICH initiative was to unify the principles and implementation of so-called Good Clinical Practice (GCP) on a worldwide basis (48).

B. Good Clinical Practice

GCP is an international ethical and scientific quality standard for designing, conducting, recording, and reporting trials that involve the participation of human subjects. Compliance with this standard provides public assurance that the rights, safety, and well-being of trial subjects are protected and that the clinical trial data are credible.

The principles of international GCP as applied by the pharmaceutical industry and regulators (47) are as follows:

> Clinical trials should be conducted in accordance with the ethical principles reflected in the Declaration of Helsinki.
> A trial should be initiated and continued only if the anticipated benefits for the individual trial subject and society outweigh the risks.
> The rights, safety, and well-being of the trial subjects should prevail over the interests of science and society.
> The available nonclinical and clinical information on an investigational product must be adequate to support the proposed clinical trial.
> Clinical trials should be scientifically sound and described in a clear, detailed protocol.
> Protocols should receive prior institutional review board (IRB) or independent ethics committee approval.
> The medical care given to, and medical decisions made on behalf of, subjects should always be the responsibility of a qualified physician.
> Each individual involved in conducting a trial should be qualified by education, training, and experience.
> Freely given informed consent should be obtained from every subject.
> Clinical trial information should be recorded, handled, and stored in a way that ensures accuracy of reporting, verification and interpretation.
> The confidentiality of records that could identify subjects should be protected.
> Investigational products should be manufactured, handled, and stored in accordance with applicable good manufacturing practice (GMP) and used only as directed by the protocol.
> Systems with procedures that assure the quality of every aspect of the trial should be implemented.

The ICH process has created many other standards and guidelines (49). These include written guidance on manufacturing, safety, and effectiveness programs aimed at improving the safety of patients and/or the efficiency of drug development.

VI. MANUFACTURING ANTITHROMBOTIC DRUGS

Unlike the early development steps for heparin, aspirin, and warfarin, contemporary manufacturing programs for antithrombotic agents are based on the recognition that effective and efficient manufacturing processes ensure product quality and performance. The design of product and process specifications is based on a mechanistic understanding of how formulation and process factors affect product performance. Such a philosophy demands continuous real-time quality assurance and a focus on the fundamental scientific aspects of the product, its storage and administration, and the patients who may be treated (50).

Quality is built into pharmaceutical products through a comprehensive understanding of a drug's (a) intended therapeutic objectives, patient population, route of administration, and pharmacological, toxicological, and pharmacokinetic characteristics and (b) its chemical, physical, and biopharmaceutic characteristics. Quality results from (c) the selection of product components and packaging based on these drug attributes and (d) the design of manufacturing processes using principles of engineering, materials science, and quality assurance that ensure acceptable and reproducible product quality and performance throughout a product's shelf life.

Adherence to these principles is by no means an academic exercise. In 1999 Abbott Laboratories received a letter from FDA outlining serious deficiencies with Abbokinase® (urokinase) and suspending sales of the product (51). FDA's concerns were related to manufacturing processes, product testing, and screening and testing of the donors of the kidney cells used to make Abbokinase.

According to FDA, during inspections of Abbott Laboratories and of BioWittaker, Inc., Abbott's supplier of human kidney cells, FDA identified deviations from current good manufacturing practice (CGMP) regulations. Deviations included inadequate screening of donors and testing of donated cells, controls for proper harvesting, storage, and handling of materials, and processes to remove or inactivate infectious agents from the product. A number of in-process lots of Abbokinase were contaminated with microorganisms. Many were found to contain various strains of reovirus and/or mycoplasma. Abbott was unable to locate the source of the problems, raising further concerns at FDA about the entire manufacturing process for Abbokinase.

Earlier, in January 1999, FDA had issued a letter to health care providers to alert them to the Abbokinase manufacturing problems (52). The letter included information about the potential risks of the product for transmitting infectious agents. It also recommended that Abbokinase be reserved only for those situations in which a physician had considered other available treatment alternatives and had determined that the use of Abbokinase was critical to the care of a specific patient in a specific situation. In addition, at FDA's request, Abbott changed the labeling of the product to include additional information reflecting these safety concerns.

However, after the January 1999 letter to health care providers, the FDA obtained additional information regarding the inadequacy of the screening and testing of the mothers and donors of the human kidney cells used to produce Abbokinase. Information was also obtained regarding seven instances of in-process lots of product being contaminated with reovirus and mycoplasma.

In the product suspension letter to Abbott, the agency detailed the steps Abbott needed to take to correct manufacturing deviations. These included:

> Completing a thorough investigation of the reovirus and mycoplasma contamination, including the source of the contamination
>
> Manufacturing Abbokinase using human kidney cells that had been obtained, processed, and tested through adequate methods
>
> Assuring that fully validated methods were used in the manufacturing process to test for and remove infectious agents

Throughout the discussion, Abbott remained steadfast in their publicly stated position (53) that Abbokinase manufacturing complied with current GMP regulations.

Whether warranted or not, it is clear, however, that action by FDA can destroy a franchise. In the case of Abbokinase, a $260 million per year revenue stream growing at 10% per year would have led to cumulative sales of $1.6 billion between 1999, the year of suspension, and 2003. Instead, Abbott revenues on Abbokinase, relaunched in 2002, have not yet reached $100 million, and competitor products, such as Genentech's CathFlow t-PA product, have been provided an attractive entry opportunity. It is hard to recover from that.

VII. MARKETING ANTITHROMBOTIC DRUGS

A. What Is Marketing?

To many, marketing means advertising and selling. This limited view understates the scope. Advertising is only a small part of marketing, and selling is a separate discipline

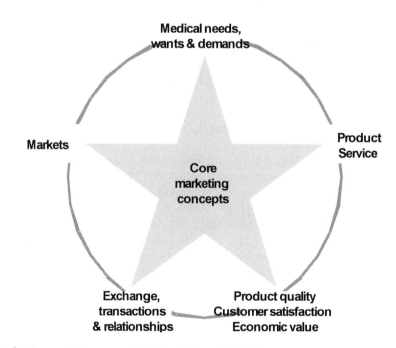

Figure 4 Core marketing concepts. (Adapted from Ref. 68.)

entirely. Effective marketing programs in pharmaceuticals, as in other industry areas, organizes around a few basic concepts and practices (Fig. 4).

B.   Medical Needs, Wants, and Demands

The fundamental concept underlying successful development and commercialization of antithrombotic drugs is an understanding of unmet medical needs, wants, and demands. At a very basic level, medical needs for antithrombotic treatment have been met by aspirin, heparin, and warfarin. Each is effective, up to a point, and each has a predictable—perhaps suboptimal—safety profile, dosage, quality, and perceived value for the low acquisition cost they generally command.

In the language of marketers, improvements that can be made to antithrombotic drugs constitute "wants." Examples of such wants include reduced gastrointestinal irritation (in the case of aspirin), improved effectiveness in high-risk patients with established thrombus (heparin), and a reduced liability for drug-drug interactions (warfarin). To some extent, wants (in contrast to needs) are influenced by issues related to medical culture. In the United States there may be an expectation that medical treatment should be taken to maximum effect for all age groups, whereas in Japan there may be greater emphasis on issues related to patient safety and comfort.

Furthermore, wants are also influenced by economic conditions. The GUSTO-I trial demonstrated a 14% relative risk reduction for mortality after acute MI in patients treated with Activase compared to streptokinase (26). The United States market bought it—literally. But many parts of the world did not; they were unwilling or unable to pay the premium price of Activase over streptokinase, and the older thrombolytic remains standard therapy in many parts of the world today (42). In the meantime, the U.S. marketplace has moved from thrombolysis to percutaneous coronary intervention, in view of further improvements in mortality (54).

Wants become demands when backed by the kind of buying power seen in the U.S. market. Most U.S. consumers, given the choice, would now select PCI over thrombolysis for acute MI. An understanding of needs, wants, and demands is developed from expert advisory boards, focus groups, and other market research—including review of the academic literature. Specific attributes of new or imaginary products are tested to determine the level of interest in each. Product performance is also monitored after market launch. Well-organized pharmaceutical companies feed this information continuously back to their drug discovery and development teams, who match plans and activities against a list of ideal product specifications. Such companies also keep close to customers in an ongoing effort to understand evolving needs, wants, and demands. Indeed, the marketplace itself has proven to be the most significant source of innovation for medical and other high-technology products (55). Remarkably, and in spite of this, most major pharmaceutical firms still base their organizational structure on functional disciplines such as research & development (R&D) versus marketing, rather than audiences.

C.   Product, Service, or Both?

Antithrombotic products are usually delivered to the pharmacy. Yet the term "product" for pharmaceutical companies usually includes the information and services associated with such delivery. For antithrombotic drugs, the services may include educational materials and events, instructions on monitoring anticoagulant effects (or even securing monitoring tests), dedicated websites for consumers or physicians, health economic tools, pharmacy in-service kits, and even practitioner education on new treatment pathways facilitated by the antithrombotic drug itself. When designed effectively, these services provide solutions to customer needs, wants, and demands. The manufacturer of a drug for PCI may be tempted to believe that the physician needs an anticoagulant, when what the physician really needs is to perform a rapid, cost-efficient, and perfectly safe procedure before going home to have dinner with the family.

D. Economic Value, Customer Satisfaction, and Quality

The economic value of an antithrombotic drug is the difference between the value the customer gains from using the product and the cost of obtaining the product. This is not as simple as it sounds. Even well-informed customers—in this case physicians, pharmacists, nurses, and others—may not always judge value objectively or accurately. They may act instead on perceived value. For example, a physician may value preventing CKMB release after PCI more highly than preventing femoral access site hemorrhage associated with a 3 g/dL fall in hemoglobin concentration or blood transfusion. For a nurse managing the hemorrhage or for a patient discharged home the next day with a 6 cm diameter hematoma in the groin, the perception of relative value may be different. Recent data suggesting that bleeding may predict 1–year mortality more accurately than CKMB elevations (56) may alter perceptions all around.

Customer satisfaction rests on the need for the antithrombotic drug to deliver performance that matches the customers' expectations. Expectations may be set, for example, by medical school education, personal experience, academic publications, or company promotional activities. If the product falls short of expectations in the hands of the physician, then there is dissatisfaction. This often-ignored phenomenon points to one of the great challenges of antithrombotic drug treatments today, namely, how to ensure that physicians and nurses follow evidence-based practice guidelines. Such guidelines are often built on data showing significant differences between two treatments in large clinical trials reporting low outcome event rates.

Consider the use of intravenous platelet GP IIb/IIIa inhibitors for the upstream treatment of non–ST elevation acute coronary syndromes. The PURSUIT, PRISM, and PRISM-PLUS trials established clinically and statistically significant treatment benefits for the new agents on top of heparin (57–59). To demonstrate such differences to his or her personal satisfaction, a physician would need to treat about 10,000 patients and observe their outcomes carefully. For most cardiologists this would take a professional lifetime. More likely, they may treat 1000 patients with non–ST segment acute coronary syndrome over 10 years.

Without GP IIb/IIIa inhibitors, the physician will likely observe 15 unnecessary end-point events, most of which will be subclinical infarcts or referrals for revascularization, over 10 years. A single major bleeding event, a strong complaint from a pharmacist about cost, or an episode of thrombocytopenia for one patient may outweigh these benefits in the mind of a physician, leading to dissatisfaction and dissuading further use. Much more work is needed to unravel the psychological complexities of physician decision making.

E. Exchange, Transactions, and Relationships

Exchange, the act of obtaining a desired object from someone by offering something in return, is a complex process in the pharmaceutical marketplace. Unlike direct markets (e.g., a customer exchanges money with a farmer for apples), pharmaceutical markets are mediated through many parties (e.g., patient, doctor, nurse, pharmacist, hospital administrator, Medicare, wholesaler, manufacturer). Each party may have different perceptions of value.

One way pharmaceutical marketers deal with this is to employ so-called relationship marketing—the process of creating, maintaining and enhancing strong, value-laden relationships with each set of customers and related stakeholders. Typically, pharmaceutical companies work with "opinion leaders" (who often, but not always, lead research programs) and create a pyramid of influential experts who act as advocates, speaking and writing about the product to the educational benefit of colleagues less well connected to the industrial system or academic college in question. Effective opinion leaders balance an expert position on several products at the same time; less effective opinion leaders become entrenched as single-product champions and lose their effectiveness. The qualities of effective advocates therefore go far beyond detailed understanding of clinical data.

The antithrombotic drug market contains vast numbers of patients at risk of venous thromboembolic disease or arterial thrombosis. Most market analysts begin with the total universe of patients and whittle the population down by exclusion. Defining the market often begins with assessment of the prevalence, incidence, and time-course of diseases and conditions associated with thrombosis. Fundamental sources of data in the United States include National Center for Health Statistics (NCHS) surveys such as the National Health and Nutrition Examination Survey (NHANES). Other sources of data in the United States include the National Heart, Lung and Blood Institute (NHLBI) and the National Institute of Neurological Disorders and Stroke (NINDS). Similar sources are available in most major European countries and Japan. Epidemiological surveys provide a view of the total potential market but overestimate the current market. Prevalence or incidence figures rarely translate directly into patients-to-treat.

But in the same way—as the saying goes—crooks rob banks because that's where the money is—the pharmaceutical industry concentrates R&D resources on large population markets. Tables 2 and 3 illustrate this concentration.

More than 50 million people in major countries suffer atrial fibrillation (AF), stable angina (SA), or peripheral arterial disease (PAD). More than half of these are in the United States. More than 10 million people experience acute coronary syndrome (ACS), venous thromboembolism (VTE), percutaneous coronary intervention (PCI), or coronary artery bypass graft (CABG) each year in these markets, with ACS dominating events. Again, the United States, with 6.5 million incident patient events, provides the lion's share of market opportunity.

Obviously, antithrombotic drug development and marketing is focused on U.S. audiences. This has led to a shift in strategic focus for EU companies such as Aventis, AstraZeneca, and Sanofi-Synthélabo, to address U.S. needs, wants, and demands.

Table 2 Prevalence of Thrombosis-Related Disorders in the United States and Five Major European Countries (Millions of Patients)

	AF	SA	PAD
United States	2.03	8.53	15.59
France	0.66	2.12	3.10
Germany	0.95	3.22	5.29
Italy	0.70	2.35	1.86
Spain	0.44	1.48	1.19
UK	0.65	2.18	3.55
Total	5.42	19.89	30.57

AF = atrial fibrillation; SA = stable angina; PAD = peripheral arterial disease.
Source: DataMonitor.

Table 3   Incidence of Cardiovascular Events (Millions of Patients)

	ACS	VTE	CVA	PCI	CABG
United States	3.48	0.40	0.73	1.12	0.77
Japan	0.47	N/A	0.46	0.17	0.02
France	0.31	0.14	0.10	0.08	0.02
Germany	0.59	0.12	0.14	0.16	0.03
Italy	0.16	0.14	0.22	0.06	0.02
Spain	0.24	0.09	0.14	0.02	0.01
UK	0.58	0.09	0.20	0.04	0.02
Total	5.82	0.98	1.99	1.65	0.89

ACS = acute coronary syndromes, including non–ST elevation ACS and ST elevation ACS (acute myocardial infarction); VTE = venous thromboembolism; CVA = cerebrovascular accident (stroke); PCI = percutaneous coronary intervention; CABG = coronary artery bypass graft surgery.
Figures are millions of incident patient events per year.
N/A = not available.
Source: DataMonitor.

Atrial fibrillation prevalence in developed western markets amounts to 5.4 million patients. A treatment value of, say, $200 equates to a $1 billion market opportunity if all patients are always treated. Stable angina and peripheral arterial disease represent another $10 billion of market opportunity on the same mathematical basis. How much could a drug company realistically aim for depends on presentation of the disease, current levels of motivation (needs) for treatment, and the readiness and willingness of consumers to pay and physicians to treat. Clearly Plavix, with sales of $2.5 billion current revenue, could look forward to significant further growth—projected by analysts to reach $5 billion over the next 5 years.

Analysis of hospital discharge data may reveal how many patients present to the health care system, how they are treated, and how they fare. Hospital discharge data include demographics, comorbidity, treatment, and outcomes—potentially important market segmentation tools. Hospital discharge data may also reveal useful geographic patterns. Prescription data may provide insight into individual physician behavior.

Following desk-based market research, live market research via telephone surveys, focus groups, and in-depth interviews may be commissioned to explore medical needs and review proposed product attributes. These forums may also be used to test product positioning.

F.   Models for Marketing Antithrombotic Drugs

Five separate models for marketing are known, and each has been adopted by pharmaceutical companies selling antithrombotics. The models, their principles, and examples are summarized in Table 4.

G.   Global Challenges

Just as aspirin became a global brand in the early 1900s, most antithrombotics are now marketed internationally (Table 5). While potentially lucrative, global branding of antithrombotics is challenging. Medical practices may differ between the major markets of Europe, Japan, and the United States, driven by cultural, economic, or legal factors.

Table 4 Marketing Models Used by Companies Selling Antithrombotic Drugs

Marketing model	Principles	Example for antithrombotics
Production	Customers favor products that are available and highly affordable; management therefore focuses on improving production and distribution efficiency	The generic drug industry—drugs such as aspirin, heparin and warfarin are freely available at low cost worldwide
Product	Customers favor products that offer the highest performance and features and that there should be focus on "building a better mousetrap"	Marketing of Activase® (Genentech) against Streptase® (Hoechst) in United States; the approach was successful until primary PCI overtook thrombolysis as the treatment of choice for acute MI; this illustrates a flaw in the product approach where emphasis is on a better mouse trap rather than the solution to many mice
Selling	Large-scale selling and promotional efforts are used to drive product utilization and increase volume	Marketing of Plavix® as an adjunct to aspirin and—shortly—Exanta® as a replacement for warfarin
Marketing	Strict focus on the needs and wants of customers and delivering these more effectively and efficiently than competitors	Angiomax® versus heparin plus GP IIb/IIIa inhibitors for PCI procedures; focus on replacing heparin to streamline PCI, increase patient throughput, and reduce cost without losing effectiveness
Societal	Determine the needs, wants, and interests of target markets, deliver the solutions efficiently to improve the consumers' and society's well-being	Almost every pharmaceutical company from Bayer to Merck to Johnson and Johnson project this approach to the outside world; execution and results have been mixed

The worldwide pharmaceutical market is growing at around 8% annually and was $406 billion in 2002. North America, Europe, Japan, and Latin America account for 85% of the world market. The 12 major markets—consisting of the United States, Japan, Germany, France, Italy, the United Kingdom, Spain, Canada, Australia, Belgium, Switzerland, and South Africa—account for over 75% of the global pharmaceutical market by value.

The U.S. pharmaceutical market is expected to exceed $330 billion in 2006 (60), and will then account for over 60% of the total major international market, up from 56% in 2001. It is also forecast that U.S. per capita expenditure on drugs will exceed $1,000, double the expenditure in Japan and three times that in the United Kingdom, by the year 2006. The next largest national pharmaceutical market, Japan, is forecast to virtually stand still, with low single-digit growth. The Japanese market was three times the size of the third biggest market (Germany) in 2001. However, in recent years, as the Japanese pharmaceutical industry has been beleaguered by continuing economic stagnation, this pharma market is forecast to be just twice the size of the third-biggest market (France) in 2006. The French and German markets will remain virtually equal in terms of value. The Italian market, with sales growth of well over 10%, will pull further ahead of the United Kingdom, where growth is only expected to be in the single digits.

Table 5 Pharmaceutical Sales Projected for Major Markets, 2000–2005

	Annual sales, 2000 (US$ billions)	Projected annual sales 2005 (US$ billions)	Projected compound annual growth rate 2000–2005 (%)	Projected 10-country market share, 2005 (%)
Belgium	2	3	5.6	0.7
Australia	3	5	9.3	1.1
Canada	6	10	10.7	2.4
Spain	6	10	9.9	2.3
Italy	11	16	8.2	3.6
UK	11	16	8.3	3.7
France	16	22	6.0	5.0
Germany	17	24	7.5	5.6
Japan	58	66	2.3	15.1
United States	150	263	11.8	60.5
Total	281	434	+9.1	100

Sales cover direct and indirect pharmaceutical channel purchases from pharmaceutical wholesalers and manufacturers in 10 key international markets. Figures include prescription and certain over-the-counter data and represent manufacturer prices.
Source: IMS HEALTH Pharma-Prognosis International, 2001–2005.

VIII. MARKET TRENDS 2003–2008

A. The Current Market for Antithrombotics

Table 6 summarizes worldwide revenues for antithrombotic drugs in 2002–2003. Individual drug revenues are listed in Table 7. Figure 5 demonstrates 2002 market share by drug category, and Figure 6 presents current sales and future projections for each.

B. Oral Antiplatelet Agents

Oral platelet inhibitors are expected to continue to grow, as further trials of Plavix are completed in new indications. Over the next 5 years there are likely to be new nonprodrug P2Y12 inhibitors, such as the Lilly/Sankyo compound CS-747 (in 2007), and AstraZeneca's AZD-6140 (in 2008).

Table 6 Worldwide Revenues for Antithrombotic Drugs

	Revenue ($ millions)		Annual growth rate (%)	Share of class revenue, 2002%
	2001	2002		
Antiplatelets	4955	5770	16.4	58
LMWH	2200	2450	11.4	25
UFH	305	260	-14.8	3
Thrombin specific inhibitors	114	220	93.0	2
Warfarins	715	685	-4.2	7
Thrombolytics	598	576	-3.7	6
Total	8887	9961	12.1	100

Table 7 Antithrombotic Products Marketed in 2003

Product	Type	Originator	US marketer	2002 Sales ($US mm)
AT antagonists				
Unfractionated heparin	Inject	Connaught	Wyeth and others	260
LMW AT antagonists				2450
Lovenox (enoxaparin)	Inject	RPR	Aventis	1500
Fragmin (dalteparin)	Inject	Pharmacia	Pharmacia	270
Fraxiparine (nadroparin)	Inject	Sanofi Synth	Sanofi Synth	315
Other LMWH	Inject			365
Other anticoagulants				220
Thrombin or Xa inhibitors				120
Angiomax (bivalirudin)	Inject	Biogen	The Medicines Co.	36
Refludan (lepirudin)	Inject	Hoechst	Berlex Laboratories	20
Argatroban	Inject	Mitsubishi	GlaxoSmithKline	57
Arixtra (fondaparinux)	Inject	Organon	Organon, Sanofi Synth	7
Protein-C antagonist				
Xigris (drotrecogin alfa)	Inject	Lilly	Lilly	100
Antiplatelet agents				5770
Aspirin (all ASA)	Oral	Bayer	Bayer and others	1790
Plavix (clopidogrel)	Oral	Sanofi Synth	Sanofi Synth	2600
Panaldine (ticlopidine)	Oral	Daiichi	Daiichi	280
Integrilin (eptifibatide)	Inject	Cor	Schering, Millenium	250
Aggrastat (tirofiban)	Inject	Merck & Co.	Merck and Co.	120
ReoPro (abciximab)	Inject	Eli Lilly	Centocor	345
Pletaal (cilostazol)	Oral	Otsuka	Otsuka	385
Prothrombin synthesis inhibitors				685
Coumadin (warfarin)	Oral	Endo	Dupont	300
Warfarin (generics)	Oral		Barr and others	385
Thrombolytics				576
Abbokinase	Inject	Abbott	Abbott	45
Activase (t-PA)	Inject	Genentech	Genentech	119
TNKase	Inject	Genentech	Genentech	89
Reteplase	Inject	Boehringer M.	Johnson & Johnson	100
Metalyse (tenectaplase)	Inject	Boehringer I.	Boehringer I.	45
All others	Inject	Various		178
Total				9961

C. Intravenous GP IIb/IIIa inhibitors

Intravenous GP IIb/IIIa inhibitor growth rates have slowed in the wake of disappointing trial results for ReoPro in ACS (GUSTO-IV and GUSTO-V) (61,62) and increasing evidence that alternative platelet inhibitors such as Plavix and the use of non–platelet agonists such as Angiomax (bivalirudin) instead of heparin may limit the need for GP IIb/IIIa inhibitors (56,63). Flat or declining worldwide sales are expected.

D. Heparins

The convenience and marginal effectiveness advantages of low molecular weight heparin (LMWH) dosing have driven impressive growth to date. Lovenox dominates the market for

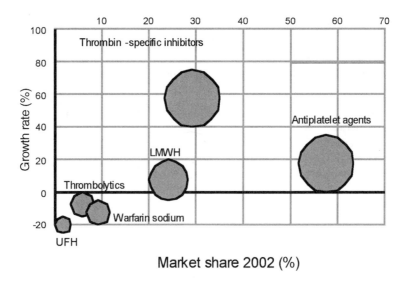

Figure 5 Growth rate and market share for major classes of antithrombotic agents in 2002.

venous thromboembolism. Results of the SYNERGY trial (64) in early 2004 will determine the further growth of Lovenox in coronary indications, where the greatest potential now lies. The entry of Arixtra® (fondaparinux), an AT-mediated factor Xa inhibitor, has not yet challenged Lovenox significantly, particularly in the United States. Fragmin® (dalteparin) has been all but abandoned by its new owner, Pfizer (via acquisition of Pharmacia in 2003), on account of the product's relatively small revenue next to Pfizer's blockbuster

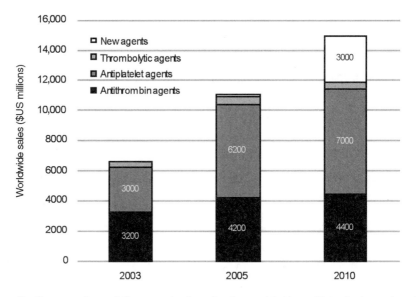

Figure 6 Current sales and future projections for the worldwide antithrombotic market. (Data from Ref. 7.)

Table 8 Antithrombotic Products in Development

Product	Type	Action	Company	Stage
Exanta (ximelagratran)	Oral	Thrombin-specific antagonist	AstraZeneca	Registration
BIBR1048MS	Oral	Thrombin-specific antagonist	Boehringer Ingel.	Phase II
SB-424323	Oral	Thrombin-specific antagonist	GlaxoSmithKline	Phase II
DX 9065a	Inject	Xa-specific antagonist	Daiichi	Phase II
DPC-423	Oral	Xa-specific antagonist	Bristol Myers	Phase I
BAY-59-7939	Oral	Xa-specific antagonist	Bayer	Phase I
N/A	Oral	Xa-specific antagonist	Tularik/Lilly	Phase I
N/A	Oral	Xa-specific antagonist	Sankyo	Phase II
Cangrelor	Inject	P2Y12 platelet antagonist	Medicines Co.	Phase II
AZD6140	Oral	P2Y12 platelet antagonist	AstraZeneca	Phase II
CS-747	Oral	P2Y12 platelet antagonist	Sankyo/Lilly	Phase I
Prolyse	Inject	Plasminogen activator	Abbott	Phase III
N/A	Inject	Plasminogen activator	Amgen	Phase III
BB-10153	Inject	Plasminogen activator	British Biotech	Phase II
N/A	Inject	Factor VIIa antagonist	Cortecs	Phase II

portfolio. Worldwide sales of unfractionated heparins, an astonishing $260 million, representing at least 20 million patient uses worldwide, are expected to continue to fall due to the continued emergence of improved alternatives.

E. Thrombin-Specific Anticoagulants

Once scrapped as ineffective after mixed trial results, this class of agent has made a significant comeback for the treatment of heparin-induced thrombocytopenia and for the management of patients undergoing PCI. Angiomax (bivalirudin) has made the most progress, with 2003 projected sales approaching $100 million in the United States alone. Further trials with Angiomax are underway in cardiac surgery and in acute coronary syndromes. Potential peak revenue has been estimated to exceed $500 million. Growth in this group of products has also been driven by the entry of Xigris™ (drotrecogin alfa activated) for sepsis, with sales of $100 million in 2002.

F. Thrombolytics

Thrombolytics have shown declining worldwide sales, as PCI has superseded drug treatment for management of AMI Price pressure in non-U.S. markets, where thrombolysis continues to be first-line treatment, is likely to restrain any further growth of this class of antithrombotics.

IX. Future Industrial Perspectives

A major shift in oral antithrombin therapy is likely to occur with the expected introduction of Astra-Zeneca's Exanta® (ximelagatran), in 2004–2005 as a replacement for warfarin in several indications. The growth of Exanta will depend on physicians' perceptions concerning moderate liver function abnormalities and the need for liver test monitoring (as opposed to INR monitoring for warfarin). Other oral thrombin-specific agents may follow, as shown in Table 8. Those that do not require monitoring of either the INR or of liver function tests are likely to dominate the market.

Further replacement of unfractionated heparin is likely in view of its failure to inhibit clot-bound thrombin and its propensity to cause clinically significant platelet aggregation via the GP IIb/IIIa receptor (65–67). Results from clinical trials being completed in 2003–2005 including SYNERGY (Lovenox in ACS), ACUITY (Angiomax vs. Lovenox in ACS), and further trials of Arixtra in ACS, will influence the ultimate shape and share of the injectable anticoagulant market.

Overall, the antithrombotic market is likely to continue to grow significantly, exceeding $13 billion within 5 years. For the medium term (10 years), a range of antiplatelet, antithrombin, and anti-Xa inhibitors are in early clinical testing. Each holds the potential for further improvement in the effectiveness, safety, ease of use, and value of antithrombotic therapy, particularly in advanced markets where increasingly sophisticated interventional approaches are likely to be used in tandem with drugs. Beyond the medium term, the identification of patients at risk for thrombosis—through the detection of abnormal coagulation genotypes and phenotypes—should refine our selection of treatment targets and interventions.

Major changes in the business environment may also impact antithrombotic drug development and commercialization. Mergers and acquisitions between pharmaceutical companies may disrupt or accelerate product investments. Price controls in Europe and increasing pressures on prices in the United States may lead to parallel importation, which accompanies globalization of markets. Over the next 25 years, novel products are likely to emerge from China and other Asian countries as their economies grow and the geographic sources of innovation diversify.

REFERENCES

1. MacFarlane RG. An enzyme cascade in the blood clotting mechanism, and its function as a biochemical amplifier. Nature 1964; 202:498–9.
2. Ammar T, Scudder LE, Coller BS. In vitro effects of the platelet glycoprotein IIb/IIIa receptor antagonist c7E3 Fab on the activated clotting time. Circulation. 1997; 95:614–617.
3. Coller BS. Blockade of platelet GPIIb/IIIa receptors as an antithrombotic strategy. Circulation. 1995; 92:2373–2380.
4. Weitz JI, Maraganore JM. The thrombin-specific anticoagulant, bivalirudin, completely inhibits thrombin-mediated platelet aggregation. Am J Cardiol. 2001; 88(suppl 5A): abstract #212.
5. Monroe DM, Hoffman M, Roberts HR. Platelets and thrombin generation. Arterioscler Thromb Biol. 2002; 22:1381–1389.
6. The Cardiovascular Market Outlook to 2008. London: Reuters Business Insight; 2003.
7. Collins B, Hollidge C. Antithrombotic drug market. Nat Rev Drug Discov. 2003; 2(1):11–12.
8. Mann CC, Plummer ML. The Aspirin Wars: Money, Medicine, and 100 Years of Rampant Competition. Boston: Harvard Business School Press, 1993.
9. Andermann AAJ. Physicians, fads, and pharmaceuticals: A history of aspirin. http://www.med.mcgill.ca/mjm/issues/v02n02/aspirin.html . Accessed November 28, 2003.
10. McTavish JR. What's in a name? Aspirin and the American Medical Association. Bull Hist Med. 1987; 61(3):343–366.
11. Smith JB, Willis AL. Aspirin selectively inhibits prostaglandin production in human platelets. Nat New Biol. 1971; 231(25):235–237.
12. Moncada S, Gryglewski R, Bunting S, Vane JR. An enzyme isolated from arteries transforms prostaglandin endoperoxides to an unstable substance that inhibits platelet aggregation. Nature. 1976; 263(5579):663–665.
13. Lewis HD Jr, Davis JW, Archibald DG, Steinke WE, Smitherman TC, Doherty JE 3rd et al. Protective effects of aspirin against acute myocardial infarction and death in men with unstable

angina. Results of a Veterans Administration Cooperative Study. N Engl J Med. 1983; 309(7):396–403.

14. Cairns JA, Gent M, Singer J, Finnie KJ, Froggatt GM, Holder DA et al. Aspirin, sulfinpyrazone, or both in unstable angina. Results of a Canadian multicenter trial. N Engl J Med. 1985; 313(22):1369–1375.

15. Rumore MM, Goldstein GS. Prevention of recurrent myocardial infarction and sudden death with aspirin therapy. Drug Intell Clin Pharm. 1987; 21(12):961–969.

16. Collins R, Baigent C, Sandercock P, Peto R. Antiplatelet therapy for thromboprophylaxis: the need for careful consideration of the evidence from randomised trials. Antiplatelet Trialists' Collaboration. BMJ. 1994; 309(6963):1215–1217.

17. Meade TW, Mellows S, Brozovic M, Miller GJ, Chakrabarti RR, North WR, et al. Fibrinolytic activity and arterial disease. Lancet. 1994; 343(8910):1442.

18. Giovannucci E, Egan KM, Hunter DJ, Stampfer MJ, Colditz GA, Willett WC et al. Aspirin and the risk of colorectal cancer in women. N Engl J Med. 1995; 333(10):609–614.

19. Rutty CJ. Miracle blood lubricant: Connaught and the story of heparin, 1928–1937. http://www.healthheritageresearch.com/Heparin-Conntact9608.html . Accessed November 28, 2003.

20. Mueller RL, Scheidt S. History of drugs for thrombotic disease. Discovery, development, and directions for the future. Circulation. 1994; 89(1):432–449.

21. Kucharski A. Medical management of political patients: the case of Dwight D. Eisenhower. Perspect Biol Med. 1978; 22 (1):115–126.

22. Frydman AM, Bara L, Le Roux Y, Woler M, Chauliac F, Samama MM. The antithrombotic activity and pharmacokinetics of enoxaparine, a low molecular weight heparin, in humans given single subcutaneous doses of 20 to 80 mg. J Clin Pharmacol. 1988; 28(7):609–618.

23. Cannon CP, Maraganore JM, Loscalzo J, McAllister A, Eddings K, George D et al. Anticoagulant effects of hirulog, a novel thrombin inhibitor, in patients with coronary artery disease. Am J Cardiol. 1993; 71(10):778–782.

24. White HD, Aylward PE, Frey MJ, Adgey AA, Nair R, Hillis WS, et al. Randomized, double-blind comparison of hirulog versus heparin in patients receiving streptokinase and aspirin for acute myocardial infarction (HERO). Circulation. 1997 Oct 7; 96(7):2155–2161.

25. The EPIC Investigators. Use of a monoclonal antibody directed against the platelet glycoprotein IIb/IIIa receptor in high-risk coronary angioplasty. N Engl J Med. 1994; 330(14):956–961.

26. The GUSTO Investigators. An international randomized trial comparing four thrombolytic strategies for acute myocardial infarction. N Engl J Med. 1993; 329(10):673–682.

27. Bahit MC, Topol EJ, Califf RM, Armstrong PW, Criger DA, Hasselblad V et al. Reactivation of ischemic events in acute coronary syndromes: results from GUSTO-IIb. Global Use of Strategies To Open occluded arteries in acute coronary syndromes. J Am Coll Cardiol. 2001; 37(4):1001–1007.

28. Miller JM, Smalling R, Ohman EM, Bode C, Betriu A, Kleiman NS, et al. Effectiveness of early coronary angioplasty and abciximab for failed thrombolysis (reteplase or alteplase) during acute myocardial infarction (results from the GUSTO-III trial). Global Use of Strategies To Open occluded coronary arteries. Am J Cardiol. 1999; 84(7):779–784.

29. Lincoff AM, Bittl JA, Harrington RA, Feit F, Kleiman NS, Jackman JD, et al. Bivalirudin and provisional glycoprotein IIb/IIIa blockade compared with heparin and planned glycoprotein IIb/IIIa blockade during percutaneous coronary intervention: REPLACE-2 randomized trial. JAMA. 2003; 289(7):853–863.

30. Stamler JS, Taber RL, Califf RM. Translation of academic discovery into societal benefit: proposal for a balanced approach—part 1. Am J Med. 2003 Nov; 115(7):596–599.

31. Stamler JS, Taber RL, Califf RM. Translation of academic discovery into societal benefit: proposal for a balanced approach-part 2. Am J Med. 200; 115(8):683–688.

32. Topol EJ, Califf RM, Van de Werf F, Simoons M, Hampton J, Lee KL et al. Perspectives on large-scale cardiovascular clinical trials for the new millennium. The Virtual Coordinating Center for Global Collaborative Cardiovascular Research (VIGOUR) Group. Circulation. 1997; 95(4):1072–1082.

33. DiMasi JA, Hansen RW, Grabowski HG. The price of innovation: new estimates of drug development costs. J Health Econ. 2003; 22:151–185.
34. DiMasi JA, Hansen RW, Grabowski HG, Lasagna L. Cost of innovation in the pharmaceutical industry. J Health Econ. 1991; 10:107–142.
35. Chew DP, Bhatt DL, Sapp S, Topol EJ. Increased mortality with oral platelet glycoprotein IIb/IIIa antagonists: A meta-analysis of phase III multicenter randomized trials. Circulation. 2001; 103:201–206.
36. The Direct Thrombin Inhibitor Trialists' Collaborative Group. Direct thrombin inhibitors in acute coronary syndromes: principal results of a meta-analysis based on individual patients' data. Lancet. 2002; 359:294–302.
37. Kong DF, Hassleblad V, Harrington RA, White HD, Tcheng JE, Kandzari DE et al. Meta-analysis of survival with platelet glycoprotein IIb/IIIa antagonists for percutaneous coronary interventions. Am J Cardiol. 2003; 92:651–655.
38. Karvouni E, Katritsis DG, Ioannidis JPA. Intravenous glycoprotein IIb/IIIa receptor antagonists reduced mortality after percutaneous coronary interventions. J Am Coll Cardiol. 2003; 41:26–32.
39. Simoons ML, GUSTO IV-ACS Investigators. Effect of glycoprotein IIb/IIIa receptor blocker abciximab on outcome in patients with acute coronary syndromes without early coronary revascularization: the GUSTO IV-ACS randomized trial. Lancet. 2001; 357:1915–1924.
40. Ottervanger JP, Armstrong P, Barnathan ES et al. Long-term results after the glycoprotein IIb/IIIa inhibitor abciximab in unstable angina: one-year survival in the GUSTO IV-ACS (Global Use of Strategies To Open Occluded Coronary Arteries IV—Acute Coronary Syndrome) Trial. Circulation. 2003; 107:437–442.
41. Topol EJ, the GUSTO V Investigators. Reperfusion therapy for acute myocardial infarction with fibrinolytic therapy or combination reduced fibrinolytic therapy and platelet glycoprotein IIb/IIIa inhibition: the GUSTO V randomised trial. Lancet. 2001; 357:1905–1914.
42. White H and Hirulog and Early Reperfusion or Occlusion (HERO)-2 Trial Investigators. Thrombin-specific anticoagulation with bivalirudin versus heparin in patients receiving fibrinolytic therapy for acute myocardial infarction: the HERO-2 randomised trial. Lancet. 2001; 358(9296):1855–1863.
43. Boersma E, Harrington RA, Moliterno DJ, White H, Theroux P. Platelet glycoprotein IIb/IIIa inhibitors in acute coronary syndromes: a meta-analysis of all major randomized clinical trials. Lancet. 2002; 359:189–198.
44. Hilts PJ. Protecting America's Health: The FDA, Business and One Hundred Years of Regulation. New York: Alfred A. Knopf; 2003:218–222.
45. The European Agency for the Evaluation of Medicinal Products. http://www.emea.eu.int/ . Accessed November 28, 2003.
46. National Institute of Health Sciences. Pharmaceuticals and Medical Devices Evaluation Center. Tokyo, Japan. http://www.nihs.go.jp/ . Accessed November 28, 2003.
47. International Conference on Harmonization. History and Future of ICH. http://www.ich.org/UrlGrpServer.jser?@_ID=276&@TEMPLATE=254 . Accessed November 28, 2003.
48. International Conference on Harmonisation. E6: Good Clinical Practice consolidated Guideline. http://www.ich.org/UrlGrpServer.jser?@_ID=276&@_TEMPLATE=254 . Accessed November 28, 2003.
49. International Conference on Harmonisation. ICH Official Web Site (home page). http://www.ich.org/UrlGrpServer.jser?@_ID=276&@_TEMPLATE=254. Accessed November 28, 2003.
50. Process Analytical Technology (PAT) Initiative. U.S. Food and Drug Administration, Center for Drug Evaluation and Research, Office of Pharmaceutical Science. http://www.fda.gov/cder/OPS/PAT.htm . Accessed November 28, 2003.
51. Serious manufacturing deficiencies with Abbokinase prompt FDA letter to Abbott Labs. FDA Talk Paper. U.S. Food and Drug Administration. http://www.fda.gov/bbs/topics/ANSWERS/ANS00964.html . Accessed November 28, 2003.

52. Important Drug Warning: Safety Information Regarding the use of Abbokinase (Urokinase). U.S. Food and Drug Administration. http://www.fda.gov/cder/biologics/ltr/abb012599.htm. Accessed November 28, 2003.

53. Warning Letter concerning "Dear Abbokinase Customer" Letter. U.S. Food and Drug Administration. http://www.fda.gov/cder/biologics/ltr/abb031999.htm . Accessed November 28, 2003.

54. Weaver WD, Simes RJ, Betriu A, Grines CL, Zijlstra F, Garcia E, et al. Comparison of primary coronary angioplasty and intravenous thrombolytic therapy for acute myocardial infarction: a quantitative review. JAMA. 1997; 278(23):2093–2098.

55. Von Hippel E. Sources of Innovation. Oxford, UK: Oxford University Press; 1988.

56. Lincoff AM, Topol EJ. Long-term efficacy of bivalirudin and provisional GP IIb/IIIa blockade compared with heparin and planned GP IIb/IIIa blockade during percutaneous coronary intervention: 6–month and 1-year results of the REPLACE-2 trial. Presented at: American Heart Association Scientific Sessions 2003, Orlando, FL, November 9–12, 2003.

57. The PURSUIT Trial Investigators. Inhibition of platelet glycoprotein IIb/IIIa with eptifibatide in patients with acute coronary syndromes. Platelet Glycoprotein IIb/IIIa in Unstable Angina: Receptor Suppression Using Integrilin Therapy. N Engl J Med 1998; 339:436–443.

58. Platelet Receptor Inhibition in Ischemic Syndrome Management (PRISM) Study Investigators. A comparison of aspirin plus tirofiban with aspirin plus heparin for unstable angina. N Engl J Med. 1998; 338:1498–505.

59. PRISM-PLUS Study Investigators. Inhibition of the platelet glycoprotein IIb/IIIa receptor with tirofiban in unstable angina and non–Q-wave myocardial infarction. N Engl J Med 1998; 338(21):1488–1497.

60. IMS Market Prognosis International 2002–2006.

61. Simoons ML and the GUSTO IV-ACS Investigators. Effect of glycoprotein IIb/IIIa receptor blocker abciximab on outcome in patients with acute coronary syndromes without early coronary revascularisation: the GUSTO IV-ACS randomised trial. Lancet. 2001; 357(9272):1915–1924.

62. Topol EJ, the GUSTO V Investigators. Reperfusion therapy for acute myocardial infarction with fibrinolytic therapy or combination reduced fibrinolytic therapy and platelet glycoprotein IIb/IIIa inhibition: the GUSTO V randomised trial. Lancet. 2001; 357(9272):1905–1914.

63. Pache J, Kastrati A, Mehilli J, Gawaz M, Neumann FJ, Seyfarth M et al. Clopidogrel therapy in patients undergoing coronary stenting: value of a high-loading-dose regimen. Catheter Cardiovasc Interv. 2002; 55(4):436–41.

64. SYNERGY Executive Committee. The SYNERGY trial: study design and rationale. Am Heart J 2002; 143:952–960.

65. Sobel M. Heparin modulates integrin function in human platelets. J Vasc Surg 2001; 33:587–594.

66. Aggarwal A, Sobel BE, Schneider DJ. Biphasic effects of hemodialysis on platelet reactivity in patients with end-stage renal disease: a potential contributor to cardiovascular risk. Am J Kidney Dis. 2002; 40(2):315–322.

67. Schneider DJ, Tracy PB, Mann KG, Sobel BE. Differential effects of anticoagulants on the activation of platelets ex vivo. Circulation. 1997; 96(9):2877–2883.

68. Kotler P, Armstrong G. Principles of Marketing. 7th ed. Englewood Cliffs, NL: Prentice Hall, 1966.

Index